THE NURSE'S DRUG HANDBOOK

THE NURSE'S DRUG HANDBOOK

FOURTH EDITION

Suzanne Loebl

George R. Spratto, Ph.D.
Professor of Pharmacology and Associate Dean
School of Pharmacy and Pharmacal Sciences
Purdue University
West Lafayette, Indiana

Nursing consultant for the fourth edition:
Barbara L. MacDermott, M.S., R.N.
Associate Professor and Assistant Dean
College of Nursing
Syracuse University
Syracuse, New York

A Wiley Medical Publication

JOHN WILEY & SONS
New York • Chichester • Brisbane • Toronto • Singapore

The authors and publisher have made a conscientious effort to ensure that the drug information and recommended dosages in this book are accurate and in accord with accepted standards at the time of publication. However, pharmacology is a rapidly changing science, so readers are advised, before administering any drug, to check the package insert provided by the manufacturer for the recommended dose, for contraindications for administration, and for added warnings and precautions. This recommendation is especially important for new, infrequently used, or highly toxic drugs.

Library of Congress Cataloging in Publication Data:

Loebl, Suzanne.
  The nurse's drug handbook.

(A Wiley medical publication)
Bibliography: p.
Includes index.
  1. Chemotherapy—Handbooks, manuals, etc. 2. Drugs—Handbooks, manuals, etc. 3. Nursing—Handbooks, manuals, etc. I. Spratto, George.
II. MacDermott, Barbara L. III. Title.
IV. Series. [DNLM: 1. Drug Therapy—nurses' instruction.
2. Drugs—nurses' instruction. QV 55 L824n]
RM 262.L63 1986   615.5'8   85-26517
ISBN 0-471-82792-4

Printed in the United States of America

10 9 8 7 6 5 4 3 2 1

PREFACE
TO THE FOURTH EDITION

As with each revision of *The Nurse's Drug Handbook*, we have tried to incorporate the latest information on new and existing drugs as well as to add features that make the book easier and more efficient to use. Over the years we have observed two groups who use the book: nursing students and practitioners. Thus, it is for these groups that the book is intended.

We believe firmly that the order of presentation of drugs should be by drug class and/or therapeutic use. This is the method by which nurses, physicians, pharmacists, and other health professionals learn pharmacology. Furthermore, we believe the grouping of the drugs in this fashion aids in learning. In addition, we are able to present general information on the disease state for which the drugs in a particular group are used.

The chapters have been regrouped and renumbered, which will make the book easier to use. Part 1 has been extensively changed, and contains eight chapters, each of which provides background information for subsequent chapters. Also, the information in these chapters allows the nurse or student to learn about the proper administration and monitoring of drugs and drug therapy. Parts 2 through 12 group the various drugs by therapeutic class or organ system on which the drugs act. There are three new parts: Part 8—Drugs Affecting the Respiratory System; Part 9—Drugs Affecting the Gastrointestinal System; and, Part 11—Agents Affecting Water and Electrolytes.

A new feature that should prove useful is the listing, inside the front cover, of the location in the book of the most commonly used drugs by trade name. Also, listed inside the back cover is the location, by both generic and trade name, of drugs that are frequently used in emergency situations.

As in the past, the drug monographs have been revised, adding and deleting information as deemed necessary. Of particular importance is the listing of Untoward Reactions by the system(s) that is most affected. This allows the user to locate quickly which of the organ systems are adversely affected by a drug as well as the specific symptoms that might be manifested. Several chapters have been reorganized so that the information is more clearly presented and thus easier to locate and use.

We have updated all trade names, action/kinetics, contraindications, uses, drug interactions, doses, and nursing implications. As in the past, we have included trade names of drugs that are available only in Canada; these are designated by an asterisk immediately following the trade name. Another new feature is the designation indicating whether the drug is available only on prescription (Rx) or can be obtained over the counter (OTC) without a prescription.

More than 50 new drug entities have been added. Among the most notable are the calcium channel blockers, several new beta-adrenergic blocking agents, new drugs for treating gastrointestinal disturbances, new agents for the treatment of hypertension, several new cephalosporins, human insulin and second generation sulfonylureas, and an oral gold dosage form for treating rheumatoid arthritis.

We have tried our best to develop a text that can be used successfully by both the registered nurse in whatever setting he or she may be practicing and the student. We wish to thank all of those who submitted suggestions to improve the book. We continue to encourge such feedback.

ACKNOWLEDGMENTS

A text of this type necessarily draws on work done by others in the fields of pharmacology, toxicology, and therapeutics. The bibliography lists frequently consulted sources used in the compilation of the material found in this text. Additional information was obtained by discussing specific questions with experts who work in a specialized field. Our thanks and admiration go to all those on whose work ours is based.

Special appreciation is extended to Estelle Heckheimer who, after many dedicated years, has decided to pursue other interests. We are deeply indebted to Barbara MacDermott of the School of Nursing, Syracuse University, who was our special consultant for nursing implications for this edition.

Colleagues at Purdue University and Syracuse University are to be thanked for their patience and constructive comments during the preparation of the fourth edition.

Special thanks go to the following people: Brenda Stevens, of Purdue University, secretary to G.S., who made helpful suggestions for word processing and who provided valuable assistance; Eric Cassel, of International Computaprint Corporation, for his help and patience as we converted to using word processing; Mary Losey, Associate Professor of Pharmacy Practice, of Purdue University who reviewed a portion of the text; and, Linda Harrison, Keith Fredericks, and William "Marty" Martin, of Computerland in West Lafayette, IN, who assisted greatly in designing and implementing a hardware system that allowed us to convert to word processing.

Our gratitude is expressed to Andy Ford, Maria Danzilo, and Andrea Stingelin of John Wiley & Sons, who have maintained great faith and encouragement for this project.

Greatest thanks, appreciation, and love go to our families for their moral support and for the unending sacrifices they made while this edition was being revised.

G.S.
S.L.

CONTENTS

PART 2   ANTI-INFECTIVES

PART 3   ANTINEOPLASTIC AGENTS

PART 4   DRUGS AFFECTING BLOOD FORMATION AND COAGULATION

PART 5 CARDIOVASCULAR DRUGS

PART 6 DRUGS AFFECTING THE CENTRAL NERVOUS SYSTEM

PART 9 DRUGS AFFECTING THE GASTROINTESTINAL SYSTEM

PART 10 HORMONES AND HORMONE ANTAGONISTS

PART 11   AGENTS AFFECTING WATER AND ELECTROLYTES

PART 12   MISCELLANEOUS AGENTS

APPENDICES

LIST OF TABLES

Part One

INTRODUCTION

Chapter One

HOW TO USE THIS HANDBOOK

The fourth edition of *The Nurse's Drug Handbook* reveals dramatic changes in the numbering of chapters and presentation of material. Realizing that drugs are classified by either their chemical or therapeutic use (and that pharmacology is most often taught by this approach), a format was developed that should increase the consistency and clarity of the information presented as well as make the text easy to use.

1

The first section discusses general information that will provide the necessary background for subsequent sections. Information on mechanism of action and pharmacokinetics (Chapter 2), untoward reactions (Chapter 3), and drug interactions (Chapter 4) is presented. In addition, comprehensive nursing implications for drug therapy (Chapter 5) and administration of medications by different routes (Chapter 6) are listed. These particular sections are of utmost importance for the nurse who administers drugs as well as the nurse who provides directions to patients on the proper administration of medication.

The pediatric, geriatric, or pregnant patient often reacts differently to drugs; these groups also manifest special problems with respect to drug therapy. These issues are discussed in Chapter 7; in addition, a presentation of nursing implications, as they relate to these special patients, will be found.

One of the most important problems that faces physicians, nurses, pharmacists, and other members of the health care team is patient compliance with the appropriate medication regimen. Helpful approaches in meeting this challenge are detailed in Chapter 8.

The major portion of the book presents information on individual drugs or drug classes. The *Handbook* is intended to be a quick reference for the practicing nurse as well as a simple text in pharmacology. With these objectives in mind, the following format was developed.

Drugs that either belong to closely related families (e.g., penicillins, sulfonamides) or are used for the treatment of a particular disease (e.g., malaria) are grouped together.

Drugs that mainly affect one physiologic system (e.g., cardiovascular) are grouped together in a section; these sections contain chapters that deal with specific conditions to be treated (e.g., hypertension, arrhythmias, angina).

Drugs that affect hormones or substitute for them (e.g., insulin, thyroid, estrogens) are presented under appropriate headings.

Drugs are arranged alphabetically within each group or subdivision with the generic name listed in bold type followed by the trade name(s).

This type of arrangement enables the nurse to locate an individual drug quickly and to find concise information about it. In addition, the introduction for specific chapters presents general information about the drugs themselves or the particular condition for which the drugs are intended. Thus, the introduction to each section should be read carefully.

Information for individual drugs is presented as follows:

DRUG NAMES   The generic name for the drug is presented first followed by one or more trade names. If the trade name is available only in Canada, the name will be followed by an asterisk (*). Also, if the drug is controlled by the U.S. Federal Controlled Substances Act, the schedule in which the drug has been placed follows the trade name (e.g., C-II, C-III, C-IV).

CLASSIFICATION   Defines type of drug unless this is self-evident. This information is most useful in learning to categorize drugs.

GENERAL STATEMENT   Presents information about the class of drug and/or what might be unusual about a particular group of drugs. In addition, information may be presented about the disease(s) for which the drugs are indicated.

ACTION/KINETICS   The action portion of this entry describes the mechanism(s) by which a drug is able to achieve its therapeutic effect, e.g., certain antibiotics interfere with the growth of bacteria. Not all mechanisms of action are known, and some are self-evident, as when a hormone is administered as a replacement. The kinetics entry lists pertinent facts, if known, about rate of drug absorption, minimum effective serum or plasma level, biologic half-life ($t\frac{1}{2}$), duration of action, metabolism, and excretion. The time it takes for half the drug to be excreted or removed from the blood, t½, is important in determining how often a drug is to be administered and how long to assess for side effects. Therapeutic serum or plasma levels indicate the desired concentration, in serum or plasma, for the drug to exert its beneficial effect. More and more drug therapy is being monitored in this fashion (e.g., antibiotics, theophyllines, cardiac glycosides). Metabolism and excretion routes may be important for patients with systemic liver or kidney disease or both. Again, information is not available for all therapeutic agents.

USES   Therapeutic application(s) for the particular agent.

CONTRAINDICATIONS   Disease states or conditions in which the drug should not be used (or used with caution). The safe use of many of the newer pharmacologic agents during pregnancy or childhood has not been established. As a general rule, the use of drugs during pregnancy is contraindicated unless specified by a physician.

UNTOWARD REACTIONS (SIDE EFFECTS)   Unwanted or bothersome effects the patient *may* experience while taking the particular agent. Untoward reactions are listed by the body organ or system affected. This feature allows easier access to information on side effects of drugs.

DRUG INTERACTIONS   Drugs that may interact with one another are listed under this entry. The study of drug interactions is a rapidly expanding area of pharmacology. The compilation of such interactions is far from complete; therefore, listings in this manual are to be considered *only* as general cautionary guidelines.

As detailed in Chapter 4, drug interactions may result from a number of different mechanisms (additive effects, interference with degradation of drug, increased speed of elimination). Such interferences may manifest themselves in a variety of ways; however, an attempt has been made throughout the text to describe these whenever possible as an increase (↑) or a decrease (↓) in the effect of the drug, followed by a brief description of the reason for the change.

It is important to realize that any side effects that accompany the administration of a particular agent may also be increased as a result of a drug interaction.

The reader should also be aware that the drug interactions are often listed for classes of drugs. Thus, the drug interaction would be likely for all drugs in that particular class.

LABORATORY TEST INTERFERENCES   These refer to the manner in which a drug may affect the laboratory test values of the patient. Some of these interferences are caused by the therapeutic or toxic effects of the drugs; others result from interference with the method itself. As detailed in Appendix 7 of Part One, interferences are described as false +, or (↑), values and as false −, or (↓), values. Many of the laboratory test interferences are also listed under the *Nursing Implications* of each drug. For quick reference, an alphabetic list of *Laboratory Test Interferences* is provided in Appendix 7.

DOSAGE   The adult and pediatric doses are presented when possible and are so indicated. The listed dosage is to be considered as a general guideline, since the exact amount of the drug to be given is determined by the physician. However, a nurse should question orders from the physician when dosages differ markedly from the accepted norm. We have tried to give complete data for drugs that are prescribed frequently.

ADMINISTRATION/STORAGE   This information provides specific pointers on how to administer and store particular agents. When in doubt, consult the extensive data given in Chapters 5 and 6.

NURSING IMPLICATIONS   Designed to assist the nurse in situations that might arise when administering the drug under consideration. The nurse must also assess the patient for the *Untoward Reactions* listed under that heading. If severe, these must be reported to the physician. Severe untoward reactions are sometimes cause for discontinuation of the drug. *Nursing Implications* are generally presented in two parts. The first part deals with such specifics as:

1. Assessment of specific physiologic functions as they might be affected by the drug.
2. Physiologic, pharmacologic, and psychologic effects of the drug and how these affect the nursing process.
3. Emergency situations that can arise as a result of the drug and how they can be handled.
4. Specific interventions that can relieve a patient's discomfort caused by the drug.
5. Measures that increase the safety of the patient when receiving a particular drug.

The second part of *Nursing Implications*, usually headed *Teach Patient and/or Family*, emphasizes the nurse's role in patient education and in promoting drug compliance. Stress is placed on helping the patient/family recognize untoward reactions, and avoiding other dangerous situations and/or feelings of anxiety that might result from taking a particular drug.

In addition, specific information on patient education is provided in the *Nursing Implications* for each drug. The proper teaching of patients is one of the most challenging aspects of nursing, but the instructions must be tailored to the needs, awareness, and sophistication of each patient.

The previous points are covered for all drugs or drug classes. When drugs are presented as a group rather than individually, the points may only be covered once for each group. In this case the nurse must look for the appropriate entry at the beginning of the group. For example, the Contraindications, Untoward Reactions, Drug Interactions, Administration, and Nursing Implications for all the penicillins are so similar that they are only listed once at the beginning of the section.

In some chapters, the drugs are presented in tabular form especially if differences between the drugs relate mainly to dosage or duration of action. The tables are constructed so that specific information for a particular drug can also be listed.

Information relevant to a particular drug, and not to the whole group, is listed under appropriate headings, such as *Additional Contraindications*, or *Additional Nursing Implications*. Such entries are *in addition to* and not *instead of* the regular entry, which must also be consulted.

A feature that will provide useful is a listing of the location of commonly used drugs by trade name (inside front cover) and a listing of the location of drugs used in emergency situations (inside back cover).

The appendices contain a wealth of information to assist the nurse in administering drugs and monitoring drug therapy appropriately. For example, information on how to treat toxicity from selected drugs and chemicals is listed in Appendix 2, and commonly prescribed combination drugs (more than one drug in the product) are presented in Appendix 3.

Although drug-drug and food-drug interactions are discussed in Chapter 4, specific interactions and nursing implications are presented in Appendices 4–6. Similarly, detailed information will be found on the effects of drugs in the geriatric patient (Appendix 8) and in pregnancy (Appendix 9).

All nurses should become proficient in the terminology used in writing prescriptions as well as the procedure to be followed in calculating doses. Information to assist the nurse with this process will be found in Appendices 10, 14, and 15.

Brief descriptions of the U.S. Federal Controlled Substances Act (Appendix 11) and Controlled Substances (Canada) (Appendix 12) are included.

A glossary of terms that some readers may find unfamiliar will be found following the appendices. Finally, a listing of resources and references that give additional information or more in-depth treatment of a topic has been included.

You are now ready to use *The Nurse's Drug Handbook*. We hope that it will become a useful text and assist you in your profession. Even though the material presented might, at first, appear overwhelming, remember that the effective drugs currently at the disposal of the health care team are the key to today's better, more effective, and efficient medical care. Certainly, the administration of drugs and the monitoring of their effects on the patient are crucial parts of the nursing process.

Chapter Two

MECHANISM OF ACTION/PHARMACOKINETICS: GENERAL PRINCIPLES

MECHANISM OF ACTION

The mechanisms by which drugs manifest the desired pharmacologic effect are sometimes clear and sometimes obscure. In some cases, the mechanism of action is obvious, for instance, when the drug replaces a missing biochemical substance, such as insulin in diabetes. In other cases, the mechanism is more complex, but known; for instance, allopurinol inhibits an enzyme necessary for the formation of uric acid. By decreasing the concentration of uric acid in the blood, allopurinol relieves gout. Sometimes the mechanism of action of a drug is unknown, even though the drug has been used for a long time. For example, the role played by phenytoin in decreasing epileptic convulsions, or the precise manner by which digitalis increases the strength of the heartbeat is not known. In this book, mechanisms of action of drugs are provided when known.

PHARMACOKINETICS

Pharmacokinetics is the study of the fate of drugs in the body. This science concerns itself with:

Drug absorption and distribution
Drug plasma concentration
Therapeutic plasma levels

Toxic plasma levels
Concentration of the active drug at the target site
Rate of metabolism
Rate of excretion

These parameters, in turn, are affected by:

Physicochemical nature of the drug (e.g., lipid solubility)
Formulation of the drug
Route of administration
Binding of the drug to plasma and/or tissue (bioavailability)
Individual characteristics of the patient
Concomitant diseases
Concomitant administration of food or other drugs

Pharmacokinetics is assuming greater importance in medicine, because large numbers of patients are currently taking an increasing number of potent drugs, often concomitantly and for prolonged periods of time. Pharmacokinetic concepts that play a major role in the administration of drugs—administration, absorption, onset of action, peak of activity, half-life, first-pass effect, drug distribution, drug elimination, therapeutic serum levels, bioavailability, therapeutic drug delivery systems—are briefly reviewed below.

Some pharmacokinetic data, as well as mechanisms of action of drugs, have been added to the discussions of individual drugs or drug classes in *The Nurse's Drug Handbook*. The information listed for the various drugs is neither complete nor entirely consistent. Pharmacokinetic data are lacking for some of the older drugs still widely used today. Moreover, data obtained from the literature and/or from drug manufacturers are often inconsistent and spotty. Onset of action is given for some drugs; time to attain peak serum levels or therapeutic serum levels is listed for others. Consistency was sacrificed for completeness of information. When available and/or known, we have listed all or some of the following: mechanism of action, onset of action, therapeutic serum levels, duration of action, metabolism/excretion, time to attain peak serum levels, and biologic half-life ($t\frac{1}{2}$).

Administration

The route used to administer drugs (Fig. 1) has a profound effect on drug absorption, distribution, metabolism, and elimination.

Oral (Enteral) Administration   Oral administration is the most economical, most widespread, but least standardizable route. Drug absorption, after oral administration, is affected by the presence of food, gastric emptying time, intestinal motility, the pH of the stomach and intestine, the nature of the drug (small, lipid-soluble molecules are absorbed more quickly than others, for example), the rate of disintegration and dissolution of the tablet (affected by physical state and coating), and blood circulation to the gastrointestinal (GI) tract. Importantly, certain drugs cannot be given orally at all (without special protective measures), since they are destroyed by stomach acid. Orally administered drugs often are partially degraded by various enzymes in the GI tract, in the intestinal mucosa, and most of all, in the liver (see *First-Pass Effect*, below). A combination of all or some of

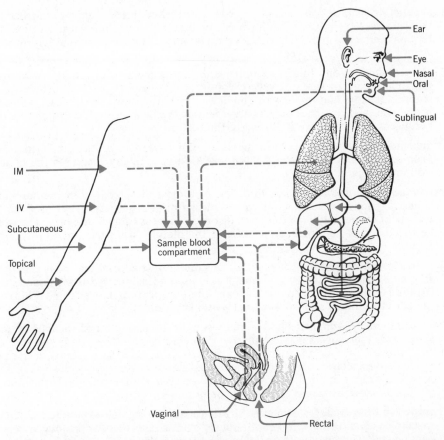

FIGURE 1 Drugs can be administered ("inputed") through a great variety of routes. When given orally, they are absorbed from the stomach and small intestine and must first pass through the liver, the organ chiefly involved in drug metabolism. (See text for a definition of first-pass effect). Reproduced with permission from Dr. Leslie Benet in E.J. Ariens (ed): *Drug Design, Volume IV*. New York: Academic Press, 1973, p. 5.

these factors could be responsible for only a fraction of orally administered drugs becoming absorbed into the bloodstream and/or reaching their site of action (see also the *Onset of Action* and *Peak of Activity* below).

Intramuscular and Subcutaneous Administration Drugs are absorbed into plasma from intramuscular (IM) or subcutaneous (SC) injection sites by simple diffusion. Larger molecules (proteins, for example) are absorbed through the lymphatic circulation. Absorption is prompt. Duration of action can be increased by the use of repository preparations that decrease the rate of absorption.

Intravenous Administration Intravenous (IV) administration ensures prompt onset of action and eliminates uncertainty associated with the incompleteness of drug absorption by other routes. Intravenous administration is the only route that can be used for certain irritating drugs or solutions, because the walls of blood vessels are relatively resistant to irritation. IV administration usually requires constant monitoring by a nurse, since this route increases the risk of toxic or untoward reactions.

Sublingual Administration   Drugs placed under the tongue are rapidly absorbed into the vena cava (venous circulation); this method of drug administration avoids the first-pass effect of the liver. This method is only suitable for certain highly active agents, such as nitroglycerin.

Rectal Administration   Rectal administration is used when oral administration is precluded (e.g., in cases of severe vomiting or unconsciousness). However, absorption is slow and uncertain. The drug is absorbed into the GI tract below the portal vein and avoids the first-pass effect of the liver. Also, the route is limited, because many drugs are irritating to the rectum.

Intracavital Administration   Intracavital administration is useful for certain antineoplastic agents. Intracavital administration specifically increases the concentration of drug at the site of action.

Intrathecal Administration   The injection of a drug directly into the spinal subarachnoid space is necessary for the administration of certain drugs used for the treatment of meningitis and related disorders; access to their site of action would be precluded or diminished, because of the blood - brain barrier. Absorption is rapid.

Mucous Membrane Administration   Mucous membrane administration is usually restricted to localized therapy, although it is used occasionally for systemic administration (antidiuretic hormone, for example). Absorption may be rapid. This route includes intranasal and intravaginal administration.

Skin (Cutaneous) Administration   Intact skin is relatively impermeable to most drugs; it is therefore a good route for achieving localized results in various skin conditions. Absorption is increased if the skin is abraded or denuded, if the drug is added to a specific solvent, or if medicated skin is covered by occlusive dressing. Also, if a drug is applied over a large surface area of the skin, and for prolonged periods of time, systemic effects may be observed.

Therapeutic Drug-Delivery Systems   In therapeutic drug-delivery systems, a pharmacologic agent is delivered continuously from a reservoir for prolonged periods of time (see *Therapeutic Drug Delivery Systems* below).

Absorption

The rate of absorption of a drug is of paramount importance, because it is reflected in the concentration of the drug in the serum and at the target site. It determines the drug's time of onset action and the time of peak effect. If absorption is too slow compared with elimination, the drug might never attain the minimum effective therapeutic serum concentration. In addition to being affected by the route of administration, absorption is also affected by:

Formulation of the drug (tablets vs. capsules, inert additives, coatings)
Character of the drug itself (e.g., acidic vs. basic)
Drug solubility
Presence (absence) of food (oral administration only)
Patient characteristics—age, body weight, individual factors, presence of concomitant disease

The customary manner of diagramming drug absorption by plotting serum concentration as a function of time is shown in Figure 2.

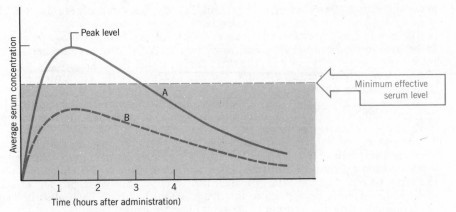

FIGURE 2   Drug absorption curve.

Onset of Action

The onset of action refers to the time interval between administration and notation of the first therapeutic effects. It depends on the route of administration, the characteristics of the drug, its rate of absorption through various membranes, and the formulation (how fast the drug is released into the system from the dosage form). The onset of action is especially variable after oral administration, depending on the presence of food in the stomach, the motility of the GI tract, and other factors.

Peak of Activity

The peak of activity—when the drug reaches its maximum effect—often coincides with peak serum concentration (Fig. 2). Many drugs cause this peak to surpass the optimally effective level, but the concentration can rapidly fall below this level as a result of biotransformation and excretion. This drop occurs especially often when a short-acting drug is given initially or intermittently.

In the treatment of diabetes, for example, insulins with various lengths of action are mixed, so as to keep insulin levels at a therapeutically effective level around the clock.

Biologic Half-Life (t½)

The time in which half the drug has been eliminated is the *biologic half-life*, or t½. (The concept of half-life was originally introduced in connection with discussion of the decay of radioactive substances.) If no additional drug is administered, it takes *two half-lives* to eliminate *75%* and *four half-lives* to eliminate *93.3% of the drug*.

In practice, most drugs are administered more than once; a subsequent **dose is** generally administered before the previous dose has been entirely eliminated. This overlap can result in drug accumulation.

The biologic half-life is an important concept in establishing dosage frequency. In general, a dosage interval equal to or less than the $t\frac{1}{2}$ is recommended for most drugs. Thus, if $t\frac{1}{2}$ is 4 hr, the drug can be given up to 6 times per day.

In practice, however, an attempt is made to consider the convenience of the patient in setting dosage schedules.

Most drugs have a short half-life (short-acting anesthetics often last only a few minutes). Other drugs, the monoamine oxidase (MAO) inhibitors, for example, have exceedingly long half-lives.

The concept of half-life is important in all aspects of drug therapy, including the treatment of drug overdosage. The narcotic antagonist naloxone, for example, has a shorter $t\frac{1}{2}$ than that of morphine; administration of the antagonist must therefore be repeated until the effects of the narcotic have worn off. The concept of half-life can only be applied to the drugs when they have been absorbed into the blood circulation—and not to those applied topically.

Half-life, as other pharmacokinetic factors, varies with the age of the patient, concomitant diseases (especially renal or hepatic impairment), and the presence of food and/or other drugs.

Sometimes a drug or its active metabolites are eliminated in two or more stages. In such cases, $t\frac{1}{2}$ is said to be biphasic or multiphasic.

First-Pass Effect

Most toxic substances, including drugs, are degraded by the microsomal enzymes of the liver. Since orally administered drugs are absorbed from the GI tract into the hepatic circulation, they must pass through the liver before they can reach the general circulation and their target. This effect often results in a considerable loss of activity of the administered drug, a phenomenon referred to as the first-pass effect. It is measured as hepatic clearance. The first-pass effect is taken into account when drugs are formulated, that is, a higher concentration must be administered orally than parenterally. Note that drugs administered sublingually or rectally do not have a first pass through the liver, but enter the general circulation directly (Fig. 1).

Distribution

The distribution of drugs in the body is governed by the physicochemical characteristics of the specific drug. The speed with which a particular agent is absorbed through the various biologic membranes depends on such factors as the size of the molecule, its solubility, and the pH of the tissues.

In general, once the drug has been injected into or has reached the bloodstream, it first attains significant concentrations in such highly perfused organs as the heart, liver, and kidneys (within minutes).

Delivery of the drug to the viscera, skin, and adipose tissue is slower (minutes to hours). Penetration of some tissues is even slower, and the distribution phase can be extremely slow for drugs that bind very strongly to serum proteins, since the complex is unable to pass out of the plasma.

Distribution of certain pharmaceutical agents to the central nervous system (CNS) is often limited, because the blood-brain barrier is selective in admitting compounds.

The ability of a drug to reach the fetus is dependent on its ability to cross the placental barrier (see Chapter 7).

Elimination

A crucial parameter from a therapeutic point of view is the time it takes for a drug to be eliminated from the body.

Elimination rates are determined experimentally on a number of test subjects, and the rate cited in the literature represents an average.

Drug elimination is a composite of drug **metabolism**, which can result in active or inactive metabolites, and drug **excretion**.

Metabolism   Metabolism is the sum total of all the reactions involved in the biotransformation of a pharmaceutical agent after it is administered. Most metabolic transformations are enzymatic and take place in the liver. This is why drug metabolism can be slowed in the presence of liver disease, thereby requiring a decrease in dosage.

In contrast, prolonged administration of certain drugs (barbiturates, phenytoin, alcohol) increases the efficacy and/or concentration of these specialized hepatic enzymes (enzyme induction); such drugs are metabolized faster than initially. In such cases, a larger dose of these drugs might be required to attain and/or maintain the drug at effective therapeutic levels.

Metabolism often increases the water solubility of the pharmaceutical agent and facilitates its renal excretion.

Sometimes metabolism is required for the drug to become active; in other instances, metabolism might convert the drug to a more toxic compound.

Excretion   The vast majority of drugs and/or their metabolites are excreted by the kidney. Some drugs are eliminated via the GI tract (feces, bile). A few agents are excreted via the lungs (gaseous anesthetics), and a fraction of some drugs appears in the saliva, sweat, or breast milk.

The rate of renal excretion is determined by the glomerular filtration rate (GFR), tubular reabsorption, and tubular secretion. In general, the more lipid-soluble a substance is, the slower its renal excretion. When elimination is slow or slowed— because of renal disease—the risk of drug accumulation and drug toxicity is increased. Note that dosage is reduced for most drugs in the presence of impaired renal function; in fact, some drugs cannot be given. When available, data on excretion are listed as percentage urinary excretion. Many drugs are excreted unchanged (chemically identical to drug administered) by the kidney.

Therapeutic Serum Levels

This term refers to the concentration of the drug in the serum at which its therapeutic action is manifested. Ideally, the optimal concentration should not be exceeded and should be maintained for prolonged periods of time. In practice, the administration of conventional dosage forms intermittently results in drug concentrations that sometimes exceed the minimal or optimal dosage levels and sometimes fall below it.

Consideration of therapeutic serum levels is particularly important for:

1. Certain antibiotics, because growth of most microorganisms is only inhibited above certain serum drug levels (minimal inhibitory concentration, or MIC).

2. When there is a narrow margin between a therapeutic effect and a toxic effect (e.g., digitalis, phenytoin).

Bioavailability

The bioavailability of a drug measures the concentration of pharmacologically active substance at the target site and/or in the serum.

Bioavailability is a function of:

The drug itself

The metabolism of the patient

The rate at which the drug is liberated from its dosage form or from storage in the body proper—many drugs, for example, bind to serum protein (plasma albumin in particular), from which they are released gradually; other drugs are stored in specific organs, in adipose tissue (lipid-soluble drugs, such as thiopental), and even in bone (tetracyclines)

Some of these factors are of such magnitude that substitution of one preparation of a specific drug for another can affect bioavailability. For example, the rate of disintegration of tablets of the same drug made by different manufacturers might be significantly different.

A drug is said not to be bioavailable if, or to the extent that it is:

Bound to protein or to any other substance that renders the drug permanently or temporarily inactive

Not released from its dosage form or site of administration

Partially or totally degraded

Protein binding plays a major role in drug interactions, because when two drugs are administered concomitantly, one drug (drug A) might have a greater affinity for protein than drug B. This action increases the concentration (bioavailability) of drug B, sometimes producing an increase in the duration and/or intensity of effect, necessitating a dosage adjustment.

Bioavailability is taken into account by the manufacturer in establishing dosage levels. In order to attain the desired therapeutic dosage levels, drugs that bind tightly to serum protein and are released slowly, for example, will have to be given at a higher concentration and less frequently than will a drug that is immediately available and that is degraded or excreted rapidly.

Therapeutic Drug-Delivery Systems

The drug serum concentration that results from drugs administered as conventional preparations (tablets, injections) undergoes wide fluctuations, especially when the pharmacologic agent is rapidly metabolized and/or excreted (i.e., has a short $t\frac{1}{2}$). Excessively high doses must be given and/or a high frequency of administration must be employed in order to maintain a drug blood concentration at or above the effective therapeutic level. Administration of high levels of medication is undesirable, however, because most drugs have toxic and/or unpleasant side effects at higher dosages. Also, patients sometimes fail to comply with orders for repeated drug administration (e.g., several times per day for a period of time).

This difficulty has been partially overcome with the development of sustained-release preparations, in which the drug is released in stages. Such preparations often consist of hundreds of small pellets coated with materials that dissolve at different rates. The development of drugs with long half-lives, which by their very nature have to be administered less frequently, is currently being emphasized.

Another mechanism of ensuring that adequate therapeutic serum levels are maintained is administration via intravenous (IV) drip. This method is used, for example, when antibiotics are administered to combat life-threatening infections.

A similar principle underlies the new therapeutic systems that deliver their drug cargo continuously for a matter of hours, weeks, or even months. Small drug reservoirs, enclosed in semipermeable membranes, are inserted into or applied near the target site. Drug diffuses out of these systems, into the body; the rate can ideally be adjusted so that input equals output (rate of excretion). Such therapeutic systems are especially suitable for drugs that have a short t½ and are required at low doses. A few of these new systems, already approved and available, are:

Progestasert delivers progesterone from an intrauterine device (IUD) for about 12 months.

Ocusert delivers pilocarpine into the conjunctival sac for 1 week.

Lacrisert delivers a moisturizing agent for dry eye syndrome.

Transderm-V delivers scopolamine for 72 hr.

Nitrodisc delivers nitroglycerin for 24 hr.

For details, see individual agents.

Chapter Three

UNTOWARD REACTIONS AND DRUG TOXICITY

DRUG ALLERGIES

Allergic responses to drugs occur in some patients and not in others. A drug allergy is an adverse response to a drug resulting from previous exposure to that drug or one closely related to it. Drug allergy is seen only after a second or subsequent exposure to the drug.

Allergic reactions to drugs differ from drug toxicity in the following ways: (1) the allergic reaction occurs in only a fraction of the population whereas drug toxicity will occur in all individuals if the dose is high enough; (2) the allergic response is unusual in that a small amount of an otherwise safe dose causes a severe reaction; (3) with allergy, the reaction is *different* from the usual pharmacologic effect of the drug; and (4) for an allergic reaction to occur, the patient must have had a previous exposure to that drug or one closely related to it.

The allergic response may be an *immediate reaction* involving antigen (in this case, the drug or part thereof) and antibody, resulting in the release of histamine. In mild cases the reaction is limited to urticaria, wheals, and itching of the skin. In severe cases, there is an *anaphylactic reaction* characterized by circulatory collapse or asphyxia due to swelling of the larynx and occlusion of the bronchial passages. Many patients are allergic to penicillin, for example. The allergic response may also be a *delayed reaction*, occurring several days or even weeks after the drug has been administered. Delayed reactions are characterized by drug fever, swelling of the joints, and reactions involving the blood-forming organs and the kidneys.

Treatment of an anaphylactic reaction may include epinephrine, oxygen, antihistamines, and corticosteroids.

DRUG IDIOSYNCRASIES

Idiosyncratic reactions are defined as those that occur in patients who have a genetically determined abnormal response to a drug. The response may be excessive or unusual. For example, succinylcholine, a muscle relaxant, is usually rapidly broken down by enzymes in the plasma and liver so that the effects of the drug last for only a few minutes. However, in a few patients, a usual dose of succinylcholine produces profound skeletal muscle relaxation and suppression of respiration, which may last several hours. Such patients have a genetic defect that produces unusual enzymes and succinylcholine is not broken down.

DRUG HYPERSENSITIVITY

Drug hypersensitivity occurs when the patient shows extreme sensitivity to an effect of the drug. The response is the usual pharmacologic effect; however, the effect is intense or exaggerated. A simple decrease in the dose may be sufficient to eliminate this type of adverse effect of a drug.

DRUG TOXICITY (POISONING)

Excess dosage of a drug, either accidental or intentional, results in an exaggerated response to that drug. Drug toxicity may be severe and lead to respiratory depression, cardiovascular collapse, and/or death if the drug is not withdrawn and adequate treatment instituted.

A relative overdose of a drug may be seen in patients who for some reason do not metabolize or excrete a particular drug rapidly enough or who are particularly sensitive to the effects of a drug due to hypersensitivity or idiosyncrasy (see above). This type of overdosage can usually be controlled by reducing the dose or by increasing the interval between doses of the drug.

Note: Elderly or debilitated patients often require smaller doses of drugs.

The nurse is responsible for prevention of accidents by teaching the care and storage of drugs, for observing and reporting signs of toxicity, for provision of first aid, and for providing emergency drugs and equipment needed for treatment while assisting the physician (see table of antidotes in *Appendix 2* for treatment of poisoning). Regardless of whether the poisoning is due to an attempted overdose or is accidental, the family members need emotional support at this time.

GENERAL UNTOWARD REACTIONS
(SIDE EFFECTS)

An unpleasant, unwanted, and/or bothersome reaction to a drug is termed either an untoward reaction or a side effect. In some cases, the untoward reaction is predictable and can occur in a large number of patients. For example, an antihistamine administered to reduce symptoms of allergy may cause drowsiness. On the other hand, other untoward reactions are not predictable in all cases and do not occur in a significant number of patients (although such untoward reactions may be quite serious). For example, only a few patients might develop a skin rash to thiazide diuretics.

Dermatologic Reactions   The skin is frequently involved in drug reactions. Although all drugs may cause dermatologic disturbances in some patients, certain pharmacologic agents are more prone to do so than others (i.e., penicillin, sulfonamides, bromides, iodides, arsenic, gold, quinine, thiazides, and antimalarials).

The dermatologic manifestations may range from pruritis and mild urticaria to all types of exanthematous eruptions, maculopapular rash, angioedema, pustular eruptions, granulomas, erythema nodosum, photosensitivity reactions, and alopecia.

In general, the administration of a drug is discontinued when the patient manifests even a mild skin reaction. The most serious types of reactions are extensive urticaria, angioedema, and those accompanied by systemic manifestations.

Some of the more serious, drug-induced skin reactions are detailed below:

1. **Exfoliative Dermatitis.** An obstinate, itchy, scaling of the skin, frequently accompanied by loss of hair and nails. Initial symptoms are a patchy or erythematous eruption accompanied by fever and malaise. Gastrointestinal symptoms are noted occasionally and are possibly caused by a similar lesion of the GI epithelium. Skin color changes from pink to dark red. The characteristic flaking begins after about 1 week. The skin remains smooth and red. New scales form as the old ones peel off. Relapses occur frequently, and death occasionally occurs as a result of secondary infection.

2. **Erythema Multiforma.** An acute or subacute eruption of the skin characterized by macules, papules, wheals, vesicles, and sometimes bullae. The lesions involve mostly the distal portions of the extremities, the face, and the mucous membranes. The condition is often accompanied by generalized malaise, arthralgia, and fever. The condition may recur and each attack usually lasts 2–3 weeks. The most serious type of erythema multiforma is the *Stevens-Johnson syndrome*. The bullous, blistery rash extends to the mucosa of the mouth, pharynx, and anogenital region. The syndrome is accompanied by high fever, severe headache, stomatitis, conjunctivitis, rhinitis, urethritis, and balanitis. It is often fatal.

3. **Photosensitivity.** A wide variety of unusual skin reactions characterized by dermatitis, urticaria, erythema multiforme-like lesions, and thickened and scaling patches may occur in some patients after a few minutes of exposure to sunlight.

Blood Dyscrasias   The bone marrow of certain patients is particularly sensitive to drugs. This may result in the insufficient manufacture of platelets, white blood cells, or red blood cells.

In principle, all drugs may cause blood dyscrasias in a particularly susceptible patient, but drugs such as the antineoplastics, certain antibiotics (including chloramphenicol), and phenylbutazone do so more frequently.

Patients who receive a drug that may cause bone marrow depression are monitored closely by frequent blood counts.

Some of the frequently observed blood dyscrasias are listed below.

1. **Agranulocytosis.** A complete absence of granulocytes associated with a marked reduction in circulating leukocytes is the most common blood dyscrasia to occur as an untoward effect of drug therapy. Early clinical signs are symptoms of infection, such as a sore throat, skin rash, fever, or jaundice.

2. **Aplastic Anemia.** Occurs when the bone marrow is damaged and blood-forming cells are replaced by fatty tissue. The result is pancytopenia, a reduction in all formed elements of blood. Aplastic anemia is usually fatal. Symptoms include anemia, leukopenia, and thrombocytopenia.

3. **Hemolytic Anemia.** Occurs when circulating red blood cells are destroyed either because of an antigen-antibody reaction or when a patient sensitive to certain chemicals has an idiosyncratic reaction. For instance, certain members of the black race or persons originating in certain regions of the Mediterranean inherit a sex-linked enzyme deficiency (glucose 6-phosphate dehydrogenase) which makes their red blood cells particularly sensitive to hemolysis by certain "oxidizing" drugs (including aspirin). Ingestion of these agents may cause acute intravascular hemolysis marked by hematuria. Treatment involves withdrawal of drug.

4. **Thrombocytopenia.** Platelet deficiency may result from destruction of the circulating platelets by pharmacologic agents or by depression of the platelet-forming elements of the bone marrow. The latter is the more serious manifestation. Severe thrombocytopenia is characterized by purpura followed by hemorrhage.

Hepatotoxicity (Liver Damage)

1. **Biliary Obstruction**. Some drugs affect the lining of the bile channels, causing them to narrow. Bile may back up into the bloodstream, and the patient appears jaundiced.

2. **Hepatic Necrosis**. Drug-induced damage of liver cells characterized by nausea, vomiting, and abdominal pain followed by jaundice.

Nephrotoxicity (Kidney Damage)

Drug-induced degeneration of renal tubules, which may interfere with further excretion of the drug. This results in increased drug toxicity. Nephrotoxicity is characterized by hematuria, anuria, casts in urine, edema, proteinuria, and uremia.

Ototoxicity (Ear Damage)

Results in damage to the vestibular and/or auditory portion of the eighth cranial nerve.

1. **Vestibular Damage**. Characterized by vertigo (sensation of turning and falling) and nystagmus (rapid, rhythmic, side-to-side movement of the eyeballs).

2. **Auditory Damage**. Characterized by tinnitus (ringing in the ears or a roaring sound) and progressive hearing loss. This effect may be caused by certain antibiotics (kanamycin, neomycin) and diuretics (ethacrynic acid, furosemide).

Central Nervous System Toxicity

Such toxicity is characterized by poor motor coordination, loss of judgment, depression of consciousness, or overstimulation including convulsions. Symptoms of depression are most likely to occur with barbiturates, other sedative-hypnotics, antianxiety agents, and alcohol.

Certain drugs also interfere with the transmission of nerve impulses at the myoneural junction. This causes muscle weakness and reduced ankle and knee reflexes. Gradually this untoward reaction can lead to apnea and cardiac arrest.

Tardive dyskinesia, characterized by the impairment of the power of voluntary movement resulting in fragmentary or incomplete movements, has been observed after long-term administration of antipsychotic drugs.

Gastrointestinal Disturbances Drug-induced nausea, diarrhea, and vomiting may result from either local irritation or systemic effects.

Drug Dependence Although not exactly an untoward reaction, drug dependence may be considered one of the problems associated with the administration of drugs.

The term "drug dependence" was developed to encompass both *psychological (psychic) dependence*, that is, drive or craving to take the drug for relief of tensions or discomfort, or for pleasure, and *physical dependence*, characterized by the appearance of physical symptoms when the administration of the drug is discontinued.

PSYCHOLOGICAL DEPENDENCE   May be mild or severe. In *mild dependence*, the person is accustomed to taking a drug that gives him a sense of well-being—for example, caffeine in coffee or nicotine in cigarettes. Such a person is said to be habituated and will not readily give up the drug. He tends to feel uneasy when deprived of it. Yet, if he so desires, the habituated person can usually, of his own accord, give up the drug without resorting to professional help. In *severe dependence* the person craves the feeling that the drug provides and will use compulsive efforts to obtain the drug (e.g., the use of heroin or amphetamines). Severe psychological dependence on drugs seems to occur in people who, once having experienced a feeling from a drug that is particularly satisfying, will continue to compulsively seek out the drug. Nurses should note patients who are asking for drugs more frequently than most patients with similar conditions. The names of such patients should be brought to the attention of the physician.

PHYSICAL DEPENDENCE   The continued ingestion of certain drugs (narcotics and depressants) results in an alteration in the body such that the drug is now required for the individual to function "normally." This is referred to as physical dependence. Discontinuation of a drug on which the patient is physically dependent may lead to *withdrawal symptoms*. These may vary with the particular drug. The withdrawal from narcotics results in increased autonomic nervous system activity and increased CNS excitability (see general statement on *Narcotics*, p. 472). Withdrawal from depressants (barbiturates, sedative-hypnotics, antianxiety agents) also results in increased excitability of certain regions of the CNS, notably those controlling motor and mental functions. The patient becomes tremulous and may suffer grand mal seizures, confusion, disorientation, and psychotic reactions.

Sexual Dysfunction Sexual function may be altered for a time by medication (e.g., tricyclic antidepressants). A change in libido or development of impotence is not necessarily permanent. Adjustment in dosage or substitution of one drug with another may relieve sexual dysfunction.

Chapter Four

DRUG INTERACTIONS: GENERAL CONSIDERATIONS AND NURSING IMPLICATIONS

DRUG–DRUG INTERACTIONS

Because many patients now receive more than one pharmacologic agent, drug interactions are a potentially major clinical problem. Indeed, in addition to having their intended, specific therapeutic effect, drugs may also influence other physiologic systems. The likelihood is high that two concomitantly administered agents influence some of the same pathways.

In most cases it is nevertheless possible to administer two interacting agents concurrently, provided that certain precautions, such as dosage adjustments, are taken. Moreover, drug interactions are not always adverse. They are sometimes taken advantage of therapeutically. For example, probenecid may be administered with penicillin to decrease the excretion rate of the penicillin and therefore result in higher blood levels.

The study of drug interactions is rapidly becoming a complex subspeciality of pharmacology. An attempt has been made throughout the text to reduce the complex explanation of drug interactions to the simplest possible terms.

A brief review of the major mechanisms that give rise to drug interactions is included in this section. This may enable the nurse to anticipate similar situations with other drug combinations.

It is important to remember that interactions apply not only to the intended therapeutic action of the drugs but also to their side effects.

It is also to be noted that the drug does not have to be a prescription one. Salicylates (aspirin) are an important interactant, as are common cathartics and constipating agents. Beverages like alcohol, and foods like tyramine-rich cheese may also play an important role.

Drug interactions often require an adjustment in dosage of one or both agents or discontinuation of one. Common major drug interactions are described under the drug or drug class.

Drugs With Opposing Pharmacologic Effects   The therapeutic effects of either or both agents may be cancelled, decreased, or abolished. An example is the combination of pilocarpine, a cholinergic drug prescribed for glaucoma, and an anticholinergic or atropine-like drug.

The interaction is usally described as "decreased effect" in the text. Correction could involve administration of only one agent, adjustment in time of administration, or increase in dosage of one or both agents.

Drugs With Similar Pharmacologic Effects   When two drugs have similar pharmacologic effects, their combined use may result in an effect equal to or even larger than the sum of that obtained if either agent were used separately. This interaction is described as "increased effect." The terms "additive," or "potentiation," might also be used to describe this interaction. An example of this interaction is the concomitant use of agents with CNS depressant actions such as alcohol, antianxiety agents, hypnotics, and antihistamines.

Changes in the Amount of Available Drug

CHANGE IN ABSORPTION FROM THE GI TRACT   The absorption of most drugs from the stomach or GI tract is pH dependent. The concomitant use of an agent that alters the pH can change the rate of absorption or the amount of drug absorbed, and thus either increase (↑) the effect or decrease (↓) the effect of the drug.

For example, the use of antacids that increase the pH of the stomach will result in a decrease in the absorption of aspirin, which is more rapidly absorbed at a lower pH.

The absorption of drugs is also affected by how long they reside in the GI tract. Drugs that affect the motility of the GI tract also affect drug absorption. The net effect of a cathartic usually is decreased absorption [decreased (↓) effect] since the drug to be absorbed in the GI tract stays there for a shorter period of time. Constipating agents, on the other hand, often result in increased absorption [increased (↑) effect].

The presence of food may also affect the absorption of drugs from the GI tract. For example, the absorption of tetracyclines is inhibited in the presence of dairy products (e.g., milk, cheese) since the calcium present in such foods complexes with the drug.

ALTERATION OF URINARY EXCRETION   Closely related to the rate at which drugs are absorbed from the GI tract is the rate at which they are eliminated in the urine or reabsorbed from the glomerular filtrate. Drugs that are eliminated more slowly because of another concomitantly administered agent stay in the body longer; thus the effect of the drug is increased.

Drugs that are eliminated faster, or are reabsorbed less, because of another concomitantly administered agent result in a decrease in the effect of the drug.

As in the case of absorption from the GI tract, elimination by the kidney is pH dependent. The pH of the urine is sometimes altered purposely by the administration of an alkalinizing agent (sodium bicarbonate) or an acidifying agent (ammonium chloride). Whether a drug will be excreted faster or more slowly with a change in pH depends on the drug. The alkalinization of the urine, for example, is sometimes taken advantage of with drugs like the sulfonamides. These agents are more soluble at a higher pH, and thus the possibility of crystallization in the kidney is reduced.

Displacement of Drugs from Protein-Binding Site   Several types of drugs bind to plasma protein. The resulting protein-bound drug is thus not free to exert a pharmacologic effect.

Protein binding is considered when dosage is established so that a given amount of drug will have the desired pharmacologic effect. This relationship, however, may be altered when another agent, which also binds to protein, is added to the therapy. If the attraction of drug B for the protein is greater than that of drug A, drug A will be displaced (or released) from the protein-binding site. This, then, will result in a greater amount of drug A available, and thus the effect of drug A will be increased. One such example is the coumarin-type anticoagulants, which are bound to protein but can be displaced by a variety of agents. A greater than expected amount of anticoagulant can have severe effects, including fatal hemorrhages.

Changes in Drug Metabolism

1. Most drugs are degraded in the liver by specific enzymes (drug-metabolizing enzymes). A change in the activity of an enzyme results in a change in the availability of the drug. Often such an interaction results in inhibition of the enzyme and hence an increased effect of the drug is observed.

However, certain drugs may stimulate the activity of enzymes involved in the breakdown of another pharmacologic agent. The barbiturates, for example, appear to stimulate certain drug-metabolizing enzymes in the liver. This results in a more rapid breakdown of the drugs normally degraded by such enzymes (e.g., steroid hormones including estrogen and progesterone, and coumarin-type anticoagulants).

2. The pharmacologic mode of action of certain drugs, such as the monoamine oxidase (MAO) inhibitors or disulfiram, consists of inhibiting a particular enzyme. An interaction may occur when this inhibited enzyme system is called upon to degrade another drug or food product.

For example, the above mechanism plays a role in the much publicized interaction of the MAO inhibitors and tyramine-rich foods like cheese. The tyramine cannot be degraded (as usual) by MAO, since the enzyme is inhibited. Tyramine accumulates and may cause severe hypertension.

Such an interaction is also taken advantage of in the treatment of alcoholics with disulfiram (Antabuse). The latter interferes with the metabolism of alcohol, leading to the accumulation of acetaldehyde, which has such unpleasant physiologic effects that the patient will refrain from alcohol ingestion while on disulfiram.

Alteration of Electrolyte Levels   Drugs that promote the loss (e.g., potassium) or retention (e.g., calcium) of electrolytes may cause the heart to become particularly sensitive to the toxic effects of digitalis. Such an interaction has been noted in the concomitant use of thiazide diuretics (which cause potassium loss) and digitalis.

Alteration of Gastrointestinal Flora   Antibiotics and other antimicrobial agents often kill the intestinal flora that synthesize vitamin K. A decrease in vitamin K concentration, which is involved in blood coagulation, increases the effect of anticoagulants and may result in hemorrhage.

FOOD–DRUG INTERACTIONS

General Considerations   Although there is increasing knowledge and concern about drug interactions, the effects of food - drug interactions are not as well known. Yet, these can produce dramatic effects, for example, when a food containing tyramine is ingested by a patient on MAO inhibitor therapy and a hypertensive crisis is precipitated. Food - drug interactions can be clinically less significant, as when the absorption of riboflavin is delayed by food ingestion. The mechanisms involved in drug - food interactions are most often attributable to effects on rate and amount of absorption, distribution, metabolism, and excretion. General interference mechanisms are discussed above. Important known food–drug interactions are identified in Appendix 4.

Nursing Implications for Maximizing Therapeutic Effect of Drugs
Teach patient and/or family

a. to take medications, the absorption of which is affected by food, on an empty stomach 1 hr before meals or 2 hr after meals, with a full glass of water.

b. which foods to include or avoid to promote the maximum therapeutic effect of medication (see Appendix 4).

c. that some foods should be either incorporated into the diet or avoided, if an alkaline or acidic urine promotes or inhibits drug action (see Appendix 4).

d. *food reactions in the body*—that the taste of the food does not indicate whether the body will metabolize it to an acid or alkaline ash. The type of ash is determined by the mineral content of the food. Acidic foods, such as coffee or citrus juices, are corrosive because they contain organic acid. They are not metabolized to an acid ash residue and therefore are not urinary acidifiers.

e. how to follow the recommended diet. Provide with written instructions, including a list of foods recommended and/or restricted. Refer for nutritional counseling, as needed.

DRUGS AND NUTRIENT UTILIZATION

Drugs can also affect the way the body uses food by hastening the excretion of certain nutrients, hindering the absorption of nutrients, or interfering with the body's ability to convert nutrients into usable forms. These drug - food interactions lead to vitamin and mineral deficiencies, particularly in children, the elderly, the chronically ill, and those on marginal diets. The diets of such patients should therefore be modified to include more foods rich in vitamins and iron.

The psychological and physical status of the client influences drug action as well. For example, malnutrition reduces the effectiveness of drugs by affecting rates of absorption and elimination of drugs, as well as tissue uptake and response. Depression reduces salivary output causing changes in nutritional uptake and possibly altering drug action.

Appendix 5 lists drugs that affect utilization of nutrients while Appendix 6 presents a compilation of foods that are acid, alkaline, or neutral.

Nursing Implications for Minimizing Nutritional Deficiencies Associated with Drug Therapy

1. *Assess*
   a. nutritional status of patient before initiating therapy and at periodic intervals during the course of therapy.
   b. subjective and objective data presented by the patient for possible negative drug effects.
   c. for malabsorption syndrome and nutritional deficiencies in those patients in poor nutritional state who are on a medication regimen with the drugs listed in Appendices 4 and 5.
2. Consult with physician regarding the need for diet supplementation.
3. *Teach patient and/or family*
   a. possible food - drug interactions that can occur with the medication the patient is taking.
   b. not to use over-the-counter medications before consulting the doctor.
   c. to practice good nutrition.
   d. where to apply for dietary funds or services, as needed (i.e., WIC, a supplemental food program for women, infants, and children).

Chapter Five

NURSING IMPLICATIONS FOR DRUG THERAPY

Nursing implications refer to the actions, precautions, and teaching that must be considered by the nurse when administering a particular drug. The nurse is not merely a drug dispenser blindly following the physician's orders; rather, the nurse is a professional, who uses knowledge of physiology, pathology, sociology, nursing, psychology, and pharmacology to participate in a team approach to disease prevention and drug therapy.

Reports from the patient, family, and other health care providers, as well as from the physician, are considered when carrying out the nursing process. Assessing and reporting to the physician both therapeutic and untoward reactions to drugs are meaningful and essential functions of the professional nurse. The initiation of appropriate nursing intervention significantly influences the success of drug therapy.

The following nursing implications are related to all types of drug therapy. They will be repeated selectively in the discussion of particular drugs to reinforce the importance of specific nursing implications related to a classification of drugs or to an individual drug.

1. Check the medication card or medication administration record with the physician's written order for patient's name, date of order, drug dosage, route, time of administration, and diet. Verify that order is not outdated by reviewing hospital policy (automatic stop orders).
2. Check whether the patient is scheduled for any diagnostic procedures that contraindicate administration of medications (e.g., gastrointestinal series, FBS). Withhold medication and check with physician if indicated.
3. Check in *Drug Handbook* for physiologic action, therapeutic use, untoward effects, contraindications, drug interactions, nursing implications, and recommended dosage for those drugs not already known. Use other references such as the *Facts and Comparisons Formulary Service* or *PDR* if necessary. Consult with pharmacist and request drug monograph if drug is not listed in reference book or is being administered for research purposes.
4. Select the specific drug ordered by the physician. Substitutes are neither acceptable nor legal. Note contraindications to interchange of brands because of potential bioavailability differences between products (e.g., phenytoin sodium).
5. Check that the dosage of the drug is within normal limits. If the dosage is not within normal limits, withhold the drug and discuss the safety of the dosage prescribed with the physician.
6. Prepare the specific dose ordered by the physician. If the strength of the solution or tablet on hand is not suitable for exact measurement, check with the pharmacist about the availability of another strength. If a more appropriate strength is not available, notify the physician, who may adjust the dosage so that medication can be measured carefully.

7. If a suitable strength tablet is unavailable, and unless contraindicated, the nurse may crush a soluble tablet and dissolve it in a small, measured amount of water. The desired fraction of the solution is then given to patient. This is not a method of choice.

8. Unless contraindicated, soluble tablets may be crushed and dissolved in a small amount of fluid and given to patients unable to swallow the tablet. Alternatively, an elixir may be provided by the pharmacy. Syrups and elixirs should not be given to diabetic patients. Tablets may also be crushed and administered with a small amount (one teaspoonful) of strained fruit unless contraindicated in diet.

9. When preparing and administering drugs, take into account the patient's name, age, sex, social background, religious preferences, diet, allergies, medical history, medical diagnosis, and nursing diagnosis.

10. Ascertain that appropriate diagnostic and baseline tests have been completed before initiating therapy. Review the results of these tests.

11. Before drug administration, identify the patient. Evaluate his emotional and physical state to determine his ability to receive the medication by the prescribed route. If the patient (e.g., a child) cannot or will not tolerate the drug by the route indicated, withhold the drug and consult with the physician, who may reduce the dosage, withdraw the drug, change the route of administration, or order another drug.

12. Take into consideration laboratory test interferences when selecting a method of testing and when using test results as a guide for administration of medication.

13. Consider the known pharmacokinetics of a drug to maximize its therapeutic effect.

14. Administer drugs as close to the designated time as possible. The recommended limits are one-half hour before or one-half hour after the designated time. Drugs ordered a.c. should usually be given 20 min before the meal. Schedule drugs and administer them at times that will maximize their therapeutic effectiveness while minimizing their untoward reactions (e.g., diuretics in the morning so that diuresis will be completed before bedtime).

15. Chart fluids taken with drugs if patient's intake and output are being monitored. Provide only liquids allowed on the diet.

16. Remain with the patient until oral drugs have been swallowed.

17. Use your knowledge of desired effects, undesired effects, and drug interactions to assess for positive and negative results. Report these observations. Untoward reactions might necessitate withholding the drug or emergency action.

18. Chart the administration of drug and related assessments immediately after administration (or if drug is withheld) to prevent duplication and errors resulting from omissions in communication.

19. Having consulted with other members of the health team, the nurse or pharmacist should teach the patient and the family the techniques and provide information necessary for successful administration of drugs in the institution or at home. This teaching is essential to promote drug compliance.

Chapter Six

NURSING IMPLICATIONS FOR THE ADMINISTRATION OF MEDICATIONS BY DIFFERENT ROUTES

There are general safety precautions that the nurse should observe for the preparation and storage of medications.

1. Double-check all mathematical calculations for preparing and administering medications. Review calculations and verify dosage of highly toxic drugs with another registered professional nurse.
2. Work with adequate lighting.
3. Be very attentive.
4. Check labels three times: (1) when taking medication from storage; (2) when preparing medication; and (3) when replacing medication in storage.
5. Check expiration date; discard medication if expiration date has passed.
6. Do not use discolored medication or medication with unexpected precipitate unless specifically directed otherwise (e.g., directions for administration may indicate that for a certain medication a change in color does not interfere with the safety of the drug).
7. Pour oral liquids from the bottle on the opposite side of the label.
8. Wipe the bottle after pouring a liquid.
9. Hold the medicine cup at eye level to pour medication. The meniscus (the lower curve of the liquid) should be at the calibration line indicating the proper dosage.
10. Pour tablets or capsules into the cap of the bottle and then empty the cap into the medication cup. Tablets or capsules are not to be poured into the nurse's hand.
11. Administer only those medications that you have prepared personally.
12. Once poured, do not return medications to the storage container.
13. Use sterile equipment and sterile technique to prepare parenteral medications.
14. Use recommended diluent for parenteral medications; follow directions for proper concentration and speed of administration of the medication.
15. Discard needles and syringes in appropriate containers after clipping shaft of needle and the tip of the syringe.
16. Discard ampules with unused portions of medication.
17. Store drugs as recommended (e.g., tablets should be kept dry and protected from light). Solutions should be stored at temperatures recommended.
18. Return bottles with damaged labels to pharmacy.
19. Do not leave medicine cabinets unlocked or medications unattended.

20. Complete a count of the controlled substances at the end of every shift with a professional registered nurse who is starting a tour of duty on the ward.

ADMINISTRATION BY ORAL ROUTE

1. Administer irritating drugs with meals or snacks to minimize their effect on the gastric mucosa.
2. If food interferes with the absorption of the drug, or if digestive enzymes destroy a significant portion of the medication, administer between meals or on an empty stomach. (See Appendix 4 for Food - Drug Interactions.)
3. Do not administer oral medications to a comatose patient.
4. If patient is vomiting, withhold medication and report to physician.

Tablets/Capsules

1. Unless a tablet is scored, it should not be broken to adjust dosage. Breaking may cause incorrect dosage, GI irritation, or destruction of drug in an incompatible pH. *Scored tablets* may be broken with a file.
2. *Time-release capsules, and enteric-coated tablets* should not be tampered with in any way. Instruct the patient to swallow whole and not to chew.
3. *Sublingual tablets* are to be placed underneath the tongue. Instruct the patient not to swallow or chew such tablets and not to drink water, all of which will interfere with effectiveness of medication.
4. *Buccal tablets* should be placed between gum and cheek (next to upper molar). Instruct the patient to avoid disturbing tablet during absorption.

Liquids

1. **Emulsions.** May be diluted with water.
2. **Suspensions.** Shake well until there is no apparent solid material.
3. **Elixirs.** Do not dilute. Diluent may cause precipitation of drug.
4. **Salty Solutions.** Unless contraindicated because of patient's diet, mix with water or fruit juice to improve taste.

ADMINISTRATION BY NASOGASTRIC TUBE

1. Place adult patient in a sitting position for administration.
2. Position an unconscious patient or an infant on the left side for administration.
3. *Check for correct placement of tube before initiating administration of medication.*
   a. Place distal end of tube in a glass of water. A few bubbles may occur as the gas in the stomach is released. *Do not administer* medication if bubbles occur with respirations, as this indicates placement of the tube in the lung.
   b. Listen to distal end of tube. No noise should be heard. *Do not administer* if a crackling sound is heard, as this also indicates placement in the lung.
   c. Attempt to withdraw a few milliliters of fluid with a syringe from the distal end. *Do not administer if there is an* absence of fluid, because this, again, indicates placement in the lung.
   d. Inject 5–10 ml of sterile water for an adult (0.5 ml for an infant) into the distal end, and listen over the epigastric area with a stethoscope for a swooshing or popping sound, indicating placement in the stomach.

4. Administration: Prevent excessive air from entering the stomach by maintaining a flow of fluid from initiation to completion of administration.
   a. Pour 5–10 ml of water into syringe at distal end of tubing and permit fluid to flow in by gravity.
   b. Before the syringe is empty, pinch off the tubing and add the medication via the syringe.
   c. As the medication is about to flow completely out of the syringe, pinch off the tubing and add 5–10 ml of water to ensure that all the medication has reached the stomach; maintain patency.
5. After completing administration of medication:
   a. Clamp nasogastric tube and remove the attached syringe.
   b. Assess for gastric distress demonstrated particularly by distention and regurgitation.
   c. Record fluid administered via nasogastric tube.

ADMINISTRATION BY INHALATION

Nursing Implications for All Methods of Administration by Inhalation
1. Administer only one medication at a time through nebulizer, unless specifically ordered to the contrary. Several drugs used together may cause undesirable reactions, or they may inactivate each other.
2. Measure medication precisely with a syringe. Dilute medication as ordered, and place in nebulizer. For home administration, ascertain that the patient has equipment necessary for preparation of medication and is able to measure accurately.
3. Discard medication left in nebulizer from previous administration.
4. Teach patient to assemble, disassemble, and clean equipment.
5. Emphasize need to clean mouthpiece and nebulizer after each administration. Other tubing is to be cleaned each day.
6. Seat patient comfortably or place in semi-Fowler position to permit greater diaphragmatic expansion.

Additional Nursing Implications for Inhalation Therapy by Nebulization
1. Types of nebulizers:
   a. Commercial metered-dose hand nebulizers.
   b. Hand nebulizers filled with diluted medication.
   c. Nebulizer connected by rubber tubing to a source of compressed air or oxygen. Midway in the rubber tubing, a Y tube is inserted; one end of the Y tube is open, and the other end is connected by more rubber tubing to the nebulizer.
2. *Test equipment* before initiating therapy:
   a. Place medication in nebulizer.
   b. Turn on either compressed air or oxygen as ordered.
   c. Occlude open end of Y tube with finger. If the equipment is working properly, a fine spray will be seen leaving the nebulizer.
3. Teach patient self-administration of medication by nebulization using the following directions:
   a. Place medication in nebulizer.

b. First exhale slowly through pursed lips.

c. Position nebulizer in mouth, but do not seal lips to it.

d. Take a deep breath through the mouth and at the same time squeeze the bulb of the nebulizer or close the end of the Y tube.

e. Hold breath for 3–4 sec at full inspiration.

f. Exhale slowly through pursed lips to create more pressure in the air passages, which will carry medication through the bronchial tree.

g. Repeat cycle for the number of times ordered to use medication in nebulizer, depending on instructions for particular medication.

Additional Nursing Implications for Inhalation Therapy by Intermittent Positive-Pressure Breathing (IPPB)

1. Select the inspiratory flow rate ordered by medical supervision. Initial treatment is often started at 5 cm of water pressure to help patient adjust to using the machine correctly; then pressure is gradually increased to the most effective level, which is usually 15–20 cm of water pressure for a 15-min treatment 3–4 times a day.

2. Encourage a slow respiratory rate, diaphragmatic breathing, and prolonged expiration through pursed lips.

3. Advise patient to take several deep breaths and to exhale as fully as possible.

4. Encourage coughing effectively several times during treatment, if clearance of secretions is the goal.

5. Administer at least 1 hour after meals to prevent nausea and vomiting.

6. Mist therapy should be provided as ordered either before or after IPPB.

Evaluate the extent of improvement after therapy by having patient breathe after all air has been pushed out. Assess respiratory rate and effort and describe any secretions that are produced.

Additional Nursing Implications After Administration of Medication by Inhalation

1. Assist patient with postural drainage or clapping and vibrating as ordered.

2. Evaluate the extent of improvement after therapy. Have patient push all air out and then breathe. Assess respiratory rate and effort, and describe any secretions that are produced.

3. Cleanse equipment thoroughly at least once daily by soaking in 1:3 solution of white vinegar and water, rinsing thoroughly, and air drying, or follow protocol of agency for cleaning equipment.

ADMINISTRATION BY IRRIGATIONS AND GARGLES

1. Throat irrigations should not be warmer than 120°F in order not to destroy or damage tissue.

2. Warn the patient that gargling with full-strength antiseptic solution may destroy normal defenses of the mouth and pharynx.

ADMINISTRATION BY NASAL APPLICATION

Nursing Implications for All Methods of Nasal Application
1. Have paper tissue available.
2. Use separate equipment for each patient to prevent spread of infection.
3. Instruct patient to blow nose gently before initiating therapy. If the patient is unable to blow his nose, then the nasal passage may be cleared with a bulb-type aspirator.
4. After completing treatment, rinse dropper or tip of spray container (be careful not to introduce water into spray container), and dry with tissue. Wipe the tip of nasal jelly tube with a damp tissue.
5. Replace cap of container as soon as treatment is completed.
6. To prevent cross-contamination, each patient should have his own dropper and medication container. If only one container is available, use an individual dropper for each patient.

Administration of Nose Drops

Additional Nursing Implications for Administration of Nose Drops
1. Instruct patient to tilt head back if the sitting or standing position is preferable during administration.
2. Instruct patient who is lying flat in bed to tilt head over the side of the bed, or place a support under neck so that it is hyperextended.
3. Insert dropper about 1/3 inch into the nares and instill the drops. Avoid touching the external nares with the dropper, since this may cause sneezing.
4. Instruct patient to maintain position for 1–2 min until the medication is absorbed.

Administration of Nasal Spray

Additional Nursing Implications for Administration of Nasal Spray
1. Instruct patient to hold head upright for spray to be administered into nares and to sniff briskly as spray container is quickly and firmly squeezed.
2. Optimally spray once or twice into each nostril.
3. Allow 3–5 min for medication to be effective.
4. Then instruct patient to blow nose gently.
5. Repeat spray if necessary.

Administration of Nasal Jelly

Additional Nursing Implications for Administration of Nasal Jelly
Teach patient to finger place jelly (about the size of a pea) into each nostril and then to sniff it well back into nose.

ADMINISTRATION OF EYE MEDICATIONS

Administration of Eye Drops

1. Instruct patient to lie down or sit with head tilted back.
2. Have a separate tissue available for each eye.
3. Wipe the lids and eyelashes clean before instillation.
4. Use an individual, squeezable plastic container or dropper for each patient. If a dropper is used, draw up only the amount of solution needed for administration.
5. Hold the applicator close to the eye, but do not touch eyelids or lashes.
6. Expose the lower conjunctival sac by drawing down the skin below the eye with a gauze pad.
7. With the same hand, use a sterile cotton ball and gently press against the lacrimal duct during and for 2 min after instillation, to prevent excessive systemic absorption of the medication as a result of draining down the lacrimal duct.
8. Place the heel of the hand administering the drops on the hand holding the gauze pad, and instill the number of drops ordered into the center of the exposed sac. Avoid dropping medication on the cornea, as this may cause tissue damage and discomfort.
9. Instruct patient to keep eye closed for 1–2 min after application to allow for absorption of medication.

Administration of Eye Ointment

1. Instruct patient to lie down or sit down with head tilted back.
2. Have a separate tissue available for each eye.
3. Expose the lower conjunctival sac as indicated above in administration of eyedrops.
4. Squeeze a strip of ointment into the conjunctival pouch—usually 1 cm (approximately ⅓ inch), unless otherwise ordered, into conjunctival pouch.
5. Instruct patient to close eyes for 1–2 min after application to permit the warmth of the body to melt the medication and spread medication over area to be treated.
6. Warn patient that vision will probably be blurred for a few minutes after application of ointment.

ADMINISTRATION OF EAR DROPS

1. Warm drops to body temperature by holding bottle in hand for a few minutes before applying.
2. Have the patient lie on side with the ear to be treated facing up.
3. For instillation in adults, pull the cartilagenous part of the pinna (the external part of the ear) back and up. Point the dropper in the direction of the eardrum, and allow the drops to fall in the direction of the external canal.

4. For instillation of drops in children under 3 years of age, pull the pinna back and down. Point the dropper in the direction of the eardrum and allow the drops to fall on the external canal.
5. Have the patient remain on side for a few minutes after instillation to allow medication to reach eardrum and be absorbed.
6. Never pack a wick tightly into the ear. On occasion, a loose cotton wick is inserted into the ear by the physician so that the medication will bathe the eardrum continuously. The wick should be changed when it appears nonabsorbent or soiled.

ADMINISTRATION OF DERMATOLOGIC PREPARATIONS

Medications can be applied to the skin by rubbing, patting, spraying, painting, or by iontophoresis (medication is driven into skin by means of an electric current).

1. Use sterile technique if there is a break in the skin.
2. Cleanse skin before medication is applied. The cleansing agent should be specified by the physician.
3. Remove ointment from jar with a tongue depressor and not with fingers.
4. If medication is to be rubbed in, apply using firm strokes.
5. Apply only a thin layer of medication unless specified otherwise.
6. Solutions should be painted on with applicator.
7. If medication stains, warn patient to take adequate precautions (use old sheets or plastic cloth).
8. Moist dressings or compresses are prepared by soaking sterile towels in solution ordered, wringing them out, and applying them to the area to be treated. Sterile gloves should be worn if sterile solution is to be applied.

RECTAL ADMINISTRATION

Retention Enemas

1. In order to avoid peristalsis, administer retention enemas slowly, using a small amount of solution (no more than 120 ml) and a small rectal tube.
2. Instruct the patient to lie on left side and to breathe through mouth to relax the rectal sphincter.
3. Retention enemas containing medication should be administered after a bowel movement to promote maximum absorption of medication in the empty rectum.
4. Have patient remain flat for 30 min after administration of enema.

Suppositories

1. As a rule, suppositories should be refrigerated, since they tend to soften at room temperature.
2. Use finger cot to protect the finger used for insertion (index finger for adults, fourth finger for infants). Instruct patient to lie on left side and to breathe through mouth to relax the sphincter. Spread the buttocks and gently insert the lubricated suppository beyond the internal sphincter (usually about 2 inches).

3. Have the patient remain on side for 20 min after insertion, to prevent expulsion. For the pediatric patient hold the buttocks together or tape them together until impulse to defecate passes.
4. If indicated, teach the patient how to self-administer enema or suppository. Observe self-administration to ensure that procedure is being done correctly.

VAGINAL ADMINISTRATION

1. Arrange douche containing medication so that container hangs just above the patient's hip. In this manner the force of the liquid does not drive the solution through the cervical os.
2. Vaginal suppository may be administered using an applicator with patient in lithotomy position.
3. If indicated, instruct the patient on how to self-administer vaginal medication. Observe self-administration to check whether procedure is done properly.
4. Instruct patient to remain with hips elevated for 5 min and then to remain in bed for at least 20 min longer, to promote absorption of medication and prevent drainage of medication after suppository has melted.

URETHRAL ADMINISTRATION

1. Cleanse area around urinary meatus as for a catheterization.
2. Insert lubricated urethral suppository using sterile technique.

ADMINISTRATION BY PARENTERAL ROUTE

Intradermal and Intracutaneous Injections These injections are made into the dermis and produce local effects. The techniques are used mainly for anesthesia and sensitivity tests.

1. The inner aspect of the forearm is the most common site for intradermal injections as it gives good visualization of the response to test media. The upper aspect of the chest or the back of the patient may be used.
2. Use a tuberculin-type syringe with a 26-gauge needle ⅜ inch long.
3. Cleanse site selected for injection using a circular motion moving outward from the projected site of insertion.
4. Stretch the skin and insert the needle with the bevel upward at a 15-degree angle until the tip of the needle is just under the outer layer of skin and inject the fluid. Withdraw the needle quickly after injection. A small blister or bleb should have been formed by the solution just below the skin.
5. After injection, observe the patient for local reactions, such as redness and swelling.

Intrasynovial and Intra-articular Injection Used for the relief of pain or the local application of medication. Be aware that local discomfort is usually intensified for several hours before palliative effect sets in.

Hypodermoclysis This technique is used primarily in patients who require parenteral fluids but whose veins do not permit IV infusion.

During the procedure, a large amount of fluid is slowly injected subcutaneously into the loose tissues on the outer side of the upper body or, more often, into the anterior aspect of the thigh.

If the tissue becomes endurated, clamp the fluid off to allow for fluid absorption. The solution may be restarted after the tissue has become more elastic.

Hyaluronidase, an enzyme that breaks down the main constituents of intracellular connective tissue, is sometimes added to the medication so that the fluid will be absorbed rapidly and cause less discomfort.

An intramuscular (IM) 20- or 22-gauge needle, 1½ inches long, is recommended for children; a 19-gauge, 2½–3 inch needle is satisfactory for adults.

At the completion of the procedure remove the needle and apply pressure; apply collodion and a small dry sterile dressing, to prevent fluid leakage.

Subcutaneous and Intramuscular Injections *For more detailed instructions about subcutaneous (SC) and intramuscular (IM) injections, see pp. 33–34 and your textbook on nursing techniques.*

1. Use sterile technique.
2. In selecting the proper gauge and length of needle for injection, consider age, weight, condition of patient, and physical properties of medication.
3. In order to promote absorption of medication and minimize pain after IM injection, palpate potential site. Choose a site that is not tender to patient and where tissue does not become firm on palpation. Alternate the sites of injection, and chart the sites used—for example, RD for right deltoid, RGM for right gluteus medius. (See Fig. 3.)
4. Cleanse site selected for injection using a circular motion, moving outward from site of insertion.
5. For SC injection, pick up tissue in selected area and hold firmly until needle has been inserted at a 45-degree angle.
6. For IM injection, stretch the skin if patient is in a normal state of nutrition. If the patient is emaciated, pinch the tissue to form a muscle bundle to ensure that the medication is injected into the muscle. Insert needle at a 90-degree angle.
7. Leave a margin of needle at least ½ inch from hub to prevent its complete disappearance in case of breakage.
8. When preparing for SC and IM injections, include a small bubble of air in syringe (0.2–0.3 ml) in addition to medication. The air bubble will help expel all solution from the needle so that irritating solutions will not leak into the tissues as the needle is withdrawn.
9. Insert the needle quickly to minimize pain. After insertion, aspirate to be sure that the needle is not in a blood vessel. If blood returns into the syringe, withdraw the needle and discard the medication. Prepare another dose using new sterile equipment, select another site, and start the injection again.
10. Administer the medication slowly to allow for absorption, and remove the needle quickly while pressing down at the point of insertion with a sterile sponge to prevent bleeding. Apply a Band-Aid if necessary.
11. Massage the area after injection to increase circulation and promote absorption of the drug. This step is contraindicated in the case of certain drugs, such as Bicillin, where absorption should be slow.

Intravenous Injections (Direct or via Continuous Infusion) The physician usually assumes responsibility for direct IV administration and starting continuous IV. The following nursing implications apply only to continuous infusion.

1. Position patient as comfortably as possible and explain procedure.

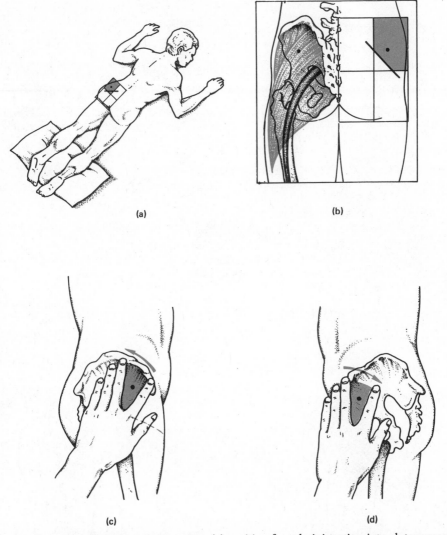

FIGURE 3 Intamuscular injection sites: (a) position for administration into gluteus maximus area; (b) detailed administration into gluteus maximus; (c) area for administration of IM into right ventrogluteal area; (d) area for administration of IM into left ventrogluteal area.

2. If area to be injected is hairy, shave it to prevent adhesive tape from causing discomfort during removal.
3. Attach additional bottles of fluid as ordered and label number of bottles used. IV fluid should be 18–24 inches above infusion site.
4. Maintain the rate of flow as ordered. Check the rate of flow by counting drops per minute at least every 30 min or more often if patient is restless and moves limb where IV is inserted. Count flow rate even if infusion pump is in use.

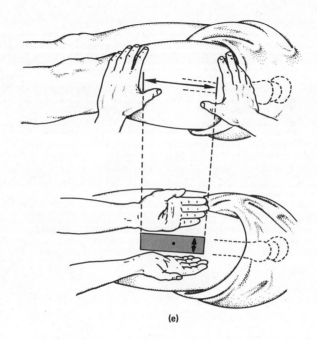

(e)

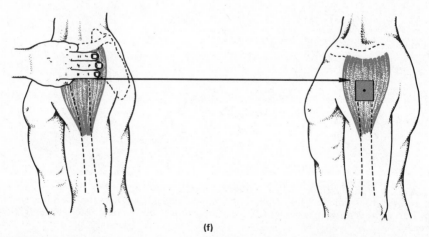

(f)

FIGURE 3 (*Continued*)   (e) area for administration of IM into vastus lateralis: top, length of area, bottom, breadth of area; and (f) area for administration of IM into the deltoid.

5. Check amount of fluid administered at least hourly.
6. Check hospital policy to ascertain which drugs a nurse may add to an IV on order by a physician. For volutrol (or pediatrol) administration, dilute as required and regulate the flow so that the medication will not damage tissue yet be absorbed before loss of potency occurs.

7. When medication is added, record the name of the drug, dosage, date and time of addition, and the nurse's signature on a label to be attached to the bottle, bag, or volutrol container.

8. If flow stops, check that the tubing is not kinked or occluded by the position of the patient. If possible, reposition the patient's extremity to reestablish flow.

9. Assess for correct placement of needle in the vein and absence of extravasation if the IV rate slows in spite of clamp or pump adjustment, if the site of injection becomes pale and/or edematous, and/or if the patient complains of pain. Three methods for assessing for correct placement of needle in the vein are commonly used:

   a. Lower the container below the level of the vein. If blood flows back into the needle and tubing, the needle is in a vein. If blood returns very slowly, the needle may have partially slipped out of the vein. If blood does not return, the needle is not in the vein. This procedure is not recommended when the IV contains a drug that may cause necrotic damage to the tissue.

   b. Use a sterile syringe with saline, and withdraw fluid from rubber at end of tubing. If blood does not return, discontinue IV.

   c. Try to stop flow by applying a tourniquet 4–6 inches above insertion site and open roller clamp wide. If IV continues to flow, needle is in SC tissue and IV is infiltrated. Discontinue IV.

10. Prevent air embolism by

   a. adding additional container of solution ordered before old container is completely emptied.

   b. checking that all connections in IV are tight.

   c. clamping off the first bottle that is empty in a Y-type set (parallel hookup), to prevent air from the empty bottle from being drawn into vein.

   d. following instructions very carefully when blood or any other type of fluid is administered under pressure.

   e. positioning the extremity receiving the infusion below the level of the heart to prevent negative pressure, venous collapse, and sucking of air into tubing.

   f. positioning the clamp or the infusion pump regulating the flow no lower than the level of the heart and no higher than 4 inches above the level of the heart to prevent the formation of negative pressure in the tubing below.

   g. allowing the tubing to fall below the level of the extremity to help prevent air from entering the vein should the infusion bottle empty before the IV is discontinued.

11. Recognize an air embolism by the occurrence of sudden vascular collapse, cyanosis, hypotension, tachycardia, venous pressure rise, and loss of consciousness.

12. Be prepared to assist with treatment should an air embolism occur. Position patient on left side and administer oxygen and other supportive measures.

13. Prevent "speed shock" by checking the rate of flow frequently and observing for untoward symptoms associated with the drug being administered.

14. Assess for symptoms of phlebitis, such as pain, tenderness, and redness along the path of the vein. Patients receiving IV for more than 24 hr are especially susceptible to phlebitis. Alcohol, hypertonic solutions with carbohydrate above 10%, and solutions with high alkaline or acid pH cause phlebitis more often. Slow IV to "keep vein open," and report immediately if symptoms of phlebitis appear.

15. Do not flush a clogged IV. The flow might have been stopped by an embolus that should not be moved into the circulation. Report the situation to physician.

16. Schedule incompatible medications to be administered at different times.
17. Remove the IV when ordered by the physician. Clamp off tubing before removing the IV so as to prevent extravasation into subcutaneous tissues. Press down with a sterile sponge at site of needle or plastic tube while it is moved to prevent bleeding. Apply bandage to former injection site to prevent bleeding and infection.
18. Chart intake and output at least hourly.

CENTRAL PARENTERAL ADMINISTRATION

1. Explain total parenteral regimen and the procedure for central parenteral administration to the patient.
2. Assist with catheter insertion.
   a. Use strict surgical asepsis (gown, mask, and gloves).
   b. Place patient in Trendelenburg position to raise venous pressure.
   c. Have local anesthetic available if ordered.
   d. Place a rolled towel lengthwise under patient's back to make the subclavian vein more prominent.
   e. Shave area of insertion and prep with acetone and Betadine.
   f. Instruct the patient to bear down (Valsalva maneuver) when the needle is inserted to prevent air from entering the vein and causing an air embolism.
   g. Assist as catheter is sutured to skin to prevent dislodgement.
   h. Assist with application of antibiotic ointment and dry sterile dressing at site of insertion.
   i. Check that patient is x-rayed to verify position of tube before total parenteral nutrition (TPN) is initiated.
3. Control sepsis.
   a. Use sterile technique in changing dressing q 2–3 days.
   b. Provide skin care at site of catheter insertion when dressing is changed. Use antibiotic ointment ordered.
   c. Use sterile technique in changing infusion tubing and filters q 24–48 hr.
   d. Use sterile technique in handling bottle of TPN solution.
   e. Observe solution for clouding, growth, or matter in the bottle. If contamination is observed, hang a new bottle and return contaminated one to pharmacy for culture.
   f. Use 5% dextrose/water (D/W) if bottle of TPN must be removed and another bottle of TPN is not readily available.
   g. Assess body temperature q 4 hr for elevation indicating infection.
   h. After hanging a new bottle, monitor for a temperature spike that would indicate contamination.
   i. If patient has chills or fever and other signs of sepsis, replace bottle and tubing and send equipment for culture. Further tests such as blood, urine, sputum, x-ray films, and physical examination are done to locate foci of infection. Should the cause of the infection be undetermined and the fever continue for 12–24 hours, assist with removal of catheter and with insertion of catheter on the other side.
4. Maintain the rate of flow.
   a. Preferably use an infusion pump or an alarm system.

    b. Use an infusion pump when a 0.22-μ filter is used. The flow with a 0.45-μ filter will continue by gravity drip so that an infusion pump is not essential.

    c. Count the drip rate at least every half-hour even if an infusion pump is used.

    d. Calculate and maintain a uniform flow rate for 24 hr.

    e. Check for kinks, and position tube meticulously.

5. Assess

    a. for signs of overload such as prominence of neck, arm, and hand veins (early symptoms), lassitude, headache, nausea, twitching, hypertension, mental fuzziness, somnolence, and convulsions.

    b. for infiltration by noting pain and swelling in shoulder, neck, or face.

    c. for an improperly placed, slipped, or broken catheter, or a leak at the tubing union, which would be indicated by a wet dressing.

    d. for glycosuria by testing fractional urines q 6 hr. Use Tes-Tape or Diastix to check urine of patient receiving cephalosporin to prevent false-positive results.

    e. daily intake and output and record.

    f. weight daily.

    g. laboratory reports for electrolyte balance and renal and liver function.

    h. caloric count of daily oral and parenteral intake and chart.

ADMINISTRATION BY INTRA-ARTERIAL INFUSION

Administration by intra-arterial infusion involves insertion of a Teflon catheter by a surgeon under fluoroscopy into the artery leading directly into the area to be treated. The arteries commonly used are the brachial, axillary, carotid, and femoral. The drug is then pumped steadily through the catheter. The tumor receives a high concentration of the chemotherapeutic agent before it is distributed to the rest of the body. The drug may be administered at varying intervals of time. Intra-arterial infusion may be performed on an ambulatory basis with a portable infusion pump, but the patient must be taught how to monitor the apparatus.

1. Assess

    a. tissue in local area for reaction, such as erythema, mild edema, blistering, and petechiae.

    b. vital signs periodically (q 15 min) when therapy is initially instituted until BP is stabilized.

    c. site of infusion for infection.

    d. intake and output to detect renal failure.

2. Describe observations completely when charting, and report to doctor.

3. Report pain since it may be indicative of severe injury to normal tissue, vasospasm, or intravasation.

4. Maintain rate of pump as ordered.

5. Do not permit infusion fluid to run through completely, because air will then enter the tubing. Add fluid as needed.

6. Clamp tubing if an air bubble is noted and call doctor.

7. *Do not disconnect the tubing between the pump and the patient to release the air bubble because hemorrhage will occur.*

8. Apply pressure if hemorrhage occurs from the artery.
9. Check tubing for kinks and prevent compression of tubing.

ADMINISTRATION BY PERFUSION (EXTRACORPOREAL OR ISOLATION PERFUSION)

Perfusion technique involves the administration of large doses of highly toxic drugs to an isolated extremity, organ, or region of the body. For perfusion in the lower extremity, the iliac, femoral, and popliteal arteries and veins are used; for upper extremity perfusion, the axillary artery and vein are injected. The abdominal aorta and vena cava are used for pelvic perfusion. The actual perfusion is accomplished in the operating room where, by means of a pump oxygenator, the patient's blood is circulated in a closed system for the part of the body involved. Efforts are made by the use of a tourniquet or ligature to prevent seepage of the concentrated drug into the systemic circulation. Seepage of the drug results in destruction of normal tissue.

Preoperative Administration

1. Explain procedure to patient, answer questions, and provide emotional support.
2. Weigh patient because dosage of chemotherapeutic agent and heparin is calculated on the basis of body weight.
3. Be certain that hematologic tests, urinalysis, and x-ray films have been done.

Postoperative Administration

1. Ascertain if hematologic tests have been made and evaluated for depression of bone marrow function, which is due to seepage of concentrated drug into systemic circulation.
2. Assess for
   a. tanning, erythema, or blistering of skin over area perfused—symptoms resemble toxic reaction to radiation.
   b. thrombosis and phlebitis of local tissue.
   c. signs of infection, such as fever and malaise, since septicemia may occur.
   d. color and warmth of extremity perfused and report untoward symptoms.
   e. pain, which may be indicative of severe tissue damage.
   f. hemorrhage, hypotension, fibrillation, arrhythmia, sudden chest pain, and pulmonary edema, all of which may be precipitated by perfusion.
3. Continue to provide comprehensive holistic nursing care, with both physical and emotional support.

Chapter Seven

DRUG RESPONSE OF THE PEDIATRIC, GERIATRIC, OR PREGNANT PATIENT

DRUG RESPONSE OF THE PEDIATRIC PATIENT

General Considerations   The safe use of many of the newer pharmacologic agents in children has not yet been established. In case of doubt, it is wise to ask the physician whether a particular agent is suitable for pediatric patients.

Pediatric dosage for individual agents is listed whenever relevant and/or available. The safe pediatric dosage can also be computed from adult dosage by means of Young's, Clark's, or Fried's rules; by calculating formulas using the surface area of child; or by calculating formulas for recommended pediatric dosage per kilogram body weight. Each of these methods of computation is detailed in Appendix 10.

The following general considerations apply to the administration of drugs to children. The pediatric patient has a different pharmacodynamic sensitivity than does the adult. Furthermore, there is often a long delay between the marketing of a drug for adults and the establishment of a rational therapeutic regimen for pediatric patients.

Many of the problems encountered in the pediatric administration of drugs are attributable to age and development related to differences in the distribution of drugs in the body and in the rates at which drugs are absorbed and eliminated.

ABSORPTION   The pH of the GI tract is higher in infants than in adults. Therefore, drugs that are absorbed in acid environment are absorbed more slowly in children (slower onset of action) than in adults. Conversely, drugs that are destroyed by acid have a longer half life (longer activity) in children than in adults.

Topical absorption is usually faster in pediatric patients, because their epidermis is thinner.

DISTRIBUTION THROUGHOUT THE BODY   A much larger proportion of body weight is water in children than in adults; the converse is true for fat. Thus, drugs that are water soluble are distributed in a smaller volume (are more concentrated) in adults than in children. Drugs that are fat soluble are more concentrated in children than in adults.

PLASMA PROTEIN BINDING   The plasma protein binding of drugs is usually less extensive in children, especially in neonates, than it is in adults because of lower percentage of plasma protein. This results in a greater concentration of free drugs (bioavailability) in children than in adults.

HEPATIC DEGRADATION AND RENAL EXCRETION   Both the liver and the kidneys of neonates and infants are immature compared with those of adults. The liver, for instance, has a lower concentration of the enzymes that participate in the degradation of drugs; for example, phenytoin, metabolized by the liver as a rule, is broken down more slowly in infants than in adults.

Renal excretion, on the other hand, which represents a complex balance between elimination and reabsorption, is often faster in infants than in adults (shorter duration of action).

All these factors are taken into consideration when a pediatric dosage is established. The administration of drugs to pediatric patients also involves many practical considerations detailed below.

Special Nursing Implications for the Administration of Pediatric Medications

1. Always wake patient before administering medication.
2. Try to gain the child's cooperation by using techniques and an approach appropriate to the level of development.
3. Indicate to the child in a firm but friendly manner that it is time to take the medication.
4. Accept a child's negative feelings and demonstrate empathy. Do not shame the child. Compliment him on positive aspects of cooperative behavior and demonstrate acceptance and liking even though the child may not have cooperated.
5. Appropriately, explain to the child the benefits of medication.
6. Realize that hospitalization and medication are regarded as punishment by some children.
7. Use diversional techniques appropriate to developmental level when giving medications to a child. For example: suggest the child count or recite the alphabet while receiving a parenteral injection or suggest that the child lie on his abdomen and turn his toes in to help relax the gluteal muscles. For a child who is quite young, play a music box or set a toy in motion and talk with the patient.
8. Crush pills for infants or children under 5 years of age, and dissolve them in syrup, water, or nonessential foods (e.g., applesauce).
9. Do not force oral medications, since aspiration pneumonia is a threat. Report to the physician if the child consistently refuses or spits out the medication so that another drug or another form of the medication can be ordered.
10. When using a plastic dropper or plastic syringe to administer medication, direct the tip toward the inner aspect of the cheek of the mouth to avoid aspiration and stimulation of the cough reflex.
11. When using a spoon to administer medication to an infant, place the spoon well back on the tongue to prevent stimulating the extrusion reflex.
12. Pouring small amounts of medication into an empty nipple from which the infant will suck can facilitate the administration of medication.
13. When administering *per os* (PO) medication to an infant, hold the child securely against your body with one arm around the child supporting his head and neck and your other hand holding his free arm while administering the medication. Elevate the infant's head to prevent aspiration.
14. When administering ear drops to a child under 3 years of age, pull the pinna of the ear back; for a child over 3 years of age, pull the pinna of the ear back and up.
15. If the child cannot, or will not, cooperate so that parenteral medication can be administered, restrain him with the help of other personnel, as necessary, and then administer medication.
16. Children under 2 years of age should receive IM injections into the vastus lateralis or rectus femoris (Fig. 4), since gluteal muscles are as yet too underdeveloped

to be used for IM administration, and damage to the sciatic nerve is likely to occur.

17. After medication, offer juice or water and verbal praise. Do not offer bribes such as candy, lollipops, or special privileges. These suggest that medications are bad and that reward is necessary for an activity that the child should learn to understand is helpful to him.

18. After insertion of suppository, either hold buttocks or tape them together until defecation impulse has passed (usually 15 min).

(continued)

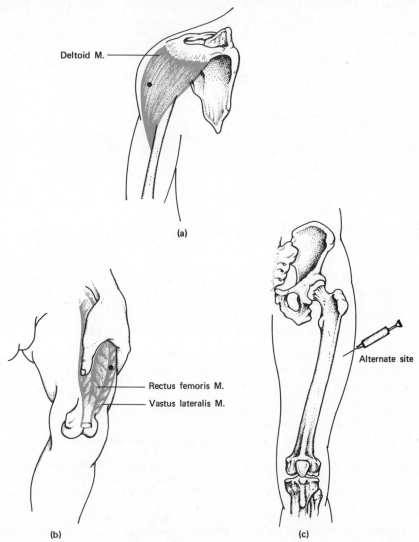

FIGURE 4   Pediatric intramuscular injection sites: (a) deltoid; (b) anterior surface of mid-lateral thigh; and (c) anterolateral surface of upper thigh.

19. Use an infusion pump whenever possible to regulate rate of flow in pediatrics. If pump is not available, adjust rate of flow while the infant is quiet (crying constricts the blood vessels and the rate will then be too rapid after he stops crying).

20. Safely and adequately restrain infant and child during IV therapy. Exercise unaffected limbs periodically to maintain circulation. Check that restraints are not inhibiting circulation. Remove tape at insertion site daily to check for tissue damage around site of insertion.

21. Assess condition of pediatric patient, rate of flow, amount absorbed, and urine output at least hourly.

22. On the pediatric floor, the medication cart and drugs should be constantly under the eyes of the nurse. She must always be alert to the possibility that children may take medications that are not theirs or may tamper with them in some way. Syringes and needles must never be left with a child to use as a toy after the nurse has left.

23. If a child does not have a name tag, identification must be made according to hospital policy before medication is administered.

24. Before beginning to pour medications the nurse should be aware of the floor plan of the ward and of the age, weight, and diagnosis of the children who are to receive the various medications.

25. Calculate dosages, and check safety of dosages ordered, using formulas in Appendix 10 p. 929. Before administration, double-check with another nurse the dosages of the following: digoxin, insulin, heparin, and blood.

DRUG RESPONSE OF THE GERIATRIC PATIENT

General Considerations Although few concrete data are available, it is generally believed that the aged population is more sensitive to both the therapeutic and toxic effects of many drugs. A comprehensive discussion of the many factors that might influence the response of the elderly patient to drugs is beyond the scope of this text; however, several points are worthy of consideration.

1. **Chronic Disease States.** Diabetes, heart disease, hypertension, chronic respiratory disease, and "senility" are diseases that require chronic drug therapy. Some of these diseases may result in an increase, while others may result in a decrease in drug response. For example, presence of chronic respiratory disease is known to exaggerate the respiratory depression observed with central nervous system (CNS) depressants.

2. **Physiological and Psychological Change As a Function of Age.** These changes result in a decrease in the functional capacity of the body leading to an alteration of drug response due to changes in absorption from the GI tract, distribution of the drug in the body (as a result of changes in blood flow or composition of body mass), biotransformation of drugs in the liver (i.e., drug-metabolizing enzymes are decreased), excretion of the drug or its metabolites (due to decreased ability of the kidney to filter or actively secrete drugs), and changes in organ or receptor sensitivity. It also is known that serum albumin decreases with age. Thus, since free drug concentration determines drug distribution and elimination, a decrease in binding of drugs to plasma proteins (or other body tissues) could result in altered responses in the elderly patient. For example, a

decreased percentage of protein-bound warfarin sodium will lead to a greater pharmacologic effect of the drug. On the other hand, reduced protein binding of phenytoin results in a greater amount of the drug available for excretion leading to a reduced pharmacologic effect and a shorter duration of action.

3. **Nutrition and Diet.** For many reasons, the elderly population often manifests dietary deficiencies either due to lack of a balanced diet or to low food intake. The resultant vitamin deficiencies or inadequate food intake may alter the response to drugs.

4. **Use of Many Medications.** It is estimated that because of the increased incidence of chronic illness in the elderly, this population uses more than two and one-half times as much medication as the rest of the population. As the number of different drugs used increases, the risk of drug interactions or adverse drug reactions increases.

5. **Lack of Compliance and Medication Errors.** It has been estimated that as much as 60% of the elderly population either fails to take their medication or takes it incorrectly. Reasons for this include (a) impaired mental capacity (patient forgets to take the medication); (b) problems with sight, hearing, or mobility, which result in failure to take the medication or errors in taking the medication; (c) complicated dosing schedules, which confuse the patient so that he fails to understand what medication to take or when to take it; (d) alteration of drug regimen based on the personal judgment of the patient, resulting in overdosage or underdosage; and (e) unavailability of medication because the patient is unable to afford it, or because the supply has been used up before appointment with the physician.

Thus, it is important for the nurse to ensure that the geriatric patient fully understands how and when to take medication and to monitor drug response carefully in the elderly. The nurse must also be aware of specific symptoms caused by an altered drug response.

Appendix 8 lists some of the more common drugs or drug classes that warrant special monitoring in the geriatric patient, the reasons for the concern, and the symptoms that may indicate an altered response.

Special Nursing Implications for the Administration of Geriatric Medications

1. Inform patient that you are administering medication, even though it may seem to him that he is only receiving food. A patient should know when he is receiving medication.

2. Assess
   a. for adverse drug reactions, recognizing that the earliest manifestation of drug toxicity in the elderly is mental confusion. For example, the initial symptoms of digitalis toxicity in the elderly are not necessarily nausea and vomiting, as in younger patients, but rather are changes in mental status due to decreased cerebral perfusion and decreased cardiac output due to secondary arrhythmias.
   b. whether failure to thrive in the elderly, characterized by insidious and progressive physical deterioration, deteriorating social competence, loss of appetite, and diminishing concentration is the result of adverse drug reactions.
   c. whether acute brain syndrome characterized by disorientation to person, place, or time, memory impairment for both remote and recent past, impairment of intellectual function, and emotional lability is the result of adverse drug reactions. If so, syndrome may be reversed by withdrawing medications.

(continued)

    d. and report to doctor whether a patient continues to manifest symptoms indicating need for continuous drug therapy or whether patient is compensating and may require less medication. Reduction in strength and number of medications, thereby minimizing adverse reactions and interactions, is a major goal of successful drug therapy in the aged.

    e. for signs of fluid overload, such as dyspnea, cough, increased respirations, and edema due to cardiac and renal dysfunction, which is more common in the elderly and alters response to drugs.

    f. tongue for signs of dehydration, characterized by furrows. Turgidity or fullness of tongue indicates hydration. Since the mucous membranes of the mouth may be chronically dry because of mouth breathing, an absence of subcutaneous fat, and the presence of atropic epidermal changes that make checking for elasticity useless, assessment of the tongue is the best indication of the hydration state of the elderly patient.

    g. patient taking insulin and oral antidiabetics for mild hypoglycemic reactions, characterized by speech disorders, confusion, and disorientation, rather than by the restlessness, tachycardia, and profuse perspiration that occur in the younger patient. Since periodic mild hypoglycemic reactions causing permanent brain damage may result from medication and patient's inability to ingest recommended dietary intake, confer with doctor regarding advisability of continued therapy.

3. Anticipate that if half-life of a medication is increased by deficient renal function, the drug may be administered less frequently or in smaller doses.

4. Combine bitter preparations, such as vitamin, mineral, and electrolyte preparations, with foods, such as applesauce or juice, to make medication more palatable and to prevent gastric irritation. The geriatric patient often loses tastebuds for sweetness and may perceive medication as bitter.

5. Recommend and/or provide, as necessary, good oral hygiene before and after administration of medication to promote ingestion and to prevent an unpleasant aftertaste.

6. Provide sufficient fluids to permit easy swallowing and to help movement of medication through the GI tract. Assist patient into a position that prevents aspiration and promotes swallowing of medication.

7. Examine oral cavity of debilitated patient to ensure that medication has not adhered to mucous membranes and, in fact, has been swallowed.

8. Administer one dose of medication each day to ensure better drug compliance, unless it is essential to use divided dose schedule.

9. Request doctor to order a slower acting diuretic for the geriatric patient if the stress of a rapid acting diuretic, such as furosemide (Lasix), is causing incontinence.

10. Administer tricyclic drugs at bedtime to minimize patient experiencing dry mouth.

11. Discourage continuous use of hypnotics, since they are of little value if taken repeatedly. Provide warm milk and backrub at bedtime, rather than medication.

12. Prevent drug-induced immobility, since this leads to perceptual changes, dehydration, and decubitus ulcer formation.

13. Remain with patient receiving a suppository until drug is absorbed. Because of the reduced body temperature of the elderly patient, it may take longer for a suppository to melt in the bowel or vagina than in a younger patient. Encourage patient to retain suppository. The desire to expel the suppository may be strong because of the extended length of time needed to dissolve medication. Consult

with doctor whether another route may be used, if patient has difficulty retaining suppository.

14. Alternate injection sites and apply a small dry sterile dressing with pressure after an injection, since the geriatric patient tends to bleed after an injection because of the loss of elasticity of tissue.

15. Avoid injection into immobile limb, if possible, because inactivity of limb will reduce rate of absorption.

16. Inspect site of injection of medication since reduction in cutaneous sensation may prevent patient being aware of pain, infection, intravasation, or other trauma.

17. Assist patient to maintain a nutritious diet to prevent dietary deficiencies, which would result in body dysfunction and may alter response to medications.

18. Encourage patient to discard drugs no longer part of the medication regimen to prevent self-medication and confusion of drugs.

19. Encourage patient to confer with doctor if he feels that medication is no longer required rather than to discontinue treatment.

20. Monitor drug compliance very closely in patient taking more than five medications, since this increases the number of adverse reactions, and interactions. See section on *Nursing Process for Teaching and Promoting Compliance with Medication Regimen*, p. 47.

DRUG RESPONSE OF THE PREGNANT PATIENT

The philosophy of drug therapy during pregnancy changed abruptly in 1961 in the wake of the thalidomide tragedy. Thalidomide, believed to be a rather innocuous sleeping medication, turned out to be a powerful teratogen, causing phocomelia, when taken by women during the first trimester of pregnancy. The teratogenic effect of drugs was again brought to the attention of the general public when it was demonstrated that the administration of diethylstilbestrol (DES) during pregnancy increased the incidence of adenocarcinoma of the vagina in female offspring of mothers who received the drug.

The Food and Drug Administration (FDA) now requires that new drugs be tested for teratogenicity in animals before they can be used in pregnant women.

Many older drugs, however, have never been tested or have been minimally tested under such circumstances. Furthermore, there is a great deal of uncertainty about applying animal data to humans.

Therefore, as a rule, a woman who is pregnant, or who is attempting to become pregnant, should not take any pharmacologic agent unless specifically so ordered or permitted by her physician, who will determine whether the *benefit of the therapy outweighs the risk of fetal malformation*.

Thus, all drugs are contraindicated in pregnancy. The warning also applies to over-the-counter agents, alcohol, street drugs, insecticides, and other environmental pollutants. Alcohol, when taken in excess, is known to induce fetal alcohol syndrome.

The implications of the effect of drugs, alcohol, street drugs, and cigarette smoking must be explained to every pregnant patient and/or woman of childbearing age. Common sense as to quantity should be used when discussing the effect of social drugs (alcohol, cigarettes); however, it has been reported that the consumption of three ounces of alcohol per day may cause congenital defects and three cigarettes per day may cause a decrease in birth weight.

The reported effects of maternal drug* ingestion on the embryo, fetus, and neonate are listed in Appendix 9. Some of the data are open to question because (1) experimental data on humans are often nonexistent and conclusions must be drawn from long-term retrospective assessment, (2) malformations also occur in patients who have not ingested these agents, and (3) malformations have been observed in patients who ingested more than one agent (epileptics, for example), and it is thus difficult to ascertain the causative agent. In spite of the "softness" of some of the data listed in Appendix 9, they should be taken into consideration, especially since there is often a choice of therapeutic agents commonly used during pregnancy, such as anti-infectives, antihypertensives, and diuretics.

Most drugs taken by a pregnant woman pass the placental barrier and may affect the embryo, fetus, and neonate. The embryo appears to be particularly sensitive to the effect of drugs during the first trimester of pregnancy, when organogenesis is taking place.

The drugs that do not cross the placental barrier usually consist of large molecules (e.g., heparin).

The decision whether to use a particular drug during pregnancy therefore requires an understanding of the pharmacodynamics of a particular agent. Insulin, for example, is known to be teratogenic when administered directly to the fetus but it does not cross the placental barrier and hence is not teratogenic. Excess insulin may, however, cause the fetus to develop hypoglycemia, which may be harmful. Insulin passes into breast milk but is destroyed in the GI tract of the nursing infant and is harmless.

LACTATION

Unless demonstrated otherwise, it must be assumed that any drug ingested by the mother will be passed along to the nursing child through the mother's milk.

As a rule, a woman who is breastfeeding should take no pharmacologic agent unless specifically so ordered or permitted by her physician.

This warning also applies to over-the-counter drugs, and the nurse should explain the reason to nursing mothers.

*The term is used here in a broad sense and includes street drugs, alcohol, nicotine, and certain pollutants.

Chapter Eight

NURSING PROCESS FOR TEACHING AND PROMOTING COMPLIANCE WITH MEDICATION REGIMEN

ASSESSMENT

Assess patient's personality, personal motivation, experiential background, ability to learn, and willingness to change by examining four factors influencing teaching and learning.

1. **Physical.** Appraise weakness, immobility, ability to swallow.
2. **Psychological.** Discuss understanding and acceptance of condition and therapy.
3. **Sociocultural.** Explore priorities, values, class, and life-style.
4. **Environmental.** Evaluate physical surroundings, family members.

PLANNING

Use assessment in all planning to promote drug compliance.

1. Set up mutually agreed goals with the patient. For example, the doctor's order is for Lente insulin 30 units o.d. before breakfast. A mutual goal might be for the patient to be able to self-administer insulin.
2. Develop a teaching plan to promote compliance.
   a. Identify behavioral objectives for the teaching-learning process. State what the patient should be able to do after the teaching-learning process. For example, after the teaching-learning process the patient will be able to self-administer insulin.
   b. Select appropriate methodology for teaching and promoting compliance (e.g., one-to-one, lecture discussion, movies, slides).

IMPLEMENTATION

1. *Do not rush patient.* Allow patient to learn at his rate.
2. Select an area without distractions, where teaching can be effective.
3. Emphasize the reward of maintained health status or improved health status

to be achieved by taking medications as ordered, since motivation is of primary importance in achieving drug compliance.

4. Explain the rationale for using the specific medication regimen and rationale for route(s) of administration.
5. Provide patient with clear, simple verbal and written directions. (Written directions must be large enough to be legible for patient.)
6. Provide clear, legible cards with information about name of drug, reason for use, untoward reactions, dosage, frequency of administration, and appropriate action to be taken for untoward reaction.
7. Provide a checkoff calendar for patient indicating day and time medication is to be taken.
8. Encourage patient to associate taking medication with daily events; for example, medication after meals.
9. Provide small containers and label for hours of day patient is to take medications. Teach patient to stock each container with appropriate medication once a day so that medications will be organized for the entire day. This technique is particularly helpful for patients with poor memory.
10. Provide containers for each day of the week, and put in medications to be taken on specific days for patient who has difficulty organizing or handling medications.
11. Arrange for financial assistance if patient is financially unable to purchase medication or equipment needed.
12. Use equipment that may be easily purchased and replaced.
13. Use equipment that is easy to handle and adaptable to home use.
14. Note number of tablets/capsules or amount of solution that patient receives from pharmacist.
15. Teach technique for administration of medication.
16. Observe return demonstration by patient. Preferably, a family member or significant other person should be present during this return demonstration.
17. Include a family member or significant other person as part of the support system for helping a patient achieve compliance with medication regimen.

EVALUATION

1. Arrange for follow-up care at appropriate intervals.
2. Evaluate
   a. patient's attitude toward self, illness, medication regimen, and compliance, by assessing verbal and nonverbal communication.
   b. for possible therapeutic effects.
   c. for possible untoward reactions.
   d. for knowledge of medication regimen and ability to administer medication correctly.
   e. for correct dosage utilization by counting the number of tablets/capsules or amount of solution remaining and comparing results to the amount issued by pharmacist.
   f. a return demonstration by patient. Preferably have a family member or significant other person present at this return demonstration. Correct as necessary.

3. Praise patient for compliance with medication regimen when success is demonstrated.
4. Refer to a home health agency, for further intervention by a community health nurse, those clients who appear to lack motivation or ability to carry out regimen as prescribed.

Part Two

ANTI-INFECTIVES

INTRODUCTION

General Statement   The beginning of modern medicine is generally related to two events: the proof by Pasteur that many diseases are caused by microorganisms and the discovery of effective anti-infective drugs. The first of these drugs were the sulfonamides (1938), followed by penicillin during the early 1940s. Since then, dozens of anti-infectives have been added to the list.

Unfortunately, the advent of the anti-infectives has not been a pure panacea. Some of the bacteria and other microorganisms have adapted to the anti-infectives, and there has been a gradual emergence of bacteria resistant to certain anti-infectives, especially the antibiotics. Fortunately, until now, most resistant strains can be eradicated by new and/or different antibiotics, antibiotic combinations, or higher dosages. Nevertheless, awareness of the problem has prompted somewhat greater scrutiny by the physician as to when and how to prescribe antibiotics.

Progress is also being made in the development of antiviral drugs.

In this handbook, the anti-infective drugs have been arranged by class (antibiotics, sulfonamides, sulfones), by disease and/or type of infectious agent: anthelmintic, antitubercular, antimalarial, amebicides, urinary germicides, and antiviral. There is considerable overlap between some of these classifications.

Some general guidelines apply to the use of most anti-infective drugs:

1. Anti-infective drugs can be divided into those that are bacteriostatic, that is, arrest the multiplication and further development of the infectious agent, or bactericidal, that is, eradicate all living microorganisms. Both time of administration and length of therapy may be affected by this difference.
2. Some anti-infectives halt the growth of or eradicate many different microorganisms and are termed broad-spectrum antibiotics. Some affect only certain very specific organisms and are termed narrow-spectrum antibiotics.
3. Some of the anti-infectives elicit a hypersensitivity reaction in some patients.

Penicillins cause more severe and frequent hypersensitivity reactions than are produced by any other drug.

4. Because of differences in susceptibility of infectious agents to anti-infectives, the sensitivity of the microorganism to the drug ordered should be determined before treatment is initiated. Several sensitivity tests are commonly used for this purpose. The most widely used test—the Kirby Bauer or disk-diffusion techniques—gives qualitative results; there are also various quantitative tests aimed at determining the minimal inhibitory concentration (MIC).

5. Certain anti-infective agents have marked side effects, some of the more serious of which are neurotoxicity, including ototoxicity, and nephrotoxicity. Care must be taken not to administer two anti-infectives with similar side effects concomitantly, nor to administer these drugs to patients in whom the side effects might be damaging (i.e., a nephrotoxic drug to a patient suffering from kidney disease). The choice of anti-infective also depends on its distribution in the body (i.e., whether it passes the blood–brain barrier).

6. Another difficulty associated with anti-infective therapy is that these drugs can eradicate the normal intestinal flora necessary for proper digestion, synthesis of vitamin K, and the control of fungi that may gain access to the GI tract (superinfection).

Action/Kinetics   The mechanism of action of the anti-infectives varies. The following modes of action have been identified.* Note that there is considerable overlap between mechanisms:

1. Interference with bacterial cell wall:
   a. Inhibition of an enzyme necessary for formation of the cell wall, resulting in cell lysis
   b. Activation of an enzyme interfering with formation of cell wall, resulting in cell wall lysis
   c. Direct action on the cell wall by agents, affecting permeability of the cell wall
2. Interference with intracellular ribosomes, and therefore with protein synthesis
3. Binding of drug to specific ribosomal subunit, which initiates the formation of abnormal polypeptides and proteins
4. Interference with nucleic acid metabolism, and therefore with protein synthesis
5. Interference with specific metabolic step essential to survival of microorganism

Nursing Implications for Anti-Infectives

1. Ask patient if he has previously experienced any unusual reaction or problem with any anti-infective, such as a rash, hives, or difficulty in breathing. Such reactions indicate an allergy or hypersensitivity.

2. Report history of allergy to any anti-infective to physician. Mark patient's chart and bed conspicuously. Inform patient not to take that drug again, unless the doctor, after having reviewed history of past allergic reactions to this medication, allows him to do so.

3. Ascertain, if indicated, that diagnostic cultures and sensitivity tests have been done before administering first dose of anti-infective. Use correct procedure for obtaining specimen and for storing and/or transporting it to laboratory.

*Sande MA, Mandell GL: Antimicrobial agents, in Gilman AG, Goodman LS, Gilman A (eds): *The Pharmacological Basis of Therapeutics*, ed 6. New York, Macmillan, 1980 pp 1080.

4. Assess patient on anti-infective therapy for hypersensitivity or allergic reactions (see *Hypersensitivity Reactions and Treatment*, p. 14). If a reaction occurs, the drug must be discontinued immediately. Epinephrine, oxygen, antihistamines, and corticosteroids must always be immediately available.

5. Anticipate reduced dosage of anti-infectives chiefly excreted by kidneys in patients with renal dysfunction. Nephrotoxic drugs are contraindicated in patients with renal dysfunction, because toxic levels of the drugs are rapidly attained when renal function is impaired.

6. Withhold medication and check with doctor when two or more anti-infectives are ordered for the same patient, especially if the drugs have similar untoward effects such as nephrotoxicity and/or neurotoxicity.

7. Administer bactericidal drugs at least 1 hr before administering bacteriostatic anti-infective when both are ordered, in order to achieve maximum effect.

8. Assess patient for therapeutic response, such as reduction of fever, increased appetite, and increased sense of well-being.

9. Assess patient for superinfections, particularly of fungal origin, characterized by black furred tongue, nausea, and diarrhea.

10. *Prevent superinfections*
    a. by limiting patient's exposure to persons suffering from an active infectious process.
    b. by rotating site of IV administration and by changing site of IV tubing every 24–48 hr.
    c. by providing and emphasizing need for good hygiene.

11. Have the order for an anti-infective administered in the hospital reviewed at least every 5–7 days for renewal or cancellation.

12. Schedule drug administration throughout 24-hr period, to maintain appropriate drug levels. A drug administration schedule is determined by the half-life ($t^{1}/_{2}$) of the drug, the severity of the infection, and the patient's need for sleep.

13. Complete drug administration before medication loses significant potency. Ensure potency of drug by diluting as recommended and by administering within the time recommended. Protect from light, if indicated. Unless contraindicated, dilute IV drugs with at least 50–100 ml, to prevent irritation to vein.

14. *Teach patient and/or family*
    a. to use anti-infectives only under medical supervision.
    b. the method and time for taking anti-infective.
    c. to report signs and symptoms of allergic reactions and superinfections.
    d. to complete recommended course of therapy even though the patient may feel well.
    e. to discard any drug remaining after course of therapy is completed.

Chapter Nine

ANTIBIOTICS

General Statement   Originally, all antibiotics were chemical substances produced by microorganisms (bacteria, fungi) that suppress the growth of, and often kill, other microorganisms. Today, many antibiotics are either partially or entirely prepared synthetically.

Antibiotics also vary in potency. Some are bacteriostatic, that is, they only inhibit the growth of an infectious agent. Others are bactericidal and kill the infectious agent outright. The bacteriostatic or bactericidal action of a particular agent is also affected by its concentration at the site of infection.

Action/Kinetics   The various mechanisms through which antibiotics interfere with the metabolism and propagation of microorganisms are listed on p. 52 (anti-infectives) and, when known, under the individual agents. Pharmacokinetic data are lacking for many agents, because effectiveness depends on site of the infection, concentration of the drug at the site, sensitivity of the specific organism to the drug, and immune defenses of the host. Dosage can often be estimated from the MIC (see p. 52) necessary to prevent visible growth (after 18–24 hr of incubation) of the infectious agent, as determined by sensitivity testing. Drug concentration at the site of infection should range from equal to 8 times MIC. Most antibiotics are well absorbed from the GI tract, although some are acid sensitive and must be administered parenterally. The vast majority of antibiotics are eliminated by the kidneys.

Uses Antibiotics, as a group, are effective against most bacterial pathogens, as well as against some of the rickettsias and a few of the larger viruses. They are ineffective against viruses that cause influenza, hepatitis, and the common cold.

The choice of the antibiotic depends on the nature of the illness to be treated, the sensitivity of the infecting agent, and the patient's previous experience with the drug. Hypersensitivity and allergic reactions (see p. 13) may preclude the use of the agent of choice.

In addition to their use in acute infections, antibiotics are given prophylactically in the following instances:

1. To protect persons exposed to a known specific organism
2. To prevent secondary bacterial infections in acutely ill patients suffering from infections unresponsive to antibiotics
3. To reduce risk of infection in patients suffering from various chronic illnesses
4. To inhibit spread of infection from a clearly defined focus, as after accidents or surgery
5. To "sterilize" the bowel or other areas of the body in preparation for extensive surgery

Instead of using a single agent, the physician may sometimes prefer to prescribe a combination of antibiotics.

Contraindications Hypersensitivity or allergic reactions to certain antibiotics are common and may preclude the use of a particular agent.

Untoward Reactions The antibiotics have few direct toxic effects. Kidney and liver damage, deafness, and blood dyscrasias are occasionally observed.

The following undesirable manifestations, however, occur frequently.

1. Antibiotic therapy often suppresses the normal flora of the body, which in turn keeps certain pathogenic microorganisms, such as *Candida albicans, Proteus*, or *Pseudomonas* from causing infections. If the flora is altered, *superinfections* (monilial vaginitis, enteritis, urinary tract infections), which necessitate the discontinuation of therapy or use of other antibiotics, can result.
2. Incomplete eradication of an infectious organism. Casual use of these agents also favors the emergence of *resistant* strains insensitive to a particular drug. Resistant strains often are either mutants of the original infectious agents that have developed a slightly different metabolic pathway and can exist in spite of the antibiotic, or are variants that have developed the ability to release a chemical substance—for instance, the enzyme penicillinase—which can destroy the antibiotic.

In order to minimize the chances for the development of resistant strains, antibiotics are usually given for a prescribed length of time after acute symptoms have subsided. Casual use of antibiotics is discouraged for the same reasons.

Laboratory Tests The bacteriologic sensitivity of the infectious organism to the antibiotic should be tested by the laboratory before initiation of therapy and during treatment.

Administration/Storage
1. Check expiration date on container.
2. Check for recommended method of storage for the drug and store accordingly.
3. Clearly mark the date of dilution and strength of solutions of all drugs. Note the length of time that the drug may be stored after dilution.

4. Complete the administration of antibiotics by volutrol before the drug loses potency.

Nursing Implications
See *Nursing Implications* for *Anti-infectives*, p. 52.

PENICILLINS

General Statement   Penicillins are distributed throughout most of the body and pass the placental barrier. They also pass into synovial, pleural, pericardial, intraperitoneal, and spinal fluids and into the fluids of the eye. Although normal meninges are relatively impermeable to penicillins, they are better absorbed by inflamed meninges.

The renal, cardiac, and hematopoietic function, as well as the electrolyte balance, of patients receiving penicillin should be monitored at regular intervals.

Action/Kinetics   Penicillins interfere with the biosynthesis of the bacterial cell wall; in particular, they affect the synthesis of dipeptidoglycan—a substance necessary to give the cell wall strength and stability. Penicillin is most effective against young, rapidly dividing organisms and has little effect on mature resting cells. Depending on the concentration of the drug at the site of infection and the susceptibility of the infectious microorganism, penicillin is either bacteriostatic or bactericidal. t½: 30–110 min; protein binding: 20–98% (see individual agents).

Uses   Gram-positive cocci including streptococci, meningococci, pneumococci, non-penicillinase-producing staphylococci, and fusospirochetal infections. Gonococci including uncomplicated gonorrhea, disseminated gonococcal infections, and gonococcal ophthalmia in neonates or adults. Rat-bite fever, anthrax, tetanus, yaws, gas gangrene, and diphtheria (treatment and prophylaxis). Subacute bacterial endocarditis due to Group A streptococci, and enterococcal endocarditis. Actinomycoses, *Pasturella*, and clostridial infections (except botulism).

Penicillins are also used for *Listeria* meningitis (in combination with gentamicin or kanamycin). Infections due to *E. coli, Proteus mirabilis, Hemophilus influenzae, Salmonella, Shigella, Proteus aeruginosa.* Syphylis including primary, secondary, latent, and congenital. Prophylaxis of rheumatic fever and bacterial endocarditis in patients with congenital or rheumatic heart disease undergoing dental work, instrumentation, or other procedures.

Note: Not all penicillins are used for the above diseases. Specific uses are indicated for each of the individually listed drugs.

Contraindications   Hypersensitivity to penicillin and cephalosporin. To be used with caution in patients with a history of asthma, hayfever, or urticaria.

Untoward Reactions   Penicillins are potent sensitizing agents; it is estimated that 15% of the American population is presently allergic to the antibiotic. Hypersensitivity reactions are reported to be on the increase in pediatric practice. Sensitivity reactions may be immediate (within 20 minutes) or delayed (as long as days or weeks after initiation of therapy).

Allergic: Skin rashes (including maculopapular and exanthematic), exfoliative dermatitis, erythema, contact dermatitis, hives, pruritus, wheezing, anaphylaxis, fever, eosinophilia. Anaphylaxis, Stevens-Johnson syndrome, angioedema, serum sickness. *GI:* Diarrhea (may be severe), abdominal cramps or pain, nausea, vomiting, bloating, flatulence, increased thirst, bitter/unpleasant taste, dark or discolored tongue, sore mouth or tongue, gastric upset, pseudomembranous colitis. *Hematologic:* Thrombocytopenia, leukopenia, agranulocytosis. *Renal:* Hematuria, pyuria, albuminuria, oliguria. Electrolyte imbalance following IV use. *Miscellaneous:* Hepatotoxicity (cholestatic jaundice), superinfection, swelling of face and ankles, labored breathing, weakness, ecchymoses, hematomas.

IM injection may cause pain and induration at the injection site while IV use may cause vein irritation and thrombophlebitis.

For **emergency treatment** of severe allergic or anaphylactic reactions, administer epinephrine (0.3–0.5 ml of a 1:1,000 sol. SC or IM or 0.2–0.3 ml diluted in 10 ml saline, given slowly by IV); corticosteroids should be on hand.

In those instances where penicillin is the drug of choice, the physician may decide to use it even though the patient is allergic, adding medication to the regimen to control the allergic response.

Drug Interactions

Interactant	Interaction
Aminoglycosides	Penicillins ↓ effect of aminoglycosides
Antacids	↓ Effect of penicillins due to ↓ absorption from GI tract
Antibiotics	↓ Effect of penicillins
Chloramphenicol	
Erythromycins	
Tetracyclines	
Anticoagulants	Penicillins may potentiate pharmacologic effect
Aspirin	↑ Effect of penicillins by ↓ plasma protein binding
Phenylbutazone	↑ Effect of penicillins by ↓ plasma protein binding
Probenecid	↑ Effect penicillins by ↓ excretion

Laboratory Test Interference   Massive doses: False + or ↑ urinary glucose, protein, and turbidity.

Dosage   Penicillin is available for oral, parenteral, inhalation, and intrathecal administration. Dosages for individual drugs are given in drug entries.

Long-acting preparations are frequently used.

Oral doses must be higher than IM or SC, because a large fraction of penicillin given orally may be destroyed in the stomach.

Administration   Intramuscular and intravenous administration of penicillin causes a great deal of local irritation. These antibiotics are thus injected slowly.

IM injections are made deeply into the gluteal muscle. IV injections are usually made through the tubing of an IV infusion.

In adults, the penicillins (diluted with additional diluent) are also given by IV drip at a rate of 100–150 drops/min.

Nursing Implications

See *Nursing Implications* for *Anti-infectives*, p. 52.

1. Assess rigorously for allergic reactions, as incidence is higher with penicillin therapy.
2. Anticipate that allergic reactions are more likely to occur in patients with a history of asthma, hay fever, urticaria, or allergy to cephalosporins.
3. Detain patient in an ambulatory care site for at least 20 min after administering a penicillin injection, to assess for the onset of anaphylaxis. Be prepared for prompt treatment of anaphylactic reaction.

4. Do not administer long-acting types of penicillin IV, because they are only for IM use. They may cause emboli or CNS or cardiac pathology, if administered IV.

5. Do not massage repository (long-acting) penicillin products after injection, because rate of absorption should not be increased.

6. Prevent rapid administration of IV penicillin, because this is locally irritating and may precipitate convulsions.

7. Administer oral penicillin on an empty stomach with a glass of water, because food delays absorption. except for penicillin V and amoxicillin.

8. *Teach patient and/or family*
    a. the signs and symptoms of allergic reaction, to stop medication when noted, and to check with medical supervision as soon as possible.
    b. to take oral penicillin with a glass of water 1 hr before meals or 2–3 hr after meals.
    c. to return for repository penicillin to complete treatment, if physician so orders.
    d. to complete entire prescribed course of therapy, even though patient may feel well; a patient with alpha-hemolytic streptococcus infection must continue with penicillin for a minimum of 10 days, and preferably 14 days, to prevent development of rheumatic fever or glomerulonephritis.

9. Most penicillins are excreted in breast milk and should be prescribed cautiously to nursing mothers.

AMDINOCILLIN   Coactin (Rx)

Classification Antibiotic, penicillin.

Uses Urinary tract infections due to *E. coli, Klebsiella,* and *Enterobacter.* Bacteremia due to *E. coli.* In conjunction with β-lactam antibiotics for severe urinary tract infections.

Dosage IM, IV. *Serious infections:* 10 mg/kg q 4 hr for 7–10 days. For severe infections, prolonged therapy may be necessary. *As adjunct with β-lactam antibiotic:* 10 mg/kg q 6 hr. In presence of renal dysfunction, reduce dose to 10 mg/kg q 6–8 hr.

Administration
1. For IV infusion, dissolve in Sterile Water for Injection and further dilute to 50 ml with 5% Dextrose Injection. Administer over 15–30 min.
2. When used with a β-lactam antibiotic, the two should be given separately.
3. IM administration should be deep into a large muscle mass as the upper, outer quadrant of the buttocks.

AMOXICILLIN (AMOXYCILLIN)   Amoxil, Larotid, Novamoxin,* Polymox, Robamax, Sumox, Trimox, Utimox, Wymox (Rx)

Classification Antibiotic, penicillin.

Action/Kinetics Semisynthetic broad-spectrum penicillin closely related to ampicillin. Destroyed by penicillinase, acid stable, and better absorbed than ampicillin.

Fifty to 80% of oral dose is absorbed from the GI tract. **Peak serum levels: PO**: 4–11 μg/ml after 1–2 hr; **t½**: 60 min. Mostly excreted unchanged in urine.

Uses   Genitourinary tract infections. Respiratory infections by *H. influenzae, S. pneumoniae*. Skin and soft tissue infections by non-penicillinase-producing staphylococci. Gram-positive streptococci. *Proteus mirabilis, Neisseria gonorrhoeae*.

Dosage   PO only: 250–500 mg q 8 hr; **pediatric under 20 kg**: 20–40 (or more) mg/kg daily in 3 equal doses. *Gonorrhea*: 3 gm, as single dose.

Administration/Storage   Dry powder is stable at room temperature for 18–30 months. Reconstituted suspension is stable for 1 wk at room temperature and for 2 wk at 2°–8°C. Chewable tablets are available for pediatric use. May be administered with food.

AMOXICILLIN AND POTASSIUM CLAVULANATE   Augmentin (Rx)

Classification   Antibiotic, penicillin.

Action/Kinetics   For details on amoxicillin, see p. 59. Potassium clavulanate inactivates lactamase enzymes, which are responsible for resistance to penicillins. Thus, this preparation is effective against microorganisms that have manifested resistance to amoxicillin. For potassium clavulanate: **Peak serum levels**: 1–2 hr; **t½**: 1 hr.

Note: Both the 250 and 500 tablets contain l25 mg potassium clavulanate.

Uses   For β-lactamase producing strains of the following organisms: *Hemophilus influenzae* causing lower respiratory tract infections, otitis media, and sinusitis; *Staphylococcus aureus, E. coli,* and *Klebsiella* causing skin and skin structure infections; *E. coli, Klebsiella,* and *Enterobacter* causing urinary tract infections.

Dosage   *Usual:* **Adults,** One '250' tablet q 8 hr; **children, less than 40 kg,** 20 mg/kg daily in divided doses q 8 hr. *Respiratory tract and severe infections:* **Adults,** one '500' tablet q 8 hr; **children, less than 40 kg,** 40 mg/kg daily in divided doses q 8 hr (this dose is also used in children for otitis media, lower respiratory tract infections, or sinusitis).

AMPICILLIN ORAL   Amcap, Amcill, Ampicin,* Ampilean,* D-Amp, Omnipen, Pfizerpen-A, Polycillin, Principen, SK-Ampicillin, Supen, Totacillin (Rx)

AMPICILLIN SODIUM, PARENTERAL   Omnipen-N, Polycillin-N, SK-Ampicillin-N, Totacillin-N (Rx)

AMPICILLIN TRIHYDRATE WITH PROBENECID   Polycillin-PRB, Principen w/Probenecid, Probampacin (Rx)

Classification   Antibiotic, penicillin.

Action/Kinetics   Synthetic, broad-spectrum antibiotic suitable for gram-negative bacteria. Acid resistant, destroyed by penicillinase. Absorbed more slowly than other penicillins. Thirty to 60% of oral dose absorbed from GI tract. **Peak serum levels: PO**: 1.8–2.9 μg/ml after 2 hr; **IM**, 4.5–7 μg/ml; **t½**: 80 min (range 50–110 min). Partially inactivated in liver; 25–85% excreted unchanged in urine.

Uses Infections of respiratory, GI, and GU tract caused by *Shigella, Salmonella, E. coli, H. influenzae, Proteus* strains, *N. gonorrhoeae, N. meningitidis,* and *Enterococcus.* Also, otitis media in children, bronchitis, rat-bite fever, and whooping cough. Penicillin G-sensitive staphylococci, streptococci, pneumococci.

Additional Drug Interactions

Interactant	Interaction
Allopurinol	↑ Incidence of skin rashes
Ampicillin	↓ Effect of oral contraceptives

Dosage   Ampicillin: PO; Ampicillin sodium: IV, IM.

Respiratory tract and soft tissue infections: **PO, 20 kg or more**: 250 mg q 6 hr; **less than 20 kg**: 50 mg/kg/day in equally divided doses q 6–8 hr. **IV, IM, 40 kg or more**: 250–500 mg q 6 hr; **less than 40 kg**: 25–50 mg/kg/day in equally divided doses q 6–8 hr.

Gastrointestinal and genitourinary tract infections: **PO, 20 kg or more**: 500 mg q 6 hr; **less than 20 kg**: 100 mg/kg/day in equally divided doses q 6–8 hr. **IV, IM, 40 kg or more**: 500 mg q 6 hr; **less than 40 kg**: 50 mg/kg/day in equally divided doses q 6–8 hr.

Urethritis (due to gonorrhea): **PO**: 3.5 gm with 1 gm probenecid (given SC) simultaneously as a single dose. **IM, IV**: 2 doses of 500 mg each within 8–12 hr.

Bacterial meningitis: **Adults/children, IV, IM**: 150–200 mg/kg/day in equally divided doses q 3–4 hr. *Bacterial endocarditis prophylaxis* (GI or GU tract surgery or instrumentation): **Adult, IM, IV**: 1 gm plus gentamicin, 1.5 mg/kg IM or IV, or streptomycin, 1 gm IM given 30–60 min before procedure with two additional doses q 8 hr with gentamicin or q 12 hr with streptomycin. **Pediatric**: ampicillin, 50 mg/kg with gentamicin, 2 mg/kg and streptomycin, 20 mg/kg. Dosage should not exceed single or daily adult dosage. *Septicemia*: **Adults/children**: 150–200 mg/kg, IV for first 3 days, then IM q 3–4 hr.

Administration/Storage

1. After reconstitution for IM or direct IV administration, the solution of sodium ampicillin must be used within the hour.
2. For IM use, dilute only with sterile water for injection or bacteriostatic water for injection.
3. For IV "piggyback," ampicillin may be reconstituted with sodium chloride injection.
4. IV injections of reconstituted sodium ampicillin should be given slowly; 2 ml should be given over a period of at least 3–5 min.
5. Administration by IV drip: Check compatability and length of time that drug retains potency in a particular solution.
6. Ampicillin chewable tablets should not be swallowed whole.
7. Give oral dosage at least 2 hr after or 1 hr before a meal.

Additional Nursing Implications
See also *Nursing Implications* for *Anti-infectives*, p. 52 and *Penicillins*, p. 58.
   Observe skin closely for rashes, as they occur more often with this drug than with other penicillins.

AZLOCILLIN SODIUM   Azlin (Rx)

Classification   Antibiotic, penicillin.

Remarks   Azlocillin is an extended-spectrum penicillin.

Uses   Lower respiratory tract infections caused by *E. coli* or *H. influenzae*. *Pseudomonas* infections including those of the respiratory tract, skin, skin structures, bones, joints, and urinary tract. Septicemia caused by *E. coli* or *Pseudomonas*. Also, upper respiratory tract infections caused by *E. coli, S. faecalis,* or *Proteus mirabilis*.

Dosage   IV (slow injection or infusion). *Upper respiratory tract infections:* 2 gm q 6 hr. *Lower respiratory tract, bone, joint, and skin infections; septicemia:* 3–4 gm q 4–6 hr (not to exceed 24 gm/day). Dosage should be reduced in renal impairment. **Pediatric:** *Acute pulmonary worsening of cystic fibrosis:* 75 mg/kg q 4 hr not to exceed 24 gm/day. Not to be used in the newborn.

Administration

1. If used in combination with other drugs, each drug should be given separately.
2. Azlocillin may be reconstituted by adding 10 ml of Sterile Water for Injection, 0.9% Sodium Chloride Injection, or 5% Dextrose Injection. This may then be diluted with the appropriate IV solution.
3. To minimize vein irritation, the concentration of azlocillin should not exceed 10%.

Additional Nursing Implications

1. Assess for signs of hypokalemia, muscular weakness, decreased or cessation of peristalsis, postural hypotension, respiratory depression, and cardiac arrhythmias.
2. Assess for bruising, hematuria, black stools, other signs of bleeding.
3. Be aware that this drug and an aminoglycoside or cephalosporin may be used simultaneously. However, do not mix together in IV solution.

BACAMPICILLIN HYDROCHLORIDE   Penglobe,* Spectrobid (Rx)

Classification   Antibiotic, penicillin.

Action/Kinetics   Bacampicillin is a semisynthetic, acid-resistant penicillin that is hydrolyzed to the active ampicillin in the GI tract. Food does not affect absorption of the drug. The drug is 98% absorbed from the GI tract and is approximately 20% plasma protein bound. **Peak serum levels**: obtained in 0.9 hr and is approximately 3 times those seen with equivalent doses of ampicillin. Seventy-five percent is excreted in the urine as active ampicillin within 8 hr.

Uses   Upper and lower respiratory tract infections caused by beta-hemolytic streptococcus, *Staphylococcus pyogenes*, pneumococci, non-penicillinase-producing staphylococci, and *Hemophilus influenzae*. Urinary tract infections caused by *E. coli, Proteus mirabilis,* and enterococci. Skin infections caused by streptococci and susceptible staphylococci. Acute uncomplicated urogenital infections caused by *Neisseria gonorrhoeae*.

Contraindications   History of penicillin allergy. Concomitant use with disulfiram (Antabuse).

Drug Interaction Bacampicillin should not be used concomitantly with disulfiram.

Laboratory Test Interferences False + reaction to Clinitest, Benedict's solution, and Fehling's solution. ↑ SGOT.

Dosage   PO. Adults (25 kg or more): 400 mg q 12 hr; **pediatric:** 25 mg/kg/day in equally divided doses q 12 hr. Dose may be doubled in lower respiratory tract infections, in cases of severe infection, or in treating less susceptible organisms. *Gonorrhea (males and females):* 1.6 gm with probenecid, 1 gm, as a single dose.

Administration May be given without regard for meals.

Additional Nursing Implications
See also *Nursing Implications* for *Anti-infectives*, p. 52 and *Penicillins*, p. 58.

1. Withhold drug and consult with doctor if patient is on disulfiram (Antabuse) therapy. Warn patient not to start disulfiram therapy while taking bacampicillin.
2. Assess patient also on allopurinol for increased incidence of skin rash.
3. Advise that diabetic patients use Labstix, Clinistix, Tes-Tape, or Diastix for testing urine, as Benedict's and Fehling's solutions result in false + reactions.

CARBENICILLIN DISODIUM   Geopen, Pyopen (Rx)

Classification Antibiotic, penicillin.

Action/Kinetics Due to high urine levels achieved, carbenicillin is especially suitable for urinary tract infections. It is acid labile and must be injected. **Peak serum levels: IM,** 10–40 μg/ml after 1 hr; **t½:** 60 min. Rapidly excreted unchanged in urine. Urinary excretion rates can be slowed by concurrent administration of probenecid.

Uses Urinary tract and systemic infections caused by *Pseudomonas aeruginosa, Proteus* sp., *E. coli, Neisseria gonorrhoeae, Streptococcus pneumoniae, Enterobacter,* and *S. faecalis.* Anaerobic bacteria causing septicemia, lung abcess, empyema, pneumonitis, peritonitis, endometritis, pelvic inflammatory disease, pelvic abscess, salpingitis, skin infections.

Additional Contraindications Pregnancy. Use with caution in patients with impaired renal function.

Additional Untoward Reactions Neurotoxicity in patients with impaired renal function. Vaginitis, increased SGOT levels.

Additional Drug Interactions

Interactant	Interaction
Gentamicin	↑ Effect of carbenicillin when used for *Pseudomonas*
Tobramycin	↑ Effect of carbenicillin when used for *Pseudomonas*; ↑ effect of both drugs when used for *Providencia* strains

Dosage *Urinary tract infections.* **Adult:** *Uncomplicated,* **IM, IV:** 1–2 gm q 6 hr; *severe,* **IV drip:** 200 mg/kg daily. **Pediatric: IM, IV,** 50–200 mg/kg/day in divided doses q 4–6 hr. *Severe systemic infections, septicemia, respiratory infections, soft tissue infections.* **Adult: IV (drip or divided doses):** 15–40 gm daily. **Pediatric: IV or IM (divided doses) or IV drip:** 250–500 mg/kg/day. *Meningitis.* **Adult: IV (drip or divided doses):** 30–40 gm daily. **Pediatric: IV (drip or divided doses):** 400–500 mg/kg/day. *Proteus or E. coli infections during dialysis or hemodialysis.* **Adult:**

IV: 2 gm q 4–6 hr. *Gonorrhea (males or females):* **IM:** 4 gm as single dose divided between 2 sites with probenecid, 1 gm **PO**, 30 min before injection.

Note: Severe systemic infections in neonates. **IM or IV infusion (15 min): over 2 kg, initial,** 100 mg/kg; **then,** for next 3 days, 75 mg/kg q 6 hr. After 3 days of age, 100 mg/kg q 6 hr. **Under 2 kg, initial,** 100 mg/kg; **then,** for next 7 days, 75 mg/kg q 8 hr. After 7 days of age, 100 mg/kg q 8 hr.

Reduce all dosages in case of renal insufficiency.

Administration/Storage

1. Minimize pain at site of deep intramuscular injection by reconstituting medication with 0.5% lidocaine (without epinephrine) or bacteriostatic water for injection containing 0.9% benzyl alcohol. Obtain a written order to use lidocaine or benzyl alcohol for dilution.
2. Do not administer more than 2 gm in any one IM injection.
3. Read directions carefully on package insert for IM and IV administration because drug is very irritating to tissue.
4. Unused reconstituted drug should be discarded after 24 hr when stored at room temperature, and should be discarded after 72 hr when refrigerated. Label with date and time when reconstituting drug.

Additional Nursing Implications

See also *Nursing Implications* for *Anti-infectives*, p. 52 and *Penicillins*, p. 58.

1. Assess patient with impaired renal function for (a) neurotoxicity manifested by hallucinations, impaired sensorium, muscular irritability, and seizures, and (b) hemorrhagic manifestations, such as ecchymosis, petechiae, and frank bleeding of gums and/or rectum.
2. Assess patient with impaired cardiac function for edema, weight gain, and respiratory distress that may be precipitated by disodium carbenicillin.
3. Provide good mouth care to minimize nausea and unpleasant aftertaste.
4. Assess patient for headaches, GI disturbances, or hypersensitivity reactions if probenecid is administered with carbenicillin.

CARBENICILLIN INDANYL SODIUM Geocillin (Rx)

Classification Antibiotic, pencillin.

Action/Kinetics The drug is acid stable. **Peak serum levels: PO,** 6.5 μg/ml after 1 hr. t½: 60 min. Rapidly excreted unchanged in urine.

Uses Urinary tract infections or bacteriuria due to *E. coli, Proteus vulgaris* and *mirabilis, Morganella, Providencia, Enterobacter, Pseudomonas,* and enterococci. Also prostatitis.

Additional Contraindications Pregnancy. Safe use in children not established. Use with caution in patients with impaired renal function.

Additional Untoward Reactions Neurotoxicity in patients with impaired renal function.

Additional Drug Interactions When used in combination with gentamicin or tobramycin for *Pseudomonas* infections, effect of carbenicillin may be enhanced.

Dosage **PO:** 382–764 mg q.i.d.

Administration/Storage
1. Protect from moisture.
2. Store at temperature of 30°C or less.

Nursing Implications
See *Nursing Implications* for *Carbenicillin Disodium*, p. 63.

CLOXACILLIN SODIUM MONOHYDRATE Bactopen,* Cloxapen, Novocloxin,* Orbenin,* Tegopen (Rx)

Classification   Antibiotic, penicillin.

Action/Kinetics   More resistant to penicillinase than is penicillin G. **Peak plasma levels:** 7–15 μg/ml after 30–60 min. **t½:** 30 min. Protein binding: 88–96%. Well absorbed from GI tract. Mostly excreted in urine, but some excreted in bile.

Uses   Infections caused by penicillinase-producing staphylococci, streptococci and pneumococci, excluding enterococci. Osteomyelitis.

Dosage   **PO:** 250–500 mg q 6 hr; **pediatric up to 20 kg:** 50–100 mg/kg daily in 4 equal doses. Older children receive adult dose.

Administration/Storage
1. Add amount of water stated on label in 2 portions; shake well after each addition.
2. Shake well before pouring each dose.
3. Refrigerate reconstituted solution and discard unused portion after 14 days.
4. Administer 1 hr before or 2 hr after meals, because food interferes with absorption of drug.

Additional Nursing Implications
See also *Nursing Implications* for *Penicillins*, p. 58.
  Assess closely for wheezing and sneezing, since they are more likely to occur with this drug.

CYCLACILLIN Cyclapen-W (Rx)

Classification   Antibiotic, penicillin.

Action/Kinetics   Semisynthetic penicillin. Better absorbed from GI tract than ampicillin and causes less diarrhea.

Uses   Especially indicated for bronchitis, pneumonia, otitis media, tonsillitis, and pharyngitis caused by *Streptococcus pneumoniae, H. influenzae* and Group A beta-hemolytic streptococci. Acute exacerbations of chronic bronchitis. Urinary tract infections caused by *E. coli* and *P. mirabilis*. Integumentary infections due to Group A beta-hemolytic streptococci and non-penicillinase-producing staphylococci.

Additional Contraindications   Children under 2 mo of age. Safe use during pregnancy and lactation not established.

Dosage   PO. *Tonsillitis/pharyngitis.* **Adults:** 250 mg q 6 hr; **pediatric (over 20 kg):** 250 mg q 8 hr; **pediatric (under 20 kg):** 125 mg q 8 hr. *Otitis media, integumental infections, bronchitis, and pneumonia.* **Adults:** 250–500 mg q 6 hr; **pediatric:** 50–100 mg/kg/day in equally spaced doses. *Genitourinary tract infections.* **Adults:** 500 mg q 6 hr; **pediatric:** 100 mg/kg/day in equally spaced doses.
    Dosage should be reduced in presence of renal failure.

Administration/Storage

1. Persistent infections may require therapy for several weeks.
2. The oral suspension should be stored in the refrigerator after reconstitution and any unused portion discarded after 14 days (after 7 days if stored at room temperature).

DICLOXACILLIN SODIUM MONOHYDRATE   Dycill, Dynapen, Pathocil, Veracillin (Rx)

Classification   Antibiotic, penicillin.

Action/Kinetics   Penicillinase resistant. **Peak serum levels: IM, PO,** 4–20 μg/ml after 1 hr. **t½:** 40 min. Chiefly excreted in urine.

Uses   Resistant staphylococcal infections. To initiate therapy in any suspected staphylococcal infection. Not indicated for meningitis.

Dosage   PO. Adults and pediatric (over 40 kg): 125–250 mg q 6 hr; **pediatric** 12.5–25 mg/kg/day in 4 equal doses. Dosage not established for the newborn.

Administration/Storage

1. To prepare oral suspension, shake container to loosen powder, measure water for reconstitution as indicated on label, add one-half the water and immediately shake vigorously because usual handling may cause lumps. Add the remainder of the water and again shake vigorously.
2. Shake well before pouring each dose.
3. Refrigerate reconstituted solution and discard after 14 days.
4. Give at least 1 hr before meals or no sooner than 2–3 hr after a meal.

HETACILLIN   Versapen (Rx)

HETACILLIN POTASSIUM   Versapen-K (Rx)

Classification   Antibiotic, penicillin.

Action/Kinetics   Is converted to the active ampicillin. Prolonged and intensive therapy at higher doses than recommended may be necessary for GI and urinary tract infections. **Peak serum levels: PO,** 0.8–2.2 μg/ml after 2–3 hr; **IM,** 1.5–3.8 μg/ml after 2–3 hr.

Uses   Infections of the respiratory, GI, genitourinary tract and of the middle ear caused by *Shigella, Salmonella, E. coli, H. influenzae, Proteus* strains, *Micrococcus* *pneumoniae*, Group A beta-hemolytic streptococcus, *Enterococcus*, non-penicillinase-producing *Staphylococcus aureus*, *Streptococcus pneumoniae*, and *Proteus mirabilis*.

Dosage   PO. Dosage varies with condition treated. **Patients weighing 40 kg or more:** 225– 450 mg q.i.d.; **patients weighing less than 40 kg:** 22.5–45 mg/kg daily in 4 equally divided doses. Infections of the GI or GU tracts may require prolonged therapy at higher doses than listed above. For severe infections therapy should be initiated with parenteral ampicillin.

Administration/Storage
1. Reconstitute pediatric drops by adding water in 2 portions and shaking thoroughly with cap on after each portion of water is added. Add amount of water specified on the label.
2. Refrigerate PO suspension after reconstitution and discard remaining portion after 14 days.
3. Administer 1 hour before or 2 hours after a meal.

METHICILLIN SODIUM   Staphcillin (Rx)

Classification   Antibiotic, penicillin.

Action/Kinetics   A semisynthetic, penicillinase-resistant salt suitable for soft tissue, penicillin G-resistant, and resistant staphylococcal infections. **Peak plasma levels: IM**, 10–20 μg/ml after 30–60 min; **IV**, 15 min. t½: 30 min. Excreted chiefly in the urine.

Additional Uses   Infections by penicillinase-producing staphylococci; osteomyelitis, septicemia, enterocolitis, bacterial endocarditis.

Additional Contraindications   Use with caution in patients with renal failure. Safe use in neonates has not been established. Periodic renal function tests are indicated for long-term therapy.

Dosage   IV. Adults: 1 gm q 6 hr; **pediatric:** 200–300 mg/kg/day; **newborns:** 50–150 mg/kg/day. **IM. Adults:** 1 gm q 4–6 hr; **infants and pediatric (less than 20 kg):** 25 mg/kg q 6 hr.

Administration/Storage
1. Do not use dextrose solutions for diluting methicillin because their low acidity may destroy antibiotic.
2. Inject medication slowly. Methicillin injections are particularly painful.
3. Inject deeply into gluteal muscle.
4. To prevent sterile abscesses at injection site, include 0.2–0.3 ml of air in syringe before starting injection so that when the needle is withdrawn the irritating solution will not leak into tissue.
5. Methicillin is very sensitive to heat when dissolved. Therefore, solutions for IM administration must be used within 24 hr, if standing at room temperatures, or within 4 days, if refrigerated. Solutions for IV use must be used within 8 hr.
6. Dilute for direct IV administration 1 gm in a minimum of 17 ml of Sterile Water for Injection or Sodium Chloride Injection USP. For continuous IV infusion dilute 1–2 gm in 50–100 ml, 4 gm in 65 ml, and 6 gm in 97 ml.

Additional Nursing Implications

See also *Nursing Implications* for *Anti-infectives* p. 52 and *Penicillins*, p. 58.

1. Do not mix methicillin with any other drug in the same syringe or IV solution.
2. *Assess*
   a. for pain along course of vein into which the drug is administered and check for redness or edema at site of injection, because drug is a vesicant.
   b. for hematuria, casts in urine, BUN, and creatinine levels.
   c. for pallor, ecchymosis, or bleeding.
   d. for fever, nausea, and other signs of hepatotoxicity, especially with prolonged therapy.
3. Be sure blood cultures and white blood cell counts with differential are taken prior to start of and weekly during therapy.

MEZLOCILLIN SODIUM   Mezlin (Rx)

Classification   Antibiotic, penicillin.

Action/Kinetics   Mezlocillin is a broad-spectrum (gram-negative and gram-positive organisms including aerobic and anaerobic strains) antibiotic used parenterally. **Therapeutic serum levels:** 35–45 μg/ml. **t½: IV,** 55 min. Excreted mostly unchanged by the kidney. Penetration to CSF is poor except if meninges are inflamed.

Uses   Septicemia and infections of the lower respiratory tract, urinary tract, abdomen, skin, and female genital tract caused by *Klebsiella, Proteus, Pseudomonas, E. coli, Bacteroides, Peptococcus, S. faecalis* (enterococcus), *Peptostreptococcus,* and *Enterobacter.* Also, *Neisseria gonorrhoeae* infections of the urinary tract and female genital system. Infections caused by *Streptococcus pneumoniae* and Group A beta-hemolytic streptococcus.

Additional Untoward Reactions   Bleeding abnormalities. Decreased hemoglobin or hematocrit values.

Laboratory Test Interferences   ↑ SGOT, SGPT, serum alkaline phosphatase, serum bilirubin, serum creatinine and/or BUN. ↓ Serum potassium.

Dosage   **IV, IM. Adults:** *Serious infections:* 200–300 mg/kg/day in 4–6 divided doses; **usual:** 3 gm q 4 hr or 4 gm q 6 hr. *Life-threatening infections:* up to 350 mg/kg/day, not to exceed 24 gm daily. *Gonococcal urethritis:* single dose of 1–2 gm with probenecid, 1 gm **PO. Infants and children:** *Serious infections:* **1 month– 12 years,** 50 mg/kg q 4 hr; **infants more than 2 kg,** 75 mg/kg q 12 hr if less than 1 week of age; otherwise, 75 mg/kg q 6 hr; **infants less than 2 kg,** 75 mg/kg q 12 hr if less than 1 week of age; otherwise, 75 mg/kg q 8 hr.

Dosage should be reduced in patients with a creatinine clearance less than 30 ml/min.

Administration/Storage

1. When given by IV infusion (including piggyback), administration of other drugs should be discontinued during administration of mezlocillin.

2. For pediatric IV administration, infuse over 30 min.
3. Vials and infusion bottles should be stored below 30°C.
4. The powder and reconstituted solution may darken slightly, but potency is not affected.
5. IM doses should not exceed 2 gm per injection. Mezlocillin should be continued for at least 2 days after symptoms of infection have disappeared.
6. For Group A beta-hemolytic streptococcus, therapy should continue for at least 10 days.

Additional Nursing Implications
See also *Nursing Implications* for *Anti-infectives*, p. 52 and *Penicillins*, p. 58.

Assess for bruising and/or bleeding from any orifice, and for drug-induced anemia manifested by fatigue, pallor, weakness, vertigo, headache, dyspnea, and palpitations.

NAFCILLIN SODIUM   Nafcil, Unipen (Rx)

Classification   Antibiotic, penicillin.

Action/Kinetics   Used for resistant staphylococcal infections. Parenteral therapy is recommended initially for severe infections. **Peak plasma levels: PO**, 7 μg/ml after 30–60 min; **IM**, 14–20 μg/ml after 30–60 min. t½: 60 min.

Uses   Infections by penicillinase-producing staphylococci; also certain pneumococci and streptococci.

Additional Untoward Reactions   Sterile abscesses and thrombophlebitis occur frequently, especially in the elderly.

Dosage   **IV, IM. Adults:** 500 mg q 4–6 hr (double IV dose in severe infections); **pediatric:** 25 mg/kg b.i.d.; **neonates:** 10 mg/kg b.i.d. **PO. Adults:** 250–500 mg q 4–6 hr (up to 1 gm q 4–6 hr for severe infections). **Pediatric:** *Pneumonia/scarlet fever:* 25 mg/kg/day in 4 divided doses. *Staphylococcal infections:* 50 mg/kg/day in 4 divided doses **(Neonates:** 10 mg/kg t.i.d.–q.i.d.) *Streptococcal pharyngitis:* 250 mg t.i.d.
IV administration not recommended for neonates or infants.

Administration/Storage
1. Reconstitute for oral use by adding powder to bottle of diluent. Replace cap tightly. Then *shake thoroughly until all powder is in solution*. Check carefully for undissolved powder at bottom of bottle. Solution must be stored in refrigerator and unused portion discarded after 1 week.
2. Reconstitute for parenteral use by adding required amount of sterile water. Shake vigorously. Date bottle. Refrigerate after reconstitution and discard unused portion after 48 hr.
3. For direct IV administration, dissolve powder in 15–30 ml of sterile water for injection or isotonic sodium chloride solution and inject over 5–10-min period into the tubing of flowing IV infusion. For IV drip, dissolve the required amount in 100–150 ml of isotonic sodium chloride injection and administer by IV drip over a period of 15–90 min.

Additional Nursing Implications

See also *Nursing Implications* for *Anti-infectives*, p. 52 and *Penicillins*, p. 58.

1. Assess patient for GI distress after oral administration.
2. Administer IM by deep intragluteal injection.
3. Do not administer IV to newborn infants.
4. Reduce rate of flow and report pain, redness, or edema at site of IV administration.

OXACILLIN SODIUM   Bactocill, Prostaphlin (Rx)

Classification   Antibiotic, penicillin.

Action/Kinetics   Penicillinase-resistant, acid stable drug. Used for resistant staphylococcal infections. **Peak plasma levels: PO**, 1.6–10 μg after 30–60 min; **IM**, 5–11 μg/ml after 30 min. **t½:** 30 min.

Uses   Infections caused by penicillinase-producing staphylococci; also certain pneumococci and streptococci.

Dosage   IM, IV. Adults and pediatric (over 40 kg): 250–500 mg q 4–6 hr (up to 1 gm q 4–6 hr in severe infections); **pediatric (less than 40 kg):** 50 mg/kg/day in equally divided doses q 6 hr (up to 100 mg/kg/day in severe infections); **neonates and premature infants:** 25 mg/kg/day. **PO. Adults and pediatric (over 40 kg):** 500 mg q 4–6 hr for minimum of 5 days. PO route should not be used initially for severe or life-threatening infections. For follow-up therapy: **Adults,** 1 gm q 4–6 hr; **pediatric:** 100 mg/kg/day in equally divided doses q 4–6 hr.

Administration/Storage

1. Administer IM by deep intragluteal injection.
2. Reconstitution: Add sterile water for injection in amount indicated on vial. Shake until solution is clear. For parenteral use, reconstituted solution may be kept for 3 days at room temperature or 1 week in refrigerator. Discard outdated solutions.
3. IV administration (two methods):
   a. For rapid, direct administration, add an equal amount of sterile water or isotonic saline to reconstituted dosage and administer over period of 10 minutes.
   b. For drip method, add reconstituted solution to either dextrose, saline, or invert sugar solution and administer over a 6-hr period, during which time drug remains potent.

Additonal Nursing Implications

See also *Nursing Implications* for *Anti-infectives*, p. 52 and *Penicillins*, p. 58. *Assess*

a. for GI distress after oral administration.
b. for pain, redness, and edema at the site of IV injection and along the course of the vein.
c. for pain and swelling at IM injection site.

PENICILLIN G BENZATHINE, ORAL   Bicillin (Rx)

PENICILLIN G BENZATHINE, PARENTERAL   Bicillin Long-Acting Suspension, Permapen (Rx)

Classification   Antibiotic, penicillin.

Action/Kinetics   The parenteral product is a long-acting (repository) form of penicillin in an aqeuous vehicle; it is administered as a sterile suspension. **Peak plasma levels: PO**, 0.16 unit/ml; **IM**, 0.03–0.05 unit/ml.

Uses   Most gram-positive (streptococci, staphylococci, pneumococci) and some gram-negative (gonococci, meningococci) organisms. Syphilis. Prophylaxis of glomerulonephritis and rheumatic fever. Surgical infections, secondary infections following tooth extraction, tonsillectomy.

Dosage   PO. Adults and pediatric over 12 years: 400,000–600,000 units q 4–6 hr. *Prophylaxis of rheumatic fever/chorea:* 200,000 units b.i.d. **Children under 12 years:** 25,000–90,000 units/day in 3–6 divided doses. **Parenteral (IM only). Adults:** 1,200,000 units as a single dose; **older children:** 900,000 units as a single dose; **pediatric under 27 kg:** 300,000–600,000 units as a single dose. *Early syphilis:* 2,400,000 units as a single dose. *Late syphilis:* 2,400,000–3,000,000 units q 7 days for total of 6,000,000–9,000,000 units. *Prophylaxis of rheumatic fever, chorea, or glomerulonephritis:* 1,200,000 units once monthly or 600,000 units q 2 weeks.

Administration/Storage

1. Shake multiple-dose vial vigorously before withdrawing the desired dose, since medication tends to clump on standing. Check that all medication is dissolved and that there is no residue at bottom of bottle.
2. Use a 20-gauge needle, and do not allow medication to remain in the syringe and needle for long periods of time before administration because the needle may become plugged and syringe "frozen."
3. Inject slowly and steadily into the muscle and *do not massage* injection site.
4. Before injection of medication, aspirate needle to ascertain that needle is not in a vein.
5. Rotate and chart site of injections.
6. *Do not administer IV*.
7. Divide between two injection sites if dose is large or available muscle mass small.

Additional Nursing Implications
See also *Nursing Implications* for *Anti-infectives*, p. 52 and *Penicillins*, p. 58. Explain to patient why he must return for repository penicillin injections.

PENICILLIN G, BENZATHINE AND PROCAINE COMBINED   Bicillin C-R, Bicillin C-R 900/300 (Rx)

Classification   Antibiotic, penicillin.

Uses   Streptococcal infections (A, C, G, H, L, and M), without bacteremia, of the upper respiratory tract, skin, and soft tissues. Scarlet fever, erysipelas, pneumo-coccal infections, and otitis media.

Dosage   IM only. *Streptococcal infections*: **Adults and children over 27 kg**: 2,400,000 units, given at a single session using multiple injection sites or alternately in divided doses on days 1 and 3; **children 13.5–27 kg**: 900,000–1,200,000 units; **infants and children under 13.5 kg**: 600,000 units. *Pneumococcal infections, except meningitis*: **Adults**, 1,200,000 units; **pediatric**: 600,000 units. Give q 2–3 days until temperature is normal for 48 hr.

Administration/Storage   See *Penicillin G Benzathine Oral and Parenteral*, p. 71.

Nursing Implications

See *Nursing Implications* for *Penicillin G Benzathine Oral and Parenteral*, p. 71.

PENICILLIN G (AQUEOUS) PARENTERAL   Penicillin G Potassium, Penicillin G Sodium, Pfizerpen (Rx)

PENICILLIN G POTASSIUM, ORAL M-Cillin B 400, P-50,* Pentids, Pfizerpen G, SK-Penicillin G (Rx)

Classification   Antibiotic, penicillin.

Action/Kinetics   The low cost of penicillin G still makes it first choice for treatment of many infections. Rapid onset makes it especially suitable for fulminating infections. Destroyed by acid and penicillinase. **Peak plasma levels: IM or SC** 6–20 units/ml after 15–30 min. **t½**: 30 min.

Additional Untoward Reactions   Rapid IV administration may cause hyperkalemia and cardiac arrhythmias. Renal damage occurs rarely.

Dosage   Parenteral (IM, IV): Depending on the infection, 1–30 million units/day. **PO. Adults:** Depending on the use, 200,000–500,000 units q 6–8 hr; **pediatric under 12 years:** 25,000–90,000 units/kg/day in 3–6 divided doses. *Prophylaxis of rheumatic fever or chorea:* **Adult:** 200,000–250,000 units b.i.d.

Administration/Storage

1. Use sterile water, isotonic saline USP or 5% D_5W and mix with volume recommended on label for desired strength.
2. Loosen powder by shaking bottle before adding diluent.
3. Hold vial horizontally and rotate slowly while directing the stream of the diluent against the wall of the vial.
4. Shake vigorously after addition of diluent.
5. Solutions may be stored at room temperature for 24 hr, or in refrigerator for 1 week. Discard remaining solution.
6. Use 1–2% lidocaine solution as diluent for IM if ordered by doctor to lessen pain at injection site. Do not use procaine as diluent for aqueous penicillin.
7. Note the long list of drugs that should *not* be mixed with penicillin during IV administration:

Aminophylline	Ascorbic acid	Chlorpromazine
Amphotericin B	Chlorpheniramine	Gentamicin

Heparin
Hydroxyzine
Lincomycin
Metaraminol
Novobiocin
Oxytetracycline
Phenylephrine
Phenytoin

Polymyxin B
Prochlorperazine
Promazine
Promethazine
Sodium bicarbonate
Sodium salts of
barbiturates

Sulfadiazine
Tetracycline
Tromethamine
Vitamin B complex
Vancomycin

Additional Nursing Implications

See also *Nursing Implications* for *Anti-infectives*, p. 52 and *Penicillins*, p. 58.

1. Drug should be ordered specifying sodium or potassium salt.
2. Assess patient for GI disturbances, which may lead to dehydration. Dehydration decreases the excretion of the drug by the kidneys and may raise the blood level of penicillin G to dangerously high levels that can cause kidney damage.

PENICILLIN G, PROCAINE, AQUEOUS Ayercillin,* Crysticillin 300 A.S. and 600 A.S., Duracillin A.S., Pfizerpen-AS, Wycillin (Rx)

Classification Antibiotic, penicillin.

Action/Kinetics Long-acting (repository) form in aqueous or oily vehicle. Destroyed by penicillinase. Because of slow onset, a soluble penicillin is often administered concomitantly for fulminating infections.

Uses Penicillin-sensitive staphylococci, pneumococci, streptococci, and bacterial endocarditis. Gonorrhea, all stages of syphilis. *Prophylaxis* : Rheumatic fever, pre- and postsurgery. Diphtheria, anthrax, fusospirochetosis (Vincent's infection), erysipeloid, rat bite fever.

Dosage **IM only, usual:** 600,000–1,000,000 units daily. *Prophylaxis against bacterial endocarditis:* **Adults:** 1,000,000 units Penicillin G with 600,000 units Penicillin G Procaine 30–60 min prior to procedure; **then,** Penicillin V, 500 mg, **PO,** q 6 hr for 8 doses. **Pediatric:** 30,000 units/kg Penicillin G with 600,000 units Penicillin G Procaine 30–60 min prior to procedure; **then,** Penicillin V, 500 mg **PO,** (250 mg **PO,** if less than 27 kg) q 6 hr for 8 doses. *Diphtheria carrier state:* 300,000 units/ day for 10 days. *Syphilis (negative spinal fluid in adults, children):* 600,000 units daily for 8 days (total 4.8 million units). *Late syphilis (positive spinal fluid):* 600,000 units daily for 10–15 days (total of 6–9 million units).

Administration/Storage

1. Note on package whether medication is to be refrigerated, since some brands require this to maintain stability.
2. Shake multiple-dose vial thoroughly to ensure uniform suspension before injection. If the medication is clumped at the bottom of the vial, it must be shaken until clump dissolves.
3. Use a 20-gauge needle and aspirate immediately after withdrawing medication from the vial; otherwise needle may become clogged and syringe may "freeze."
4. Administer into 2 sites if dose is large or available muscle mass is small.
5. Aspirate to check that the needle is not in a vein.
6. Inject deep into muscle at a slow rate.

7. Do not massage after injection.
8. Rotate and chart injection sites.

Additional Nursing Implications
See also *Nursing Implications* for *Anti-infectives*, p. 52 and *Penicillins* p. 58.
   Observe for wheal or other skin reactions at site of injection that may indicate a reaction to procaine as well as to penicillin.

PENICILLIN V (PHENOXYMETHYL PENICILLIN) (Rx)

PENICILLIN V POTASSIUM (PHENOXYMETHYL PENICILLIN POTASSIUM) Beepen-VK, Betapen-VK, Deltapen-VK, Ledercillin VK, Novopen-VK,* Penapar VK, Penicillin VK, Pen-Vee K, Pfizerpen VK, PVF,* PVF K,* Repen-VK, Robicillin VK, SK-Penicillin-VK, Uticillin VK, V-Cillin K, Veetids (Rx)

Classification Antibiotic, penicillin.

Action/Kinetics These preparations are closely related to penicillin G. They are acid stable and resist inactivation by gastric secretions. They are well absorbed from GI tract and are not affected by foods.
   Peak plasma levels: Penicillin V, **PO**: 2.7 μg/ml after 30–60 min; Penicillin V potassium, **PO**: 1–9 μg/ml after 30–60 min. **t ½**: 30 min.
   Periodic blood counts and renal function tests are indicated during long-term usage.

Uses Penicillin-sensitive staphylococci, pneumococci, streptococci, gonococci. Vincent's infection of the oropharynx. *Prophylaxis*: Rheumatic fever, chorea, bacterial endocarditis, pre- and postsurgery. Should *not* be used as prophylaxis for genitourinary instrumentation or surgery, sigmoidoscopy, or childbirth.

Additional Drug Interactions

Interactant	Interaction
Neomycin, oral	↓ Absorption of penicillin V
Oral Contraceptives	↓ Effectiveness of oral contraceptives

Dosage **PO. Adults and children over 12 years:** *Streptococcal infections:* 125–250 mg q 6–8 hr for 10 days. *Pneumococcal or staphylococcal infections, fusospirochetosis of oropharynx:* 250–500 mg q 6–8 hr. *Prophylaxis of rheumatic fever/chorea:* 125–250 mg b.i.d. **Children under 12 years: Usual,** 25,000–90,000 units/kg/day in 3–6 divided doses.
   Prophylaxis of bacterial endocarditis. **PO. Adults and children over 27 kg:** 2 gm 30–60 min prior to procedure; **then,** 500 mg q 6 hr for 8 doses. **Pediatric:** 1 gm 30–60 min prior to procedure; **then,** 250 mg q 6 hr for 8 doses. See also, Penicillin G Procaine, Aqueous.

Administration

1. Administer without regard to meals.
2. Do not administer at the same time as neomycin, because malabsorption of penicillin V may occur.

PIPERACILLIN SODIUM   Pipracil (Rx)

Classification   Antibiotic, penicillin.

Action/Kinetics   Piperacillin is a semisynthetic, broad-spectrum penicillin for parenteral use. The drug penetrates cerebrospinal fluid in the presence of inflamed meninges.

Peak serum level: 244 µg/ml. **t½:** 36–72 min. Excreted unchanged in urine and bile.

Additional Uses   Intra-abdominal infections, gynecologic infections, septicemia, skin and skin structure infections, bone and joint infections, mixed infections. Prophylaxis in surgery including GI, biliary, hysterectomy, cesarean section.

Additional Untoward Reactions   Rarely, prolonged muscle relaxation.

Laboratory Test Interference   BUN, creatinine.

Dosage   IM, IV. *Serious infections,* **IV:** 3–4 gm q 4–6 hr (12–18 gm/day). *Complicated urinary tract infections,* **IV:** 8–16 gm/day in divided doses q 6–8 hr. *Uncomplicated urinary tract infections and most community-acquired pneumonias,* **IM, IV:** 6–8 gm/day in divided doses q 6–12 hr. *Uncomplicated gonorrhea infections:* 2 gm **IM** with 1 gm probenecid **PO** 30 min before injection (both given as single dose). *Prophylaxis in surgery:* **First dose: IV,** 2 gm prior to surgery; **second dose:** 2 gm either during surgery (abdominal) or 4–6 hr after surgery (hysterectomy, cesarean); **third dose:** 2 gm at an interval depending on use. Dosage should be decreased in renal impairment. Dosages have not been established in infants and children under 12 years of age.

Administration

1. No more than 2 gm should be administered IM at any one site.
2. For IM, use upper, outer quadrant of gluteus or well-developed deltoid muscle. Do not use lower or mid-third of upper arm.
3. Reconstitute each gram with at least 5 ml diluent, such as sterile or bacteriostatic water for injection, sodium chloride for injection, or bacteriostatic sodium chloride for injection. Shake until dissolved.
4. Inject IV slowly over a period of 3–5 min to avoid vein irritation.
5. Administer by intermittent IV infusion in at least 50 ml over a period of 20–30 min via "piggyback" or soluset.
6. After reconstitution, solution may be stored at room temperature for 24 hours, refrigerated for 1 week, or frozen for 1 month.

TICARCILLIN DISODIUM   Ticar (Rx)

Classification   Antibiotic, penicillin.

Action/Kinetics   Parenteral, semisynthetic antibiotic with an antibacterial spectrum resembling carbenicillin. Primarily suitable for treatment of gram-negative organisms, but also effective for mixed infections. Combined therapy with gentamicin or tobramycin is sometimes indicated for treatment of *Pseudomonas* infections. *The drugs should not be mixed during administration because of gradual mutual inactivation.*

Peak plasma levels: **IM,** 25–35 µg/ml after 1 hr; **IV,** 15 min. **t½:** 70 min. Elimination complete after 6 hr.

Uses   Bacterial septicemia, skin and soft tissue infections, acute and chronic respiratory tract infections caused by susceptible strains of *Pseudomonas aeruginosa*, *Proteus* species, *E. coli*, and other gram-negative organisms.

Genitourinary tract infections caused by above organisms and *Enterobacter* and *Streptococcus faecalis*.

Anaerobic bacteria causing empyema, anaerobic pneumonitis, lung abscess, bacterial septicemia, peritonitis, intra-abdominal abscess, skin and soft tissue infections, salpingitis, endometritis, pelvic inflammatory disease, pelvic abscess.

Additional Contraindications Pregnancy. Use with caution in presence of impaired renal function and for patients on restricted salt diets.

Additional Untoward Reactions Neurotoxicity and neuromuscular excitability, especially in patients with impaired renal function. Elevated alkaline phosphatase, SGOT, and SGPT values.

Additional Drug Interactions Effect of carbenicillin may be enhanced when used in combination with gentamicin or tobramycin for *Pseudomonas* infections.

Dosage *Systemic infections.* **IV infusion, Adults and children less than 40 kg:** 200–300 mg/kg daily in divided doses q 3–6 hr for adults and q 4–6 hr for children. **IV infusion, IM, Neonates (over 2 kg, 0–7 days of age):** 75 mg/kg q 12 hr; **if over 7 days:** 75 mg/kg q 8 hr. *Urinary tract infections.* **IV infusion (complicated infections), Adults and children (less than 40 kg):** 150–200 mg/kg daily in divided doses q 4–6 hr. **IM or Direct IV (uncomplicated infections): Adults,** 1 gm q 6 hr; **pediatric (less than 40 kg):** 50–100 mg/kg daily in divided doses q 6–8 hr.

Patients with renal insufficiency should receive a loading dose of 3 gm **(IV)** and subsequent doses as indicated by creatinine clearance.

Administration/Storage
1. Discard unused reconstituted solutions after 24 hr when stored at room temperature, and after 72 hr when refrigerated.
2. Reconstitute with 1% lidocaine HCl (without epinephrine) or with bacteriostatic water for injection containing 0.9% benzyl alcohol to prevent pain and induration.
3. Use dilute solution of 50 mg/ml or less for IV use, and administer slowly to prevent vein irritation and phlebitis.
4. Do not administer more than 2 gm of the drug in each IM site.

Additional Nursing Implications
See also *Nursing Implications* for *Anti-infectives*, p. 52 and *Penicillins*, p. 58. *Assess*
a. for signs of hemorrhagic manifestations, such as petechiae, ecchymosis, or frank bleeding. Check bleeding time.
b. patient with cardiac history for edema, weight gain, or respiratory distress precipitated by sodium in drug.
c. patient on high doses for signs of electrolyte imbalance, especially with regard to sodium and potassium.

ERYTHROMYCINS

General Statement The erythromycins are produced by strains of *Streptomyces erythreus* and have bacteriostatic and occasionally bactericidal activity (at high concentrations, or if microorganism is particularly susceptible).

The erythromycins are absorbed from the upper part of the small intestine. Erythromycin for oral use is coated with an acid-resistant material to avoid destruction by gastric juice.

Erythromycin diffuses into body tissues, the peritoneal, pleural, ascitic and amniotic fluids, the saliva, the placental circulation, and across the mucous membrane of the tracheobronchial tree. It diffuses poorly into the spinal fluid.

Action/Kinetics The erythromycins inhibit protein synthesis of microorganisms by binding to a ribosomal subunit (50S) thus interfering with the transmission of genetic information. The drugs are only effective against rapidly multiplying organisms. **Peak serum levels: PO**, attained after 1–4 hr. **t½**: 1.5–2 hr, *but prolonged in patients with renal impairment*. The drug is partially metabolized by liver and primarily excreted in bile. Drugs are excreted in breast milk.

Uses Mild to moderate infections of the upper and lower respiratory tracts, skin, and soft tissue infections caused by *Streptococcus pyogenes, S. pneumoniae*, and *Listeria monocytogenes*. Erythrasma caused by *Corynebacterium*. Pharyngitis, pertussis, adjunct for treatment of diphtheria, acne, conjunctivitis, genitourinary tract infections, prophylaxis of rheumatic fever. Erythromycins have also been used to treat pneumonia caused by *Mycoplasma pneumoniae*, for Legionnaire's disease either alone or in combination, and for skin infections caused by *Staphylococcus aureus*. Prophylaxis before tooth extraction or surgery in patients with history of rheumatic fever or congenital heart disease.

The drugs are used as alternatives to penicillins or tetracyclines to treat all stages of syphilis, for disseminated gonococcal infections, and pelvic inflammatory disease. In combination with penicillin or spectinomycin for chlamydial infections in pregnant women.

Many erythromycins are available in ointment and solutions for ophthalmic, otic, and dermatologic use.

Contraindication Hypersensitivity to erythromycin, in utero syphilis.

Untoward Reactions Erythromycins have a low incidence of untoward reactions (except for the estolate salt). *GI* (most common): Nausea, vomiting, diarrhea, cramping, abdominal pain, stomatitis, anorexia, melena, heartburn, pruritus ani. *Allergic:* Skin rashes, urticaria, anaphylaxis (rare). *Miscellaneous:* Superinfection. *Following topical use:* Itching, burning, irritation, or stinging of skin. Dry, scaly skin.

IV use may result in venous irritation and thrombophlebitis; IM use produces pain at the injection site with development of necrosis or sterile abscesses.

Drug Interactions

Interactant	Interaction
Carbamazepine	↑ Effect of carbamazepine due to ↓ breakdown by liver
Digoxin	Erythromycin ↑ bioavailability of digoxin
Methylprednisolone	↑ Methylprednisolone due to ↓ breakdown by liver
Penicillin	Effect ↓ by erythromycins
Sodium bicarbonate	↑ Effect of erythromycin in urine due to alkalinization
Theophylline	↑ Effect of theophylline due to ↓ breakdown in liver
Warfarin	Erythromycin ↑ effect of warfarin

Laboratory Test Interferences False + or ↑ values of urinary catecholamines, urinary steroids, and SGOT and SGPT.

Dosage **PO** and **IM** (painful); some preparations can be given **IV**. (See Table 1, p. 78.)

TABLE 1 ERYTHROMYCINS

Drug	Main Uses	Dosage	Remarks
Erythromycin (E-Mycin, Eryc, Ery-Tab, Erythromid,* Erythromycin Base Film-tabs, Ilotycin, Ilotycin Ophthalmic, Robimycin, RP-Mycin) Rx	Respiratory infections, beta-hemolytic streptococci, amebiasis	**PO: initially, 500 mg; then,** 250 mg q 6 hr, can increase to 4 gm/day; **pediatric:** 30–50 mg/kg/day in 3–4 divided doses. *Primary Syphilis:* 20–40 gm in divided doses over a period of 10–15 days.	Food does not affect absorption.
Erythromycin estolate (Ilosone, Novorythro*) Rx	Sensitive staphylococci, pneumococci, and streptococci in penicillin-sensitized patients; Legionnaire's disease	**Adults and children over 25 kg, PO:** 250 mg q 6 hr; **children 4.5–11.5 kg:** 11 mg/kg q 6 hr; **children 11.5–25 kg:** 125 mg q 6 hr	Most active form of erythromycin with relatively long-lasting activity. Special contraindications: cholestatic jaundice or preexisting liver dysfunction; not recommended for treatment of chronic disorders such as acne and furunculosis or for prophylaxis of rheumatic fever. *Additional Untoward Reactions* Cholestatic jaundice—usually after 10–14 days of therapy; alteration of certain laboratory tests. *Administration/Storage* 1. Shake oral suspension well before pouring. 2. Do not store suspension longer than 2 weeks at room temperature. 3. Chewable tablets must be chewed or crushed.
Erythromycin ethylsuccinate (E.E.S., E-Mycin E, EryPed, Pediamycin, Wyamycin E) Rx	Sensitive staphylococci, pneumococci and streptococci in penicillin-sensitized patients. Topical: skin infections by susceptible organisms	**Adults and older children, PO:** 400 mg q 6 hr; **pediatric:** 30–50 mg/kg/day in 3–4 divided doses. *Primary Syphilis:* 48–64 gm in divided doses over 10–15 days. *Dysenteric Amebiasis:* 400 mg q.i.d. for 10–14 days. *Before surgery, to prevent alpha-hemolytic streptococci-induced endocarditis:* 800 mg before procedure and 400 mg q 6–8	The injectible form contains 2% butylbenzocaine and is contraindicated in patients allergic to the "caine" (e.g., procaine, benzocaine) type of local anesthetic *Administration/Storage* 1. Inject into large muscle mass. 2. Rotate site of injections. 3. Do not administer to infants, as muscle mass is too small. 4. Do not mix with other medications in same syringe. 5. Avoid accidental IV administration.

79

6. Refrigerate aqueous suspensions and store for maximum of 1 week.
7. Chewable tablets must be chewed or crushed.

Drug Interactions
Drug for IV administration is incompatible with amikacin, aminophylline, cefazolin, cephalothin, cephaloridine, metaraminol, novobiocin, oxytetracycline, pentobarbital, secobarbital, streptomycin, tetracycline.
Administration/Storage
1. Follow directions on vial for dilution.
2. Concentrate, which must be diluted further before administration, will remain stable in refrigerator for 7 days.
3. Administer slowly over period of 20–60 min or infuse IV over 24 hr.
Change to oral therapy as soon as possible.
Additional Untoward Reactions
Transient deafness
Drug Interactions
Some recommend that no drugs be added to IV solutions of erythromycin lactobionate.

Drug causes more allergic reactions, such as skin rash and urticaria, than other erythromycins.
Administration
Do not administer with meals, because food decreases absorption.

Drug	Uses	Dosage
		hr for 4 doses after procedure.
Erythromycin gluceptate (Ilotycin Gluceptate IV) Rx	Primarily for unconscious, vomiting, or gravely ill patients with serious infections of gram-positive bacteria, especially hemolytic streptococci, pneumococci or staphylococci, gonococci; Legionnaire's disease	**Adults and children, IV only:** 250–1,000 mg q 6 hr. *Acute pelvic inflammatory disease caused by gonorrhea:* 500 mg q 6 hr for 3 days, followed by 250 mg erythromycin stearate PO q 6 hr for 7 days. *Legionnaire's disease:* 1–4 gm/day in divided doses.
Erythromycin lactobionate (Erythrocin Lactobionate IV, Erythrocin Piggyback) Rx	For seriously ill or vomiting patients suffering from infections by susceptible organisms; acute pelvic inflammatory disease from gonorrhea; Legionnaire's disease	**Adults and children: IV,** 15–20 mg/kg/day up to 4 gm/day in severe infections. *Acute pelvic inflammatory disease caused by gonorrhea:* 500 mg q 6 hr for 3 days followed by 250 mg erythromycin stearate, **PO,** q 6 hr for 7 days. *Legionnaire's disease:* 1–4 gm/day in divided doses.
Erythromycin stearate (Apo-Erythro-S,* Eramycin, Erypar, Erythrocin Stearate, Ethril, SK-Erythromycin, Wyamycin S) Rx	Sensitive staphylococci, pneumococci, and streptococci in penicillin-sensitized patients	**PO, buffered tablets:** 250 mg q 6 hr or 500 mg q 12 hr. **Pediatric:** 30–50 mg/kg daily in 4–6 equally divided doses.

Administration/ Storage

1. Inject deep into muscle mass. Injections are painful and irritating.
2. Do not administer with or immediately prior to fruit juice or other acid drinks because acidity may decrease activity of drug.
3. Do not routinely administer PO medication with meals because food decreases the absorption of most erythromycins. However, physician may order medication to be given with food to reduce GI irritation.

Nursing Implications

See *Nursing Implications* for *Anti-infectives*, p. 52.

Erythromycins are often administered in combination with sulfonamides. In that case, observe all the precautions indicated for both groups of drugs when erythromycin is administered with a sulfonamide drug.

Nursing Implications for Erythromycin Antibiotic Ointments

1. If skin reactions occur, discontinue use and report to physician.
2. Clean affected area before applying ointment.

Nursing Implications for Ophthalmic Solutions

Assess for mild reaction which, although generally transient, must be reported to physician.

Nursing Implications for Otic Solutions

1. Instill at room temperature.
2. Pull pinna of ear down and back for children under 3 years of age, and up and back for patients over 3 years of age.

TETRACYCLINES

General Statement   Tetracyclines are well absorbed from the stomach and upper small intestine. They are well distributed throughout all tissues and fluids and diffuse through noninflamed meninges and the placental barrier. They become deposited in the fetal skeleton and calcifying teeth.

Action/Kinetics   The tetracyclines inhibit protein synthesis by microorganisms by binding to a crucial ribosomal subunit (50S), thereby interfering with the transmission of genetic information, via the same mechanism as for the erythromycins. The drugs are mostly bacteriostatic and are only effective against multiplying bacteria. t½ ranges from 7 to 18.6 hr (see individual agents) and is increased in the presence of renal impairment. The drugs bind to serum protein (range 20–

93%; see individual agents). The drugs are concentrated in the liver and mostly excreted in the bile.

Uses   Used mainly for infections caused by *Rickettsia, Chlamydia,* and *Mycoplasma.* Due to development of resistance, tetracyclines are usually not used for infections by common gram-negative or gram-positive organisms.

Tetracyclines are the drugs of choice for rickettsial infections such as Rocky Mountain spotted fever, endemic typhus, and others. They are also the drugs of choice for psittacosis, lymphogranuloma venerum, and urethritis due to *Mycoplasma hominis* and *Ureoplasma urealyticum.* Epididymo-orchitis due to *Chlamydia trachomatis* and/or *Neisseria gonorrheae.* Atypical pneumonia caused by *Mycoplasma pneumoniae.* Adjunct in the treatment of trachoma.

Tetracyclines are the drugs of choice for gram-negative bacteria causing bartonellosis, brucellosis, granuloma inguinale, cholera. They are used as alternatives for the treatment of plague, tularemia, chancroid, or *Campylobacter fetus* infections. Prophylaxis of plague after exposure. Infections caused by *Acinetobacter, Bacteroides, Enterobacter aerogenes, E. coli, Shigella.* Respiratory and/or urinary tract infections caused by *Hemophilus influenzae,* or *Klebsiella pneumoniae.*

As an alternative to penicillin for uncomplicated gonorrhea or disseminated gonococcal infections especially with penicillin allergy. Acute pelvic inflammatory disease. Tetracyclines are also useful as an alternative to penicillin for early syphilis.

Although not generally used for gram-positive infections, tetracyclines may be beneficial in anthrax, *Listeria* infections, and actinomycosis. They have also been used in conjunction with quinine sulfate for chloroquine-resistant *Plasmodium falciparum* malaria and as an intracavitary injection to control pleural or pericardial effusion caused by metastatic carcinoma.

Topical uses include skin granulomas caused by *Mycobacterium marinum;* ophthalmic bacterial infections causing blepharitis, conjunctivitis, or keratitis; and, as an adjunct in the treatment of ophthalmic chlamydial infections such as trachoma or inclusion conjunctivitis. Tetracyclines are used as an alternative to silver nitrate for prophylaxis of neonatal gonococcal ophthalmia. Vaginitis. Severe acne.

Contraindications   Hypersensitivity; avoid drug during tooth development stage (last trimester of pregnancy, neonatal period, and childhood up to 8 years), because tetracyclines interfere with enamel formation and dental pigmentation.

Use with caution and at reduced dosage in patients with impaired kidney function.

Never administer intrathecally.

Untoward Reactions   *GI* (most common): Nausea, vomiting, thirst, diarrhea, anorexia, flatulence, epigastric distress, bulky loose stools. Less commonly, stomatitis, dysphagia, black hairy tongue, glossitis, or inflammatory lesions of the anogenital area. Rarely, pseudomembranous colitis. *Allergic* (rare): Dermatoses, skin rashes, pruritus, urticaria, eosinophilia, angioedema, asthma-like symptoms, anaphylaxis, serum sickness, pericarditis. *Skin:* Paresthesia, photosensitivity, discoloration of nails. *CNS:* Dizziness, lightheadedness, unsteadiness. *Hematologic:* Atypical lymphocytes, leukocytosis, leukopenia, hemolytic anemia, neutropenia, thrombocytopenia, thrombocytopenic purpura. *Miscellaneous:* Candidal superinfection including oral and vaginal candidiasis, discoloration of infants' and children's teeth, bone lesions, delayed bone growth, increased urination, hepatotoxicity.

IV administration may cause thrombophlebitis; IM injections are painful and may cause induration at the injection site.

The administration of deteriorated tetracyclines may result in Fanconi-like syndrome characterized by nausea, vomiting, acidosis, proteinuria, glycosuria, aminoaciduria, polydipsia, polyuria, hypokalemia.

Drug Interactions

Interactant	Interaction
Aluminum salts	↓ Effect of tetracyclines due to ↓ absorption from GI tract
Antacids, oral	↓ Effect of tetracyclines due to ↓ absorption from GI tract
Anticoagulants, oral	IV tetracyclines ↑ hypoprothrombinemia
Bismuth salts	↓ Effect of tetracyclines due to ↓ absorption from GI tract
Bumetanide	↑ Risk of kidney toxicity
Calcium salts	↓ Effect of tetracyclines due to ↓ absorption from GI tract
Cimetidine	↓ Effect of tetracyclines due to ↓ absorption from GI tract
Contraceptives, oral	↓ Effect of oral contraceptives
Digoxin	Tetracyclines ↑ bioavailability of digoxin
Diuretics, thiazide	↑ Risk of kidney toxicity
Ethacrynic acid	↑ Risk of kidney toxicity
Furosemide	↑ Risk of kidney toxicity
Iron preparations	↓ Effect of tetracyclines due to ↓ absorption from GI tract
Magnesium salts	↓ Effect of tetracyclines due to ↓ absorption from GI tract
Methoxyflurane	↑ Risk of kidney toxicity
Penicillins	Tetracyclines may mask bactericidal effect of penicillins
Sodium bicarbonate	↓ Effect of tetracyclines due to ↓ absorption from GI tract
Zinc salts	↓ Effect of tetracyclines due to ↓ absorption from GI tract

Laboratory Test Interferences   False + or ↑ urinary catecholamines, urinary protein (degraded), coagulation time. False − or ↓ urinary urobilinogen, glucose tests (see *Nursing Implications*). Prolonged use or high doses may change liver function tests, and white blood counts.

Dosage   PO, IM, IV, and topical. (For details see Table 2, p. 84.)

Administration/ Storage

1. Do not use outdated or deteriorated drugs, as a Fanconi-like syndrome may occur (see *Untoward Reactions*).
2. Discard unused capsules to prevent use of deteriorated medication.
3. Administer IM into large muscle mass to avoid extravasation into subcutaneous or fatty tissue.
4. Administer on an empty stomach. Withhold antacids, iron salts, dairy foods, and other foods high in calcium for at least 2 hr after PO administration. Do not administer milk with tetracyclines.

Nursing Implications

See *Nursing Implications* for *Anti-infectives*, p. 52.

1. *Assess*
   a. for gastric distress following administration of medication. Report to physician, who may order a light meal with medication or reduce individual dose of the medication and increase the frequency of administration.
   b. for maintenance of adequate intake and output, because renal dysfunction may result in drug accumulation, leading to toxicity.
   c. patient with impaired kidney function for increased BUN, acidosis, anorexia, nausea, vomiting, weight loss, and dehydration. Continue assessment after cessation of therapy, because symptoms may appear later.
   d. patient on IV therapy for nausea, vomiting, chills, fever, and hypertension, resulting from too rapid administration or an excessively high dose. Slow IV and report if symptoms occur.
   e. infant for bulging fontanel, which may be caused by too-rapid IV infusion Slow IV rate and report.
   f. patient with impaired hepatic or renal function for impairment of consciousness or other CNS disturbances, because drug can interfere with respiration of brain tissue.
   g. for symptoms of enterocolitis, such as diarrhea, pyrexia, abdominal distention, and scanty urine. These symptoms may necessitate discontinuance of drug and substitution of another antibiotic.
   h. for sore throat, dysphagia, fever, dizziness, hoarseness, and inflammation of mucous membranes of the body, indicating an untoward reaction.
   i. for onycholosis (loosening or detachment of the nail from the nail bed).
2. Prevent or treat pruritis ani by cleansing of the anal area with water several times a day and/or after each bowel movement.
3. Advise patient to avoid direct or artificial sunlight, which can cause a severe sunburnlike reaction, and to report erythema if it occurs.
4. Advise patient that zinc tablets or vitamin preparations containing zinc may interfere with absorption of tetracyclines.
5. If GI disturbances occur, do not use antacids that contain calcium, magnesium, or aluminum.
6. Tetracyclines should not be taken with milk, cheese, ice cream, or other foods containing calcium. If dose is taken with meals, avoid these foods until 2 hours after meals.

CEPHALOSPORINS

General Statement   The cephalosporins are semisynthetic antibiotics derived from cultures of *Cephalosporium acremonium*. They resemble the penicillins both chemically and pharmacologically.

Some cephalosporins are rapidly absorbed from the GI tract and quickly reach effective concentrations in the urinary, GI, and respiratory tracts except in patients with pernicious anemia or obstructive jaundice. The drugs are eliminated rapidly in patients with normal renal function.

TABLE 2   TETRACYCLINES

Drug	Dosage	Remarks
Chlortetracycline hydrochloride (Aureomycin Ophthalmic, Aureomycin Ointment)	**Ophthalmic, 1%:** Small amount in lower conjunctival sac q 3–4 hr. **Topical, 3%:** Apply to affected area 1–5 times daily.	
Demeclocycline hydrochloride (Declomycin) Rx	**PO. Adult:** 600 mg daily in 2–4 divided doses. **Children over 8 yr:** 6–12 mg/kg daily in 2–4 divided doses. *Gonorrhea:* **Initial,** 600 mg; **then,** 300 mg q 12 hr for 4 days to a total of 3 gm. *GU or rectal Chlamydia trachomatis infections:* 300 mg q.i.d. for 7 days.	**t½:** 10–17 hr; 40–50% excreted unchanged in urine. Causes photosensitivity more frequently than other tetracyclines. May cause increased pigmentation of skin. Antihistamines and corticosteroids may be useful in treatment of hypersensitivity. Also used to treat chronic inappropriate ADH secretion. *Aditional Untoward Reactions* Reversible diabetes insipidus syndrome.
Doxycycline calcium (Vibramycin) Rx Doxycycline hyclate (Doxy-Caps, Doxychel, Hyclate, Doxy-Lemmon, Doxy-Tabs, Vibramycin, Vibra-Tabs) Rx Doxycycline monohydrate (Vibramycin) Rx	**PO, IV. Adult: 1st day,** 100 mg q 12 hr; **then,** depending on severity of infection, 100–200 mg daily administered in 1–2 doses. **Children, over 8 yr; 45 kg or less: 1st day,** 4.4 mg/kg in 1–2 doses. PO. *Acute gonorrhea:* 200 mg at once; **then,** 100 mg h.s. on 1st day followed by 100 mg b.i.d. for 3 days. *Syphilis (primary/secondary):* 300 mg daily in divided doses for 10 days. *GU or rectal Chlamydia trachomatis infections:* 100 mg b.i.d. for minimum of 7 days. *Prophylaxis of "traveler's diarrhea":* 100 mg daily.	**t½:** 14.5–22 hr; 30–40% excreted unchanged in urine. More slowly absorbed, and thus more persistent than other tetracyclines. Preferred for patients with impaired renal function for treating infections outside urinary tract. *Drug Interaction* Carbamazepine, phenytoin, and barbiturates ↓ effect of doxycycline by ↑ breakdown by the liver. *Additional Untoward Reactions* Esophagitis, esophageal ulceration. *Administration/Storage* 1. Powder for suspension has expiration date of 12 months from date of issue. 2. Solution stable for 2 weeks when stored in refrigerator. 3. Follow directions on vial for dilution. Concentrations should be no lower than 0.1 mg/ml or higher than 1.0 mg/ml. 4. During infusion protect solution from light. 5. Complete solutions diluted with NaCl Injection, and D₅W, Ringer's Injection, and 10% invert sugar within 12 hr. 6. Complete solutions diluted with Lactated Ringer's In-

TABLE 2 *(Continued)*

Drug	Dosage	Remarks
		jection or 5% Dextrose in Lactated Ringer's within 6 hr.
Meclocycline sulfosalicylate (Meclan) Rx	**Topical use only.** Apply 1% cream to affected areas b.i.d. in AM and PM.	Used to treat acne vulgaris. Poorly absorbed through skin. Rarely, causes skin irritation, contact dermatitis. Long-term use may cause follicular staining. May stain fabrics. *Administration* 1. Apply solution until skin is thoroughly wet. 2. Avoid excessive use of cream to prevent staining of fabric. *Additional Nursing Implications* 1. Check for history of hypersensitivity. 2. *Teach patient:* a. not to allow medication to enter eyes, nose or mouth b. that stinging or burning after application is transient. c. that yellow tinge to skin may be removed by washing. d. that cosmetics may be used. e. that fluorescence of treated areas under ultraviolet light may occur.
Methacycline hydrochloride (Rondomycin) Rx	**PO. Adult:** 600 mg daily in 2–4 divided doses. **Children over 8 years:** 6–12 mg/kg daily in 2–4 doses. *Gonorrhea:* **initially,** 900 mg; **then,** 300 mg q.i.d. for a total of 5.4 gm. *Syphilis:* 18–24 gm in divided doses over 10–15 days. *Eaton agent (PPLO) pneumonia:* 900 mg daily for 6 days.	t½: 11–14.7 hr. 40–50% excreted unchanged in urine. Pediatric dosage should not be administered with milk formulas or calcium-containing foods.
Minocycline hydrochloride (Minocin, Minocin IV) Rx	**PO, IV, Adult: initial,** 200 mg; **then,** 100 mg q 12 hr (not to exceed 400 mg/day). **Children over 8 years: initial,** 4 mg/kg; **then,** 2 mg/kg q 12 hr. *Meningococcal carrier state:*	t½: 11–18.6 hr. 5–10% excreted unchanged in urine. Absorption less affected by milk or food than other tetracyclines. Also used to treat asymptomatic carriers of *N. meningitidis.* *Additional Untoward Reaction*

TABLE 2 (Continued)

Drug	Dosage	Remarks
	100 mg b.i.d. for 5 days. *Mycobacterium marinum infections:* 100 mg b.i.d. for 6–8 wk. *GU or rectal Chlamydia trachomatis or Ureaplasma urealyticum infections:* 100 mg b.i.d. for minimum of 7 days. *Gonorrheal urethritis in males:* 100 mg b.i.d. for 5 days. *Gonorrhea sensitive to penicillin:* **initially,** 200 mg; **then,** 100 mg for minimum of 4 days.	Blue-gray pigmentation areas of cutaneous inflammation, vertigo, ataxia, drowsiness, vestibular symptoms. *Administration/Storage* 1. Do not dissolve in solutions containing calcium because precipitate may form. 2. After dissolving medication in vial, further dilute to 500–1,000 ml. 3. Start administration of final dilution immediately. 4. Discard solution after 24 hr at room temperature.
Oxytetracycline (Oxymycin, Terramycin, Terramycin IM) Rx Oxytetracycline hydrochloride (E.P. Mycin, Terramycin, Terramycin IV, Uri-Tet) Rx	**PO, IV, IM: See** Tetracycline hydrochloride.	t½: 5.6 hr. 40–70% excreted unchanged in urine. Do not give with food or antacid. Pediatric dosage should not be administered with milk or calcium-containing foods. Check dilutions for IV administration.
Oxytetracycline and nystatin (Terrastatin) Rx	**PO.** See Tetracycline.	Used for candidal infections. Also, see p 136. for nystatin information.
Tetracycline (Achromycin V, Cefracycline,* Panmycin, Retet-S, Robitet, Sumycin, SK-Tetracycline, Tetracyn) Rx Tetracycline hydrochloride (Achromycin IM and IV, Achromycin Ophthalmic, Achromycin V, Apo-Tetra*, Cyclopar, Cyclopar 500, Medicycline*, Neo-Tetrine*, Nor-Tet, Novo-Tetra*, Panmycin, PMS Tetracycline*, Retet, Retet 500, Robitet '250' and '500', SK-Tetracycline, Sumycin '250' and '500', Tetra-C, Tetra-Cap, Tetracyn, Tetralan-250 and -500, Tetram) Rx	**PO. Adult: Usual,** 250–500 mg q 6 hr. **Children over 8 years:** 25–50 mg/kg daily in 2–4 equal doses. *Brucellosis:* 500 mg q.i.d. for 3 wk with 1 gm streptomycin IM b.i.d. for 1st week and once/day the 2nd wk. *Syphilis:* Total of 30–40 gm over 10–15 days. *Gonorrhea, uncomplicated:* 500 mg q 6 hr for 5 days (total: 10 gm). *Gonorrhea sensitive to penicillin:* **initially,** 1.5 gm; **then,** 500 mg q 6 hr for 4 days (total: 9 gm). *GU or rectal Chlamydia trachomatis infections:* 500 mg q.i.d. for minimum of 7 days. *Severe acne:* **initially,** 1 gm daily; **then,** 125–250 mg daily (long-term). **IM. Adult: Usual,** 250	t½: 7–11 hr; 60% excreted unchanged in urine. Dosage always expressed as the hydrochloride salt. **Administer IV very slowly.** Rapid administration may cause thrombophlebitis. **Do not administer the phosphate complex intravenously.** *Additional Untoward Reactions* Esophagitis, esophageal ulceration.

TABLE 2 (*Continued*)

Drug	Dosage	Remarks
	mg once daily or 300 mg/day in divided doses q 8–12 hr. Up to 800 mg daily may be used. **Children over 8 yr:** 15–25 mg/kg up to maximum of 250 mg in single daily injection. **IV. Adult:** 250–500 mg q 12 hr, not to exceed 500 mg q 6 hr. **Children over 8 yr:** 12 mg/kg/day in 2 divided doses. **Ophthalmic:** 1–2 gtts solution b.i.d.–q.i.d. or small amount ointment in lower conjunctival sac q 3–4 hr.	
Tetracycline hydrochloride and amphotericin B (Mysteclin-F) Rx	**PO.** See Tetracycline.	Used for candidal infections. Also, see p. 127 for amphotericin B information.

The cephalosporins are broad-spectrum antibiotics that have been classified into first, second, and third generation drugs. The difference between generations is based on antibacterial spectrum in that third generation cephalosporins have more activity against gram-negative organisms and resistant organisms and less activity against gram-positive organisms than first generation drugs. Third generation cephalosporins are also stable against beta-lactamases. Cephalosporins can be destroyed by cephalosporinase.

Action/Kinetics The cephalosporins interfere with a final step in the formation of the bacterial cell wall (inhibition of mucopeptide biosynthesis) resulting in unstable cell membranes that undergo lysis (same mechanism of actions of penicillins). The cephalosporins are most effective against young, rapidly dividing organisms. The t½ ranges from 69 to 132 min, and serum protein binding ranges from 5 to 86%. The cephalosporins are rapidly excreted by the kidneys.

Uses Cephalosporins are effective against infections of the biliary tract, gastrointestinal tract, genitourinary system, bones, joints, upper and lower respiratory tract, skin, and skin structures. Also, gynecologic infections, meningitis, osteomyelitis, endocarditis, intra-abdominal infections, peritonitis, otitis media, gonorrhea, peritonitis, septicemia, and prophylaxis prior to surgery. A listing of the organisms against which cephalosporins are effective follow.

First Generation Cephalosporins. Gram-positive cocci including *Staphylococcus aureus, S. epidermis, S. pyogenes, Streptococcus pneumoniae*, Group A and B streptococci, viridans streptococci, and anaerobic streptococci. Also, *Clostridium perfringens, Listeria monocytogenes, Corynebacterium diphtheriae*. Limited activity against gram-negative bacteria.

Second Generation Cephalosporins. Spectrum similar to first generation cephalosporins. Also, active against *Hemophilus influenzae*. Some activity against gram-negative bacteria including *E. coli, Klebsiella pneumoniae, Proteus mirabilis, Shigella*.

Third Generation Cephalosporins. Less active against gram-positive cocci. Effective against *Hemophilus meningitidis* and *H. influenzae*. Also, *Citrobacter, Enterobacter, E. coli, Klebsiella, Neisseria gonorrheae, Proteus, Morganella, Providencia, Serratia.* Some activity against *Bacteroides fragilis* and *Pseudomonas.*

Contraindications Hypersensitivity to cephalosporins. Patients hypersensitive to penicillin may occasionally cross-react to cephalosporins. Safe use in pregnancy and lactation has not been established.

Use with caution in the presence of impaired renal or hepatic function or together with other nephrotoxic drugs. Creatinine clearances should be performed on all patients with impaired renal function who receive cephalosporins. Use with caution in patients over 50 years of age.

Untoward Reactions *GI:* Nausea, vomiting, diarrhea, abdominal cramps or pain, dyspepsia, glossitis, heartburn, sore mouth or tongue. Pseudomembranous colitis. *Allergic:* Urticaria, rashes (maculopapular, morbilliform, or erythematous), pruritus (including anal and genital areas), fever, chills, eosinophilia, erythema, angioedema, serum sickness, joint pain, exfoliative dermatitis, anaphylaxis. *Note:* Cross allergy may be manifested between cephalosporins and penicillins. *Hematologic:* Positive direct and indirect Coomb's test. Rarely, neutropenia, thrombocytopenia, agranulocytosis, leukopenia. *CNS:* Headache, malaise, fatigue, vertigo, dizziness. Intrathecal use may result in hallucinations, nystagmus, or seizures. *Miscellaneous:* Hepatic toxicity (increased SGOT and SGPT values). Superinfection including oral candidiasis and enterococcal infections.

IV use may manifest thrombophlebitis. IM use may cause pain and induration with sterile abscesses at the site of administration. Nephrotoxicity may occur in patients over 50 and in young children.

Drug Interactions

Interactant	Interaction
Aminoglycosides	↑ Risk of renal toxicity
Anticoagulants	Cephalosporins ↑ prothrombin time
Bacteriostatic agents	↓ Effect of cephalosporins
Bumetanide	↑ Risk of renal toxicity
Colistin	↑ Risk of renal toxicity
Ethacrynic acid	↑ Risk of renal toxicity
Furosemide	↑ Risk of renal toxicity
Polymyxin B	↑ Risk of renal toxicity
Probenecid	↑ Effect of cephalosporins by ↓ excretion by kidney
Vancomycin	↑ Risk of renal toxicity

Laboratory Test Interferences False + for urinary glucose with Benedict's solution, Fehling's solution or Clinitest. Enzyme tests (Clinistix, Tes-Tape) are unaffected. False + Coombs' test.

Administration Can be administered without regard to meals.

Nursing Implications
See *Nursing Implications* for *Anti-infectives*, p. 52.
1. Assess patient with a history of hypersensitivity reaction to penicillin for cross-sensitivity to cephalosporins.
2. Assess for impaired renal function characterized by casts, proteinuria, reduced urinary output, increased BUN, and serum creatinine, or reduced creatinine clearance.

3. Anticipate lower doses for patients with renal impairment.
4. Advise patient that medication may cause positive Coombs' test. This would be of concern if patient is being cross-matched for blood transfusions or in newborns whose mothers have had cephalosporins during pregnancy.
5. Pseudomembranous colitis may occur with cephalosporins. If diarrhea develops, report to physician immediately and continue to monitor for signs and symptoms of electrolyte imbalance.

CEFACLOR Ceclor (Rx)

Classification   Antibiotic, cephalosporin (second generation).

Action/Kinetics   Peak serum levels: 5–15 μg/ml after 1 hr. **t½: PO**, 36–54 min. Well absorbed from GI tract. Sixty to 85% excreted in urine within 8 hr.

Uses   Otitis media. Infections of the upper and lower respiratory tract, urinary tract, skin, and skin structures.

Additional Untoward Reactions   Transient lymphocytosis.

Dosage   Adult: 250 mg q 8 hr. Dose may be doubled in more severe infections or those caused by less susceptible organisms. Total daily dose should not exceed 4 gm. **Children**: 20 mg/kg/day in divided doses q 8 hr. Dose may be doubled in more serious infections, otitis media, or for infections caused by less susceptible organisms. Total daily dose should not exceed 1 gm. Safety for use in infants less than 1 month of age not established.

CEFADROXIL MONOHYDRATE Duricef, Ultracef (Rx)

Classification   Antibiotic, cephalosporin (first generation).

Action/Kinetics   Peak serum levels: PO, 15–33 μg/ml after 90 min. **t½: PO**, 70–80 min. Ninety percent of drug excreted unchanged in urine within 24 hr.

Uses   Pharyngitis, tonsillitis. Infections of the urinary tract, skin, and skin structures.

Contraindications   Safe use in children (and during pregnancy) not established. Creatinine clearance determinations must be carried out in patients with renal impairment.

Dosage   PO. Adults: 1–2 gm daily in single or divided doses. **Children:** 30 mg/kg daily in divided doses q 12 hr. **For patients with creatinine clearance rates below 50 ml/min: initial,** 1 gm; **maintenance**, 500 mg at following dosage intervals: q 36 hr for creatinine clerance rates of 0–10 ml/min; q 24 hr for creatinine clearance rates of 10–25 ml/min; q 12 hr for creatinine clearance rates of 25–50 ml/min.

CEFAMANDOLE NAFATE Mandol (Rx)

Classification   Antibiotic, cephalosporin (second generation).

Action/Kinetics   Cefamandole nafate has a particularly broad spectrum of activity.

Peak serum levels: IM, 12–36 μg/ml after 30–120 min. **t½: IM**, 60 min; **IV**, 30 min. Sixty-five to 85% excreted unchanged in urine.

Uses Infections of the urinary tract, lower respiratory tract, bones, joints, skin, and skin structures. Mixed infections of the respiratory tract, skin, and in pelvic inflammatory disease. Peritonitis, septicemia, prophylaxis in surgery. Also, with aminoglycosides in gram-positive or gram-negative sepsis.

Additional Untoward Reactions Hypoprothrombinemia leading to bleeding and/or bruising.

Additional Drug Interaction Concomitant use with ethanol produces a disulfiram-type reaction and hypotension.

Dosage **IV or deep IM injection only** (in gluteus or lateral thigh to minimize pain). **Adult**, usual 0.5–1 gm q 4–8 hr. *Severe infections*: Up to 2 gm q 4 hr. **Infants and children**: 50–100 mg/kg/day in equally divided doses q 4–8 hr. *Severe*: Up to 150 mg/kg/day (not to exceed adult dose) divided as above. *Preoperative:* **Adults, initial,** 1–2 gm 30–60 min prior to surgery; **then,** 1–2 gm q 6 hr for 2–3 days. **Pediatric (3 months and older):** 50–100 mg/kg daily in divided doses using same schedule as adults. *Impaired renal function:* **initial,** 1–2 gm, then a maintenance dosage is given, depending on creatinine clearance according to schedule provided by manufacturer.

Administration/Storage

1. Consult package insert for details on how to reconstitute drug.
2. Reconstituted solutions of cefamandole nafate are stable for 24 hr at room temperature, and 96 hr when stored in the refrigerator. Cefamandole solutions reconstituted with dextrose or sodium chloride are stable for 6 months when frozen immediately after reconstitution.
3. Carbon dioxide gas forms when reconstituted solutions are kept at room temperature. This gas does not affect the activity of the antibiotic and may be dissipated or used to aid in the withdrawal of the contents of the vial.
4. Use separate IV fluid containers and separate injection sites for each drug when cefamandole is administered concomitantly with another antibiotic such as an aminoglycoside.

CEFAZOLIN SODIUM   Ancef, Kefzol (Rx)

Classification Antibiotic, cephalosporin (first generation).

Action/Kinetics **Peak serum concentration: IM** 17–76 μg/ml after 1 hr. **t½: IM, IV:** 69–132 min. Eighty to 100% excreted unchanged in urine.

Uses Infections of the urinary tract, biliary tract, respiratory tract, bones, joints, soft tissue, and skin. Endocarditis, septicemia, prophylaxis in surgery.

Additional Untoward Reactions Nephrotoxicity, pseudomembranous colitis.

Dosage **IM, IV only . Adult**: 250 mg q 8 hr to 1 gm q 6 hr. Rarely, up to 12 gm daily for serious infections as endocarditis or septicemia. **Children over 1 month**: 25–50 mg/kg daily in 3–4 doses. *For severe infections*, up to 100 mg/kg daily may be used. *Preoperative:* 1 gm 30–60 min prior to surgery. *During surgery:* 0.5–1 gm. *Postoperative:* 0.5–1 gm q 6–8 hr for up to 5 days. *Impaired renal function:* **initial,** 0.5 gm; **then,** maintenance doses are given depending on creatinine clearance according to schedule provided by manufacturer. Safety in patients under 1 month of age not determined.

Administration/Storage
1. Dissolve the solute by shaking vial.
2. Discard reconstituted solution after 24 hr at room temperature and after 96 hr when refrigerated.

CEFONICID SODIUM Monocid (Rx)

Classification Antibiotic, cephalosporin (second generation).

Uses Infections of the lower respiratory tract, urinary tract, bones, joints, skin, and skin structures. Septicemia. Prophylaxis in surgery.

Dosage IV, Deep IM. *Infections:* **Adults,** 0.5–2 gm once daily, depending on the seriousness of condition. *Prophylaxis in surgery:* **Adults,** 1 gm 1 hr prior to surgery; dosage may be repeated for 2 more days if required. Dosage should be decreased in renal impairment.

Administration
1. If 2 gm is required IM, one-half the dose should be given in different large muscle masses.
2. For IV bolus, cefonicid should be given slowly over 3–5 min either through IV tubing or directly.
3. For IV infusion, reconstitute in 50–100 ml of appropriate diluent (see package insert). Solutions are stable for 24 hr at room temperature and 72 hr if refrigerated.

CEFOPERAZONE SODIUM Cefobid (Rx)

Classification Antibiotic, cephalosporin (third generation).

Uses Infections of skin, skin structures, respiratory tract. Intra-abdominal infections including peritonitis. Bacterial septicemia, pelvic inflammatory disease, endometritis, other infections of the female genital tract.

Additional Untoward Reactions Hypoprothrombinemia resulting in bleeding and/ or bruising.

Additional Drug Interaction Concomitant use with ethanol may cause an Antabuse-like reaction.

Dosage IM, IV. Adult, usual: 2–4 gm daily in divided doses q 12 hr (up to 12–16 gm daily has been used in severe infections or for less sensitive organisms).
Note: This drug is significantly excreted in the bile; thus, the daily dose should not exceed 4 gm in hepatic disease or biliary obstruction.

Administration
1. Following reconstitution, the solution should be allowed to stand for dissipation of any foaming and to determine if complete solubilization has occurred. Vigorous shaking may be necessary for solubilization of higher concentrations.
2. Reconstituted drug may be frozen; however, after thawing, the unused portion should be discarded.
3. The unreconstituted powder should be protected from light and stored in the refrigerator.

4. If used for neonates, cefoperazone should not be reconstituted with diluents containing benzyl alcohol.

Additional Nursing Implications
1. Patient should avoid alcohol for 72 hours after the last dose. An Antabuse-like reaction may occur with the ingestion of alcohol.
2. Assess for bruising, hematuria, black stools, or other signs of bleeding.

CEFORANIDE   Precef (Rx)

Classification   Antibiotic, cephalosporin (second generation).

Uses   Infections of the lower respiratory tract, urinary tract, bones, joints, skin, and skin structures. Endocarditis, prophylaxis in surgery.

Dosage   IM, IV. Adults: 0.5–1 gm q 12 hr; **pediatric:** 20–40 mg/kg daily in equally divided doses q 12 hr. *Prophylaxis in surgery:* 0.5–1 gm 60 min before surgery; may be repeated for 2 days after surgery. For all uses, dosage should be reduced in renal impairment.

Administration
1. IM injections should be made into a deep muscle mass.
2. Ceforanide should be used IV in serious or life-threatening infections such as septicemia.
3. Should be administered over 3–5 minutes if given by direct IV injection or over 30 minutes if IV infusion used.

CEFOTAXIME SODIUM   Claforan (Rx)

Classification   Antibiotic, cephalosporin (third generation).

General Statement   Cefotaxime sodium is a cephalosporin for parenteral use. Treatment should be continued for a minimum of 10 days for Group A beta-hemolytic streptococcal infections to minimize the risk of glomerulonephritis or rheumatic fever. The IV route is preferable for patients with severe or life-threatening infections or for patients manifesting malnutrition, trauma, surgery, malignancy, heart failure, or diabetes, especially if shock is present or possible.

Uses   Infections of the genitourinary tract, lower respiratory tract (including pneumonia), skin, skin structures, bones, joints, and central nervous system (including ventriculitis and meningitis). Intra-abdominal infections (including peritonitis), gynecologic infections (including endometritis and pelvic inflammatory disease), septicemia, bacteremia, and prophylaxis in surgery. Used with aminoglycosides for gram-positive or gram-negative sepsis where the causative agent has not been identified.

Dosage   IV, IM. Adults. *Uncomplicated infections:* 1 gm q 12 hr. *Moderate to severe infections:* 1–2 gm q 6–8 hr. *Septicemia:* **IV**, 2 gm q 6–8 hr. *Life-threatening infections:* **IV**, 2 gm q 4 hr up to 12 gm daily. *Preoperative prophylaxis:* 1 gm 30–

90 min prior to surgery; **then,** after 30–120 min, 1 gm, and 1 gm within 2 hr following surgery. **Pediatric, 1 month to 12 years:** 50–180 mg/kg daily in 4–6 divided doses; **1–4 weeks:** 50 mg/kg q 8 hr; **0–1 week:** 50 mg/kg q 12 hr.

Note: Use adult dose in children 50 kg or over.

Dosage should be reduced in patients with impaired renal function.

Administration/Storage

1. Cefotaxime should not be mixed with aminoglycosides for continuous IV infusion. If they are to be given to the same patient, each should be given separately.
2. Cefotaxime is maximally stable at a pH value of 5–7; solutions should not be prepared with diluents having a pH value greater than 7.5 (e.g., sodium bicarbonate injection).
3. Dry cefotaxime should be stored below 30°C and should be protected from excess heat and light to prevent darkening.
4. Add recommended amount of diluent, shake to dissolve, and observe for particles or discoloration of solution. Do not administer if particles are present or if solution is discolored. The normal color of solution ranges from light yellow to amber.
5. For IM use, reconstitute with Sterile Water for Injection or Bacteriostatic Water for Injection. Inject deeply into large muscle. Divide doses of 2 gm and administer into different sites.
6. For intermittent IV administration, 1 or 2 gm cefotaxime should be mixed with 10 ml Sterile Water for Injection and administered over 3–5 min.
7. Discontinue IV administration of other solutions during administration of cefotaxime.
8. After reconstitution, the drug remains stable for 24 hr at room temperature, 5 days refrigerated, and 13 weeks frozen. Thaw frozen samples at room temperature before use. Do not refreeze unused portions.

CEFOXITIN SODIUM   Mefoxin (Rx)

Classification   Antibiotic, cephalosporin (second generation).

Action/Kinetics   Broad-spectrum cephalosporin that is penicillinase- and cephalosporinase-resistant and is stable in the presence of beta-lactamases. **Peak serum concentration: IM**, 20–30 min. t½: **IM, IV**, 41–65 min. Eighty-five percent of drug excreted unchanged in urine after 6 hr.

Uses   Infections of the urinary tract (including gonorrhea), bones, joints, lower respiratory tract (including lung abscesses and pneumonia), skin, and skin structures. Intra-abdominal infections (including intra-abdominal abscesses and peritonitis), gynecologic infections (including pelvic inflammatory disease, pelvic cellulitis, and endometritis), septicemia, and prophylaxis in surgery.

Dosage   **IM, IV. Adult**: 1–2 gm q 6–8 hr up to 12 gm daily in serious infections. *Gonorrhea*: 2 gm IM with 1 gm probenecid PO. *Prophylaxis in surgery*: 2 gm 30–60 min before surgery followed by 2 gm q 6 hr after first dose for 24 hr only.*Impaired renal function:* **initial,** 1–2 gm; **then,** follow maintenance schedule provided by manufacturer. **Children over 3 mo**: 80–160 mg/kg daily in 4–6 divided doses. Total daily dosage should not exceed 12 gm. *Prophylaxis*: 30–40 mg/kg q 6 hr.

Administration/Storage

1. Do not mix with other antibiotics during administration.
2. Reconstituted solutions are stable for 24 hr at room temperature, 1 week in refrigerator, and 26 weeks when frozen.
3. Store drug vials below 30°C.
4. Reconstituted solutions are white to light amber. Color does not affect potency.
5. For IM injections lidocaine hydrochloride 0.05% (without epinephrine) may be used as diluent, by doctor's order, to reduce pain at injection site.
6. Do not administer cefoxitin rapidly because it is irritating to veins.

Additional Nursing Implications

See also *Nursing Implications* for *Anti-infectives*, p. 52.

1. Monitor intake and output and withhold medication and report to doctor if there is transient or persistent reduction of urinary output.
2. Assess site of infusion for pain and redness because medication can cause thrombophlebitis.

CEFTIZOXIME SODIUM Cefizox (Rx)

Classification   Antibiotic, cephalosporin (third generation).

Uses   Infections of the urinary tract, lower respiratory tract, skin, skin structures, bones, and joints. Intra-abdominal infections, septicemia, meningitis (caused by *Hemophilus influenzae* or *S. pneumoniae*), gonorrhea (including uncomplicated cervical and urethral gonorrhea caused by *Neisseria*).

Dosage   **IM, IV. Adults.** *Uncomplicated urinary tract and other infections:* 0.5 gm q 12 hr. *Severe or resistant infections:* 1 gm q 8 hr or 2 gm q 8–12 hr. *Life-threatening infections:* up to 3–4 gm q 8 hr **IV.** *Gonorrhea, uncomplicated:* 1 gm as single dose **IM. Pediatric, over 6 months:** 50 mg/kg q 5–8 hr up to 200 mg/kg daily (not to exceed the maximum adult dose).
   Dosage should be reduced in impaired renal function.

Administration

1. For IM doses of 2 gm, divide the dose equally and give in different large muscle masses.
2. For direct IV administration, give slowly over 3–5 minutes.
3. Reconstituted solutions are stable at room temperature for 8 hr and, if refrigerated, for 48 hr.

CEFTRIAXONE SODIUM Rocephin (Rx)

Classification   Antibiotic, cephalosporin (third generation).

Action/Kinetics   t½: Approximately 6–8 hr. Significantly protein bound.

Uses   Infections of the lower respiratory tract, urinary tract, skin, skin structures, bone, joints, abdomen. Also, uncomplicated gonorrhea, pelvic inflammatory disease, meningitis, prophylaxis of infections in surgery.

Additional Untoward Reactions   Increase in serum creatinine, presence of casts in the urine.

Dosage   **IV, IM. Adults: usual,** 1–2 gm daily in single or divided doses q 12 hr, not to exceed 4 gm/day. Therapy is maintained for 4–14 days, depending on the infection. **Pediatric:** *other than meningitis,* 50–75 mg/kg/day not to exceed total daily dose of 2 gm given in divided doses q 12 hr. *Meningitis:* 100 mg/kg/day not to exceed total daily dose of 4 gm given in divided doses q 12 hr. A loading dose of 75 mg/kg may be used. *Prophylaxis of infection in surgery:* 1 gm 30–120 min prior to surgery. *Uncomplicated gonorrhea:* **IM,** 250 mg as a single dose.

Administration

1. IM injections should be deep into the body of a large muscle.
2. IV injections should be by infusion of concentrations ranging from 10–40 mg/ml.
3. The drug should not be mixed with other antibiotics.
4. Stability of solutions for IM or IV use varies depending on the diluent used; the package insert should be carefully checked.

CEFUROXIME SODIUM   Zinacef (Rx)

Classification   Antibiotic, cephalosporin (second generation).

Uses   Infections of the urinary tract, lower respiratory tract (including pneumonia), skin, and skin structures. Septicemia, meningitis, gonorrhea, prophylaxis in surgery.

Additional Untoward Reactions   Decrease in hemoglobin and hematocrit.

Dosage   **IM, IV. Adults.** *Uncomplicated infections:* 0.75 gm q 8 hr. *Severe, complicated, or life-threatening infections:* 1.5 gm q 6–8 hr. *Bacterial meningitis:* 3 gm q 8 hr. *Gonorrhea (uncomplicated):* 1.5 gm as single IM dose. *Prophylaxis in surgery:* **IV,** 1.5 gm 30–60 min before surgery; if procedure is of long duration, **IV, IM,** 0.75 gm q 8 hr. **Pediatric, over 3 months.** *Uncomplicated infections:* 50–100 mg/kg daily in divided doses q 6–8 hr (not to exceed adult dose). *Bacterial meningitis:* **initial IV,** 200–240 mg/kg daily in divided doses q 6–8 hr; **then,** after clinical improvement, 100 mg/kg daily **IV.**
Dosage should be reduced in impaired renal function.

Administration

1. Use IV route for severe or life-threatening infections such as septicemia.
2. For direct IV injection, give over 3–5 minutes.
3. For IM use, inject deep into a large muscle mass.
4. Prior to reconstitution, protect the drug from light. The powder and reconstituted drug may darken without affecting potency.
5. Cefuroxime should not be added to solutions of aminoglycosides; if both drugs are required, each should be given separately to the patient.

Additional Nursing Implication
Monitor hemoglobin and hematocrit if signs of anemia develop.

CEPHALEXIN Ceporex,* Keflex, Novolexin* (Rx)

Classification Antibiotic, cephalosporin (first generation).

Action/Kinetics **Peak serum levels: PO**, 9–39 μg/ml after 1 hr. Absorption delayed in children. **t½ (PO):** 30–72 min. Ninety percent of drug excreted unchanged in urine within 8 hr.

Uses Infections of the respiratory tract, skin, soft tissues, bones, and genitourinary tract (including acute prostatitis). Otitis media.

Additional Untoward Reactions Nephrotoxicity, pseudomembranous colitis.

Dosage **PO. Adult** : 250 mg q 6 hr up to 4 gm daily. **Pediatric:** 25–50 mg/kg daily in 4 equally divided doses (up to 100 mg/kg for otitis media). Dosage may have to be reduced in patients with impaired renal function or increased for very severe infections. Action of drug can be prolonged by the concurrent administration of oral probenecid (Benemid).

Administration/Storage After reconstitution the drug should be refrigerated and the unused portion discarded after 14 days.

CEPHALOTHIN SODIUM Ceporacin,* Keflin Neutral (Rx)

Classification Antibiotic, cephalosporin (first generation).

Action/Kinetics Poorly absorbed from GI tract; must be given parenterally. **Peak serum levels: IM**, 6–21 μg/ml after 30 min. **t½ (IM, IV):** 30–60 min; 55–90% excreted unchanged in urine.

Its low nephrotoxicity, ototoxicity, and neurotoxicity make the drug suitable for patients with impaired renal function.

Uses Infections of the genitourinary tract, gastrointestinal tract, respiratory tract, abdomen (including peritonitis), skin, soft tissues, bones, and joints. Meningitis, septicemia (including endocarditis), and prophylaxis in surgery.

Additional Untoward Reactions Nephrotoxicity, severe phlebitis, hemolytic anemia, increased prothrombin time.

Laboratory Test Interferences Large doses may produce false + results in urinary protein tests that use sulfosalicylic acid. Cephalothin may also falsely elevate urinary 17-ketosteroid values.

Dosage **IM, IV. Adults: usual,** 0.5–1 gm q 4–6 hr. *Severe infections:* 2 gm q 4 hr (up to 12 gm daily). *Preoperative and during surgery:* 1–2 gm 30–60 min prior to surgery and during surgery. *Postoperative:* 1–2 gm q 6 hr for 24 hr. *Impaired renal function:* **initial,** 1–2 gm; **then,** use manufacturer's guidelines for maintenance doses. **Pediatric:** 80–160 mg/kg daily in divided doses. *Prophylaxis in surgery:* 20–30 mg/kg using adult schedule.

Administration/Storage

1. Dilute according to directions on package insert.
2. Discard reconstituted solution after 12 hr at room temperature and after 96 hr when refrigerated.
3. Dissolve precipitate by warming in hand and shaking. Do not overheat.

4. Replace medication and IV solution after 24 hr.

5. For direct IV administration, use a small needle into larger veins.

CEPHAPIRIN SODIUM   Cefadyl (Rx)

Classification Antibiotic, cephalosporin (first generation).

Action/Kinetics **Peak serum levels: IM**, 9.4 μg/ml after 30 min. t½ **(IM, IV)** : 21–47 min. Virtually entirely excreted in the urine within 6 hr with 41–60% excreted unchanged.

Uses Infections of the respiratory tract, urinary tract, skin, and skin structures. Septicemia, endocarditis, osteomyelitis, prophylaxis in surgery.

Additional Untoward Reactions   Increase in serum bilirubin.

Dosage   **IM, IV only. Adults:** 0.5–1 gm q 4–6 hr up to 12 gm daily for serious or life-threatening infections. *Preoperatively:* 1–2 gm 30–60 min before surgery. *During surgery:* 1–2 gm. *Postoperatively:* 1–2 gm q 6 hr for 24 hr. **Pediatric, over 3 months:** 40–80 mg/kg daily in 4 equally divided doses.

Administration   Discard after 12 hr when kept at room temperature and after 10 days, when refrigerated at 4°C.

CEPHRADINE   Anspor, Velosef (Rx)

Classification Antibiotic, cephalosporin (first generation).

Action/Kinetics Similar to cephalexin. Rapidly absorbed from GI tract or IM injection site (30 min to 2 hr); 60–90% excreted after 6 hr. **Peak Serum Levels: PO**, 8–24 μg/ml after 30–60 min; **IM**, 5.6–13.6 μg/ml after 1–2 hr. t½ : 42–120 min; 80–95% excreted in urine unchanged.

Uses Infections of the respiratory tract (including lobar pneumonia, tonsillitis, pharyngitis), urinary tract (including prostatitis and enterococcical infections), skin, skin structures, and bone. Otitis media, septicemia, prophylaxis in surgery, following cesarean section to prevent infection.
  In severe infections, therapy is usually initiated parenterally.

Contraindications Safe use in children under 1 year of age and in pregnancy has not been established.

Additional Untoward Reactions   Increase in serum bilirubin, hepatomegaly, pseudomembranous colitis, tightness in chest.

Dosage   **PO. Adults: usual,** 250 mg q 6 hr or 500 mg q 12 hr. Double the dose in lobar pneumonia, prostatitis, or severe urinary tract infections (up to 1 gm q 6 hr may be required for certain infections). **Pediatric, over 9 months:** 25–50 mg/kg daily in equally divided doses q 6–12 hr (75–100 mg/kg/day for otitis media).
  Deep IM, IV. Adults: 2–4 gm daily in equally divided doses q.i.d. *Surgical prophylaxis:* 1 gm 30–90 min before surgery; **then,** 1 gm q 4–6 hr for 1–2 doses (or up to 24 hr postoperatively). **Pediatric, over 1 year:** 50–100 mg/kg/day in equally divided doses q.i.d.
  Dosage should be reduced in impaired renal function.

Administration/Storage

1. Dilute according to directions on package insert.
2. Do not mix with Lactated Ringer's injection.
3. Discard reconstituted solution after 10 hr at room temperature and after 48 hr when refrigerated at 5°C.
4. Retain for use slightly yellow solution.
5. Be especially careful to inject IM into muscle, since sterile abscesses from accidental subcutaneous injection have occurred.
6. Protect before and after reconstitution from excessive heat and light.
7. Replace medication in prolonged IV administration after 10 hr.
8. Administer PO medication without regard to meals.

MOXALACTAM DISODIUM   Moxam (Rx)

Classification   Antibiotic, cephalosporin (third generation).

Action/Kinetics   Broad-spectrum semisynthetic cephalosporin stable in the presence of beta lactamase, penicillinase, and cephalosporinase. Cross-sensitivity with penicillin has not been observed; in selected cases, it can be used instead of chloramphenicol or aminoglycosides.

Well absorbed into pleural, interstitial, and cerebrospinal (both normal and inflamed meninges) fluids, aqueous humor. **Peak serum concentrations (dose-dependent): IM**, 15 μg/ml 1–2 hr after 500 mg; **IV infusion**, 57 μg/ml after 500 mg. **t½ (IM)**: 2.1 hr (longer in patients with impaired renal function). Sixty to 90% of drug is excreted by the kidneys within 24 hr.

Uses   Infections of the urinary tract, central nervous system (including ventriculitis and meningitis), bones, joints, and lower respiratory tract (including pneumonia). Intra-abdominal infections (including endometritis, pelvic cellulitis, peritonitis), bacterial septicemia, *Pseudomonas* infections. Used concomitantly with aminoglycosides in gram-positive or gram-negative sepsis or other serious infections in which the causative organism is not known.

Contraindications   Hypersensitivity to drug. Safe use in pregnancy not established. Use with caution in individuals with history of sensitivity to penicillins or other cephalosporins.

Additional Untoward Reactions   Hypoprothrombinemia resulting in bleeding and/or bruising.

Laboratory Test Interferences   ↑ SGOT, SGPT, BUN, alkaline phosphatase, serum creatinine.

Drug Interactions   Moxalactam may induce an Antabuse-like reaction if used with alcohol.

Dosage   **Deep IM, IV. Adults**: *Mild to moderate infections*, 0.5–2 gm q 12 hr. *Mild skin and skin-structure infections, uncomplicated pneumonia*: 0.5 gm q 8 hr. *Mild, uncomplicated urinary tract infections*: 0.25 gm q 12 hr. *Persistent or serious urinary tract infections:* 0.5 gm q 8–12 hr. *Life-threatening infections or infections due to less susceptible organisms*: up to 4 gm q 8 hr may be required. **Neonates, up to 1 week of age**: 50 mg/kg q 12 hr; **1–4 weeks of age**: 50 mg/kg q 8 hr. **Infants**: 50 mg/kg q 6 hr. **Children**: 50 mg/kg q 6–8 hr. Pediatric dosage may be increased up to 200 mg/kg, but should not exceed the maximum adult dosage. *For pediatric gram-negative meningitis*: initial loading dose, 100 mg/kg; **then,**

follow above dosage regimen. *For patients with impaired renal function*: Initially, 1–2 gm; **maintenance:** see recommendations of manufacturer.

Administration/Storage

1. **IM:** 1 gm moxalactam should be diluted with 3 ml of either Sterile Water for Injection, Bacteriostatic Water for Injection, 0.9% Sodium Chloride Injection, Bacteriostatic Sodium Chloride Injection, or 0.5% Lidocaine Injection.
2. **Intermittent IV:** 1 gm moxalactam should be diluted with 10 ml Sterile Water for Injection, 5% Dextrose Injection, or 0.9% Sodium Chloride Injection. Inject slowly over 3–5 min, or give in tubing of other IV. (*Note:* IV solutions containing alcohol should be avoided.) If a Y-tube administration set is used, the other solution should be discontinued while moxalactam is being given.
3. **Continuous IV Infusion:** 1 gm moxalactam should be diluted with 10 ml Sterile Water for Injection and added to appropriate IV solution.
4. Reconstituted moxalactam is stable for 96 hr when refrigerated (5°C) and 24 hr at room temperature.

Additional Nursing Implications

See also *Nursing Implications* for *Anti-infectives*, p. 52.

1. *Assess*
   a. for bleeding caused by eradication of intestinal bacteria that produce vitamin K.
   b. for phlebitis at site of IV administration.
2. Question concomitant use of aminoglycosides. If administered with aminoglycosides, assess renal function carefully for potentiation of nephrotoxic effect.
3. *Teach patient and/or family* that alcohol should not be ingested while on therapy with moxalactam, because an Antabuse-like reaction may occur.

CHLORAMPHENICOL

CHLORAMPHENICOL Chloromycetin (Cream, Kapseals, and Otic), Chloroptic,* Fenicol,* Mychel, Novochlorocap,* Pentamycetin* (Rx)

CHLORAMPHENICOL OPHTHALMIC Antibiopto, Chloromycetin, Chloroptic S.O.P., Econochlor, Ophthochlor, Sopamycetin* (Rx)

CHLORAMPHENICOL PALMITATE Chloromycetin Palmitate (Rx)

CHLORAMPHENICOL SODIUM SUCCINATE Chloromycetin Sodium Succinate, Mychel-S (Rx)

General Statement This antibiotic was originally isolated from *Streptomyces venezuellae* and is now produced synthetically. The antibiotic can be extremely toxic (due to protein synthesis inhibition in rapidly proliferating cells, as in bone marrow) and should not be used for trivial infections.

Action/Kinetics Chloramphenicol inhibits protein synthesis in bacteria by binding to ribosomes (50S subunit, an essential link in the protein synthesis machinery of the cell), thus interfering with peptide bond synthesis. Therapeutic concentration 5–20 μg/ml serum (less for neonates). **Peak serum concentration: IM**, 2 hr. t½: 2.7 hr. Drug is metabolized in liver; 75–90% of drug excreted in urine within 24 hr, as parent drug (8–12%) and inactive metabolites. The drug is mostly bacteriostatic. Chloramphenicol is well absorbed from the GI tract and is distributed to all parts of the body, including CSF, pleural and ascitic fluids, saliva, milk, and aqueous and vitreous humor.

Uses *Not to be used for trivial infections, prophylaxis of bacterial infections, or to treat colds, flu, or throat infections.* Treatment of choice for typhoid fever but not for typhoid carrier state. Serious infections caused by *Salmonella, Rickettsia, Chlamydia,* and lymphogranuloma-psittacosis group. Meningitis due to *H. influenzae.* Brain abscesses due to *Bacteroides fragilis.* Cystic fibrosis anti-infective. Meningococcal or pneumococcal meningitis. Used topically for bacterial ocular infections, otitis externa, and skin infections.

Contraindications Hypersensitivity to chloramphenicol; pregnancy, especially near term and during labor; nursing mother. Avoid simultaneous administration of other drugs that may depress bone marrow.

Untoward Reactions *Hematologic* (most serious): Aplastic anemia, thrombocytopenia, granulocytopenia, hemolytic anemia, pancytopenia. *Hematologic studies should be undertaken before and every 2 days during therapy. GI:* Nausea, vomiting, diarrhea, glossitis, stomatitis, unpleasant taste, enterocolitis, pruritus ani. *Allergic:* Fever, skin rashes, angioedema, macular and vesicular rashes, hemorrhages of the skin, intestine, bladder, mouth. Anaphylaxis. *CNS:* Headache, delirium, confusion, mental depression. *Neurologic:* Optic neuritis, peripheral neuritis. *Following topical use:* Burning, itching, irritation, redness of skin. *Miscellaneous:* Superinfection. Jaundice (rare). Herxheimer-like reactions when used for thyphoid fever (may be due to release of bacterial endotoxins).

Gray syndrome in infants: Rapid respiration, ashen gray color, failure to feed, abdominal distention with or without vomiting, progressive pallid cyanosis, vasomotor collapse, death. Can be reversed when drug is discontinued.

Note: Neonates should be observed closely since the drug accumulates in the bloodstream and the infant is thus subject to greater hazards of toxicity.

Drug Interactions

Interactant	Interaction
Acetaminophen	↑ Effect of chloramphenicol
Anticoagulants, oral	↑ Effect of anticoagulants due to ↓ breakdown by liver
Antidiabetics, oral	↑ Effect of antidiabetics due to ↓ breakdown by liver
Barbiturates	↑ Effect of barbiturates due to ↓ breakdown by liver
Cyclophosphamide	↑ Effect of cyclophosphamide due to ↓ breakdown by liver
Iron preparations	Chloramphenicol ↓ response to iron therapy
Penicillins	Possible ↓ effect of penicillins
Phenytoin	↑ Effect of phenytoin due to ↓ breakdown by liver
Vitamin B$_{12}$	Chloramphenicol ↓ response to vitamin B$_{12}$ therapy

Dosage **PO, IV.** Chloramphenicol, chloramphenicol palmitate, **Adults and chil-**

dren, 50 mg/kg daily in 4 equally divided doses q 6 hr. Can be increased to 100 mg/kg daily in very severe infections, but dosage should be reduced as soon as possible. **Neonates and children with immature metabolic function**: 25 mg/kg daily in divided doses q 12 hr.

Chloramphenicol sodium succinate—**IV only**, same dosage as above; switch to **PO** as soon as possible.

Chloramphenicol Ophthalmic Ointment 1%: ½ inch ribbon placed in lower conjunctival sac 2–6 times daily depending on severity of infection.

Chloramphenicol Ophthalmic Solution 0.5%: 1–2 drops in lower conjunctival sac 2–6 times daily (or more for acute infections).

Chloramphenicol Otic Solution 0.5%: 2–3 drops in ear t.i.d.

Chloramphenicol Topical Cream 1%: Apply 1–5 times daily.

Administration/Storage   Administer IV as a 10% solution over at least a 60-sec interval.

Nursing Implications

See also *Nursing Implications* for *Anti-infectives*, p. 52.

1. Arrange for patient to be closely assessed for untoward reactions. After baseline hematologic studies are completed, further hematologic studies should be done every 2 days to detect early signs of bone marrow depression.

2. Administer only as long as necessary, and avoid repeated courses of therapy with chloramphenicol, as the drug is highly toxic.

3. Anticipate reduced dosage in patients with impaired renal function and in newborn infants.

4. Avoid concomitant administration of drugs that also cause bone marrow depression.

5. *Assess*

   a. for bone marrow depression characterized by weakness, fatigue, sore throat, and bleeding. Discontinuation of drug may be indicated.

   b. for optic neuritis, characterized by bilaterally reduced visual acuity, an indication for immediate discontinuation of drug.

   c. for peripheral neuritis, characterized by pain and disturbance of sensation, indications for immediate discontinuation of drug.

   d. premature and newborn infants for development of gray syndrome, characterized by rapid respiration, failure to feed, abdominal distention with or without vomiting, loose green stools, progressive cyanosis, and vasomotor collapse. Withhold drug, if any such symptoms are noted.

   e. for toxic and irritative effects, such as nausea, vomiting, unpleasant taste, diarrhea, and perineal irritation following PO administration. Differentiation of drug-induced diarrhea and that caused by a superinfection is critical and may be accomplished by assessment and analysis of all symptoms presented.

6. Use Lab-Stix to test the urine of diabetic patients, because chloramphenicol may produce a false + reaction with Fehling's or Benedict's solutions, both of which contain copper sulfate.

7. Be alert to drug interactions of chloramphenicol with dicumarol, phenytoin, chlorpropamide, and tolbutamide. Such interactions may result in severe toxicity, because concurrent administration with chloramphenicol can increase their half-life (t½), leading to an increased pharmacologic effect.

CLINDAMYCIN AND LINCOMYCIN

General Statement   Clindamycin is a semisynthetic antibiotic. Lincomycin is isolated from *Streptomyces lincolnensis*. The spectrum of these antibiotics resembles that of the erythromycins and includes a variety of gram-positive, particularly staphylococci, streptococci, and pneumococci, and some gram-negative organisms. Both drugs are rapidly absorbed from the GI tract and widely distributed. They should not be used for trivial infections.

Action/Kinetics   Suppresses protein synthesis by microorganism by binding to ribosomes (50S subunit), which is essential for transmittal of genetic information. Drugs are both bacteriostatic and bactericidal.

Uses

CLINDMYCIN   Serious respiratory tract infections (e.g., empyema, lung abscess, pneumonia) caused by staphylococci, streptococci, and pneumococci. Serious skin and soft-tissue infections, septicemia, intra-abdominal infections, pelvic inflammatory disease, female genital tract infections. May be the drug of choice for *Bacteroides fragilis*. In combination with aminoglycosides for mixed aerobic and anaerobic bacterial infections. Staphylococci-induced acute hematogenous osteomyelitis. Adjunct to surgery for chronic bone/joint infections. Used topically for inflammatory acne vulgaris.

Investigational: Endocarditis caused by gram-positive cocci or anaerobic organisms; acne vulgaris in patients resistant to tetracyclines or erythromycins.

LINCOMYCIN   Not a first-choice drug for any of the above infections but useful for patients allergic to penicillin. Used for serious respiratory tract, skin, and soft tissue infections due to staphylococci, streptococci, or pneumococci. Septicemia. In conjunction with diphtheria antitoxin, in the treatment of diphtheria.

Contraindications   Hypersensitivity to drugs. Use with caution in patients with GI disease, liver or renal disease, history of allergy or asthma. Not for use in treating viral and minor bacteria infections.

Untoward Reactions   *GI:* Nausea, vomiting, diarrhea, abdominal pain, tenesmus, flatulence, bloating, anorexia, weight loss, esophagitis. Nonspecific colitis, pseudomembranous colitis (may be severe). *Allergic:* Morbilliform rash (most common). Also, maculopapular rash, urticaria, pruritus, fever, hypotension. Rarely, polyarteritis, anaphylaxis, erythema multiforme. *Hematologic:* Leukopenia, neutropenia, eosinophilia, thrombocytopenia, agranulocytosis. *Miscellaneous:* Superinfection. *Following IV use:* Thrombophlebitis, erythema, pain, swelling. IV lincomycin may cause hypotension, syncope, and cardiac arrest (rare). *Following IM use:* Pain, induration, sterile abscesses. *Following topical use:* Erythema, irritation, dryness, peeling, itching, burning, oiliness. Also, sore throat, fatigue, urinary frequency, headache.

Drug Interactions

Interactant	Interaction
Antiperistaltic antidiarrheals (opiates, Lomotil)	↑ Diarrhea due to ↓ removal of toxins from colon
Erythromycin	Cross interference → ↓ effect of both drugs
Kaolin (e.g., Kaopectate)	↓ Effect due to ↓ absorption from GI tract
Neuromuscular blocking agents	↑ Effect of blocking agents

Laboratory Test Interferences   ↓ Levels of SGOT, SGPT, NPN, alkaline phosphatase, bilirubin, BSP retention, and ↓ platelet count.

Nursing Implications

See *Nursing Implications* for *Anti-infectives*, p. 52.

1. *Assess*
   a. for GI disturbances, such as abdominal pain, diarrhea, anorexia, nausea, vomiting, bloody or tarry stools, and excessive flatulence. Discontinuation of drug may be indicated.
   b. for drug interactions caused by concurrent administration of neuromuscular blocking agents. Be alert to hypotension, bronchospasms, cardiac disturbances, hyperthermia, and respiratory depression.
2. Be prepared to manage colitis, which can occur 2–9 days or several weeks after initiation of therapy, by providing fluids, electrolytes, protein supplements, systemic corticosteroids, and vancomycin.
3. Do not administer, and caution patient against using, antiperistaltic agents, if diarrhea occurs, because these can prolong or aggravate condition.
4. Do not use any acne or topical mercury preparations containing a peeling agent in an area affected by medication, as severe irritation can occur.
5. Do not administer kaolin concomitantly, because this will reduce absorption of antibiotic. If kaolin is required, administer 3 hr before antibiotic.
6. Administer on an empty stomach to assure optimum absorption. Drug should be administered only as long as necessary.

CLINDAMYCIN HYDROCHLORIDE HYDRATE   Cleocin Hydrochloride (Rx)

CLINDAMYCIN PALMITATE HYDROCHLORIDE   Cleocin Pediatric (Rx)

CLINDAMYCIN PHOSPHATE   Cleocin Phosphate, Cleocin T, Dalacin* (Rx)

Classification   Antibiotic, clindamycin and lincomycin.

Action/Kinetics   **Peak serum concentration: PO,** 2.5 μg/ml after 45 min. **t½:** 2.4 hr. In serious infections the rate of IV administration is adjusted so as to maintain appropriate serum drug concentrations: 4–6 μg/ml.

Dosage   **PO Only. Adults,** Clindamycin HCl hydrate, Clindamycin palmitate HCl: 150–450 mg q 6 hr depending on severity of infection. **Pediatric,** Clindamycin HCl hydrate: 8–20 mg/kg daily divided into 3–4 equal doses; clindamycin palmitate HCl: 8–25 mg/kg daily divided into 3–4 equal doses. **Children less than 10 kg:** Minimum recommended dose is 37.5 mg t.i.d.
   IV. Clindamycin Phosphate. **Adults:** 0.6–2.7 gm daily in 2–4 equal doses depending on severity of infection. *Life-threatening infections:* 4.8 gm. **Pediatric over**

1 month: 15–40 mg/kg daily in 3–4 equal doses depending on severity of infections. *Severe infections:* No less than 300 mg daily, regardless of body weight. Dosage should be reduced in severe renal impairment.

Administration/Storage

1. Give parenteral clindamycin only to hospitalized patients.
2. Dilute IV injections to maximum concentration of 6 mg/ml with no more than 1,200 mg administered in 1 hr.
3. Single IM injections greater than 600 mg are not advisable.
4. Do not refrigerate; otherwise, solution will become thickened.
5. Administer IV over a period of 20–60 min, depending on dose and therapeutic serum concentration to be attained.
6. Administer oral form with a full glass of water so as to prevent esophageal ulceration.
7. Inject deeply into muscle to prevent induration, pain, and sterile abscesses.
8. Food does not affect absorption to any significant extent.

Additional Nursing Implications

See also *Nursing Implications* for *Clindamycin* and *Lincomycin*, p. 103.

1. *Assess*
   a. for rash as this is the most frequently reported adverse reaction.
   b. patient with renal and/or hepatic impairment and newborns for organ function.
2. Withhold drug and report toxic blood levels when drug is administered at high dosage levels.

LINCOMYCIN HYDROCHLORIDE   Lincocin (Rx)

Classification   Antibiotic, clindamycin and lincomycin.

Action/Kinetics   **Peak plasma levels: PO**, 2–4 hr. **IM**, 30 min. t½: 5.4 hr.

Dosage   PO, adults: 500 mg t.i.d.–q.i.d.; **children over 1 mo of age:** 30–60 mg/kg/day in 3–4 divided doses depending on severity of infection. **IM, adults:** 600 mg q 12–24 hr; **children over 1 mo of age:** 10 mg/kg/day q 12–24 hr depending on severity of infection. **IV, adults;** 0.6–1.0 gm q 8–12 hr up to 8 gm daily, depending on severity of infection; **children over 1 mo of age:** 10–20 mg/kg/day depending on severity of infection. **Subconjunctival injection:** 0.75 mg/0.25 ml.

In impaired renal function, reduce dosage by 70–75%. Total blood counts and liver function tests should be done periodically during long-term therapy.

Administration/Storage

1. Prepare drug for administration as directed on package insert.
2. Administer on an empty stomach between meals, and not with a sugar substitute.
3. Administer slowly IM to minimize pain.
4. For IV use, carefully follow recommended concentration and rate of administration to prevent severe cardiopulmonary reactions.

Additional Nursing Implications

See also *Nursing Implications* for *Clindamycin* and *Lincomycin*, p. 103.

1. *Assess and report*
   a. for generalized aches and pains.
   b. for transient flushing and sensations of warmth and cardiac disturbances, which may accompany IV infusions. Monitor pulse before, during, and after infusion until stable at levels normal for patient.
2. Do not administer kaolin concomitantly with lincomycin, because this will reduce absorption of antibiotic. If kaolin is needed, administer 3 hr before antibiotics.

POLYMYXINS

Action/Kinetics Polymyxins act like detergents in that they increase the permeability of the plasma cell membrane of the bacterium, causing leakage of essential metabolites and ultimately inactivation.

Untoward Reactions *Nephrotoxicity:* Albuminuria, cylinduria, azotemia, hematuria, proteinuria, leukocyturia, electrolyte loss. *Neurologic:* Dizziness, flushing of face, mental confusion, irritability, nystagmus, muscle weakness, drowsiness, paresthesias, blurred vision, slurred speech, ataxia, coma, seizures. Neuromuscular blockade may lead to respiratory paralysis. *GI:* Nausea, vomiting, diarrhea, abdominal cramps. *Miscellaneous:* Fever, urticaria, skin exanthemata, eosinophila, anaphylaxis.

Following intrathecal use: Meningeal irritation with fever, stiff neck, headache, increase in leukocytes and protein in the CSF. Nerve root irritation may result in neuritic pain and urine retention. *Following IM use:* Irritation, severe pain. *Following IV use:* Thrombophlebitis.

COLISTIMETHATE SODIUM   Coly-Mycin M (Rx)

COLISTIN SULFATE (POLYMYXIN E)   Coly-Mycin S (Rx)

Classification Antibiotic, polymyxin.

General Statement This antibiotic is derived from *Bacillus polymyxa* var. *colistinus*. It is both bactericidal and bacteriostatic. It is not absorbed from the GI tract.

Action/Kinetics **Peak serum concentration of colistimethate (IM):** 5 µg/ml after 1–2 hr. **t½:** 2–3 hr.

Uses **Colistimethate.** Acute or chronic infections (urinary tract, septicemia, burns, wounds, respiratory tract) due to gram-negative organisms including *E. aerogenes, E. coli, K. pneumoniae, Pseudomonas aeruginosa.* Other more effective and less toxic drugs are available, however. Not useful for *Neisseria* or *Proteus* infections.

Colistin. Diarrhea in infants and children caused by enteropathogenic *E. coli* (effectiveness is questioned, however). Gastroenteritis due to *Shigella.*

Contraindications Hypersensitivity to the drug. Minor infections.

Dosage *Colistimethate*: **IV or IM, Adults and children**: 2.5–5 mg/kg/day in 2–4 divided doses. **For IV use**, direct intermittent administration: one-half daily dose q 12 hr; inject over a 3–5-min period. Dosage by all routes should be reduced in patients with renal impairment. *Colistin sulfate*: **PO**: 5–15 mg/kg/day in 3 divided doses, although higher doses may be required. Reduce dosage in patients with renal impairment.

Administration/Storage

1. Prepare both the solution for injection and the suspension for PO administration according to instructions on package insert.
2. Refrigerate reconstituted medications and discard after 7 days.
3. Administer IM medications deep into the muscle.
4. Protect solution from light.
5. Oral suspensions of the drug are stable for 2 weeks, if refrigerated.

Nursing Implications

See *Nursing Implications* for *Anti-infectives*, p. 52.

1. Assess for nephrotoxicity demonstrated by albuminuria, hematuria, anuria, casts, edema, and uremia.
2. Monitor intake and output.
3. Instruct patient to report tingling sensation about mouth and tongue, visual and speech disturbances, pruritis, and ototoxic effects.
4. Warn patients to avoid hazardous tasks, since drug may cause speech disturbances, dizziness, vertigo, and ataxia.
5. Have available equipment for assisted respiration, oxygen, and calcium chloride for parenteral injection in case of apnea.

POLYMYXIN B SULFATE, PARENTERAL   Aerosporin (Rx)

POLYMYXIN B SULFATE STERILE OPHTHALMIC (Rx)

Classification Antibiotic, polymyxin.

General Statement Polymyxin B sulfate is derived from the spore-forming soil bacterium *Bacillus polymyxa*. It is bactericidal against most gram-negative organisms; rapidly inactivated by alkali, strong acid, and certain metal ions. It is virtually nonabsorbed from the GI tract except in newborn infants. After parenteral administration, polymyxin B seems to remain in the plasma.

Action/Kinetics **Peak serum levels: IM**, 2 hr. t½: 4.3–6 hr. Longer in presence of renal impairment. Sixty percent of drug excreted in urine.

Uses Acute infections of the urinary tract and meninges, septicemia caused by *Pseudomonas aeruginosa*. Meningeal infections caused by *H. influenzae*, urinary tract infections caused by *E. coli*, bacteremia caused by *E. aerogenes* or *Klebsiella* *pneumoniae.* Combined with neomycin for irrigation of the urinary bladder to prevent bacteriuria and bacteremia from indwelling catheters.

Topical: Conjunctival and corneal infections. Blepharitis and keratitis due to bacterial infections. Used with systemic agents for anterior intraocular infections and corneal ulcers caused by *Pseudomonas aeruginosa.* Alone or in combination for ear infections.

Contraindications   Hypersensitivity. Polymyxin B sulfate is a potentially toxic drug to be reserved for the treatment of severe, resistant infections in hospitalized patients. The drug is not indicated for patients with severely impaired renal function or nitrogen retention.

Drug Interactions

Interactant	Interaction
Aminoglycoside antibiotics	Additive nephrotoxic effects
Cephalosporins	↑ Risk of renal toxicity
Phenothiazines	↑ Risk of respiratory depression
Skeletal muscle relaxants (surgical)	Additive muscle relaxation

Laboratory Test Interferences   False + or ↑ levels of urea nitrogen, and creatinine. Casts and RBCs in urine.

Dosage   **IV: Adults and children**, 15,000–25,000 units/kg/day (maximum) in divided doses q 12 hr. **Infants:** up to 40,000 units/kg/day. **IM** (not usually recommended due to pain at injection site): **Adults and children**, 25,000–30,000 units/ kg/day in divided doses q 4–6 hr. **Infants:** up to 40,000 units/kg/day. Both IV and IM doses should be reduced in renal impairment. **Intrathecal** (*meningitis*): **Adults and children over 2 yr**, 50,000 units once daily for 3–4 days, then 50,000 units every other day until 2 weeks after cultures are negative; **Children under 2 yr**, 20,000 units once daily for 3–4 days, or 25,000 units once every other day; dosage of 25,000 units should be continued every other day for 2 weeks after cultures are negative. **Ophthalmic Solution:** 1–2 drops 2–6 times daily depending on severity of infection.

Administration/Storage

1. Store and dilute as directed on package insert.
2. Pain on IM injection can be lessened by reducing drug concentration as much as possible. It is preferable to give drug more frequently in more dilute doses. If ordered, procaine hydrochloride (2.0 ml of a 0.5–1.0% solution per 5 units of dry powder) may be used for mixing the drug for IM injection.
3. **Never use preparations containing procaine hydrochloride for IV or intrathecal use**.

Nursing Implications
See *Nursing Implications* for *Anti-infectives*, p. 52.

1. Do not administer with other nephrotoxic or neurotoxic agents.
2. *Assess*
   a. for nephrotoxicity characterized by albuminuria, casts, nitrogen retention, and hematuria. Monitor intake and output.

(continued)

b. for drug fever and neurologic disturbances, demonstrated by dizziness, blurred vision, irritability, circumoral and peripheral numbness and tingling, weakness, and ataxia. Usually, these symptoms disappear within 24 to 48 hr after the drug is discontinued.

c. for muscle weakness, an early sign of muscle paralysis and impending apnea. Withhold drug when signs of muscle weakness appear. Be prepared to assist respiration and have calcium gluconate on hand for emergency use in case of respiratory difficulties.

3. Use safety precautions for ambulatory or bedridden patients with neurologic disturbances.

4. Anticipate a prolonged regimen of topical application of polymyxin B solution, because drug is not toxic when used in wet dressings, and the physician may wish to avoid emergence of resistant strains.

AMINOGLYCOSIDES

General Statement   The aminoglycosides are broad-spectrum antibiotics, primarily used for the treatment of serious gram-negative infections caused by *Pseudomonas, E. coli, Proteus, Klebsiella*, and *Enterobacter.*. The mechanism of action of the antibiotics is the inhibition of protein synthesis of the infecting microorganism.

Aminoglycoside antibiotics are distributed in the extracellular fluid, cross the placental barrier, but not the blood–brain barrier. Penetration of the CSF is increased when the meninges are inflamed.

The aminoglycosides are excreted, largely unchanged, in the urine. This makes the drugs suitable for urinary tract infections. Concomitant administration of bicarbonate (alkalinization of urine) improves treatment of such infections. There is considerable cross-allergenicity between the individual aminoglycosides. The aminoglycosides are powerful antibiotics that can induce serious side effects. They should not be used for minor infections. Except for streptomycin, resistance of the organisms to aminoglycosides develops slowly. Whenever possible, the sensitivity of the infectious agent should be determined before instituting therapy.

Action/Kinetics   Believed to inhibit protein synthesis by binding to ribosomes (30S subunit), thereby interfering with the transmission of genetic information crucial to the life of the microorganism. The aminoglycosides are usually bactericidal.

The aminoglycosides are poorly absorbed from the GI tract and are therefore usually administered parenterally, the only occasional exception being some enteric infections of the GI tract and prior to surgery. They are also absorbed from the peritoneum, bronchial tree, wounds, denuded skin, and joints.

The aminoglycosides are rapidly absorbed after IM injection. **Peak plasma levels:** usually attained $1/2$–2 hr after IM administration. Measurable levels persist for 8–12 hr after a single administration. **t½:** 2–3 hr. This value increases sharply in patients with impaired kidney function. Ranges of t½ from 24 to 110 hr have been observed. Excreted mainly unchanged in urine.

Uses   Gram-negative bacteria causing bone and joint infections, septicemia (including neonatal sepsis), skin and soft tissue infections (including those from burns), respiratory tract infections, postoperative infections, intra-abdominal infections (including peritonitis), urinary tract infections. In combination with clindamycin for mixed aerobic-anaerobic infections. Also, see individual drugs.

They should be used for gram-positive bacteria only when other less toxic drugs are either ineffective or contraindicated. Their use in CNS *Pseudomonas* infections such as meningitis or ventriculitis is questionable.

Contraindications Hypersensitivity of aminoglycosides, long-term therapy (except streptomycin for tuberculosis). Use with extreme caution in patients with impaired renal function or preexisting hearing impairment. Safe use in pregnancy and during lactation not established.

Untoward Reactions

OTOTOXICITY Both auditory and vestibular damage have been noted. The risk of ototoxicity and vestibular impairment is increased in patients with poor renal function and the elderly. Auditory symptoms include tinnitus and hearing impairment while vestibular symptoms include dizziness, nystagmus, vertigo, and ataxia.

RENAL IMPAIRMENT This may be characterized by cylindruria, oliguria, proteinuria, azotemia, hematuria, increase or decrease in frequency of urination, increased BUN, NPN, or creatinine and increased thirst.

Other symptoms include: *Neurotoxicity:* Neuromuscular blockade, headache, tremor, lethargy, paresthesia, peripheral neuritis (numbness, tingling, or burning of face/mouth), arachnoiditis, encephalopathy, acute organic brain syndrome. CNS depression characterized by stupor, flaccidity and rarely coma and respiratory depression in infants. Optic neuritis with blurred vision or loss of vision. *GI:* Nausea, vomiting, diarrhea, increased salivation, anorexia, weight loss. *Allergic:* Rash, urticaria, pruritus, burning, fever, stomatitis, eosinophilia. Rarely, agranulocytosis and anaphylaxis. Cross allergy among aminoglycosides has been observed. *Miscellaenous:* Joint pain, laryngeal edema, pulmonary fibrosis, superinfection.

Drug Interactions

Interactant	Interaction
Bumetanide	↑ Risk of ototoxicity
Capreomycin	↑ Muscle relaxation
Cephalosporins	↑ Risk of renal toxicity
Cisplatin	Additive renal toxicity
Colistimethate	↑ Muscle relaxation
Digoxin	Possible ↑ or ↓ effect of digoxin
Ethacrynic acid	↑ Risk of ototoxicity
Furosemide	↑ Risk of ototoxicity
Methoxyflurane	↑ Risk of renal toxicity
Penicillins	↓ Effect of aminoglycosides
Polymyxins	↑ Muscle relaxation
Skeletal muscle relaxants (surgical)	↑ Muscle relaxation
Vancomycin	Additive ototoxicity and renal toxicity
Vitamin A	↓ Effect of vitamin A due to ↓ absorption from GI tract

Laboratory Test Interferences   ↑ BUN, BSP retention, creatinine, SGOT, SGPT, bilirubin. ↓ Cholesterol values.

Dosage   See individual agents.

Administration

1. Inject drug deep into muscle mass to minimize transient pain.
2. Administer for only 7–10 days and avoid repeating course of therapy unless serious infection is present that does not respond to other antibiotics.
3. Withhold drug and report toxic serum levels.
4. Administer IV solution diluted and at rate ordered, to prevent excessive serum concentrations.
5. Renal, auditory, and vestibular function should be assessed regularly during drug administration.

Nursing Implications

See also *Nursing Implications* for *Anti-infectives*, p. 52.

1. Weigh patient for correct calculation of dosage.
2. Do audiometry for baseline assessment.
3. Be sure baseline kidney function tests have been ordered and results reported before administering first dose.
4. *Assess for nephrotoxicity*
   a. those patients who have renal dysfunction because they are more susceptible to developing toxicity. Ascertain that a pretreatment audiogram is done and repeated during therapy, if administration of aminoglycosides is to exceed 5 days.
   b. for presence of cells or casts in urine, oliguria, proteinuria, lowered specific gravity, or increasing BUN, NPN, or creatinine.
5. Maintain intake and output.
6. Hydrate patient well unless contraindicated.
7. *Assess*
   a. for signs of ototoxicity.
   b. for tinnitus and vertigo, signs of vestibular injury more common with gentamicin and streptomycin.
   c. for subjective hearing loss or loss of high tones on the audiometer, indicating auditory damage more common with kanamycin and neomycin.
   d. for neuromuscular blockade with muscular weakness leading to apnea when aminoglycoside is administered together with a muscle relaxant or after anesthesia. Have calcium gluconate or neostigmine available, to reverse blockade.
8. Protect patient with vestibular dysfunction by supervising ambulation and providing side rails if necessary.
9. Continue monitoring for ototoxicity because the onset of deafness may occur several weeks after aminoglycoside has been discontinued.
10. Withhold medication and check with medical supervision if signs of toxicity are noted. Doctor will either reduce dosage or discontinue medication.
11. Do not administer concurrently or sequentially with a topical or systemic nephrotoxic or ototoxic drug; for example, potent diuretics, such as ethacrynic acid or furosemide.
12. Assess closely premature infants, neonates, and older patients receiving aminoglycosides because they are particularly sensitive to their toxic effects.

AMIKACIN SULFATE   Amikin (Rx)

Classification   Antibiotic, aminoglycoside.

Action/Kinetics   Amikacin is derived from kanamycin. Its spectrum is somewhat broader than that of other aminoglycosides, including *Gerratia* and *Acinetobacter* species, as well as certain staphylococci and streptococci. Amikacin is effective against both penicillinase and non-penicillinase-producing organisms. **Therapeutic serum levels: IM**, 8–16 μg/ml after 45–120 min. t½: 0.8–2.8 hr.

Dosage   **IM** (preferred) and **IV, adults, children, and older infants:** 15 mg/kg/day in 2–3 equally divided doses q 8–12 hr for 7–10 days; **maximum daily dose:** 15 mg/kg. *Uncomplicated urinary tract infections* 250 mg b.i.d.; **newborns:** loading dose of 10 mg/kg followed by 7.5 mg/kg q 12 hr. *Impaired renal function:* normal loading dose of 7.5 mg/kg; **then** administration should be monitored by serum level of amikacin (35 μg/ml max) or creatinine clearance rates.
   Duration of treatment: **Usual:** 7–10 days.

Administration/Storage (for IV Administration)

1. Add 500 mg vial to 200 ml of sterile diluent, such as normal saline or D₅W.
2. Administer over a 30–60 min period for children and adults.
3. Administer to infants in the amount of fluid ordered by the doctor. The IV administration to infants should be 1–2 hr.
4. Store colorless liquid at room temperature no longer than 2 years.
5. Potency is not affected if the solution turns a very light yellow.

GENTAMICIN SULFATE   Apogen, Apogen Pediatric, Cidomycin,* Garamycin, Garamycin Intrathecal, Garamycin IV Piggyback, Garamycin Ophthalmic, Garamycin Pediatric, Genoptic Ophthalmic, Genoptic S.O.P. Ophthalmic, Gentacidin, Gentamicin, Gentamicin Ophthalmic, Gentamicin Sulfate IV Piggyback, Jenamicin, Pediatric Gentamicin Sulfate (Rx)

Classification   Antibiotic, aminoglycoside.

Action/Kinetics   **Therapeutic serum levels: IM**, 4–10 μg/ml. Prolonged serum levels above 12 μg/ml should be avoided. t½: 1.2–5.0 hr.
   The drug can be used concurrently with carbenicillin for the treatment of serious *Pseudomonas* infections. However, the drugs should not be mixed in the same flask because carbenicillin will inactivate gentamicin.

Additional Uses   Gentamicin is the drug of choice for hospital-acquired gram-negative sepsis (including neonatal sepsis). In combination with carbenicillin for life-threatening infections caused by *Pseudomonas aeruginosa*. Serious staphylococcal infections.

Additional Untoward Reactions   Muscle twitching, numbness, seizures, increased blood pressure, alopecia, purpura, pseudotumor cerebri.

Additional Drug Interaction   With carbenicillin or ticarcillin, gentamicin may result in increased effect when used for *Pseudomonas* infections.

Dosage   **IM** (Usual), **IV. Adults with normal renal function:** 1 mg/kg q 8 hr, up to 5 mg/kg daily in life-threatening infections; **children:** 2–2.5 mg/kg q 8 hr; **infants and neonates:** 2.5 mg/kg q 8 hr; **premature infants or neonates less than 1 week of age:** 2.5 mg/kg q 12 hr. *Prevention of bacterial endocarditis:* **Adults:**

1.5 mg/kg gentamicin (not to exceed 80 mg) plus penicillin G, 2,000,000 units or ampicillin, 1 gm, all IM or IV 30–60 min before the procedure; two additional doses can be given at 8-hr intervals. **Children:** 2 mg/kg gentamicin plus penicillin G, 30,000 units/kg or ampicillin, 50 mg/kg in same dosage interval as adults. Pediatric dosage should not exceed single or 24-hr adult doses. **Adults with impaired renal function:** to calculate interval (hours) between doses, multiply serum creatinine level (mg/100 ml) by 8. **Intrathecal** (*for meningitis*): **Use only the intrathecal preparation. Adults, usual:** 4–8 mg once daily; **children and infants, 3 months and older:** 1–2 mg once daily.

   Ophthalmic solution (0.3%): 1–2 drops in lower conjunctival sac 2–6 times daily. **Ophthalmic ointment (0.3%):** ½ inch ribbon in lower conjunctival sac 2–6 times daily. **Topical cream/ointment (0.1%):** Apply 1–5 times/day to affected area.

   Duration of treatment: **Usual,** 7–10 days.

Administration (of Cream or Ointment)

1. Remove the crusts of impetigo contagiosa before applying ointment to permit maximum contact between antibiotic and infection.
2. Apply ointment gently and cover with gauze dressing if desirable.
3. Avoid further contamination of infected skin.

KANAMYCIN SULFATE   Anamid,* Kantrex, Klebcil (Rx)

Classification   Antibiotic, aminoglycoside.

Action/Kinetics   The activity of kanamycin resembles that of neomycin and streptomycin. **Therapeutic serum levels: IM,** 8–16 μg/ml. **t½:** 2–2.5 hr.

Additional Uses   Adjunct in treatment of tuberculosis. Orally for hepatic encephalopathy to inhibit ammonia-forming bacteria in the GI tract. Orally to prepare the intestine prior to surgery. Peritoneally to irrigate infected wounds, cavities, surgical sites. As an aerosol for respiratory tract infections.

Additional Untoward Reactions   Sprue-like syndrome with steatorrhea, malabsorption, and electrolyte imbalance.

Additional Drug Interaction   Procainamide ↑ muscle relaxation.

Dosage   **PO**. *Intestinal bacteria suppression:* 1 gm q hr for 4 hr; **then,** 1 gm q 6 hr for 36–72 hr. *Hepatic coma:* 8–12 gm/day in divided doses. **IM, IV. Adults and children:** 15 mg/kg/day in 2–3 equal doses. Maximum daily dose should not exceed 1.5 gm regardless of route of administration. For calculating dosage interval (in hours) in patients with impaired renal function, multiply serum creatinine (mg/100 ml) ×9. **Intraperitoneal:** 500 mg diluted in 20 ml sterile distilled water. **Inhalation** : 250 mg in saline—nebulize b.i.d.–q.i.d. **Irrigation of abscess cavities, pleural space, ventricular cavities:** 0.25% solution.

Administration

1. Do not mix with other drug medication in IV bottle. Administer IV slowly and at concentrations not exceeding 2.5 mg/ml.
2. Unopened vials may change color, but this does not affect potency of drug.
3. Do not mix with other drugs in same syringe for IM injection.
4. Inject deep into large muscle mass to minimize pain and local irritation. Rotate sites of injection. Local irritation may occur with large doses.

5. IV administration is rarely used and must not be used for patients with renal impairment.
6. Drug should not be administered for more than 12 to 14 days.

NEOMYCIN SULFATE   Mycifradin Sulfate, Neobiotic (Rx)

Classification   Antibiotic, aminoglycoside.

Action/Kinetics   **Peak plasma levels: PO**, 1–4 hr; **Therapeutic serum level**: 5–10 μg/ml. **t½**: 3 hr.

Additional Uses   PO: Hepatic coma, sterilization of gut prior to surgery, inhibition of ammonia-forming bacteria in GI tract in hepatic encephalopathy. Therapy of intestinal infections due to pathogenic strains of *E. coli*, primarily in children. *Investigational:* Hypercholesterolemia. **Topical**: Widely used for infections of the skin, eyes, and ears, including skin wounds and ulcers.

Additional Contraindication   Intestinal obstruction (PO).

Additional Untoward Reactions   Sprue-like syndrome with steatorrhea, malabsorption, and electrolyte imbalance. Skin rashes after topical or parenteral administration.

Additional Drug Interactions

Interactant	Interaction
Digoxin	↓ Effect of digoxin due to ↓ absorption from GI tract
Penicillin V	↓ Effect of penicillin due to ↓ absorption from GI tract
Procainamide	↑ Muscle relaxation produced by neomycin

Dosage   PO. *Preoperatively in abdominal surgery:* **Adults and children:** 88 mg/kg/day in 6 equally divided doses for 1–3 days. *Hepatic coma:* **Adults**, 4–12 gm/day in divided doses for 5–6 days; **children:** 50–100 mg/kg/day in divided doses for 5–6 days. *Infectious diarrhea:* **Adults** 3 gm/day; **infants and children**, 50 mg/kg/day for 2–3 days. **IM. Adults:** 15 mg/kg/day in 4 equal doses, not to exceed 1 gm/day. The IM preparation should not be used in infants and children.

Maximum course of therapy is 10 days. The drug is also administered by instillation in case of emergency abdominal surgery or peritonitis.

TOPICAL APPLICATION   Neomycin alone or in combination with other antibiotics (bacitracin or gramicidin) and/or an anti-inflammatory agent (corticosteroid) is used for a variety of topical infections.

OPHTHALMIC   A small amount of a 0.5% ointment is instilled into the conjunctival sac one or more times daily. One to 2 drops of a 0.1–0.5% solution is instilled into the eye 2 to 4 times daily. **Severe infections:** Solution may be applied more frequently.

OTIC   For external otitis, chronic otitis media, and various dermatoses of the external auditory canal. Instill 3 to 5 drops 3 to 4 times daily. Alternatively, a gauze wick moistened with the preparation may be loosely inserted into the external canal.

DERMATOLOGIC   Used for itching, burning, inflamed skin conditions that are threatened by, or complicated by, a secondary bacterial infection. Apply cream to affected area 2 to 3 times daily.

Additional Nursing Implications

See also *Nursing Implications* for *Anti-infectives*, p. 52 and *Aminoglycosides*, p. 110.

1. Have on hand neostigmine to counteract renal failure, respiratory depression and arrest, which may occur when neomycin is administered intraperitoneally.
2. Anticipate a slight laxative effect produced by oral neomycin. Withhold the drug and consult with physician in case of suspected intestinal obstruction.
3. Provide low-residue diet for preoperative disinfection and, unless contraindicated, a cathartic immediately preceding PO administration of neomycin sulfate, 1.0 gm q 1–4 hr for 24 to 72 hr.
4. Apply ointment or solution of neomycin after cleaning the affected area. Solution is apparently more effective than ointment and is used in wet dressings.

NETILMICIN SULFATE   Netromycin (Rx)

Classification   Antibiotic, aminoglycoside.

Action/Kinetics   Netilmicin is a semisynthetic aminoglycoside that may be effective in infections resistant to other aminoglycosides. t½: 2–2.5 hr. **Peak serum levels after IM:** 30–60 min. **Therapeutic serum levels:** 0.5–10 µg/ml.

Additional Uses   Effective against *Salmonella, Shigella,* and *Serratia* species.

Dosage   IM, IV. Adults: 1.5–2 mg/kg q 12 hr (complicated upper respiratory tract infections); for serious systemic infections: 1.3–2.2 mg/kg q 8 hr or 2–3.25 mg/kg q 12 hr. **Pediatric, 6 weeks–12 years:** 1.8–2.7 mg/kg q 8 hr or 2.7–4 mg/kg q 12 hr; **neonates, less than 6 weeks:** 2–32.5 mg/kg q 12 hr.

   Patients with impaired renal function: Dose individualized based on creatinine clearance; check package insert carefully.

Administration

1. Measure blood levels carefully in burn patients as they often have altered pharmacokinetics to netilmicin.
2. The usual course of therapy is 7–14 days.
3. For IV administration, the dose can be diluted in 50–200 ml of a parenteral solution and given over a period of 30–120 min. For infants and children, the volume of fluid is less.
4. Diluted netilmicin is stable for 72 hr when stored in glass containers either at room temperature or refrigerated.

Additional Nursing Implication

Since drug can cause neuromuscular blockade, check rate and quality of respiration at least every 4 hours around the clock.

PAROMOMYCIN SULFATE   Humatin (Rx)

Classification   Antibiotic, aminoglycoside.

Action/Kinetics Paromomycin is obtained from *Streptomyces rimosus forma paromomycina*. Its spectrum of activity resembles that of neomycin and kanamycin. The drug is poorly absorbed from the GI tract and is ineffective against systemic infections when given orally.

Additional Uses Inhibition of ammonia-forming bacteria in GI tract in hepatic encephalopathy, intestinal amebiasis, preoperative suppression of intestinal flora. *Investigational:* Anthelmintic.

Contraindications Intestinal obstruction. To be used with caution in the presence of GI ulceration because of possible systemic absorption.

Additional Untoward Reactions Diarrhea or loose stools. Heartburn, emesis, and pruritus ani. Superinfections, especially by monilia.

Drug Interaction Penicillin is inhibited by paromomycin.

Dosage **PO**: *Hepatic coma*: **Adults,** 4 gm daily in divided doses for 5–6 days. *Intestinal amebiasis*: **Adults and children,** 25–35 mg/kg/day administered in 3 doses with meals for 5–10 days. *Anthelmintic*: **Adults,** 1 gm q 15 min for 4 doses; **pediatric:** 11 mg/kg q 15 min for 4 doses.

Administration

1. Do not administer parenterally.
2. Administer before or after meals.

Additional Nursing Implications
See *Nursing Implications* for *Anti-infectives*, p. 52 and *Aminoglycosides*, p. 110. Assess for and report diarrhea, dehydration, and general weakness.

STREPTOMYCIN SULFATE (Rx)

Classification Antibiotic, aminoglycoside.

Action/Kinetics Like other aminoglycoside antibiotics, streptomycin is rapidly distributed throughout most tissues and body fluids including necrotic tubercular lesions. **Therapeutic serum levels: IM,** 25 μg/ml. **t½:** 2–3 hr.

Additional Uses Tuberculosis in conjunction with other antitubercular agents. Emergence of resistant strains has greatly reduced the usefulness of streptomycin; also tularemia, glanders (*Actinobacillus mallei*), bubonic plague (*Pasteurella pestis*), brucellosis, cholera, and bacterial endocarditis caused by *H. influenzae*.

Additional Contraindications Hypersensitivity, contact dermatitis, and exfoliative dermatitis. Do not give to patients with myasthenia gravis.

Additional Laboratory Test Interference False urine glucose determinations with Benedict's solution and Clinitest.

Dosage **IM only.** *Tuberculosis (adjunct):* **initial,** 1 gm daily with other tuberculostatic drugs; **then,** reduce streptomycin dosage to 1 gm 2–3 times/week for minimum of 1 year. **Pediatric:** in combination with other drugs, 20 mg/kg once daily (not to exceed 1 gm/day). Older, debilitated patients should receive lower dosages. *Bacterial endocarditis due to penicillin-sensitive alpha and nonhemolytic streptococci (with penicillin):* 1 gm b.i.d. for 1 week; **then,** 0.5 gm b.i.d. for 2nd week.

Enterococcal endocarditis (with penicillin): 1 gm b.i.d. for 2 weeks; **then,** 0.5 gm b.i.d. for 4 weeks. *Bacterial endocarditis prophylaxis:* **IM,** Streptomycin, 1 gm with aqueous penicillin G, 1 million units and procaine penicillin G, 600,000 units, 30–60 min prior to procedure. *Plague:* 0.5–1 gm q 6 hr. *Tularemia:* 0.25–0.5 gm q 6 hr for 7–10 days. *Other infections:* **Adults,** 1–4 gm/day in divided doses q 6–12 hr, depending on severity of infections; **pediatric:** 20–40 mg/kg/day in divided doses q 6–12 hr.

Administration/Storage

1. Protect hands when preparing drug. Wear gloves if drug is prepared often because it is irritating.
2. In a dry form, the drug is stable for at least 2 years at room temperature.
3. Aqueous solutions prepared without preservatives are stable for at least 1 week at room temperature and for at least 3 months under refrigeration.
4. Use only solutions prepared freshly from dry powder for intrathecal, subarachnoid, and intrapleural administration because commercially prepared solutions contain preservatives harmful to tissues of the CNS and pleural cavity.
5. Commercially prepared, ready-to-inject solutions are for IM use only. These solutions are prepared with phenol and are stable at room temperature for prolonged periods of time.
6. Administer deep into muscle mass to minimize pain and local irritation.
7. Solutions may darken after exposure to light, but this does not necessarily cause a loss in potency.
8. When injection into the subarachnoid space is required for treatment of meningitis, only solutions made freshly from the dry powder should be used. Commercial solutions may contain preservatives toxic to the CNS.

Additional Nursing Implications

See also *Nursing Implications* for *Anti-infectives* p. 52 and *Aminoglycosides*, p. 110. Use Tes-Tape for urine glucose test because Benedict's and Fehling's solution can give false + reactions.

TOBRAMYCIN SULFATE   Nebcin, Tobrex Ophthalmic (Rx)

Classification   Antibiotic, aminoglycoside.

Action/Kinetics   This aminoglycoside is very similar to gentamicin and can be used concurrently with carbenicillin. **Therapeutic serum levels: IM,** 4–8 µg/ml. t½: 1–2 hr.

Additional Uses   Meningitis; neonatal sepsis.

Additional Drug Interactions   With carbenicillin or ticarcillin, tobramycin may have an increased effect when used for *Pseudomonas* infections.

Dosage   IM, IV. Adults: 3 mg/kg/day in 3 equally divided doses q 8 hr; *for life-threatening infections* up to 5 mg/kg/day in 3 or 4 equal doses. **Pediatric:** Either 2–2.5 mg/kg q 8 hr or 1.5–1.9 mg/kg q 6 hr; **neonates 1 week of age or less:** up to 4 mg/kg/day in 2 equal doses q 12 hr.

Impaired renal function: **initial,** 1 mg/kg; **then,** maintenance dose calculated according to information supplied by manufacturer.

Administration/Storage

1. Prepare IV solution by diluting calculated dose of tobramycin with 50–100 ml of IV solution.
2. Infuse over 20 to 60 min.
3. Use proportionately less diluent for children than for adults.
4. Do not mix with other drugs for parenteral administration.
5. Store drug at room temperature—no longer than 2 years.
6. Discard solution of drug containing up to 1 mg/ml after 24 hr at room temperature.

MISCELLANEOUS ANTIBIOTICS

BACITRACIN INTRAMUSCULAR   Bacitin,* Bacitracin, Bacitracin Sterile (Rx)

BACITRACIN OINTMENT   Baciquent (OTC)

BACITRACIN OPHTHALMIC   Baciquent Ophthalmic (Rx)

Classification   Antibiotic, miscellaneous.

General Statement   Antibiotic produced by *Bacillus subtilis*. Bactericidal for many gram-positive organisms and *Neisseria*. Not absorbed from the GI tract. When given parenterally, drug is well distributed in pleural and ascitic fluids.

Bacitracin has a very high nephrotoxicity. Its systematic use is restricted to infants (see *uses*). Renal function must be carefully evaluated prior to and daily during use.

Action/Kinetics   Interferes with synthesis of cell wall, preventing incorporation of amino acids and nucleotides. Bacitracin is bactericidal and bacteriostatic and active against protoplasts. **Peak plasma levels: IM,** 0.2–2 μg/ml after 2 hr. Ten to 40% is excreted in urine after IM administration.

Uses   Bacitracin is used locally during surgery for cranial and neurosurgical infections caused by susceptible organisms.

As an ointment (preferred) or solution, bacitracin is prescribed for superficial pyoderma-like impetigo and infectious eczematoid dermatitis, for secondary infected dermatoses (atopic dermatitis, contact dermatitis), and for superficial infections of the eye, ear, nose, and throat by susceptible organisms.

Parenteral use is limited to the treatment of staphylococcal pneumonia and staphylococcal-induced empyema in infants.

Contraindications   Hypersensitivity or toxic reaction to bacitracin. Pregnancy.

Untoward Reactions   Nephrotoxicity due to tubular and glomerular necrosis, renal failure, toxic reactions, nausea, vomiting.

Drug Interactions

Interactant	Interaction
Aminoglycosides	Additive nephrotoxicity and neuromuscular blocking activity
Anesthetics	↑ Neuromuscular blockade → possible muscle paralysis
Neuromuscular blocking agents	Additive neuromuscular → muscle paralysis

Dosage   **IM only. Infants, 2.5 kg and below:** 900 units/kg/day in 2–3 divided doses; **infants over 2.5 kg:** 1,000 units/kg/day in 2–3 divided doses. **Ophthalmic ointment (500 units/gm):** ½ inch in lower conjunctival sac 2–6 times daily. **Topical ointment (500 units/gm):** Apply 1–5 times daily to affected area.

Administration

1. Do not mix bacitracin with glycerin or other polyalcohols that cause drug to deteriorate. Bacitracin unguentin base is anhydrous, consisting of liquid and white petrolatum.
2. Cleanse area before applying bacitracin as a wet dressing or ointment.
3. Adequate fluid intake must be maintained with parenteral use.

Nursing Implications

See *Nursing Implications* for *Anti-infectives*, p. 52.

1. Check that renal function tests have been done before initiating therapy and daily during therapy.
2. Assess intake and output.
3. Maintain adequate fluid intake and output with parenteral use of drug.
4. Withhold drug and consult with doctor when fluid output is inadequate.
5. Test pH of urine daily, because it should be kept at pH 6 or greater, to decrease renal irritation.
6. Have available sodium bicarbonate or another alkali to administer should pH drop below a value of 6.
7. Do not administer concurrently or sequentially with a topical or systemic nephrotoxic drug.

FURAZOLIDONE   Furoxone (Rx)

Classification   Antibacterial, miscellaneous.

Action/Kinetics   Acts by interfering with crucial enzyme systems. Bactericidal against many pathogens of GI tract, but affects normal flora minimally. Poorly absorbed from and inactivated in intestine.

Uses   Bacterial or protozoal diarrhea; enteritis caused by *Salmonella, Shigella, Staphylococcus, Escherichia, Enterobacter aerogenes, Vibrio cholerae,* and *Giardia lamblia.*

Contraindications   Nursing mothers and infants under 1 month of age.

Untoward Reactions   *GI:* Nausea, vomiting, colitis, proctitis, anal pruritus. *Allergic:* Urticaria, rashes, hypotension, fever, arthralgia. *Other:* Headache, malaise, Antabuse-like reaction, hemolysis in glucose-6-phosphate dehydrogenase deficient patients.

Drug Interactions

Interactant	Interaction
Alcohol, ethyl	Antabuse-like reaction possible
Antidepressants, tricyclic	↑ Effects (including toxicity) of furazolidone
Antihistamines	↑ Chance of hypotension and hypoglycemia
CNS depressants	Furazolidone ↑ depressant effects
Guanethidine	Hypotensive effect ↓ by furazolidone
Hypoglycemics, oral	↑ Hypoglycemic effect
Insulin	↑ Hypoglycemic effect
Meperidine	Concomitant use may cause unpredictable CNS and cardiovascular effects
Monoamine oxidase inhibitors	↑ Effect due to monoamine oxidase inhibitor activity of furazolidone
Narcotics	↑ Chance of hypotension and hypoglycemia
Sympathomimetics, indirect acting	↑ Effect due to monoamine oxidase inhibitor activity of furazolidone

Laboratory Test Interference False + urine glucose values.

Dosage PO. **Adults**: 100 mg. q.i.d.; **children 5 years and older**: 25–50 mg q.i.d.; **1–4 years**: 17–25 mg q.i.d. (use liquid); **1 month to 1 year**: 8–17 mg q.i.d. (use liquid). Daily dosage for all ages should not exceed 8.8 mg/kg.

Administration/Storage Store liquid in amber-colored bottles.

Nursing Implications

See also *Nursing Implications* for *Anti-infectives*, p. 52.

1. *Assess*
   a. for hypersensitivity reactions demonstrated by a drop in blood pressure, arthralgia, fever, and urticaria. Withhold drug if any of these symptoms is observed.
   b. for GI symptoms, malaise, or headache that subsides when dosage is reduced or drug is withdrawn.
2. Anticipate withdrawal of drug if clinical response does not occur within 7 days.
3. *Teach patient and/or family*
   a. not to eat food containing tyramine (such as broad beans, strong unpasteurized cheeses, yeast extracts, beer, pickled herring, chicken livers, bananas, avocados, or fermented food) because furazolidone is a monoamine oxidase inhibitor. These reactions are more likely to occur in patients receiving doses larger than those usually recommended or who receive the drug for more than 5 days.
   b. to use sedatives, antihistamines, tranquilizers, and narcotic drugs concurrently with therapy only with the knowledge of the physician.
   c. not to drink alcohol during therapy or for 4 days after because an Antabuse-like reaction, characterized by flushing, palpitation, dyspnea, hyperventilation, tachycardia, nausea, vomiting, drop in blood pressure, and even profound collapse, may occur. Drug may color urine brownish.

NITROFURAZONE   Furacin, Furazyme (Rx)

Classification   Antibiotic, miscellaneous (topical germicide).

Action/Kinetics   Nitrofurazone is a broad-spectrum, mostly bactericidal, agent for both aerobic and anaerobic gram-positive organisms. Nitrofurazone's activity has been attributed to its interference with enzyme systems necessary for carbohydrate metabolism.

Uses   Adjunctive therapy for patients with second- and third-degree burns or skin grafts. Skin grafting if bacterial contamination may cause rejection of graft or infection of donor site.

Untoward Reactions   Overgrowth by nonsusceptible microorganisms including fungi. Very low incidence of contact dermatitis.

Dosage   **Powder**: Apply directly. **Soluble dressing/cream**: Apply directly or place on gauze. Used once daily or every few days.

Administration/Storage

1. Store in light-resistant containers and prevent exposure to light, heat, and/or alkaline materials.
2. Discard cloudy solutions because they suggest microbial contamination of the drug.
3. Discoloration does not indicate a loss in strength of the material.
4. Reautoclaving may be done at 121°C for 30 min at 15–20 pounds of pressure, but discoloration usually occurs and the consistency of the base (particularly an ointment) is changed.

Nursing Implications

See also *Nursing Implications* for *Anti-infectives*, p. 52.

1. Protect skin adjacent to chronic stasis ulcers by covering the skin with zinc oxide ointment and using Furacin only on the lesion.
2. Assess and report rash, pruritus, and/or irritation, which are indications for termination of treatment with Furacin.
3. Minimize adverse effects by removing medication by irrigation at the first sign of irritation.
4. Flush dressing with sterile saline at time of removal to prevent dressing adhering to wound.

Nursing Implications for Furacin Soluble Dressing and Powder

FURACIN SOLUBLE DRESSING

1. Either apply directly with a tongue blade or place first on gauze.
2. To prepare sterile impregnanted gauze:
   a. Place sterile gauze strips in a tray and cover with Furacin soluble dressing.
   b. Repeat above adding several layers of gauze for each layer of soluble dressing.
   c. To minimize discoloration caused by autoclaving, sprinkle sterile water on each layer of dressing.
   d. Cover the tray loosely and autoclave at 121°C for 30 min at 15–20 pounds of pressure.

3. Impregnate bandage rolls by putting some soluble dressing in the bottom of the glass jar. Stand rolls on end and place more dressing on top. Then autoclave as above.

FURACIN SOLUBLE POWDER   Apply directly from shaker top of a nonmetallic powder insufflator.

NOVOBIOCIN SODIUM   Albamycin (Rx)

Classification   Antibiotic, miscellaneous.

General Statement   Novobiocin is derived from *Streptomyces niveus* and is primarily bacteriostatic. It is readily absorbed from the GI tract and diffuses well into pleural, joint, and ascitic fluids. Because of the high incidence of adverse reactions and rapid development of resistance, the drug should be used only for serious infections. Frequent total and differential blood counts and liver function tests should be performed during prolonged therapy.

Jaundice, hyperbilirubinemia, or sulfobromophthalein retention is an indication for discontinuance of drug.

Action/Kinetics   Inhibits protein and nucleic acid synthesis and interferes with formation of bacterial cell wall, probably affecting its stability. The drug is mainly bacteriostatic. Well absorbed from GI tract. **Peak plasma concentration**: 2 hr. Excreted primarily in feces.

Uses   Infections by susceptible strains of staphylococci and *Proteus*. Indicated for the treatment of enteritis, postoperative wound infections, cellulitis, abscesses and ulcers, and resistant urinary tract infections.

Contraindications   Hypersensitivity to drug. Avoid use in newborn or premature infants.

Untoward Reactions   Novobiocin is a potent sensitizing agent and can cause skin rash, urticaria, fever, pruritus, swollen joints, and blood dyscrasias, which can be fatal. Liver damage, jaundice, nausea, vomiting, anorexia, abdominal distress, and lightheadedness have also been reported. The drug may also cause superinfections and favors the emergence of resistant strains, particularly staphylococci. It can cause neonatal hyperbilirubinemia.

Drug Interaction   Tetracyclines ↓ effect of novobiocin.

Dosage   PO. Adult: 250 mg q 6 hr or 500 mg q 12 hr (in severe infections, can increase dose to maximum of 1 gm q 12 hr). **Children**: 15 mg/kg/day in divided doses q 6–12 hr (up to 45 mg/kg/day for severe infections).

Nursing Implications
See also *Nursing Implications* for *Anti-infectives*, p. 52.
Assess

a. for allergic reactions, since drug is a potent sensitizing agent. Have emergency equipment available.

(continued)

b. for symptoms of blood dyscrasias, such as anemia, purpura, paleness, and bleeding.

c. newborn infants for jaundice, which may lead to kernicterus and subsequent brain damage. Withhold drug if jaundice is noted.

d. whether patient is able to tolerate oral intake, and report to physician so that drug may be ordered PO as soon as possible.

PENTAMIDINE ISOETHIONATE   Pentam 300 (Rx)

Classification   Miscellaneous antibiotic (antiprotozal).

Action/Kinetics   The drug inhibits synthesis of DNA, RNA, and proteins, thereby interfering with cell metabolism. Up to two-thirds of the dose may be excreted unchanged in the urine.

Uses   Pneumonia caused by *Pneumocystis carnii. Investigational:* Trypanosomiasis, visceral leishmaniasis.

Contraindications   Safety and efficacy in pregnancy have not been established. Use with caution in patients with hepatic or kidney disease, hypertension or hypotension, hyperglycemia or hypoglycemia, hypocalcemia, and hematologic problems such as leukopenia, anemia, or thrombocytopenia.

Untoward Reactions   *Cardiovascular:* Severe hypotension, ventricular tachycardia, phlebitis, cardiac arrhythmias. *GI:* Nausea, anorexia, bad taste in mouth. *CNS:* Dizziness, confusion, hallucinations. *Hematologic:* Leukopenia, anemia, thrombocytopenia. *Other:* Hypoglycemia (may be severe), hypocalcemia, acute renal failure (elevated serum creatinine), Stevens Johnson syndrome, fever, rash, neuralgia, hyperkalemia, elevated liver function tests.

Dosage   **IV, Deep IM. Adults and children:** 4 mg/kg once daily for 14 days. Dosage should be reduced in renal disease.

Administration

1. To prepare IM solution, dissolve one vial in 3 ml of Sterile Water for Injection.
2. To prepare IV solution, dissolve one vial in 3–5 ml of Sterile Water for Injection or 5% Dextrose Injection. May then be further diluted in 50–250 ml of 5% Dextrose solution. This can then be slowly infused over 60 min. IV solutions are stable for 24 hr at room temperature.

Nursing Implications

1. Check IV site at least every 8 hours for signs of phlebitis.
2. *Assess*
   a. for bruising, hematuria, black stools, and other signs of bleeding.
   b. for signs and symptoms of hypoglycemia, which may be severe.
3. Take vital signs every 4 hours around the clock and report any significant change, especially a drop in blood pressure or increase in pulse.
4. If patient is not on a cardiac monitor, take apical pulse for possible arrhythmia by auscultation.

SPECTINOMYCIN HYDROCHLORIDE PENTAHYDRATE Trobicin (Rx)

Classification Antibiotic, miscellaneous.

General Statement Spectinomycin is produced by *Streptomyces spectabilis* and is effective against a wide variety of gram-negative and gram-positive organisms, including those causing gonorrhea. It is ineffective against syphilis, and this is why it is a poor choice of drug when mixed infections are present.

Action/Kinetics Inhibits bacterial protein synthesis by binding to ribosome (30S subunit) thereby interfering with transmission of genetic information crucial to life of microorganism. Spectinomycin is mainly bacteriostatic. Spectinomycin is not absorbed from GI tract and is only given IM. **Peak plasma concentration:** 100 μg/ml after 1 hr. t½: 1.2–2.8 hr. Not significantly bound to protein. Excreted in urine.

Uses Acute gonorrhea in infections resistant to penicillin or in patients allergic to penicillin.

Contraindication Sensitivity to drug.

Untoward Reactions A single dose of spectinomycin has caused soreness at the site of injection, urticaria, dizziness, nausea, chills, fever, and insomnia.

Multiple doses have caused a decrease in hemoglobin, hematocrit, and creatinine clearance and an increase in alkaline phosphatase, blood urea nitrogen, and serum glutamic pyruvic transaminase (SGPT).

Dosage **IM Only:** 2 gm. In areas where antibiotic resistance is known to be prevalent, give 4 gm divided between 2 gluteal injection sites.

Administration/Storage
1. Powder is stable for 3 years.
2. Use reconstituted solution within 24 hr.
3. Inject deeply into the upper outer quadrant of the gluteus muscle.
4. Injections may be made in 2 sites for patients requiring 4 gm.

Nursing Implications
See *Nursing Implications* for *Anti-infectives*, p. 52.
Advise patients treated with spectinomycin and suspected of having syphilis to return for serologic tests monthly for at least 3 months.

TROLEANDOMYCIN Tao (Rx)

Classification Antibiotic, miscellaneous.

General Statement Troleandomycin is a broad-spectrum antibiotic salt prepared from cultures of *Streptomyces antibioticus*. Its spectrum of activity resembles that of erythromycin, being bacteriostatic and effective against gram-negative bacteria. Troleandomycin is widely distributed in body tissues and fluids but not in spinal fluid unless the meninges are inflamed.

Periodic liver function tests are indicated. Troleandomycin may alter some liver function tests for periods of up to 5 weeks. When used for acute gonococcal infection in patients with suspected lesions of syphilis, dark-field examination should precede initiation of therapy and serologic tests should be made at monthly intervals for 3 months.

Action/Kinetics Believed to inhibit protein synthesis of bacteria. **Peak plasma concentration: PO**, 2 hr. Excreted in urine (10–25%) and in feces.

Uses Severe, acute infections by susceptible staphylococci, streptococci, pneumococci, clostridium, and corynebacterium. Single doses of troleandomycin are effective against acute gonococcal urethritis.

Contraindications Hypersensitivity to drug. Liver dysfunction or known sensitivity toward hepatotoxic drugs. Not recommended for prophylaxis or therapy for longer than 10 days. Occasional cross-sensitivity with erythromycin.

Untoward Reactions Hepatotoxicity: hyperbilirubinemia and jaundice. Superinfections. Local irritation at site of injection. Nausea, vomiting, esophagitis, rectal burning, diarrhea, headache, and skin rash. Rarely, anaphylactoid reactions.

Drug Interactions

Interactant	Interaction
Carbamazepine	↑ Effect of carbamazepine due to ↓ breakdown by liver
Contraceptives, oral	Additive jaundice
Ergotamine	Ischemic reactions
Theophylline	↑ Effect of theophylline

Dosage **PO. Adults:** 250–500 mg q 6 hr; **pediatric:** 6.6–11 mg/kg q 6 hr. Continue therapy for 10 days for streptococcal infections.

Nursing Implications

See *Nursing Implications* for *Anti-infectives*, p. 52.
  Assess for jaundice, as drug should be discontinued at first signs of hepatotoxicity.

VANCOMYCIN HYDROCHLORIDE Vancocin (Rx)

Classification Antibiotic, miscellaneous.

Action/Kinetics This antibiotic, derived from *Streptomyces orientalis*, diffuses in pleural, pericardial, ascitic, and synovial fluids after parenteral administration. Appears to bind to bacterial cell wall, arresting its synthesis and damaging the cytoplastic membrane, by a mechanism that is different from the damage inflicted by penicillin. Drug is bactericidal and bacteriostatic. Poorly absorbed from GI tract. **Peak plasma levels, IV:** 33 μg/ml after 5 min following 0.5 gm. **t½:** 4–8 hr for adults and 2–3 hrs for children. The half-life is markedly increased in the presence of renal impairment (240 hr has been noted). Primarily excreted in urine unchanged. Auditory and renal function tests are indicated before and during therapy.

Uses Agent should be reserved to treat life-threatening infections where other treatments have been ineffective. Patients with severe staphylococci infections resistant or allergic to penicillin or cephalosporins such as endocarditis, osteomyelitis, pneumonia, and septicemia. Oral administration is useful in treatment of enterocolitis and pseudomembranous colitis.

Contraindications Hypersensitivity to drug. Minor infections. Use with extreme caution in the presence of impaired renal function or previous hearing loss.

Untoward Reactions Ototoxicity (may lead to deafness), nephrotoxicity (may lead to uremia). *Red-neck syndrome:* Chills, erythema of neck and back, fever, paresthesia. *Dermatologic:* Urticaria, macular rashes. *Allergic:* Drug fever, hypersensitivity, anaphylaxis. *Other:* Nausea, tinnitus, eosinophilia, neutropenia, hypotension (due to rapid administration). Thrombophlebitis at site of injection. Deafness may progress after drug is discontinued.

Drug Interactions Never give with other ototoxic or nephrotoxic agents especially aminoglycosides and polymyxins.

Dosage **IV, PO**: **Adults,** 0.5–1 gm q 6–12 hr; **pediatric**, 44 mg/kg/day in divided doses. *Prophylaxis of bacterial endocarditis* (in combination with other antibiotics): **IV, Adults**, 1 gm 30–60 min before procedure; **IV, pediatric**, 20 mg/kg 30–60 min before procedure. *Pseudomembranous colitis:* **PO, Adults**, 0.5–2 gm daily in 3–4 divided doses for 7–10 days; **pediatric,** 44 mg/kg daily in divided doses. Dosage must be reduced in patients with renal disease.

Administration/Storage

1. Mix as indicated on package insert.
2. Intermittent infusion is the preferred route, but continuous IV drip may be used.
3. Avoid rapid IV administration, as this may result in nausea, warmth, and generalized tingling.
4. Avoid extravasation during injections.
5. Reduce risk of thrombophlebitis by rotating injection sites or adding additional diluent.
6. Dilute one 500-mg vial in 1 oz of water for oral administration. Patient may drink solution or it may be administered by nasogastric tube.
7. Aqueous solution is stable for 2 weeks.
8. Once rubber stopper is punctured, ampule should be refrigerated to maintain stability.

Nursing Implications
See *Nursing Implications* for *Anti-infectives*, p. 52.
Assess

a. for ototoxicity demonstrated by tinnitus, progressive hearing loss, dizziness, and/or nystagmus.
b. for nephrotoxicity demonstrated by albuminuria, hematuria, anuria, casts, edema, and uremia.
c. intake and output.

Chapter 10

ANTIFUNGAL AGENTS

General Statement   Several types of fungi or yeasts are pathogenic for humans. Some fungal infections are systemic, and others are limited to the skin, hair, or nails. A third group infects mostly moist mucous membranes, including the GI tract and vagina. *Candida* organisms belong to this last group.

Drug therapy depends both on the infectious agent and on the type of infection. An accurate diagnosis of the infection, before therapy, is most important for the choice of the therapeutic agents.

As in other infections, it is important that drug therapy be continued until the infectious agent has been completely eradicated to avoid the emergence of resistant strains.

ACRISORCIN Akrinol (Rx)

Classification   Antifungal, topical.

Uses   Superficial fungal (tinae versicolor) infections characterized by multiple macular patches caused by *Malassezia furfur*.

Contraindications   Hypersensitivity to drug or to any component of preparation. Avoid use around eyes. Patient should avoid exposure to prolonged sunlight.

Untoward Reactions   *Dermatologic:* Hypersensitivity, photosensitivity, blisters, erythematous vesicular eruptions, hives.

Dosage   Rub gently a small amount of 0.2% cream to affected area b.i.d. (AM and PM) for a minimum of 6 weeks.

Additional Nursing Implications

See *Nursing Implications* for *Anti-infectives*, p. 52.

1. Assist with establishing diagnosis by describing lesions and obtaining scrapings of lesions, because a technique for culture of organism does not exist.

2. *Teach patient and/or family to*
   a. avoid exposure of affected area to sun or ultraviolet light.
   b. report symptoms of sensitivity, such as blisters or erythema.
   c. report any worsening of symptoms.
   d. take warm, soapy bath and to scrub lesion with stiff brush before evening dose.
   e. remove soap completely and dry lesion with towel before applying cream, because soap can reduce the antifungal activity of drug.
   f. launder clothing daily and change linen in contact with lesion.

AMPHOTERICIN B   Fungizone, Fungizone IV (Rx)

Classification   Antibiotic, antifungal.

General Statement   This antibiotic is produced by *Streptomyces nodosus* and is the drug of choice for deep infections. It can be administered IV, instilled into cavities (intrathecally), and used topically. Depending on the dose, amphotericin B is fungistatic or fungicidal. It is effective against most pathogenic fungi, including North American blastomycosis.

The drug is very toxic and should only be used for patients under close medical supervision with a relatively certain diagnosis of deep mycotic infections. IV administration is usually reserved for life-threatening disease.

Action/Kinetics   Amphotericin B binds to specific chemical structures—sterols—of fungal cellular membrane, increasing cellular permeability and promoting loss of potassium and other substances. Amphotericin B is poorly absorbed from GI tract. It is highly bound to serum protein (90%). t½: 24 hr. **Peak plasma levels**: 2–4 μg/ml. Slowly excreted by kidneys.

Uses   Disseminated North American blastomycosis, cryptococcosis, and other systemic fungal infections, including coccidioidomycosis, paracoccid ioidomycosis, histoplasmosis, aspergillosis, disseminated candidiasis, and monilial overgrowth resulting from oral antibiotic therapy. Topical: cutaneous and mucocutaneous infections of *Candida (Monilia)* infections.

Contraindication   Hypersensitivity to drug.

Untoward Reactions   **After topical use.** Irritation, pruritus, dry skin. **After systemic use.** *GI:* Nausea, vomiting, diarrhea, dyspepsia, anorexia, abdominal cramps, melena, gastroenteritis. *CNS:* Fever, chills, headache, malaise, vertigo, seizures (rare). *CV:* Thrombophlebitis, phlebitis. Rarely, arrhythmias, hyper- or hypotension, ventricular fibrillation, cardiac arrest. *Renal:* Anuria, oliguria, azotemia, hypokalemia, renal tubular acidosis, nephrocalcinosis, hyposthenuria. *Hematologic:* Anemia, thrombocytopenia, leukopenia, agranulocytosis, eosinophila, leukocytosis. *Other:* Muscle and joint pain, weight loss, tinnitus, blurred or double vision, peripheral neuropathy, hearing loss, hepatic failure, pruritus, rashes, flushing, anaphylaxis.

Side effects may be reduced by aspirin, antiemetics, antihistamines, and corticosteroids. Sodium balance should be maintained.

Drug Interactions

Interactant	Interaction
Aminoglycosides	Additive nephrotoxicity and/or ototoxicity
Corticosteroids, Corticotropin	↑ K depletion caused by amphotericin B

Interactant	Interaction
Digitalis glycosides	↑ K depletion caused by amphotericin B; ↑ Incidence of digitalis toxicity
Flucytosine	Synergistic antifungal effect
Miconazole	Amphotericin B ↓ effect of miconazole
Rifampin	Synergistic antifungal effect
Skeletal muscle relaxants (surgical) Succinylcholine d-Tubocurarine	↑ Muscle relaxation
Tetracyclines	Synergistic antifungal effect

Laboratory Test Interferences ↑SGPT, SGOT, alkaline phosphatase, creatinine, BUN, NPN, BSP retention values.

Dosage   Slow IV infusion, initial: 0.25 mg/kg/day. May be increased gradually by 0.1–0.2 mg/kg/day, up to a maximum dose of 1.0 mg/kg/day to 1.5 mg/kg every other day. A test dose (1 mg) should be given first to assess patient tolerance. Depending on use, treatment may be required for several months. **Topical (lotion, cream, ointment—each 3%)**: apply liberally to affected areas b.i.d.–q.i.d.

Administration/Storage

1. Follow directions on vial for dilution. Only use distilled water without a bacteriostatic agent or 5% dextrose as diluent in order to avoid precipitation of drug.
2. Strict aseptic technique must be used in preparation as there is no bacteriostatic agent in the medication.
3. Use sterile #20 gauge needle every time entrance is made into the vial.
4. Do not use saline solution or distilled water with bacteriostatic agent as a diluent, since a precipitate may result.
5. Do not use the initial concentrate if there is any precipitate.
6. An in-line membrane filter with a pore diameter > 1 micron may be used.
7. Protect from light during administration and storage.
8. Minimize local inflammation and danger of thrombophlebitis by administering the solution below the recommended dilution of 0.1 mg.
9. Initiate therapy in the most distal veins.
10. Have on hand 200–400 units of heparin sodium, since it may be ordered for the infusion to prevent thrombophlebitis.
11. Administer the IV for 6 hr.
12. Amphotericin may be stored after reconstitution for 24 hr in a dark room or in a refrigerator for 1 week without significant loss of potency.
13. Use dilutions of 0.1 mg/ml immediately after preparation.

Additional Nursing Implications

See *Nursing Implications* for *Anti-infectives*, p. 52.

1. Interrupt IV and notify physician should patient develop adverse reaction during administration.
2. Ascertain whether physician wants patient to have antipyretics, antihistamines, or antiemetics prior to IV therapy.

3. Check that weekly BUN, NPN, and potassium levels have been determined. Ascertain that the physician is aware of any untoward results.
4. *Assess*
   a. patient also on digitalis therapy, for muscle weakness, a sign of hypokalemia; have potassium chloride available to treat hypokalemia.
   b. vital signs every half-hour during IV administration and at least daily while patient is on therapy.
   c. intake and output and report reduction in urine output and blood sediment, or cloudiness in the urine.
   d. for signs of malnutrition and dehydration; weigh patient twice weekly.
   e. for sensory loss or foot drop in patients receiving intrathecal amphotericin, because inflammation of the spinal roots may occur.

Administration   (Creams and Lotions) Rub into lesion.

Additional Nursing Implications
See *Nursing Implications* for *Anti-infectives*, p. 52.
Teach patient and/or family
   a. that drug does not stain skin when it is rubbed into lesion.
   b. that any discoloration of fabric caused by cream or lotion may be removed by washing with soap and water.
   c. that any discoloration caused by ointment may be removed with a standard cleaning fluid.

CICLOPIROX OLAMINE   Loprox (Rx)

Classification   Antifungal, topical.

Action/Kinetics   Broad-spectrum fungicide effective against dermatophytes, yeast, *Malassezia furfur, Trichophyton rubrum, T. mentagrophytes, Epidermophyton floccosum, Microsporu canis,* and *Candida albicans.* A small amount of drug is absorbed through the skin; it also penetrates into the hair.

Uses   Tinea pedis, tinea corporis, tinea cruris, candidiasis (moniliasis), tinea versicolor.

Contraindications   Safety and efficacy in pregnancy, lactation, and children under 10 years of age not established.

Untoward Reactions   Rarely, pruritus or exacerbation of condition.

Dosage   Apply morning and evening into the affected and surrounding skin. If no improvement after 4 weeks, diagnosis should be reevaluated.

Administration
   1. Even though symptoms have improved, the drug should be used for the full prescribed time.

2. The physician should be notified if the area of application shows blistering, burning, itching, oozing, redness, or swelling.
3. Occlusive dressings or wrappings should not be used.

Nursing Implications

If drug is used for suspected *Malassezia furfur* infection, assist with establishing diagnosis by describing lesions and obtaining scraping of lesion because a technique for culture of organism does not exist.

CLOTRIMAZOLE   Canesten,* Gyne-Lotrimin, Lotrimin, Mycelex, Mycelex-G, Myclo* (Rx)

Classification   Antifungal.

Action/Kinetics   Broad-spectrum antifungal effective against *Malassezia furfur, Trichophyton rubrum, T. mentagrophytes, Epidermophyton floccosum, Microsporum canis, Candida albicans.*

Uses   Tinea pedis, tinea cruris, tinea corporis, tinea versicolor, and candidiasis.

Contraindications   Hypersensitivity. First trimester of pregnancy.

Untoward Reactions   *Skin:* Irritation of skin including stinging, pruritus, urticaria, erythema, peeling, blistering, edema. *Vaginal:* Lower abdominal cramps, urinary frequency, bloating.

Dosage   Topical: Massage into affected skin and surrounding areas b.i.d. in AM and PM. Diagnosis should be reevaluated if no improvement in 4 weeks. **Vaginal Tablets:** One tablet/day at bedtime for 7 days; or, 1 tablet b.i.d. for 3 days. **Vaginal Cream:** 5 gm (1 applicatorful)/day at bedtime for 7–14 days.

Administration
1. Unless directed by physician to do otherwise, apply after cleaning the affected area.
2. If treating vaginal infections, the patient should not engage in intercourse; or, to prevent infection, the partner should wear a condom.
3. To prevent staining of clothes, a sanitary napkin should be used with vaginal tablets or cream.

ECONAZOLE NITRATE   Ecostatin,* Spectazole (Rx)

Classification   Antifungal, topical.

Action/Kinetics   Broad-spectrum fungicide effective against *Microsporum audouini, M. canis, M. gypseum, Epidermophyton floccosum, Trichophyton mentagrophytes, T. rubrum, T. tonsurans, Candida albicans, Pityrosporum oriculare,* and some gram positive bacteria. Effective concentrations are found in the stratum corneum, epidermis, and the dermis.

Uses   Tinea cruris, tinea corporis, tinea pedis, cutaneous candidiasis, tinea versicolor.

Contraindications   Use with caution in pregnancy and lactation.

Untoward Reactions   *Topical:* Burning, erythema, itching, stinging.

Dosage   Except for tinea versicolor, cream should be applied in the morning and evening. *Tinea versicolor:* Apply once daily. If no improvement after recommended treatment period, diagnosis should be reevaluated.

Administration

1. To reduce chance of reinfection, tinea pedis should be treated for 1 month and tinea cruris, tinea corporis, and candidial infections should be treated for 2 weeks.
2. The drug should be used for the full prescribed time even though symptoms have improved.
3. The physician should be notified if condition worsens or symptoms of burning, itching, redness, and stinging occur.
4. Unless otherwise directed, cream should be applied after cleaning the affected area.

FLUCYTOSINE   Ancobon, Ancotil* (Rx)

Classification   Antibiotic, antifungal.

Action/Kinetics   Indicated only for serious systemic fungal infections. The drug is less toxic than amphotericin B. Liver, renal system, and hematopoetic system must be closely monitored.

Flucytosine appears to penetrate the fungal cell and then, after metabolism, to act as an antimetabolite interfering with nucleic acid and protein synthesis. Well absorbed from GI tract. **Peak plasma concentration**: 2–6 hr. **Therapeutic serum concentration**: 20–25 μg/ml. **t½**: 2.5–6 hr, higher in presence of impaired renal function. Ninety percent of drug excreted unchanged in urine.

Uses   Serious systemic infections by susceptible strains of *Candida* or *Cryptococcus*.

Contraindications   Hypersensitivity to drug. Use with extreme caution in patients with kidney disease or history of bone marrow depression.

Untoward Reactions   *GI:* Nausea, vomiting, diarrhea. *Hematologic:* Anemia, leukopenia, thrombocytopenia. *CNS:* Headache, vertigo, drowsiness, confusion, hallucinations. *Other:* Increase in BUN, creatinine, and liver enzymes.

Dosage   **PO, adult and children** : 50–150 mg/kg daily in 4 divided doses. Patients with renal impairment receive lower dosages.

Administration   Reduce or avoid nausea by administering capsules a few at a time over a 15 min period.

Additional Nursing Implications

See *Nursing Implications* for *Anti-infectives*, p. 52.

1. Before administering first dose, check that culture has been taken.
2. Ascertain that weekly cultures are taken to determine that strains have not become resistant. Strain is considered resistant if MIC (minimal inhibitory concentration) value is greater than 100.
3. Monitor input and output. Report reduction in urine output as well as blood, sediment, or cloudiness in the urine.

GRISEOFULVIN MICROSIZE   Fulvicin-U/F, Grifulvin V, Grisactin (Rx)

GRISEOFULVIN ULTRAMICROSIZE   Fulvicin-P/G, Grisactin Ultra, Gris-Peg (Rx)

Classification   Antibiotic, antifungal.

General Statement   Griseofulvin is a natural antibiotic derived from a species of *Penicillium*. It is the only oral drug effective against dermatophytic (tinae ringworm) infections. When taken systemically, the drug is deposited in the newly formed skin and nails, which are then resistant to reinfection by the tinae. The drug is not effective against *Candida*. Susceptibility of the infectious agent should be established before treatment is begun.

Action/Kinetics   Believed to interfere with cell division (metaphase) or DNA replication. Absorbed from duodenum. **Peak plasma concentration**: 0.37–2 μg/ml after 4 hr. **t½**: 9–24 hr. Levels may be increased by giving the drug with a high-fat diet.

Uses   Tinae (ringworm) infections of skin including athlete's foot, and infections of the scalp, groin, and nails.

Contraindications   Porphyria or history thereof, hepatocellular failure, and hypersensitivity to drug. Exposure to artificial or sunlight.

Untoward Reactions   *Hypersensitivity:* Rashes, urticaria, angioneurotic edema, allergic reactions. *GI:* Nausea, vomiting, diarrhea, epigastric pain. *CNS:* Dizziness, headache, tiredness, confusion, insomnia. *Other:* Oral thrush, acute intermittent porphyria, paresthesias of extremities, proteinuria, leukopenia.

Drug Interactions

Interactant	Interaction
Alcohol, ethyl	Tachycardia and flushing with griseofulvin
Anticoagulants, oral	↓ Effect of anticoagulants due to ↑ breakdown in liver
Barbiturates	↓ Effect of griseofulvin due to ↓ absorption from GI tract

Laboratory Test Interferences   ↑SGPT, SGOT, alkaline phosphatase, BUN, and creatinine level values.

Dosage   PO. Adults: *Tinea corporis, cruris, or capitis:* 0.5 gm griseofulvin microsize daily in single or divided doses. *Tinea pedis or unguium:* 0.75–1 gm daily of griseofulvin microsize. After response, decrease dose to 0.5 gm daily. **Pediatric, 30–50 lb:** 125–250 mg griseofulvin microsize daily; **pediatric, over 50 lb:** 250–500 mg microsize daily.

Administration   Length of treatment varies from 1 month to 1 year.

Additional Nursing Implications
See *Nursing Implications* for *Anti-infectives*, p. 52.
Teach patient and/or family to

a. eat a diet high in fat, since this enhances the absorption of griseofulvin from the intestines.

b. take all medication prescribed, to prevent recurrence of infection.

c. practice appropriate hygiene to prevent reinfection.

d. avoid exposure to intense natural and artificial light, since photosensitivity reactions may occur.

e. report fever, sore throat, and malaise, which are all symptomatic of leukopenia.

f. understand that to be considered cured repeated cultures and scrapings of affected site(s) must be negative.

HALOPROGIN   Halotex (Rx)

Classification   Antifungal, topical.

Uses   Topical treatment of fungal infections of feet (tinea pedis), male genital region (tinea cruris), smooth skin surfaces (tinea corporis), and hand (tinea manuum) caused by *Trichophyton rubrun, T. tonsurans, T. mentagrophytes, Microsporum canis,* and *Epidermophyton floccosum.* Also, multiple macular patches (tinea versicolor) caused by *Malassezia furfur.*

   If drug ineffective after 4 weeks of treatment, reevaluate diagnosis and therapy. Presence of mixed infections or resistant fungi may indicate need for systemic therapy.

Contraindications   Hypersensitivity to drug or to any component of preparations. *Avoid contact around eyes.* Safe use during pregnancy not established.

Untoward Reactions   *Topical:* Local irritation, burning sensation, pruritus, exacerbation of preexisting lesions.

Dosage   Apply 1% cream or solution liberally to lesions b.i.d. for 2–3 weeks. Interdigital lesions may require therapy for 4 weeks.

Additional Nursing Implications
See *Nursing Implications* for *Anti-infectives*, p. 52.
Teach patient and/or family to

a. discontinue application of cream and to report to doctor if local irritation, burning sensation, or worsening of condition is noted.

b. use proper technique of application.

c. continue both haloprogin and additional anti-infective if ordered concomitantly.

d. return to medical supervision if drug is ineffective after 4 weeks.

IODOCHLORHYDROXYQUIN   Torofor, Vioform (OTC)

Classification   Antibacterial, antifungal.

Uses   Topical fungal infections including athlete's food and eczema.

Untoward Reactions   Itching, irritation, redness, swelling of skin.

Laboratory Test Interference   Thyroid function tests if absorbed through skin.

Dosage   Apply b.i.d.–t.i.d. not over 1 week.

Administration   The drug may stain skin, hair, or clothing.

KETOCONAZOLE   Nizoral (Rx)

Classification   Broad-spectrum antifungal.

Action/Kinetics   Ketoconazole inhibits synthesis of ergosterol, a vital component of cell membranes of fungi. **Peak plasma levels**: 3.5 μg/ml after 1-2 hr. **t½** (biphasic): first, 2 hr; second, 8 hr. Requires acidity for dissolution. Metabolized in liver and most excreted through feces.

Uses   Candidiasis, chronic mucocutaneous candidiasis, candiduria, histoplasmosis, chromomycosis, oral thrush, coccidioidomycosis, paracoccidioidomycosis. Should not be used for fungal meningitis due to poor penetration to the CSF.

Contraindications   Hypersensitivity, fungal meningitis.

Untoward Reactions   *GI:* Nausea, vomiting, abdominal pain, diarrhea. *CNS:* Headache, dizziness, somnolence, fever, chills. *Other:* Hepatotoxicity, photophobia, pruritus, gynecomastia, impotence, thrombocytopenia.

Drug Interactions

Interactant	Interaction
Antacids, Anticholinergics, Cimetidine	↓ Absorption of ketoconazole due to ↑ pH induced by these drugs

Laboratory Test Interference   Transient ↑ serum liver enzymes.

Dosage   **PO. Adults:** 200-400 mg as single dose/day. **Pediatric, over 2 yr:** 3.3-6.6 mg/kg daily. Pediatric dosage in children less than 2 yr of age not established.

Administration

1. Minimum treatment for candidiasis is 1-2 weeks, while minimum treatment for other systemic mycoses is 6 months.
2. Ketoconazole should be given a minimum of 2 hr before administration of drugs that increase gastric pH (such as antacids, anticholinergics, or H_2 blockers).
3. Teach patient with achlorhydria to dissolve each tablet in 4 ml aqueous solution of 0.2 N HCl, and to use a straw (glass or plastic) to take this solution so as to avoid contact with teeth. This is followed by drinking a glass of tap water.

Additional Nursing Implications
See *Nursing Implications* for *Anti-Infectives*, p. 52.
Teach patient and/or family

a. to use caution when driving or performing hazardous tasks because drug can cause headaches, dizziness and drowsiness.
b. to report persistent fever, pain or diarrhea.

MICONAZOLE   Micatin, Monistat 7, Monistat-Derm, Monistat I.V. (Rx except for Micatin which is OTC)

Classification   Antifungal agent.

Action/Kinetics   Miconazole is a broad-spectrum fungicide that alters the permeability of the fungal membrane. **Peak blood levels**: 1 μg/ml. The drug is eliminated in 3 phases; **t½ of each phase**: 0.4, 2.1, and 24 hr. More than 90% of miconazole is bound to serum proteins. Excretion of the drug is unaltered in patients with renal insufficiency, including patients on hemodialysis.

Uses Systemic fungal infections caused by coccidioidomycosis, candidiasis, cryptococcosis, paracoccidioidomycosis, chronic mucocutaneous candidiasis. When used for the treatment of either fungal meningitis or urinary bladder infection, IV infusion must be supplemented with intrathecal administration or bladder irrigation of the drug. *Investigationally*: As ointment for treatment of athlete's foot, and vaginal infections.

Contraindications Hypersensitivity. Safe use in pregnancy and in children less than 1 year of age has not been established.

Untoward Reactions **Following topical use:** Burning, irritation, maceration. **Following systemic use.** *GI:* Nausea, vomiting, diarrhea, anorexia. *Hematologic:* Thrombocytopenia, aggregation of erythrocytes, rouleau formation on blood smears. Transient decrease in hematocrit. *Dermatologic:* Pruritus, rash, flushing. *CV:* Transient tachycardia or arrhythmias following rapid injection of undiluted drug. *Other:* Fever, drowsiness, transient decrease in serum sodium values. Hyperlipemia due to the vehicle (PEG 40 and castor oil).

Drug Interactions

Interactant	Interaction
Amphotericin B	Amphotericin B ↓ activity of miconazole
Coumarin anticoagulants	Miconazole ↑ anticoagulant effect

Dosage **IV infusion, adults**: 200–3,600 mg/day in divided doses depending on the specific organism; **pediatric**: total daily dose, 20–40 mg/kg in divided doses; a dose of 15 mg/kg/infusion should not be exceeded. **Intrathecal**: 20 mg/dose of the undiluted solution as an adjunct to **IV** therapy. **Bladder instillation**: 200 mg of diluted solution as adjunct treatment of fungal infections of urinary bladder. **Topical**: Apply to cover affected areas in AM and PM (once daily for tinea versicolor). **Vaginal**: One applicatorful daily at bedtime for 7 days.

Administration

1. IV therapy may be required from 1 to more than 20 weeks, depending on the organism.
2. For IV infusion, the drug should be diluted in at least 200 ml of either 0.9% sodium chloride or 5% dextrose solution and administered over a period of 30 to 60 min.
3. Succeeding intrathecal injections should be alternated between lumbar, cervical, or cisternal punctures every 3 to 7 days.

Nursing Implications
See *Nursing Implications* for *Anti-infectives*, p. 52.

1. Provide symptomatic treatment for nausea, vomiting, diarrhea, dizziness, and pruritus.
2. Assess for redness and pain at site of IV infusion.

NATAMYCIN   Natacyn (Rx)

Classification   Antifungal (ophthalmic).

General Statement   Natamycin is an antifungal antibiotic derived from *Streptomyces natalensis*. It is active against a variety of yeasts and filamentous fungi including *Candida, Aspergillus, Cephalosporium, Fusarium*, and *Penicillium*. Before initiating therapy, it is advisable to determine susceptibility of infectious organism to drug in smears and cultures of corneal scrapings. Since experience with natamycin is still limited, tolerance to drug should be assessed twice weekly. Discontinue drug if toxicity is suspected. Review therapy if no improvement noted after 7 to 10 days.

Action/Kinetics   Binding of drug to fungal cell membrane resulting in alteration of metabolism of infectious agent. Fungicidal. The drug reaches therapeutic levels, after topical administration, in the corneal stroma, but not in the intraocular fluid. Not absorbed systemically.

Uses   For ophthalmic use only. Drug of choice for *F. solani* keratitis. For treatment of fungal blepharitis, conjunctivitis, and keratitis caused by susceptible organisms. Effectiveness of natamycin for use as single agent in fungal endophthalmitis not established.

Contraindications   Hypersensitivity to drug. Safe use in pregnancy not established.

Untoward Reaction   Occasional allergies.

Dosage   Ophthalmic: *Fungal keratitis*: Initial, 1 gtt of 5% suspension in conjunctival sac q 1–2 hr; can usually be reduced, after 3–4 days, to 1 gtt 6–8 times/day. Continue therapy for 14–21 days, during which dosage can be reduced gradually at 4–7-day intervals. *Blepharitis/conjunctivitis*: 1 gtt 4–6 times daily.

Administration/Storage   Store natamycin at room temperature or in refrigerator. Shake well before using. Avoid contamination of dropper.

Additional Nursing Implications
See also *Nursing Implications* for *Anti-infectives*, p. 52.
Teach patient and/or family

a. initially to return for medical supervision at least twice weekly.
b. proper administration technique.
c. to continue therapy for 14–21 days as ordered, even though condition might appear to be under control.

NYSTATIN   Candex, Korostatin, Mycostatin, Nadostine,* Nilstat, Nyaderm,* O-V Statin (Rx)

Classification   Antibiotic, antifungal.

General Statement   This natural antifungal antibiotic is derived from *Streptomyces noursei* and is both fungistatic and fungicidal against all species of *Candida*. The drug is too toxic for systemic infections. It can be given PO for intestinal moniliasis infections but is not absorbed from the GI tract. These infections occur rarely, however.

Note: Nystatin is combined with tetracycline to prevent fungal superinfections from the latter. An example is the product Terrastatin.

Action/Kinetics   Nystatin binds to fungal cell membranes (sterols), resulting in altered cellular permeability and leakage of potassium and other essential intracellular components. Nystatin is excreted in the feces.

Uses   *Candida albicans* infections of the skin, mucous membranes, GI tract, vagina, and mouth (thrush).

Untoward Reactions   Nystatin has few toxic effects. Large oral doses may cause epigastric distress, nausea, vomiting, and diarrhea.

Dosage   PO. *Intestinal candidiasis:* **Tablets,** 500,000–1,000,000 units t.i.d.; continue treatment for 48 hr after cure to prevent relapse. *Oral candidiasis:* **Oral suspension, adults and children:** 400,000–600,000 units q.i.d. (½ dose in each side of mouth held as long as possible before swallowing); **infants:** 200,000 units q.i.d. (same procedure as adults); **premature or low birth weight infants:** 100,000 units q.i.d. **Vaginal tablets:** 100,000 units (1 tablet) inserted in vagina each day for 2 weeks. **Topical (ointment, cream, lotion, powder**—contains 100,000 units/ml or gm): apply to affected areas b.i.d.–t.i.d., or as indicated until healing is complete; continue use for 1 week after clinical cure.

Administration/Storage

1. Protect drug from heat, light, moisture, and air.
2. Do not mix oral suspension in foods since the medication will be inactivated.
3. The suspension can be stored for 7 days at room temperature or for 10 days in the refrigerator without loss of potency.
4. Apply nystatin ointment to mycotic lesions with a swab.
5. Drop 1 ml of oral suspension in each side of mouth or apply with a swab to treat oral moniliasis. Instruct patient to keep medication in mouth as long as possible before swallowing.
6. Insert vaginal tablets high in vagina with an applicator.

Additional Nursing Implications

See *Nursing Implications* for *Anti-infectives*, p. 52.

1. Continue administration of medication for at least 48 hr after symptoms have disappeared. Anticipate that vaginal tablets may be continued in the gravid patient for 3 to 6 weeks before term to reduce incidence of thrush in the newborn.
2. *Teach patient and/or family to*
   a. continue using vaginal tablets even when menstruating since the treatment should be continued for 2 weeks.
   b. discontinue medication and to report to physician, should vaginal tablets cause irritation.

TOLNAFTATE   Aftate, Tinactin (OTC)

Classification   Topical antifungal.

Uses   Tinea pedis, tinea cruris, tinea corporis, tinea manuum, and tinea versicolor.

Contraindications   Scalp and nail infections. *Avoid getting into eyes.*

Untoward Reactions Mild skin irritation.

Dosage Apply b.i.d. for 2–3 weeks although treatment for 4–6 weeks may be necessary in some instances. Available in a number of forms including: *Aerosol (Liquid or Powder), Cream, Gel, Liquid, Powder, Solution.*

Administration
1. Discontinue use if improvement not noted within 10 days.
2. Concomitant therapy should be used if bacterial or *Candida* infections are also present.
3. The choice of vehicle is important for effective therapy.
   a. Powders are used in mild conditions, as adjunctive therapy, with creams, liquids, or ointments.
   b. For prophylaxis, creams, liquids or ointments are used, especially if the area is moist.
   c. Liquids and solutions are used if the area is hairy.

TRIACETIN Enzactin, Fungacetin, Fungoid (Rx: Fungoid; OTC: Enzactin, Fungacetin)

Classification Antifungal.

Uses Topical fungal infections including athlete's foot.

Dosage Apply to affected area b.i.d.

Administration
1. Use dilute alcohol or mild soap and water to clean affected areas prior to use.
2. After symptoms disappear, use for an additional week.

UNDECYLENIC ACID AND DERIVATIVES Caldesene, Cruex, Decylenes, Desenex, Devine's Kool Foot, NP-27, Quinsana Plus, Ting, Undoguent (OTC)

Classification Antibacterial, antifungal.

Uses Minor skin irritations including diaper rash, burning, prickly heat, chafing, jock itch. Athlete's foot, ringworm.

Contraindictions Use on pustular or broken skin. In diabetics or in impaired circulation unless directed by the physician. *Avoid contact with eyes and mucous membranes.*

Dosage Apply as needed to affected area. Available in a number of forms including: *Cream, Foam, Liquid, Ointment, Powder, Soap, Solution.*

Administration
1. Affected area should be clean and dry prior to application of medication.
2. The choice of vehicle is important for effective therapy. (See Administration, Tolnaftate).

Chapter Eleven

SULFONAMIDES/SULFONES

SULFONAMIDES

General Statement   The sulfonamides are synthetic, bacteriostatic agents that have a wide range of antimicrobial activity against gram-positive and gram-negative organisms. At high concentrations, some are bactericidal.

Sulfonamides are poorly soluble, weak acids. They form salts with bases. The sodium salts are very soluble in water.

It is always desirable to determine the susceptibility of the pathogen before, or soon after, initiation of therapy.

Sulfonamides have the advantage of being relatively inexpensive.

Action/Kinetics   The sulfonamides interfere with the utilization of para-aminobenzoic acid (PABA), required by bacteria for growth; thus sulfonamides halt multiplication of bacteria but do not kill fully formed microorganisms.

The various sulfonamides are absorbed and excreted at widely differing rates. This has an important bearing on their therapeutic use. For instance agents that are poorly absorbed from the GI tract are particularly indicated for intestinal infections because they remain localized in the intestine for a long time.

Sulfonamides are absorbed into the bloodstream and distributed throughout all tissues, including the CSF, where concentrations attain 50 to 80% of that found in the blood. The sulfonamides are primarily excreted by the kidneys.

Uses   The range of usefulness of the sulfonamides has been greatly reduced by the emergence of resistant strains of bacteria and the development of more effective antibiotics.

Acute, nonobstructive urinary tract infections caused by *E. coli, Klebsiella, Enterobacter, S. aureus, P. mirabilis, P. vulgaris.* Drug of choice for nocardiosis. Elimination of meningococci from the nasopharynx in asymptomatic *N. meningitidis* carriers. As an alternative to penicillin for prophylaxis of rheumatic fever.

As an alternative to tetracyclines for chlamydial infections or for trachoma and inclusion conjunctivitis. In conjunction with pyrimethamine for toxoplasmosis. In combination with quinine sulfate and pyrimethamine for chloroquine-resistant *Plasmodium falciparum.* In combination with penicillin for otitis media. Also, see individual drugs.

Contraindications   Except for hypersensitivity reactions, there are few absolute contraindications. Sulfonamides, however, are potentially dangerous drugs and cause a 5% overall incidence of major and minor untoward reactions.

Sulfonamides should be used with caution, and in reduced dosage, in patients with impaired liver or renal function, intestinal or urinary tract obstructions, blood dyscrasias, allergies, asthma, and hereditary glucose 6-phosphate dehydrogenase deficiency.

Sulfonamides may cause mental retardation and should never be administered during the third term of pregnancy, to nursing mothers, or infants under 2 months of age, except for the treatment of congenital toxoplasmosis (a serious parasitic disease that can cause brain inflammation) or in life-threatening situations.

Untoward Reactions   *GI:* Nausea, vomiting, diarrhea, abdominal pain, glossitis, stomatitis, anorexia, pancreatitis. *Allergic:* Rash, pruritus, photosensitivity, erythema nodosum or multiforme, Stevens–Johnson syndrome, conjunctivitis, rhinitis, balanitis. Serum sickness, disseminated lupus erythematosis, periarteritis nodosa, arteritis. *CNS:* Headaches, dizziness, mental depression, ataxia, confusion, psychoses, drowsiness, restlessness. *Renal:* Renal damage due to precipitation of sulfonamide or its acetyl derivative in the tubules. Manifested by crystalluria, hematuria, oliguria. *Hematologic:* Acute hemolytic anemia especially in glucose 6-phosphate dehydrogenase deficiency, aplastic anemia, granulocytopenia, leukopenia, eosinophilia, agranulocytosis, thrombocytopenia, methemoglobinemia. *Miscellaneous:* Jaundice, hypoglycemia, arthralgia, acidosis, periorbital edema, purpura, superinfection.

By killing the intestinal flora, the sulfonamides also reduce the bacterial synthesis of vitamin K. This may result in hemorrhage. Administration of vitamin K to patients on long-term sulfonamide therapy is recommended.

Drug Interactions

Interactant	Interaction
Anesthetics, local	↓ Effect of sulfonamides
Antacids	↓ Effect of sulfonamides due to ↓ absorption from GI tract
Anticoagulants, oral	↑ Effect of anticoagulants due to ↓ in plasma protein binding
Antidiabetics, oral	↑ Hypoglycemic effect due to ↓ in plasma protein binding
Cyclosporine	↓ Effect of cyclosporine and ↑ nephrotoxicity
Methenamine	↑ Chance of sulfonamide crystalluria due to acid urine
Methotrexate	↑ Effect of methotrexate due to ↓ in plasma protein binding and ↓ renal tubular excretion
Oxacillin	↓ Effect of oxacillin due to ↓ absorption from GI tract
Paraldehyde	↑ Chance of sulfonamide crystalluria
Phenylbutazone	↑ Effect of sulfonamide by ↑ blood levels
Phenytoin	↑ Effect of phenytoin due to ↓ breakdown in liver

Interactant	Interaction
Probenecid	↑ Effect of sulfonamides by ↓ in plasma protein binding
Salicylates	↑ Effect of sulfonamides by ↑ blood levels

Laboratory Test Interferences False + or ↑ liver function tests (amino acids, bilirubin, BSP), renal function (BUN, NPN creatinine clearance), blood counts, prothrombin time, Coombs' test. Urine glucose (copper reduction methods, such as Benedict's or Clinitest), protein, urobilinogen.

Dosage See Table 3, p. 142. Sulfonamides are usually given PO. Dosage is adjusted individually. An initial loading dose is usually recommended. Short-acting compounds must be given every 4–6 hr.

Topical application of sulfonamides is rarely ordered today, except for Sulfamylon (mafenide), which is used as a 10% ointment to treat burn infections.

Creams of triple sulfa or sulfisoxazole are used for vaginitis.

When sulfonamides are given as adjuncts to GI surgery, medication is usually started 3–5 days before surgery, and for 1–2 weeks postoperatively, after peristalsis has resumed.

Nursing Implications
See *Nursing Implications* for *Anti-infectives*, p. 52.

1. Assess patient for the following untoward reactions that require the withdrawal of drug:
    a. skin rash.
    b. blood dyscrasias characterized by sore throat, fever, pallor, purpura, jaundice, or weakness.
    c. serum sickness characterized by eruptions of purpuric spots and pain in limbs and joints. Serum sickness may develop 7 to 10 days after initiation of therapy.
    d. early symptoms of Stevens–Johnson syndrome characterized by high fever, severe headaches, stomatitis, conjunctivitis, rhinitis, urethritis, and balanitis (inflammation of the tip of the penis).
    e. jaundice, which may indicate hepatic involvement, 3–5 days after initiation of therapy.
    f. renal involvement characterized by renal colic, oliguria, anuria, hematuria, and proteinuria.
    g. ecchymosis and hemorrhage caused by decreased synthesis of vitamin K by intestinal bacteria.
2. Test pH level of urine once a day with Labstix. Excess acidity, or administration of a particularly insoluble sulfonamide, may require alkalinization of urine. The drug of choice for this purpose is sodium bicarbonate.
3. Encourage adequate fluid intake to prevent crystalluria. Measure intake and output. Minimum output of urine should be 1,500 ml daily. For long-acting sulfonamides, adequate fluid intake must be maintained 24–48 hr after discontinuation of drug.
4. Question patient as to what other drugs are taken since numerous drug interference reactions have been reported. Check on possible interactions.
5. Question unusual order for long-acting sulfonamides.

(Continued on page 146)

TABLE 3 SULFONAMIDES

Drug	Main Use	Dosage	Remarks
Mafenide acetate (Sulfamylon Acetate) Rx	Topical application in the treatment of second- and third-degree burns (prevention of infections)	**Cream:** ¹⁄₁₆-in.-thick film applied over entire surface of burn with gloves once or twice daily until healing is progressing satisfactorily or until site is ready for grafting.	Do not use for already established infections. Unlike other sulfonamides, mafenide is not inhibited by pus or body fluids. *Additional Untoward Reactions* Burns treated with Sulfamylon are to be covered only with a thin dressing. Causes pain on application.
Silver sulfadiazine (Flamazine,* Silvadene) Rx	Topically for prevention and treatment of sepsis in second- and third-degree burns	Same as mafenide acetate.	*Administration* With a sterile glove apply ¹⁄₁₆-in. layer to all debrided, cleansed, burned areas 1–2 times daily or when ung. is accidentally removed. Dressings are not required. Continue application until healing occurs. The drug is absorbed from burn areas; thus, plasma concentration may reach therapeutic levels.
Sulfacetamide sodium (AK-Sulf, AK-Sulf Forte, Bleph-10 Liquifilm, Cetamide, Isopto Cetamide, Ophthacet, Sebizon, Sulf-10, Sulfacel-15, Sulten-10) Rx	Topically for ophthalmic infections including trachoma; seborrheic dermatitis; cutaneous bacterial infections	**Ophthalmic Solution:** 1–2 drops of 10%, 15%, or 30% solution in conjunctival sac several times daily. **Ophthalmic ointment (10%):** Apply 1–3 times daily in conjunctival sac. *For cutaneous infections:* Apply lotion (10%) to affected area b.i.d.–q.i.d. *Seborrheic dermatitis:* apply 1–2 times per day (for mild cases, apply overnight).	*Administration* When used for seborrheic dermatitis of the scalp, medication should be applied at bedtime and allowed to remain overnight. If hair and scalp are oily or if there is debris, precede application by shampooing.
Sulfacytine (Renoquid) Rx	Used only for acute nonobstructive urinary tract infections	**PO initial:** 500 mg: **maintenance:** 250 mg. q.i.d. for 10 days.	Short-acting. Protect tablets from heat, light, and moisture. Do not use in children under 14 years. t½: 4–4.5 hr
Sulfadiazine (Microsulfon) Rx Sulfadiazine Sodium Rx	Urinary tract infections, bacillary dysentery, rheumatic fever prophylaxis	**PO, Adults, initial:** 2–4 gm; **maintenance:** 2–4 gm daily in 3–6 divided doses; **pediatric over 2 months:** 75 mg/kg/day; **maintenance:** 150	Short acting. Often combined with other anti-infectives.

Drug	Use	Dose	Remarks
		mg/kg/day in 4–6 divided doses. *Rheumatic fever prophylaxis,* **under 30 kg:** 0.5 gm/day; **over 30 kg:** 1 gm/day.	Intermediate-acting.
Sulfamerazine Rx	Rarely used other than in combination with other sulfonamides	**PO, initial:** 3–4 gm; **maintenance:** 3–4 gm daily in 3–6 equally divided doses; **pediatric 3–10 years,** 1.5 gm initially; **then** 1 gm q 12 hr; **infants 6 months to 3 years:** 1 gm initially; **then** 0.5 gm q 12 hr; **infants under 6 months:** 0.5 gm initially; **then,** 0.25 gm q 12 hr.	
Sulfamethazine Rx	Rarely used other than in combination with other sulfonamides		Short-acting. Use of this agent alone for treatment of infections is at present uncommon.
Sulfamethizole (Microsul, Proklar, Thiosulfil, Thiosulfil Forte, Urifon) Rx	Urinary tract infections	**PO. Adults:** 0.5–1 gm t.i.d–q.i.d.; **pediatric over 2 months:** 30–45 mg/kg/day in 4 divided doses.	Short-acting. *Additional Drug Interaction* Sulfamethizole ↑ effects of tolbutamide, phenytoin, and chlorpropamide due to ↓ breakdown by liver.
Sulfamethoxazole (APO-Sulfamethoxazole, Gantanol, Gantanol DS, Urobak) Rx	Urinary and upper respiratory tract infections, lymphogranuloma venereum	**PO, Adults, initial:** 2 gm; **then,** 1 gm in AM and PM (for severe infections, give 3 gm daily). **Pediatric, (over 2 months), initial:** 50–60 mg/kg; **then,** 25–30 mg/kg AM and PM, not to exceed 75 mg/kg/day. *Lymphogranuloma venereum:* 1 gm b.i.d. for 2 weeks.	Intermediate-acting. (t½: 8.6 hrs) Also found in Bactrim, Bactrim DS, Septra, and Septra DS (*see* Appendix 3)
Sulfapyridine (Dagenan*) Rx	Dermatitis herpetiformis	**PO, initial:** 500 mg q.i.d., when improvement is noted, decrease by 500 mg daily at 3-day intervals, until symptom-free maintenance is	Intermediate-acting. Slowly and incompletely absorbed from GI tract. More toxic than other sulfonamides; seldom used.

TABLE 3 (*Continued*)

Drug	Main Use	Dosage	Remarks
Sulfasalazine (Azulfidine, Azulfidine En-Tabs, PMS Sulfasalazine,* Salazopyrin,* S.A.S.,* S.A.S.-500, Sulfadyne) Rx	Ulcerative colitis	achieved. Increase dosage if symptoms return. **PO. Adults: initial, 3–4 gm** daily in divided doses; **maintenance: 500 mg q.i.d.; pediatric, initial: 40–60 mg/kg** daily in 3–6 equally divided doses. **Maintenance: 30 mg/kg** daily in 4 equally divided doses. *For desensitization to sulfasalazine:* Reinstitute at level of 50–250 mg daily; **then,** double dose q 4–7 days until desired therapeutic level reached. Use oral suspension.	About ⅓ of the dose of sulfasalazine passes to the colon where it is split to 5-aminosalicylic acid and sulfapyridine. Intermittent therapy (2 wk on/2 wk off) is recommended. Drug does not affect microflora. *Additional Contraindications* Children below 5 years, persons with marked sulfonamide and salicylate hypersensitivity. *Additional Drug Interaction* 1. Sulfasalazine may ↓ effect of digoxin by ↓ its absorption. 2. Ferrous sulfate will ↓ blood levels of sulfasalazine.
Sulfisoxazole (Gantrisin, Koro-Sulf, Novosoxazole,* SK-Soxazole, Sulfizin) Rx Sulfisoxazole acetyl (Gantrisin, Lipo Gantrisin) Rx	Urinary tract infections, topical and ophthalmic infections	**PO, Adults, initial: 2–4 gm; maintenance: 4–8 gm daily** in 4–6 divided doses. **Pediatric over 2 months, initial: 75 mg/kg/day; maintenance: 150 mg/kg/day in 4–6** doses, up to maximum of 6 gm/day. Vaginal cream (10%): 2.5–5 gm inserted	Short acting. t½: 5.9 hr. Also found in Azo-Gantrisin *see* Appendix 3. Lipo-Gantrisin contains sulfisoxazole acetyl in a homogenized vegetable oil mixture. *Additional Drug Interaction:* Sulfisoxazole may ↑ effects of thiopental due to ↓ plasma protein binding. Switch to PO administration as soon as possible. For SC administration, dilute com-

mercial solution containing 400 mg/ml with sterile water for injection, to obtain solution containing 50 mg/ml.

Drug	Use	Dosage
Sulfisoxazole diolamine (Gantrisin Diolamine) Rx	Ophthalmic infections including trachoma	into vagina b.i.d. for 2 weeks. May be repeated. **IM, IV (slow injection or drip), SC: Initial,** 50 mg/kg; **then,** 100 mg/kg in 2–4 divided doses. **Ophthalmic solution (4%):** 1–2 drops into conjunctival sac several times daily. **Ophthalmic ointment (4%):** Small amount in conjunctival sac 1–3 times daily and at bedtime.
Sulfadiazine, Sulfamerazine, Sulfamethazine, (Neotrizine, Sulfaloid, Sul-Trio MM #2, Triple Sulfa #2) Rx	See individual drugs	**PO. Adults: initially,** 2–4 gm; **then,** 2–4 gm daily in divided doses. **Pediatric, over 2 months: initially,** 75 mg/kg; **then,** 150 mg/kg/day in 4–6 doses, not to exceed 6 gm daily.
Sulfathiazole, Sulfacetamide, Sulfabenzamide, (Sulfa-Gyn, Sultrin Triple Sulfa, Triple Sulfa, Trysul) Rx	Prophylaxis or treatment of cervical and vaginal infection	**Vaginal tablets:** 1 tablet inserted into the vagina b.i.d. for 10 days (may be repeated). **Vaginal cream:** One applicatorful b.i.d. for 4–6 days; **then,** reduce dosage to ¼–½.

6. *Teach patient and/or family*
    a. to report side effects and untoward symptoms.
    b. to take drug on time.
    c. that certain sulfonamides may color urine orange-red.
    d. to remain under medical supervision during course of therapy.
    e. to take medication with 6–8 oz (180–240 ml) of water and to maintain adequate fluid intake for 24–48 hr after discontinuation of drug.

SULFONE

DAPSONE (DDS) (Rx)

Action/Kinetics Dapsone is a synthetic agent with both bacteriostatic and bactericidal activity especially against *Mycobacterium leprae* (Hansen's bacillus). Although the exact mechanism is not known, dapsone is thought to act similarly to sulfonamides in that it interferes with the metabolism of the infectious organism. Widely distributed throughout the body. **Peak plasma levels:** 4–8 hr. t½: About 28 hr. The drug is acetylated in the liver and metabolites are excreted in the urine.

Uses Lepromatous and tuberculoid types of leprosy, dermatitis herpetiformis, and malaria prophylaxis. *Investigational:* Relapsing polychondritis.

Contraindications Advanced amyloidosis of kidneys. Lactation. Appears to be well tolerated during pregnancy.

Untoward Reactions *Hematologic:* Hemolytic anemia, aplastic anemia, agranulocytosis. *GI:* Nausea, vomiting, anorexia, abdominal discomfort. *CNS:* Headache, insomnia, vertigo, paresthesia, psychoses. *Dermatologic:* Photosensitivity, lupuslike syndrome, hyperpigmented macules. *Hypersensitivity:* Severe skin reactions including exfoliative dermatitis, erythema multiforme, urticaria, erythema nodosum. *Other:* Peripheral neuropathy, muscle weakness, hypoalbuminemia, albuminuria, nephrotic syndrome, blurred vision, tinnitus, male infertility, fever.

A leprosy reactional state may occur in large numbers of patients taking dapsone. Symptoms include skin reactions, fever, swelling of joints, depression, orchitis, neuritis, iritis, malaise, epistaxis, and skin nodules. This is not an indication to discontinue therapy, however. Steroids and analgesics may be used to reduce symptoms.

Drug Interaction

Interactant	Interaction
Para-aminobenzoic acid	↓ Effect of dapsone
Probenecid	↑ Effect of dapsone due to inhibition of renal excretion.
Rifampin	↓ Effect of dapsone due to ↑ excretion

Laboratory Test Interference Altered liver function tests.

Dosage *Leprosy:* 6–10 mg/kg/week. (**Adults,** 50–100 mg/day.) The full dose should be initiated and continued without interuption. *Dermatitis herpetiformis:* **Adults, initial:** 50 mg/day; dosage may be increased to 300 mg/day. **Maintenance:** Reduce dosage (by as much as 50%) after 6 months on a gluten-free diet. Dosage should be correspondingly less in children.

Administration

1. For tuberculoid and indeterminate patients, dosage should be continued for at least 3 years.
2. For lepromatous patients, full dosage may be necessary for life.
3. Possible resistance to dapsone should be carefully evaluated.

Nursing Implications

See *Nursing Implications* for *Anti-infectives*, p. 52.

1. *Assess*
   a. for improvement of inflammation and ulceration of the mucous membranes during the first 3–6 months of therapy. Lack of response may indicate need for other therapy.
   b. for allergic dermatitis, which usually appears before the tenth week of therapy. Allergic dermatitis may develop into fatal exfoliative dermatitis.
   c. for psychoses, GI disturbances, lepra reaction, headaches, dizziness, lethargy, severe malaise, tinnitus, paresthesias, deep aches, neuralgic pains, and ocular disturbances.
   d. patients in whom there are other concurrent chronic conditions particularly closely and anticipate reduction in dosage of sulfones.
   e. for symptoms of anemia. Report RBC below $2,500,000/mm^3$ or if RBC remains low during first 6 weeks of therapy.
   f. WBC and report when below $5000/mm^3$.
2. Dosage is increased slowly during initiation period.
3. Check whether doctor wishes patient to receive hematinics.
4. Use strict medical asepsis, because patient may have leukopenia.
5. Teach lactating mothers to report cyanosis of nursing infant, as this indicates high sulfone levels, and withdrawal of drug may be indicated.

Chapter Twelve

ANTHELMINTICS

General Statement   Helminthiasis, or infestation of the body by parasites, is a very common affliction. About 20 million Americans are said to harbor pinworms, for instance. Therefore, anthelmintics are very important drugs; their purpose is to rid the body of parasitic worms, eggs, and larvae.

Humans can become infested by a great variety of worms. Some of the more common worms are described below.

FILARIA   This infestation is transmitted by mosquitoes. The parasite is a very tiny roundworm that migrates into the lymphatic system and bloodstream. Living and dead worms can obstruct the lymphatics, causing elephantiasis. Mosquito control is the chief means of combating this infestation. **Drug treatment:** Results are poor. The drug used is diethylcarbamazine.

HOOKWORM   Infestation with hookworm is quite common. These worms cause debilitation resulting in iron-deficiency anemia, characterized by fatigue, lassitude, and apathy. Several variants of hookworm exist. **Drug treatment:** Tetrachloroethylene, thiabendazole, and mebendazole.

PINWORMS   These infestations are common in school-age children. Complications are rare, although heavy infestations may cause abdominal pain, weight loss, and insomnia. **Drug treatment:** Piperazine citrate, pyrvinium pamoate, pyrantel pamoate, thiabendazole, mebendazole.

ROUNDWORMS   Cause a serious parasitic infestation because the worms can penetrate other tissues. They can obstruct the respiratory and gastrointestinal tracts, as well as the bile duct or appendix. **Drug treatment:** Piperazine, pyrantel pamoate, thiabendazole, mebendazole, diethylcarbamazine.

SCHISTOSOMIASIS   This parasitic infestation of the liver occurs most often in Asia and some parts of Africa. Called schistosomiasis or bilharziasis, it is transmitted by certain species of snails and is very difficult to eradicate. **Drug treatment:** Oxamniquine; niridazole, available from Centers for Disease Control (CDC), see p. 156.

TAPEWORM   The tapeworm consists of a scolex or head that hooks into a segment of intestine. The body is that of a segmented flatworm, sections of which are found in the stools. Tapeworm infestations are difficult to eradicate but have few side effects. **Drug treatment:** Quinacrine; niclosamide, available from the CDC, see p. 156.

THREADWORMS   This parasite infests the upper GI tract. Heavy infestations can cause malabsorption syndrome, diarrhea, and general discomfort. **Drug treatment:** Thiabendazole, hexylresorcinol (for heavy infestations only—PO and retention enemas), pyrvinium pamoate.

WHIPWORM   This threadlike parasite lodges in the mucosa of the cecum. **Drug treatment:** Thiabendazole, mebendazole.

TRICHINOSIS   These parasites are transmitted by the consumption of raw or inadequately cooked pork. The infection is serious; larvae burrow into the bloodstream and form cysts in skeletal muscle. No effective therapeutic agent exists that will eradicate the larvae. **Drug treatment:** Corticosteroids to control the inflammation caused by systemic infestation; thiabendazole. Parasites that infest only the intestinal tract can be eradicated by locally acting drugs. Other parasites enter tissues and must be treated by drugs that are absorbed from the GI tract.

Accurate diagnosis is extremely important before treatment is started because its success depends on selecting the drug best suited for the eradication of a specific infestation.

Since many parasitic infestations are transmitted by persons sharing bathroom facilities, the physician may wish to examine the entire household for parasitic infestation. Treatment is often accompanied or followed by repeated laboratory examinations to determine whether the parasite has been eradicated.

Untoward Reactions Since the anthelmintics do not belong to any one chemical group, their untoward reactions are related to specific compounds. However, nausea, vomiting, cramps, and diarrhea are common to most.

Additional Nursing Implications

See also *Nursing Implications* for *Anti-infectives*, p. 52.

1. Provide the patient or family with written instructions regarding diet, cathartics, enemas, medications, and follow-up tests when treatment is to be carried out at home.
2. Review these instructions with patient or family member to be sure they are understood by the person responsible for the patient's treatment and care. *Good hygienic practices reduce the incidence of helminthiasis.*
3. Emphasize the need for follow-up examinations to check the results of treatment.
4. Specific practices are as follows:

PINWORMS

1. Instruct responsible family member how to prevent infestation with pinworms:
   a. wash hands after toileting and before meals.
   b. keep nails short.
   c. wash ova from anal area in the morning.
   d. apply antipruritic ointment to anal area to reduce scratching, which transfers pinworms.
2. Alert family that physician may wish all members to be examined for pinworms.
3. After the end of the treatment course, swab the perianal area each morning with Scotch tape until no further eggs are found on microscopic examination for 7 consecutive days.

ROUNDWORMS Two to 3 weeks after therapy, stools should undergo microscopic examination to determine fecal egg count. Stools must be examined daily until no further roundworm ova are found.

HOOKWORM/TAPEWORM After administration of medication, cathartics, and enema, examine the results of the enema for the head of the worm, which will appear bright yellow.

DIETHYLCARBAMAZINE CITRATE   Hetrazan (Rx)

Note This drug is no longer available commercially but can be obtained from the Center for Disease Control.

Classification Anthelmintic.

Action/Kinetics Diethylcarbamazine apparently damages the threadlike microfilaria and their larvae so that they are readily destroyed by the defense systems of the body. Adult worms of most species are killed. The drug is readily absorbed from the GI tract and rapidly distributed throughout the body fluids and tissues.

Peak plasma concentrations: 3–4 hr. Metabolized, 95% excreted in urine within 30 hr.

Uses   Systemic parasitic disease caused by filaria, especially of the *Wucheria bancrofti*, *W. malayi*, and *Loa loa* types. These infections are transmitted by certain mosquitoes. Also, onchocerciasis, roundworm, and tropical eosinophilia.

Contraindications and Cautions   Patients with onchocerciasis—the filarial worm infestation—have violent reactions, including an allergic eye inflammation, within 15 hr.

Untoward Reactions   Transient headache, general malaise, weakness, joint pain, anorexia, nausea, and vomiting.

Dosage   *Filariasis, onchocerciasis, loiasis*: 2–4 mg/kg t.i.d. after meals for 3–4 weeks. *Ascariasis*, **adults**: 13 mg/kg/day for 7 days; **children**, 6–10 mg/kg t.i.d. for 7–10 days. An additional course of therapy may be necessary in difficult cases.

Additional Nursing Implications

See also *Nursing Implications* for *Anthelmintics*, p. 149.

1. Anticipate that the concomitant administration of antihistamines and corticosteroids may be ordered for the treatment of onchocerciasis.
2. Have hydrocortisone eyedrops, 5% solution, on hand in case of ocular complications.
3. Administer drug after meals.

MEBENDAZOLE   Vermox (Rx)

Classification   Anthelmintic.

Action/Kinetics   Mebendazole exerts its anthelmintic effect by blocking the glucose uptake of the organisms, thereby depleting their energy until death results. **Peak plasma levels**: 2–4 hr. Excreted in feces.

Uses   Whipworm, pinworm, roundworm, common and American hookworm infections; in single or mixed infections.

Contraindications   Hypersensitivity to mebendazole. Pregnancy. Use with caution in children under 2 years of age.

Untoward Reactions   Transient abdominal pain and diarrhea.

Dosage   *Whipworm, roundworm, and hookworm*, **PO, adults and children**: 1 tablet morning and evening on 3 consecutive days. *Pinworms*: 1 tablet, 1 time. All treatments can be repeated after 3 weeks.

Administration

1. Tablet may be chewed, crushed, and/or mixed with food.
2. No prior fasting, purging, or other procedures required.

NICLOSAMIDE   Niclocide (Rx)

Classification   Anthelmintic.

Action/Kinetics   Niclosamide acts by inhibiting oxidative phosphorylation in the mitochondria of the helminth. The proximal segments and scolex are killed following contact with the drug.

Uses Beef tapeworm (*Taenia saginata*), dwarf tapeworm (*Hymenolepsis nana*), fish tapeworm (*Diphyllobothrium latum*).

Contraindications Safety and efficacy in pregnancy, lactation, and children under 2 years of age have not been established.

Untoward Reactions *GI:* Nausea and vomiting (most common), loss of appetite, abdominal discomfort, diarrhea, constipation, rectal bleeding, bad taste in mouth, irritation of oral mucosa. *Topical:* Skin rashes, alopecia. *CNS:* Dizziness, drowsiness, headache, weakness. *Miscellaneous:* Backache, irritability, fever, palpitations, sweating.

Dosage PO. *Beef and fish tapeworm.* **Adults:** 2 gm as single dose. **Pediatric, over 75 lb:** 1.5 gm as single dose; **pediatric, 25–75 lb:** 1.0 gm as single dose. *Dwarf tapeworm:* **Adults,** 2.0 gm as single daily dose for 7 days. **Pediatric, over 75 lb:** 1.5 gm on first day; **then,** 1.0 gm daily for next 6 days. **Pediatric, 25–75 lb:** 1.0 gm on first day; **then,** 0.5 gm daily for next 6 days.

Administration
1. Tablets should be chewed thoroughly and swallowed with a little water. For small children, a paste may be made by crushing the tablets with a small amount of water.
2. The drug should be taken after a light meal. GI upset may occur.
3. If constipation occurs, a mild laxative may be used.
4. The scolex (head) of the tapeworm may be digested in the intestine and thus may not be found in the feces.
5. The stool must be negative for 3 months before the patient is considered cured.

OXAMNIQUINE   Vansil (Rx)

Classification Anthelmintic, antischistosomiasis.

General Statement Oxamniquine is effective against one species of schistosomes, *Schistosoma mansoni*, which causes systemic infection of liver and spleen. *S. mansoni* is found in Egypt, elsewhere in Africa, South America, and the West Indies, including Puerto Rico. The agent is found in water and is transmitted by snails. Oxamniquine is more effective against male than against female schistosomes, but females cease laying eggs following treatment; thus the infection eventually subsides due to decreased reproduction.

Action/Kinetics **Peak plasma concentration:** 1–1.5 hr; t½: 1–2.5 hr. Well absorbed after PO administration. Inactive metabolites excreted in urine.

Uses All stages of *S. mansoni* infections (acute and chronic).

Contraindications None known. Safe use in pregnancy not known; use only when potential benefits outweigh unknown danger to fetus.

Untoward Reactions Well tolerated. *CNS:* Transient drowsiness and dizziness, headaches. Convulsions have been observed, but mostly in epileptics; therefore, closely monitor patients with history of convulsive disorders. *GI:* Nausea, vomiting, abdominal pain, anorexia. *Dermatologic:* Urticaria.

Dosage PO. **Adults:** 12–25 mg/kg as single oral dose. **Children (under 30 kg):** 10 mg/kg followed in 2–8 hr with a second 10 mg/kg dose.

Administration Administer after food to minimize GI distress.

Additional Nursing Implications
See also *Nursing Implications* for *Anthelmintics*, p. 149.

Inform patient not to drive a car or operate hazardous machinery, because drug may cause dizziness and/or drowsiness.

PIPERAZINE CITRATE   Antepar Citrate, Vermizine (Rx)

Classification   Anthelmintic.

Action/Kinetics   The drug is believed to paralyze the muscles of parasites; this dislodges the parasites and promotes their elimination. The drug is readily absorbed from the GI tract, partially metabolized by liver, the remainder excreted in urine. Rate of elimination differs in patients.

Uses   Pinworm (oxyuriasis) and roundworm (ascariasis) infestations. Particularly recommended for pediatric use.

Contraindications   Impaired liver or kidney function, seizure disorders, hypersensitivity.

Untoward Reactions   Piperazine has a low toxicity. *GI:* Nausea, vomiting, diarrhea, cramps. *CNS:* Tremors, headache, vertigo, decreased reflexes, paresthesias, seizures, ataxia, chorea, memory decrement. *Ophthalmologic:* Nystagmus, blurred vision, cataracts, strabismus. *Allergic:* Urticaria, fever, skin reactions, purpura, lacrimation, rhinorrhea, arthralgia, bronchospasm, cough. *Other:* Muscle weakness.

Drug Interactions   Concomitant administration of piperazine and phenothiazines may result in an increase in extrapyramidal effects (including violent convulsions) caused by phenothiazines.

Laboratory Test Interference   False − or ↓ uric acid values.

Dosage   **PO.** *Pinworms:* **Adults and children,** 65 mg/kg as single daily dose for 7 days up to a maximum daily dose of 2.5 gm. *Roundworms:* **Adults,** 1 dose of 3.5 gm/day for 2 consecutive days; **pediatric,** 1 dose of 75 mg/kg/day for 2 consecutive days not, to exceed 3.5 gm daily. For severe infections, repeat therapy after 1 week.

Administration   Administer drug after breakfast or in 2 divided doses.

Additional Nursing Implications
See also *Nursing Implications* for *Anthelmintics*, p. 149.

Teach patient or responsible other to keep pleasant-tasting medication out of reach of children.

PRAZIQUANTEL   Biltricide (Rx)

Classification   Anthelmintic.

Action/Kinetics   Praziquantel causes increased cell permeability in the helminth, resulting in a loss of intracellular calcium with massive contractions and paralysis of musculature with breakdown of the integrity of the organism. Thus, phagocytes can attack the parasite and death follows. t½: 0.8–1.5 hr. **Maximum serum levels:** 1–3 hr. Significant first-pass effect.

Uses Schistosomal infections due to *Schistosoma japonicum, S. mansoni, S. mekongi,* and *S. hematobium.* Investigational: Liver flukes, neurocysticercosis.

Contraindications Ocular cysticercosis. Use with caution in pregnancy. Safety in children less than 4 years of age not established.

Untoward Effects *GI:* Nausea, abdominal discomfort. *CNS:* Malaise, headache, dizziness, drowsiness. *Other:* Fever, urticaria (rare).

Note: These symptoms may also be due to the helminth infection itself.

Dosage Three doses of 20 mg/kg with an interval between doses of not less than 4 or more than 6 hr.

Administration
1. Due to dizziness and drowsiness, caution should be exercised while driving or performing tasks requiring alertness.
2. The tablets should be taken during meals with liquids. The tablets should not be chewed.
3. The patient should be hospitalized for treatment if the schistosomiasis or fluke infection is accompanied by cerebral cysticercosis.

PYRANTEL PAMOATE   Antiminth, Combantrin* (Rx)

Classification Anthelmintic.

Action/Kinetics The anthelmintic effect is attributed to the neuromuscular blocking effect of this agent. Poorly absorbed from GI tract. **Peak plasma levels**: 0.05–0.13 μg/ml after 1–3 hr. Partially metabolized in liver. Fifty percent excreted unchanged in feces and 7% in urine.

Uses Pinworm and roundworm infestations.

Contraindications Use with caution in presence of liver dysfunction.

Untoward Reactions *GI effects* (most frequent): Anorexia, nausea, vomiting, cramps, diarrhea. *Hepatic:* Transient elevation of SGOT. *CNS:* Headache, dizziness, drowsiness, insomnia. *Other:* Skin rashes.

Drug Interactions Use with piperazine for ascariasis results in antagonism of the effect of both drugs.

Dosage **PO, adults and children**: 1 dose of 11 mg/kg (maximum). **Maximum total dose**: 1.0 gm.

Administration
1. Drug may be taken without regard to food intake.
2. Purging not necessary prior to or during treatment.
3. May be taken with milk or fruit juice.

PYRVINIUM PAMOATE   Povan, Vanquin* (Rx)

Classification Anthelmintic.

Action/Kinetics The drug appears to inhibit respiration of, and glucose absorption by, parasitic worms. Not absorbed to great extent in GI tract.

Uses Pinworm infestations.

Contraindications Intestinal obstruction, acute abdominal disease, and other conditions in which there might be GI absorption. To be used with caution in patients with renal or hepatic disease.

Untoward Reactions *GI:* Nausea, vomiting, cramping, diarrhea. *Hypersensitivity:* Photosensitivity, Stevens-Johnson syndrome.

Dosage **PO. Adults and children**: 1 dose of 5 mg/kg body weight. Dose may be repeated in 2–3 weeks.

Administration

1. Instruct patient to swallow tablet whole to prevent staining of teeth.
2. Administer tablets, rather than liquid, because this reduces the chance of emesis.

Additional Nursing Implications

See also *Nursing Implications* for *Anthelmintics*, p. 149.

1. Pour liquid medication carefully, because it stains materials.
2. Advise patients and parents that the drug stains teeth, underclothing, stools, and vomitus a bright red.

QUINACRINE HYDROCHLORIDE   Atabrine Hydrochloride (Rx)

Classification Anthelmintic, antimalarial.

Action/Kinetics Believed to interfere with DNA synthesis of infectious organism and also to release their grip on intestinal wall, allowing parasites to be removed by purging. Well absorbed from GI tract. **Peak plasma concentrations**: 1–3 hr. Widely distributed in body tissues and is highly bound to tissue and plasma proteins. Metabolized and slowly excreted in urine. Remnants of drug are noted 2 months after cessation of therapy.

Uses Effective against beef, pork, fish, and dwarf tapeworms. Used for giardiasis. Antimalarial. *Investigational:* Intrapleurally in cystic fibrosis to prevent recurrent pneuomothorax.

Contraindications History of psychosis, pregnancy, in patients with psoriasis or those receiving the antimalarial primaquine, porphyria. Use with caution in hepatic disease, alcoholism, and in patients over 60 years of age.

Untoward Reactions *CNS:* Headache, dizziness, seizures, vertigo, nervousness, irritability, psychoses, nightmares. *GI:* Nausea, vomiting, diarrhea, anorexia, cramps. *Dermatologic:* Exfoliative dermatitis, contact dermatitis. *Ophthalmologic:* Corneal deposits or edema leading to blurred vision, visual difficulties, halos. Retinopathy. *Other:* Aplastic anemia, hepatitis, lichen planus-like eruptions.

Drug Interactions

Interactant	Interaction
Alcohol	Antabuse-like reaction
Primaquine	↑ Toxicity of primaquine; concomitant use contraindicated

Laboratory Test Interferences   False + or ↑ values for diagenex blue (gastric function test).

Dosage   PO. *Beef, pork, fish tapeworm*: **Adults,** 4 doses of 200 mg 10 min apart with sodium bicarbonate (600 mg with each dose); **children, 5–14 years**: 400–600 mg in 3–4 divided doses 10 min apart with sodium bicarbonate (300 mg with each dose). *Dwarf tapeworm*: **Adults,** 3 doses of 300 mg 20 min apart on day 1; **then,** 100 mg t.i.d. for 3 days. **Children, 4–8 years: initially,** 200 mg; **maintenance,** 100 mg after breakfast for 3 days. **8–10 years: initially,** 300 mg; **then,** 100 mg b.i.d. for 3 days. **11–14 years: initially,** 400 mg; **then** 100 mg t.i.d. for 3 days. *Giardiasis*: **Adults,** 100 mg t.i.d. for 5–7 days; **children:** 7 mg/kg in 3 divided doses after meals for 5 days. *Antimalarial*: **Adults and children over 8 years**: 200 mg with 1 gm sodium bicarbonate every 6 hr for 5 doses; **then,** 100 mg t.i.d. for 6 days; **children 4–8 years**: 200 mg every 8 hrs the first day, **then** 100 mg 2 times daily for 6 days; **children 1–4 years**: 100 mg every 8 hr the first day, **then** 100 mg daily for 6 days. *Suppression of malaria*: **Adults,** 100/mg/day; **children**: 50 mg/day. Drug should be taken for 1–3 months.

Administration

1. Maintain patient on low fat diet for 24–48 hr before medication to minimize systemic absorption.
2. Omit lunch and supper on day before drug is given.
3. Administer a saline cathartic on evening before medication.
4. Administer quinacrine hydrochloride with 600 mg of sodium bicarbonate to minimize nausea and vomiting.
5. Administer a saline cathartic 1 hr after medication is given.
6. Follow by a soap suds enema to be sure the bright yellow head of the tapeworm is expelled.
7. Administer the drug through a duodenal tube, if ordered, to reduce gastric irritation.

THIABENDAZOLE   Mintezol (Rx)

Classification   Anthelmintic.

Action/Kinetics   The drug interferes with an enzyme specific to several helminths. It is readily absorbed from the GI tract. **Peak plasma levels**: 1–2 hr. Most excreted within 24 hr.

Uses   Cutaneous larva migrans, pinworms, threadworms, large roundworms, hookworms, and whipworms. Particularly useful for the treatment of mixed infestations. To reduce symptoms of trichinosis during the invasive phase.

Contraindications   To be used with caution in patients with hepatic disease or impaired hepatic function.

Untoward Reactions   *GI:* Nausea, vomiting, anorexia, diarrhea, epigastric distress. *CNS:* Dizziness, drowsiness, headache, irritability, seizures. *Allergic:* Pruritus, angioedema, flushing of face, chills, fever, skin rashes, Stevens-Johnson syndrome, anaphylaxis, lymphadenopathy. *Hepatic:* Jaundice, cholestasis, liver damage, transient increase in SGOT. *Renal:* Crystalluria, hematuria, enuresis, foul odor of urine. *Other:* Tinnitus, blurred vision, hypotension, collapse, hyperglycemia, leukopenia, perianal rash.

Dosage   PO: 25 mg/kg body weight b.i.d. up to a maximum of 3.0 gm/day.

Administration

1. Administer drug preferably after meals.
2. For strongloidiasis, cutaneous larva migrans, hookworm, whipworm, or round-worm, 2 doses/day are given for 2 days. For trichinelliasis, give 2 doses/day for 2–4 days. For pinworm, give 2 doses for one day repeated again after 7–14 days.

Nursing Implications

See also *Nursing Implications* for *Anthelmintics*, p. 149.

Caution patient and responsible family member about the CNS disturbances, including muscular weakness and loss of mental alertness that might be caused by the drug. Warn that the patient should neither go to school or work nor operate hazardous machinery after taking the medication.

Note: A number of drugs are investigational for certain infections but can be obtained from the Center for Disease Control (CDC). The drugs may be requested from the Parasitic Disease Drug Service, Bureau of Epidemiology, CDC, Atlanta, Georgia. The following drugs are available:

Drug	Disease
Bayer 2502	Chagas' disease
Bithionol	Paragonimiasis
Dehydroemetine	Amebiasis
Diloxanide furoate (Furamide)	Amebiasis due to *E. histolytica*
Melarsoprol (Mel B, Arsobal)	Sleeping sickness
Niclosamide (Yomesan)	Tapeworm infestations
Niridazole (Ambilhar)	Schistosomiasis
Pentamidine isethionate (Lomidine)	Pneumocystis pneumonia, Gambian sleeping sickness
Sodium antimony dimercaptosuccinate (Astiban)	Schistosomiasis
Sodium antimony gluconate (Pentostam)	Leishmaniasis
Suramin	Rhodesian sleeping sickness, onchocerciasis

Reprinted with permission from *Facts and Comparisons*, 1981, p. 444. (Facts and Comparisons, Inc., St. Louis, Missouri.)

Chapter Thirteen

ANTITUBERCULAR AGENTS

General Statement   Tuberculosis is rarely treated by a single drug because this usually leads to the emergence of resistant strains. However, when only one drug is used, the drug of choice is isoniazid.

The primary agents for the treatment of tuberculosis are isoniazid, streptomycin, ethambutol, and para-aminosalicylic acid (PAS). A combination of isoniazid–streptomycin–ethambutol is currently favored by many clinicians for advanced cavitary pulmonary tuberculosis. For noncavitous disease, ethambutol has replaced PAS as the drug of first choice.

Nursing Implications

See *Nursing Implications* for *Anti-infectives*, p. 52.

1. Anticipate that more than one antitubercular agent will be given concomitantly to prevent the emergence of a resistant strain.
2. Do not administer concomitantly antitubercular agents that are highly ototoxic.
3. Assess for nephrotoxicity, ototoxicity, and hepatotoxicity, caused by most antitubercular agents.
4. Protect the patient manifesting vestibular difficulties during ambulation to prevent falls and injury.
5. Teach patient the importance of taking drugs as ordered.

AMINOSALICYLATE SODIUM   Nemasol Sodium,* P.A.S. Sodium, Teebacin (Rx)

Classification   Tertiary antitubercular agent.

Action/Kinetics   Aminosalicylic acid interferes with folic acid synthesis of susceptible tubercle microorganisms. The drug is bacteriostatic. The various salts are readily absorbed from the GI tract and are well distributed in body tissues. t½: 1 hr. The metabolized drug is mostly excreted in urine.

Uses   Adjuvant to other tuberculostatic agents in the treatment of pulmonary and extrapulmonary tuberculosis. Often used concurrently with isoniazid and/or streptomycin.

Contraindications Hypersensitivity to PAS. To be administered with caution to patients with impaired renal function.

Untoward Reactions *GI:* Nausea, vomiting, diarrhea, abdominal pain. *Allergic:* Fever, skin rashes, hepatitis. *Hematologic:* Agranulocytosis, thrombocytopenia, hemolytic anemia, leukopenia. *Other:* Jaundice, vasculitis, encephalopathy, syndrome resembling infectious mononucleosis, goiter.

Drug Interactions

Interactant	Interaction
Ammonium chloride	↑ Chance of aminosalicylic acid crystalluria
Anticoagulants, oral	Additive effect on prothrombin time
Ascorbic acid	↑ Chance of aminosalicylic acid crystalluria
Isoniazid	↑ Effect of isoniazid due to ↓ metabolism
Para-aminobenzoic acid (PABA)	Inhibits activity of aminosalicylic acid
Phenytoin	↑ Effect of phenytoin
Potassium aminosalicylate	↑ Chance of arrhythmias in patients on diuretics or digitalis
Probenecid	↑ Effect of aminosalicylic acid by ↓ excretion by kidney
Pyrazinamide	↓ Pharmacologic effect of pyrazinamide
Rifampin	↓ Effect of rifampin due to ↓ absorption from GI tract
Salicylates	Possible ↑ effect of PAS due to ↓ excretion by kidney or ↓ plasma protein binding

Laboratory Test Interference Discolors urine. False + acetoacetic acid test.

Dosage **PO. Adults:** 14–16 gm/day in 2–3 divided doses. **Pediatric:** 275–420 mg/kg daily in 3–4 divided doses.

Administration/Storage

1. Store in a light-resistant dry jar at a cool temperature.
2. Solutions for oral administration should be used within 24 hr and under no circumstances if color is darker than that of a freshly prepared solution.
3. Reduce GI disturbance by administering the drug after meals or with 5–10 ml of aluminum hydroxide, as ordered by the physician.

Additional Nursing Implications

See also *Nursing Implications* for *Anti-infectives*, p. 52 and *Antitubercular agents*, p. 157.

1. *Assess*
   a. for GI distress, which usually disappears after several days of therapy. Persistence may require cessation of therapy.
   b. for hypersensitivity reaction characterized by rise in body temperature (102–104°F; 39–40°C) in previously afebrile patients.

c. for goiter and hypothyroidism. Anticipate physician ordering thyroid therapy if conditions appear.

d. for electrolyte imbalance in patients with cardiac or renal disease.

2. Use Tes-Tape, Clinistix, or Diastix to evaluate glycosuria since a false-positive reaction may be obtained with Benedict's solution, Clinitest tablets, or Fehling's solution.

CAPREOMYCIN SULFATE   Capastat Sulfate (Rx)

Classification Tertiary antitubercular agent.

Action/Kinetics Action unknown. Capreomycin is bactericidal. Must be administered parenterally. **Peak plasma concentations: IM,** 20–47 μg/ml after 1–2 hr. t½: 4–6 hr. Primarily excreted in urine.

Uses Resistant-type tubercle bacillus. Should always be given in combination with other antitubercular agents.

Contraindications Hypersensitivity to drug. Use with caution in renal insufficiency or auditory impairment. Never use together with streptomycin.

Untoward Reactions Nephrotoxicity, hepatic toxicity, ototoxicity (tinnitus, vertigo). *Hematologic:* Leukopenia, leukocytosis, eosinophilia. *Allergic:* Urticaria, skin rashes, fever. *Other:* Pain at injection site, sterile abscesses, bleeding at injection site. Hypokalemia.

Dosage **IM deep:** 1.0 gm daily (not to exceed 20 mg/kg/day) for 60–120 days, followed by 1.0 gm every 2–3 weeks. Therapy should be maintained for 18–24 months.

Administration/Storage

1. Reconstituted solutions are stable for 48 hours at room temperature and for 14 days when refrigerated.

2. Capreomycin sulfate injections may develop a pale straw color and darken, but this does not affect the efficacy of the product.

3. Administer deep into large muscle mass to minimize pain, induration, excessive bleeding, and sterile abscesses at site of injection.

Additional Nursing Implications

See also *Nursing Implications* for *Anti-infectives*, p. 52 and *Antitubercular agents*, p. 157.

1. *Assess*

a. for otoxocity manifested by damage to vestibular and auditory portion of eighth cranial nerve, tinnitus, deafness, dizziness, ataxia.

b. for symptoms of nephrotoxicity evidenced by decreasing renal function. If decreased, patient must be evaluated and the drug either reduced or discontinued.

2. Protect patient with vertigo or ataxia during ambulation.

CYCLOSERINE   Seromycin (Rx)

Classification   Tertiary antitubercular agent.

Action/Kinetics   Broad-spectrum antibiotic produced by a strain of *Streptomyces orchidaceus* or *Garyphalus lavendulae*. Disturbs cell wall synthesis by interfering with the incorporation of the amino acid alanine. The drug is bactericidal and bacteriostatic. Well absorbed from the GI tract and widely distributed in body tissues. **Peak plasma concentration**: 3–4 hr. t½: 10 hr. Sixty to 70% excreted unchanged in urine.

Uses   Active pulmonary and extrapulmonary tuberculosis. Indicated only when primary therapy with streptomycin, isoniazid, and para-aminosalicylic acid cannot be used. Also useful in the treatment of acute urinary infections caused by susceptible organisms, especially *E. coli* and *Enterobacter*.

Contraindications   Hypersensitivity to cycloserine, epilepsy, depression, severe anxiety, psychosis, severe renal insufficiency, and alcoholism. Safe use in pregnancy and children has not been established.

Untoward Reactions   *CNS:* Drowsiness, dizziness, headache, mental confusion, tremors, vertigo, loss of memory, psychoses, aggression, increased reflexes, seizures, paresthesias, paresis, dysarthria, coma. *Other:* Skin rashes, increased transaminase.

Neurotoxic effects depend on blood levels of cycloserine. Hence, frequent determinations of cycloserine blood levels are indicated, especially during the initial period of therapy.

Drug Interaction   Ethionamide potentiates the CNS toxicity of cycloserine.

Dosage   **PO.** *Tuberculosis:* **initial,** 250 mg q 12 hr for first two weeks; **then,** 0.5–1 gm daily in divided doses based on blood levels. Dosage should not exceed 1 gm daily. *Urinary tract infections:* 250 mg q 12 hr for patients with normal renal function.

Additional Nursing Implications

See also *Nursing Implications* for *Anti-infectives*, p. 52 and *Antitubercular agents*, p. 157.

1. *Assess*
   a. for sudden development of congestive heart failure in patients receiving high doses of cycloserine.
   b. for untoward reactions, especially neurologic, as these will necessitate withdrawing the drug at least for a short period of time. Have emergency equipment available for convulsions (pyridoxine, anticonvulsants, sedatives, oxygen, IV, gastric lavage, respirator, means of maintaining body temperature, mouth gag, and side rails).
2. Caution patient against operating any machinery as the drug promotes lethargy, drowsiness, and dizziness.

ETHAMBUTOL HYDROCHLORIDE   ETIBI,* Myambutol (Rx)

Classification   Secondary antitubercular agent.

Action/Kinetics   Tuberculostatic. Arrests multiplication of tubercle bacilli but does not affect those microorganisms during their resting state. Probably interferes with RNA synthesis. Readily absorbed after oral administration. Widely distributed in body tissues. **Peak plasma concentration**: 2–5 μg/ml after 2–4 hr. **t½**: 3.3 hr. About 60% of metabolized and unchanged drug excreted in urine. Drug accumulates in patients with renal insufficiency.

Uses Secondary drug for pulmonary tuberculosis. Always use in combination with other tuberculostatic drugs.

Contraindications Hypersensitivity to ethambutol, preexisting optic neuritis, and children under 13 years of age. Should be used with caution and in reduced dosage in patients with gout, impaired renal function, and in pregnant patients.

Untoward Reactions *Ophthalmologic:* Optic neuritis, decreased visual acuity, loss of color (green) discrimination, temporary loss of vision or blurred vision. *GI:* Nausea, vomiting, anorexia, abdominal pain. *CNS:* Fever, headache, dizziness, confusion, disorientation, malaise, hallucinations. *Allergic:* Pruritus, dermatitis, anaphylaxis. *Other:* Peripheral neuropathy (numbness, tingling), precipitation of gout, thrombocytopenia, joint pain, toxic epidermal necrolysis.
 Renal damage. Also anaphylactic shock, peripheral neuritis (rare), hyperuricemia, and decreased liver function.
 Adverse symptoms usually appear during the early months of therapy and disappear thereafter. Periodic renal and hepatic function tests as well as uric acid determinations are recommended.

Dosage **PO, initial treatment**: 15 mg/kg per day given once daily until maximal improvement noted; **for retreatment**: 25 mg/kg daily as a single dose with at least one other tuberculostatic drug; **after 60 days**: 15 mg/kg administered once daily.

Additional Nursing Implications

See also *Nursing Implications* for *Anti-infectives*, p. 52 and *Antitubercular agents*, p. 157.

1. Ascertain that patient has had visual acuity test before ethambutol therapy and that patient does not have preexisting visual problems. Also check that patient has vision test every 2 to 4 weeks while on therapy.

2. Reassure patient that effects on eyes generally disappear within several weeks to several months after therapy has been discontinued.

3. Teach female patient that, should she become pregnant, to discontinue use of the drug and report immediately to physician.

ETHIONAMIDE Trecator-SC (Rx)

Classification Tertiary antitubercular agent.

Action/Kinetics Believed to interfere with peptide synthesis of susceptible organisms. Bacteriostatic and bactericidal. Well absorbed after oral administration. Widely distributed in body tissues. **Peak plasma concentration**: 3 hr: **t½**: 3 hr. Extensively metabolized by liver. Excreted primarily in urine.

Use Active tuberculosis (any form). Should be given only with other antituberculosis drugs.

Contraindication Children under 12 years of age. Use with caution in pregnancy.

Untoward Reactions *GI:* Nausea, vomiting, anorexia, diarrhea, stomatitis, metallic taste. *CNS:* Asthenia, drowsiness, depression, seizures, dizziness, headache, tremors, restlessness, psychoses. *Ophthalmologic:* Blurred vision, double vision, optic neuritis. *Hepatic:* Jaundice, hepatitis. *Other:* Peripheral neuropathy, neuritis, alopecia, acne, skin rashes, postural hypotension, impotence, gynecomastia, menorrhagia, thrombocytopenia, diabetic control more difficult.

Drug Interactions

Interactant	Interaction
Alcohol, ethyl	↑ CNS toxicity of ethionamide
Cycloserine	Ethionamide potentiates CNS toxicity of cycloserine with possibility of convulsions

Dosage   **PO. Adults: usual,** 0.5–1 gm daily in divided doses together with pyridoxine. Given with at least one other tuberculostatic drug.

Administration

1. Do not administer to children under 12 years of age unless primary therapy has failed.
2. Administer after meals to minimize gastric irritation.

Additional Nursing Implications

See also *Nursing Implications* for *Anti-infectives*, p. 52 and *Antitubercular agents*, p. 157.
Assess

    a. for toxic effects, particularly severe nausea, which can be treated with antiemetics.

    b. for potentiation of toxic effects of cycloserine (congestive heart failure) if given concomitantly.

    c. urine of diabetic patients more frequently and also assess for untoward symptoms related to diabetes. The latter condition is more difficult to control in patients with tuberculosis.

ISONIAZID   INH, Isonicotinic Acid Hydrazide, Isotamine,* Laniazid, Nydrazid, PMS Isoniazid,* Rimifon,* Teebaconin (Rx)

Classification   Primary antitubercular agent.

General Statement   Isoniazid is the most effective tuberculostatic agent. Patients on isoniazid fall into two groups depending on the manner in which they metabolize isoniazid.

1. **Slow inactivators:** Show earlier, favorable response, but have more toxic reactions, i.e. neuropathies because of higher blood levels of drug.
2. **Rapid inactivators:** Possibly have poor clinical response due to rapid inactivation. This group requires an increased daily dose of the drug. More likely to develop hepatitis.

The metabolism of isoniazid is genetically determined and involves the level of a hepatic enzyme. As a rule, 50% of whites and blacks inactivate the drug slowly, whereas the majority of American Indians, Eskimos, Japanese, and Chinese are rapid inactivators.

Action/Kinetics   Isoniazid probably interferes with lipid and nucleic acid metabolism of growing bacteria resulting in alteration of bacterial wall. The drug is tuberculostatic. It is readily absorbed after oral and parenteral (IM) administration and is widely distributed in body tissues. **Peak plasma concentration: PO**, 1–2 hr; t½: 1–4 hr. These values are increased in association with liver and kidney impairment. Drug is metabolized in liver and excreted primarily in urine.

Uses   Tuberculosis caused by human, bovine, and BCG strains of *Mycobacterium tuberculosis*. The drug should not be used as the sole tuberculostatic agent. Preventive therapy.

Contraindications   Severe hypersensitivity to isoniazid. Extreme caution should be exercised in patients with convulsive disorders, in which case the drug should be administered only when the patient is adequately controlled by anticonvulsant medication. Also, use with caution for the treatment of renal tuberculosis and, in the lowest dose possible, in patients with impaired renal function and in alcoholics.

Untoward Reactions   Peripheral neuritis, muscle twitches. *CNS:* Ataxia, stupor, seizures, toxic encephalopathy, euphoria, impaired memory, dizziness, toxic psychoses. *GI:* Nausea, vomiting, epigastric distress, xerostomia. *Hypersensitivity:* Fever, skin rashes, vasculitis, lymphadenopathy. *Hepatic:* Liver dysfunction, jaundice, bilirubinemia, hepatitis (rarely fatal). Increases in serum SGOT and SGPT. *Hematologic:* Agranulocytosis, eosinophilia, thrombocytopenia, methemoglobinemia, anemias. *Other:* Tinnitus, optic neuritis, optic atrophy, hyperglycemia, metabolic acidosis, urinary retention, gynecomastia in males, lupus-like syndrome, arthralgia.

   Note: Pyridoxine, 10–50 mg/day, may be given concomitantly with isoniazid to decrease CNS side effects. Ophthalmologic and liver function tests are recommended periodically.

Drug Interactions

Interactant	Interaction
Aminosalicylic acid	↑ Effect of isoniazid by ↑ blood levels
Atropine	↑ Side effects of isoniazid
Ethanol	↑ Chance of isoniazid-induced hepatitis
Disulfiram (Antabuse)	↑ Side effects of isoniazid (esp. CNS)
Meperidine	↑ Side effects of isoniazid
Phenytoin	↑ Effect of phenytoin due to ↓ breakdown in liver
Rifampin	Additive liver toxicity

Laboratory Test Interferences   Altered liver function tests. False + or ↑ K, SGOT, SGPT, urine glucose (Benedict's, Clinitest).

Dosage   **PO (usual).** *Active tuberculosis:* **Adults,** 5 mg/kg daily (up to 300 mg total) as a single dose; **children and infants:** 10–20 mg/kg/day (up to 300–500 mg total) in a single dose. *Prophylaxis:* **Adults,** 300 mg/day in a single dose; **children and infants:** 10 mg/kg/day (up to 300 mg total) in a single dose.

Administration/Storage

1. Store in dark, tightly closed containers.
2. Solutions for IM injection may crystallize at low temperature and should be allowed to warm to room temperature if precipitation is evident.
3. Teach patient to take drug on empty stomach or 1 hr before or 2 hr after meals.
4. Isoniazid should be coadministered with pyridoxine, 6–50 mg/day, in malnourished, alcoholic, or diabetic patients.

Additional Nursing Implications

See *Nursing Implications* for *Anti-infectives*, p. 52 and *Antitubercular agents*, p. 157.

1. Have on hand parenteral sodium phenobarbital for the control of isoniazid-induced neurotoxic symptoms, particularly convulsions.
2. Anticipate that cholinergic drugs, atropine, and certain narcotics (meperidine) may aggravate side reactions.
3. Withhold drug and consult with physician in case of marked CNS stimulation.
4. Explain to patient that pyridoxine is given to prevent neurotoxic effects of isoniazid.
5. Assess diabetic patients closely because diabetes is more difficult to control when isoniazid is administered. Alert patients to this fact.
6. Anticipate that lower doses of the drug are to be given to patients with renal problems and check intake and output of fluids to ascertain that renal output is adequate to prevent systemic accumulation of the drug.
7. Provide patient with only a 1-month supply of the drug as he should be examined and evaluated monthly while on isoniazid.
8. Anticipate slight local irritation at site of injection.
9. Teach patient and/or family to withhold drug and report fatigue, weakness, malaise, and anorexia immediately because they are prodromal signs of hepatitis.

KANAMYCIN   Kantrex, Klebcil (Rx)

Classification   Tertiary antitubercular agent and aminoglycoside antibiotic.

Dosage   IM. Adults: 15 mg/kg once daily. Not recommended for use in children. For all information on kanamycin, *see* p. 112.

PYRAZINAMIDE   (Rx)

Classification   Secondary antitubercular agent.

Action/Kinetics   Bacteriostatic and bactericidal. Well absorbed from GI tract, widely distributed in tissues. **Peak plasma concentration:** 2 hr; t½: 9–10 hr, longer in presence of impaired renal and hepatic function. Metabolized in liver and chiefly excreted in urine.

Use   Active tuberculosis, any form. Suitable for short-term use in selected patients. Not suitable for either initial therapy or long-term use. This drug should only be used in conjunction with other antituberculosis agents.

Contraindication   Preexisting liver malfunction.

Untoward Reactions   *Hepatic:* Cellular damage, hepatomegaly, jaundice, tenderness. *GI:* Nausea, vomiting, diarrhea, anorexia. *CNS:* Fever, malaise. *Other:* Gout, disturbances in blood clotting, arthralgia, skin rashes, photosensitivity, splenomegaly. Frequent liver function tests are required.

Drug Interactions

Interactant	Interaction
Aminosalicylic acid	↓ Pharmacologic effect of pyrazinamide
Probenecid	↓ Pharmacologic effect of pyrazinamide
Salicylates	↓ Pharmacologic effect of pyrazinamide

Dosage   PO. Adults, usual: 20–35 mg/kg daily in 3–4 divided doses. Maximum daily dose is 3.0 gm.

Additional Nursing Implications

See also *Nursing Implications* for *Anti-infectives*, p. 52 and *Antitubercular agents*, p. 157.

1. Question doses that exceed 35 mg/kg/day as higher doses tend to promote hepatic damage.
2. Administer only under close medical supervision.
3. *Assess*
   a. for jaundice.
   b. diabetic patients closely for hypo- or hyperglycemia because drug affects sugar metabolism.
   c. for fatigue, poor appetite, weakness, irritability, signs of anemia and prodromal signs of hepatitis.
4. Schedule for frequent liver function tests.

RIFAMPIN   Rifadin, Rimactane, Rofact* (Rx)

Classification   Primary antitubercular agent.

Action/Kinetics   Semisynthetic antibiotic derived from *Streptomyces mediterranei*. Rifampin suppresses RNA synthesis, thereby interfering with bacterial replication. The drug is both bacteriostatic and bactericidal and is most active against rapidly replicating organisms. The drug is well absorbed from the GI tract and is widely distributed in body tissues. **Peak plasma concentration:** 4–32 μg/ml after 2–4 hr. t½: 3 hr (higher in patients with hepatic impairment). In normal patients t½ decreases with usage. Drug metabolized in liver, 60% excreted in feces.

Uses   Pulmonary tuberculosis. Must be used in conjunction with at least one other tuberculostatic drug (such as isoniazid, ethambutol) but is the drug of choice for retreatment. Also for treatment of asymptomatic meningococcal carriers. *Investigational:* In combination for infections due to *Staphylococcus aureus* and *epidermis;* Legionnaire's disease; in combination with dapsone for leprosy; prophylaxis of meningitis due to *H. influenzae*.

Contraindications   Hypersensitivity; not recommended for intermittent therapy. Safe use in pregnancy and lactation has not been established. Use with extreme caution in patients with hepatic dysfunction.

Untoward Reactions   *GI:* Nausea, vomiting, diarrhea, cramps, heartburn, flatulence. *CNS:* Headache, drowsiness, fatigue, ataxia, dizziness, confusion, fever, difficulty in concentration. *Hepatic:* Jaundice, hepatitis. Increases in SGOT, SGPT, bilirubin, alkaline phosphatase. *Hematologic:* Thrombocytopenia, leukopenia, hemolytic anemia. *Allergic:* Flulike symptoms, dyspnea, wheezing, purpura, pruritus, urticaria, skin rashes, sore mouth and tongue, conjunctivitis. *Renal:* Hematuria, hemoglobinuria, renal insufficiency, acute renal failure. *Other:* Visual disturbances, muscle weakness or pain, arthralgia, adrenocortical insufficiency, increases in BUN and serum uric acid.

Note: Body fluids and feces may be red-orange in color.

Drug Interactions

Interactant	Interaction
Aminosalicylic acid	↓ Effect of rifampin due to ↓ absorption from GI tract
Anticoagulants, oral	↓ Effect of anticoagulant due to ↑ breakdown by liver
Barbiturates	↓ Effect of barbiturate due to ↑ breakdown by liver
Contraceptives, oral	↓ Effect of contraceptives due to ↑ breakdown of estrogen by liver
Corticosteroids	↓ Effect of corticosteroids due to ↑ breakdown by liver
Digitoxin	↓ Effect of digitoxin due to ↑ breakdown by liver
Hypoglycemics, oral	↓ Effect of hypoglycemic due to ↑ breakdown by liver
Isoniazid	Additive liver toxicity
Methadone	↑ Chance of methadone withdrawal symptoms due to ↑ breakdown by liver
Quinidine	↓ Effect of quinidine due to ↑ breakdown by liver

Laboratory Test Interferences   ↑ in SGOT, SGPT, alkaline phosphatase, BUN, bilirubin, uric acid, BSP retention values. False + Coombs' test.

Dosage   PO. *Pulmonary tuberculosis*: **Adults,** single dose of 600 mg daily; **children over 5 years**: 10–20 mg/kg daily, not to exceed 600 mg/day. *Meningococcal carriers*: 600 mg daily for 4 days; **children over 5 years**: 10–20 mg/kg daily for 4 days, not to exceed 600 mg/day.

Administration

1. Administer once daily 1 hr before or 2 hr after meals to ensure maximum absorption.
2. Check to be sure there is a desiccant in the bottle containing capsules of rifampin as these are relatively moisture sensitive.
3. If administered concomitantly with PAS, drugs should be given 8–12 hr apart, as the acid interferes with the absorption of rifampin.

Additional Nursing Implications

See also *Nursing Implications* for *Anti-infectives*, p. 52 and *Antitubercular agents*, p. 157.
Access

1. for GI disturbance, impaired renal function, auditory nerve impairment, blood dyscrasias, and liver dysfunction.
2. Inform the patient that rifampin imparts an orange color to urine, feces, saliva, sputum, and tears.

STREPTOMYCIN SULFATE   (Rx)

Classification   Aminoglycoside, secondary antitubercular agent. See *Aminoglycoside Antibiotics*, p. 115.

Chapter Fourteen

ANTIMALARIALS

General Statement   A knowledge of the life cycle of the causative agent is helpful in understanding the mode of action of the antimalarial drugs.

Malaria is transmitted by the anopheles mosquito. The causative organism is a parasite known as *Plasmodium*, of which there are several species infective to humans: *P. falciparum, P. vivax, P. malariae,* and *P. ovale*.

Plasmodia pass through a complex life cycle, part of which takes place in the gut of the mosquito and part in humans. In the sporozoite stage of development, the organism is transmitted to humans by a mosquito bite. The sporozoite migrates to the human liver where it grows and divides (exoerythrocytic, fixed-tissue stage), emerging as a merozoite. The merozoite enters various tissues, including the red blood cells (asexual erythrocytic stage), causing them to burst. This results in a rise in body temperature. Some merozoites develop into male parasites and others into females. At this stage they are known as gametocytes, which infect the mosquito again when it bites a human carrier. It then reproduces in the gut of the mosquito and develops to the sporozoite stage, to complete the cycle.

Clinical manifestations of malaria are not evident during all stages of the life cycle, and no single drug can eradicate the parasite at all stages. Treatment is divided into six categories, according to the end result obtained and the stage at which the malaria is being treated. The categories of treatment are as follows:

1. *Causal prophylaxis*: eradication of the parasite during the primary exoery-throcytic state (killing of sporozoites). This prevents the disease from spreading.
2. *Suppressive prophylaxis*: prevents parasites from developing into erythrocytic state (inhibition of erythrocytic stage). This form of treatment prevents clinical manifestations of malaria. Suitable drugs: chloroquine, chloroguanide, pyrimethamine. Symptoms reappear if drug therapy is stopped. When antimalarials are used prophylactically, the drug is administered up to 2 weeks before entering the malarious area and is continued for varying periods of time (depending on the drug) after the person leaves the area.
3. *Clinical cure*: halts further development of erythrocytic stage and terminates a clinical attack. Suitable drugs: chloroquine, amodiaquine, quinine.
4. *Suppressive cure*: complete elimination of malarial parasite from affected individual. Suitable drug: pyrimethamine.
5. *Radical cure*: eradication of erythrocytic and exoerythrocytic forms of the parasite and relief of symptoms. Suitable drug: primaquine.
6. *Gametocytocidal therapy*: destruction of sexual form of malarial parasite. Suitable drug: primaquine.

Nursing Implications

See *Nursing Implications* for *Anti-infectives*, p. 52.

4-AMINOQUINOLINES

General Statement Two 4-aminoquinolines—chloroquine (Aralen), and hydroxychloroquine (Plaquenil)—are widely used for the treatment of malaria. They are all synthetic agents that resemble quinine. They also are used as amebicides and in the treatment of rheumatic diseases.

Action/Kinetics The 4-aminoquinolines are believed to complex with DNA and therefore to interfere with the replication of the infectious organism. The aminoquinolines are rapidly and almost completely absorbed from the GI tract. **Peak plasma levels**: 1–3 hr. They are metabolized and excreted extremely slowly, and the presence of some drug has been demonstrated in the bloodstream weeks and months after the drug has been discontinued.

Urinary excretion is increased by acidifying the urine and slowed by alkalinization.

Uses Suppression or prophylaxis of malaria caused by *Plasmodium falciparum, P. vivax, P. ovale, P. malariae.* Will cause a radical cure of falciparum malaria but will not prevent relapses of vivax. The drugs are only effective against the erythrocytic stages and therefore will not prevent infections.

Extraintestinal amebiasis caused by *E. histolytica.* Lupus erythematosus. As an alternative to gold salts or penicillamine in rheumatoid arthritis patients resistant to salicylates or nonsteroidal anti-inflammatory agents.

Contraindications To be used with extreme caution in the presence of hepatic, severe GI, neurologic, and blood disorders.

Unless deemed essential, the drugs should not be used in the presence of psoriasis, porphyria, and pregnancy. Not to be used concomitantly with gold or phenylbutazone or in patients receiving drugs that depress blood-forming elements of bone marrow.

Untoward Reactions   *GI:* Nausea, vomiting, diarrhea, cramps, anorexia, epigastric distress, stomatitis, dry mouth. *CNS:* Headache, fatigue, nervousness, anxiety, irritability, agitation, apathy, confusion, personality changes, depression, psychoses, seizures. *Dermatologic:* Pruritus, changes in pigment of skin and mucous membranes, dermatoses, bleaching of hair. *Hematologic:* Neutropenia, aplastic anemia, thrombocytopenia, agranulocytosis. *Ocular:* Retinopathy, which may be permanent and lead to blindness. Blurred vision, difficulty in focusing or in accommodation, chronic use may lead to corneal deposits or keratopathy. *Miscellaneous:* Hypotension, ECG changes, peripheral neuritis, ototoxicity, neuromyopathy manifested by muscle weakness.

Drug Interactions

Interactant	*Interaction*
Acidifying agents—urinary (Ammonium chloride, etc.)	↑ Urinary excretion of antimalarial and thus ↓ its effectiveness
Alkalinizing agents—urinary (Bicarbonate, etc.)	↓ Excretion of antimalarial and thus ↑ amount of drug in system
Antipsoriatics (Anthralin, Resorcinol)	4-Aminoquinolines inhibit antipsoriatic drugs
MAO inhibitors	↑ Toxicity of 4-aminoquinolines due to ↓ breakdown in liver

Laboratory Test Interference   Colors urine brown.

Dosage   See individual drug entries.

Administration/Storage

1. For suppressive therapy, give drug on same day each week. Give immediately before or after meal so as to minimize gastric irritation.
2. For discoid lupus erythematosus, give with evening meal.
3. Store in amber-colored containers.

Nursing Implications

See also *Nursing Implications* for *Anti-infectives*, p. 52.

1. *Assess*
   a. for retinopathy manifested by visual disturbances. Retinal changes are not reversible. Regular ophthalmologic examinations are mandatory during prolonged therapy.
   b. for acute toxicity, which may occur in accidental overdosage in children or in suicidal patients. Symptoms of acute toxicity develop within 30 min of ingestion. Death may occur within 2 hr.
      (1) *Symptoms of acute toxicity* are headache, drowsiness, visual disturbances, cardiovascular collapse, convulsions, and cardiac arrest.
      (2) Have on hand emergency equipment, including setup for gastric lavage, barbiturates, vasopressors, and oxygen. Observe for 6 hours after acute toxicity has been treated.
      (3) Check TPR and BP as well as intake and output and state of consciousness at frequent intervals.
      (4) Anticipate that fluids will have to be forced and ammonium chloride ad-

(continued)

ministered for weeks to months to acidify urine and promote renal excretion of the drug.

(5) Warn patients to keep drug out of children's reach.

2. Check toxic effects of other drugs being used as the combination with chloroquine may reinforce toxic effects.

CHLOROQUINE HYDROCHLORIDE   Aralen HCL (Rx)

CHLOROQUINE PHOSPHATE   Aralen Phosphate (Rx)

Classification   4-Aminoquinoline—Antimalarial, amebecide.

Note: See *Malaria*, p. 167 and 4-*Aminoquinolines*, p. 168.

Additional Untoward Reactions   Chloroquine may exacerbate psoriasis and precipitate an acute attack.

Dosage   PO *(Phosphate). Acute malarial attack*: **Adults, initial**, 600 mg; **then, 300** mg after 6 hr and 300 mg/day for next 2 days. **Children, initial**, 10 mg/kg; **then**, 5 mg/kg after 6 hr and 5 mg/kg for next 2 days. Children's dose should not exceed 600 mg for initial dose or 300 mg for subsequent doses. *Suppression of malaria*: **Adults**, 5 mg (base)/kg, not to exceed 300 mg/week; **children less than 1 year**: do not exceed 62 mg/week; **1–3 years**: do not exceed 125 mg/week; **4–6 years**: do not exceed 165 mg/week; **7–10 years**: do not exceed 250 mg/week; **11–16 years**: do not exceed 375 mg/week. *Amebiasis*: **Adults**, 1 gm/day for 2 days; **then**, 500 mg/day for 2–3 weeks (combine with an intestinal amebicide). **IM** *(Hydrochloride). Acute malarial attack*: **Adults, initial**, 200–250 mg; repeat dosage in 6 hr if necessary. Total daily dose in first 24 hr should not exceed 800 mg (base). Begin PO therapy as soon as possible. **Children and infants**: 5 mg (base)/kg repeated in 6 hr; dose should not exceed 10 mg (base)/kg/day. *Amebiasis*: **Adults**, 200–250 mg daily for 10–12 days. Begin PO therapy as soon as possible.

HYDROXYCHLOROQUINE SULFATE   Plaquenil Sulfate (Rx)

Classification   4-Aminoquinoline.

Note: See *Malaria*, p. 167 and 4-*Aminoquinolines*, p. 168. Also used as an antirheumatic.

Additional Untoward Reactions   The appearances of skin eruptions or of misty vision and visual halos are indications for withdrawal.

Drug Interaction   Concomitant use with phenylbutazone or gold salts may cause dermatitis and ↑ risk of severe skin reactions.

Dosage   PO. *Acute malarial attack*: **Adults, initial**, 620 mg; **then**, 310 mg after 6 hr and 310 mg/day for next 2 days. **Children, initial**, 10 mg/kg; **then**, 5 mg/kg after 6 hr and 5 mg/kg for next 2 days. Children's dose should not exceed daily adult dose. *Suppression of malaria*: **Adults**, 5 mg (base)/kg not to exceed 310 mg (base)/week; **children less than 1 year** : not to exceed 50 mg/week; **1–3 years**:

do not exceed 100 mg/week; **4–6 years**: do not exceed 130 mg/week; **7–10 years**: do not exceed 200 mg/week; **11–16 years**: do not exceed 290 mg/week. *Rheumatoid arthritis*: **Adults**, 400–600 mg daily taken with milk or meals; *maintenance* (usually after 4–12 weeks): 200–400 mg daily. (*Note:* Several months may be required for a beneficial effect to be seen). *Lupus erythematosus*: **Adults, usual,** 400 mg once or twice daily; **prolonged maintenance**: 200–400 mg daily.

8-AMINOQUINOLINE

PRIMAQUINE PHOSPHATE   (Rx)

Classification   8-Aminoquinoline, antimalarial.

General Statement   See also *General Statement* at beginning of section. Primaquine is active against primary exoerythrocytic forms of vivax and falciparum malaria. It produces radical cure of vivax malaria by eliminating both exoerythrocytic and erythrocytic forms. It cures suppressed infections after the patient leaves endemic areas and prevents relapse. For this reason, the drug is administered concurrently with quinine or chloroquine.

Action/Kinetics   Believed to interfere with mitochondria of parasite, resulting in a profound alteration of metabolism of cell (decreased protein synthesis). Well absorbed from GI tract. **Peak plasma levels**: 2 hr. Poorly distributed in body tissues.

Uses   Exoerythrocytic forms of vivax malaria—radical cure.

Contraindications   Very active forms of vivax and falciparum malaria.

Untoward Reactions   *GI:* Abdominal cramps, epigastric distress, nausea, vomiting. *Hematologic:* Methemoglobinemia. Blacks and members of certain Mediterranean ethnic groups (Sardinians, Sephardic Jews, Greeks, Iranians), manifest a high incidence of glucose 6-phosphate dehydrogenase deficiency and as a result have a low tolerance for primaquine. These individuals manifest marked hemolytic anemia following primaquine. *Miscellaneous:* Headache, pruritus, interference with visual accomodation, cardiac arrhythmias, hypertension.

Drug Interactions

Interactant	Interaction
Bone marrow depressants, hemolytic drugs	Additive untoward reactions
Quinacrine (Atabrine)	Quinacrine interferes with metabolic degradation of primaquine and thus enhances its toxic side reactions. **Do not give primaquine** to patients who are receiving or have received quinacrine within the past 3 months.

Dosage   **PO**: *Radical cure of vivax malaria*: 26.3 mg daily for 14 days. *Suppression of malaria*: **Adults**, 26.3 mg daily for 14 days or 79 mg once a week for 8 weeks; **children**: 0.3 mg (base)/kg/day for 14 days or 0.9 mg (base)/kg/week for 8 weeks.

Administration/Storage
1. Administer drug with meals or antacids, as ordered. This reduces or prevents GI distress.

2. Store in tightly closed containers.
3. Therapy is initiated during the last 2 weeks of or after suppressive therapy with chloroquine or a similar drug.

Nursing Implications
See *Nursing Implications* for *Anti-infectives*, p. 52.

1. *Assess*
   a. for dark urine indicating hemolysis, and a marked fall in hemoglobin, or erythrocyte count as these are indications for withdrawal of drug. Monitor intake and output.
   b. dark-skinned patients. Because of a possible inborn deficiency of glucose 6-phosphate dehydrogenase, these patients are particularly susceptible to hemolytic anemia while on primaquine.
2. Teach patients to monitor color of urine and to report immediately any darkening or brown color.
3. For suppressive therapy, give drug on same day each week. Give immediately before or after meal so as to minimize gastric irritation.

MISCELLANEOUS ANTIMALARIALS

PYRIMETHAMINE   Daraprim (Rx)

Classification   Antimalarial, antitoxoplasmotic, folic acid antagonist.

General Statement   Because of slow onset a faster-acting antimalarial, such as chloroquine or amodiaquine, should be used during acute attacks. Pyrimethamine has some antitoxoplasmotic activity. For treatment of toxoplasmosis, drug is given together with a sulfonamide.

Action/Kinetics   Interferes with nucleic acid metabolism of parasite (folic acid antagonists). Completely absorbed from GI tract. Very slowly excreted in urine. Drug is detectable in urine 30 or more days after administration.

Uses   Falciparum malaria: causal prophylaxis, suppressive prophylaxis, radical cure, primary attacks, and relapses.
Vivax malaria: suppressive cure and possibly some causal prophylaxis. Toxoplasmosis (a sulfonamide is usually given concomitantly).

Contraindication   Not recommended for treatment of resistant parasites.

Untoward Reactions   Few toxic effects at usual dosage. Occasional dermatoses. Large doses may cause *GI:* Anorexia, vomiting, atrophic glossitis. *Hematologic:* Megaloblastic anemia, leukopenia, thrombocytopenia, pancytopenia. *CNS:* Very large doses and overdosage may cause convulsions.

Drug Interactions

Interactant	Interaction
Folic acid	↓ Effect of pyrimethamine
PABA	↓ Effect of pyrimethamine
Quinine	↑ Effect of quinine due to ↓ in plasma protein binding

Dosage   PO. *Acute malarial attack* (used with other antimalarials): **Adults,** 50 mg/ day for 2 days; **pediatric, 4–10 years:** 25 mg/day for 2 days. *Prophylaxis of malaria*: **Adults and children over 10 years**: 25 mg once weekly; **children 4–10 years**: 12.5 mg once weekly; **infants and children under 4 years**: 6.25 mg once weekly. *Toxoplasmosis*: **initial,** 50–75 mg daily with 1–4 gm sulfapyrimidine for 1–3 weeks; **then,** reduce dosage of each drug by one-half and continue treatment for an additional 4–5 weeks. **Pediatric: initial,** 1 mg/kg/day divided into 2 equal doses for 2–4 days; **then,** reduce dosage to one-half and continue for 1 month (also use sulfonamide).

Nursing Implications

See *Nursing Implications* for *Anti-infectives*, p. 52.

1. Anticipate slow onset of action. A faster-acting drug is usually used for an acute malarial attack.
2. Administer for suppressive prophylaxis during the seasons of malarial transmission.
3. Administer at weekly intervals in recommended dosages to avoid interference with blood cell formation and the development of resistance, both of which necessitate changes in therapy.
4. Anticipate that with high doses, as given to patients with toxoplasmosis, signs of folic acid deficiency, such as megaloblastic anemia, thrombocytopenia, leukopenia, or GI side effects, may develop. The drug should be discontinued or reduced, and folic acid (Leucovorin) administered.
5. Have available barbiturates and folic acid for emergency treatment for convulsions resulting from ingestion of large overdoses.
6. Assess patients for symptoms of malaria as resistance to the drug can develop.

QUINACRINE HYDROCHLORIDE   Atabrine Hydrochloride (Rx)

See *Anthelmintics*, p. 154.

QUININE SULFATE   Coco-Quinine, QM-260, Quinamm, Quine, Quiphile, Strema (Rx)

Classification   Antimalarial.

General Statement   This drug is a natural alkaloid obtained from the bark of the cinchona tree. In addition to its antimalarial properties, it has antipyretic and analgesic properties similar to those of the salicylates. It relieves muscle spasms and is used as a diagnostic agent for myasthenia gravis. Quinine has been used increasingly in the last several years since resistant forms of vivax and falciparum were observed in Southeast Asia. No resistant forms of the parasite have been found for quinine.

Action/Kinetics   Quinine is presumed to have a variety of toxic effects on parasites, including decreasing its respiration and affecting DNA replication. Quinine is rapidly and completely absorbed from GI tract, widely distributed in body tissues.

The drug is highly bound to protein, and about 10% is excreted unchanged in urine.

Uses   In combination with pyramethamine and sulfadiazine or tetracycline for resistant forms of *P. falciparum*. Nocturnal leg cramps.

Contraindications   Patients with tinnitus. To be used with caution in patients with optic neuritis.

Untoward Reactions   Use of quinine may result in symptoms referred to as cinchonism. Mild cinchonism is characterized by tinnitus, headache, nausea, slight visual disturbances. Larger doses, however, may cause severe CNS, cardiovascular, gastrointestinal, or dermatologic effects.

Allergic: Flushing, rashes, fever, facial edema, pruritus, dyspnea, tinnitus, gastric upset. *GI:* Nausea, vomiting, gastric pain. *Ophthalmologic:* Blurred vision, photophobia, diplopia, night blindness, decreased visual fields, impaired color perception. *CNS:* Headache, confusion, restlessness, vertigo, syncope, fever. *Hematologic:* Thrombocytopenia, hypoprothrombinemia. *CV:* Symptoms of angina, ventricular tachycardia, conduction disturbances. *Miscellaneous:* Sweating.

Drug Interactions

Interactant	Interaction
Anticoagulants, oral	Additive hypoprothrombinemia
Digoxin	Quinine ↑ effect of digoxin
Heparin	Effect ↓ by quinine
Pyramethamine	↑ Effect of quinine due to ↓ in plasma protein binding
Skeletal muscle relaxants (surgical) Succinylcholine *d*-Tubocurarine	↑ Respiratory depression and apnea

Dosage   **PO**. *Chloroquine–resistant malaria*: **Adults**, 650 mg q 8 hr for 10–14 days; **children**: 25 mg/kg/day divided into 3 doses, for 10–14 days. *Nocturnal leg cramps*: 200–300 mg at bedtime.

Nursing Implications
See *Nursing Implications* for *Anti-infectives*, p. 52.
Assess
   a. for cinchonism (ringing of ears, blurring of vision, and headache, which may be followed by digestive disturbances,impairment of hearing and sight, confusion, and delirium), indicating overdosage. Quinine overdosage should be treated by thorough gastric lavage or induced emesis.
   b. for tremor and palpitation, tinnitus, impaired hearing, dizziness, which may appear with therapeutic doses.

SULFADOXINE AND PYRIMETHAMINE   Fansidar (Rx)

Classification   Antimalarial

Action/Kinetics   Sulfadoxine completes with para-aminobenzoic acid for synthesis of folic acid while pyrimethamine inhibits the formation of tetrahydrofolate from dihydrofolate. These reactions are necessary for one-carbon transfer reactions in the synthesis of nucleic acids. **Peak plasma levels:** sulfadoxine, 2.5–6 hr; pyrimethamine, 1.5–8 hr. Both drugs are long-acting.

For specific information regarding pyrimethamine, see p. 172.

Uses   Malaria, especially chloroquine-resistant strains.

Contraindications   Megaloblastic anemia. Infants less than 2 months old. Pregnancy (near term) and lactation. Use with caution in patients with glucose 6-phosphate dehydrogenase deficiency.

Untoward Reactions   See sulfonamides, p. 140 and pyrimethamine, p. 172.

Dosage   PO. Tablets contain pyrimethamine, 25 mg, and sulfadoxine, 500 mg. *Acute malaria (in combination with other drugs)*: **Adults,** 2–3 tablets. **Pediatric, 9–14 years:** 2 tablets; **4–8 years:** 1 tablet; **under 4 years:** ½ tablet. *Prophylaxis:* Drug is taken either once weekly or once every 2 weeks. **Adults,** weekly, 1 tablet; biweekly, 2 tablets. **Pediatric, 9–14 years:** weekly, ¾ tablet; biweekly, 1½ tablets. **4–8 years:** weekly, ½ tablet; biweekly, 1 tablet. **Under 4 years:** weekly, ¼ tablet; biweekly, ½ tablet.

Administration
1. High intake of fluid should occur to prevent precipitation in the urine.
2. For prophylaxis, therapy should be initiated 1–2 days before entering endemic area and should continue during stay and for 4–6 weeks after leaving. Primaquine should be given after this time.

Chapter Fifteen

AMEBICIDES AND TRICHOMONACIDES

General Statement   Amebiasis is a widely distributed disease caused by the protozoan *Entamoeba histolytica*. The disease has a high incidence in areas with low standards of hygiene. In the United States, the average rate of infestation is generally from 1 to 10%; however, in certain southern localities the incidence is as high as 40%.

Entamoeba histolytica has two forms: (1) an active motile form known as the trophozoite form, and (2) a cystic form that is very resistant to destruction and responsible for the transmission of the disease.

The overt manifestations of amebiasis vary. Some patients manifest violent acute dysentery (sudden development of severe diarrhea, cramps, and passage of bloody, mucoid stools), while others have few overt symptoms or are even completely asymptomatic.

Diagnosis is made on the basis of microscopic examination of fresh, or at least moist, stools by a trained examiner. More than one sample of stool must be negative before amebiasis can be ruled out.

Amebae often migrate from the GI tract to other parts of the body (extraintestinal amebiasis). The spleen, lungs, or liver are frequently affected. The amebae colonize in these organs and form abscesses that may rupture and thereby serve as infectious foci.

Drugs used for the treatment of this disease fall into two main categories; some are more suitable for the treatment of intestinal forms of the disease, while others are required for extraintestinal infestations. At present, no one drug can cure all types of amebic infestations, and many physicians prefer to use a combination of several therapeutic agents. Often the more effective, but very toxic agents, are used initially for a short period of time, while long-term eradication or prophylaxis is carried out with less toxic agents.

Since many of the agents used in the treatment of amebiasis are also used for trichomoniasis, nursing implications and dosages for the treatment of *Entamoeba histolytica* will be given in this section.

Infestation with the parasite *Trichomonas vaginalis* causes vaginitis characterized by an irritating, profuse, creamy or frothy vaginal discharge associated with severe itching and burning. Diagnosis is made on the basis of demonstrating the presence of the trichomonad microscopically in the vaginal secretion.

Vaginitis caused by *Trichomonas vaginalis* is treated by various locally applied antitrichomonal agents—often effective amebicides—and also by the oral administration of metronidazole (Flagyl). This drug is usually prescribed for both sexual partners so as to prevent reinfection.

Acid douches (vinegar or lactic acid) are a helpful adjunct to treatment.

Eradication of the infectious agent—which frequently becomes resistant—should be ascertained for 3 months after treatment has ceased. The examination usually is made after menstruation, since trichomonas infections often flare up during menstruation.

The incidence of infections by another protozoan organism, *Giardia lambia*, is increasing in North America. The organism is transmitted in the feces. Infections are characterized by mucous diarrhea, abdominal pain, and weight loss. Drugs of choice are metronidazole and quinacrine.

Nursing Implications

See *Nursing Implications* for *Anti-infectives*, p. 52.

AMEBICIDES

1. Assess patients on therapy for acute dysentery or extraintestinal amebiasis closely because the agents of choice are highly toxic.
2. Anticipate that the patient frequently will be on a combination of drug therapy for amebiasis and must be observed for toxic reactions to all drugs.
3. Be prepared to give intensive supportive nursing care to patients having acute dysentery; assist in the effort to control diarrhea, maintain electrolyte balance, and prevent complications caused by malnutrition. The patient's activity may have to be curtailed during the acute phase of the disease.

4. Administer drugs only for the period of time ordered and allow for rest periods between courses of therapy. Advise patients against self-medication.

5. *Teach*
   a. carriers to continue with drug therapy, stressing the benefit to themselves, their families, and co-workers.
   b. the necessity for thorough handwashing, especially in industry, schools, and other institutions where disease is likely to be spread.
   c. the need for food handlers to be particularly conscientious about handwashing after toileting. Emphasize the need for the availability of soap, water, and towels.
   d. patient and carriers to have regular stool examinations to check for recurrence.

TRICHOMONACIDES

1. *Teach patient and/or family*
   a. the proper method of douching and good feminine hygiene.
   b. the methods of insufflation or insertion of vaginal suppository, depending on drug regimen.
   c. to wear a pad to prevent clothing or bed linen from becoming stained by the medication in vaginal suppositories, especially if they contain iodine, which has a tendency to stain. Stress that the pad must be changed frequently and must not be worn moist for any length of time because it may serve as a growth medium for the infecting organism.
   d. that sexual partner may be an asymptomatic carrier and also may require therapy to prevent reinfection of woman.

CARBARSONE (Rx)

Classification   Amebicide.

Action/Kinetics   Carbarsone is an organic arsenical, effective against both the motile and cystic forms of amebae. It appears to be selectively more toxic for protozoa than for mammalian cells and it seems to inhibit sulfhydryl enzymes. The drug is readily absorbed from GI tract and is excreted slowly by kidneys.

Uses   Acute and chronic intestinal amebiasis including trophozoite form of *Entamoeba histolytica*. Particularly suitable for the treatment of carriers.

Contraindications   Renal and hepatic disease, including amebic hepatitis or amebic abscesses of the liver. Also, patients with arsenic intolerance or previous loss of vision.

Untoward Reactions   *Dermatologic:* Pruritus, skin eruptions. *GI:* GI upset, hepatitis. *Other:* Sore throat, neuritis, visual problems, splenomegaly, edema, icterus.

Note: Deaths have resulted from hepatic necrosis, hemorrhagic encephalitis, and exfoliative dermatitis. Toxicity may be treated with dimercaprol (BAL).

Symptoms of overdosage include: *GI:* Nausea, vomiting, diarrhea, abdominal pain. *CNS:* Seizures, coma. *Other:* Skin and mucous membrane ulceration, renal damage.

Dosage   **PO. Adult**: 250 mg b.i.d.–t.i.d. for 10 days. Dosage can be repeated after a rest period of 10–14 days. **Pediatric, 2–4 years**: 2 gm total dose over a 10-day period (66 mg t.i.d.); **5–8 years**: 3 gm total dose over 10 days (100 mg t.i.d.); **9–12 years**: 4 gm total dose over 10 days (133 mg t.i.d.); **12 years and older**: 5 gm total dose over 10 days (167 mg t.i.d.). For pediatric dosage, divide contents of a capsule and give in food or liquid.

Additional Nursing Implications

See also *Nursing Implications* for *Anti-infectives*, p. 52 and *Amebicides*, p. 176.

AMEBIASIS

1. Assess for dermatitis, CNS inflammation, and visual disturbances, which are all signs of arsenic intoxication.
2. Have dimercaprol (BAL) on hand as an antidote to arsenic poisoning.
3. Maintain patient on light diet and allow only moderate activity.

CHLOROQUINE   Aralen (Rx)

See *Antimalarials*, p. 170.

EMETINE HYDROCHLORIDE   (Rx)

Classification   Amebicide.

Action/Kinetics   Emetine is an alkaloid that kills the motile (trophozoite) form of ameba but not amebic cysts. It acts locally on the intestinal wall and in the liver and blocks protein synthesis in the parasite. It tends to accumulate in tissues and is excreted very slowly by the kidneys being detected in the urine 40–60 days after administration.

Uses   Acute amebic dysentery, amebic hepatitis, and extraintestinal amebiasis. Also for balantidiasis, fascioliasis, and paragonimiasis.

Contraindications   Emetine is potentially a very toxic compound, not to be used for minor cases, for prophylaxis, or for carriers. Its main toxic effect is on the cardiovascular system. It is contraindicated for patients with cardiac or renal disease; aged, debilitated persons; children; or during pregnancy, unless the condition does not respond to other therapy.

Untoward Reactions   *CV:* Tachycardia, ECG irregularities, congestive heart failure, hypotension, precordial pain, cardiac dilation, gallop rhythm. *GI:* Nausea, vomiting, diarrhea (common). *CNS:* Headache, dizziness. *Dermatologic:* Urticaria, eczema, purpura. *Other:* Dyspnea; muscle weakness, stiffness, and pain.

Dosage   *Amebiasis.* **Deep SC or IM (DO NOT USE IV). Adults**: 65 mg daily in single or two divided doses for 3–5 days (until acute symptoms subside). Some recommend a dose of 1 mg/kg/day, not to exceed 65 mg/day. Period of treatment should not exceed 10 days, and a rest period of 6 weeks should be observed before treatment is repeated. The dose should be halved in underweight or debilitated patients. **Pediatric (only in severe dysentery not responsive to other amebicides): 8 years and older**: no more than 20 mg/day; **8 years and younger**: no more than 10 mg/day. *Amebic hepatitis or abscess*: 65 mg/day for 10 days.

For acute fulminating amebic dysentery, emetine should be administered long enough to control diarrhea or other dysenteric symptoms (usually 3–5 days).

Administration

1. Injection may cause local irritation, induration,and swelling. Keep record of injection site and rotate.
2. Apply heat to relieve pain and hasten absorption of drug.
3. Aspirate syringe before injecting because accidental IV administration of emetine is dangerous.

Additional Nursing Implications

See also *Nursing Implications* for *Anti-infectives*, p. 52 and *Amebecides*, p. 176.

1. Maintain patient at bedrest during the course of treatment and for several days after therapy has been completed.
2. Assess blood pressure and pulse rate several times daily during the course of therapy. Report a rise in pulse rate above 110 beats/min, tachycardia, and a fall in blood pressure, because such symptoms require that the drug be discontinued.
3. *Teach patient and/or family*
   a. physician's specific recommendations concerning limited activity after a course of therapy so that activities can be planned.
   b. to report promptly any unusual symptoms experienced during the posttreatment period.

ERYTHROMYCIN (Rx)

See Chapter 9, p. 76. See also Table 1.

GENTIAN VIOLET Genapax (Rx)

Classification Vaginal anti-infective.

Action/Kinetics This traditional rosaniline dye is effective against some gram-positive bacteria, many fungi (yeasts and dermatophytes) and many strains of *Candida*. Treatment should continue until symptoms subside and cultures are negative.

Uses Infections caused by *Candida albicans,* topical geotropics.

Contraindications Hypersensitivity to gentian violet, presence of other vaginal infections, extensive vaginal excoriation, and ulceration. Use with caution in patients suspected of having diabetes mellitus, because vaginal infections often are the first symptoms of this disease. Ulcerative lesions of the face.

Untoward Reactions *Topical:* Irritation, hypersensitivity, ulceration of mucous membranes, permanent staining if applied to granulation tissue. *GI:* Following use for oral candidiasis, esophagitis, laryngitis, tracheitis, laryngeal obstruction.

Dosage One tampon (5 mg) inserted for 3–4 hr once or twice daily for 12 consecutive days. An additional tampon may be used overnight in resistant cases.

Administration

Tampon should be inserted high into vagina. During last trimester of pregnancy, the suppository should be inserted partially into vagina, preferably by hand.

Nursing Implications

Teach patient

a. good skin care and proper hygiene, to prevent further infection.

b. to keep exposed areas as dry as possible.

c. to wear clean panties with a cotton crotch.

d. to protect skin and clothing from dye.

e. to ask doctor for instructions about douching.

f. that male partner should wear a condom.

IODOQUINOL (DIIODOHYDROXYQUIN)   Moebiquin, Yodoxin (Rx)

Classification   Amebicide, trichomonacide, and local anti-infective.

Action/Kinetics   Mostly unabsorbed from the GI tract. Appearance of free iodine in blood or urine indicates that some of the drug is absorbed.

Uses   Acute and chronic intestinal amebiasis.

Contraindications   Hepatic or renal damage or iodine intolerance. Severe thyroid conditions. Nonspecific diarrhea in children.

Untoward Reactions   *GI:* Nausea, vomiting, diarrhea, cramps, anal pruritus. *Dermatologic:* Pruritus, urticaria, skin rashes. *Ophthalmologic:* Optic neuritis or atrophy. *CNS:* Fever, chills, headache, vertigo. *Other:* Peripheral neuropathy, thyroid enlargement.

Laboratory Test Interference   Certain thyroid function tests ($\downarrow$ uptake of ^{131}I) for up to 6 months after discontinuance of therapy.

Dosage   **PO. Adults:** 650 mg b.i.d.–t.i.d. after meals for 20 days; **pediatric:** 40 mg/kg/day in 3 divided doses for 20 days.

Additional Nursing Implications

See also *Nursing Implications* for *Anti-infectives* p. 52.

AMEBIASIS   *Assess* for symptoms of iodism, such as furunculosis, dermatitis, sore throat, chills, and fever.

METRONIDAZOLE   Apo-Metronidazole,* Flagyl, Metryl, Neo-Tric,* Novonidazol,* PMS Metronidazole,* Protostat, Satric (Rx)

Classification   Systemic trichomonacide, amebicide.

Action/Kinetics   Effective against anaerobic bacteria and protozoa. Specifically inhibits growth of *trichomonae* and *amebae* by binding and degrading DNA. Well absorbed from GI tract and widely distributed in body tissues. **Peak serum concentration: PO**, 5–40 μg/ml after 1–2 hr.; t½: **PO**, 6–8 hr. Eliminated primarily in urine, which may be red-brown in color following either PO or IV use.

Uses   Amebiasis. Symptomatic and asymptomatic trichomoniasis; to treat asymptomatic partner. Amebic dysentery and amebic liver abscess. To reduce postoperative anaerobic infection following colorectal surgery, elective hysterectomy, and emergency appendectomy. Anaerobic bacterial infections of the abdomen, female genital system, skin or skin structures, bones and joints, lower respiratory tract, and CNS. Also, septicemia, endocarditis. Orally for Crohn's disease and pseudomembranous colitis. *Investigational:* giardiasis, *Gardnerella vaginalis.*

Contraindications   Blood dyscrasias, active organic disease of the CNS, pregnancy, especially during the first trimester and near term.

Untoward Reactions   *GI:* Following PO use, nausea, dry mouth, metallic taste, vomiting, diarrhea, abdominal discomfort, constipation. *Nervous system:* Headache, dizziness, vertigo, incoordination, ataxia, confusion, irritability, depression, weakness, insomnia, syncope, seizures, peripheral neuropathy including paresthesias. *Hematologic:* Leukopenia, bone marrow aplasia. *GU:* Burning, dysuria, cystitis, polyuria, incontinence, dryness of vagina or vulva, dyspareunia, decreased libido. *Allergic:* Urticaria, pruritus, erythematous rash, flushing, nasal congestion, fever, joint pain. *Other:* Furry tongue, glossitis, stomatitis (due to overgrowth of *Candida*). ECG abnormalities, thrombophlebitis.

Drug Interactions

Interactant	Interaction
Alcohol, ethyl	Antabuse-like reaction possible
Anticoagulants, oral	↑ Anticoagulant effect due to ↓ breakdown by liver
Disulfiram (Antabuse)	Additive effects

Dosage   **PO.** *Amebiasis: Acute amebic dysentery or amebic liver abscess:* **Adult,** 500–750 mg t.i.d. for 5–10 days; **pediatric:** 35–50 mg/kg daily in 3 divided doses for 10 days. *Trichomoniasis, Female*: 250 mg t.i.d. for 7 days; or, 2 gm given on 1 day in single or divided doses. **Pediatric:** 5 mg/kg t.i.d. for 7 days. An interval of 4–6 weeks should elapse between courses of therapy. *Note:* Pregnant patients should not be treated during the first trimester. *Male*: Individualize dosage; usual, 250 mg t.i.d. for 7 days. *Giardiasis:* 250 mg t.i.d. for 7 days. *Gardnerella vaginalis:* 500 mg b.i.d. for 7 days. **IV.** *Anaerobic bacterial infections:* **Initial:** 15 mg/kg infused over 1 hr; **then,** after 6 hrs, 7.5 mg/kg q 6 hrs for 7–10 days (daily dose should not exceed 4 gm). *Anaerobic bacterial infections:* **IV, Adults, initial,** 15 mg/kg; **then,** 7.5 mg/kg q 6 hr (maximum daily dose: 4 gm). Treatment may be necessary for 2–3 weeks although PO therapy should be initiated as soon as possible. *Prophylaxis of anaerobic infection during surgery:* **IV,** 0.5–1 gm 1 hr prior to surgery and 0.5 gm 8 and 16 hr after surgery.

Administration

1. If used IV, drug should not be given by IV bolus.
2. Syringes with aluminum needles or hubs should not be used.
3. If a primary IV fluid set-up is used, discontinue the primary solution during infusion of metronidazole.
4. The order of mixing to prepare the Powder for Injection is important:
   a. Reconstitution.
   b. Dilution in IV solutions (glass or plastic containers).
   c. Neutralization of pH with sodium bicarbonate solution. Neutralized solutions should not be refrigerated.

Additional Nursing Implications

See also *Nursing Implications* for *Anti-infectives*, p. 52.

1. Assess for symptoms of CNS toxicity, such as ataxia or tremor, which necessitate withdrawal of drug.
2. *Teach patient and/or family*
   a. the necessity for male partner to have therapy since organism may also be located in the male urogenital tract.
   b. that the drug may turn urine brown.
   c. not to drink alcohol when on metronidazole therapy because an Antabuse-like reaction may occur. Symptoms include abdominal cramps, vomiting, flushing, and headache.

PAROMOMYCIN SULFATE   Humatin (Rx)

See *Aminoglycosides*, p. 114.

POVIDONE-IODINE   Acu-Dyne, Aerodine, Betadine, BPS, Bridine,* Efodine, Final Step, Frepp, Frepp/Sepp, Isodine, Mallisol, Operand, Pharmadine, Polydine, Povadyne, Proviodine,* Sepp, Surgi-Sep (OTC)

Classification   Antiseptic/germicide.

Action/Kinetics   This product is a nonstinging, nonstaining iodine complex with all the antiseptic properties of iodine but without skin and mucous membrane irritation. Bactericidal for gram-positive and gram-negative bacteria, antibiotic-resistant organisms, fungi, viruses, protozoa, and yeasts. It is only used topically. After product application the coloration of skin is an indication of area of antimicrobial activity.

Uses   Topical dressing; degerming of skin; antiseptic for wounds, burns, abrasions, or preoperatively. Treatment of dandruff.

Contraindications   Rare cases of skin sensitivity.

Dosage   All solutions and ointments are used full strength, and all pads, swabs, and other means of application are used only once. Treated area can be bandaged. The following products are available: *Aerosol, Antiseptic Gauze Pads or Solution, Antiseptic Lubricating Gel, Applicators, Cleansing Bar, Foam Skin Cleanser, Helafoam Solution, Mouthwash/Gargle, Ointment, Perineal Wash Concentrate, Prep Solution, Scrub (including Applicators or Swab Sticks), Shampoo, Skin Cleanser, Solution (including Prep Pads, Prep Swabs, Swabs, Swab Aid, Swab Sticks, Wipes), Spray, Surgical Scrub (including Sponge/Brush), Whirlpool Concentrate.*

Additional Nursing Implications

See also *Nursing Implications* for *Anti-infectives*, p. 52.

1. Assess for skin sensitivity.
2. Inform patient that drug stains wash off easily.
3. Allow exposed areas to dry before bandaging.

TETRACYCLINES (Rx)

See Chapter 9, p. 80.

Chapter Sixteen

URINARY GERMICIDES/ ANALGESICS

Urinary tract infections are commonly treated by several of the antimicrobial agents considered in other sections (*Miscellaneous Antibiotics, Sulfonamides*). Agents used specifically for urinary tract infections are listed in this section.

See *Nursing Implications* for *Anti-infectives*, p. 52.

ACETOHYDROXAMIC ACID   Lithostat (Rx)

Classification   Inhibitor of urease.

Action/Kinetics   This drug inhibits the enzyme urease, which decreases the hydrolysis of urea to ammonia. It is especially useful in urinary tract infections of urea-splitting organisms. Following administration of acetohydroxamic acid, urinary pH decreases, leading to increased efficacy of antibiotics. The drug is not antibacterial itself. **Peak blood levels:** 15–60 min. **t½:** 5–10 hr. To be effective the drug must be excreted unchanged in the urine (approximately 35–65%).

Uses   As an adjunct in urinary tract infections due to urea-splitting organisms.

Contraindications   Should not be used instead of surgery or antibiotic therapy. Renal dysfunction. In females not using contraception. Pregnancy, lactation.

Untoward Reactions   *GI:* Nausea, vomiting, anorexia. *CNS:* Headaches (common), malaise, depression, tremors, nervousness. *Hematologic:* Hemolytic anemia, reticulocytosis without anemia. *Other:* Phlebitis in the legs; nonpruritic, macular skin rash; alopecia.

Drug Interactions

Interactant	Interaction
Alcohol	Nonpruritic, macular skin rash within 30–60 min
Iron	↓ Absorption of iron due to chelation by acetohydroxamic acid

Dosage   PO. Adults: 250 mg t.i.d.–q.i.d. up to a maximum of 1.5 gm daily. **Pediatric: initial,** 10 mg/kg/day; **then,** adjust dose depending on response and hematologic picture. **Serum creatinine greater than 1.8 mg/dl:** maximum of 1 gm/day in divided doses at 12 hr intervals.

Nursing Implications

1. While the drug has been used in a limited number of patients, the incidence of adverse effects is high (30%).
2. Complaints of headaches, especially during the first 2–3 days of therapy, are common and respond well to aspirin.
3. Assure patient that nausea, vomiting, anorexia, and malaise are usually transient. Drug therapy is rarely terminated for these symptoms.
4. Teach patient to inspect lower legs for redness and tenderness, pain, signs of superficial phlebitis. Report these to physician.
5. If loss of body hair is severe, wigs and eye makeup can be recommended.
6. Warn patient to forego ingestion of alcohol while on this drug, as rash may develop.
7. Because drug chelates iron, iron deficiency anemia may result. Supplemental iron tablets may be suggested.

CINOXACIN   Cinobac (Rx)

Classification   Urinary anti-infective.

Action/Kinetics   Cinoxacin acts by inhibiting DNA replication resulting in a bactericidal action. It is rapidly absorbed after oral administration; a 500-mg dose results in a urine concentration of 300 μg/ml during the first 4 hr and 100 μg/ml during the second 4-hr period. Within 24 hr, 97% is excreted in the urine, 60% unchanged. **Mean serum t½:** 1.5 hr.

Uses   Initial and recurrent urinary tract infections caused by *E. coli, P. mirabilis, P. vulgaris, Klebsiella,* and *Enterobacter* species.

Contraindications   Prepubertal children. Anuric patients. Pregnancy and lactation. Use with caution in patients with hepatic or kidney disease. Hypersensitivity.

Untoward Effects   *GI*: Nausea, vomiting, anorexia, cramps, diarrhea. *CNS*: Headache, dizziness, insomnia, confusion, nervousness. *Dermatologic*: Rash, pruritus, urticaria, edema. *Other*: Tingling sensation, photophobia, perineal burning, tinnitus.

Laboratory Test Interference   Abnormal BUN, SGOT, SGPT, serum creatinine, and alkaline phosphatase.

Dosage   PO. Adults: 1 gm/day in 2–4 divided doses for 7–14 days. *In patients with impaired renal function:* **Initial,** 500 mg; **then,** dosage schedule based on creatinine clearance (See package insert).

Additional Nursing Implications

See *Nursing Implications* for *Anti-infectives*, p. 52.

1. Ascertain that renal and hepatic function tests are completed before initiating therapy.
2. Do not administer to anuric patient.

FLAVOXATE HYDROCHLORIDE Urispas (Rx)

Classification Urinary tract antispasmodic.

Action/Kinetics Acts directly on smooth muscle of urinary tract causing muscle relaxation and increasing urinary bladder capacity. (Mechanism similar to that of papaverine.) Flavoxate also has anticholinergic, local anesthetic, and analgesic properties. Well absorbed from GI tract. Ten to 30% excreted in urine.

Uses Symptomatic relief of urinary tract irritation, dysuria, urgency, nocturia, suprapubic pain, incontinence associated with cystitis, prostatitis, urethritis, urethrocystitis, and other urinary tract disorders. Compatible for use with urinary tract germicides.

Contraindications Obstructive disorders of urinary tract, including pyloric or duodenal obstructions, intestinal lesions, ileus, achalasia (absence of gastric acid), and GI hemorrhage. Use with caution in glaucoma. Safe use in pregnancy or in children under 12 years of age not established.

Untoward Reactions *GI:* Nausea, vomiting, xerostomia. *CNS:* Drowsiness, headache, vertigo, nervousness, mental confusion (especially in the elderly). *CV:* Tachycardia, palpitations. *Hematologic:* Eosinophilia, leukopenia. *Ophthalmologic:* Blurred vision, increased ocular tension, accommodation disturbances. *Other:* Urticaria, skin rashes, fever, dysuria.

Dosage **Adults and children over 12 years**: 100 or 200 mg t.i.d. or q.i.d. Dose may be reduced when symptoms decrease.

Additional Nursing Implications

See also *Nursing Implications* for *Cholinergic Blocking Agents*, p. 594. *Teach patient and/or family*

a. not to drive a car or operate hazardous machinery as drug may cause drowsiness and blurred vision.
b. good oral hygiene to relieve dryness of mouth.

METHENAMINE (OTC)

METHENAMINE HIPPURATE Hip-Rex,* Hiprex, Urex (Rx)

METHENAMINE MANDELATE Mandelamine (Rx)

Classification Urinary tract anti-infective.

Action/Kinetics   This drug is converted in an acid medium into ammonia and formaldehyde (the active principle), which denatures protein. It is thus most effective when the urine has a pH value of 5.5 or less. Readily absorbed from GI tract. To be effective, urinary formaldehyde concentration must be greater than 25 μg/ml. Seventy to 90% of drug and metabolites excreted in urine within 24 hr.

Uses   Acute, chronic, and recurrent urinary tract infections by susceptible organisms, especially gram-negative organisms including *E. coli.* As a prophylactic before urinary tract instrumentation. Never used as sole agent in the treatment of acute infections.

Contraindications   Renal insufficiency, severe liver damage, or severe dehydration.

Untoward Reactions   *GI:* Nausea, vomiting, diarrhea, anorexia, cramps, stomatitis. *GU:* Hematuria, albuminuria, crystalluria, dysuria, urinary frequency or urgency, bladder irritation. *Dermatologic:* Skin rashes, urticaria, pruritus. *Other:* Tinnitus, muscle cramps, headache, dyspnea, edema, lipoid pneumonitis.

Drug Interactions

Interactant	Interaction
Acetazolamide (Diamox)	↓ Effect of methenamine due to ↑ alkalinity of urine by acetazolamide
Sodium bicarbonate	↓ Effect of methenamine due to ↑ alkalinity of urine by sodium bicarbonate
Sulfonamides	↑ Chance of sulfonamide crystalluria due to acid urine produced by methenamine
Thiazide diuretics	↓ Effect of methenamine due to ↑ alkalinity of urine produced by thiazides

Laboratory Test Interference   False-positive urinary glucose with Benedict's solution. Drug interferes with determination of urinary catecholamines and estriol levels by acid hydrolysis technique (enzymatic techniques not affected).

Dosage   **PO**. *Methenamine*: **Adults,** 1 gm q.i.d.; **children 6–12 years**: 500 mg q.i.d.; **children under 6 years**: 50 mg/kg/day in 3 divided doses. *Hippurate*: **Adults and children over 12 years**: 1 gm b.i.d.; **children 6–12 years**: 0.5–1 gm b.i.d. *Mandelate*: **Adults**: 1 gm q.i.d. after meals and at bedtime; **children 6–12 years**: 0.5 gm q.i.d.; **children under 6 years**: 18.3 mg/kg q.i.d.

Administration   Administer with one-half glass of water after meals and at bedtime.

Nursing Implications

See also *Nursing Implications* for *Anti-infectives*, p. 52.

1. *Assess*
   a. for skin rash, which is an indication for drug withdrawal.
   b. patients on high dosage for bladder irritation, painful and frequent micturition, albuminuria, and hematuria.
   c. for idiosyncratic effect characterized by nausea, vomiting, dermatologic reaction, tinnitus, and muscle cramps.
2. Clearly indicate on chart that patient is receiving drug because drug will interfere with urinary estriol, catecholamines, and HIAA tests.
3. Maintain an adequate fluid intake (between 1,500 and 2,000 ml daily).
4. Monitor intake and output.

5. Use Labstix or Nitrazine paper daily to test that pH of urine is 5.5 or lower.
6. Teach patient and/or family that urine may become turbid and full of sediment when mandelamine is administered concomitantly with sulfamethizole.

METHYLENE BLUE   Urolene Blue (Rx)

Classification   Urinary germicide, antidote, oxidizing agent.

Action/Kinetics   Methylene blue is a dye possessing bacteriostatic activity. High doses oxidize Fe^{2+} (ferrous ion) of reduced hemoglobin to Fe^{3+} (ferric ion) resulting in methemoglobinemia (basis for use in cyanide poisoning). Lower doses increase the conversion of methemoglobin to hemoglobin.

Uses   Mild GU tract antiseptic, drug-induced methemoglobinemia, antidote for cyanide poisoning, treatment of urinary tract calculi (oxalate). *Investigational:* Diagnosis of ruptured amniotic membranes; by its dye effect can determine body structures and fistulas.

Contraindications   Hypersensitivity to drug. Renal insufficiency. Use with caution in patients with glucose 6-phosphate dehydrogenase deficiency, as hemolysis may result.

Untoward Reactions   *GI*: Nausea, vomiting, diarrhea. *GU*: Dysuria, bladder irritation. *Other*: Anemia, fever, cyanosis, CV abnormalities.

Dosage   **PO:** *GU antiseptic*: 65–130 mg t.i.d. after meals with a full glass of water. **IV:** *Antidote:* 1–2 mg/kg slowly over several minutes.

Nursing Implications
1. Assess for symptoms of GI or GU dysfunction.
2. Teach patient and/or family that medication may turn urine and stools blue-green and will stain tissue.

NALIDIXIC ACID   Neg Gram (Rx)

Classification   Urinary germicide.

Action/Kinetics   Nalidixic acid is believed to inhibit the DNA synthesis of the microorganism. The drug is either bacteriostatic or bactericidal. Nalidixic acid is rapidly absorbed from the GI tract. **Peak plasma concentration**: 20–40 μg/ml after 1–2 hr; **peak urine levels**: 150–200 μg/ml after 3–4 hr. t½: 1.1–2.5 hr, increased to 21 hr in anuric patients. The drug is extensively protein bound, partially metabolized in liver and rapidly excreted in urine.

Sensitivity determinations are recommended before and periodically during prolonged administration of nalidixic acid. Renal and liver function tests are advisable if course of therapy exceeds 2 weeks.

Uses   Acute and chronic urinary tract infections caused by susceptible gram-negative organisms, including *E. coli, Proteus, Enterobacter,* and *Klebsiella*.

Contraindications To be used with caution in patients with liver disease, severely impaired kidney function, epilepsy, and severe cerebral arteriosclerosis. Safety in pregnancy has not been established.

Untoward Reactions *GI:* Nausea, vomiting, diarrhea, pain. *CNS:* Drowsiness, headache, dizziness, weakness, vertigo, toxic psychoses, seizures (rare). *Allergic:* Photosensitivity, skin rashes, arthralgia, pruritus, urticaria, angioedema, eosinophilia. *Hematologic:* Leukopenia, thrombocytopenia, hemolytic anemia (especially in patients with glucose 6-phosphate dehydrogenase deficiency). *Other:* Metabolic acidosis, cholestatic jaundice, paresthesia.

Drug Interactions

Interactant	Interaction
Antacids, oral	↓ Effect of nalidixic acid due to ↓ absorption from GI tract
Anticoagulants, oral	↑ Effect of anticoagulants due to ↓ in plasma protein binding
Nitrofurantoin	↓ Effect of nalidixic acid

Laboratory Test Interferences False + for urinary glucose with Benedict's solution, Fehling's solution, or Clinitest Reagent tablets. Falsely elevated 17-ketosteroids.

Dosage **PO. Adults: initially**, 1 gm q.i.d. for 1–2 weeks; **maintenance**, if necessary, 2 gm daily. **Children 12 years and younger: initially**, 55 mg/kg/day administered in 4 equal doses; **maintenance**, if necessary, 33 mg/kg/day. Not for use in infants less than 3 months of age.

Nursing Implications

See also *Nursing Implications* for *Anti-infectives*, p. 52.
   Use Clinistix Reagent Strips or Tes-Tape for urinary tests, as other methods may result in a false-positive reaction.

NITROFURANTOIN   Apo-Nitrofurantoin,* Furadantin, Furalan, Furan, Furanite, Furatoin, Nephronex,* Nitrofan, Novofuran,* (Rx)

NITROFURANTOIN MACROCRYSTALS   Macrodantin (Rx)

Classification Urinary germicide.

Action/Kinetics Nitrofurantoin interferes with bacterial carbohydrate metabolism by inhibiting acetylcoenzyme A; also, the drug interferes with bacterial cell wall synthesis. It is bacteriostatic at low concentrations and bactericidal at high concentrations. Tablets are readily absorbed from the GI tract. Nitrofurantoin macrocrystals (Macrodantin) are available; this preparation maintains effectiveness while decreasing GI distress.

Uses Severe urinary tract infections refractory to other agents. Useful in the treatment of pyelonephritis, pyelitis, or cystitis caused by susceptible organisms, including *E. coli*, *Staphylococcus aureus*, and *Streptococcus faecalis*, and certain strains of *Enterobacter*, *Proteus*, and *Klebsiella*.

Contraindications Anuria, oliguria, and patients with impaired renal function (creatinine clearance below 40 ml/min); pregnant women, especially near term; infants below 3 months of age; and nursing mothers. To be used with extreme caution in patients with anemia, diabetes, electrolyte imbalance, avitaminosis B, or a debilitating disease.

Untoward Reactions Nitrofurantoin is a potentially toxic drug with many side effects. *GI:* Nausea, vomiting, anorexia, diarrhea, abdominal pain, parotitis, pancreatitis. *CNS:* Headache, dizziness, vertigo, drowsiness, nystagmus. *Hematologic:* Leukopenia, thrombocytopenia, eosinophilia, megaloblastic anemia, agranulocytosis, granulocytopenia, hemolytic anemia (especially in patients with glucose 6-phosphate dehydrogenase deficiency). *Allergic:* Drug fever, skin rashes, pruritus, urticaria, angioedema, anaphylaxis, arthralgia, asthma symptoms in susceptible patients. *Hepatic:* Hepatitis, cholestatic jaundice, cholestatic hepatitis, liver dysfunction. *Other:* Peripheral neuropathy, alopecia, superinfections of the genitourinary tract, hypotension, muscle pain.

Drug Interactions

Interactant	Interaction
Acetazolamide (Diamox)	↓ Effect of nitrofurantoin due to ↑ alkalinity of urine produced by acetazolamide
Antacids, oral	↓ Effect of nitrofurantoin due to ↓ absorption from GI tract
Anticholinergic drugs	↑ Effect of nitrofurantoin due to ↑ absorption from stomach
Nalidixic acid	Nitrofurantoin ↓ effect
Sodium bicarbonate	↓ Effect of nitrofurantoin due to ↑ alkalinity of urine produced by sodium bicarbonate

Dosage **PO. Adults:** 50–100 mg q.i.d., not to exceed 400 mg/day; **prolonged therapy:** 25–50 mg q.i.d. **Children:** 5–7 mg/kg/day in 4 equal doses; **prolonged therapy:** 1 mg/kg/day in 1–2 doses. Contraindicated in children less than one month of age. **IV (only). Patients over 54.5 kg:** 180 mg b.i.d.; **patients less than 54.5 kg:** 6.6 mg/kg/day in 2 equal doses.

Administration/ Storage

1. Slow IV administration to relieve nausea and vomiting.
2. Administer oral medication with meals or milk to reduce gastric irritation.
3. Preferably, administer capsules containing crystals, instead of tablets, because crystals cause less GI intolerance.
4. Store oral medications in amber-colored bottles.
5. Mix, store, and administer parenteral preparations, as ordered on vial.

Additional Nursing Implications

See also *Nursing Implications* for *Anti-infectives*, p. 52.

1. *Assess*
   a. for acute or delayed anaphylactic reaction and have emergency equipment available.
   b. for peripheral neuropathy, manifested by numbness and tingling in the extremeties. These are indications for drug withdrawal, since the condition may become worse and irreversible.

(continued)

c. for superinfection of the GI tract.

d. blacks and ethnic groups of Mediterranean and Near-Eastern origin for symptoms of anemia.

2. Label chart showing patient is on drug, because it may alter certain laboratory determinations.

3. Anticipate severe pain at site of injection. This may require that the drug be discontinued. The IM route should not be used for more than 5 days.

4. *Teach patient and/or family* that drug may turn urine brown.

OXYBUTYNIN CHLORIDE Ditropan (Rx)

Classification Spasmolytic.

Action/Kinetics Oxybutynin causes increased vesicle capacity and delay of initial urgency to void. Has no effect at either the neuromuscular junction or autonomic ganglia. Has 4–10 times the antispasmodic effect of atropine but only one-fifth the anticholinergic activity. **Onset**: rapid; **peak effect**: 3–4 hr; **duration**: 6–10 hr.

Use Neurogenic bladder disease characterized by urinary retention, urinary overflow, or incontinence.

Contraindications Glaucoma, GI obstruction, paralytic ileus, intestinal atony, megacolon, severe colitis, myasthenia gravis, obstructive urinary tract disease, massive hemorrhage. *Use with caution when increased cholinergic effect is undesirable and in the elderly.*

Untoward Reactions *GI*: Nausea, vomiting, constipation, bloated feeling. *CNS*: Drowsiness, insomnia, weakness. *EENT*: Dry mouth, blurred vision, dilation of pupil, cycloplegia, increased ocular tension. *CV*: Tachycardia, palpitations. *Other*: Decreased sweating, urinary hesitancy and retention, impotence, suppression of lactation, severe allergic reactions, drug idiosyncrasies, urticaria, and other dermal manifestations.

OVERDOSAGE Intense CNS disturbances (restlessness, psychoses), circulatory changes (flushing, hypotension) and failure, respiratory failure, paralysis, coma.

TREATMENT OF OVERDASAGE Stomach lavage, physostigmine (0.5–2 mg IV; repeat as necessary up to maximum of 5 mg). Supportive therapy, if necessary. Counteract excitement with sodium thiopental (2%) or chloral hydrate (100–200 ml of 2% solution) rectally. Artificial respiration may be necessary if respiratory muscles become paralyzed.

Dosage **PO. Adults**: 5 mg b.i.d.–t.i.d.; maximum dosage, 20 mg daily. **Children (over 5 yr)**: 5 mg t.i.d.; maximum dosage, 15 mg daily.

Administration/Storage Store in tight containers at 15°–30°C.

Additional Nursing Implications

See also *Nursing Implications* for *Cholinergic Blocking Agents*, p. 594.

1. Be prepared to assist with treatment of overdosage, as noted in *Untoward Reactions*.

2. *Teach patient and/or family*

a. to report side effects noted in *Untoward Reactions* to doctor.

b. to use caution in driving a car or operating dangerous machinery, as drug may cause drowsiness and blurred vision.

c. to consult with doctor before continuing with medication if diarrhea occurs (especially in patients with an ileostomy or colostomy), as this may be an early symptom of intestinal obstruction.

d. to avoid overexposure to heat and need for increased fluids in hot weather, because sweating is inhibited by drug and heat stroke may occur.

e. to rinse mouth with water and increase fluids, unless contraindicated to relieve dryness of mouth.

f. to return for cystometry to evaluate response to therapy and need for continuation of medication.

PHENAZOPYRIDINE HYDROCHLORIDE   Azodine, Azo-Standard, Baridium, Di-Azo, Phenazo,* Phenazodine, Phenylazo Diamino Pyridine HCL, Pyridiate, Pyridium, Pyronium* (Rx)

Classification   Urinary anesthetic.

Action/Kinetics   Phenazopyridine hydrochloride is an azo dye with local anesthetic properties on the urinary tract.

Uses   Pain relief in chronic urinary tract infections or irritation, including cystitis, urethritis and pyelitis, trauma, surgery, or urinary tract instrumentation. May also be used as an adjunct to antibacterial therapy.

Contraindications   Renal insufficiency

Untoward Reactions   *GI:* Nausea. *Hematologic:* Methemoglobinemia, hemolytic anemia (especially in patients with glucose 6-phosphate dehydrogenase deficiency). *Dermatologic:* Yellowish tinge of the skin or sclerae may indicate accumulation of drug due to renal insufficiency. *Other:* Renal and hepatic toxicity.

Laboratory Test Interferences   Clinistix or Tes-Tape, colorimetric laboratory test procedures.

Dosage   **PO. Adult**: 100–200 mg t.i.d.

Treatment of Overdosage   To treat methemoglobinemia, administer methylene blue (IV: 1–2 mg/kg) or ascorbic acid (PO: 100–200 mg).

Administration   Give with or after meals to prevent GI upset.

Nursing Implications

1. *Assess* patient for cyanosis, a symptom of methemoglobenemia that indicates a toxic reaction.
2. Have ascorbic acid/methylene blue available for treatment of overdosage.
3. *Teach patient and/or family*
   a. to stop drug and report to doctor if skin or sclera become yellow tinged and/or skin or mucous membrane blueish.

Chapter Seventeen

ANTIVIRAL DRUGS

General Statement   Viruses, sometimes called naked genes, are the most elementary of the infectious agents. They consist of a core of nucleic acid and a coat of protein. To replicate, viruses must penetrate suitable cells whose machinery they take over to make copies of themselves. Viruses do not have cell walls, whose synthesis is usually interfered with by antibiotics like penicillin. This is why most antibiotics are ineffective against viruses.

Many virus infections (measles, small pox, polio) are prevented by means of immunization. Others, like influenza, just run their natural course. Recently several drugs have been developed that are moderately effective against certain viruses.

Nursing Implications
See *Nursing Implications* for *Anti-infectives*, p. 52.

ACYCLOVIR (ACYCLOGUANOSINE)   Zovirax (Rx)

Classification   Antiviral anti-infective.

Action/Kinetics   Acyclovir is converted to acyclovir triphosphate, which interferes with herpes simplex virus DNA polymerase thereby inhibiting DNA replication. Systemic absorption is minimal following topical administration. **Peak levels after PO:** 1.5–2 hr. **t½, PO:** 3.3 hr. Metabolites and unchanged drug are excreted through the kidney. Dosage should be reduced in patients with impaired renal function. Dosage forms include capsules, ointment, and injection.

Uses   **PO.** Initial and recurrent genital herpes. **Parenteral.** Initial therapy for severe genital herpes; initial and recurrent mucosal and cutaneous HSV-1 and HSV-2 infections in immunocompromised individuals. **Topical.** Acyclovir decreases healing time and duration of viral shedding in initial herpes genitalis. Also for limited non-life-threatening muocutaneous herpes simplex virus infections in immunocompromised patients. The drug does not seem to be beneficial in recurrent herpes genitalis or in herpes labialis in nonimmunocompromised patients.

Contraindications   Hypersensitivity to formulation. Use in the eye, during pregnancy, lactation. Use with caution with concomitant intrathecal methotrexate or interferon. Safety and efficacy of oral form not established in children.

Untoward Reactions   **PO.** *Short-term treatment. GI:* Nausea, vomiting, diarrhea, anorexia, sore throat, taste of drug. *CNS:* Headache, dizziness, fatigue. *Other:* Edema, skin rashes, leg pain, inguinal adenopathy. *Long-term treatment. GI:* Nausea, vomiting, diarrhea, sore throat. *CNS:* Headache, vertigo, insomnia, fatigue, fever, depression, irritability. *Other:* Arthralgia, rashes, palpitations, superficial thrombophlebitis, muscle cramps, menstrual abnormalities, acne, lymphadenopathy, alopecia.

Parenteral. *At injection site:* Phlebitis, inflammation. *CNS:* Encephalopathic changes, jitters, headache. *Other:* Skin rashes, urticaria, sweating, hypotension, nausea, thrombocytosis.

Topical. Transient burning, stinging, pain. Pruritus, rash, vulvitis.

Note: All of these effects have also been reported using a placebo preparation.

Dosage   PO. *Initial genital herpes:* 200 mg q 4 hr (while awake) for a total of 5 capsules/day for 10 days. *Chronic genital herpes:* 200 mg t.i.d. for up to 6 months. Up to 5 200 mg capsules/day may be required. *Intermittent therapy:* 200 mg q 4 hr (while awake) for a total of 5 capsules/day for 5 days. **IV infusion.** *All uses:* **Adults,** 5 mg/kg q 8 hr for 7 days. **Pediatric, less than 12 years:** 250 mg/m^2 q 8 hr for 7 days. Dose should be given over 1 hr. **Topical (5% ointment):** Lesion should be covered with sufficient amount of ointment (½ in. ribbon per 4 sq in. of surface area) every 3 hr 6 times per day for 7 days.

Storage
1. Reconstituted solution should be used within 12 hr.
2. If refrigerated, reconstituted solution may show a precipitate which dissolves at room temperature.
3. Store ointment in a dry place at room temperature.

Nursing Implications
See also *Nursing Implications* for *Anti-infectives,* p. 52.
Teach patient and/or family

1. to cover all lesions with acyclovir as ordered but not to exceed the frequency or length of time that treatment is recommended.
2. to apply acyclovir ointment in the amount directed with a finger cot or rubber glove to prevent transmission of infection.
3. to report burning, stinging, itching, and rash if they occur due to application of acyclovir.
4. to complete examination and tests to rule out possible presence of other sexually transmitted diseases.
5. to return for medical supervision if there is a recurrence of herpes simplex virus as acyclovir is ineffective for treatment of reinfection.
6. acyclovir will not prevent transmission of disease to others or prevent reinfection.
7. that total dose and dosage schedule differ depending on whether the infection is initial or chronic and whether intermittent therapy regimen is being used. Therefore, following prescribed dosage and duration of treatment is extremely important.

AMANTADINE HYDROCHLORIDE   Symmetrel (Rx)

Classification   Antiviral and antiparkinson agent.

Action/Kinetics   Amantadine is believed to prevent penetration of virus into cells, possibly by inhibiting uncoating of the RNA virus. Well absorbed from GI tract.

Peak serum concentration: 0.2 mg/ml after 1–4 hr. **t½**: range of 9–37 hr, longer in presence of renal impairment. Ninety percent excreted unchanged in urine.

Use Influenza A viral infections of the respiratory tract (prophylaxis and treatment of high-risk patients). Parkinsonism and drug-induced extrapyramidal effects.

Contraindications Hypersensitivity to drug. Use with caution in epilepsy, congestive heart disease, renal dysfunction, the elderly, pregnancy. Safety in lactation and in children less than one year has not been established.

Untoward Reactions *GI:* Nausea, vomiting, constipation, anorexia, xerostomia. *CNS*: Depression, psychosis, convulsions, hallucinations, confusion, ataxia, irritability, anxiety, headache, dizziness, fatigue, insomnia. *CV*: Congestive heart failure, orthostatic hypotension, peripheral edema. *Other*: Urinary retention, leukopenia, neutropenia, mottling of skin of the extremities due to poor peripheral circulation (livedo reticularis), skin rashes, visual problems, slurred speech, oculogyric episodes.

Drug Interaction When used concomitantly with anticholinergic drugs, may ↑ incidence of atropine-like side effects.

Dosage **PO. Adults**: 200 mg daily as a single or divided dose. **Children, 1–9 years**: 4.4–8.8 mg/kg/day up to a maximum of 150 mg/day in 2–3 divided doses (use syrup); **9–12 years**: 100 mg b.i.d. *Prophylactic treatment*: institute before or immediately after exposure and continue for 10–21 days if used concurrently with vaccine or for 90 days without vaccine. *Symptomatic management*: initiate as soon as possible and continue for 24–48 hr after disappearance of symptoms. Dose should be decreased in renal impairment (see package insert). *For Antiparkinson dosage*, see p. 438.

Treatment of Overdosage Gastric lavage or induction of emesis followed by supportive measures. Ensure that patient is well hydrated; give fluids by IV if necessary.

Administration/Storage Protect capsules from moisture.

Additional Nursing Implications
See also *Nursing Implications* for *Anti-infectives*, p. 52.

1. *Assess*
   a. patients with history of epilepsy or other seizures for an increase in seizure activity and take appropriate precautions.
   b. patient with a history of CHF or peripheral edema for increased edema and/or respiratory distress and report promptly.
   c. patient with renal impairment for crystalluria, oliguria, and increased BUN or creatinine levels and report promptly.
2. *Teach patient and/or family*
   a. not to drive a car or work in a situation where alertness is important, because medication can affect vision, concentration, and coordination.
   b. to rise slowly from a prone position, because orthostatic hypotension may occur.
   c. to lie down if he feels dizzy or weak, to relieve the orthostatic hypotension.
   d. to report any exposure to rubella, because drug may increase susceptibility to disease.

IDOXURIDINE   Herplex Liquifilm, Stoxil (Rx)

Classification   Antiviral agent.

Action/Kinetics   Idoxuridine resembles thymidine. It interferes with the replication of certain DNA viruses in the cell.

Uses   Herpes simplex keratitis, especially for initial epithelial infections characterized by the presence of threadlike extensions.

Note: Idoxuridine will control infection but will not prevent scarring, loss of vision, or vascularization. Alternative form of therapy must be instituted if no improvement is noted after 7 days, or if complete reepithelialization fails to occur after 21 days of therapy. Corticosteroids can be used concurrently.

Contraindications   Hypersensitivity; deep ulcerations involving stromal layers of cornea. Safe use in pregnancy not established.

Untoward Reactions   Localized to eye: Temporary visual haze, irritation, pain, pruritus, inflammation, folicular conjunctivitis with preauricular adenopathy, mild edema of eyelids and cornea, allergic reactions (rare), photosensitivity, corneal clouding and stippling, small punctate defects.

Drug Interactions   Concurrent use of boric acid may cause irritation.

Dosage   **Ophthalmic (0.1%) soln: initial**, 1 drop q hr during day and q 2 hr during night; **following improvement**: 1 drop q 2 hr during day and q 4 hr at night. Continue for 3–5 days after healing is complete. **Ophthalmic (0.5%) ointment**: Insert in conjunctival sac 5 times/day q 4 hr with last dose at bedtime; continue for 3–5 days after healing is complete.

Administration/Storage

1. Store idoxuridine solution at 2°–8°C and protect from light.
2. Do not mix with other medications.
3. Store idoxuridine ointment 2°–15°C.
4. Administer ophthalmic medication as scheduled even during the night.
5. Do not use drug that was improperly stored, because of loss of activity and increased toxic effects.
6. Topical corticosteroids may be used with idoxuridine in the treatment of herpes simplex with corneal edema, stromal lesions, or iritis.
7. To control secondary infections, antibiotics may be used with idoxuridine.

Additional Nursing Implications

See also *Nursing Implications* for *Anti-infectives*, p. 52.

1. *Assess* patient for symptoms of vision loss.
2. Reassure patients that hazy vision that follows instillation of medication will be of short duration.
3. *Do not* apply boric acid to the eye when patient is on idoxuridine therapy because it may cause irritation.
4. Encourage patients to wear dark glasses if they suffer from photophobia.
5. Anticipate that if idoxuridine has been used concurrently with corticosteroids, the idoxuridine will be continued longer than the steroid to prevent reinfection.

TRIFLURIDINE   Viroptic (Rx)

Classification   Antiviral, topical ophthalmic.

Action/Kinetics   Probably interferes with DNA synthesis and virus replication.

Uses   Primary keratoconjunctivitis and recurrent epithelial keratitis caused by herpes simplex virus types 1 and 2. Epithelial keratitis resistant to idoxuridine. Is especially indicated for infections resistant to idoxuridine or vidarabine.

Contraindications   Hypersensitivity or chemical intolerance to drug. Safe use in pregnancy not established.

Untoward Reactions   *Ophthalmic*: Local, usually transient; irritation of conjunctiva and cornea including burning or stinging and edema of eyelids. Increased intraocular pressure. *Other*: Superficial punctate keratopathy, epithelial keratopathy, hypersensitivity, stromal edema, irritation, keratitis sicca, hyperemia.

Dosage   One drop of 1% solution q 2 hr onto cornea up to maximum of 9 drops/eye/day during acute stage (presence of corneal ulcer). Following reepithelialization, decrease dosage to 1 drop q 4 hr (or minimum of 5 drops/eye/day) for 7 days. Do not use for more than 21 days.

Administration/Storage

1. Instill drop onto cornea. Apply finger pressure lightly to lacrimal sac for 1 minute after instillation.
2. Maybe used concomitantly in the eye with antibiotics (chloramphenicol, bacitracin, polymyxin B sulfate, erythromycin, neomycin, gentamicin, tetracycline, sulfacetamide sodium), corticosteroids, anticholinergics, epinephrine HCl, and sodium chloride.
3. Drug is heat sensitive. Store in refrigerator at 2°–8°C.

Additional Nursing Implications
See also *Nursing Implications* for *Anti-infectives*, p. 52.

1. *Teach patient and/or family*
   a. administration and storage of trifluridine recommended above.
   b. that mild, transient burning sensation may occur on instillation.
   c. to report untoward symptoms to doctor, but not to stop medication without specific instructions to do so.
   d. to arrange with doctor for regular supervision by an ophthalmologist.
   e. that improvement should occur within 7 days, healing in 14 days. Thereafter, 7 more days of therapy are necessary to prevent recurrence.
   f. to report to doctor if no improvement is noted within 7 days.
   g. not to administer drug longer than 21 days, because toxicity may occur (remaining medication should be discarded after 21 days.)

VIDARABINE   Vira-A (Rx)

Classification   Antiviral agent.

Action/Kinetics   Vidarabine specifically interferes with the propagation of a number of viruses within the cell. It is effective against herpes simplex, probably by inhibiting DNA synthesis. Vidarabine is rapidly metabolized to ara-HX, which has a decreased antiviral activity. **Peak plasma levels**: vidarabine, 0.2–0.4 μg/ml; ara-HX, 3–6 μg/ml. **t½: IV**, vidarabine, 1.5 hr; ara-HX, 3.3. hr. Drug and metabolites excreted by kidneys.

Uses   *Systemic:* Herpes simplex viral encephalitis. *Topical:* Primary keratoconjunctivitis and recurrent epithelial keratitis caused by herpes simplex virus types 1 and 2. Epithelial keratitis resistant to idoxuridine. It is more effective than idoxuridine for deep recurrent infections.

Contraindications   Hypersensitivity to drug. Safe use in pregnancy not established. *Systemic:* use with caution in patients susceptible to fluid overload, cerebral edema, or with impaired renal or hepatic function. *Topical:* hypersensitivity to drug or any component of mixture.

Untoward Reactions   Systemic. *GI:* Nausea, vomiting, diarrhea, hematemesis. *CNS:* Tremor, dizziness, ataxia, confusion, hallucinations, psychoses, encephalopathy (may be fatal). *Hematologic:* Decrease in reticulocytes, hemoglobin, and hematocrit. *Other:* Weight loss, malaise, rash, pruritus, pain at injection site. *Topical:* Photophobia, lacrimation, conjunctival injection, foreign body sensation, temporal visual haze, burning, irritation, superficial punctate keratitis, pain, punctal occlusion, sensitivity.

Laboratory Test Interference   ↑ Bilirubin, SGOT.

Dosage   IV infusion: 15 mg/kg/day for 10 days. **Ophthalmic ointment**: ½ inch of 3% ointment applied into lower conjunctival sac 5 times daily at 3 hr intervals. Continue therapy for 7 days after complete reepithelialization but at reduced dosage (e.g., twice daily).

Administration

1. Systemic: slowly infuse total daily dose at constant rate over 12 to 24 hr.
2. 2.2 ml of IV solution is required to dissolve 1 mg of medication. A maximum of 450 mg may be dissolved in 1 liter. Should be used within 48 hr after dilution. Do not refrigerate solution.
3. Any carbohydrate or electrolyte solution is suitable as diluent. Do not use biologic or colloidal fluids.
4. Shake vidarabine vial well before withdrawing dosage. Add to prewarmed (35°–40°C) infusion solution. Shake mixture until completely clear.
5. For final filtration use an in-line filter (0.45-micron).
6. Dilute just before administration and use within 48 hr.
7. Topical corticosteroids or antibiotics may be used concomitantly with vidarabine but benefits vs. risks must be assessed.

Additional Nursing Implications
See also *Nursing Implications* for *Anti-infectives*, p. 52.

1. *Assess*
   a. patient on systemic therapy for fluid overload.
   b. patient for renal, liver, and hematologic dysfunction, precipitated by vidarabine.
2. *Teach patient and/or family*
   a. to continue under close supervision of an ophthalmologist while receiving therapy for optic problem.
   b. that ophthalmic ointment will cause a haze after application.

Part Three
ANTINEOPLASTIC AGENTS

Chapter Eighteen
ANTINEOPLASTIC AGENTS

Natural Products and Miscellaneous Agents

Hormonal and Antihormonal Agents

Radioactive Isotopes

Alphabetic Summary of Antineoplastic Agents (Table 4).

General Statement Much progress, at last, has been made in the drug therapy of neoplastic diseases, and a few forms of cancer can now be considered "curable" by chemotherapy alone. In many other forms of cancer, especially in cases of suspected metastatic disease, chemotherapy is an important adjunct in treatment. Recent progress can be partially attributed to the more judicious use of an increasing number of combination regimens of antineoplastic agents (see Summary Table 5), the composition and time of administration of which are based on a better understanding of the characteristics of a specified neoplastic disease and on the kinetics of the cell cycle (see *Action/Kinetics*). Some of the principles underlying successful cancer chemotherapy are reviewed below. Extensive nursing implications to increase the comfort of the patient during cancer therapy are provided.

General Impact of Antineoplastic Agents With rare exceptions, neoplastic disease cannot yet be cured by drugs. However, there are many compounds that slow down the disease process or induce a remission.

All antineoplastic agents are cytotoxic (i.e., cell poisons) and therefore interfere with normal cells as well as with neoplastic cells. However, neoplastic cells are much more active and multiply more rapidly than normal cells and are thus more affected by the antineoplastic agents.

Normal tissue cells, such as those of the bone marrow and the GI mucosal epithelium, are naturally very active and particularly susceptible to antineoplastic agents. The margin between the dose of antineoplastic drug needed to destroy the neoplastic cells and that needed to cause bone marrow damage is very narrow. Thus, patients who receive antineoplastic agents are closely watched for signs of bone marrow depression, which is characterized by low blood counts (leukocytes, erythrocytes, platelets). Since white blood cells (WBC) or platelets show the effect of an overdose more rapidly than do erythrocytes, the platelet and WBC count is often used as a guide to dosage. If a blood or marrow test indicates a precipitous fall in the WBC or platelet count, the antineoplastic agent may have to be discontinued or the dosage modified significantly. Sometimes the effect of the antineoplastic drugs on the bone marrow is cumulative, with the depression of WBCs and

TABLE 4 ANTINEOPLASTIC AGENTS

Agent	Abbreviation	Type	Disease	Toxicity
Asparaginase	L-ASP	Enzyme (natural product)	Acute lymphocytic leukemia	*Acute:* Nausea, fever, anaphylaxis *Delayed:* Hypersensitivity, abdominal pain, coagulation defects, renal and hepatic damage, pancreatitis, hyperglycemia, CNS depression, others
Bleomycin	BLM	Antibiotic	Testes, ovary, bladder, head, neck, thyroid, cervix, endometrium, neuroblastoma, osteogenic sarcoma, Hodgkin's disease, lymphomas	*Acute:* Nausea, vomiting, anaphylaxis, hypotension *Delayed:* Pneumonitis, pulmonary fibrosis, skin reactions, alopecia, stomatitis
Busulfan	BUS	Alkylating, alkyl sulfonate type	Chronic granulocytic leukemia, primary thrombocytosis	*Acute:* Mild nausea and vomiting *Delayed:* Bone marrow depression, hyperpigmentation, pulmonary fibrosis, acute leukemia
Carmustine	BCNU	Alkylating agent, nitrosourea type	Hodgkin's, non-Hodgkin's lymphomas, primary brain tumor, renal cell, stomach, colon, malignant melanoma	*Acute:* Nausea, vomiting, local phlebitis *Delayed:* Bone marrow depression, alopecia
Chlorambucil	CHL	Alkylating agent, nitrogen mustard	Chronic lymphocytic leukemia, primary macroglobinemia, Hodgkin's disease, non-Hodgkin's lymphomas, breasts, ovary, testes	*Acute:* Mild nausea and vomiting *Delayed:* Bone marrow depression, acute leukemia
Chromic Phosphate ^{32}P	^{32}P	Radioactive isotope	Peritoneal or pleural effusions of metastatic cancer; localized disease	*Acute:* Radiation sickness *Delayed:* Bone marrow depression
Cisplatin	CPDD	Platinum coordination complexes	Testes, ovary, bladder, head, neck, thyroid, cervix, endometrium, neuroblastoma	*Acute:* Nausea, vomiting *Delayed:* Bone marrow depression, renal damage, ototoxicity

TABLE 4 (Continued)

Agent	Abbreviation	Type	Disease	Toxicity
Cyclophosphamide	CYC	Alkylating agent, nitrogen mustard	Acute, chronic lymphocytic leukemia, Hodgkin's, non-Hodgkin's lymphomas, multiple myeloma, neuroblastoma, breast, ovary, lung, Wilms' tumor, rhabdomyosarcoma	*Acute:* Nausea, vomiting *Delayed:* Bone marrow depression, alopecia, hemorrhagic cystitis
Cytarabine	Ara-C	Antimetabolite, pyrimidine analog	Acute granulocytic and lymphocytic leukemias, erythroleukemia, meningeal leukemia	*Acute:* Nausea and vomiting *Delayed:* Bone marrow depression, megaloblastosis, diarrhea, hepatic damage
Dacarbazine	DTIC	Alkylating agents, triazene type	Malignant melanoma, insulinoma, malignant carcinoid	*Acute:* Nausea, vomiting, local irritation *Delayed:* Bone marrow depression, flulike syndrome, alopecia, renal damage, ↑ liver enzymes
Dactinomycin (Actinomycin D)	DACT	Antibiotic	Choriocarcinoma, Wilms' tumor, rhabdomyosarcoma, testes, osteogenic sarcoma	
Daunorubicin (Daunomycin)	DNR	Antibiotic	Acute nonlymphocytic leukemia, solid tumors in children	*Acute:* Nausea, vomiting, local irritation *Delayed:* Cardiotoxicity, bone marrow supression
Doxorubicin		Antibiotic	Soft tissue osteogenic and related sarcomas, Hodgkin's and non-Hodgkin's lymphomas, acute leukemias, breast, GU, thyroid, lung, stomach, neuroblastomas, Wilm's tumor	*Acute:* Nausea, vomiting, local irritation *Delayed:* Bone marrow depression, cardiotoxicity, stomatitis, diarrhea, erythema in irritated area
Dromostanolone		Androgen	Breast cancer in women, premenopausal women	*Delayed:* Edema, masculinization, hypercalcemia
Etoposide	VP-16-213	Inhibitor of mitosis	Refractory testicular tumors	*Acute:* Nausea, vomiting, hypotension, anaphylaxis *Delayed:* Leukopenia, thrombocytopenia, alopecia, peripheral neuropathy

Drug	Abbreviation	Class	Indications	Toxicity
Floxuridine	FUDR	Antimetabolite	Palliative treatment of localized cancer of head, neck, brain, liver, gallbladder, or bile ducts; GI adenocarcinoma to liver	*Acute:* Nausea, vomiting. *Delayed:* Bone marrow depression, stomatitis, diarrhea, alopecia, pigmentation, cerebellar ataxia
Fluorouracil	5-FU	Antimetabolite, pyrimidine analog	Breast, colon, stomach, pancreas, ovary, head, neck, urinary bladder, premalignant skin lesions (topical)	*Acute:* Nausea, vomiting. *Delayed:* See under *Floxuridine*
Hydroxyurea	HYD	Miscellaneous	Melanoma, resistant chronic myelocytic leukemia, metastatic cancer of ovary, carcinoma of head and neck	*Acute:* Mild nausea and vomiting. *Delayed:* Bone marrow depression, hyperkeratosis, hyperpigmentation, stomatitis
Lomustine	CCNU	Alkylating agent, nitrosourea type	Hodgkin's, non-Hodgkin's lymphomas, primary brain tumors, renal cell, stomach, colon, oat cell	*Acute:* Nausea and vomiting. *Delayed:* Bone marrow depression, alopecia
Mechlorethamine	HN 2	Alkylating agent, nitrogen mustard	Hodgkin's, non-Hodgkin's lymphoma, breast, ovary	*Acute:* Mild nausea and vomiting, local irritation. *Delayed:* Bone marrow depression, alopecia, hemorrhagic cystitis
Medroxyprogesterone acetate		Progesterone	Palliation of endometrial, renal cancer	*Delayed:* Edema
Megestrol acetate		Synthetic progestin	Palliation of endometrial or breast cancer	*Delayed:* Edema
Melphalan	MPL	Alkylating agent, nitrogen mustard	Plasma cell myeloma, breast, ovary	*Acute and Delayed:* See under *Mechlorethamine*
Mercaptopurine	6-MP	Antimetabolite, purine analog	Acute lymphocytic and granulocytic and chronic granulocytic leukemias; acute myelogenous and myelomonocytic leukemias	*Acute:* Nausea and vomiting. *Delayed:* Bone marrow depression, liver damage, oral ulcers potentiated by allopurinol
Methotrexate	MTX	Antimetabolite, folic acid analog	Acute lymphocytic leukemia, choriocarcinoma, mycosis fungoides, breast, testes, head and neck, lung, osteogenic sarcoma	*Acute:* Nausea and vomiting. *Delayed:* Bone marrow depression, stomatitis, ulcerations, diarrhea, hepatic and renal toxicity, pulmonary infiltrates, osteoporosis, alopecia

TABLE 4 (Continued)

Agent	Abbreviation	Type	Disease	Toxicity
Mitomycin	MTC	Antibiotic	Stomach, cervix, colon, breast, pancreas, bladder	*Acute:* Nausea, vomiting, local irritation *Delayed:* Bone marrow depression (cumulative), stomatitis, alopecia, renal toxicity
Mitotane	op'DDD	Adrenal suppressant	Adrenal cortex carcinoma	*Acute:* Nausea, vomiting *Delayed:* CNS depression, dermatitis, visual disturbances, adrenal insufficiency, diarrhea
Pipobroman		Alkylating agent	Polycythemia vera, chronic granulocytic leukemia	*Acute:* Nausea, vomiting, abdominal cramps *Delayed:* Skin rash, diarrhea, bone marrow depression
Plicamycin (Mithramycin)		Antibiotic	Testes, malignant hypercalcemia	*Acute:* Nausea, vomiting, local irritation *Delayed:* Bone marrow depression, hemorrhagic diathesis, stomatitis, diarrhea, hepatic damage, hypocalcemia
Polyestradiol phosphate		Estrogen	Palliation of prostatic cancer	*Acute:* Nausea, vomiting, headaches *Delayed:* Edema, gynecomastia, loss of libido, testicular atrophy, inhibition of anterior pituitary function
Prednisone	PRED	Corticosteroid		See *Corticosteroids* p. 735
Procarbazine	PCB	Miscellaneous methyl hydrazine derivative	Hodgkin's disease	*Acute:* Nausea, vomiting *Delayed:* Bone marrow depression, stomatitis, dermatitis, neuropathy, CNS depression
Semustine[a]	MCCNU	Alkylating agent, nitrosourea type	Hodgkin's and non-Hodgkin's lymphoma, primary brain tumors, renal cell, stomach, colon, malignant melanoma	See under *Lomustine*

Drug	Classification	Disease	Toxicity
Sodium iodide ^{131}I	Radioactive isotope	Thyroid	*Acute:* Radiation sickness
Sodium Phosphate ^{32}P	Radioactive isotope	Polycythemia vera, chronic lymphocytic and granulocytic leukemias, multiple skeletal metastases	*Acute:* Radiation sickness *Delayed:* Bone marrow depression
Streptozocin	Alkylating agent, nitrosourea type	Metastatic islet cell pancreatic carcinoma	*Acute:* Nausea, vomiting, confusion, depression, lethargy *Delayed:* Hematologic toxicity, glucose intolerance, renal toxicity
Tamoxifen	Anti-ESTR	Antiestrogen	Advanced breast cancer in postmenopausal women	*Acute:* Occasional nausea *Delayed:* Hot flashes, vaginal bleeding, pruritus vulvae
Testolactone		Androgen	Advanced or disseminated breast cancer	*Delayed:* Edema, masculinization, hypercalcemia
Thioguanine	6-TG	Antimetabolite, purine analog	Acute granulocytic, myelogenous, lymphocytic, chronic granulocytic leukemias	*Acute:* Occasional nausea and vomiting *Delayed:* Bone marrow depression, possible liver damage
Triethylenethiophosphoramide	THIO	Alkylating agent, ethyleneamine derivative	Hodgkin's and non-Hodgkin's lymphomas, retinoblastoma, breast, ovary	*Acute:* Mild nausea, vomiting *Delayed:* Bone marrow depression
Uracil mustard		Alkylating agent, nitrogen mustard	Chronic lymphocytic leukemia, Hodgkin's and non-Hodgkin's lymphoma, ovary, thrombocytosis, chronic myelogenous leukemia	*Acute:* Mild nausea, vomiting *Delayed:* Bone marrow depression
Vinblastine	VBL	Plant alkaloid	Hodgkin's and non-Hodgkin's, breast, renal cells, testes, lymphoma, mycosis fungoides	*Acute:* Nausea, vomiting, local irritation *Delayed:* Bone marrow depression, alopecia, stomatitis, loss of deep tendon reflexes, jaw pain, paralytic ileus
Vincristine	VCR	Plant (vinca) alkaloid	Acute lymphocytic leukemia, neuroblastoma, Wilms' tumor, rhabdomyosarcoma, Hodgkin's and non-Hodgkin's lymphoma, breast, oat cell	*Acute:* Local irritation *Delayed:* Peripheral neuropathy, neuritic pain, alopecia, constipation, paralytic ileus, mild bone marrow depression

TABLE 5   COMMONLY USED ANTINEOPLASTIC COMBINATIONS

ABVD	Bleomycin Dacarbazine Doxorubicin Vinblastine	CISCA	Cisplatin Cyclophosphamide Doxorubicin
AC	Cyclophosphamide Doxorubicin	CMC-High dose	Cyclophosphamide Lomustine Methotrexate
A-COPP	Cyclophosphamide Doxorubicin Prednisone Procarbazine Vincristine	CMF	Cyclophosphamide Fluorouracil Methotrexate
		CMFP	Cyclophosphamide Fluorouracil Methotrexate Prednisone
Adria + BCNU	Carmustine Doxorubicin		
Ara-C + ADR	Cytarabine Doxorubicin	CMFVP(Cooper's Regimen)	Cyclophosphamide Fluorouracil Methotrexate Prednisone Vincristine
Ara-C + DNR + PRED + MP	Cytarabine Daunorubicin Mercaptopurine Prednisone		
Ara-C +6-TG	Cytarabine Thioguanine	COP	Cyclophosphamide Prednisone Vincristine
BCVPP	Carmustine Cyclophosphamide Prednisone Procarbazine Vinblastine	COPP or "C" MOPP	Cyclophosphamide Prednisone Procarbazine Vincristine
		CVP	Cyclophosphamide Prednisone Vincristine
CAF	Cyclophosphamide Doxorubicin Fluorouracil		
CAMP	Cyclophosphamide Doxorubicin Methotrexate Procarbazine	CY-VA-DIC	Cyclophosphamide Dacarbazine Doxorubicin Vincristine
CAV	Cyclophosphamide Doxorubicin Vincristine	FAC	Cyclophosphamide Doxorubicin Fluorouracil
CAVe	Doxorubicin Lomustine Vinblastine	FAM	Doxorubicin Fluorouracil Mitomycin
		M-2 Protocol	Carmustine Cyclophosphamide Melphalan Prednisone Vincristine
CHL + PRED	Chlorambucil Prednisone		
CHOP	Cyclophosphamide Doxorubicin Prednisone Vincristine		
CHOR	Cyclophosphamide Doxorubicin Vincristine	MACC	Cyclophosphamide Doxorubicin Lomustine Methotrexate

TABLE 5 (*Continued*)

MOPP	Mechlorethamine Prednisone Procarbazine Vincristine	Cycle 2 Cycle 3	Same as cycle 1 without radia- tion therapy *Month 1*
MOPP-LO-BLEO	Bleomycin Mechlorethamine Prednisone Procarbazine Vincristine		Dactinomycin Doxorubicin *Month 2* Cyclophosphamide Vincristine
MPL + PRED (MP)	Melphalan Prednisone		*Month 3* No drugs for 28 days
MTX-MP	Mercaptopurine Methotrexate	Cycle 4	Repeat Cycle 3
MTX + MP + CTX	Cyclophosphamide Mercaptopurine Methotrexate	VAC Pulse	Cyclophosphamide Dactinomycin Vincristine
POCC	Cyclophosphamide Lomustine Procarbazine Vincristine	VAC Standard	Cyclophosphamide Dactinomycin Vincristine
T-2 Protocol Cycle 1	*Month 1* Dactinomyci Doxorubicin Radiation therapy *Month 2* Cyclophosphamide Doxorubicin Vincristine Radiation therapy *Month 3* Cyclophosphamide Vincristine	VBP VP VP-L-Asparagi- nase	Bleomycin Cisplatin Vinblastine Prednisone Vincristine L-Asparaginase Prednisone Vincristine

platelets occurring weeks or months after initiation. Thus patients must be followed carefully.

Drugs are usually withheld when the WBC count falls below 2,000/mm³ and the platelet count falls below 100,000/mm³.

Antineoplastic agents should only be administered by people knowledgeable in their management. Facilities must be available for frequent laboratory evaluations, especially total blood counts and bone marrows. Intravenous medications must be administered by the physician.

The toxicity of the antineoplastic agents is also manifested in the lining of the GI tract. Oral ulcers, intestinal bleeding, and diarrhea are warning signs of excess toxicity.

Finally, since hair follicles are also rapidly proliferating tissue, alopecia often accompanies the treatment of antineoplastic disease.

Antineoplastic agents fall into several broad categories: Alkylating Agents, Antimetabolites, Antibiotics, Natural Products and Miscellaneous Agents, Hormonal and Antihormonal Agents, and Radioactive Isotopes.

In the current edition of *The Nurse's Drug Handbook*, the chemotherapeutic agents have been separated into these specific classes.

The choice of the chemotherapeutic agent(s) depends both on the type of the tumor and on its site of growth. Although it has been said that cancer is not one disease but many, a simpler major subdivision involves separation into solid tumors and hematologic malignancies. The former are confined to a specific tissue or organ site initially and usually involve surgery and/or irradiation. Chemotherapy is used to eradicate remaining cells or metastases, or when primary treatment is insufficient or impossible.

Chemotherapy is usually the major form of therapy in hematologic malignancies; some cures have been achieved, notably in Hodgkin's disease and the leukemias of childhood.

In this edition of *The Nurse's Drug Handbook*, currently used antineoplastic drugs are classified according to type of agent (see above). The individual drug monographs list mode of action and kinetics, dosage, and administration. For quick reference, agents are also listed alphabetically in Table 4. Included are the abbreviations by which the antineoplastic agents are known and the combination regimens in which they are often included (Table 5). Dosage for the combinations is not given because these values are highly individualized.

General information applying to all antineoplastic agents (action, contraindications, untoward reactions, use, administration, and extensive nursing implications) is presented below.

Action During division, cells go through a definite number of stages during which they are more or less susceptible to various chemotherapeutic agents (see *Action/ Kinetics* of various agents). Some agents, notably the alkylating agents, have been shown to be effective during all stages of the cycle, while others, the antimetabolites, for example, are only effective during stages of DNA synthesis.

The various cell stages are described in Figure 5.

Uses Most of the drugs discussed in this section are used exclusively for neoplastic

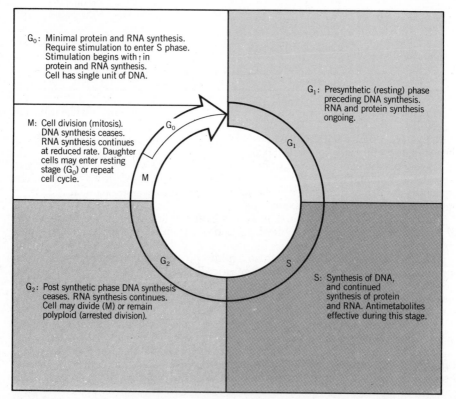

G_0: Minimal protein and RNA synthesis. Require stimulation to enter S phase. Stimulation begins with ↑ in protein and RNA synthesis. Cell has single unit of DNA.

M: Cell division (mitosis). DNA synthesis ceases. RNA synthesis continues at reduced rate. Daughter cells may enter resting stage (G_0) or repeat cell cycle.

G_1: Presynthetic (resting) phase preceding DNA synthesis. RNA and protein synthesis ongoing.

G_2: Post synthetic phase DNA synthesis ceases. RNA synthesis continues. Cell may divide (M) or remain polyploid (arrested division).

S: Synthesis of DNA, and continued synthesis of protein and RNA. Antimetabolites effective during this stage.

FIGURE 5.

disease. A few are used for patients on an experimental basis for some of the rheumatic diseases.

Contraindications   Hypersensitivity to drug. Most antineoplastic agents are contraindicated for a period of 4 weeks after radiation therapy or chemotherapy with similar drugs. Use with caution, and at reduced dosages, in patients with preexisting bone marrow depression, malignant infiltration of bone marrow or kidney, or liver dysfunction.

The safe use of these drugs during pregnancy has not been established; they are contraindicated during the first trimester.

Untoward Reactions   *Bone marrow depression* (leukopenia, thrombocytopenia, agranulocytosis, anemia) *is the major danger of antineoplastic therapy. Bone marrow depression can sometimes be irreversible. It is mandatory that the patient have frequent total blood counts and bone marrow examinations. Precipitous falls must be reported to a physician*.

Other untoward reactions include: *GI*: Nausea, vomiting (may be severe), anorexia, diarrhea (may be hemorrhagic), stomatitis, enteritis, abdominal cramps, intestinal ulcers. *Hepatic*: Hepatic toxicity including jaundice and changes in liver enzymes. *Dermatologic*: Dermatitis, erythema, various dermatoses including maculopapular rash, alopecia (reversible), pruritus, urticaria, cheilosis. *Immunologic*: Immunosuppression with increased susceptibility to viral, bacterial, or fungal infections. *CNS*: Depression, lethargy, confusion, dizziness, headache, fatigue, malaise, fever, weakness. *Genitourinary*: Acute renal failure, reproductive abnormalities including amenorrhea and azoospermia. **Note**: Alkylating agents, in particular, may be both carcinogenic and mutagenic.

Administration
1. Preparation of antineoplastics:
   a. Use gloves to protect skin when reconstituting antineoplastics.
   b. Use caution in preparation, particularly to prevent skin reactions.
   c. Wash immediately if solution comes in contact with skin or mucous membranes.
   d. Should material accidentally enter the eyes, wash eyes out well and see an ophthalmologist for further care.
2. Use piggyback setup with an electric IV pump.
3. Start infusion with the solution not containing the vesicant drug.
4. Preferably, do not use the dorsum of the hand, wrist, or antecubital fossa as the site of infusion.
5. Avoid administering medication through a previously used site.
6. After IV has been started and unmedicated solution is infusing, check for blood return and for pain, redness, or edema before starting solution containing medication.
7. During administration of medication, constantly observe for reduction of IV flow rate, redness, pain, or swelling.
8. Discontinue IV medication if these signs occur or patency cannot be established and start unmedicated solution at KVO rate. Report to physician immediately.
9. *Teach patient and/or family* to report pain, redness, or edema near the injection site during or after treatment.
10. Due to effects on the reproductive system, patient should be advised to practice contraception.
11. Report extravasation to doctor and follow protocol of institution to minimize effects of extravasation.
12. Charting of antineoplastic administration:
    a. Record patient's drug protocol on medication sheet.

b. Day 1 is the first day of the first dose.

c. Number each day after that in sequence, even though patient might not receive drug daily.

d. Indicate when the nadir (the time of most severe physiologic depression) is likely to occur, so that possible complications, such as infection and bleeding, can be anticipated and treated early.

e. When the drug regimen is repeated, the first day of therapy is charted as day 1.

Nursing Implications for Antineoplastic Agents

1. Establish a team approach involving the patient, family, nurse, doctor, social worker, and other health workers to develop a therapeutic plan with a holistic approach to the patient's physical, emotional, social, and spiritual concerns.

2. Use the nursing process to provide physical and psychosocial holistic care to both patient and family as they experience the effects and associated difficulties of chemotherapy administered for palliation, remission, or cure.

3. Reassure patient that the occurrence of untoward effects does not necessarily represent a setback, but rather indicates that the chemotherapeutic agent is also effectively destroying tumor cells.

Nursing Implications before Initiation of Chemotherapy

Assess for baseline data

a. nutritional status.

b. skin condition.

c. oral condition.

d. degree of mobility.

e. emotional status.

f. history of hypersensitivity.

g. history of surgery, x-ray, or chemotherapy.

Nursing Implications for Bone Marrow Depression

LEUKOPENIA

1. *Assess*

a. WBC (normal values: 5,000–10,000/mm³).

b. differential (normal values: neutrophils 60–70%, lymphocytes 25–30%, monocytes 2–6%, eosinophils 1–3%, basophils 0.25–0.5%).

c. sudden sharp drop in WBC or a reduction in WBC below 2,000/mm³, because these findings might necessitate reduction in dosage or withdrawal of the drug. Withhold drug and report.

d. temperature q 4 hr, and recheck in 1 hr if there is a slight elevation. Report fever above 38°C (100°F) because patient has limited resistance to infection resulting from leukopenia and immunosuppression.

e. skin and orifices of body for signs of infection. Early identification is extremely important, because due to the absence of granulocytes, local abscesses do not form with pus, but infection becomes systemic as a septicemia.

2. *Prevent infection by*
   a. using strict medical asepsis.
   b. providing good body care.
   c. using pHisohex or an antiseptic to wash patient with a tendency toward skin eruption.
   d. providing mouth care q 4–6 h, with either normal saline or hydrogen peroxide diluted to half strength with water. Follow with a substrate of milk of magnesia. (Make substrate of magnesia by discarding the clear liquid in the top of the bottle and then use the thick white liquid that remains for coating the oral mucosa.) Do not use lemon or glycerin, because they tend to reduce the production of saliva and change the pH of the mouth. Mucosal deterioration occurs if mouth care is not provided at least q 6 hr.
   e. cleaning and drying rectal area after each bowel movement. Apply A&D ointment if there is irritation.
   f. being prepared to initiate reverse isolation if WBC falls below 1,500–2,000/mm^3 by
      (1) maintaining patient in private room.
      (2) using gloves, masks, and gowns as ordered.
      (3) limiting articles brought into room.
      (4) providing private bathroom or bedside commode.
      (5) minimizing unnecessary traffic in and out of room.
      (6) screening visitors for infection before they enter room.
   g. preventing nosocomial infections from invasive procedures by
      (1) cleansing skin with an antiseptic before procedure.
      (2) changing tubing of IV infusion q 24 hr.
      (3) changing site of IV infusion q 48 hr.

THROMBOCYTOPENIA

1. *Assess*

   a. platelet count (normal values: 200,000–300,000/mm^3). Patient with a platelet count below 150,000/mm^3 should be monitored in the hospital.
   b. urine for blood cells.
   c. stool for guaiac.
   d. skin for petechiae or bruising.
   e. all orifices for bleeding.
   f. blood pressure q.d. on hospitalized patient.

2. *Prevent bleeding by*

   a. minimizing SC or IM injections. If they are necessary, apply pressure for 3–5 min to prevent leakage or hematoma. Report unusual bleeding after injection.
   b. not applying a blood pressure cuff or other tourniquet for excessive periods of time.

(continued)

    c. advising patient to use safety measures to prevent bleeding from a minor trauma that might cause cuts or bruises, by

      (1) cautioning not to pick nose, as bleeding may result.

      (2) recommending use of electric razor for shaving rather than a blade.

      (3) providing a soft-bristled toothbrush or having patient massage gums with finger to limit irritation.

3. *Assist with treatment of bleeding*

    a. for epistaxis by pinching nose for 10 min and applying pressure to upper lip to stop nosebleed.

    b. with transfusion (usually ordered if platelet count falls below 150,000/mm³). Take baseline vital signs before start of transfusion and then q 15 min after transfusion is started. Monitor vital signs for at least 2 hr after transfusion is completed. Assess for histoincompatability indicated by chills, fever, and urticaria. Stop transfusion, provide supportive care, and report. (See *Nursing Implications* for *Blood*, p. 281 and 283.)

ANEMIA

1. *Assess*

    a. hemoglobin (normal values: 14–16 gm/100 ml blood).

    b. hematocrit (normal values: Men, 40–54%; women, 37–47%).

    c. patient for pallor, lethargy, or unusual fatigue.

2. *Minimize anemia by*

    a. providing a nutritious diet that patient can tolerate.

    b. administering or instructing patient to take vitamins and iron supplementation as ordered.

3. *Assist with treatment of anemia by*

    a. administering diet high in iron that patient can tolerate.

    b. administering vitamins and iron supplements, as ordered.

    c. assisting with transfusion as noted above with treatment of thrombocytopenia.

Nursing Implications for Gastrointestinal Toxicity

NAUSEA/VOMITING

1. *Assess*

    a. for anorexia and/or refusal of food.

    b. nutritional status and compare with baseline.

    c. frequency, character, and amount of vomitus.

2. *Prevent nausea and vomiting by*

    a. premedicating with antiemetic as ordered before administering antineoplastic drug. Usually the antiemetic is ordered to be administered ½ hr before or just after administration of antineoplastic agent.

    b. administering antineoplastic on an empty stomach, with meals, or at bedtime, so as to minimize nausea and vomiting and produce the most therapeutic effect for the patient.

    c. teaching patient and/or family how to insert an antiemetic suppository.

    d. providing ice chips at onset of nausea.

e. providing carbonated beverages to counteract nausea.

f. encouraging ingestion of dry carbohydrates, such as toast and dry crackers before initiating activity.

g. waiting for nausea and vomiting to pass before serving food.

h. providing small nutritious snacks and planning meal schedules to coincide with patient's best tolerance time.

i. providing nourishing foods that the patient likes.

j. encouraging intake of a high-protein diet.

k. freezing dietary supplements and serving them like ice cream to make them more palatable.

l. avoiding serving foods with overpowering aroma.

m. encouraging patient to chew foods well.

n. providing good oral hygiene both before and after meals.

3. *Assist with treatment of nausea and vomiting by*

a. administering antiemetic, as ordered, or contacting doctor if antiemetic has not been ordered. All vomiting should be reported to doctor, as change in chemotherapeutic regimen or correction of electrolyte balance might be required.

b. providing supportive care to maintain patient as comfortable, clean, and free from odor as possible.

c. explaining to patient that GI discomfort is actually a sign that the drug is also affecting tumor cells.

d. assisting with correction of electrolyte balance and provision of hyperalimentation, as necessary.

DIARRHEA/ABDOMINAL CRAMPING

1. *Assess*

a. frequency and severity of cramping caused by hypermotility.

b. frequency, color, consistency, and amount of diarrhea, all of which indicate amount of tissue destruction occurring.

c. for signs of dehydration and acidosis indicating electrolyte imbalance.

2. *Prevent diarrhea/abdominal cramping by*

a. providing a bland low-roughage diet.

b. increasing constipating foods, such as hard cheeses in the diet.

3. *Assist with treatment of diarrhea by*

a. administering antidiarrheal, if ordered, or contacting doctor if antidiarrheal has not been ordered. Diarrhea or abdominal cramping should be reported, as change in chemotherapeutic regimen or correction of electrolyte balance may be required.

b. increasing fluids, unless contraindicated.

c. assisting with correction of electrolyte balance.

d. providing good skin care, especially to the perianal area to prevent skin breakdown. Apply A&D ointment for perianal tenderness.

STOMATITIS (MUCOSAL ULCERATION)

1. *Assess*

a. for dryness of mouth, erythema, and white patchy areas of the oral mucous

(continued)

membranes that indicate developing stomatitis. Assessment should be done each time the drug is administered.

2. *Prevent stomatitis by*

   a. assessing mouth q.d. and reporting bleeding gums or burning sensation when acid liquids such as juice are ingested.

   b. setting up a regular schedule for oral care.

   c. providing good mouth care as detailed under *Prevent Infection*, p. 211.

   d. applying Vaseline to lips at least b.i.d.

3. *Assist with treatment of stomatitis by*

   a. continuing to provide good oral care.

   b. applying topical viscous anesthetic, such as lidocaine (Xylocaine) before meals or providing a swish of lidocaine to anesthetize oral mucosa. Patient may swallow lidocaine after swishing it around oral cavity. A doctor's order is required for the use of lidocaine.

   c. providing bland foods at medium temperatures.

Nursing Implications for Neurotoxicity

1. *Assess*

   a. for symptoms of minor neuropathies, such as tingling in hands and feet and loss of deep tendon reflexes.

   b. for symptoms of serious neuropathies, such as weakness of hand strength, ataxia, loss of coordination, foot drop or wrist drop, and paralytic ileus.

2. *Prevent functional loss due to neurotoxicity by*

   a. reporting symptoms of neuropathies early, because the doctor may decide to change the medication regimen to prevent functional loss that may be irreversible.

   b. practicing and teaching seizure precautions.

3. *Assist with treatment of neuropathies by*

   a. using appropriate safety measures in caring for patient with a functional loss.

   b. maintaining good body alignment by correct positioning.

   c. obtaining medical orders for stool softeners and laxatives, as needed.

Nursing Implications for Ototoxicity

1. *Assess* for hearing difficulties before initiating therapy.

2. *Teach patient* to report tinnitus or alteration in hearing.

Nursing Implications for Hepatotoxicity

1. *Assess*

   a. liver function tests

      (1) Serum bilirubin (normal values: 0.3–1.0 mg/dl). An elevation may indicate there is liver disease or an increased rate of red cell hemolysis.

      (2) SGOT (normal values 5–40 units/ml). Elevation is indication of changes in the liver, skeletal muscles, lungs, pancreas, and heart. Hepatitis produces striking elevation in the SGOT.

      (3) SGPT (normal values: 5–35 units/ml). Elevation is indicative of conditions leading to hepatic necrosis.

      (4) LDH (normal values: 100–225 units/ml). Elevation may be indicative of hepatitis, pulmonary infarction, and CHF.

  b. for signs of liver involvement, such as abdominal pain, high fever, diarrhea, and yellowing of skin and sclera.

2. *Prevent further hepatotoxicity by*

  a. reporting elevations in liver function tests and signs of liver involvement to doctor, as these are indications for changing medication regimen.

3. *Assist with treatment for hepatotoxicity by*

  a. providing supportive nursing care to relieve symptoms, such as pain, fever, diarrhea, and jaundice.

Nursing Implications for Renal Toxicity

1. *Assess*

  a. renal function tests.

      (1) BUN (normal values: 10–20 mg/100 ml)

      (2) Serum uric acid (normal values: 2.0–7.8 mg/100 ml)

      (3) Creatinine clearance (normal values: women 0.8–1.7 gm/24 hr, men 1.0–1.9 gm/24 hr)

      (4) Quantitative uric acid (normal values: 250–750 mg/day)

  b. for stomach pain, swelling of feet or lower legs, shakiness, unusual body movement, and stomatitis.

  c. intake and output.

2. *Limit hyperuricemia by*

  a. encouraging extra fluid intake to speed excretion of uric acid and decrease hazard of crystal and urate stone formation.

  b. assisting with alkalinization of urine, as ordered.

Nursing Implications for Immunosuppression

1. *Assess*

  a. for fever, chills, or sore throat.

  b. WBC and differential.

2. *Assist with treatment of patient with immunosuppression by*

  a. preventing infection as noted above under leukopenia.

  b. advising delay of active immunizations for several months after therapy is completed, as there may be either a hypo- or hyperactive response.

Nursing Implications for Genitourinary Alterations

1. *Assess*

  a. for alterations in GU functioning.

  b. whether patient understands that most symptoms, such as amenorrhea, cease after medication is discontinued.

(continued)

c. before initiation of therapy, by consulting with physician as to whether he has informed patient that sterility might be a permanent result of therapy.

2. *Prevent teratogenesis by*

a. teaching patient/partner of childbearing age to use contraceptive measures to avoid pregnancy, both during and for several months after therapy, as drug could have a teratogenic effect on the fetus if the woman were to conceive during this period.

Nursing Implications for Alopecia

1. Ascertain that patient understands that body hair might fall out during therapy, but that hair will grow back. Hair may be of a different texture or color, but will start to regrow about 8 weeks after therapy is completed.

2. *Minimize alopecia by*

a. assisting with application of scalp tourniquet during and for 10–15 min after medication is administered.

b. applying ice packs to scalp during administration of medication and then for the next 15 min.

3. *Alternatives for managing alopecia include*

a. shaving head, if hair starts to fall out in large clumps, and using a wig or scarf until scalp hair regrows.

b. using a wig or scarf while hair is falling out and regrowing.

c. encouraging expression of feelings related to changes in self-image.

Nursing Implications for Alterations in Skin

1. Assess skin for breakdown.

2. Maintain cleanliness of skin and prevent dryness.

3. Prevent excessive exposure to sun or artificial ultraviolet light.

4. *Teach patient and/or family*

a. to use principles for *Teaching and Promoting Compliance*, p. 47.

b. to provide patient with appropriate literature, such as *Chemotherapy and You*, published by the U. S. Department of Health and Human Services, NIH Publication 81-1136, to be used as a guide to self-help during treatment.

ALKYLATING AGENTS

Action/Kinetics The alkylating agents include nitrogen mustards, the oldest known anticancer agents. Nitrogen mustard gases were used during World War I for chemical warfare.

The compounds are highly reactive; under physiologic conditions they donate an alkyl group (carbonium ion) to biologically important macromolecules, such as DNA. These reactions inactivate the molecule, bringing *cell division* to a halt. This cytotoxic activity is not limited to cancerous cells, but affects replication of the other cells of an organism, especially that of rapidly proliferating tissues, such as the bone marrow, intestinal epithelium, and hair follicles.

The toxic effects of the alkylating agents are cell cycle specific. The specific effect on cell division becomes apparent when the cell enters the S phase and cell division is blocked at the G_2 phase (premitotic phase), resulting in cells having a double complement of DNA.

Resistance of cancer cells to alkylating agents usually develops slowly and gradually. The resistance seems to be the sum total of several minor adaptations and not a reaction to a single one. Such mechanisms include decreased permeability of the cells, increased production of noncancer receptors (nucleophilic subtances), and increased efficiency of the DNA repair system.

BUSULFAN (BUSULPHAN)   Myleran (Abbreviation: BUS) (Rx)

Classification   Antineoplastic, alkylating agent.

Action/Kinetics   Increased appetite and sense of well-being may occur a few days after therapy is started. WBC drops during second or third week. Issue no more than 3 or 4 days' supply to a patient at one time, since close medical supervision, including laboratory tests, is mandatory. Sometimes administered with allopurinol to prevent symptoms of clinical gout. Busulfan may cause severe bone marrow depression.

Rapidly absorbed from GI tract; appears in serum 0.5–2 hr after PO administration. Ten to 50% excreted by kidney in 24 hr.

Uses   Chronic myelocytic, granulocytic, or myeloid leukemia (drug of choice).

Additional Untoward Reactions   Pancytopenia (more severe than other agents), bronchopulmonary dysplasia, pulmonary fibrosis, cataracts (after prolonged use), hyperpigmentation, adrenal insufficiency-like syndrome, gynecomastia, cholestatic jaundice, myasthenia gravis.

Laboratory Test Interference   ↑ Uric acid in blood and urine.

Dosage   **PO**. Individualized according to WBC count. **Initial, usual dose**: 4–8 mg daily until leukocyte count falls below 15,000/mm³; **maintenance**: 1–3 mg daily if remission is shorter than 3 months. Discontinue therapy if there is a precipitous fall in WBC count.

CARMUSTINE   BiCNU (Abbreviation: BCNU) (Rx)

Classification   Antineoplastic, alkylating agent.

Action/Kinetics   Similar to lomustine; thus cross-resistance may develop. Drug rapidly cleared from plasma and metabolized. Crosses blood-brain barrier (concentration in CSF 15–70% greater than in plasma). t½: 15–30 min. Thirty percent excreted in urine after 24 hr, 60–70% after 96 hr.

Uses   Palliative treatment of primary and metastatic brain tumors. Multiple myeloma (in combination with prednisone). Advanced Hodgkin's disease and non-Hodgkin's lymphomas (in combination with other agents).

Additional Untoward Reactions   Nausea and vomiting within 2 hr after administration, lasting 4 to 6 hr. Rapid IV administration may produce transitory intense flushing of skin and conjunctiva (onset: after 2 hr; duration: 4 hr). Pulmonary fibrosis, ocular toxicity including retinal hemorrhage.

Drug Interaction Additive bone marrow depression when used with cimetidine.

Dosage **IV**: 200 mg/m² q 6 weeks as a single or divided dose (on consecutive days). Subsequent dosage should only be given if platelet levels are greater than 100,000/mm³ and leukocytes are greater than 4,000/mm³.

Administration/Storage

1. Discard vials in which powder has become an oily liquid.
2. Store unopened vials at 2°–8°C and protect from light. Store diluted solutions at 4°C and protect from light.
3. Reconstitute powder with absolute ethyl alcohol (provided); then add sterile water. For injection, these dilutions are stable for 24 hr when stored as noted above.
4. Stock solutions diluted to 500 ml with 0.9% sodium chloride for injection or 5% dextrose for injection are stable for 48 hr when stored as noted above.
5. Administer by IV over 1- to 2-hr period, as faster injection may produce intense pain and burning at site of injection.
6. *Do not use vial for multiple doses*, since there is no preservative in vial.

Additional Nursing Implications

See also *Nursing Implications*, p. 210.

1. *Assess* for extravasation, if patient complains of burning or pain at site of injection. Discomfort may be due to alcohol diluent.
2. If there is no extravasation, reduce rate of flow if patient complains of burning at site of injection.
3. Slow IV rate if patient demonstrates intense flushing of skin and/or redness of conjunctiva.

CHLORAMBUCIL   Leukeran (Abbreviation: CHL) (Rx)

Classification Antineoplastic, alkylating agent.

Action/Kinetics Relatively nontoxic agent. Rapidly absorbed from the GI tract. Plasma t½: about 90 min. Sixty percent of the drug is excreted through the urine 24 hr after drug administration, and 40% is bound to tissues, including fat.

Uses Chronic lymphocytic leukema, malignant lymphomas (including lymphosarcoma), giant follicular lymphomas, and Hodgkin's disease.

Additional Untoward Reactions Keratitis, pulmonary fibrosis, bronchopulmonary dysplasia.

Laboratory Test Interference ↑ Uric acid levels in serum and urine.

Dosage **PO**: *Individualized* according to response of patient; **initial usual dose**: 0.1–0.2 mg/kg body weight (or 4–10 mg) daily for 3–6 weeks; **maintenance**: 0.03–0.1 mg/kg daily. **Alternative for chronic lymphocytic leukemia: initial,** 0.4 mg/kg; **then,** repeat this dose every 2 weeks increasing by 0.1 mg/kg until either toxicity or control observed.

Administration

1. The drug should be taken 1 hr before breakfast or 2 hr after the evening meal.
2. From 80–96 oz fluid should be consumed each day.
3. During therapy contraception should be practiced.

CYCLOPHOSPHAMIDE   Cytoxan, Neosar, Procytox* (Abbreviation: CYC) (Rx)

Classification   Antineoplastic, alkylating agent.

Action/Kinetics   t½ (after IV administration): 4–6.5 hr, but remnants of drug and/or metabolites detectable in serum after 72 hr. Metabolized in liver; 36–99% of drug excreted in urine within 48 hr. Excreted in milk.

Uses   Multiple myeloma. Malignant lymphomas: Hodgkin's disease, follicular lymphoma, lymphocytic lymphosarcoma, reticulum cell sarcoma, lymphoblastic lymphosarcoma, Burkitt's lymphoma. Mycosis fungoides. Leukemias: Chronic lymphocytic and granulocytic leukemia, acute myelogenous and monocytic leukemia, acute lymphoblastic leukemia in children. Neuroblastoma, adenocarcinoma of ovary, retinoblastoma. Carcinoma of lung and breast. *Investigational:* Rheumatic diseases.

Additional Untoward Reactions   Hemorrhagic cystitis. Bone marrow depression appears frequently during ninth to fourteenth day of therapy. Alopecia occurs more frequently than with other drugs. Secondary neoplasia (especially of urinary bladder), pulmonary fibrosis, cardiotoxicity, darkening of skin or fingernails.

Drug Interactions

Interactant	Interaction
Allopurinol	↑ Chance of bone marrow toxicity
Insulin	Insulin ↑ hypoglycemia
Phenobarbital	↑ Rate of metabolism in liver of cyclophosphamide
Succinylcholine	↑ Succinylcholine-induced apnea due to ↓ breakdown in plasma
Thiazide diuretics	↑ Chance of bone marrow toxicity

Laboratory Test Interference   ↑ Uric acid in blood and urine; false-positive Pap test; ↓ serum pseudocholinesterase. Suppression of certain skin tests.

Dosage   **Loading dose: IV**: 40–50 mg/kg in divided doses over 2–5 days. **PO**: 1–5 mg/kg depending on patient tolerance. **Maintenance** (various schedules): **PO**: 1–5 mg/kg/day; **IV**: 10–15 mg/kg q 7–10 days or **IV**: 3–5 mg/kg 2 times a week. Attempt to maintain leukocyte count at 3,000–4,000/mm³. Dosage should be adjusted for kidney or liver disease.

Administration/Storage

1. IV: Dissolve 100 mg cyclophosphamide in 5 ml sterile water. Let solution stand until it clears but use within 3–4 hr after preparation.
2. PO: Administer preferably on empty stomach. Give with meals in case of GI disturbance.
3. Store in tightly closed containers, preferably in refrigerator.

Additional Nursing Implications

See also *Nursing Implications*, p. 210.

1. Keep patient well hydrated to help prevent hemorrhagic cystitis due to excessive concentration of drug in urine.
2. Encourage frequent voiding.
3. *Assess* for dysuria and hematuria.

(continued)

4. Reassure patient with alopecia that hair will grow back when drug is stopped or a maintenance dosage is given.

5. Advise women that drug may cause a false + Pap test.

6. Advise diabetic patient that signs and symptoms of hypoglycemia may be precipitated by drug interaction with insulin, and to consult with doctor for possible insulin dosage adjustment.

7. See *Nursing Implications* for *Neuromuscular Blocking Agents*, p. 604, if patient is also receiving succinylcholine, as apnea may be induced.

DACARBAZINE   DTIC, DTIC-Dome, Imidazole Carboxamide (Abbreviation: DTIC) (Rx)

Classification   Antineoplastic, alkylating agent.

Action/Kinetics   The drug acts by alkylation, antimetabolite activity, and combination with sulfhydryl groups. t½: 35–75 min. Drug probably localizes in liver. Limited amounts (14% of plasma level) enter CSF. Thirty to 46% of drug excreted in urine within 6 hr, one-half of it unchanged.

Uses   Metastatic malignant melanoma. Hodgkin's disease (with other agents). *Investigational:* soft tissue sarcoma, and neuroblastoma.

Additional Untoward Reactions   Especially serious (fatal) hematologic toxicity. More than 90% of patients develop nausea, vomiting, and anorexia 1 hour after initial administration, persisting for 12 to 48 hours. Rarely, diarrhea, stomatitis, and intractable nausea. Also, flulike syndrome, severe pain along injected vein, facial flushing, alopecia. Elevation of SGOT, SGPT and other enzymes, CNS symptoms.

Dosage   **IV only.** *Malignant melanoma:* 2–4.5 mg/kg daily for 10 days; may be repeated at 4-week intervals; or 250 mg/m²/day for 5 days; may be repeated at 3-week intervals. *Hodgkin's disease:* 150 mg/m²/day for 5 days; or 375 mg/m² on day 1 with other drugs repeated every 15 days.

Administration/Storage

1. In order to minimize GI effects, antiemetics, fasting (4–6 hr preceding treatment), and good hydration (1 hr before treatment) have been suggested.

2. Extreme care should be taken to avoid extravasation.

3. Drug can be given by IV push over 1-min period or further diluted and administered by IV infusion (preferred) over 15–30-min period.

4. Protect dry vials from light and store at 2°–8°C.

5. Reconstituted solutions are stable for up to 72 hr at 4°C or 8 hr at 20°C. More dilute solutions for IV infusions are stable for 24 hr when stored at 2°–8°C.

Additional Nursing Implications

See also *Nursing Implications*, p. 210.

1. Ascertain whether doctor wishes patient to fast 4–6 hr before treatment to reduce emesis or to maintain good hydration by allowing fluids up to 1 hr before administration to minimize dehydration following treatment.

2. Report nausea and vomiting, which may last 1–12 hr after injection.

3. Have available phenobarbital and/or prochlorperazine (Compazine) for palliation of vomiting following administration of dacarbazine.

4. Reassure patient that after the first 1–2 days of administration of dacarbazine,

vomiting ceases because tolerance develops to the drug.

5. Alert patient to report to doctor flulike syndrome with fever, myalgia, and malaise, which may occur after treatment.

6. Advise patient to avoid prolonged exposure to sun or ultraviolet light as photosensitivity reaction may occur.

LOMUSTINE   CeeNu (Abbreviation: CCNU) (Rx)

Classification   Antineoplastic, alkylating agent.

Action/Kinetics   Similar to carmustine; thus cross-reactivity with carmustine has been observed. Rapidly absorbed from GI tract. Metabolized within 1 hr. **Peak plasma level:** 1–6 hr. **t½:** biphasic: initial 6 hr; postdistribution 1–2 days. 15–20% of drug remains in body after 5 days. Crosses blood - brain barrier, concentration in CSF higher than in plasma. Fifty percent of drug excreted within 12 hr, 75% within 4 days. Metabolites present in milk.

Uses   Primary and metastatic brain tumors. Disseminated Hodgkin's disease (in combination with other antineoplastics).

Additional Untoward Reactions   High incidence of nausea and vomiting 3–6 hr after administration and lasting 24 hr. Renal and pulmonary toxicity. Dysarthria.

Laboratory Test Interference   Elevated liver function tests (reversible).

Dosage   **PO. Adults** and **children: initial,** 130 mg/m^2 as a single dose q 6 weeks. If reduced bone marrow function, decrease dose to 100 mg/m^2 q 6 weeks. Subsequent dosage based on blood counts of patient (platelets above 100,000/mm^3 and leukocytes above 4,000/mm^3). Blood tests should be undertaken weekly.

Administration/Storage

1. Reduce GI distress by the administration of antiemetics before drug, or by giving drug to fasting patient.

2. Teach patient that medication comes in capsules of 3 strengths and that a combination of capsules will make up the correct dose, and that this combination is to be taken at one time.

3. Store below 40°C.

Additional Nursing Implications

See also *Nursing Implications*, p. 210.

1. Anticipate that patient may have nausea and vomiting up to 36 hr after treatment; this may be followed by 2 to 3 days of anorexia. Administer antiemetic as ordered.

2. Emphasize to patient the benefit to be derived from lomustine as he is often depressed by prolonged nausea and vomiting.

3. Explain to patient that intervals of 6 weeks are necessary between doses for optimum effect with minimal toxicity.

MECHLORETHAMINE HYDROCHLORIDE   Mustargen Hydrochloride, Nitrogen Mustard (Abbreviation: HN 2) (Rx)

Classification   Antineoplastic, alkylating agent.

Action/Kinetics Drug is inactivated within minutes.

Uses Malignant lymphomas, including Hodgkin's disease, lymphosarcomas, chronic lymphocytic or myelocytic leukemia, mycosis fungoides, polycythemia vera, generalized neoplastic disease, inoperable localized tumors, and bronchogenic carcinoma. One of the drugs used in MOPP therapy.

Additional Untoward Reactions High incidence of nausea and vomiting. Petechiae, subcutaneous hemorrhages, tinnitus, deafness, herpes zoster, or temporary amenorrhea. Extravasation into subcutaneous tissue causes painful inflammation.

Drug Interaction Amphoterecin B: combination increases possibility of blood dyscrasias.

Dosage **IV**, *total dose*: 0.4 mg/kg/course of therapy given as single dose or in 2–4 divided doses over 2–4 days. Drug can also be given by the intracavitary route. Depending on blood cell count, a second course may be given after 3 weeks.

Administration

1. Since drug is highly irritating, and contact with skin should be avoided, plastic or rubber gloves should be worn during preparation.
2. Drug is best administered through tubing of a rapidly flowing IV saline infusion.
3. Prepare solution immediately before administration.
4. Medication is available in a rubber-stoppered vial to which 10 ml of sterile distilled water should be added.
5. Insert the needle and keep it inserted until the medication is dissolved and the required dose withdrawn. Carefully discard the vial with the remaining solution so that no one will come in contact with it.
6. For intracavitary administration turn patient every 60 sec for 5 min to the following positions: prone, supine, right side, left side, and knee-chest. Lack of effect often results from failure to move the patient often enough.

Additional Nursing Implications
See also *Nursing Implications*, p. 210.

1. Administer phenothiazine and/or sedative as ordered prior to medication and as needed to control severe nausea and vomiting, which usually occur 1–3 hr after administration of nitrogen mustard.
2. Administer in late afternoon, and follow with sedation (sleeping pill) at an appropriate time so as to control untoward symptoms and induce sleep.
3. Monitor IV closely because extravasation causes swelling, erythema, induration, and sloughing.
4. In case of extravasation, remove IV and assist in infusion of area with isotonic sodium thiosulfate (4.14% solution of USP salt) and apply cold compresses. If sodium thiosulfate is not available, use isotonic sodium chloride solution.
5. Irrigate eye copiously with saline solution and consult with an ophthalmologist should there be accidental contact with eye.
6. Irrigate skin with water for 15 min and then with 2% solution of thiosulfate in the event of accidental contact.

MELPHALAN Alkeran, Pam, L-Pam, L-Phenylalanine Mustard, L-Sarcolysin (Abbreviation: MPL) (Rx)

Classification Antineoplastic, alkylating agent.

Action/Kinetics   Well absorbed from GI tract. $t^{1/2}$: 90 min. Highly toxic, marked bone marrow depression. Acute, nonlymphatic leukemia has been reported in patients with multiple myeloma who have received melphalan.

Uses   Multiple myeloma. Epithelial carcinoma of ovary (nonresectable).

Laboratory Test Interference   ↑ Uric acid and urinary 5-hydroxyindole acetic acid levels.

Dosage   **PO.** *Multiple myeloma:* **initial**, 6 mg daily. Adjust as required on the basis of frequent (1–3 per week) blood counts. Discontinue after 2–3 weeks for up to 4 weeks. When WBC increases, reinstitute maintenance therapy. **Usual maintenance:** 2 mg/day. Discontinue if leukocyte count falls below 3,000/mm³ or if platelet count falls below 100,000/mm³. **Alternative therapy: initial**, 10 mg/day for 7 to 10 days; **maintenance** (usual: 2 mg/day) based on leukocyte and platelet counts. *Epithelial ovarian cancer:* 0.2 mg/kg/day for 5 days as a single course. Repeat every 4–5 weeks depending on leukocyte and platelet counts.

PIPOBROMAN   Vercyte (Rx)

Classification   Antineoplastic, alkylating agent.

Action/Kinetics   Well absorbed from the GI tract.

Uses   Polycythemia vera; chronic granulocytic leukemia.

Additional Contraindication   Children under 15 years of age.

Dosage   **PO.** *Polycythemia vera:* 1 mg/kg daily. When hematocrit has been reduced to 50% – 55%, **maintenance dosage** of 100–200 μg/kg is instituted. *Chronic granulocytic leukemia:* **initial**, 1.5–2.5 mg/kg daily; **maintenance:** 7–175 mg daily to be instituted when leukocyte count approaches 10,000/mm³.

Administration   Administer in divided doses.

Additional Nursing Implications
See also *Nursing Implications*, p. 210.
  Be alert to the persistence of adverse reactions, because they may necessitate withdrawal of the drug.

STREPTOZOCIN   Zanosar (Rx)

Classification   Antineoplastic, alkylating agent.

Action/Kinetics   **$t^{1/2}$ after rapid IV use:** 35 min. Unchanged drug and metabolites excreted in urine.

Uses   Metastatic islet cell pancreatic carcinomas (functional and nonfunctional).

Additional Untoward Reactions   Renal toxicity (up to ²/₃ of patients) manifested by anuria, azotemia, glycosuria, hypophosphatemia, and renal tubular acidosis. Toxicity is dose-related and cumulative and may be fatal. Glucose intolerance (reversible) or insulin shock with hypoglycemia, depression.

Dosage   **IV:** *Daily schedule:* 500 mg/m² for 5 consecutive days every 6 weeks (until maximum benefit or toxicity). Dose should not be increased. *Weekly schedule:* **Initial,** 1,000 mg/m² weekly for 2 weeks; **then,** if no response or no toxicity, dose can be increased not to exceed a single dose of 1,500 mg/m². Response should be seen in 17–35 days.

Administration

1. Drug should be reconstituted with dextrose injection or 0.9% sodium chloride injection.
2. No preservatives are found in the product; thus, total storage time for reconstituted drug is 12 hr. The ampule is not considered to be multiple dose.

Additional Nursing Implications

See also Nursing Implications, p. 210.

1. Measure fluid intake and urinary output. If urine output decreases, report to physician as drug can cause anuria.
2. Test urine for glucose at least once a day.
3. Watch for symptoms of hypoglycemia.
4. Monitor kidney function tests.

TRIETHYLENETHIOPHOSPHORAMIDE   Tespa, Thiotepa, Tspa
(Abbreviation: THIO) (Rx)

Classification   Antineoplastic, alkylating agent.

Action/Kinetics   The effect of Thiotepa is cumulative and delayed, especially if excretion is delayed. Report when WBC count falls below 4,000/mm³ or platelet level below 150,000/mm³. This usually requires reduction in dosage or withdrawal of drug. Prophylactic antibiotics are sometimes ordered when WBC count falls below 3,000/mm³.

The drug disrupts DNA bonds. Eighty-five percent is excreted unchanged in urine.

Uses   Adenocarcinoma of the breast or ovary. Control of serious effusions of pleural, pericardial, and peritoneal cavities. Urinary bladder tumors. Cerebral metastases, chronic granulocytic and lymphocytic leukemia, malignant lymphomas including Hodgkin's disease, and bronchogenic cancer. *Investigational*: Prevention of pterygium recurrences after surgery.

Additional Contraindication   Acute leukemia.

Additional Untoward Reactions   Anorexia or decreased spermatogenesis.

Drug Interaction   Thiotepa increases the pharmacologic and toxic effect of succinylcholine due to a decrease in breakdown by the liver.

Dosage   **IV** (may be rapid): 0.3–0.4 mg/kg at 1- to 4-week intervals. **Intratumor or intracavitary administration**: 0.6–0.8 mg/kg; **maintainance (intratumor)**: 0.07–0.8 mg/kg at 1- to 4-week intervals, depending on condition of patient. *Carcinoma of bladder*: 60 mg in 30–60 ml distilled water instilled into the bladder and retained for 2 hr. Give once a week for 4 weeks.

Administration/Storage

1. Minimize pain on injection and retard rate of absorption by simultaneous administration of local anesthetics. Drug may be mixed with procaine HCl 2% or epinephrine HCl 1:1,000 or both, upon order of the physician.
2. Store vials in the refrigerator. Reconstituted solutions may be stored for 5 days

in the refrigerator without substantial loss of potency.

3. Since Thiotepa is not a vesicant, it may be injected quickly and directly into the vein with the desired volume of sterile water. Usual amount of diluent is 1.5 ml.

4. Do not use normal saline as a diluent.

5. Discard solutions grossly opaque or with precipitate.

Additional Nursing Implications

See also *Nursing Implications*, p. 210.

1. Encourage patients who receive drug as bladder instillations to retain fluid for 2 hr.

2. Reposition patient with a bladder instillation every 15 min for maximum contact.

URACIL MUSTARD (Rx)

Classification   Antineoplastic, alkylating agent.

Action/Kinetics   Complete blood counts should be done once or twice weekly during therapy and 1 month thereafter. Effect of drug sometimes takes 3 months to become apparent, and drug should be given that long unless precluded by toxicity reaction.

Uses   Chronic lymphocytic leukemia, lymphomas including Hodgkin's disease, lymphosarcoma, lymphoblastoma, giant follicular lymphomas, and reticulum cell sarcoma. Chronic myelogenous leukemia. Cancer of ovary, polycythemia vera, and mycosis fungoides.

Untoward Reactions   During therapy significant decreases in leukocyte and platelet counts occur.

Laboratory Test Interference   ↑ Serum uric acid levels.

Dosage   PO. Adults: 0.15 mg/kg once weekly for 4 weeks. **Children:** 0.30 mg/kg once weekly for 4 weeks.

Administration   Adequate fluid intake during therapy.

Additional Nursing Implications

See also *Nursing Implications*, p. 210.

1. Encourage continuation with therapy, as beneficial effect could be delayed by as long as 3 months.

2. Warn patient/family not to have smallpox immunization during therapy with uracil mustard, as vaccinia could result as a complication of immunosuppression.

3. Encourage large fluid intake to prevent hyperuricemia.

ANTIMETABOLITES

Action/Kinetics   Antimetabolites are able to disrupt DNA replication by interfering with an essential step in its synthesis and/or metabolism. Antimetabolites are thought to interfere with important enzymatic reactions in the synthesis of nucleic acids, purines, pyrimidines, and their prescursors. Antimetabolites may also be incorporated into nucleic acids in place of corresponding nucleotides resulting in alterations in important cellular functions and inhibition of DNA synthesis. Antimetabolites are usually cell cycle specific, being effective during the S and G_2 phases.

The antimetabolites fall into several categories: folic acid antagonists, pyrimidine antagonists, purine analogs, and miscellaneous agents.

CYTARABINE   Ara-C, Cytosar-U, Cytosine Arabinoside (Rx)

Classification   Antineoplastic, antimetabolite.

Action/Kinetics   Probably inhibits conversion of cytidine to deoxycytidine during DNA synthesis. Well absorbed from GI tract, rapidly removed from blood (5–20 min). Crosses blood–brain barrier. Metabolized in liver. Ninety percent eliminated in urine in 24 hr.

Uses   Acute myelocytic leukemia in adults and children, acute lymphocytic leukemia, chronic myelocytic leukemia, erythroleukemia, and meningeal leukemia. In combination with other drugs for non-Hodgkin's lymphoma in children.

Additional Untoward Reactions   "Cytarabine syndrome" (6–12 hr following drug administration) manifested by bone pain, fever, maculopapular rash, conjunctivitis, chest pain, or malaise. Nephrotoxicity, neuritis, skin ulceration, sepsis, acute pancreatitis, pneumonia, hyperuricemia. Thrombophlebitis at injection site.

The incidence of side effects is higher in patients receiving rapid IV injection than in those receiving drug by IV infusion.

Dosage   Cytarabine is frequently used in combination with other drugs; thus, dosage varies and must be carefully checked. *Acute myelocytic leukemia:* **IV infusion,** 200 mg/m²/day for 5 days (total dose: 1,000 mg/m²); repeat every 2 weeks. *Meningeal leukemia or acute lymphocytic leukemia in children:* **intrathecal,** 30 mg/m² with hydrocortisone sodium succinate and methotrexate, each at a dose of 15 mg/m². The drug should be discontinued if platelets fall to 50,000/mm³ or less or polymorphonuclear granulocytes fall to 1,000/mm³ or less.

Administration/Storage
1. Until reconstituted, cytarabine must be stored in refrigerator.
2. Reconstituted solution should be stored at room temperature and used within 48 hr.
3. Discard hazy solution.
4. Use water containing 0.9% benzyl alcohol for reconstitution of drug.
5. Elliot's B solution may be used as a diluent for intrathecal use.

FLOXURIDINE   FUDR (Abbreviation: FUDR) (Rx)

Classification   Antineoplastic, antimetabolite.

Action/Kinetics   Pyrimidine antagonist rapidly metabolized to fluorouracil (see below). Inhibits thymidylate synthetase and thus formation of thymidylate and DNA. Also affects RNA synthesis. Sixty to 80% excreted as respiratory CO_2 (8–12 hr); small amount (15%) excreted in urine (1–6 hr).

Uses   Palliative management of certain cancers in selected patients believed to profit from intra-arterial therapy, including carcinomas of the neck, head, brain, liver, gallbladder, and bile ducts. Used in patients with disease limited to an area capable of infusion by a single artery. Also for GI adenocarcinoma metastatic to liver.

Additional Untoward Reactions   Esophagopharyngitis, myocardial ischemia, angina, acute cerebellar syndrome, photophobia, lacrimation, decreased vision. Complications of intra-arterial administration are arterial aneurism, arterial ischemia, arterial thrombosis, bleeding at catheter site, occluded, displaced or leaking catheters, embolism, fibromyositis, infection at catheter site, thrombophlebitis.

Laboratory Test Interference   ↑ Excretion of 5-hydroxyindoleacetic acid. ↑ Serum transaminase and bilirubin, lactic dehydrogenase, alkaline phosphatase. ↓ Plasma albumin.

Dosage   **Intra-arterial infusion:** 0.1–0.6 mg/kg/day.

Administration   Higher doses (0.4–0.6 mg) are best given by hepatic artery infusion because the liver metabolizes the drug, reducing the possibility of systemic toxicity.

Nursing Implications

See *Nursing Implications* for Administration by Intra-arterial Infusion, p. 37 and *Antineoplastic agents*, p. 210.

FLUOROURACIL   Adrucil, Efudex, 5-Fluorouracil, 5-FU, Fluoroplex (Abbreviation: 5-FU) (Rx)

Classification   Antineoplastic, antimetabolite.

Action/Kinetics   Pyrimidine antagonist inhibiting thymidylate desoxyuridylic acid, hence DNA, and to a lesser degree, RNA synthesis. Sixty to 80% eliminated as respiratory CO_2 (8–12 hr); small amount (15%) excreted in urine (1–6 hr).

Highly toxic, initiate in hospital. Initially, topical creams cause ulceration, which might heal only 1–2 months after cessation of therapy.

Uses   Systemic: palliative management of certain cancers of the GI tract, rectum, liver, ovaries, colon, pancreas, and breast. Relieves pain and reduces size of tumor. Topical (as solution or cream): actinic or solar keratosis, superficial basal cell carcinoma.

Additional Contraindications   Systemic: patients in poor nutritional state, with severe bone marrow depression, severe infection, or recent (4-week-old) surgical intervention. To be used with caution in patients with hepatic or liver dysfunction. Pregnancy.

Additional Untoward Reactions   Esophagopharyngitis, myocardial ischemia, angina, acute cerebellar syndrome, photophobia, lacrimation, decreased vision.

Dosage   Individualize dosage. **IV: initial,** 12 mg/kg/day for 4 days not to exceed 800 mg/day. If no toxicity seen, administer 6 mg/kg on days 6, 8, 10, and 12. Discontinue therapy on day 12. **Maintenance:** repeat dose of first course every 30 days or when toxicity from initial course of therapy is gone; or, give 10–15 mg/kg/week as a single dose. Do not exceed 1 gm/week. **If patient is debilitated:** 6 mg/kg/day for 3 days; if no toxicity, give 3 mg/kg on days 5, 7, and 9 (daily dose should not exceed 400 mg). **Topical:** *Actinic or solar keratoses:* Apply 1–5% cream or solution to cover lesion b.i.d. for 2–6 weeks. *Superficial basal cell carconima:* Apply 5% cream or solution to cover lesion b.i.d. for 3–6 weeks.

Administration/Storage

IV

1. Store in a cool place (50°–80°F, or 10°–27°C). Do not freeze. Excessively low temperature causes precipitation.
2. Do not expose the solution to light.
3. Solution may discolor slightly during storage, but potency and safety are not affected.
4. If precipitate forms, resolubilize by heating to 140°F with vigorous shaking. Allow to return to room temperature and allow air to settle out before withdrawing and administering medication.
5. Further dilution is not needed, and solution may be injected directly into the vein with a 25-gauge needle.
6. Drug can be administered by IV infusion for periods of ½–8 hr. This method has been reported to produce less systemic toxicity than rapid injection.

TOPICAL

1. Apply with fingertips, nonmetallic applicator, or rubber gloves. Wash hands immediately thereafter.
2. Avoid contact with eyes, nose, and mouth.
3. Limit occlusive dressings to lesions, since they are responsible for increased incidence of inflammatory reactions in normal skin.
4. Complete healing in keratoses may require 2 months.

Additional Nursing Implications

See also *Nursing Implications*, p. 210.

1. Observe for intractable vomiting, stomatitis, and diarrhea, all of which are early signs of toxicity and cause for immediate discontinuance of drug. Drug should also be discontinued if WBC and platelet counts are depressed below 3,500/mm³ and 100,000/mm³, respectively.
2. Practice reverse isolation when WBC is below 2,000/mm³.
3. Prevent exposure to strong sunlight and other ultraviolet rays, because they intensify skin reaction to the drug.

HYDROXYUREA   Hydrea (Abbreviation: HYD) (Rx)

Classification   Antineoplastic, antimetabolite.

Action/Kinetics   Believed to interfere with DNA, but not RNA synthesis. Most active in inhibiting incorporation of thymidine into DNA. Rapidly absorbed from GI tract. **Peak serum concentration:** 2 hr. Degraded in liver; 50% excreted as respiratory CO_2, remainder unchanged in urine.

Uses   Melanoma, resistant chronic myelocytic (granulocytic) leukemia, inoperable ovarian carcinoma, and squamous cell carcinomas of head and neck.

Additional Contraindications   Give with caution to patients with marked renal dysfunction. Dosage has not been established in children.

Additional Untoward Reactions   Erythrocyte abnormalities including megaloblastic erythropoiesis. Constipation, redness of the face.

Laboratory Test Interference   ↑ Uric acid in serum; ↑ BUN and creatinine.

Dosage PO: Individualized. *Solid tumors, intermittent therapy or when used to-gether with irradiation*: 80 mg/kg as a single dose q third day; *solid tumors, continuous therapy*: 20–30 mg/kg daily as a single dose. Intermittent dosage offers advantage of reduced toxicity. If effective, maintain patient on drug indefinitely unless toxic effects preclude such a regimen. *Resistant chronic myelocytic leukemia*: 20–30 mg/kg/day in a single dose. Therapy should be discontinued if WBC drops below, 2,500/mm³ or platelet count below 100,000/mm³.

Administration

1. If the patient cannot swallow a capsule, contents may be given in glass of water that should be drunk immediately, even though some material may not dissolve and may float on top of glass.
2. Hydroxyurea should be started 7 days before irradiation.

Additional Nursing Implications

See also *Nursing Implications*, p. 210.

1. Check for exacerbation of postirradiation erythema.
2. Anticipate that the dosage for the elderly will be smaller.

MERCAPTOPURINE 6-Mercaptopurine, 6-MP, Purinethol (Abbreviation: 6-MP) (Rx)

Classification Antimetabolite, purine analog.

Action/Kinetics Metabolized to purine antagonist, which inhibits DNA and RNA synthesis. About 50% absorbed from GI tract. **Maximum serum levels**: 2 hr; disappearance from serum complete in 8 hr. Excreted in urine. Cross-resistance with thioguanine has been observed.

Uses Drug of choice for acute lymphocytic or lymphoblastic leukemia, especially in children. Also chronic granulocytic leukemia. Acute myelogenous and myelomonocytic leukemia. Effectiveness varies depending on use.

Additional Contraindication Use with caution in patients with impaired renal function.

Additional Untoward Reactions Produces less GI toxicity than folic acid antagonists, and side effects are less frequent in children than in adults.

Drug Interaction Allopurinol potentiates mercaptopurine by ↓ breakdown. Requires reduction of antineoplastic agent by 25–33⅓%.

Dosage PO. *Highly individualized*: 2.5 mg/kg/day. **Usual, adults**: 100–200 mg; **children**: 50 mg. Dosage may be increased to 5 mg/kg daily after 4 weeks, if beneficial effects are not noted. Dosage is increased until symptoms of toxicity appear. **Maintenance after remission**: 1.5–2.5 mg/kg daily.

Administration

1. Since the maximum effect of mercaptopurine on the blood count may be delayed and blood counts may drop for several days after drug has been discontinued, therapy should be discontinued at first sign of abnormally large drop in leukocyte count.
2. Administer drug in one dose daily at any convenient time.
3. Limit intake of alcoholic beverages.

Additional Nursing Implications
See also *Nursing Implications*, p. 210.
Advise patient to limit use of alcohol.

METHOTREXATE, METHOTREXATE SODIUM   Amethopterin, Folex, Mexate, MTX (Abbreviation: MTX) (Rx)

Classification   Antimetabolite, folic acid analog.

Action/Kinetics   Inhibition of dihydrofolate reductase, which results in decreased synthesis of purines and consequently DNA. Fair absorption from GI tract. **Peak serum levels**: $1/2$–4 hr, depending on route. Accumulates in body. Not metabolized. Excreted by kidney (55–92% in 24 hr).

Renal function tests are recommended before initiation of therapy; daily leukocyte counts should be taken during therapy.

Uses   Uterine choriocarcinoma (curative), hydatidiform mole, acute lymphocytic and lymphoblastic leukemia, lymphosarcoma, and other disseminated neoplasms in children; meningeal leukemia, some beneficial effect in regional chemotherapy of head and neck tumors, breast tumors, and lung cancer. Advanced mycosis fungoides. Severe or disabling psoriasis.

Contraindications   Psoriasis patients with kidney or liver disease, blood dyscrasias, or if pregnant.

Additional Untoward Reactions   Severe bone marrow depression. Hemorrhagic enteritis, intestinal ulceration or perforation, acne, ecchymosis, hematemesis, melena, increased pigmentation, diabetes, chronic interstitial obstructive pulmonary disease. Intrathecal use may result in chemical arachnoiditis, transient paresis, or seizures. Concomitant exposure to sunlight may aggravate psoriasis.

Drug Interactions

Interactant	Interaction
Alcohol, ethyl	Additive hepatotoxicity; combination can result in coma
Anticoagulants, oral	Additive hypoprothrombinemia
Chloramphenicol	↑ Effect of methotrexate by ↓ plasma protein binding
Folic acid-containing vitamin preparations	↓ Response to methotrexate
PABA	↑ Effect of methotrexate by ↓ plasma protein binding
Phenylbutazone	↑ Effect of methotrexate by ↓ plasma protein binding
Phenytoin	↑ Effect of methotrexate by ↓ plasma protein binding
Probenecid	↑ Effect of methotrexate by ↓ renal clearance
Pyrimethamine	↑ Methotrexate toxicity
Salicylates (aspirin)	↑ Effect of methotrexate by ↓ plasma protein binding; also, salicylates ↓ renal excretion of methotrexate

Interactant	Interaction
Smallpox vaccination	Methotrexate impairs immunologic response to smallpox vaccine
Sulfonamides	↑ Effect of methotrexate by ↓ plasma protein binding
Tetracyclines	↑ Effect of methotrexate by ↓ plasma protein binding

Dosage *Methotrexate is administered* **PO**; *methotrexate sodium is administered* **IM, IV, intra-arterially,** *or* **intrathecally.** *Dose individualized. Choriocarcinoma,* **PO, IM:** 15–30 mg/day for 5 days. May be repeated 3 to 5 times with 1 week rest period between courses. *Leukemia,* **initial:** 3.3 mg/m² (with prednisone 60 mg/ m² daily); **maintenance: PO, IM,** 30 mg/m² 2 times weekly or **IV,** 2.5 mg/kg q 14 days. *Meningeal leukemia,* **intrathecal:** 12 mg/m² q 2–5 days until cell count returns to normal. *Lymphomas,* **PO:** 10–25 mg/day for 4–8 days for several courses of treatment with 7- to 10-day rest periods between courses. *Mycosis fungoides:* **PO,** 2.5–10 mg/day for several weeks or months; **alternatively, IM,** 50 mg once per week or 25 mg twice weekly. *Lymphosarcoma:* 0.625–2.5 mg/kg/day in combination with other drugs.

Administration

1. Use only sterile water, without preservatives, to reconstitute powder for parenteral administration.
2. Prevent inhalation of particles of medication and skin exposure.

Additional Nursing Implications
See also *Nursing Implications*, p. 210.

1. Monitor intake and output, and encourage fluid intake to facilitate excretion of drug.
2. Report oliguria, since this may require discontinuing drug.
3. *Assess* for oral ulcerations, one of the first signs of toxicity.
4. Calcium leucovorin—a potent antidote for folic acid antagonists—should be on hand in case of overdosage. If necessary, 3–6 mg is usually injected intramuscularly. Antidotes are ineffective if not administered within 4 hr of overdosage. Corticosteroids are sometimes given concomitantly with initial dose of methotrexate.
5. Advise patient not to ingest alcohol when receiving methotrexate, as coma may result.
6. Do not vaccinate for smallpox when the patient is receiving methotrexate, because the impaired immunologic response could result in vaccinia.
7. Anticipate reduction in anticoagulant dosage if administered concomitantly.
8. Question doctor as to whether patient is receiving other organic acids, such as aspirin, phenylbutazone, probencid, and/or sulfa drugs, as they affect renal clearance of methotrexate and increase thrombocytopenic and GI side effects of methotrexate.

THIOGUANINE TG, 6-Thioguanine (Abbreviation: 6-TG) (Rx)

Classification Antimetabolite, purine analog.

Action/Kinetics Purine antagonist, which inhibits DNA and RNA synthesis. Partially absorbed from GI tract. **Peak serum levels**: 10–12 hr, partially detoxified by liver, excreted in urine and feces.

More effective in children than in adults. Cross-resistance with mercaptopurine. Perform platelet counts weekly; discontinue if abnormally large fall in blood count is noted, indicating severe bone marrow depression. Effect of drug is cumulative.

Uses   Acute lymphocytic, lymphoblastic, or myelogenous leukemias in adults and children. Chronic granulocytic leukemia.

Additional Untoward Reactions   Loss of vibration sense, unsteadiness of gait. Adults tend to show a more rapid WBC fall than do children.

Laboratory Test Interference   ↑ Uric acid in blood and urine.

Dosage   PO: *Individualized* and determined by hematopoietic response; **adult and pediatric: initial**: 2 mg/kg daily. From 2 to 4 weeks may elapse before beneficial results become apparent. Compute dose to nearest multiple of 20 mg. If no response, dosage may be increased to 3 mg/kg daily. **Usual maintenance** (even during remissions): 2 mg/kg daily.

Additional Nursing Implications

See also *Nursing Implications* p. 210.

1. Provide assistance to ambulatory patients who may experience loss of vibration sense and thus have unsteady gait (may be unable to rely on canes).
2. Encourage increased fluid intake to minimize hyperuricemia and hyperuricosuria.
3. Monitor liver function tests as a baseline before therapy is instituted and then monthly.
4. Teach patient to withhold drug and report jaundice to doctor if it occurs.
5. Emphasize to adult patients that contraceptive measures are advised with this drug.

ANTIBIOTICS

Action/Kinetics   A number of antineoplastic antibiotics are very effective chemotherapeutic agents. Most of these agents are cell cycle specific and interfere with the replication of DNA, RNA, and protein synthesis. A number of the antineoplastic antibiotics are specific for certain tissues or organs, and many are part of combination therapy (Table 5).

BLEOMYCIN SULFATE   Blenoxane, (Abbreviation: BLM) (Rx)

Classification   Antineoplastic, antibiotic.

Action/Kinetics   Glycopeptide antibiotic produced by *Streptomyces verticillus*. Drug currently used is mostly mixture of bleomycin A_2 and B_2. Drug has relatively low bone marrow depressant activity, localizes in certain tissues, and is an important component of some combination regimens.

Believed to cause DNA scission (chelation, oxidation, complex formation, intercalation). **Peak plasma levels** (after 4–5 days of therapy): 50 ng/ml. **t½**: Biphasic: initial, 1.3 hr; distribution, 9 hr. Two-thirds excreted in urine.

Uses   Palliative treatment of certain solid tumors, lymphomas, Hodgkin's disease, and squamous cell carcinomas. Some effectiveness in testicular carcinomas.

Additional Contraindications Renal or pulmonary diseases.

Additional Untoward Reactions Pulmonary fibrosis, especially in older patients. Mucocutaneous toxicity and hypersensitivity reactions. In approximately 1% of lymphoma patients, an idiosyncratic reaction manifested by hypotension, fever, chills, mental confusion, and wheezing has been reported.

Dosage **SC, IM, IV.** *Squamous cell carconima, sarcomas, testicular carcinoma*: 0.25– 0.5 units/kg (10–20 units/m²) once or twice weekly. *Hodgkin's disease*: **SC, IM, IV**, 0.25–0.5 units/kg once or twice weekly; **maintenance** (after a 50% response): **IM, IV**, 1 unit daily or 5 units weekly.

Administration/Storage
1. Reconstituted bleomycin is stable for 2 weeks when stored at room temperature and for 4 weeks when stored at 2°–8° C.
2. Administer IV slowly over 10 min.
3. Hodgkin's disease and testicular tumors should respond within 2 weeks while squamous cell cancers require at least 3 weeks.

Additional Nursing Implications
See also *Nursing Implications*, p. 210.

1. *Assess* patient for basilar rales, cough, dyspnea on exertion, and tachypnea, all of which are dose-related symptoms of pulmonary toxicity.
2. *Teach patient and/or family* about idiosyncratic reaction noted in untoward reactions that may occur in patient with lymphoma.

DACTINOMYCIN Actinomycin D, ACT, Cosmegen (Rx)

Classification Antineoplastic, antibiotic.

General Statement Chromopeptide antibiotic produced by *Streptomyces parvullus*. Potent antitumor agent inducing marked bone marrow depression. During therapy, leukocyte counts should be performed daily, platelet counts q 3 days. Frequent liver and kidney function tests are recommended. Appearance of toxic manifestations may be delayed by several weeks. Irreversible bone marrow depression may occur in patients with preexisting renal, hepatic, or bone marrow impairment. The drug is corrosive to soft tissue.

Action/Kinetics Cell cycle specific (M phase). Links to DNA, blocking effect of RNA polymerase and transcription of DNA. Disappears rapidly from blood. **Plasma t½:** 36 hr. Animal studies indicate 50% excreted unchanged in bile and urine.

Uses In combination with surgery and/or irradiation for treatment of Wilms' tumor (nephroblastoma) and its metastases; tumors of the uterus and testes. Osteogenic sarcoma. Has some effect in rhabdomyosarcoma in children. Ewing's sarcoma, sarcoma botryoides.

Contraindications Concurrent infection with chickenpox or herpes zoster.

Additional Untoward Reactions Anaphylaxis. Due to corrosiveness, extravasation causes severe damage to soft tissues. Hypocalcemia. When combined with radiation, increased severity of skin reactions, GI toxicity, and bone marrow depression.

Dosage **IV, Individualized. Adults, usual,** 0.5 mg/day for maximum of 5 days. **Pediatric:** 15 μg/kg daily for 5 days; **alternatively**, a total dose of 2.5 mg/m² over 1 week. Total daily dosage for both adults and children should not exceed 15 μg/kg. Course of treatment may be repeated after 3 weeks unless contraindicated due to toxicity. If no toxicity, second course can be given after 3 weeks. **Isolation-perfusion**: 0.05 mg/kg for pelvis and lower extremities and 0.035 mg/kg for upper extremities.

Administration

1. For IV use, dactinomycin is available in a lyophilized dactinomycin–mannitol mixture that turns a gold color upon reconstitution with sterile water. Use only sterile water without a preservative to reconstitute the drug for IV use as it will precipitate. Solutions should not be exposed to direct sunlight.
2. *The drug is extremely corrosive.* It is most safely administered through the tubing of a running IV. It may be given directly into the vein, but the needle used to draw up the solution should be discarded and another sterile needle attached, before injection, to prevent subcutaneous reaction and thrombophlebitis.
3. Any portion of the solution not used for the injection should be discarded.

Additional Nursing Implications
See also *Nursing Implications*, p. 210.

1. Report erythema of the skin, which can lead to desquamation sloughing, particularly in areas previously affected by radiation.
2. Warn patient of the possibility of delayed toxic reactions and stress importance of returning for blood tests.
3. Assess and report if patient is pregnant, lactating, or infected with herpes, all of which are contraindications for dactinomycin.
4. Anticipate that dactinomycin may be administered intermittently if nausea and vomiting persist, even when an emetic is given.
5. Anticipate that penicillin will not be used if patient contracts an infection, because dactinomycin inhibits the action of penicillin.

DAUNORUBICIN   Cerubidine (Abbreviation: DNR) (Rx)

Classification   Antineoplastic, antibiotic.

General Statement   Anthracycline antibiotic produced by *Streptomyces coeruleo-rubidus*. Cross-resistance with doxorubicin (produced by similar microorganism) and vinca alkaloids. Because of cardiotoxicity, baseline and regular ECGs are indicated during therapy and for several months thereafter.

Action/Kinetics   Binds to DNA, thereby interfering with cell replication and perhaps causing DNA chain scission. Rapidly cleared from plasma. $t^{1/2}$: triphasic: initial, 12 min; intermediate, 3.3 hr; terminal, 30 hr. Drug rapidly taken up by heart, kidneys, lung, liver, and spleen. Metabolized to daunorubinicol. Latter chiefly excreted in bile (40%) and unchanged in urine (25%). Does not pass blood-brain barrier.

Uses   Acute nonlymphocytic leukemia in adults (myelogenous, erythroid, monocytic). When combined with cytarabine, increased effectiveness. Acute lymphocytic leukemia in children (increased effectiveness when combined with vincristine and prednisone).

Contraindications   Use with caution in preexisting heart disease or bone marrow depression, pregnancy (teratogenic), renal or hepatic failure.

Additional Untoward Reactions   *Myocardial toxicity*: Potentially fatal congestive heart failure. Mucositis (3–7 days after administration), red-colored urine, hyperuricemia. Severe tissue necrosis if extravasation occurs.

Dosage   IV infusion (rapid). *Acute nonlymphocytic leukemia*. **As sole agent:** 60 mg/ m^2/day on days 1, 2, and 3 every 3–4 weeks. **With cytosine arabinoside:** *daunorubicin*, 45 mg/m^2/day on days 1, 2, and 3 of first course and days 1 and 2 of additional courses; *cytosine arabinoside (Ara-c)*, **IV infusion**, 100 mg/m^2/day for 7 days during first course and for 5 days during any additional courses of treatment. Up to 3 courses may be required. *Acute lymphocytic leukemia in children:* daunorubicin, 25 mg/m^2 and vincristine, 1.5 mg/m^2 each **IV** on day 1 every week with prednisone, 40 mg/m^2 **PO** daily. Usually 4 courses will induce remission. Dosage should be reduced in patients with renal or hepatic disease.

Administration/Storage
1. Dilute in vial with 4 ml Sterile Water for Injection USP. Agitate gently until dissolved (solution contains 5 mg daunorubicin/ml). Withdraw desired dose into syringe containing 10–15 ml isotonic saline; inject into tubing of rapidly flowing 5% glucose or normal saline IV. *Never administer daunorubicin IM or SC.*
2. Reconstituted solution stable for 24 hr at room temperature; for 48 hr when refrigerated.
3. Protect from sunlight.
4. Do not mix with other drugs or heparin.

Additional Nursing Implications
See also *Nursing Implications*, p. 210.

1. *Assess* patient during and after termination of therapy for myocardial toxicity manifested by changes in baseline ECG, edema, dyspnea, and cyanosis. Patients with a cardiac history who receive doses above 550 mg/m^2 are more susceptible to CHF.
2. Have digitalis preparations, and diuretics available; be aware that physician may order a sodium-restricted diet and bed rest to treat CHF.
3. *Teach patient*
   a. to report signs and symptoms of cardiac toxicity.
   b. that urine may appear red due to drug.

DOXORUBICIN HYDROCHLORIDE   ADR, Adriamycin (Rx)

Classification   Antineoplastic, antibiotic.

General Statement   Anthrocycline antibiotic produced by *Streptomyces peucetius*. Cross-resistance with daunorubicin produced by similar microorganism. Because of cardiotoxicity of drug, baseline and monthly ECGs are indicated during therapy and for several months thereafter.

Action/Kinetics   Disrupts DNA replication. Metabolized to the active doxorubicinol and inactive compounds. See also *Daunorubicin*, p. 234.

Uses   Acute lymphoblastic leukemia, acute myeloblastic leukemia, Wilms' tumor, soft tissue and osteogenic sarcoma, neuroblastoma, cancer of the breast, ovaries, lungs, bladder, and thyroid, lymphomas (Hodgkin's and non-Hodgkin's).

Additional Contraindications   Depressed bone marrow or cardiac disease.

Additional Untoward Reactions   *Myocardial toxicity:* Potentially fatal congestive heart failure. Mucositis, lacrimation, conjunctivitis. Hyperpigmentation of nailbeds. Facial flushing if injection too rapid. Hyperuricemia, red-colored urine (initially). Extravasation may cause severe cellulitis and tissue necrosis. Drug may reactivate previous cardiac, skin, mucosa, and liver radiation damage.

Drug Interactions   Doxorubicin potentiates the toxicity of cyclophosphamide and 6-mercaptopurine.

Dosage   IV, *highly individualized*: 60–75 mg/m² of body surface q 21 days, or 30 mg/m² of body surface for 3 successive days q 4 weeks. Total dose by either regimen 550 mg/m² of body surface. Use reduced dosage in patients with hepatic dysfunction, depending on serum bilirubin level: if bilirubin is 1.2–3 mg/100 ml, give 50% of usual dose; if bilirubin is greater than 3 mg/100 ml, give 25% of usual dose.

Administration

1. Initiate therapy only in hospitalized patients.
2. *Do not administer SC or IM as severe necrosis of tissue may result. In order to minimize danger of extravasation, inject into tubing of free-flowing IV infusion.*
3. If stinging or burning occurs during IV administration, stop and restart infusion at another site.
4. Should not be mixed with heparin, dexamethasone sodium phosphate, or cephalothin since a precipitate may form.

Additional Nursing Implications

See also *Nursing Implications*, p. 210.

1. Observe patient for cardiac arrhythmias and/or respiratory difficulties, which could be indicative of cardiac toxicity.
2. If medication reactivates previous radiotherapy damage, such as erythema, edema, and desquamation, reassure the patient that these symptoms will disappear after 7 days.
3. Inform the patient that urine will turn red for 1–2 days after initiation of therapy.
4. Advise the patient that alopecia will occur; reassure him that hair will grow back 2–3 months after discontinuation of therapy.
5. Monitor IV administration carefully. Stinging, burning, or edema at injection site are indicative of extravasation. Administration should be stopped, and injection site moved, so as to avoid tissue necrosis.
6. Be prepared with an injectable corticosteroid for local infiltration and flood site with normal saline. Examine area frequently for ulceration, which might necessitate early wide excision followed by plastic surgery.

MITOMYCIN   Mutamycin (Abbreviation: MTC) (Rx)

Classification   Antineoplastic, antibiotic.

Action/Kinetics   Antibiotic produced by *Streptomyces caespitosus*. Not recommended as single agent for primary treatment or instead of surgery and/or radiotherapy.

Formation of a mitomycin-DNA complex that inhibits RNA synthesis. Most active during late G_1 and early S stages. Rapidly cleared from blood (50% removed in 17 min). Metabolized in liver, 10% excreted unchanged in urine, more when dose is increased.

Uses Palliative treatment and adjunct to surgical or radiologic treatment of disseminated adenocarcinoma of the stomach, and pancreas. Used in combination with other agents. *Investigational:* Superficial bladder cancer.

Additional Contraindications Use with extreme caution in presence of impaired renal function.

Additional Untoward Reactions Severe bone marrow depression, especially leukopenia and thrombocytopenia. Pulmonary toxicity including dyspnea with nonproductive cough. Microangiopathic hemolytic anemia with renal failure and hypertension especially when used long-term in combination with fluorouracil. Extravasation causes severe necrosis of surrounding tissue.

Dosage **IV only**: 20 mg/m² as a single dose via infusion or 2 mg/m²/day for 5 days. After 2-day rest period, 2 mg/m²/day for 5 more days. Subsequent courses of treatment are based on hematologic response and should not be repeated until leukocyte count is at least 3,000/mm³ and platelet is at least 75,000/mm³.

Administration/Storage

1. Drug is very toxic, and extravasation is to be avoided.
2. Reconstitute 5- or 20-mg vial with 10–40 ml as indicated on label. Medication will dissolve if allowed to remain at room temperature.
3. Drug at concentration of 0.5 mg/ml is stable for 14 days under refrigeration or for 7 days at room temperature.
4. Diluted to a concentration of 20–40 µg/ml, the drug is stable for 3 hr in D_5W, 12 hr in isotonic saline, and 24 hr in sodium lactate injection.
5. Mitomycin (5–15 mg) and heparin (1,000–10,000 units) in 30 ml of isotonic saline is stable for 48 hr at room temperature.

Additional Nursing Implications
See also *Nursing Implications*, p. 210.
Monitor IV closely to prevent extravasation and subsequent cellulitis.

PLICAMYCIN (MITHRAMYCIN) Mithracin (Abbreviation: MTH) (Rx)

Classification Antineoplastic, antibiotic

General Statement Antibiotic produced by *Streptomyces plicatus*. Drug affects calcium metabolism, leading to a decrease in blood calcium levels. Should be used only for hospitalized patients. Therapy should be interrupted if WBC count goes below 3,000/mm³ or if prothrombin time is more than 4 sec higher than that of the control. Daily platelet count should be performed on patients who had x-ray films taken of abdomen and mediastinum.

Action/Kinetics Mechanism similar to dactinomycin, p. 233. Forms plicamycin-DNA complex, inhibiting cellular and enzymatic RNA synthesis and bringing cell replication to a halt.

Uses Malignant testicular tumors usually associated with metastases. Hypercalcemia and hypercalciuria associated with advanced malignancy and not responsive to other therapy.

Additional Contraindications Thrombocytopenia, coagulation disorders, and increased tendency to hemorrhage. Do not use for children under 15 years of age.

Additional Untoward Reactions Severe thrombocytopenia, hemorrhagic tendencies. Facial flushing. Hepatic and renal toxicity. Extravasation may cause irritation or cellulitis.

Laboratory Test Interferences ↑ BUN and serum creatinine; ↓serum calcium, potassium, and phosphorus; ↑ serum SGOT, SGPT, alkaline phosphatase, bilirubin, isocitric dehydrogenase, ornithine carbamyl transferase, lactic dehydrogenase; ↑ BSP retention.

Dosage **IV only.** *Individualized. Testicular tumor:* 25–30 (maximum) μg/kg daily for 8–10 (maximum) days. A second approach is 50 μg/kg on alternate days for an average of 6 doses. *Hypercalcemia, hypercalciuria:* 25 μg/kg daily for 3 to 4 days. Additional courses of therapy may be warranted at weekly intervals if initial course is unsuccessful.

Administration/Storage

1. *Store vials of medication in refrigerator at temperature below 10°C (36–46° F). Discard unused portion of drug.*
2. Reconstitute fresh for each day of therapy.
3. Drug is unstable in acid solution (pH 5 and below) and in reconstituted solutions (pH 7) and thus deteriorates rapidly.
4. Add sterile water to the vial as recommended on the package insert, and shake the vial to dissolve the drug.
5. Add the calculated dosage of the drug to the IV solution ordered (recommended 1 liter of D₅W) and adjust the rate of flow as ordered (recommended time is 4–6 hr for 1 liter).

Additional Nursing Implications

See also *Nursing Implications*, p. 210.

1. *Assess* patients for any sign of hemorrhage, such as epistaxis, hemoptysis, hematemesis, purpura, or ecchymoses.
2. If antiemetic drugs are ordered, administer before or during therapy with mithramycin.
3. Check IV closely for extravasation. Stop IV if extravasation occurs; apply moderate heat to disperse drug and reduce pain and tissue damage. Restart IV at another site.
4. Prevent excessively rapid flow, as this precipitates more severe GI side efects.

NATURAL PRODUCTS AND MISCELLANEOUS AGENTS

Some of the more potent antineoplastic agents do not belong to any specific group. Two—vinblastine and vincristine—are alkaloids, produced by the periwinkle plant; a third is the natural enzyme asparaginase, which breaks down one of the amino acids required for protein synthesis; and the fourth, procarbazine, is believed to inhibit RNA and DNA synthesis by an oxidative process.

ASPARAGINASE   Elspar, Kidrolase* (Abbreviation: L-ASP) (Rx)

Classification   Antibiotic, miscellaneous.

Action/Kinetics   Drug isolated from *E. coli*. Cell cycle specific (G_1 phase). Neoplastic cells seem unable to synthesize enough asparagine, an amino acid, to meet their metabolic needs. The supply of asparagine is further decreased by the enzyme asparaginase, which converts asparagine to aspartic acid. **t½:** ranges from 8 to 30 hr. The drug accumulates in plasma and tissue, and a small amount (1%) appears in CSF. Excretion is unknown. More toxic in adults than in children.

Use   Acute lymphocytic leukemia mostly used in combination with other drugs.

Contraindications   Anaphylactic reactions to asparaginase, acute hemorrhagic pancreatitis. Institute retreatment with great care. Also use with caution in presence of liver dysfunction. Maintenance therapy.

Additional Untoward Reactions   Hypersensitivity reaction including those with negative skin tests. Hyperglycemia, uricemia, azotemia, acute hemorrhagic pancreatitis, fatal hyperthermia. Hallucinations, Parkinson-like syndrome (rare).

Drug Interactions

Interactant	Interaction
Methotrexate	Asparaginase ↓ effect of methotrexate
Prednisone	Even though used with asparaginase, may cause ↑ toxicity
Vincristine	Even though used with asparaginase, may cause ↑ toxicity; ↑ hyperglycemic effect

Laboratory Test Interferences   ↑ Blood ammonia, BUN, glucose, and uric acid. ↓ Serum calcium and albumin. Interference with interpretation of thyroid function tests.

Dosage   **IV, IM**, *individualized*. **When used as sole agent: Adults and children,** 200 IU/kg/day **IV** for 28 days. **In combination with prednisone and vincristine: asparaginase,** 1,000 IU/kg/day **IV** for 10 days beginning on day 22 of course of therapy; **vincristine:** 2 mg/m² **IV** once weekly on days 1, 8, and 15 of course of treatment (single dosage should not exceed 2 mg); **prednisone:** 40 mg/m²/day **PO** in 3 doses for 15 days; **then,** 20 mg/m² for 2 days, 10 mg/m² for 2 days, 5 mg/m² for 2 days, and 2.5 mg/m² for 2 days, followed by discontinuance of therapy. **Alternative regimen: asparaginase,** 6,000 IU/m² **IM** on days 4, 7, 10, 13, 16, 19, 22, 25, and 28 of course of treatment; **vincristine:** 1.5 mg/m² **IV** weekly on days 1, 8, 15, and 22 of course of treatment (maximum single dose should not exceed 2 mg); **prednisone:** 40 mg/m²/day **PO** in 3 divided doses for 28 days followed by gradual discontinuation over a two-week period.

Administration

1. An intradermal skin test (0.1 ml of a 20-IU/ml solution) is to be done at least 1 hr before initial administration of drug and when 1 week or more has elapsed between treatments.
2. A desensitization procedure, with increasing amounts of asparaginase, is sometimes carried out in patients hypersensitive to drug.
3. Treatment should be initiated only in hospitalized patients.
4. When used IV, give over at least 30 minutes in side of arm; use an infusion of either sodium chloride injection or dextrose injection (5%).
5. When used IM, no more than 2 ml should be given at a single injection site.

Additional Nursing Implications

See also *Nursing Implications*, p. 210.

1. Have emergency equipment ready to counteract anaphylactic shock (oxygen, epinephrine, and corticosteroids) at each administration of asparaginase since a severe reaction is more likely to occur with this drug.
2. Ascertain that serum amylase determinations are done as a baseline and periodically during therapy to detect pancreatitis.
3. Advise patient to report promptly to the doctor any stomach pain, nausea, and vomiting since these are symptoms of pancreatitis.
4. Monitor patient for hyperglycemia, glycosuria, and polyuria, which may be precipitated by asparaginase.
5. Have IV fluids and regular insulin available should hyperglycemia occur. Anticipate discontinuation of asparaginase.
6. Monitor intake and output, assessing patient for renal failure.
7. Assess patient for peripheral edema due to hypoalbuminemia triggered by asparaginase.
8. Caution the patient and/or family that the drug may cause drowsiness, even several weeks after administration; therefore, the patient should not drive a car or operate hazardous machinery.
9. Assess for shakiness or unusual body movements, a Parkinson-like condition that may be precipitated by asparaginase.
10. Alert patient to report hyperthermia.
11. Administer vincristine and prednisone, if ordered, before asparaginase to reduce the toxic effect.
12. Anticipate administration of asparaginase 9–10 days before or within 24 hr after methotrexate to prevent reduction in effect of methotrexate and to reduce the GI and hematologic effects of methotrexate.

CISPLATIN   Platinol (Abbreviation: CPDD) (Rx)

Classification   Antineoplastic, miscellaneous.

Action/Kinetics   Cisplatin interferes with DNA replication by forming complexes with DNA. t½: initial; 25–49 min; **postdistribution**, 58–73 hr. Incomplete urinary excretion (only 27–43% after 5 days). Drug concentrates in liver, kidneys, large and small intestines, with low penetration of CNS.

Uses   Treatment of metastatic testicular (in combination with bleomycin and vinblastine) and ovarian (in combination with doxorubicin) tumors in patients with prior radiotherapy or surgery. Advanced bladder cancer.

Additional Contraindications   Preexisting renal impairment, bone marrow suppression, hearing impairment, and allergic reactions to platinum.

Additional Untoward Reactions   Severe cumulative renal toxicity. Ototoxicity characterized by tinnitus, especially in children, anaphylactic reactions, neurotoxicity.

Dosage   **IV.** *Metastatic testicular tumors:* **usual dosage,** cisplatin, 20 mg/m² daily for 5 days q 3 weeks for 3 courses; bleomycin sulfate, **IV (rapid infusion)**: 30 units weekly (on day 2 of each week) for 12 consecutive weeks; vinblastine sulfate, **IV**: 0.15–0.2 mg/kg twice weekly (days 1 and 2) q 3 weeks for 4 courses (i.e., 8 doses total). *Metastatic ovarian tumor, as single agent*: 100 mg/m² once q 4 weeks. *In combination with doxorubicin hydrochloride,* cisplatin: 50 mg/m² once q 3 weeks (on day 1); doxorubicin hydrochloride: 50 mg/m² once q 3 weeks (on day 1). The drugs are given sequentially. *Advanced bladder cancer:* 50–70 mg/m² once q 3–4 weeks.

Note: Repeat courses should not be administered until (1) serum creatinine is below 1.5 mg/100 ml and/or the BUN is below 25 mg/100 ml; (2) platelets are equal to or greater than 100,000/mm³ and white blood cells are equal to or greater than 4,000/mm³; and (3) auditory activity is within the normal range.

Administration/Storage

1. Store unopened vials of dry powder in refrigerator at 2°–8°C to maintain stability for 2 years.
2. Reconstitute 10- and 50-mg vials with 10 or 50 ml of sterile water for injection as instructed on package insert.
3. Do not refrigerate reconstituted vials, as a precipitate will form. Reconstituted solution is stable at room temperature for 20 hr.
4. Use of a 0.45-μm filter is advised.
5. Before administration of cisplatin, hydrate patient with 1–2 liters of fluid by IV over a period of 8–12 hr.
6. Add dosage recommended from reconstituted vial to 2 liters of 5% dextrose in one-half or one-third N saline containing 37.5 gm mannitol. Infuse over a period of 6–8 hr. Furosemide is ordered by some practitioners instead of mannitol.
7. Do not use any equipment with aluminum for preparing or administering, as a black precipitate will form and loss of potency will occur.

Additional Nursing Implications

See also *Nursing Implications*, p. 210.

1. Have emergency equipment available to treat the occurrence of an anaphylactic reaction to cisplatin.
2. *Assess*
   a. for facial edema, bronchoconstriction, tachycardia, and shock.
   b. for tremors that may progress to seizures due to hypomagnesia.
   c. for tetany, confusion, or signs of hypocalcemia associated with hypomagnesia.
3. Ascertain that baseline renal tests are performed before therapy is instituted, as cisplatin may cause severe cumulative renal toxicity.
4. Hydrate well and monitor intake and output for adequate hydration and output for 24 hr after treatment. Report oliguria.
5. Anticipate that additional doses of cisplatin will not be administered until the patient's renal function has returned to baseline value.
6. Schedule patient for audiometry before initiating therapy and before administering subsequent doses to ascertain that patient's hearing has not been affected.
7. Be alert to complaints of ringing in ears, difficulty in hearing, edema of lower extremities, and decreased urination.

ETOPOSIDE (VP-16-213)   Vepesid (Rx)

Classification   Antineoplastic, miscellaneous.

Action/Kinetics   Etoposide is a semisynthetic derivative of podophyllotoxin. Etoposide acts as a mitotic inhibitor at the G_2 portion of the cell cycle to inhibit DNA synthesis. **t½: Adult,** 7 hr; **children,** approximately 5.7 hr. **Effective plasma levels:** 0.3–10 μg/ml.

Uses   With combination therapy to treat refractory testicular tumors.

Contraindications   Safety and efficacy in children have not been established.

Additional Untoward Reactions   Anaphylactic-type reactions, hypotension, peripheral neuropathy, somnolence.

Dosage   **IV:** 50–100 mg/m^2/day on days 1–5 or 100 mg/m^2/day on days 1, 3, and 5, every 3 weeks. Used in combination with other agents.

Administration
1. Slow IV infusion over 30–60 min will decrease the chance of hypotension.
2. The drug should be diluted with either 5% dextrose or 0.9% sodium chloride injection for a final concentration of 0.2 or 0.4 mg/ml.

Additional Nursing Implications
See also Nursing Implications, p. 210.
1. Be prepared for anaphylactic reaction by having corticosteroids, pressor agents, antihistamines, and plasma expanders readily available.
2. Be sure reports of baseline hemoglobin and white cell count with differential are available before drug is administered.
3. Monitor for signs of infection and bleeding, which are more likely to occur with this drug than with most alkylating agents.
4. Record blood pressure at least twice a day, and note any significant drop in reading.
5. Report tingling, numbness, and other signs of peripheral neuropathy.
6. Be aware that patient may feel fatigued and be sleepy during and after drug administration. Schedule nursing activities accordingly.

PROCARBAZINE HYDROCHLORIDE   Matulane, N-Methylhydrazine, MIH, Natulan* (Abbreviation: PCB) (Rx)

Classification   Antineoplastic, miscellaneous.

Action/Kinetics   Inhibits synthesis of protein, RNA, and DNA, possibly because of autooxidation (production of hydrogen peroxide). Well absorbed from GI tract. Drug equilibrates between plasma and CSF. Twenty-five to 40% eliminated in urine, mostly as metabolites, after 24 hr. Procarbazine is mostly used in combination with other drugs (MOPP therapy).

Use   As an adjunct in Hodgkin's disease.

Additional Contraindications   Hypersensitivity to drug. Depressed bone marrow. Low white and red blood cell or platelet count.

Additional Untoward Reactions   *GI:* Dysphagia, constipation or diarrhea. *CNS:* Psychosis, manic reactions, insomnia, nightmares, foot drop, decreased reflexes, tremors, coma, delirium, convulsions. *Dermatologic:* Hyperpigmentation, photosensitivity. *Miscellaneous:* Petechiae, purpura, arthralgia.

Drug Interactions

Interactant	Interaction
Alcohol	Antabuse-like reaction
Antihistamines	Additive CNS depression
Antihypertensive drugs	Additive CNS depression
Barbiturates	Additive CNS depression
Guanethidine	Excitation and hypertension
Hypoglycemic agents, oral	↑ Hypoglycemic effect
Insulin	↑ Hypoglycemic effect
Levodopa	Excitation and hypertension
Monoamine oxidase inhibitors	Possibility of hypertensive crisis
Methyldopa	Excitation and hypertension
Narcotics	Additive CNS depression
Phenothiazines	Additive CNS depression; also, possibility of hypertensive crisis
Reserpine	Excitation and hypertension
Sympathomimetics	Possibility of hypertensive crisis
Tricyclic antidepressants	Possibility of hypertensive crisis
Tyramine-containing foods	Possibility of hypertensive crisis

Dosage   **PO. Adults**: 2–4 mg/kg daily for first week; **then**, 4–6 mg/kg/day until leukocyte count falls below 4,000/mm³ or platelets fall below 100,000/mm³. If toxic symptoms appear, discontinue drug and resume treatment at 1–2 mg/kg/day; **maintenance**: 1–2 mg/kg/day. **Children**: *highly individualized*, 50 mg/day for first week; then 100 mg/m² (to nearest 50 mg) until maximum response obtained.

Additional Nursing Implications

See also *Nursing Implications*, p. 210.

1. Assess patient closely and alert family to observe and report untoward CNS reactions, which may necessitate withdrawal of the drug as noted in untoward reactions.
2. Instruct patients on procarbazine therapy not to drink alcohol, as an Antabuse-type reaction may occur.
3. Advise the patient not to take any other medication before consulting with physician, as procarbazine has monoamine oxidase inhibitory activity. This would contraindicate the use of sympathomimetic drugs and foods that have a high tyramine content during therapy and for 2 weeks after discontinuing therapy.
4. Teach diabetic patient that procarbazine increases effect of insulin and oral hypoglycemics. Hypoglycemic symptoms should be reported to doctor because adjustment of antidiabetic medication may be necessary.
5. Teach patient to avoid exposure to sun or to ultraviolet rays, as a photosensitive skin reaction may occur.

VINBLASTINE SULFATE   Velban, Velbe* (Abbreviation: VBL) (Rx)

Classification   Antineoplastic, plant alkaloid.

Action/Kinetics   Alkaloid, isolated from the periwinkle plant, is believed to inhibit mitosis (M phase in cell cycle). Rapidly cleared from tissue. Almost completely metabolized in the liver after IV administration. Metabolites are excreted in the bile. No cross-resistance with vincristine.

Uses   Palliative treatment of Hodgkin's disease, lymphocytic lymphoma, mycosis fungoides, advanced carcinoma of testis, histiocytic lymphoma, Kaposi's sarcoma, Letterer-Siwe disease. Less responsive are choriocarcinoma resistant to other agents, carcinoma of the breast. Usually administered in combination with other drugs.

Additional Untoward Reactions   Toxicity is dose related and more pronounced in patients over age 65 or in those suffering from cachexia (profound general ill health) or skin ulceration. *GI:* Ileus, rectal bleeding, hemorrhagic enterocolitis, vesiculation of the mouth, bleeding from a former ulcer. *Dermatologic:* Total epilation, skin vesiculation. *Neurologic:* Paresthesias, neuritis, mental depression, loss of deep tendon reflexes, seizures. Extravasation may result in phlebitis and cellulitis with sloughing.

Drug Interactions

Interactant	Interaction
Bleomycin sulfate	Combination of bleomycin and vinblastine may produce signs of Raynaud's disease in patients with testicular cancer
Glutamic acid	Inhibits effect of vinblastine
Tryptophan	Inhibits effect of vinblastine

Dosage   **IV**, *individualized, using WBC as guide*. Vinblastine is administered once every 7 days. **Adults: initial**, 3.7 mg/m^2 ; **then**, after 7 days, graded doses of 5.5, 7.4, 9.25, and 11.1 mg/m^2 at intervals of 7 days (maximum dose should not exceed 18.5 mg/m^2). **Children: initial**, 2.5 mg/m^2; **then**, after 7 days, graded doses of 3.75, 5.0, 6.25, and 7.5 mg/m^2 at intervals of 7 days (maximum dose should not exceed 12.5 mg/m^2). **Maintenance** doses are calculated based on WBC—at least 4,000/mm^3.

Administration/Storage

1. Dilute vinblastine with 10 ml of sodium chloride injection.
2. Inject into flowing infusion or directly into vein.
3. If extravasation occurs, move infusion to other vein. Treat affected area with injection of hyaluronidase and application of moderate heat so as to decrease local reaction.
4. Remainder of solution may be stored in refrigerator for 30 days.
5. If the drug gets into the eye, wash eye thoroughly with water immediately to prevent irritation and ulceration.

Additional Nursing Implication

See also *Nursing Implications*, p. 210.

Assess patient for cyanosis and pallor of extremities and for signs of Raynaud's disease if patient is also receiving bleomycin.

VINCRISTINE SULFATE   Oncovin (Abbreviation: VCR) (Rx)

Classification   Antineoplastic, plant alkaloid.

Action/Kinetics   See *Vinblastine Sulfate*, p. 244. When combined with corticosteroids, it is currently the drug of choice for childhood leukemia. Less bone marrow depression than with other vinca alkaloids. No cross-resistance with vinblastine. Frequently used in combination therapy.

Uses   Acute leukemia in children. Hodgkin's disease, Wilms' tumor, neuroblastoma, lymphosarcoma, rhabdomyosarcoma, reticulum cell sarcoma. *Investigational:* Idiopathic thrombocytopenic purpura.

Additional Untoward Reactions   *Neurologic:* Paresthesias, depression of deep tendon reflexes, footdrop, seizures, difficulties in gait. *GI:* Intestinal necrosis or perforation. Constipation, paralytic ileus. *Renal:* Inappropriate antidiuretic hormone secretion (polyuria or dysuria). *Ophthalmic:* Blindness, ptosis, diplopia, photophobia.

Drug Interactions

Interactant	Interaction
Glutamic acid	Inhibits effect of vincristine
Methotrexate	Combination may cause hypotension

Dosage   IV (direct, infusion), *individualized with extreme care as overdose can be fatal*. **Adults: usual, initial,** 1.4 mg/m^2 1 time a week; **children**: 2 mg/m^2 1 time a week. *For hepatic insufficiency:* if serum bilirubin is 1.5–3, administer 50% of the dose; if serum bilirubin is more than 3.1 or SGOT is more than 180, dose should be omitted.

Administration/Storage
1. Dissolve powder in sterile water or isotonic saline injection to a concentration ranging from 0.01 mg to 1 mg/ml. Medication is injected either directly into a vein or into the tubing of a flowing IV infusion over a period of 1 min.
2. Store in refrigerator. Dry powder is stable for 6 months. Solutions are stable for 2 weeks under refrigeration. Protect drug from exposure to light.
3. If extravasation occurs, move infusion to another vein. Treat affected area with injection of hyaluronidase and application of moderate heat so as to decrease local reaction.

Additional Nursing Implications
See also *Nursing Implications*, p. 210.

1. Assess early signs and symptoms of neuromuscular side effects, such as sensory impairment and paresthesia, before neuritic pain and motor difficulties are apparent, as neuromuscular manifestations are irreversible.
2. Prevent constipation by encouraging fluids and high-fiber diet.
3. Assess for absence of bowel sounds indicative of paralytic ileus, which requires symptomatic care as well as temporary discontinuance of vincristine.
4. Be prepared to relieve high colon impaction caused by vincristine with laxatives and high enemas.

HORMONAL AND ANTIHORMONAL ANTINEOPLASTIC AGENTS

The growth of cancers affecting sex organs or sex glands—notably the breasts, uterus, prostate, and testes—seems to be enhanced by the presence of the hormone normally controlling the function of these tissues. Administration of an antihormone or a different hormone, which alters the hormonal milieu by competing for hormone receptors, seems to inhibit neoplastic growth. Hormones are usually not used as primarily chemotherapeutic agents. Estrogens may also exacerbate certain tumors.

Mitotane is a drug included with these antineoplastic agents. It is not a hormone as such, but suppresses, by a yet unknown mechanism, the production of adrenocortical hormones by the adrenal cortex and is useful in the treatment of inoperable cancer of the adrenals.

Additional Nursing Implications

See *Nursing Implications* for *Antineoplastic Agents*, p. 210.

1. Assess for insomnia, lethargy, anorexia, nausea, vomiting, coma, and vascular collapse—symptoms of hypercalcemia.
2. Ascertain that serum calcium concentrations are routinely done; assess results. (Normal: 4.5–5.5 mEq/liter.) The effect of the steroid and osteolytic metastases may result in hypercalcemia.
3. Withhold drug and report high serum calcium levels.
4. Encourage high fluid intake to minimize hypercalcemia.
5. Be prepared to assist with administration of IV fluids, diuretics, adrenocorticosteroids, and phosphate supplementation for severe hypercalcemia.
6. Closely monitor patients who resume therapy after drug-induced hypercalcemia is corrected.

DIETHYLSTILBESTROL DIPHOSPHATE Honvol,* Stilphostrol (Abbreviation: DES) (Rx)

Classification Synthetic estrogen.

Action/Kinetics Synthetic estrogen, which competes with androgen receptors.

Uses Palliative treatment of prostatic cancer.

Contraindications Known or suspected breast cancer, estrogen-dependent neoplasia, active thrombophlebitis, thromboembolic disease, markedly impaired liver function. Use with caution in presence of hypercalcemia, epilepsy, migraine, asthma, cardiac and renal disease.

Untoward Reactions Thrombophlebitis, pulmonary embolism, cerebral thrombosis, neuro-ocular lesions. *GI*: Nausea, vomiting, anorexia. *CNS*: Headaches, malaise, irritability. *Skin*: Allergic rash, itching. *GU*: Gynecomastia, changes in libido. *Other*: Porphyria, backache, pain and sterile abscess at injection site, postinjection flare. See also *Estrogens*, p. 743.

Dosage **PO:** 50 mg t.i.d.; increase to 200 mg t.i.d. or more, depending on response. **IV:** Day 1, 0.5 gm; **then**, 1 gm daily for 5 or more days. **Maintenance: IV**, decrease to 0.25–0.5 gm 1 to 2 times weekly. (Maintenance dose may also be given orally.)

Administration
1. Dissolve IV dose in 300 ml normal saline or 5% dextrose.
2. Administer slowly by drip (20–30 drops/min for first 10–15 min); then adjust flow for a total administration of 1 hr.

Additional Nursing Implications
See *Nursing Implications* for *Hormonal and Antihormonal Antineoplastic Agents*, p. 246.
1. *Assess* patient with poor cardiac function for edema.
2. Anticipate that gynecomastia in men may be prevented with low doses of radiation before therapy with diethylstilbestrol is initiated.
3. *Teach patient and/or family*
   a. to report nausea, vomiting, abdominal pain, and painful swelling of breasts to doctor.
   b. that solid foods often relieve nausea.
   c. to be alert for increased complications and/or edema in patients with poor cardiac function.

DROMOSTANOLONE PROPIONATE   Drolban (Rx)

Classification   Androgen.

Action/Kinetics   Synthetic steroid related to testosterone. May protect cell from action of progesterone.

Uses   Palliative treatment of inoperable, advanced, or disseminated mammary cancer in postmenopausal or ovariectomized women.

Contraindications   Breast cancer in men, premenopausal women.

Additional Untoward Reactions   Mild virilization, hypercalcemia, edema, increased libido. Local irritation at injection site. See also *Androgens*, p. 771.

Drug Interactions   Dromostanolone may ↑ effect of oral anticoagulants.

Dosage   IM: 100 mg 3 times/week. Other treatment should be instituted if the disease *progresses* during the first 6 to 8 weeks of therapy.

Administration   Do not refrigerate.

Nursing Implications
See *Nursing Implications*, p. 246.

ESTRAMUSTINE PHOSPHATE SODIUM   Emcyt (Rx)

Classification   Hormonal agent, alkylating agent.

Action/Kinetics   Estramustine is a water-soluble drug that combines estradiol and a nitrogen mustard. Chronic estramustine administration results in plasma levels and effects of estradiol similar to those of conventional estradiol therapy. It is well absorbed from the GI tract and dephosphorylated before reaching the general circulation.

Uses Palliative treatment of metastatic and/or progressive prostatic carcinoma.

Contraindications Active thrombophlebitis or thromboembolic disease unless the tumor mass is causing the thromboembolic disorder. Use with caution in presence of cerebral vascular disease, coronary artery disease, diabetes, hypertension, congestive heart failure, impaired liver or kidney function, metabolic bone diseases associated with hypercalcemia.

Additional Untoward Reactions *Cardiovascular:* Myocardial infarction, cardiovascular accident, thrombosis, congestive heart failure, increased blood pressure, thrombophlebitis, leg cramps, edema. *Respiratory:* Pulmonary embolism, dyspnea, upper respiratory discharge, hoarseness. *GI:* Flatulence, burning sensation of throat, thirst. *Dermatologic:* Easy bruising, flushing, peeling of skin or fingertips. *Miscellaneous:* Chest pain, tearing of eyes, breast tenderness or enlargement, decreased glucose tolerance.

Laboratory Test Interferences ↑ Bilirubin, SGOT, LDH.

Dosage **PO:** 14 mg/kg/day in 3–4 divided doses (range: 10–16 mg/kg/day). Treat for 30–90 days before assessing beneficial effects; continue therapy as long as the drug is effective.

Administration/Storage Capsules should be stored in the refrigerator although they may be at room temperature for 1–2 days without affecting potency.

Additional Nursing Implications

See also *Nursing Implications*, p. 246.

1. *Assess*
   a. diabetic patients for hyperglycemia because glucose tolerance may be decreased.
   b. periodically for hypertension because elevated blood pressure has occurred in conjunction with therapy.
2. Explain to patient that the impotence he may have experienced due to previous estrogen therapy may be reversed. Since estramustine phosphate sodium may cause genetic mutation, contraceptive measures should be practiced to prevent teratogenesis.

MEDROXYPROGESTERONE ACETATE Depo-Provera (Rx)

Classification Progesterone. See *Progesterones*, p. 749.

Action/Kinetics Prevents stimulation of endometrium by pituitary gonadotropins.

Use Adjunct in palliative treatment of inoperable, recurrent, or metastatic endometrial or renal carcinoma.

Dosage **IM only: initial**, 400–1,000 mg/week; **maintenance**: 400 mg/month. Medroxyprogesterone is not intended to be the primary therapy.

Nursing Implications

See *Nursing Implications* for *Hormonal and Antihormonal Antineoplastic Agents*, p. 246; also for *Progestins*, p. 749 and *Medroxyprogesterone Acetate*, p. 754.

MEGESTROL ACETATE   Megace, Pallace (Rx)

Classification   Synthetic progestin.

Action/Kinetics   The antineoplastic activity is due to suppression of gonadotropins (antiluteinizing effect). For general information on *Progestins*, see *Hormones, Progestins*, p. 749.

Drug contains tartrazine, which can cause allergic-type reactions, including asthma, often occurring in patients sensitive to aspirin.

Uses   Palliative treatment of endometrial or breast cancer. Should not be used as sole treatment.

Additional Contraindications   Not to be used for diagnosis of pregnancy.

Untoward Reactions   *Few*: Abdominal pain, headache, nausea, vomiting, breast tenderness, carpal tunnel syndrome (soreness, weakness, and tenderness of muscles of thumbs), deep vein thrombosis, alopecia.

Dosage   **PO**. *Breast cancer*: 40 mg q.i.d. *Endometrial cancer*: 40–320 mg/day in divided doses. To determine efficacy, treatment should be continued for at least 2 months.

Nursing Implications

See *Nursing Implications* for *Hormonal and Antihormonal Antineoplastic Agents*, p. 246 and *Progestins*, p. 750.

MITOTANE   Lysodren, O', P'-DDD (Abbreviation: OP' DDD) (Rx)

Classification   Antihormone.

Action/Kinetics   Related to DDT; suppresses activity of adrenal cortex. About 40% of drug absorbed from GI tract, detectable in serum for long periods of time (6–9 weeks after administration). Drug, however, mostly stored in adipose tissue.

Steroid replacement therapy may have to be instituted (i.e., increased) to correct adrenal insufficiency. Therapy is continued as long as drug seems effective. Beneficial results might not become apparent until after 3 months of therapy.

Use   Inoperable cancer of the adrenal cortex.

Contraindications   Hypersensitivity to drug. Discontinue temporarily after shock or severe trauma. Use with caution in the presence of liver disease other than metastatic lesions. Long-term usage may cause brain damage and functional impairment.

Additional Untoward Reactions   Adrenal insufficiency. *CNS:* Sedation, vertigo, lethargy. *Ophthalmic:* Blurring, diplopia, retinopathy, opacity of lens. *Renal:* Hemorrhagic cystitis, hematuria, proteinuria. *Cardiovascular:* Flushing, orthostatic hypotension, hypertension. *Miscellaneous:* Hyperpyrexia.

Laboratory Test Interference   ↓ PBI and urinary 17-hydroxycorticosteroids.

Dosage   **PO: initial**, 9–10 gm/day in 3 to 4 equally divided doses. Adjust dosage upward or downward according to severity of side effects or lack thereof. **Usual maintenance**: 8–10 gm/day. **Range**: 2–19 gm/day.

Administration

1. Institute treatment in hospital until stable dosage schedule is achieved.
2. Treatment should be continued for 3 months to determine beneficial effects.

Additional Nursing Implications

See also *Nursing Implications*, p. 246.

1. Assess for symptoms of adrenal insufficiency, such as weakness, increased fatigue, lethargy, and GI symptomatology.
2. Assess for brain damage by participating in behavioral and neurologic assessments of patient.
3. Withhold medication and report to doctor if shock or severe trauma occurs because of drug-induced suppression of adrenal function.
4. To counteract shock or trauma, be prepared to administer steroid medications in high doses, because depressed adrenals may not produce sufficient steroids.
5. Stress importance of wearing Medic Alert identification to patients on mitotane in case of trauma or shock.

POLYESTRADIOL PHOSPHATE   Estradurin (Rx)

Classification   Estrogen

Action/Kinetics   Estradiol is slowly split off from the parent compound thus providing continuous levels for long periods of time. The estradiol combines with androgen receptors; 90% of dose leaves plasma in 24 hr and is stored in the reticuloendothelial system and slowly released. For general information on estrogens, see *Hormones, estrogens* p. 742.

Use   Palliation of cancer of the prostate.

Dosage   IM: 40–80 mg q 2 to 4 weeks. Response should be noted in approximately 3 months and drug continued until the disease begins progressing again.

Administration/Storage

1. Add sterile diluent as directed by manufacturer. Swirl *gently* to dissolve.
2. Inject deeply IM. Painful, and may require concomitant administration of local anesthetic.
3. Stable at room temperature for 10 days. Shield from light.
4. Do not use solutions that have deposit or are cloudy.

Nursing Implications

See *Nursing Implications* for *Hormonal and Antihormonal Agents*, p. 246; see also *Nursing Implications for Estrogens*, p. 744.

TAMOXIFEN   Nolvadex (Rx)

Classification   Antiestrogen.

Action/Kinetics   Antiestrogen is believed to occupy estrogen binding sites in target tissue (breast). **Peak serum levels**: 0.06–0.14 μg/ml attained after 7–14 hr. **t½,**

biphasic: initial, 7–14 hr; distribution, 4 or more days. Objective response may be delayed 4–10 weeks with bone metastases.

Uses Palliative treatment of advanced breast cancer in postmenopausal women, especially in cases of recent positive estrogen receptor tests.

Untoward Reactions Hot flashes, nausea, vomiting (25%). Also, vaginal bleeding and discharge, menstrual irregularities, skin rash. Rarely, hypercalcemia, peripheral edema, distaste for food, pruritus vulvae, depression, dizziness, lightheadedness, headaches, increased bone and tumor pain, anorexia, pulmonary embolism, mild to moderate thrombocytopenia, and leukopenia. Ophthalmologic effects.

Laboratory Test Interference ↑ Serum calcium (transient).

Dosage **PO**: 10–20 mg b.i.d. (AM and PM).

Additional Nursing Implications
See also *Nursing Implications*, p. 246.

1. Advise patient to report side effects to doctor, because reduction in dosage may be indicated.
2. Explain to patient experiencing increased bone and lumbar pain and local disease flares that these symptoms may be associated with a good response to medication.
3. Be certain that patient with increased pain has adequate orders for analgesics and provide them as needed.
4. Advise patients to have regular ophthalmologic examinations if doses of drug are much higher than recommended for antihormonal antineoplastic agent.

TESTOLACTONE Teslac (Rx)

Classification Androgen.

Action/Kinetics Synthetic steroid related to testosterone. May protect cell from action of progesterone. Does not cause virilization.

Uses Palliative treatment of advanced or disseminated mammary cancer in postmenopausal women or in premenopausal ovariectomized patients.

Additional Contraindication Breast cancer in men; premenopausal women with intact ovaries.

Additional Untoward Reactions Inflammation and irritation at injection site; increases BP during parenteral administration. Hypercalcemia. Numbness or tingling of fingers, toes, face. See also *Androgens*, p. 770.

Drug Interactions Testolactone may ↑ effect of oral anticoagulants.

Dosage **PO**: 250 mg q.i.d. **IM**: 100 mg 3 times weekly. Therapy usually should be continued for 3 months.

Additional Nursing Implications
See also *Nursing Implications*, p. 246.
Anticipate a reduction in dose of anticoagulants if on concomitant therapy.

RADIOACTIVE ISOTOPES

Two radioactive isotopes are used as antineoplastic agents. The first, sodium iodine ^{131}I, concentrates in the thyroid and is used for the treatment of cancer of the thyroid. The other, radioactive phosphorus, concentrates in rapidly proliferating cells, preferentially destroying neoplastic cells. Refer to other sources for more detailed information on use of radioactive agents.

Additional Nursing Implications
See also *Nursing Implications*, p. 210.

1. For radiation protection, observe the procedure used in the hospital in which the medication is administered.
2. Provide supportive care to patient for malaise and abdominal cramping caused by radiation.

CHROMIC PHOSPHATE ^{32}P   Phosphocol ^{32}P (Rx)

Classification   Radioactive isotope.

Action/Kinetics   The particles emitted by the radioactive chromic phosphate impede the growth of neoplastic cells. t½: 495 hr.

Uses   Treatment of peritoneal or pleural effusions caused by metastatic disease (intracavitary) or localized disease (interstitial).

Additional Contraindications   Ulcerative tumors. Exposed cavities.

Additional Untoward Reactions   Transitory radiation sickness, pleuritis, peritonitis, bone marrow depression, nausea and abdominal cramping. Radiation damage when injected accidentally interstitially or into a loculation (small space).

Dosage   For average (70 kg) patient:

Intraperitoneal instillation	10–20 mCi (millicurie)
Intrapleural instillation	6–12 mCi
Interstitial use	0.1–0.5 mCi/gram of tumor

Administration
1. Administered by physician.
2. Measure patient's dose using suitable radioactive calibration system immediately before administration.

SODIUM IODIDE ^{131}I   Iodotope, Sodium Iodide ^{131}I

See *Thyroid* and *Antithyroid Drugs*, p. 699

SODIUM PHOSPHATE ^{32}P

Classification   Radioactive isotope.

Action/Kinetics The radioactive phosphorus of the drug concentrates in rapidly proliferating tissue. Upon decay, it emits beta particles. t½: 14.3 days. Initially the radioactivity decreases rapidly (25–50% in 4–6 days), then much more slowly (more than 1% a day). Remaining radioactivity concentrates in osseous tissue.

Uses Polycythemia vera, chronic myelocytic leukemia, and chronic lymphocytic leukemia. Palliative treatment of multiple skeletal metastases.

Additional Contraindications Pregnancy, nursing mothers, children younger than 18 years of age, or acute episodes of leukemia. Polycythemia vera in patients with leukocyte count of less than 5,000/mm³, platelet count of less than 150,000/mm³, or reticulocyte count of less than 0.2%. Chronic myelocytic leukemia with a leukocyte count of less than 20,000/mm³. Skeletal metastases with a leukocyte count of less than 5,000/mm³ or platelet count of less than 100,000/mm³. Sequential therapy with a chemotherapeutic agent.

Additional Untoward Reaction Radiation sickness (rare).

Dosage **PO, IV.** *Polycythemia vera:* 1–8 mCi (usually **IV**); doses may be repeated. *Leukemias:* 6–15 mCi (with hormone manipulation).

Administration/Storage
1. Store at room temperature in containers suitable for absorption of radiation.
2. Solution and container may darken, but this does not affect efficacy.
3. Note expiration date—should be 2 months after date of standardization.
4. Have patient fast for 2 hr before and 6 hr after administration of drug to minimize the amount of unabsorbed radioactive material.
5. Avoid using milk and milk products, iron, bismuth, and soft drinks for patients on sodium phosphate ³²P.

Additional Nursing Implications
See *Nursing Implications* for *Radioactive Isotopes*, page 252.
For radiation protection, observe the procedure of the hospital in which medication is administered.

Part Four

DRUGS AFFECTING BLOOD FORMATION AND COAGULATION

Chapter Nineteen

ANTIANEMIC DRUGS

General Statement   Anemia refers to the many clinical conditions in which there is a deficiency in the number of red blood cells (RBCs) or in the hemoglobin level within those cells. Hemoglobin is a complex substance consisting of a large protein (globin) and an iron-containing chemical referred to as heme. The hemoglobin is contained inside the red cells. Its function is to combine with oxygen in the lungs and transport it to all tissues of the body, where it is exchanged for carbon dioxide (which is transported back to the lungs).

A lack of either RBCs or hemoglobin may result in an inadequate supply of oxygen to various tissues. The average life span of a RBC is 120 days; thus, new ones have to be constantly formed. They are produced in the bone marrow, with both vitamin B_{12} and folic acid playing an important role in their formation. In addition, a sufficient amount of iron is necessary for the formation and maturation of RBCs. This iron is supplied in a normal diet and also is salvaged from old RBCs.

There are many types of anemia. However, the two main categories are (1) iron deficiency anemias, resulting from greater than normal loss or destruction of blood cells, and (2) megaloblastic anemias, resulting from deficient production of blood cells. Iron deficiency anemia can result from hemorrhage or blood loss; the bone marrow is unable to replace the quantity of red cells lost even when working at maximum capacity (due to iron-deficient diet or failure to absorb iron from the GI tract). The RBCs in iron deficiency anemias (also called microcytic or hypochromic anemias) contain too little hemoglobin. When examined under the microscope, they are paler and sometimes smaller than normal. The cause of the iron deficiency must be determined before therapy is started.

Therapy consists of administering compounds containing iron so as to increase the body's supplies. Such drugs are discussed in this chapter (Table 6).

Megaloblastic anemias may result from insufficient supplies of the necessary vitamins and minerals needed by the bone marrow to manufacture blood cells. Pernicious anemia, for example, results from inadequate vitamin B_{12}. The RBCs characteristic of the megaloblastic anemias are enlarged and particularly rich in hemoglobin. However, the blood contains fewer mature RBCs than normal and usually contains a relatively higher number of immature red cells (megaloblasts) that have been prematurely released from the bone marrow.

IRON PREPARATIONS   These agents are usually a complex of iron and another substance and are normally taken by mouth. The amount absorbed from the GI tract depends on the dose administered; therefore the largest dose that can be tolerated without causing side effects is given. Under certain conditions, iron compounds must be given parenterally, particularly (1) when there is some disorder limiting the amount of drug absorbed from the intestine, or (2) when the patient is unable to tolerate oral iron.

Iron preparations are only effective in the treatment of anemias specifically resulting from iron deficiency. Blood loss is almost always the only cause of iron deficiency in adult males and postmenopausal females. The daily iron requirement is increased by growth and pregnancy, and iron deficiency, therefore, is particularly common in infants and young children on diets low in iron. Pregnant women and women with heavy menstrual blood loss may also be deficient in iron.

Iron is available for therapy in two forms: bivalent and trivalent. Bivalent (ferrous) iron salts are administered more often than trivalent (ferric) salts because they are less astringent and less irritating than ferric salts and are better absorbed.

Iron preparations are particularly suitable for the treatment of anemias in infants and children, in blood donors, during pregnancy, and in patients with chronic blood loss. Optimum therapeutic responses are usually noted in 2 to 4 weeks of treatment.

The RDA for iron is 90–300 mg daily.

Action/Kinetics   Iron is an essential mineral normally supplied in the diet. Iron salts and other preparations supply additional iron to meet the needs of the patient. Iron is absorbed from GI tract, transported by transferrin and incorporated into hemoglobin. Absorption kinetics depend on the iron salt ingested. Under normal circumstances iron is very well conserved by the body.

TABLE 6   ANTIANEMICS

Drug	Dosage	Remarks
Ferrous fumarate (Feostat, Feco-T, Fersamyl,* Fumasorb, Fumerin, Hemacyte, Ircon, Neo-Fer,* Neo-Fer-50,* Novofumar,* Palafer,* Palmiron) OTC	*Tablets, chewable tablets, extended release, suspension.* **PO. Adults:** 100–400 mg (equivalent to 33–133 mg elemental iron) daily in divided doses. **Pediatric, 6–12 years:** 100–300 mg (33–100 mg elemental iron) daily in divided doses (use suspension); **pediatric, 1–5 years: initial,** equivalent of 15 mg elemental iron daily; **then,** increase to maximum of 45 mg elemental iron daily in divided doses; **infants:** 10–20 mg elemental iron daily in divided doses.	Better tolerated than ferrous gluconate or sulfate; 33% elemental iron.
Ferrous gluconate (Apo-Ferrous Gluconate,* Fergon, Ferralet, Fertinic,* Novoferrogluc,* Simron) OTC	*Capsules, elixir, tablets,* **PO:** 320–640 mg (equivalent to 38–77 mg elemental iron) t.i.d.; **Infants and children less than 6 years:** 120–300 mg daily; **children 6–12 years:** 100–300 mg t.i.d.	Particularly indicated for patients who cannot tolerate ferrous sulfate because of gastric irritation; 11.6% elemental iron.
Ferrous sulfate (Apo-Ferrous Sulfate,* Feosol, Fero-Grad,* Fero-Grad-500,* Fero-Gradumet, Fer-in-Sol, Fer-Iron, Ferospace, Fersofor,* Hematinic, Mol-Iron, Novoferrosulfa,* PMS Ferrous Sulfate,* Slow-Fe*) OTC	**PO; Adults:** 300–1,200 mg (equivalent to 60–240 mg elemental iron) daily in divided doses; **children less than 6 years:** 15–45 mg elemental iron daily in divided doses using the pediatric preparation; **children, 6–12 years:** 24–120 mg elemental iron daily in divided doses using the elixir or syrup; **infants:** 10–25 mg elemental iron daily using divided doses of the pediatric preparation. *Prophylaxis for premature or poorly developed infants:* 1–2 mg/kg daily. *Pregnancy, lactation:* 10–20 mg elemental iron daily.	Least expensive, most effective iron salt for oral therapy; 20% elemental iron.
Ferrous sulfate exiccated (Feosol, Fer-in-Sol, Ferralyn, Iromal, Slow-Fe) OTC		Is more stable in air; contains 30% elemental iron.

TABLE 6   (*Continued*)

Drug	Dosage	Remarks
Iron dextran injection (Imferon) Rx See drug entry in text, p. 260.	IM use not recommended. **IV; Adults and children:** 100 mg of undiluted drug daily at a rate not to exceed 50 mg/min. Larger doses may be given as an infusion after being diluted with 500–1,000 ml of saline. Rate of infusion: 1 liter over 4–6 hr.	A test dose of 1–2 drops followed by 25 mg in 15 min should be administered before initiation of additional therapy. Used mainly for patients intolerant to oral iron.
Polysaccharide-Iron Complex (Hytinic, Niferex, Nu-Iron)	*Tablets, capsules, elixir,* **PO:** 100—300 mg; **children 6–12 years:** 100 mg/day; **2–6 years:** 50 mg/day; **under 2 years:** 25 mg.	Easily absorbable iron-polysaccharide complex with relatively low toxicity and little GI disturbance; does not stain teeth; tablets contain 50–150 mg elemental iron, elixir 100 mg elemental iron/5cc.
Soy Protein-Iron Complex (Fe-Plus) OTC	**PO:** 50 mg t.i.d.	Easily absorbably iron-soy protein complex; take with meals; swallow with water

Uses   Prophylaxis and treatment of iron deficiency anemia.

Contraindications   Patients with hemosiderosis, hemachromatosis, peptic ulcer, regional enteritis, and ulcerative colitis. Hemolytic anemia, pyridoxine-responsive anemia, and cirrhosis of the liver.

Drug Interactions

Interactant	Interaction
Allopurinol	May ↑ hepatic iron levels
Antacids, oral	↓ Effect of iron preparations due to ↓ absorption from GI tract
Chloramphenicol	Chloramphenicol ↓ iron clearance from plasma and ↓ iron uptake into red blood cells
Cholestyramine	↓ Effect of iron preparations due to ↓ absorption from GI tract
Pancreatic extracts	↓ Effect of iron preparations due to ↓ absorption from GI tract
Penicillamine	↓ Effect of penicillamine due to ↓ absorption from GI tract
Tetracyclines	↓ Effect of tetracyclines due to ↓ absorption from GI tract
Vitamin E	Vitamin E ↓ response to iron therapy

Untoward Reactions   *GI effects:* Constipation, gastric irritation, mild nausea, abdominal cramps, and diarrhea. These effects may be minimized by administering preparations as a coated tablet. Soluble iron preparations may stain teeth.

Toxic reactions are more likely to occur after parenteral administration and include nausea and vomiting, fever, peripheral vascular collapse, and fatal anaphylactoid reactions. These symptoms may occur within 60 sec of a toxic dose. Symptoms may then disappear for 6 to 24 hr, followed by a second crisis. Symptoms including nausea and diarrhea or constipation may occur after use of oral preparations.

TREATMENT OF IRON TOXICITY   The treatment of iron intoxication is symptomatic. It concentrates on removing iron from the body and combating shock and acidosis. Vomiting should be induced immediately, followed by the administration of eggs and milk. Other measures include gastric lavage with aqueous solutions of sodium bicarbonate or sodium phosphate, followed by oral bismuth subcarbonate as a protectant and IV dextrose and sodium chloride injection to correct dehydration. Plasma, whole blood, calcium disodium edetate, deferoxamine, methionine, oxygen, and antibiotics may be ordered.

Some patients may report late manifestations 1 to 2 months after toxic overdosage. These late manifestations include GI distress caused by necrotic alterations of the gastric or intestinal mucosa. Residual effects may also include pyloric stenosis, fibrosis of the liver, and dilatation of the right side of the heart with pulmonary congestion and hemorrhage.

Laboratory Test Interference   Iron-containing drugs may affect electrolyte balance determinations.

Dosage   **PO: usual,** 90–300 mg elemental iron per day. Duration of therapy: 2–4 months longer than the time anemia is reversed, usually 6 or more months. For specific agents, see Table 6, p. 257.

Administration

1. Administer iron preparations with meals to reduce gastric irritation.
2. Administer with citrus juice to enhance absorption of iron.
3. Do not administer the drug with milk or an antacid as these will interfere with the absorption of iron (except for ferrous lactate, which may be given with milk).
4. Administer liquid preparations well diluted with water or fruit juice through a straw to prevent staining the teeth. To infants and young children, administer liquid preparation with a dropper. Deposit liquid well back against the cheek.

Nursing Implications

1. Encourage anyone with symptoms of anemia to seek medical supervision rather than medicating himself with iron.
2. Be prepared to assist with treatment of poisoning, as discussed under *Untoward Reactions.*
3. Monitor vital signs of patients suffering from iron poisoning for at least 48 hr, particularly, since a second crisis may occur within 12 to 48 hr.
4. *Teach patient and/or family*
   a. possible untoward effects, such as constipation, gastric irritation with abdominal cramps, and diarrhea. Encourage patient to report these symptoms since they can be relieved by a change in medication, dosage, or time of administration.
   b. to eat a nutritious diet. Stress the intake of foods high in iron, such as liver, raisins, apricots, and green vegetables.
   c. to keep iron preparations out of the reach of children.

IRON DEXTRAN INJECTION   Feostat, Feronim, Hematran, Hydextran, I.D.-50, Imferon, Irodex, K-Feron, Nor-Feran, Proferdex, Rocyte (Rx)

Classification   Iron preparation, parenteral.

General Statement   Parenteral iron is indicated only when the patient cannot tolerate oral iron or is suffering from very severe anemia (hemoglobin less than 7.5 gm/100 ml).

Iron dextran is absorbed slowly from the injection site, that is, 1% to 15% is absorbed within 2 hours; 60% to 68% within several days; and the remainder over a period of up to 6 months.

Iron dextran usually is given IM but can be given IV (this route is not recommended). Also, iron dextran injection can cause fatal anaphylactoid reactions; therefore, a small test dose is recommended. Iron dextran should not be given concurrently with oral iron and should be discontinued unless the hemoglobin level increases by at least 2 gm/100 ml in 3 weeks.

Additional Contraindications   Pernicious anemia, acute leukemia in the absence of iron depletion by blood loss, anemia associated with chronic leukemia or bone marrow depression, and other anemias not resulting from iron deficiency. Hypersensitivity to drug. Siderosis, hemochromatosis, or severe renal or hepatic failure.

Additional Untoward Reactions   Headache, fever, malaise, nausea, vomiting, aching of lower limbs, arthralgia, transient loss of taste, lymphadenopathy, local pain, persistent staining of skin at site of injection, mild urticaria, severe anaphylactic reactions, or transient leukocytosis.

SIDE EFFECTS AFTER IV INJECTION   Local phlebitis, dyspnea, shock, cyanosis, urticaria, edema of the face, photophobia, joint pain, and thrombosis in veins remote from the site of infusion.

Dosage   **Test dose prior to therapeutic regimen: IM, IV:** 25 mg (0.5 ml); observe patient for at least 1 hr. *Iron deficiency anemia:* IM: Use dosage formula. **Maximum daily doses of iron: Adults over 50 kg:** 250 mg; **adults and children 9–50 kg:** 100 mg; **infants 3.5–9 kg:** 50 mg; **infants under 3.5 kg:** 25 mg. **IV:** Calculate dosage according to formula and dilute needed dose in 200–250 ml saline. If no reaction to test dose, give needed dose over 1–2 hrs.

Administration

1. Prevent staining skin by using a separate needle to withdraw medication from the container and by using the Z-track method of injection.
2. Insert the solution deeply with at least a 2-inch needle, 19–20 gauge, into the upper outer quadrant of the gluteus muscle.
3. Withdraw syringe to check that the needle is not in a blood vessel before injecting medication.
4. Injection sites should be alternated. Chart the site of injection to facilitate alternating sites.
5. Instruct the patient standing for the injection to bear weight on the leg opposite the injection site. If he is in bed, position so that patient is in a lateral position with the injection site uppermost.

Additional Nursing Implications
See also *Nursing Implications*, p. 259.

1. Anticipate that medication will be discontinued and illness further investigated if 500 mg iron daily does not cause a rise of at least 2 gm/100 ml of hemoglobin in 3 weeks.
2. Check that a small test dose is ordered before initiating therapy.
3. Do not administer iron products and tetracyclines within 2 hr of each other because iron reduces absorption of tetracycline.
4. Do not administer antacids together with iron compounds because former decreases absorption of iron.

Chapter Twenty

ANTICOAGULANTS AND HEMOSTATICS

General Statement Blood coagulation is a precise mechanism that can be broken down as follows:

1. It is initiated when an inactive precursor escapes from the damaged platelets and activates *thromboplastin*.
2. The activated thromboplastin helps convert the protein *prothrombin* into *thrombin*.

3. *Thrombin* mediates the formation of the threadlike *fibrin* —an insoluble protein—from the soluble *fibrinogen*. The latter forms a clot, trapping blood cells and platelets. Vitamin K, calcium, and various accessory factors manufactured in the liver are essential for blood coagulation.

Once formed, the blood clot is dissolved by another enzymatic chain reaction involving a substance called fibrinolysin.

Blood coagulation can be affected by a number of diseases. An excessive tendency to form blood clots is one of the main factors involved in cardiovascular disorders, and a defect in the clotting mechanism is the cause of hemophilia and related diseases.

Since several of the factors that participate in blood clotting are manufactured by the liver, severe liver disease can also affect blood clotting, as does vitamin K deficiency.

Drugs that influence blood coagulation can be divided into three classes: (1) *anticoagulants*, or drugs that prevent or slow blood coagulation; (2) *thrombolytic agents*, which increase the rate at which an existing blood clot dissolves; and (3) *hemostatics*, which prevent or stop internal bleeding. Protamine sulfate, whose sole use is to correct heparin overdosage, is listed at the end of the anticoagulant section.

The dosage of all agents discussed in this chapter must be very carefully adjusted since overdosage can have serious consequences.

ANTICOAGULANTS

General Statement   There are three major types of anticoagulants: (1) coumarin or coumarin-type drugs (bishydroxycoumarin, warfarin); (2) indandione derivatives (anisindione); and (3) heparin. The following considerations are pertinent to all types.

Anticoagulant drugs are used mainly in the management of patients with thromboembolic disease; they do not dissolve previously formed clots, but they do forestall their enlargement and prevent new clots from forming.

Some physicians also prescribe anticoagulants prophylactically. However, there is still considerable controversy about the long-term use of these agents.

Action/Kinetics   These drugs interfere with hepatic synthesis of prothrombin and related clotting factors, thus decreasing blood levels of prothrombin. **Onset**: slow, **Duration**: 1–6 days (see individual agents). t½: long. As a rule, the indandiones have a faster onset and a shorter t½ than is found with coumarins. Therapy is aimed at keeping prothrombin time at 10–30% of normal—determined before and after start of therapy.

Uses   Venous thrombosis, pulmonary embolism, acute coronary occlusions with myocardial infarctions, and strokes caused by emboli or cerebral thrombi.

Prophylactically for rheumatic heart disease, atrial fibrillation, traumatic injuries of blood vessels, vascular surgery, major abdominal, thoracic, and pelvic surgery, prevention of strokes in patients with transient attacks of cerebral ischemia, or other signs of impending stroke.

Contraindications   Patients with possible defects in the clotting mechanism (hemophilia) or with frail or weakened blood vessels, peptic ulcer, chronic ulcerations of the GI tract, hepatic and renal dysfunction, subacute bacterial endocarditis, or severe hypertension. Also after neurosurgery or recent surgery of the eye, spinal cord, or brain, or in the presence of drainage tubes in any orifice. Alcoholism.

Coumarin and Indandione-type Anticoagulants

Uses Prophylaxis and treatment of intravascular clotting, postoperative thrombophlebitis, pulmonary embolism, acute embolic and thrombotic occlusions of the peripheral arteries, acute coronary thrombosis, and recurrent idiopathic thrombophlebitis. Atrial fibrillation with embolization. *Investigational:* Prophylaxis of recurrent myocardial infarction.

Heparin is often used concurrently during the therapeutic initiation period.

Contraindications Hemorrhagic tendencies, blood dyscrasias, ulcerative lesions of the GI tract, diverticulitis, colitis, subacute bacterial endocarditis, threatened abortion, recent operations on the eye, brain, or spinal cord, regional anesthesia and lumbar block, vitamin K deficiency, leukemia with bleeding tendencies, thrombocytopenic purpura, open wounds or ulcerations, acute nephritis, impaired hepatic or renal function, or severe hypertension.

The drugs should be used with caution in menstruating women, in pregnant women (because they may cause hypoprothrombinemia in the infant), in nursing mothers, during postpartum, and following cerebrovascular accidents.

Untoward Reactions Hemorrhagic accidents are the chief danger of anticoagulant therapy. Frequent prothrombin time determinations should be performed for patients on long-term therapy to ascertain that values remain within safe levels.

Blood in urine may be a first warning of impending hemorrhage.

ANTIDOTES Coumarin-type drugs can be counteracted by oral (100–200 mg) or IV administration (50–100 mg) of vitamin K (phytonadione).

Fresh whole blood or plasma transfusions may be required in emergencies.

Dosage PO: *individualized*. See Table 7, below.

TABLE 7 ANTICOAGULANTS

Drug	Dosage	Remarks
Anisindione (Miradon) Rx	**PO: Day 1:** 300 mg Day 2: 200 mg, Day 3: 100 mg. **Maintenance: Usual:** 25–150 mg daily; up to 250 mg daily may be required	Indandione type; long acting; **time to peak:** 2–3 days; **duration of action:** 1–3 days; t½: 3–5 days.
Bishydroxycoumarin (Dicumarol) Rx	**PO: Day 1:** 200–300 mg; then, 25–200 mg/day on subsequent days, depending on prothrombin time	Coumarin type; onset delayed. **time to peak:** 3–5 days; **duration of action:** 2–10 days; t½: 1–2 days. *Additional Nursing Implications* Explain to patient need for prothrombin times since effect of drug is cumulative and persistent.
Phenprocoumon (Liquamar) Rx	**PO: Day 1:** 21–30 mg, Day 2: 2–12 mg, Day 3: 1–4 mg. **Maintenance:** 0.75–6 mg daily	Coumarin type; **time to peak:** 2–3 days; **duration:** 7–14 days; t½: 4–9 days. Cumulative effect noticeable up to 14 days after withdrawal. Adjust dosage carefully (difficult; check prothrombin time often) in patients with uncontrolled congestive heart failure or those re-

TABLE 7   *(Continued)*

Drug	Dosage	Remarks
		ceiving large doses of salicylates, barbiturates, phenothiazines, antibiotics, corticosteroids, or corticotropin. *Additional Untoward Reaction* Diarrhea. Recovery may take up to 7 days.
Warfarin potassium (Athrombin-K) Rx Warfarin sodium (Coufarin, Coumadin sodium, Panwarfin, Warfilone,* Warnerin Sodium*) Rx	**PO:** *potassium salt;* **PO, IM, IV:** *sodium salt.* Doses are identical, regardless of salt or route. **Initial loading dose:** 40–60 mg daily. *Debilitated patients:* 20–30 mg daily. **Maintenance:** 2–10 mg daily regulated according to prothrombin time. If no loading dose, give 10–15 mg daily until desired prothrombin time is achieved.	Only coumarin-type drug suitable for parenteral administration; **time to peak:** 0.5–3 days; **duration:** 2–5 days; **t½:** 1.5–2.5 days. Response to drug more uniform than with other anticoagulants. Daily prothrombin time recommended during initial week, weekly thereafter. *Additional Contraindications* Liver or kidney disease. *Administration* After reconstitution, sodium warfarin injection may be stored for several days at 4° C. Discard solution if precipitate becomes noticeable. Store in light-resistant containers.

Drug Interactions   These drugs are responsible for more adverse drug interactions than are found with any other group. Patients on anticoagulant therapy must be monitored very carefully each time a drug is added or withdrawn.

Monitoring usually involves determination of prothrombin time. In general, a lengthened prothrombin time means potentiation of the anticoagulant. Since potentiation may mean hemorrhages, a lengthened prothrombin time warrants **reduction of the dosage of the anticoagulant**. However, the anticoagulant dosage must again be increased when the second drug is discontinued.

A shortened prothrombin time means inhibition of the anticoagulant and may require an increase in dosage.

Interactant	Interaction
Acetaminophen	Slight ↑ in hypoprothrombinemia
Alcohol, ethyl	↑ or ↓ Effect of oral anticoagulants
Allopurinol	↑ Effect of anticoagulants due to ↓ breakdown by liver
Aminoglycoside antibiotics	Potentiate pharmacologic effect of anticoagulants
Anabolic steroids	Potentiate pharmacologic effect of anticoagulants

Interactant	Interaction
Antacids, oral	↓ Effect of anticoagulants due to ↓ absorption from GI tract
Antidepressants, tricyclic	↑ Effect of anticoagulants due to ↓ breakdown by liver
Barbiturates	↓ Effect of anticoagulants due to ↑ breakdown by liver
Carbamazepine	↓ Effect of anticoagulants due to ↑ breakdown by liver
Cephalorsporins	↑ Effect of anticoagulants due to ↑ prothrombin time
Chloral hydrate	↑ Effect of anticoagulants by ↓ plasma protein binding
Chloramphenicol	↑ Effect of anticoagulant due to ↓ breakdown by liver
Cholestyramine	↓ Anticoagulant effect due to binding in and ↓ absorption from GI tract
Cimetidine	↑ Anticoagulant effect due to ↓ breakdown by liver
Clofibrate	↑ Anticoagulant effect by ↓ plasma protein binding
Colestipol	↓ Effect of anticoagulants due to ↓ absorption from GI tract
Contraceptives, oral	↓ Anticoagulant effect by ↑ activity of certain clotting factors (VII and X)
Contrast media containing idodine	↑ Effect of anticoagulants by ↑ prothrombin time
Corticosteroids, corticosterone	↓ Effect of anticoagulants by ↓ hypoprothrombinemia; also ↑ risk of GI bleeding due to ulcerogenic effect of steroids
Danazol	↑ Effect of anticoagulants
Dextrothyroxine	↑ Effect of anticoagulants
Disulfiram (Antabuse)	↑ Effect of anticoagulants by ↓ breakdown by liver
Estrogens	↓ Anticoagulant response by ↑ activity of certain clotting factors
Ethchlorvynol	↓ Effect of anticoagulants due to ↑ breakdown by liver
Glucagon	↑ Effect of anticoagulants by ↑ hypoprothrombinemia
Glutethimide	↓ Effect of anticoagulants due to ↑ breakdown by liver
Griseofulvin	↓ Effect of anticoagulants due to ↑ breakdown by liver
Haloperidol	↓ Effect of anticoagulants due to ↑ breakdown by liver
Heparin	↑ Effect by ↑ prothrombin time
Hypoglycemics, oral	↑ Effect of anticoagulants due to ↓ plasma protein binding; also, ↑ effect of sulfonylureas
Indomethacin	↑ Effect of anticoagulants by ↓ plasma protein

Interactant	Interaction
	binding; also indomethacin is ulcerogenic and may inhibit platelet function leading to hemorrhage
Methotrexate	Additive hypoprothrombinemia
Mineral oil	↑ Hypoprothrombinemia by ↓ absorption of vitamin K from GI tract; also mineral oil could ↓ absorption of anticoagulants from GI tract
Methylthiouracil	Additive hypoprothrombinemia
Metronidazole	↑ Effect of anticoagulants due to ↓ breakdown by liver
Penicillin	Penicillin may potentiate the pharmacologic effect of anticoagulants
Phenylbutazone	↑ Effect of anticoagulants by ↓ plasma protein binding and ↓ breakdown by liver; phenylbutazone may also produce GI ulceration and therefore ↑ chance of bleeding
Phenytoin	↑ Effect of phenytoin due to ↓ in breakdown by liver; also possible ↑ in anticoagulant effect by ↓ plasma protein binding
Propylthiouracil	Additive hypoprothrombinemia
Quinidine, quinine	Additive hypoprothrombinemia
Rifampin	↓ Anticoagulant effect due to ↑ breakdown by liver
Salicylates	↑ Effect of anticoagulants by ↓ plasma protein binding, ↓ plasma prothrombin, and ↓ platelet aggregation; also, ↑ risk of GI bleeding due to ulcerogenic effect of salicylates
Sulfinpyrazone	↑ Anticoagulant effect due to ↓ breakdown by liver and inhibition of platelet aggregation
Sulfonamides	↑ Effect of sulfonamides by ↑ blood levels; also ↑ anticoagulant effect due to ↓ plasma protein binding and ↓ breakdown by liver
Sulfonylureas	↑ Effect of anticoagulant due to ↓ plasma protein binding; also, ↑ effect of sulfonylureas
Sulindac	↑ Effect of anticoagulants
Tetracyclines	IV tetracyclines ↑ hypoprothrombinemia
Thyroid hormones	↑ Anticoagulant effect due to ↑ breakdown of clotting factors
Triclofos	↑ Effect of anticoagulants due to ↓ plasma protein binding
Xanthines	↓ Effect of anticoagulants by ↑ plasma prothrombin and factor V

Laboratory Test Interferences False ↓ levels of serum theophylline determined by Schack and Waxler UV method (warfarin and dicumarol). Metabolites of indandione derivatives may color alkaline urine red; color disappears upon acidification.

Nursing Implications

1. Assist the health team in evaluating the patient's reliability, which is essential in coumarin therapy. The aged, psychotics, and alcoholics often cannot be relied on to take medication without supervision.
2. Ask a reliable relative or friend of the patient to report any untoward effects and to make sure that the patient takes medication and comes in for blood tests.
3. Ascertain that prothrombin levels are checked at prescribed intervals and reported promptly.
4. Monitor prothrombin levels more closely; anticipate dose adjustment of the anticoagulant if the patient is also receiving one of the many drugs noted to interact with anticoagulants.
5. Assess closely for evidence of bleeding (bleeding gums, hematuria, tarry stools, hematemesis, ecchymosis and/or petechiae) during initial therapy and if the patient is also receiving other medication that increases anticoagulant effect.
6. Report the sudden appearance of lumbar pain in patients receiving anticoagulant therapy since this may indicate retroperitoneal hemorrhage.
7. Report symptoms of GI dysfunction in a patient on anticoagulant therapy, since these may indicate intestinal hemorrhage. Anticipate that a patient with a history of ulcers of the GI tract or who recently underwent surgery should have frequent laboratory tests for blood in urine or feces to assess for GI bleeding.
8. Have vitamin K available for parenteral emergency use.
9. *Teach patient and/or family*
   a. about the possibility of bleeding and symptoms of impending hemorrhage. Avoid causing undue anxiety.
   b. that in the event of bleeding (e.g., from the gums, or in the form of black and blue areas on the skin, or blood in urine), to stop taking medication and to call physician for further instructions.
   c. that for those receiving indandione-type anticoagulants, medication turns alkaline urine red-orange. Discoloration resulting from the drug can be differentiated from hematuria by acidifying urine.
   d. that for those receiving coumarin-type therapy, a card should be carried stating that the patient is on anticoagulant therapy, in order to alert medical or paramedical personnel should an accident or excessive bleeding occur or surgery be required.
   e. the necessity for remaining under medical supervision for blood tests and adjustment of dosage.
   f. that other medications, changes in diet, and physical state may affect the action of the anticoagulant. Illness should be promptly reported to the physician.
   g. to carry Vitamin K capsules at all times.
   h. not to take nonprescription drugs, particularly aspirin, alcohol, or vitamin preparations high in vitamin K, without checking with the physician responsible for coumarin therapy.
   i. to use an electric razor rather than a razor blade for shaving.

Heparin and Protamine Sulfate

HEPARIN CALCIUM Calciparine Subcutaneous (Rx)

HEPARIN SODIUM Hepalean,* Lipo-Hepin, Lipo-Hepin/BL, Liquaemin Sodium, Minihep* (Rx)

Classification Anticoagulant, natural.

General Statement Heparin is a naturally occurring substance isolated from porcine intestinal mucosa or bovine lung tissue. Must be given parenterally. Heparin does not interfere with wound healing. Leukocyte counts should be performed in heparinized blood within 2 hr after adding heparin. Heparinized blood should not be used for complement, isoagglutin, erythrocyte fragility test, or platelet counts.

Action/Kinetics At low doses heparin prevents conversion of prothrombin to thrombin; at high doses it increases the rate at which thrombin and activated coagulation factor are neutralized. This prevents conversion of fibrinogen to fibrin and thus decreases or inhibits blood coagulation. **Onset: IV,** immediate; **deep SC:** 20–60 min. **t½:** 60–90 min in healthy persons. **t½** increases with dose, severe renal disease, anephric patients, cirrhosis, and decreases with pulmonary embolism and liver impairment other than cirrhosis. *Metabolism:* probably by reticuloendothelial system. Clotting time returns to normal within 2 to 6 hr.

Uses As an anticoagulant, heparin is used to prevent the extension of clots or to prevent thrombi and emboli from recurring. It is also used prophylactically in the management of thromboembolic disease and to prevent complications after many kinds of surgery including cardiac and vascular surgery. To treat hyperlipemia and in renal dialysis and blood transfusions to prevent clotting. Diagnosis and treatment of disseminated intravascular coagulation (DIC). Prophylaxis of cerebral thrombosis in stroke. Coronary occlusion following myocardial infarction. Atrial fibrillation with embolization.

Contraindications Active bleeding, blood dyscrasias (or other disorders characterized by bleeding tendencies such as hemophilia), purpura, thrombocytopenia, liver disease with hypoprothrombinemia, suspected intracranial hemorrhage, suppurative thrombophlebitis, inaccessible ulcerative lesions (especially of the GI tract), open wounds, extensive denudation of the skin, and increased capillary permeability (as in ascorbic acid deficiency).

The drug should not be administered during surgery of the eye, brain, or spinal cord or during continuous tube drainage of the stomach or small intestine. Use is also contraindicated in subacute endocarditis, shock, advanced kidney disease, threatened abortion, severe hypertension, or hypersensitivity to drug.

Use with caution during menstruation, pregnancy, and postpartum, as well as in patients with a history of asthma, allergies, mild liver or kidney disease, or in alcoholics.

Untoward Reactions Hemorrhage ranging from minor local ecchymoses to major hemorrhagic complications. Such reactions are more likely to occur in prophylactic administration during surgery than in the treatment of thromboembolic disease. Thrombocytopenia.

Rare allergic reactions characterized by chills, fever, pruritus, urticaria, burning feet, rhinitis, conjunctivitis, lacrimation, asthma-like reactions, hyperemia, arthralgia, or anaphylactoid reactions have been noted. Use a test dose of 1,000 units in patients with a history of asthma or allergic disease. Long-term therapy may cause osteoporosis and/or spontaneous fractures and hypoaldosteronism.

Discontinuance of heparin has resulted in rebound hyperlipemia, priapism, transient alopecia, and decreased aldosterone synthesis.

Heparin resistance has been observed in some elderly patients. In these cases, large doses may be required.

IM injections of heparin may produce local irritation, hematoma, and tissue sloughing.

OVERDOSAGE Symptoms: nosebleeds, hematuria, tarry stools, petechiae, and easy bruising may be the first signs. Treatment: Drug withdrawal is usually sufficient to correct heparin overdosage. In some cases, blood transfusion or the administration of a heparin antagonist (protamine sulfate) may be necessary.

Drug Interactions

Interactant	Interaction
ACTH	Heparin antagonizes effect of ACTH
Anticoagulants, oral	Additive ↑ prothrombin time
Antihistamines	↓ Effect of heparin
Aspirin	Additive ↑ prothrombin time
Corticosteroids	Heparin antagonizes effect of corticosteroids
Dextran	Additive ↑ prothrombin time
Diazepam	Heparin ↑ plasma levels of diazepam
Digitalis	↓ Effect of heparin
Dipyridamole	Additive ↑ prothrombin time
Hydroxychloroquine	Additive ↑ prothrombin time
Ibuprofen	Additive ↑ prothrombin time
Indomethacin	Additive ↑ prothrombin time
Insulin	Heparin antagonizes effect of insulin
Phenylbutazone	Additive ↑ prothrombin time
Quinine	Additive ↑ prothrombin time
Tetracyclines	↓ Effect of heparin

Laboratory Test Interference ↑ SGOT and SGPT.

Dosage Adjusted for each patient on the basis of laboratory tests. **Deep SC: initial loading dose**, 10,000–20,000 units (preceded by 5,000 units IV); **maintenance**: 8,000–10,000 units q 8 hr or 15,000–20,000 20,000 units q 12 hr. *Use concentrated solution.* **Intermittent IV: initially**, 10,000 units undiluted or in 50–100 ml saline; **then**, 5,000–10,000 units q 4 to 6 hr undiluted or in 50–100 ml saline. **Continuous IV infusion**: 20,000–40,000 units/day in 1,000 ml saline. *Prophylaxis of postoperative thromboembolism*: **Deep SC**: 5,000 units of concentrated solution 2 hr before surgery and 5,000 units q 8 to 12 hr thereafter for 7 days or until patient is ambulatory. *Surgery of heart and blood vessels*: **initial**, 150–400 units/kg (dose depends on estimated length of surgery); to prevent clotting in the tube system, add heparin to fluids in pump oxygenator. *Extracorporeal renal dialysis*: See instructions on equipment. *Blood transfusion*: 400–600 units/100 ml whole blood. *Laboratory samples*: 70–150 units/10–20-ml sample to prevent coagulation.

Administration/Storage

1. Patient must be hospitalized for heparin therapy.
2. Protect solutions from freezing.
3. Heparin should not be administered IM.
4. Administer by deep SC injection to minimize local irritation, hematoma, and tissue sloughing and to prolong action of drug.

a. Z-track method: Use any fat roll, but abdominal fat rolls are preferred. Use a ½-inch or ⅝-inch needle. Grasp the skin layer of the fat roll and lift it upward. Insert the needle at about a 45-degree angle to the skin surface and then administer the medication. With this medication it is not necessary to check whether or not the needle is in a blood vessel. Rapidly withdraw the needle while releasing the skin.

b. "Bunch technique" method: Grasp the tissue around the injection site creating a tissue roll of about ½ inch in diameter. Insert the needle into the tissue roll at a 90-degree angle to the skin surface and inject the medication. It is not necessary to check whether or not the needle is in a blood vessel. Remove the needle rapidly when the skin is released.

c. Do not administer within 2 inches of the umbilicus because of increased vascularity of area.

5. Do not massage before or after injection.

6. Change sites of administration.

7. Caution should be used to prevent negative pressure (with a roller pump), which would increase the rate at which heparin is injected into the system. Administer with a constant rate infusion pump.

Nursing Implications

1. Ensure that activated partial thromboplastin times (APTT) are performed as ordered and the results are reported to the physician promptly. With full-dose heparin administered by continuous IV the APTT should be done before onset of therapy, q 4 hr during the early stages, and then daily. With full-dose intermittent IV heparin therapy the APPT should be done before the initiation of therapy, before each dose during the early stages, and then daily. During full-dose therapy the accepted therapeutic range for the APPT is 1.5–2.5 times the control value in seconds. The activated coagulation time (ACT) may be used also. Because the test can be done at the bedside, it is very convenient for monitoring the degree of anticoagulation in patients having extracorporeal circulation. The accepted therapeutic range for the ACT is 2–3 times the control values.

2. Anticipate that each dose of heparin will be ordered on an individual basis after coagulation test has been reviewed by the physician except when small doses are administered for prophylaxis.

3. Anticipate dosage adjustment if patient is also receiving one of the many drugs that interact with anticoagulants.

4. Assess patient closely for signs of bleeding such as bleeding gums, hematuria, tarry tools, hematemesis, ecchymosis and/or petechiae.

5. Instruct patient to report any signs of active bleeding.

6. Have protamine sulfate available for emergency use to stop bleeding.

7. Teach patient and/or family
   a. to report any signs of active bleeding.
   b. that for a woman of childbearing age, any excessive menstrual flow should be reported, since this may be caused by the drug and would necessitate a reduction in dosage.
   c. that for a patient with alopecia the condition is only temporary.
   d. that alterations in GU function and spontaneous fractures should be immediately reported to physician prescribing heparin.

HEPARIN LOCK FLUSH SOLUTION   Hepalean-Lok,* Hep-Lock (Rx)

Classification   Anticoagulant flushing agent.

Use   Dilute solutions of heparin sodium (100 USP units/ml) are used to maintain patency of indwelling catheters used for IV therapy or blood sampling. Not to be used therapeutically. See *Heparin*, p. 268 for all other information.

Nursing Implications
1. Maintain patency by injecting 1 ml of heparin lock flush solution into the diaphragm of the device after each use. This dose should maintain patency for up to 4 hr.
2. When a drug incompatible with heparin is to be administered, flush the device with sterile water for injection or 0.9% sodium chloride injection before and immediately after the incompatible drug is administered. After the second flush, inject another dose of heparin lock flush solution.
3. When repeated blood samples are drawn from the venipuncture device, the presence of heparin or normal saline may cause laboratory test interference. Clear the heparin lock flush solution by aspirating and discarding 1 ml of fluid from the device before withdrawing the blood sample. Inject another 1 ml of heparin lock flush solution into device after bloods are drawn.

PROTAMINE SULFATE (Rx)

Classification   Antiheparin agent.

Action/Kinetics   Protamine sulfate is a strongly basic polypeptide that complexes with strongly acidic heparin forming an inactive stable salt. **Onset:** 30–60 sec. **Duration:** 2 hr. Upon metabolism, may liberate heparin (heparin rebound).

Use   Treatment of heparin overdose only. Not suitable for treating spontaneous hemorrhage, postpartum hemorrhage, menorrhagia, or uterine bleeding. Heparin rebound may occur during or after transfusion, extracorporeal dialysis, or cardiopulmonary bypass procedures. This may be corrected by administering more protamine sulfate.

Contraindication   Patients previously shown to have intolerance.

Untoward Reactions   *CV:* Sudden fall in blood pressure, bradycardia, dyspnea, transitory flushing, warm feeling. To minimize, administer slowly (over 1–3 minutes). *GI:* Nausea, vomiting. *CNS:* Lassitude. As a result of its weak anticoagulant effect, overdoses may cause hemorrhage.

Dosage   **Slow IV.** Dosage is determined by venous coagulation studies. No more than 50 mg of protamine sulfate should be given in any 10-min interval.
    It is estimated that 1 mg of protamine sulfate will neutralize about 90 USP units of heparin derived from lung tissue, or approximately 115 USP units of heparin derived from intestinal mucosa.

Administration/Storage
1. Note expiration date, which is 2 yr after manufacture.
2. Store at 2°–15° C .
3. After reconstitution, solution may be stored in refrigerator for 24 hr.

Nursing Implications

1. Anticipate that the patient may show a sudden fall in blood pressure, bradycardia, dyspnea, transitory flushing, and a feeling of warmth if the drug is administered too rapidly. Reassure the patient that these symptoms will pass. Slow IV administration and report.
2. Monitor blood pressure before and closely after administration of drug until pressure is stable. Then check hourly or as indicated by medical supervision.
3. Assess patient closely and report signs of heparin rebound, characterized by increased bleeding and lowered blood pressure, and/or shock.
4. Anticipate need for repeated doses of protamine sulfate if heparin has been administered in a repository form.

HEMOSTATICS

General Statement   These drugs are used to control excessive bleeding in persons who have an inborn clotting defect, who suffer from a disease that affects the clotting mechanism, or who exhibit continuous leakage from a capillary that cannot be controlled by other (physical, surgical) means.

The mechanism of blood coagulation was detailed at the beginning of this section. Defects in clotting are difficult to treat because excessive, drug-induced blood coagulation is far more dangerous than the hemorrhage itself.

Hemostatic agents are divided into (1) topically active agents, and (2) systemic agents.

Topical Agents

CELLULOSE, OXIDIZED   Oxycel, Novocell, Surgicel (Rx)

Classification   Hemostatic, topical.

Action/Kinetics   Upon contact with blood, oxidized cellulose (cellulosic acid) forms a tenacious, almost black mass that adheres to bleeding surfaces. This mass becomes gelatinous after 1–2 days. *Systemic absorption:* oxidized cellulose 2–7 days; if soaked with blood: 6 weeks or more. Oxidized cellulose also possesses antibacterial activity against a number of gram-positive and gram-negative organisms.

Uses   Surgery, to control moderate bleeding when suturing or ligation is impractical (such as biliary tract surgery), partial hepatectomy, resections or injuries of the pancreas, spleen, or kidneys, and bowel resections. Dental and oral surgery.

Contraindications   The material should not be used on open, external wounds because it interferes with new skin formation. It also should not be used for permanent packing because it interferes with bone regeneration. Vascular surgery; around optic nerve and chiasm.

Untoward Reactions   Retention of fluid, infection, foreign body reaction. *Following topical use:* burning, stinging. *When used in the nose:* burning, headache, sneezing, stinging, necrosis or perforation if material packed too tightly. Obstruction of intestine or urethra when used in these areas.

Dosage   Minimum amount necessary. Pellets are especially indicated in dentistry.

Administration
1. Use sterile technique in removing from containers.
2. Apply minimal amount necessary to control hemorrhage.
3. Apply in dry form.
4. Oxidized cellulose can not be resterilized; thus unused material should be discarded.
5. Never pull oxidized cellulose from wound without irrigating material. Otherwise, fresh bleeding may be initiated.
6. Artificial scab can be removed after it becomes gelatinous.

GELATIN SPONGE, ABSORBABLE   Gelfoam (OTC)

Classification   Hemostatic, topical.

Action/Kinetics   Specially prepared gelatin that absorbs approximately 50% of its weight in blood or other fluid. *Onset*: instantaneous. Absorbed systemically within 4–6 weeks. When applied to bleeding surfaces or mucosal membranes (nasal, rectal, or vaginal), liquefies within 2–5 days.

Uses   During surgery to control capillary bleeding including dental, oral, and prostatic surgery.

Contraindications   Frank infection, sole agent in presence of blood dyscrasias or abnormal bleeding, postpartum bleeding, menorrhagia. To close skin incisions.

Untoward Reactions   Infection, abscess formation.

Dosage   Enough of the sponge, pack, or dental pack used dry or saturated with sterile isotonic saline to cover bleeding surface. Prostatectomy cones are also available for use with the Foley bag catheter.

Administration
1. Moisten material with sterile isotonic sodium chloride before applying to bleeding surface. Squeeze to remove air bubbles and replace in the solution so material can swell to original size prior to application.
2. Resterilization by heating changes the absorption time.

GELATIN FILM, ABSORBABLE STERILE Gelfilm, Gelfilm Ophthalmic (OTC)

Classification   Hemostatic, topical.

Action/Kinetics   This is a thin, absorbable gelatin film that takes up to 50 times its weight of blood and water. Like absorbable gelatin sponge (see above), it can be left in place and is absorbed within 8 days to 6 months.

Uses   Neurosurgery, thoracic surgery, and ocular surgery.

Dosage   *Topical*: as required; after soaking, cut to desired size and shape.

Administration
1. Moisten gelatin with sterile isotonic saline solution before applying it to bleeding surface.
2. Use immediately upon withdrawal from package to ensure sterility.

MICROFIBRILLAR COLLAGEN HEMOSTAT   Avitene (Rx)

Classification   Hemostatic, topical.

Action/Kinetics   Attracts platelets, which then release clotting factors that initiate formation of a fibrinous mass. Absorbable, water insoluble.

Uses   During surgery to control capillary bleeding and as an adjunct to hemostasis when conventional procedures are ineffectual or insufficient.

Contraindications   Closure of skin incisions, because preparation may interfere with healing. On bone surfaces to which prosthetic materials will be attached.

Untoward Reactions   Potentiation of infections, abscess formation, hematomas, wound dehiscence, mediastinitis. Formation of adhesions, foreign body reaction.

Dosage   *Individualized*: depending on severity of bleeding. *Usual for capillary bleeding*: 1 gm for 50-cm area. More for heavier flow.

Administration

1. Before applying dry product, compress surface to be treated with dry sponge. Use dry smooth forceps to handle.
2. Apply hemostat directly to source of bleeding.
3. After hemostat is in place, apply pressure with a dry sponge, and not a gloved hand.
4. When controlling oozing from porous (cancellous) bone, pack hemostat tightly into affected area.
5. Tease off excess material after 5–10 min.
6. Apply more hemostat in case of breakthrough bleeding.
7. Avoid spillage on nonbleeding surfaces, especially in the abdomen or thorax.
8. Remove excess material after a few minutes.
9. Do not reautoclave. Discard unused portion.
10. Avoid contacting nonbleeding surfaces with microfibrillar collagen hemostat.

Nursing Implication
Assess for shock while monitoring BP and pulse because hemostat may mask a deeper hemorrhage by sealing off its exit site.

NEGATOL   Negatan (Rx)

Classification   Hemostatic and astringent, topical.

Action/Kinetics   Negatol is an acidic material that causes coagulation of blood proteins.

Use   Suppuration, bleeding, ulceration, and oozing of skin and mucous membranes including those of the mouth, vagina, and cervix.

Contraindication   Hypersensitivity to drug. Will not control bleeding from large vessels.

Untoward Reactions   Rarely: local irritation of the skin surrounding the vaginal orifice. Also imparts a transitory grayish hue to treated mucous membranes.

Dosage   Paint surface with full strength product or dilute (1:10).

Administration
1. Cleanse and dry affected area.
2. Paint area with negatol.
3. For oral ulceration: dry affected area, apply topical anesthetic as ordered, apply negatol with applicator. Hold latter in place for 1 min. Rinse with copious amounts of water to neutralize.
4. For cervical use: use 1:10 dilution of product to establish tolerance of patient to negatol. Insert a 1-inch gauze pack, dipped into dilute or full strength negatol, into cervical canal. For vaginal involvement: pack vagina with gauze soaked in 1:10 dilution of negatol. Remove all packing within 24 hr and follow with a 2-quart douche of dilute negatol or vinegar.

Nursing Implication
Advise patient to wear a perineal pad to prevent soiling of clothing by the highly acid substance.

THROMBIN, TOPICAL Thrombinar, Thrombostat (Rx)

Classification   Hemostatic, topical.

Action/Kinetics   Catalyzes conversion of fibrinogen to fibrin. It is most effective when thrombin can mix with blood as soon as it reaches the surface. *Onset:* less than 1 min.

Use   During surgery, to control capillary bleeding. May be used with absorbable gelatin sponges.

Contraindications   Thrombin should never be injected, particularly IV. IV injections may be fatal.

Dosage   **Topical: usual,** 100 units/ml solution; if bleeding profuse, 1,000–2,000 units/ml may be needed. Also, may be applied dry to oozing surfaces.

Administration/Storage
1. Dry powder may be stored indefinitely.
2. Thrombin solution may be applied by a spray or with a sterile syringe and needle.
3. If used with absorbable gelatin sponge, the sponge strips should be soaked in the thrombin solution, then compressed to remove air bubbles, and then saturated with the solution. When applied to the area, the sponge should be held in place 10–15 seconds.
4. Thrombin solutions should be used the same day they are prepared. If preservatives are added, the solution should be used within 48 hrs.

Systemic Agents

AMINOCAPROIC ACID Amicar (Rx)

Classification   Hemostatic, systemic.

Action/Kinetics   Inhibits action of plasminogen (clotting factor), thereby preventing fibrinolysis (clot dissolution). **Peak plasma levels:** 2 hr. **Effective plasma levels:** 0.13 mg/ml. **Duration (after IV):** 3 hr or less; 40–60% excreted unchanged in kidney after 12 hr.

Uses Excessive bleeding associated with systemic hyperfibrinolysis and urinary fibrinolysis. Surgical complications following heart surgery and portacaval shunt in cancer of the lung, prostate, cervix, stomach, and other types of surgery associated with heavy postoperative bleeding. Aplastic anemia.

Contraindications Patients with active, intravascular clotting possibly associated with fibrinolysis and bleeding. Use with caution, or not at all, in patients with uremia or cardiac, renal, or hepatic disease. First and second trimester of pregnancy.

Untoward Reactions *GI:* Nausea, cramping, diarrhea. *CNS:* Dizziness, malaise, headache. *CV:* Hypotension, thrombophlebitis. *Other:* Tinnitus, conjunctival suffusion, myopathies, nasal stuffiness, skin rash, prolongation of menses, reversible acute renal failure.

Drug Interactions

Interactant	Interaction
Anticoagulants, oral	↓ Anticoagulant effects
Contraceptives, oral (Estrogen)	Combination with aminocaproic acid may lead to hypercoagulable condition

Laboratory Test Interferences ↑ Serum aldolase, SGOT, creatinine phosphokinase, and potassium.

Dosage PO, IV. **Initial priming dose:** 4–5 gm during first hour; **then,** 1 gm q hr for 8 hr or until bleeding is controlled. **Maximum daily dose:** 30 gm.

Administration

1. For IV use, may be mixed with saline, 5% dextrose, sterile water, or Ringer's solution. It should never be injected undiluted.
2. For IV, priming dose is dissolved in 250 ml; continuous infusion is at the rate of 1 gm/hr in 50 ml of diluent.

Nursing Implications

1. Assess baseline BP and pulse before starting IV.
2. Assess patient frequently for hypotension, bradycardia, and arrhythmias, which indicate that the IV administration is too fast. Slow IV and report if such symptoms occur.
3. With all systemic hemostatics, observe carefully for signs and symptoms of thrombosis, such as leg pain, chest pain, or respiratory distress.
4. Have vitamin K or protamine sulfate available for emergency use.

ANTIHEMOPHILIC FACTOR (AHF, FACTOR VIII) Factorate, Factorate Generation II, Hemofil, Hemofil T, Koate, Profilate (Rx)

Classification Hemostatic, systemic.

Action/Kinetics Antihemophilic factor (AHF) is isolated from pooled normal human blood and is essential for blood coagulation. The potency and purity of preparation varies but each lot is standardized. Details on the package should be noted. Plasma protein (factor VIII) accelerates abnormally slow transformation of prothrombin to thrombin. t½: 8–24 hr. One AHF unit is the activity found in 1 ml of normal pooled human plasma that is less than 1 hr old.

Use Control of bleeding in patients suffering from hemophilia A (Factor VIII deficiency and acquired factor VIII inhibitors).

Untoward Reactions *GI:* Nausea, vomiting. *CNS:* Headaches, paresthesia, clouding or loss of consciousness. *CV:* Tachycardia, flushing, hypotension. *Other:* Disturbance of vision, constriction of chest, or rigor. Jaundice and viral hepatitis.

Antihemophilic factor contains traces of blood group A and B isohemagglutins. These may cause intravascular hemolysis in patients with types A, B, or AB blood.

Dosage **IV only. Individualized,** depending on severity of bleeding, degree of deficiency, body weight, and presence of inhibitors of factor VIII.

Note: Dosages given are only guidelines. *Overt bleeding:* **initial,** 15–25 units/kg; **then,** 8–15 units/kg q 8–12 hr for 3–4 days. *Joint hemorrhage, without aspiration:* 8–10 units/kg at 8–12 hr intervals for 1 or more days; *with aspiration:* 8 units/ kg prior to aspiration; **then,** 8 units/kg 8 hr later (repeat if necessary). *Muscle hemorrhage:* 8–10 units/kg q 12–24 hr for 2–3 days, depending on severity of bleeding. *Muscle hemorrhage in vicinity of vital organs:* **initial,** 15 units/kg; **then,** 8 units/kg q 8 hr for 48 hr followed by 4 units/kg q 8 hr for 48 additional hr (or longer). *Bleeding from massive wounds:* **initial,** 40–50 units/kg; **then,** 20–25 units/ kg q 8–12 hr to achieve AHF level 80–100% of normal. *Surgery:* 20–30 units/kg before surgery and 15 units/kg q 8 hr after surgery for 10 days. Postinfusion level of AHF should be 60% and maintained at 30% for at least 10–14 days postoperatively. *Prophylaxis in hemophilia A:* **patients weighing 50 kg or less:** 250 units once daily in the morning; **patients weighing 50 kg or more:** 500 units once daily in the morning.

Administration/Storage

1. Antihemophilic factor is very labile and is inactivated rapidly: within 10 min at 56° C and within 3 hr at 49° C. Store vials at 2°–8° C. Check expiration date. **Do not freeze.**
2. Warm the concentrate and diluent to room temperature before reconstitution.
3. Place one needle in the concentrate to act as an airway and then aseptically with a syringe and needle add the diluent to the concentrate.
4. Gently agitate or roll the vial containing diluent and concentrate to dissolve the drug. **Do not shake vigorously.**
5. Administer drug within 3 hr of reconstitution, to avoid incubation if contamination occurred during mixing.
6. Do not refrigerate drug after reconstitution, because the active ingredient may precipitate out.
7. Keep reconstituted drug at room temperature during infusion because, at a lower temperature, precipitation of active ingredients may occur.
8. *Medication should not be administered faster than 10 ml/min.*

Nursing Implications

1. *Assess*
   a. baseline pulse and blood pressure before starting IV.
   b. pulse and blood pressure during administration. Slow IV and report tachycardia and hypotension.
2. Slow IV and report if patient complains of headaches, flushing, numbness, back pain, visual disturbances, or chest constriction.

ANTI-INHIBITOR COAGULANT COMPLEX   Autoplex, Feiba Immuno (Rx)

Classification   Hemostatic, systemic.

Action/Kinetics   Product is prepared from pooled human plasma containing various concentrations of activated and precursor clotting factors including some of the kinin generating system. Considerable variation between batches occurs; however, each bottle is labeled with the units of factor VIII correction activity that it contains. One unit of factor VIII correction activity is that amount of activated prothrombin complex that when added to an equal volume of factor VIII–deficient or inhibitor plasma, will correct the clotting time to 35 sec (normal).

Overcomes absence or insufficient blood coagulation caused by an inhibitor of blood clotting factor VIII.

Uses   The drug is indicated only for patients in whom the presence of factor VIII inhibitor has been ascertained. Specifically, for hemophiliacs (approximately 10%) with presence of factor VIII inhibitors, patients with factor VIII inhibitor levels greater than 10 Bethesda units or in whom factor VIII inhibitor levels increase to greater than 10 Bethesda units after treatment with AHF, and for selected patients in whom factor VIII inhibitor levels are normally less than 10 Bethesda units after being treated with AHF.

Contraindications   Signs of fibrinolysis, disseminated intravascular coagulation (DIC).

Untoward Reactions   Viral hepatitis, intravascular coagulations (see *Nursing Implications*). Hypersensitivity reactions including fever, chills, changes in blood pressure, indications of protein sensitivity.

Drug Interactions   The concomitant use of anti-inhibitor coagulation complex is not recommended with highly activated prothrombin complex products, with aminocaproic acid, or with tranexamic acid.

Dosage   **IV only**. Dosage range: 25–100 factor VIII correctional units/kg, depending on the severity of hemorrhage. Dosage should be repeated if no improvement is seen 6 hr after the initial dose.

Administration/Storage

1. Reconstitute solution according to directions.
2. The rate of administration can be as high as 10 ml/min; however, if the patient reports headache, or if there is evidence of flushing, changes in pulse rate, or blood pressure, discontinue and reinitiate at a rate of 2 ml/min.
3. Store unreconstituted complex under refrigeration (2°–8° C). Avoid freezing.
4. In children, fibrinogen levels should be measured before the initial infusion and monitored during therapy.

Additional Nursing Implications

1. Assess baseline BP and pulse before starting IV.
2. Stop IV and assist with monitoring patient for DIC by prothrombin and thromboplastin test if alterations in blood pressure and pulse, respiratory distress, cough, chest pain, or headache occur.
3. Ascertain that postinfusion prothrombin time is at least two-thirds of the preinfusion value before initiating additional therapy.

FACTOR IX COMPLEX (HUMAN)   Konyne, Profilnine, Proplex, Proplex SX (Rx)

Classification   Hemostatic, systemic.

Action/Kinetics   This is a concentrate of several human coagulation factors (II, VII, IX, and X) prepared from normal human plasma that are essential to the clotting mechanism. Thus, it replaces factors essential to initiation of blood clotting. **t½ (biphasic):** 4–6 hr and 22.5 hr. Readily cleared from plasma. A unit is the activity present (as factor IX) in 1 ml of normal plasma less than 1 hr old.

Uses   For patients with factor IX deficiency, especially hemophilia B and Christmas disease. Patients with inhibitors to factor VIII.

Contraindications   Liver disease with suspected intravascular coagulation or fibrinolysis. Assess benefit vs. risk prior to use in liver disease or elective surgery.

Untoward Reactions   Transient fever, chills, headaches, flushing, and tingling. Most of these side effects disappear when rate of administration is slowed. Viral hepatitis. The preparation also contains trace amounts of blood groups A and B and isohemagglutins, which may cause intravascular hemolysis when administered in large amounts to patients with blood groups A, B, and AB.

Dosage   **IV. Individualized,** depending on severity of bleeding, degree of deficiency, body weight, and level of factor required. Minimum factor IX level required in surgery or following trauma is 25% of normal, which is maintained for 1 week after surgery. **Maintenance, usual:** 10–20 units/kg/day. *Bleeding in hemophilia A patients with factor VII inhibitor:* 75 units/kg in a single dose; a second dose may be given after 8–12 hr if necessary. *Prophylaxis of bleeding in factor IX–deficient patients:* 500 units weekly.

Administration/Storage

1. Store at 2°–8° C.
2. Avoid freezing the diluent provided with drug.
3. Discard 2 years after date of manufacture.
4. Before reconstitution, warm diluent to room temperature but not above 40° C.
5. Agitate the solution gently until the powder is dissolved.
6. Administer drug within 3 hr of reconstitution to avoid incubation in case contamination occurred during preparation.
7. Do not refrigerate after reconstitution, because the active ingredient may precipitate out.
8. Administer at the rate of flow ordered.

Nursing Implications

1. Assess baseline BP and pulse before starting IV.
2. Reduce rate of flow if patient reports a tingling sensation, chills, fever, and headache; report to physician.

Chapter Twenty-one

BLOOD, BLOOD COMPONENTS, AND BLOOD SUBSTITUTES

General Statement   Blood, blood fractions, and blood extenders are not drugs in the ordinary sense. However, since they are often administered and monitored by nurses, they are discussed here briefly.

Blood transfusions have become a reality since it was discovered that blood coagulation can be prevented through the addition of anticoagulants (citrate, heparin) and that blood falls into certain well-defined groups that can be exchanged relatively freely between members of the same group. Nevertheless, the transfusion of whole blood is associated with a certain risk (hypersensitivity, hepatitis), and the recent advent of blood components represents a major advance in therapy because the patient can now receive only the components necessary for treatment. The type of blood or blood substitute to be administered is determined by the need of the patient and the availability of the most suitable preparation.

Uses   Replacement of blood loss resulting from trauma, surgery, or disease. Plasma volume expansion, severe clotting defects, and hemostasis (disease or drug-induced), and agranulocytosis. Burns, hypoproteinemia.

Untoward Reactions   These depend on the blood or blood fraction being administered. *Viral hepatitis* (onset 4 weeks to 6 months after transfusion): Characterized by anorexia, nausea, fever, malaise, tenderness and enlargement of liver, jaundice, and GI and skin reactions. *Hypersensitivity reactions*: Mild: urticaria, pruritus. Severe: bronchospasms. *Febrile reactions*: Characterized by fever (103°–104° F, or 39.4°–40.0° C), tremors, chills, and headaches. Onset: during initial 15 min of transfusion. *Hemolysis*: Potentially fatal complication caused by mismatching or mislabeling of blood or other human errors. Characterized by flushing, tachycardia, restlessness, dyspnea, chills, fever, headache, sharp pain in lumbar region, pressure feeling in chest, feeling of head fullness, nausea, and vomiting. Also hemoglobinuria and hemoglobinemia, and oliguria and acute renal failure. Usual onset: after administration of 100–200 ml incompatible blood. Shock and/or death occasionally occurs within min after initiation of transfusion. *Jaundice*: Caused by larger than normal number of hemolyzed RBCs that may be present in blood approaching its expiration date. Occurs more frequently in patients with inadequate liver function. *Hypervolemia* (*overexpanded blood volume*): Characterized by labored breathing, cough, dyspnea, cyanosis, and pulmonary edema. Occurs more frequently in the very young, in the elderly, or in patients with cardiac or pulmonary disease. *Pyrogenic febrile reaction from contamination products* (*especially bac-*

teria): Characterized by chills, fever, profound shock, coma, convulsions, and often death. Onset: after transfusion of 50–100 ml.

Administration

1. Use normal saline as part of the Y setup (parallel setup) for blood transfusion. Do not use dextrose injection since this will cause clumping of RBCs. **Never use distilled water as this will cause hemolysis**.
2. Never add medication to blood or plasma.
3. Whenever possible, use plastic bags for transfusion to reduce danger of air embolism.

Nursing Implications for Blood, Blood Expanders, Fractions, and Substitutes

1. Regulate IV to 20 drops/min for the first 10 min and remain with the patient to assess for untoward reactions. **Stop the IV at once and notify medical supervision should any of the following untoward reactions occur:**

   a. *Anaphylactic reaction*: Urticaria, tightness of chest, wheezing, hypotension, nausea, and vomiting. Have epinephrine, antihistamines, corticosteroid, and resuscitative equipment available.

   b. *Circulatory embarrassment*: Dyspnea, cyanosis, persistent cough (early sign), frothy sputum (late sign). Position the patient upright with lower extremities dependent. Obtain rotating tourniquets to be used as ordered.

   c. *Febrile (pyrogenic) reaction*: Sudden chilling, fever, headache, nausea, and vomiting. Take temperature every half-hour after chill; repeat until within the normal range.

   d. *Bacterial contamination*: Severe chills, high fever, hypotension, and shocklike state. Take temperature every half-hour after chill; repeat until within normal range.

   e. *Hemolytic reaction*: Chills, feeling of fullness in head, pressure feeling in the chest, flushing of face, sharp pain in lumbar region, distention of neck veins, hypotension, and circulatory collapse. Have mannitol available. Encourage oral fluids for next few hours. Measure and save all urine voided. Monitor intake and output. Have citrated blood tube available for bloods to be drawn to check for free hemoglobin in plasma.

2. Send the remainder of the material and the equipment used for the infusion to the laboratory for analysis if an untoward reaction has occurred.
3. Increase to rate of flow ordered if no reaction is evident after the first 10 min.
4. Anticipate that the rate of flow for elderly and cardiac patients will be slower.
5. Check blood pressure and pulse every half-hour during the infusion and report lack of response to therapy or significant deviations from patient's baseline whether elevated or depressed.

ALBUMIN, NORMAL HUMAN SERUM   Albuminar-5 and -25, Albutein 5% and 25%, Buminate 5% and 25%, Plasbumin-5 and -25 (Rx)

Classification   Blood volume expander.

Action/Kinetics   Prepared from whole blood, serum, plasma, or placentas from healthy human donors. It is supplied as a 5% (isotonic and isosmotic with normal human plasma) and 25% (salt-poor solution of which each 50 ml is osmotically equivalent to 250 ml of citrated plasma) strength. It contains sodium, 130–160 mEq/liter.

Uses Blood volume expander in shock, following surgery, hemorrhage, burns, or other trauma. Hypoproteinemia due to toxemia of pregnancy, anuria, acute hepatic cirrhosis or coma, acute nephrotic syndrome, tuberculosis, and premature infants. As an adjunct to exchange transfusions in hyperbilirubinemia and erythroblastosis fetalis. Prophylaxis and treatment of cerebral edema, shock, or hypotension in fluid-overloaded hemodialysis patients.

Contraindications Severe anemia or cardiac failure.

Untoward Reactions Pulmonary edema, circulatory overload, chills, fever, urticaria, nausea, dehydration, or heart failure.

Laboratory Test Interference ↑ Serum alkaline phosphatase.

Dosage **IV infusion, individualized. 5%.** *Hypoproteinemia*: rate not to exceed 5–10 ml/min. *Burns*: 500 ml initially; supplement as necessary. *Shock*: **adults and children**, 250–500 ml initially; repeat after 15–30 min if response inadequate. **25%.** *Hypoproteinemia with or without edema*: Adults, 50–75 gm/day; **pediatric**: 25 gm/day. Rate should not exceed 2 ml/min. *Nephrosis*: 100–200 ml (25–50 gm) at intervals of 1–2 days. *Burns*: determined by extent; dose must be sufficient to maintain plasma albumin levels of approximately 2.5 gm/100 ml with a plasma oncotic pressure of 20 mm Hg. *Shock*: dose determined by condition of patient. *Pediatric, emergencies:* **initial**, 25 gm; *nonemergencies:* 1/4–1/2 the adult dose. *Premature infants:* 1 gm/kg. *Hyperbilirubinemia and erythroblastosis fetalis*: 4 ml/kg (1 gm/kg) 1–2 hr before transfusion of blood.

Administration/Storage

1. Do not use turbid or sedimented solution.
2. Preparation does not contain preservatives. Use each opened bottle at once.
3. May be given as rapidly as needed initially. However, as plasma volume approaches normal, the 5% solution should not be given faster than 2–4 ml/min and the 25% solution should not be given faster than 1 ml/min.
4. In hypoproteinemia, the 5% solution should not be given faster than 5–10 ml/min and the 25% solution should not be given faster than 2–3 ml/min in order to minimize the possibility of circulatory overload and pulmonary edema.

Additional Nursing Implications

See also *Nursing Implications*, p. 281.

1. *Assess*
   a. for pulmonary edema demonstrated by cough, dyspnea, cyanosis, and rales. **Stop** administration of albumin immediately should any of these symptoms appear.
   b. intake and output.
   c. for diuresis and reduction of edema if present.
   d. for dehydration necessitating further administration of IV fluids.
   e. blood pressure and pulse closely.
   f. for hemorrhage or shock that may occur because of rapid increase in blood pressure causing bleeding in severed blood vessels that had not been previously noted.
2. Anticipate that after administration of albumin for treatment or prevention of cerebral edema, fluids should be withheld completely during the next 8 hr. Provide the patient with adequate mouth care.

BLOOD, WHOLE

Classification Blood replacement.

Note: Because of the danger of hepatitis, mismatching errors, and allergic reactions, whole blood is only given when absolutely necessary.

Uses Anemia, severe blood loss, and hypovolemia.

Untoward Reactions Serum hepatitis and hemolytic (chills, fever, flushing, restlessness, headache, nausea, vomiting) and allergic (bronchospasms) reactions.

Dosage IV: 500 ml; repeat as necessary.

Additional Nursing Implications
See *Nursing Implications* for Blood, Blood Expanders, p. 281.

1. Obtain one unit of blood from blood bank just before transfusion unless there is an emergency situation.
2. Do not store blood in the ward refrigerator as temperature fluctuations make storage unsuitable (Blood should be stored at 1°–10° C).
3. Do not infuse cold blood. Preferably warm it at room temperature for 20–30 min before infusion.
4. Check patient name band with blood identification slip to verify name and hospital number; check blood type on blood bag with lab report on patient chart. Check for blood expiration date (21 days for citrated and 4 days for heparinized blood).
5. Gently invert blood bag to remix plasma and RBC before starting transfusion.
6. Use an in-line micron filter to prevent microembolization, particularly pulmonary and cerebral embolization from microaggregates present in stored blood.
7. Assess vital signs before transfusion is started to use as a baseline. Take vital signs ½ hourly during transfusion and then at the end of the transfusion.
8. Allow a maximum of 4 hr for infusion of a unit of whole blood. Adjust flow according to patient's age and condition. Consult with physician regarding speed of transfusion.
9. Do not add any medication to blood bag or blood line.
10. Review agency policy for administration of blood.

DEXTRAN 40   10% LMD, Gentran 40, Rheomacrodex (Rx)

DEXTRAN 70   Hyskon,* Macrodex (Rx)

DEXTRAN 75   Gentran 75 (Rx)

Classification Blood volume expander.

Action/Kinetics Dextran is a biosynthesized, water-soluble, large molecule (polymer) which is available in various molecular weights (sizes). Dextran 40 has a lower molecular weight than that of dextran 70 or 75. The lower molecular weight products cause fewer allergic reactions. The preparation is a blood volume expander but is not a substitute for whole blood or its fractions.

Uses *Dextran 40:* Fluid replacement, treatment of shock due to surgery, hemorrhage, burns, or other trauma. As a priming fluid, alone or with other agents, in pump oxygenators for perfusing during extracorporeal circulation. Prophylaxis of acute thrombosis and pulmonary embolism in high risk surgical patients (i.e., hip surgery). *Investigational:* Increase circulation in myocardial infarction or sickle cell crisis. Prophylaxis of nephrotoxicity associated with contrast media, transplantation/graft procedures.

Dextran 70/75: Fluid replacement, treatment of shock. *Investigational:* Nephrosis, toxemia of late pregnancy, prophylaxis of postoperative deep-vein thrombosis.

Contraindications Severe CHF, renal failure, severe bleeding disorders, and known hypersensitivity. Use with caution in presence of renal, hepatic, or myocardial disease.

Untoward Reactions Anaphylactic reaction, urticaria, transient acidosis, pulmonary edema (chest tightness, angioedema), circulatory overload, increased clotting time, hypotension, tubular stasis, or blockage of kidney. Dextran 70/75 may also cause nausea, vomiting, fever, arthralgia, or involuntary defecation (in anesthetized patients).

Laboratory Test Interference ↓ Immunoglobulins A, G, and M. ↑ SGOT and SGPT.

Dosage *Dextran 40*, **adults and children, IV: First day,** 2 gm/kg (20 ml of 10% solution/kg); **then,** daily dose should not exceed 1 gm/kg for more than 5 days. *Priming fluid:* 1–2 gm/kg, not to exceed 2 gm/kg. *Prophylaxis of venous thrombosis, pulmonary embolism:* On day of surgery, 50–100 gm (10 ml/kg) of the 10% solution; **then,** 50 gm (500 ml) daily for 2–3 days followed by 50 gm (500 ml) q 2–3 days up to 14 days. *Dextran 70 and Dextran 75,* **Individualized, adults, usual:** 500 ml of 6% solution; total dose for first 24 hr should not exceed 1.2 gm/kg (20 ml/kg). Beyond 24 hr, dosage should not exceed 0.6 gm/kg (10 ml/kg). **Pediatric:** total dose should not exceed 20 ml/kg.

Administration/Storage

1. Do not administer unless solution is clear.
2. Dissolve flakes in solution by heating the solution in water bath at 100° C for 15 min or by autoclaving at 110° C for 15 min.
3. Store unopened solution bottles at constant temperature, preferably 25° C, to prevent flake formation.
4. Discard partially used bottles, since they do not contain preservatives.
5. In emergencies, Dextran 70 or 75 may be administered to adults at a rate of 20–40 ml/min. In patients with normal or nearly normal plasma volume, the rate of infusion should not exceed 4 ml/min.

Additional Nursing Implications
See also *Nursing Implications*, p. 281.

1. Complete drawings of samples for blood test before administration of dextran because values are affected by drug.
2. *Assess*
   a. for dehydration before initiation of therapy. Additional fluids may be necessary if dehydration develops.
   b. specific gravity of urine (normal 1.005–1.025), because low values may indicate that dextran is not being eliminated and might mandate discontinuance of drug.

c. output for oliguria or anuria, which may necessitate withdrawal of drug.

d. sudden increase in central venous pressure (CVP), which is indicative of circulatory overload. Slow IV and report.

e. salt-restricted patients closely for edema, elevated BP, cough, cyanosis, and moist rales. Dextran solutions contain sodium, which may precipitate pulmonary edema.

f. for signs of bleeding (especially 3–9 hr after administration) from orifices, site of trauma, or purpura.

g. hematocrit after completing administration.

h. anesthesized patients on Dextran 70 or 75 for vomiting or for involuntary defecation.

HETASTARCH   Hespan (Rx)

Classification   Plasma expander.

Action/Kinetics   This synthetic water-soluble large molecule (polymer) resembles glycogen. Its action is similar to dextran, but it produces fewer allergic reactions and does not interfere with blood cross-matching. Hetastarch is not a substitute for whole blood or its fractions.

Use   Shock (burns, hemorrhages, sepsis, and surgery). Fluid replacement, plasma volume expansion. Adjunct in removal of WBCs (leukopheresis). *Investigational:* Cryoprotective agent for long-term storage of whole blood. Plasma volume expansion during cardiopulmonary bypass surgery. Priming fluid in pump oxygenation for perfusion during extracorporeal circulation.

Contraindications   Severe bleeding disorders, severe CHF, or renal failure with oliguria or anuria.

Untoward Reactions   *Hematologic:* Prolonged prothrombin, partial thromboplastin, and clotting times. *Allergic:* Vomiting, fever, itching, chills, influenza-like syndrome, headache, edema of lower extremities, myalgia, anaphylaxis. *Miscellaneous:* Circulatory overload.

Dosage   **IV infusion only. Individualized, usual,** *plasma expansion:* 500–1,000 ml (30–60 gm) of 6% solution up to maximum of 1,500 ml (90 gm)/day. *For acute hemorrhage:* rapid rate up to 20 ml/kg/hr (1.2 gm/kg/hr). Use slower rates for burns and septic shock. *Leukopheresis:* 250–500 ml infused at a constant ratio, usually 8:1 to venous whole blood.

Administration   Discard partially used bottles.

Nursing Implications

1. *Assess*

   a. output for oliguria or anuria necessitating withdrawal of hetastarch.

   b. specific gravity of urine (normal 1.005–1.025), because low values indicate that hetastarch is not being excreted and might mandate discontinuance of plasma expander.

(continued)

c. hematocrit after administration of 500 ml of hetastarch, because values lower than 30% by volume should be avoided.

d. sudden rise in central venous pressure (CVP), indicating a circulatory overload.

e. salt-restricted patient closely for edema, elevated BP, cough, cyanosis, and moist rales, because sodium in hetastarch may precipitate pulmonary edema in patients with cardiac or kidney dysfunction.

f. for purpura or other signs of bleeding from orifices or wounds, especially 3–9 hr after administration, because hetastarch may temporarily prolong bleeding time.

PLASMA, NORMAL HUMAN (Rx)

PLASMA PROTEIN FRACTION Plasmanate, Plasma-Plex, Plasmatein, Protenate (Rx)

Classification Blood volume expander.

Action/Kinetics The cell-free portion of the blood, or a 5% solution of human plasma proteins in sodium chloride injection, is used when whole blood is unnecessary or unavailable. Preparations contain albumin, globulins, and electrolytes. Contains sodium 130–160 mEq/liter.

Plasma, normal human, which is available in fresh, frozen, and dried form, contains clotting factor; plasma protein fraction does not.

Uses Hypovolemic shock, burn patients, hypoproteinemia, hemorrhages when whole blood is unavailable, and dehydration in infants and small children. Hyperbilirubinemia and erythroblastosis fetalis.

Contraindications Cardiopulmonary bypass surgery, severe anemia. Use with caution in renal, hepatic, or cardiac failure.

Untoward Reactions *CV:* Flushing, erythema, vascular overload. Hypotension (from rapid IV infusion or intra-arterial use). *GI:* Nausea, vomiting. *Other:* Urticaria, chills, headache, back pain, fever.

Dosage Individualized. **Plasma, normal human, IV infusion:** 250–500 ml. **Plasma protein fraction (5%), IV infusion:** *hypovolemic shock,* 250–500 ml (12.5–25 gm protein) at a rate not to exceed 10 ml/min; **pediatric, infants and young children: initial,** 4.5–6.8 ml/kg (225–340 mg protein/kg) at a rate not to exceed 10 ml/min. Subsequent dosage depends on response. *Hypoproteinemia:* 1,000–1,500 ml (50–75 gm protein) at a rate not to exceed 5–8 ml/min.

Administration/Storage

1. Note expiration date. Preparations are stable for a long time when refrigerated.

2. Check administration rate with physician. Usual rate of administration: adult and infants, 5–10 ml/min. As plasma volume approaches normal, rate should not exceed 5–8 ml/min.

3. Not to be given near any site of infection or trauma.

RED CELLS, PACKED

Classification   Blood replacement.

Action/Kinetics   Packed red blood cells or concentrates are prepared by removing plasma from whole blood. The preparation sometimes goes through a freeze-thaw process that yields a purer product. Administration of packed red cells reduces the risk of circulatory overload and the amount of transfused blood antibodies and electrolytes (sodium, potassium, citrate). Other dangers associated with blood transfusions (hepatitis, allergic reactions, mismatching) are not reduced.

Uses   Aplastic anemia, hemorrhages, and when it is desirable to replace red cells without expanding blood volume. Especially suitable for the elderly, infants, and patients with cardiopulmonary or renal disease.

Untoward Reactions   See *Blood, Whole,* p. 283.

Dosage   Equivalent of indicated amount of whole blood.

Administration/Storage
1. Store between 1°–6° C.
2. Check label for expiration date and to ascertain typing and cross-matching blood and patient.
3. Allow 45–90 minutes for administration of packed cells.

Additional Nursing Implications
See *Nursing Implications* for *Blood*, pp. 281 and 283.

Chapter Twenty-two

THROMBOLYTIC AGENTS

General Statement   Streptokinase and urokinase are used to promote the dissolution (lysis) of the insoluble fibrin trapped in intravascular emboli and thrombi. By activating the patient's own fibrinolytic system, the thrombolytic enzymes increase the degradation of the fibrin clots in the blood vessels. In thrombolytic therapy the enzymes interfere with the clotting mechanism of the body, the most serious complication of which is hemorrhage. Anticoagulant therapy is contraindicated during treatment with thrombolytic enzymes. However, heparin therapy usually follows treatment with these agents.

Action/Kinetics   Promote thrombolysis by stimulating conversion of plasminogen to plasmin (fibrinolysin).

Uses   Acute, massive pulmonary embolism, pulmonary emboli accompanied by unstable hemodynamics, coronary artery thrombosis associated with myocardial infarction.

Contraindications   Any condition presenting a risk of hemorrhage, such as recent surgery or biopsies, delivery withing 10 days, pregnancy, ulcerative disease. Also hepatic or renal insufficiency, TB, recent cerebral embolism, thrombosis, hemorrhage, subacute bacterial endocarditis, rheumatic valvular disease, thrombocytopenia. The use of the drugs in septic thrombophlebitis may be hazardous. Safe use in children has not been established.

Untoward Reactions   Hemorrhage, decreased hematocrit, fever, allergic reactions, phlebitis near site of IV infusion, increased tendency to bruise.

Drug Interactions

Interactant	Interaction
Anticoagulants, oral	
Aspirin	
Heparin	↑ Chance of bleeding
Indomethacin	
Phenylbutazone	

Dosage   When administering thrombolytic agents, monitor thrombin time q 4–12 hr. It should lie between 2 and 5 times the normal control value. Dosage of thrombolytic enzyme should be decreased when values are lower than 2 times normal, increased when they exceed 5 times normal.

Nursing Implications

1. Avoid unnecessary handling of patient to prevent bruising.
2. Avoid intramuscular, intra-arterial, and intravenous injections to prevent bleeding at site of these invasive procedures.
3. Should IM injection be necessary, apply pressure after withdrawing needle, to prevent a hematoma and bleeding from puncture.
4. Use an infusion pump for IV administration.
5. Should intra-arterial injection be necessary, do not use femoral artery but rather use either the radial or brachial artery.
6. Apply manual pressure and a pressure dressing for 15 min after intra-arterial or IV injection. Retain pressure dressing in place for the next hour, and check frequently for bleeding.
7. Check that patient has had blood typed and cross-matched when receiving thrombolytic therapy.
8. Discontinue therapy if bleeding from an invasive procedure is serious, and call for packed red cells and plasma expanders (other than dextran). Have corticosteroids and aminocaproic acid (Amicar) on hand.
9. Check that thrombin time is less than 2 times normal control value (10–15 sec) before starting an infusion. After therapy with thrombolytic agents, heparin should not be started until the thrombin time again is less than 2 times the normal control value. Take blood for thrombin time to laboratory in ice bath.
10. Anticipate the use of IV heparin and oral anticoagulants after thrombolytic therapy is concluded, to prevent rethrombosis.

11. *Assess*
    a. sites of injection and postoperative wounds for bleeding during thrombolytic therapy.
    b. for allergic reactions ranging from anaphylaxis to moderate and mild reactions, usually controlled with antihistamines and corticosteroids.
    c. for redness and pain at site of IV infusion. If necessary, dilute solution further to prevent phlebitis.
12. Do not administer drugs such as indomethacin, phenylbutazone, or aspirin, which alter platelet function, without consulting medical supervision.
13. Provide symptomatic treatment for fever reaction. Acetaminophen rather than aspirin is recommended when thrombolytic agents are being administered.

STREPTOKINASE Kabikinase, Streptase (Rx)

Classification Thrombolytic agent.

Action/Kinetics Most patients have a natural resistance to streptokinase that must be overcome with the loading dose before the drug becomes effective. Thrombin time and streptokinase resistance should be determined before initiation of the therapy.

Acts by enhancing the conversion of plasminogen to plasmin; also, the streptokinase-plasminogen complex is converted to streptokinase-plasmin, which itself can convert plasminogen to plasmin. **Onset**: rapid; **duration**: 12 hr. **t½ (biphasic)**: *initial*, 18 min; *final*, 83 min.

Additional uses Lysis of deep vein thrombi, clearing occluded arteriovenous cannulae.

Additional Contraindications History of significant allergic response. Streptokinase resistance in excess of 1 million IU.

Dosage **IV**. *Venous or arterial thrombosis, arterial embolism*: **initially**, 250,000 IU over 30 min; **maintenance**: 100,000 IU/hr for 24 hr for pulmonary embolism, up to 72 hr for deep vein or arterial thrombosis. May be followed by continuous IV heparin infusion to prevent recurrent thrombosis (start only after thrombin time has decreased to less than twice the normal, control value, usually 3–4 hr). *Coronary artery thrombosis*: **initial, within 6 hr of symptoms of acute myocardial infarction**, 20,000 IU; **then**, 2,000 IU/min for 1 hr. *Arteriovenous cannula occlusion*: 250,000 IU in 2 ml IV solution into each occluded limb of cannula; **then**, after 2 hr aspirate cannula limbs, flush with saline, and reconnect cannula.

Administration/Storage
1. Sodium chloride injection USP or 5% dextrose injection is the preferred diluent.
2. Reconstitute gently as directed by manufacturer without shaking vial.
3. Use within 24 hr after reconstitution.

UROKINASE Abbokinase, Winkinase* (Rx)

Classification Thrombolytic agent.

Action/Kinetics   **Onset:** rapid; **duration:** 12 hr. **t½:** 10–15 min, although effect on coagulation disappears after a few hours.

Additional Use   To clear IV catheters.

Dosage   **IV infusion only: loading dose,** 4,400 IU/kg administered over 10 min; **maintenance, IV:** 4,400 IU/kg administered continuously over 12 hr. Total volume should not exceed 200 ml. May be followed by continuous IV heparin infusion to prevent recurrent thrombosis (start only after thrombin time has decreased to less than twice the normal control value). *Clear IV catheter:* See manufacturers' instructions.

Additional Administration/Storage

1. Reconstitute only with sterile water for injection USP without preservatives. Do not use bacteriostatic water.
2. Reconstitute immediately before using.
3. Discard any unused portion.
4. Dilute reconstituted urokinase before IV administration in 0.9% normal saline.
5. Total volume of fluid administered not to exceed 200 ml.

Part Five

CARDIOVASCULAR DRUGS

Chapter Twenty-three

CARDIAC GLYCOSIDES

Cardiac Glycosides

Deslanoside *296*

Digitalis, glycosides mixture *296*

Digitalis Leaf, powdered *296*

Digitoxin *296*

Digoxin *297*

Other

Amrinone *298*

General Statement Cardiac glycosides, such as digitalis, are plant alkaloids. They are probably the oldest, yet still the most effective drugs for treating congestive heart failure (CHF). By improving myocardial contraction, they improve blood supply to all organs, including the kidney, thus improving function. This action results in diuresis, thereby correcting the edema often associated with cardiac insufficiency. Digitalis glycosides are also used for the treatment of cardiac arrhythmias, since they decrease pulse rate as well.

The cardiac glycosides are cumulative in action. This effect is partially responsible for the difficulties associated with their use.

Action/Kinetics Cardiac glycosides increase the force of myocardial contraction. They also increase the refractory period of the atrioventricular (A-V) node, increase total peripheral resistance, and slow ventricular rate. The main action is attributed to inhibition of Na-K-activated ATPase which, in turn, increases intracellular sodium concentration. Sodium is then exchanged for extracellular calcium, thereby increasing muscle contraction. The cardiac glycosides are absorbed from the GI tract. Absorption varies from 40% to 90%, depending on the preparation and *brand*. With most preparations, peak plasma concentrations are reached within 2–3 hr. t½ ranges from 1.7 days for digoxin to 7 days for digitoxin. The drugs are primarily excreted through the kidneys either unchanged (digoxin) or metabolized (digitoxin). The initial dose of digitalis glycosides is larger (loading dose) and is traditionally referred to as the digitalizing dose (DD); subsequent doses are referred to as maintenance doses (MD).

Uses Congestive heart failure especially secondary to hypertension, coronary artery or atherosclerotic heart disease, valvular heart disease. Control of rapid ventricular contraction rate in patients with atrial fibrillation or flutter. Slow heart rate in sinus tachycardia due to congestive heart failure. Supraventricular tachycardia. Prophylaxis and treatment of recurrent paroxysmal atrial tachycardia with paroxysmal A-V junctional rhythm. In conjunction with propranolol for angina. Cardiogenic shock (value not established).

Contraindications Coronary occlusion or angina pectoris in the absence of CHF or hypersensitivity to cardiogenic glycosides. Use with caution in patients with ischemic heart disease, acute myocarditis, ventricular tachycardia, hypertrophic subaortic stenosis, hypoxic or myxedemic states, Adams-Stokes or carotid sinus syndromes, cardiac amyloidosis, or cyanotic heart and lung disease, including emphysema and partial heart block.

Electric pacemakers may sensitize the myocardium to cardiac glycosides.

The cardiac glycosides should also be given cautiously and at reduced dosage to elderly debilitated patients, pregnant women and nursing mothers, and to newborn, term, or premature infants who have immature renal and hepatic function. Similar precautions also should be observed for patients with reduced renal and/or hepatic function, since such impairment retards excretion of cardiac glycosides.

Untoward Reactions Cardiac glycosides are extremely toxic and have caused death even in patients who have received the drugs for long periods of time. There is a very narrow margin of safety between an effective therapeutic dose and a toxic dose. Overdosage caused by the cumulative effects of the drug is a constant danger in therapy with cardiac glycosides. Digitalis toxicity is characterized by a wide variety of symptoms, which are hard to differentiate from the cardiac disease itself.

CV: Changes in the rate, rhythm, and irritability of the heart and the mechanism of the heartbeat. Extrasystoles, bigeminal pulse, coupled rhythm, ectopic beat, and other forms of arrhythmias have been noted. Death most often results from ventricular fibrillation. Cardiac glycosides should be discontinued in adults when pulse rate falls below 60 beats per minute. All cardiac changes are best detected by electrocardiogram (ECG), which is also most useful in patients suffering from intoxication. Acute hemorrhage.

GI: Anorexia, nausea, vomiting, excessive salivation, epigastric distress, abdominal pain, diarrhea, bowel necrosis. Patients on digitalis therapy may experience two vomiting stages: The first is an early sign of toxicity and is a direct effect of digitalis on the GI tract. Late vomiting indicates stimulation of the vomiting center of the brain, which occurs after the heart muscle has been saturated with digitalis.

CNS: Headaches, fatigue, lassitude, irritability, malaise, muscle weakness, insomnia, stupor. Psychotomimetic effects (especially in elderly or arteriosclerotic patients or neonates) including disorientation, confusion, depression, aphasia, delirium, hallucinations, and rarely, convulsions. *Neuromuscular:* Neurologic pain involving the lower third of the face and lumbar areas, paresthesia. *Visual disturbances:* Blurred vision, flickering dots, white halos, borders around dark objects, diplopia, amblyopia, color perception changes. *Hypersensitivity (5–7 days after starting therapy):* Skin reactions (urticaria, fever, pruritus, facial and angioneurotic edema). *Other:* Chest pain, coldness of extremities.

Children: Atrial arrhythmias and atrial tachycardia with AV block are the most common signs of toxicity; in neonates excessive slowing of sinus rate, sinoatrial (S-A) arrest, and prolongation of P-R interval occur.

Patients suffering from digitalis intoxication should be admitted to the intensive care area for continuous monitoring of ECG. Administration of digitalis should be halted. If serum potassium is below normal, potassium salts should be administered. Antiarrhythmic drugs, such as phenytoin or lidocaine, can be given if ordered by the physician.

Drug Interactions One of the most serious side effects of digitalis-type drugs is hypokalemia (lowering of serum potassium levels). This may lead to cardiac arrhythmias, muscle weakness, hypotension, and respiratory distress. Other agents causing hypokalemia reinforce this effect and increase the chance of digitalis toxicity. Such reactions may occur in patients who have been on digitalis maintenance for a very long time.

Interactant	Interaction
Aminoglycosides	↓ Effect of digitalis glycosides due to ↓ absorption from GI tract
Aminosalicylic acid	↓ Effect of digitalis glycosides due to ↓ absorption from GI tract
Amphotericin B	↑ K depletion caused by digitalis: ↑ incidence of digitalis toxicity
Antacids	↓ Effect of digitalis glycosides due to ↓ absorption from GI tract
Barbiturates	↓ Effect of digitalis glycosides due to ↑ breakdown by liver
Calcium preparations	Cardiac arrhythmias if parenteral calcium given with digitalis
Chlorthalidone	↑ K and Mg loss with ↑ chance of digitalis toxicity
Cholestyramine	Cholestyramine binds digitoxin in the intestine and ↓ its absorption
Colestipol	Colestipol binds digitoxin in the intestine and ↓ its absorption
Ephedrine	↑ Chance of cardiac arrhythmias
Epinephrine	↑ Chance of cardiac arrhythmias

Interactant	Interaction
Ethacrynic acid	↑ K and Mg loss with ↑ chance of digitalis toxicity
Furosemide	↑ K and Mg loss with ↑ chance of digitalis toxicity
Glucose infusions	Large infusions of glucose may cause ↓ in serum K and ↑ chance of digitalis toxicity
Hypoglycemic drugs	↓ Effect of digitalis glycosides due to ↑ breakdown by liver
Methimazole	↑ Chance of toxic effects of digitalis
Penicillamine	↓ Effect of digoxin
Phenylbutazone	↓ Effect of digitalis glycosides by ↑ breakdown by liver
Phenytoin	↓ Effect of digitalis glycosides by ↑ breakdown by liver
Procainamide	↑ Effect of digitalis glycosides
Propranolol	Propranolol potentiates digitalis-induced bradycardia
Quinidine	↑ Effect of cardiac glycosides
Reserpine	↑ Chance of cardiac arrhythmias
Rifampin	↓ Effect of digitoxin due to ↑ breakdown by the liver
Succinylcholine	↑ Chance of cardiac arrhythmias
Sympathomimetics	↑ Chance of cardiac arrhythmias
Thiazides	↑ K and Mg loss with ↑ chance of digitalis toxicity
Thyroid hormones	↑ Effectiveness of digitalis glycosides

Laboratory Test Interferences   May ↓ prothrombin time. Alters tests for 17-ketosteroids and 17-hydroxycorticosteroids.

Dosage   **PO, IM, or IV.**   *Highly individualized.* See Table 8, p. 296 for usual dosages.
Initially the drugs are usually given at higher ("digitalizing" or loading) doses. These are reduced as soon as the desired therapeutic effect is achieved or undesirable toxic reactions develop. The response of the patient to cardiac glycosides is gauged by clinical and ECG observations.

There are considerable differences in the rates at which patients become digitalized. Patients with mild signs of congestion can often be digitalized gradually over a period of several days. Patients suffering from more serious congestion, for example, those showing signs of acute left ventricular failure, dyspnea, or lung edema, can be digitalized more rapidly by parenteral administration of a fast-acting cardiac glycoside.

Once digitalization has been attained (pulse 68–80 beats/min) and symptoms of CHF have subsided, the patient is put on maintenance dosage. Depending on the drug and the age of the patient, the daily maintenance dose is often approximately 10% of the digitalizing dose.

Administration
1. Check the order, the medication card, and the bottle label of the medication to be given, since many of the cardiac glycosides have similar names. Their dosage and duration of effect differ markedly.

2. Measure all PO liquid cardiac medications precisely with a calibrated dropper or a syringe.
3. Administer after meals to lessen gastric irritation.

Nursing Implications

FOR PATIENTS STARTING ON A DIGITALIZING DOSE

1. Ascertain that the following laboratory tests have been completed and reviewed before administering medication: hemoglobin, hematocrit, serum electrolytes, and liver and renal function tests. The findings of these tests serve as a baseline in making a differential diagnosis and in determining the course of therapy. Laboratory tests should be repeated periodically and the results reviewed.
2. Ascertain that an ECG has been completed and reviewed before administration. Be prepared to assist by connecting patient to a cardiac monitor, which must be closely assessed.

FOR PATIENTS BEING DIGITALIZED AND FOR PATIENTS ON A MAINTENANCE DOSE OF CARDIAC GLYCOSIDE

1. *Assess*
   a. for bradycardia and/or arrhythmias by monitoring cardiac monitor, or count the apical rate for at least 1 min before administering the drug. If the adult pulse rate is below 60 beats/min (children, 90–110) or an arrhythmia not previously noted occurs, withhold the drug and consult immediately with the physician. Obtain written doctor's orders, indicating the pulse rates—both high and low—at which cardiac glycoside is to be withheld. Be aware that *any* change in rate *or* rhythm can indicate digitalis toxicity.
   b. for pulse deficit, by taking the apical radial pulse simultaneously for 1 minute with another nurse. Withhold drug and report pulse deficit, as this is indicative of an adverse effect.
   c. for persistent cough, dyspnea, and chest rales, indicating CHF.
   d. for edema. Weigh patient q.d. and report significant weight gain. Measure calf for edema 5 cm above the medial malleolus, and measure abdomen for ascites at the level of the umbilicus. Compare measurements daily while patient is being digitalized. Assess dependent areas, such as the posterior calves and sacrum, for pitting edema.
   e. for adequate intake and output to ensure adequate hydration and elimination, which will help prevent a cumulative toxic effect.
   f. for symptoms of toxicity noted in *Untoward Reactions*.
2. Provide patient with food high in potassium, such as orange juice and bananas. Explain to patient the necessity for taking oral potassium supplement if ordered by the doctor. Request the pharmacy to provide the most palatable preparation of potassium available. (Potassium preparations are usually bitter.)
3. Anticipate that patient on non-potassium-sparing diuretics and a cardiac glycoside will require potassium supplementation.
4. Space doses of antacids (if ordered) containing aluminum or magnesium and kaolin/pectin mixtures at least 6 hr apart from cardiac glycosides to prevent decreased therapeutic effect of glycoside.
5. Use cardiac monitor for newborns to identify early toxicity manifested by excessive slowing of sinus rate, sinoatrial arrest, and prolongation of P-R interval.

(continued on page 298)

TABLE 8 CARDIAC GLYCOSIDES[a]

Drug	Digitalizing Dose(DD) and Maintenance Dose(MD)	Onset (ON) and Duration (DR)	Remarks
Deslanoside (Cedilanid,* Cedilanid-D, Desacetyl-lanatoside-C) Rx	**DD: IM** or **IV**, 1.6 mg in 1–2 equal doses; **pediatric, IM** or **IV:** 0.022 mg/kg body weight. **MD:** Switch to **PO** preparation.	**ON:** 10–30 min **DR:** 3–6 days. t½: approx. 33–36 hr. Peak effect: 20 min.	Used for rapid digitalization in emergency situations (acute cardiac failure with pulmonary edema, atrial arrhythmias). Injection vehicle contains ethyl alcohol and glycerin. Protect from light.
Digitalis, glycosides mixture (Digiglusin) Rx	**DD (rapid): PO, initially, 6 USP** units; **then,** 4 USP units 4–6 hr later followed by 2 USP units q 4–6 hr until therapeutic effect reached. **DD (slow):** 2 USP units b.i.d. for 4 days. **MD:** 0.5–3 USP units/day.	**ON:** 25 min to 2 hr; maximum effect: 4–12 hr. **DR:** 2–3 weeks. (See *Digitoxin*)	
Digitalis leaf, powered Rx	**DD: PO:** 50–150 mg 3–4 times daily for 3–4 days to a maximum of 1.2 gm. **MD: Usual,** 100–200 mg daily (range: 30–400 mg daily).	**ON:** 25 min to 2 hr; maximum effect: 4–12 hr. **DR:** 2–3 weeks (See *Digitoxin*)	This preparation contains standardized amounts of dried leaves of *Digitalis purpurea* plant for PO use
Digitoxin (Crystodigin, Purodigin) Rx	**Adults. DD: DD: IV, PO (rapid):** 0.6 mg followed by 0.4 mg in 4–6 hr; **then,** 0.2 mg q 4–6 hr until therapeutic effect reached. **DD: PO (slow):** 0.2 mg b.i.d.for 4 days. **MD: PO:** 0.05–0.3 mg/day **(usual):** 0.15 mg/day). **Pediatric. DD: PO, IV** (give in 3–4 doses, with 6 hr between doses), **premature and newborn:** 0.022 mg/kg;	**ON: PO,** 1.5–6 hr; maximum effect: 6–12 hr; **IV,** 25–120 min; maximum effect: 1.5–3 hr. **DR:** 2–3 weeks; t½: 7–9 days; therapeutic plasma levels: 10–25 ng/ml	Most potent of digitalis glycosides. Its slow onset of action makes it unsuitable for emergency use. Drug of choice for maintenance. 1 mg digitoxin is therapeutically equivalent to 1 gm digitalis leaf. Is almost completely absorbed from GI tract. Withhold drug and check with doctor if plasma level exceeds 34 ng/ml, indicating toxicity. *Administration:* Inject deeply into gluteal muscle. *Storage:* Incompatible with acids and alkali. Protect from light

| Digoxin (Lanoxicaps, Lanoxin) Rx | **under 1 year:** 0.045 mg/kg; **1–2 years:** 0.04 mg/kg; **over 2 years:** 0.03 mg/kg. **MD:** 1/10 of the digitalizing dose.

Adults and children over 10 yr. DD: IV, 0.5–1 mg in divided doses q 4–6 hr. **DD: PO (rapid),** initially, 0.5–0.75 mg; **then,** 0.25–0.5 mg q 6–8 hr until therapeutic effect achieved. **MD:** 0.125–0.5 mg/day; **for elderly,** 0.125–0.25 mg/day. **Children under 10 yr. DD: IV,** in divided doses, **Premature and newborn (up to 2 weeks):** 0.025–0.040 mg/kg; **2 weeks to 2 years:** 0.025–0.050 mg/kg; **2–10 years:** 0.025–0.040 mg/kg. Initially, one-fourth to one-half the calculated dose; then, one-fourth the total dose q 6 hr until dosage completed. **DD: PO:** in divided doses, **up to 30 days of age:** 0.040–0.060 mg/kg; **1–24 months:** 0.060–0.080 mg/kg; **2–10 years:** 0.040–0.060 mg/kg. **MD:** 20–30% of the digitalizing dose/day. In all patients reduce dosage in impaired renal function. | **ON: PO,** 0.5–2 hr; maximum effect: 2–6 hr; **IV,** 5–30 min; maximum effect: 1.5–3 hr. **DR:** 2–6 days. **t½:** 35 hr; therapeutic plasma level: 0.8–2.0 ng/ml. | Action more prompt and shorter than digitoxin. Injection vehicle contains propylene glycol, sodium phosphate, and citric acid. May be drug of choice for CHF because of (1) rapid onset, (2) relatively short duration, (3) can be administered PO, IV. *Storage:* Incompatible with acids and alkali. Protect from light.
Additional Drug Interactions
1. The following drugs increase serum digoxin levels leading to possible toxicity: anticholinergics, erythromycin, hydroxychloroquine, tetracyclines, verapamil.
2. Penicillamine decreases serum digoxin levels. |

[a] Abbreviations: DD, digitalizing dose; MD, maintenance dose; ON, onset; DR duration; USP, United States Pharmacopeia.

6. Be alert to cardiac arrhythmias in children, as they occur more frequently as signs of toxicity.

7. Assess the patient for positive response to digitalization, as shown by improvement in rate and rhythm of heartbeat, improvement in breathing, reduction in weight, and diuresis.

8. Refer patient and/or family requiring assistance in health maintenance to a community health agency.

9. *Teach patient and/or family*

   a. why regular medical supervision is essential.

   b. to continue same brand of cardiac glycoside on which patient was stabilized in hospital.

   c. to follow directions for taking medication.

   d. to check with doctor if one dose is accidentally missed and not to double up on the following dosage of medication. Develop a checklist that the patient can mark when taking medication. This technique is particularly useful for elderly patients with memory loss.

   e. to take medication after meals.

   f. to discard any previously prescribed cardiac glycosides, to avoid mistakes.

   g. how to count pulse before taking the medication. Emphasize guidelines for withholding and reporting to doctor.

   h. how to recognize toxic symptoms. Provide a list of toxic symptoms; stress need for early recognition of toxicity and prompt reporting, especially anorexia, often the earliest symptom.

   i. to record weight every morning before breakfast. Report rapid weight gain. Bring written record of weights to doctor at time of appointment.

   j. how to maintain a low-salt (sodium) diet. Encourage intake of foods rich in potassium as well as ingestion of potassium preparations, if ordered.

   k. not to take any other medication before consulting with doctor, because drug interactions occur frequently with cardiac glycosides.

   l. to be alert to persistent cough, difficulty in breathing, and edema, all signs of CHF that must be promptly reported to doctor.

   m. to adhere to written instructions. Review these instructions with the patient and/or family at least several days before discharge.

AMRINONE LACTATE   Inocor I.V. (Rx)

Classification   Cardiac inotropic agent.

Action/Kinetics   Amrinone causes an increase in cardiac output by increasing the force of contraction of the heart as well as by vasodilation. It reduces afterload and preload by directly relaxing vascular smooth muscle. **t½:** 3.6 hr. **Plasma levels:** 3.0 μg/ml. **Peak effect:** 10 min. **Duration:** 30 min–2 hr.

Uses   Congestive heart failure (short-term therapy in patients unresponsive to digitalis, diuretics, and/or vasodilators). Can be used in digitalized patients.

Contraindications   Hypersensitivity to bisulfites. Severe aortic or pulmonary valvular disease in lieu of surgery. Acute myocardial infarction. Safety and efficacy in pregnancy, lactation, and in children not established.

Untoward Reactions   *GI:* Nausea, vomiting, abdominal pain, anorexia. *CV:* Hypotension, arrhythmias. *Other:* Thrombocytopenia, hepatotoxicity, fever, chest pain, burning at site of injection, hypersensitivity reactions.

Drug Interactions   Excessive hypotension when used with disopyramide.

Dosage   **IV. Initial:** 0.75 mg/kg as bolus slowly over 2–3 min. **Maintenance, IV infusion:** 5–10 μg/kg/min. Depending on response, an additional bolus of 0.75 mg/kg may be given 30 min after initiation of therapy. Daily dose should not exceed 10 mg/kg although up to 18 mg/kg/day has been used in some patients for short periods.

Administration

1. Amrinone should not be diluted with solutions containing dextrose (glucose) prior to injection. However, the drug may be injected into running dextrose (glucose) infusions through a Y-connector or directly into the tubing.
2. Protect from light and store at room temperature.

Nursing Implications

1. Be aware that patient will be on a cardiac monitor while on this drug.
2. Monitor serum potassium levels.
3. Note any drop in blood pressure; drug can cause hypotension.
4. Monitor platelet counts and report any bruises or bleeding.
5. Be aware drug has unusual hypersensitivity reactions including pericarditis, pleuritis, and ascites.

Chapter Twenty-four

CORONARY VASODILATORS (ANTIANGINAL DRUGS)

Nitrites/Nitrates

Calcium Channel Blocking Drugs

Other Vasodilators

General Statement   Most coronary vasodilating drugs are either nitrites or nitrates. Their chemical, pharmacologic, and clinical actions are closely related, and they are treated here as a group.

Drugs that improve the peripheral circulation specifically used for the treatment of peripheral vascular disease are discussed under *Peripheral Vasodilators*, p. 311.

Organic nitrites and nitrates are the oldest and still the most widely used vasodilating drugs.

In addition to lowering the oxygen requirement of the myocardium, the nitrates probably redistribute blood flow in the heart in favor of regions that require more oxygen, selectively dilating large coronary vessels. The latter effect results in a drop in blood pressure and a decrease in the cardiac stroke volume.

The action of the nitrites on the coronary vessels of the heart (dilation, redistribution of blood flow) and the decrease in cardiac work abolish the acute oxygen shortage (hypoxia) of the heart muscle. This relieves the acute pain characteristic of angina pectoris.

The dilation of the capacitance vessels (veins) peripherally may cause syncope in a standing subject.

Action/Kinetics   Systemically, the primary effect of the cardiac glycosides is to reduce the oxygen requirements of the myocardium. The various nitrates have different durations of action. (See Table 9.) Onset is usually very rapid, and duration short, when the drugs are given sublingually, the usual route of administration. Oral administration results in slower onset and a prolonged activity. Several systems for prolonged transdermal administration have been developed.

TABLE 9   CORONARY VASODILATORS (ORGANIC NITRITES)

Drug	Amyl nitrite (Amyl Nitrite Aspirols, Amyl Nitrite Vaporoles) Rx
Pharmacokinetics	**ON**: Nasal inhalation, 30 sec; **DUR**: 3–5 min.
Dosage	*Angina Pectoris*: 0.18–0.3 ml (1 container crushed). *Cyanide poisoning*: inhalation, q 30 to 60 sec until patient regains consciousness and at increasingly longer intervals for the next 24 hr; **then**, switch to IV sodium nitrite as soon as possible.
Remarks	Also used for acute cyanide poisoning. Administer by inhalation only. *Additional Nursing Implications* *1. Amyl nitrite vapors are highly flammable. Do not use near flame or intense heat* *2. Teach patient and/or family* a. to enclose fabric-covered ampule in a handkerchief or piece of cloth and to crush by hand. b. to sit down during inhalation to avoid hypotension. c. that drug has a pungent odor, but several deep breaths must nevertheless be taken.
Drug	Erythrityl tetranitrate (Cardilate) Rx
Pharmacokinetics	**Sublingual, Chewable: ON**: 5 min; maximum effect; 30–45 min. **DUR**: 2 hrs. **PO. ON**: 30 min; maximum effect: 1–1½ hr; **DUR**: 4–6 hr.
Dosage	**Sublingual**: 5–10 mg; **PO: initial**, 10–30 mg t.i.d.

TABLE 9 (*Continued*)

Remarks	*Uses*: Prophylaxis and chronic treatment of angina. Diffuse esophageal spasm.
	May improve exercise tolerance. Not indicated for acute attacks of angina pectoris. Tolerance may develop.
	Additional Nursing Implications
	1. Report headache and/or GI upset, which may require dosage reduction early in therapy.
	2. Administer analgesic for headache as ordered
	3. *Teach patient and/or family*
	a. that all activity restrictions cannot be removed even though drug may permit more normal activity.
	b. that sublingual tingling sensations may be relieved by placing tablet in buccal pouch.

Drug	Isosorbide dinitrate chewable (Isordil, Onset-5 and -10, Sorate-5 and -10, Sorbitrate) Rx
	Isosorbide dinitrate oral (Apo-ISDN, Coronex,* Dilatrate-SR, Iso-Bid, Isonate, Isonate TR, Isordil Tembids, Isordil Titradose, Isotrate Timecelles, Novosorbide,* Sorate-40, Sorbide T.D., Sorbitrate, Sorbitrate SA) Rx
	Isosorbide dinitrate sublingual (Coronex,* Isonate 2.5 mg SL and 5 mg SL, Isordil, Sorate-2.5 and -5, Sorbitrate) Rx
Pharmacokinetics	**Sublingual chewable. On**: 3 min. **DUR**: 1–2 hr. **PO. ON**: 15–30 min. **DUR**: 4–6 hr. **Extended release. ON**: 30 min; **DUR**: 12 hr.
Dosage	**Chewable tablets**: 5 mg as often as tolerated for acute attack or q 4–6 hr for prophylaxis. **Oral tablets: Prophylaxis,** 5–30 mg q.i.d. **Sustained release**: 40 mg q 6–12 hr. **Sublingual**: *Acute attack*, 2.5–10 mg. (up to 40 mg may be necessary) as often as tolerated, or q 4–6 hr for prophylaxis.
Remarks	*Additional Use*: Diffuse esophageal spasm. Oral tablets are only for prophylaxis while sublingual and chewable forms may be used to terminate acute attacks of angina. Vascular headaches occur especially frequently. Administer with meals to eliminate or reduce headaches; otherwise, take on an empty stomach.

Drug	Nitroglycerin intravenous (Nitro-Bid IV, Nitrol IV, Nitrostat IV, Tridil) Rx
Pharmacokinetics	**ON**: Immediate; **DUR**: 3–5 min.
Dosage	**IV infusion only. Initial**: 5 µg/min delivered by precise infusion pump. May be increased by 5 µg/min q 3–5 min until response seen. If no response seen at 20 µg/min, dose can be increased by 10–20 µg/min until response noted. Monitor continously to titrate each patient to desired level of response.
Remarks	Also used for hypertension associated with surgery and congestive heart failure associated with acute myocardial infraction.
	Administration
	1. Use only a glass IV bottle and administration set provided by the manufacturer because nitroglycerin is readily adsorbed onto many plastics. Avoid adding unneccssary plastic to IV system.
	2. Aspirate medication into a syringe and then inject immediately into a glass bottle (or polyolefin bottle) to minimize contact with plastic.

(continued)

TABLE 9 (*Continued*)

3. Administer with a volumetric infusion pump rather than a peristaltic pump to regulate flow more accurately.
4. Do not administer with any other medications in the IV system.
5. Do not interrupt IV nitroglycerin for administration of a bolus of any other medication.
6. To provide correct dosage, remove 15 ml from tubing if concentration of solution is changed.
7. Dilute with 5% dextrose, USP, or 0.9% sodium chloride injection.

Nursing Implications

1. Monitor continuously heart rate, blood pressure, central venous pressure, and pulmonary artery pressure to ensure maintenance of adequate vital signs with systemic perfusion.
2. Anticipate that after initial positive response, dosage increments will be smaller and adjustments will be made at longer intervals.
3. Be prepared with volume expanders for borderline hypotensive patients.
4. Be alert to hypotension, sweating, nausea and vomiting, and tachycardia/bradycardia, which indicate that the dose is more than the patient can tolerate. Elevate legs to restore blood pressure and be prepared to reduce solution rate or administer additional IV fluids.
5. Have propranolol available to counteract sinus tachycardia, which may occur in a patient with angina pectoris while he is receiving a maintenance dose of nitroglycerin. A heart rate of 80 or less is preferred to reduce myocardial demand.
6. Assess for thrombophlebitis at IV site. Be prepared to remove IV from reddened area and assist with reinsertion.
7. Check that topical, oral, or sublingual doses are adjusted if patient is on concomitant therapy with IV nitroglycerin.
8. Anticipate that patient will be weaned from IV nitroglycerin by tapering doses to avoid pretherapy or cardiovascular distress. Tapering is usually initiated when the patient is receiving the peak effect from oral or topical vasodilators. The IV flow is usually reduced, and the patient is monitored for hypertension and angina, which would require increased titration.

Drug	Nitroglycerin sublingual (Nitrostat) Rx
	Nitroglycerin sustained release (Klavikirdal, N-G-C, Niong, Nitro-Bid Plateau Caps, Nitrocap 6.5 and T.D., Nitroglyn, Nitrolin, Nitro-Long, Nitronet, Nitrong, Nitrospan, Nitrostat SR, Trates Granucaps) Rx
	Nitroglycerin, topical (Nitro-Bid, Nitrol, Nitrong, Nitrostat) Rx
Pharmacokinetics	**Sublingual. ON**: 2 min. **DUR**: up to 30 min. **Topical. ON**: 20–60 min. **DUR**: 2–12 hr. **Sustained Release. ON**: 40 min. **DUR**: 8–12 hr.
Dosage	**Sublingual**: 150–600 μg q 2–3 hr, as required. For *acute attacks*: 150–600 μg 5 min until pain relieved. **Sustained release**: 1 capsule or tablet (1.3–9 mg) q 8–12 hr on an empty stomach. **Topical ointment** (2%): 1–2 inches q 8 hr (up to 5 inches q 4 hr may be necessary). One inch = approximately 15 mg nitroglycerin. Determine optimum

TABLE 9 (*Continued*)

	dosage by starting with ½ inch q 8 hr and increasing by ½ inch each successive dose until headache occurs; then, decrease to largest dose that does not cause headache. When ending treatment, reduce both the dose and frequency of administration over 4-6 weeks to prevent sudden withdrawal reactions.
Remarks	Drug of choice for prophylaxis and treatment of angina pectoris. Sustained release and ointment preparations are used to prevent anginal attacks. *Additional Nursing Implications* (topical administration) 1. Squeeze ointment onto dose measuring application papers, which are packaged with the medicine, and spread with applicator. 2. Use the paper to spread the ointment onto a nonhairy area of skin. Many patients find application to chest psychologically helpful, but it may be applied to other nonhairy areas. Rotate sites to prevent irritation. 3. Apply in a thin, even layer covering an area of skin 5-6 inches in diameter. 4. Either tape the application paper over the area or place a piece of plastic wrap-type material to cover medicated area. A clear plastic covering leaks less ointment, decreases skin irritation, and increases amount absorbed. 5. Once the dose is established, use the same type of covering to ensure that the same amount of drug is absorbed during each application. 6. Tighten cap of tube after use. 7. The nurse should protect her skin from contact with the ointment to prevent absorption into her system. Wash hands after application.
Drug	Nitroglycerin transdermal system [Nitrodisc 5 mg/24 hr (16 mg) and 10 mg/24 hr (32 mg); Nitro-Dur 5 cm² (26 mg), 10 cm² (51 mg), 15 cm² (77 mg), 20 cm² (104 mg), 30 cm² (154 mg); Transderm-Nitro 2.5 (12.5 mg), 5 (25 mg), 10 (50 mg), 15 (75 mg).] Rx **ON**: 30–60 min; **DUR**: 24 hr. For every square centimeter of Nitro-Dur, 0.5 mg nitroglycerin is released every 24 hr. For Nitrodisc and Transderm-Nitro, the amount released is indicated by the name (e.g., Nitrodisc 5 mg releases 5 mg/day and Transderm-Nitro 2.5 releases 2.5 mg/day).
Dosage	**Initial**: 1 pad applied each day to skin site free of hair and free of excessive movement (e.g., chest, upper arm). **Maintenance**: Additional systems may be added depending on the clinical response.
Remarks	To avoid skin irritation, the application site should be slightly different each day. Do not apply to distal areas of extremities. If the pad loosens, apply a new pad. Follow instructions for specific products on package insert.
Drug	Nitroglycerin transmucosal (Nitrogard-SR*, Susadrin) Rx
Pharmacokinetics	**ON**: 3 min; **DUR**: 6 hr.
Dosage	**Initial**: 1 mg on arising, after lunch, and after evening meal; **then**, increase dose (use 2 mg tablet) if angina occurs while tablet is in place or increase to 4 tablets daily if angina occurs between tablet use. *Acute prophylaxis*: Do not use more than 1 tablet q 2 hr.
Remarks	Tablet should be placed either between the lip and gum above the upper incisors or between the gum and cheek

TABLE 9   (*Continued*)

	in the buccal area. Three to 5 hr are required for tablet dissolution. Allow tablet to dissolve in mouth; do not swallow. Store in tightly closed container below 30°C (86°F).
Drug	Pentaerythritol tetranitrate (Duotrate Plateau and 45 Plateau, Naptrate, Pentol, Pentol S.A., Pentraspan SR, Pentritol, Pentylan, Peritrate, Peritrate SA, P.E.T.N., Vaso-80 Unicelles) Rx
Pharmacokinetics	**ON:** 20–60 min. **DUR:** 4–5 hr. **t½:** 10 min. **Sustained release: ON:** slow; **DUR:** 12 hr. Excreted in urine and feces.
Dosage	**PO. Initial,** 10–20 mg t.i.d.–q.i.d.; **then,** up to 40 mg q.i.d. **Extended release:** 30-80 mg b.i.d.
Remarks	Available in combination with rapid-acting nitrates (e.g., Peritrate with nitroglycerin). Used for prophylaxis of angina attacks but not to be used to terminate acute attacks. Long-term use may induce tolerance to nitroglycerin. *Additional Untoward Reactions* Severe rash, exfoliative dermatitis. *Administration/Storage* Drug is taken ½ hr before or 1 hr after meals as well as at bedtime. Sustained release tablets are taken on an empty stomach.

Uses   Acute attacks of angina pectoris and prophylactic therapy aimed at reducing their number and severity. *IV nitroglycerin:* Decrease blood pressure in surgical procedures resulting in hypertension. *Investigational:* Reduce workload of heart in acute myocardial infarction (MI) and CHF. *Nitroglycerin ointment:* Adjunct in treating Raynaud's disease.

Contraindications   Sensitivity to nitrites, which may result in severe hypotensive reactions, MI, or tolerance to nitrites. Use with caution in patients with glaucoma, head trauma, cerebral hemorrhage, or anemia.

Untoward Reactions   Severe toxicity is rarely encountered with therapeutic use. *CNS:* Headaches (most common), syncope, dizziness, weakness. *CV:* Postural hypotension (common), tachycardia, transient flushing, cardiovascular collapse. *GI:* Nausea, vomiting, dry mouth. *Miscellaneous:* Rash, skin pallor, cold sweating, involuntary urination and/or defecation, blurred vision. **Topical use:** Peripheral edema, contact dermatitis.

Tolerance can occur following chronic use. Nitrites convert hemoglobin to methemoglobin, which impairs the oxygen-carrying capacity of the blood, resulting in anemic hypoxia. This interaction is dangerous in patients with preexisting anemia.

Drug Interactions

Interactant	Interaction
Alcohol, ethyl	Hypotension due to vasodilator effect of both agents
Antihypertensive drugs	Additive hypotension
Dihydroergotamine	↑ Effect dihydroergotamine due to increased blood levels
Phenothiazines	Additive hypotension

Laboratory Test Interference   ↑ Urinary catecholamines.

Dosage   See Table 9, p. 300.

Administration   Nitrites and nitrates are available in a variety of dosage forms including sublingual, chewable, topical, transdermal, oral, inhalation, and parenteral. It is important to understand the appropriate use of each of these dosage forms.

Storage   Avoid exposure to air, heat, and moisture.

Nursing Implications

1. Allow the hospitalized patient to keep sublingual tablets at bedside, but note
   a. how much of the drug the patient requires to relieve angina.
   b. how frequently the drug is taken.
   c. whether the relief is partial or complete.
   d. length of time before relief.
   e. whether side effects are occurring. Chart observations.
2. *Assess*
   a. for tolerance, which may begin several days after treatment is started and which is manifested by absence of response to the usual dose. Nitrites may be discontinued temporarily until such tolerance is lost and then reinstituted. During the interim, other vasodilators may be ordered.
   b. patients taking nitrites that have prolonged effects; observe for nausea, headache, vomiting, drowsiness, and visual disturbances during long-term prophylaxis.
   c. for sensitivity to the hypotensive effects of nitrites, symptoms of which include nausea, vomiting, pallor, restlessness, and collapse.
   d. patients on additional therapy with other drugs that cause hypotension; potentiation of hypotension would mandate dosage adjustment.
3. *Teach patient and/or family*
   a. to carry sublingual tablets for use in aborting an attack, to observe the expiration date on the bottle, and to obtain a fresh bottle when needed.
   b. to carry sublingual tablets in a *glass* bottle, tightly capped. Do not use plastic containers or bottles with child proof caps as patient must get to the tablets quickly.
   c. if anginal pain is not relieved in 5 min by first sublingual tablet, to take up to 2 more at 5-min intervals. If pain has not subsided 5 min after third tablet, patient should be taken to emergency room by family or ambulance. Patient should **not** drive himself.
   d. to take sublingual tablets 5–15 min prior to any situation likely to cause anginal pain: climbing stairs, sexual intercourse, exposure to cold weather.
   e. to take sublingual tablet while sitting or lying down, to prevent postural hypotension.
   f. not to drink alcohol, because nitrite syncope, a severe shocklike state, may occur.
   g. how to apply topical nitroglycerin (see p. 303).

CALCIUM CHANNEL BLOCKING DRUGS

Action/Kinetics   Calcium ions are important for generation of action potentials and for excitation/contraction of muscles. For contraction of cardiac and smooth muscle to occur, extracellular calcium must move into the cell through openings called calcium channels. The calcium channel blocking agents (also called slow channel blockers or calcium antagonists) inhibit the influx of calcium through the cell membrane, resulting in a depression of automaticity and conduction velocity in both smooth and cardiac muscle. This leads to a depression of contraction in these tissues.

In the myocardium, these drugs dilate coronary vessels and inhibit spasms of coronary arteries. They also decrease total peripheral resistance, thus reducing energy and oxygen requirements of the heart. These effects benefit various types of angina.

These agents also are effective against certain cardiac arrhythmias by slowing AV conduction and prolonging repolarization. In addition, they depress the amplitude, rate of depolarization, and conduction in atria.

Treatment of Overdosage

1. Hypotension: IV isoproterenol, metaraminol, norepinephrine, calcium.
2. Ventricular tachycardia: IV procainamide or lidocaine; also, cardioversion.
3. Bradycardia, asystole, A–V block: IV atropine sulfate, calcium, isoproterenol, norepinephrine; also, cardiac pacing.

DILTIAZEM HCI   Cardizem (Rx)

Classification   Calcium channel blocker: antianginal and antiarrhythmic.

Action/Kinetics   See information under *Calcium Channel Blocking Drugs.* **Onset:** 30 min. **Time to peak plasma levels:** 2–3 hr. **t½:** 3.5–9 hr. **Therapeutic serum levels:** 0.04–0.2 μg/ml.

Uses   Chronic stable angina, angina due to coronary artery spasm. *Investigational:* Essential hypertension.

Contraindications   Hypotension, second- or third-degree A–V block, sick sinus syndrome. Use with caution in hepatic disease. Safety for use in pregnancy, lactation, and children has not been established.

Untoward Reactions   *CV:* AV block, bradycardia, congestive heart failure, hypotension, peripheral edema, arrhythmias. *GI:* Nausea, diarrhea, constipation. *CNS:* Fatigue, weakness, nervousness, dizziness, lightheadedness, disturbances in sleep. *Dermatologic:* Rashes, pruritus, urticaria. *Other:* Photosensitivity, joint pain or stiffness, elevated liver enzymes.

Dosage   **PO. Initial:** 30 mg q.i.d. before meals and at bedtime; **then,** increase gradually to total daily dose of 240 mg given in 3–4 divided doses q 1–2 days.

Administration

1. Sublingual nitroglycerin may be given concomitantly for acute angina.
2. Diltiazem may be given together with long-acting nitrates.

Nursing Implications

Teach patient and/or family

1. to take pulse and blood pressure at home at the same time of day at least twice a week and to report to the physician a drop in pulse rate of more than 10 beats/min or a drop in blood pressure of more than 20 mm either systolic or diastolic.
2. to continue carrying short-acting nitrites (nitroglycerin) at all times as directed by the physician.

NIFEDIPINE Adalat,* Procardia (Rx)

Classification Calcium channel blocker: antianginal and antiarrhythmic.

Action/Kinetics See information under *Calcium Channel Blocking Drugs.* **Onset:** 20 min. **Time to peak plasma levels:** 0.5 hr. **t½:** 2–5 hr. **Therapeutic serum levels:** 0.025–0.1 μg/ml.

Uses Vasospastic angina, chronic stable angina (effort-associated angina). *Investigational:* PO or sublingually in hypertensive emergencies, Raynaud's phenomenon, primary pulmonary hypertension and asthma.

Contraindications Hypersensitivity. Safety for use in pregnancy and lactation not established.

Untoward Reactions *CV:* Peripheral and pulmonary edema, myocardial infarction, ventricular arrhythmias, conduction disturbances, hypotension, palpitations, syncope, congestive heart failure. *GI:* Nausea, diarrhea, constipation, flatulence, abdominal cramps. *CNS:* Dizziness, lightheadedness, nervousness, sleep disturbances, headache, weakness, disturbances in equilibrium. *Dermatologic:* Rash, urticaria, pruritus. *Respiratory:* Dyspnea, cough, wheezing, throat, nasal congestion. *Musculoskeletal:* Muscle cramps, joint pain or stiffness. *Other:* Fever, chills, sweating, blurred vision, sexual difficulties, hepatitis.

Drug Interactions

Interactant	Interaction
Beta-adrenergic blocking agents	↑ Risk of congestive heart failure, severe hypotension, or exacerbation of angina
Cimetidine	↑ Effect of nifedipine
Digoxin	↑ Effect digoxin by ↓ excretion by kidney
Quinidine	Possible ↓ effect of quinidine

Dosage PO. **Individualized.** Initial: 10 mg t.i.d.; **maintenance:** 10–30 mg t.i.d.–q.i.d. Doses greater than 180 mg daily are not recommended.

Administration

1. Before increasing the dose, blood pressure should be carefully monitored.
2. A single dose should not exceed 30 mg.
3. Concomitant therapy with beta-adrenergic blocking agents may be undertaken; however, note drug interaction above.
4. Sublingual nitroglycerin and long-acting nitrates may be used concomitantly with nifedipine.
5. Protect capsules from light and moisture and store at room temperature in original container.

Nursing Implications

1. *Assess*
   a. during titration period for excessive hypotensive response and increased heart rate due to peripheral vasodilation. These untoward effects may precipitate angina.
   b. patient who is also receiving a beta-adrenergic blocking agent for development of severe hypotension, heart failure, or exacerbation of angina.

(continued)

c. patient who has recently terminated therapy with a beta-blocker for withdrawal syndrome characterized by increased angina.

d. patient for peripheral edema that may result from arterial vasodilation precipitated by nifedipine or may indicate increasing ventricular dysfunction. If peripheral edema is noted, assess further for signs of congestive failure such as weakness, breathlessness, and abdominal discomfort.

2. If therapy with a beta-blocker is to be discontinued, taper dosage to prevent withdrawal syndrome.

3. *Teach patient and/or family* to take pulse and blood pressure at home at the same time of day at least twice a week and to report to the physician any significant change, especially an increase in pulse rate and a decrease in blood pressure.

VERAPAMIL   Calan, Isoptin (Rx)

Classification   Calcium channel blocker: antianginal and antiarrhythmic.

Action/Kinetics   See information under *Calcium Channel Blocking Drugs.* **Onset: PO,** 30 min; **IV,** 3–5 min. **Time to peak plasma levels (PO):** 1–2 hr. **t½:** 3–7 hr. **Therapeutic serum levels:** 0.08–0.3 µg/ml.

Uses   Angina pectoris due to coronary artery spasm, chronic stable angina, preinfarction angina (unstable, crescendo), supraventricular tachyarrhythmias (IV), to control rapid ventricular rate in atrial flutter or fibrillation. *Investigational:* Prophylaxis of migraine.

Contraindications   Severe hypotension, second- or third-degree A–V block, cardiogenic shock, severe congestive heart failure, sick sinus syndrome (unless patient has artificial pacemaker). Use with caution in hypertrophic cardiomyopathy and impaired renal function. Safety in pregnancy and lactation not established.

Untoward Reactions   *CV:* Congestive heart failure, A–V block, bradycardia, asystole, premature ventricular contractions (after IV use), peripheral and pulmonary edema, hypotension, syncope. *GI:* Nausea, constipation, abdominal discomfort. *CNS:* Dizziness, headache, fatigue, sleep disturbances, depression, drowsiness, vertigo. *Other:* Blurred vision, alopecia, sexual difficulties, muscle cramps or fatigue, spotty menstruation, sweating, rotary nystagmus.

Drug Interactions

Interactant	Interaction
Anticoagulants, oral	↑ Anticoagulant effect due to ↓ plasma protein binding
Antihypertensive agents	Additive hypotensive effect
Beta-adrenergic blocking agents	Additive depressant effects on myocardial contractility and A–V conduction
Calcium salts	↓ Effect of verapamil
Disopyramide	Additive depressant effects on myocardial contractility and A–V conduction
Digoxin	↑ Risk of digoxin toxicity
Theophyllines	↑ Effect of theophyllines
Vitamin D	↓ Effect of verapamil

Note: Since verapamil is significantly bound to plasma proteins, interaction with other drugs bound to plasma protein may occur.

Dosage   **PO.** *Angina.* **Individualized. Adults: initial,** 80 mg q 6–8 hr; **then,** increase dose to total of 240–480 mg/day. **Slow IV.** *Supraventricular tachyarrhythmias.* **Adults: initial,** 5–10 mg over 2 min (over 3 min in older patients); **then,** 10 mg 30 min later if response not adequate. **Pediatric, up to 1 year:** 0.1–0.2 mg/kg over 2 min; **1–15 years:** 0.1–0.3 mg/kg (not to exceed 5 mg total dose) over 2 min. If response to initial dose is inadequate it may be repeated after 30 min.

Administration

1. Give as a slow IV bolus over 2 min (3 min to geriatric patients to minimize toxic effects).
2. IV dosage should be administered under continuous ECG monitoring with resuscitation equipment available.
3. Ampules should be stored at 15° - 30° C and protected from light.
4. Before administration, ampules should be inspected for particulate matter or discoloration.

Nursing Implications

1. Have available ECG, BP monitoring, and resuscitation equipment when administering verapamil IV.
2. *Assess*
   a. for achievement of normal sinus rhythm (attained usually 10 minutes after IV administration).
   b. for bradycardia and hypotension, which may indicate need for treatment of overdosage.
3. Do not administer concurrently with IV beta-adrenergic blocking agents (i.e., propranolol).
4. Do not administer disopyramide (Norpace) 48 hr before or 24 hr after verapamil administration.
5. Unless treating verapamil overdosage, withhold medication, and check with physician, before administering any medication that elevates serum calcium levels.

OTHER VASODILATORS

DIPYRIDAMOLE   Apo-Dipyridamole,* Persantine, Pyridamole (Rx)

Classification   Coronary vasodilator.

Action/Kinetics   Selectively dilates small resistance vessels of coronary vascular bed, probably by increasing tissue concentration of adenosine diphosphate (ADP), a powerful vasodilator. The drug also decreases clotting time (platelet aggregation).

Uses   Chronic angina pectoris (long-term treatment). Not indicated for acute attacks. *Investigational:* In combination with aspirin for prevention of myocardial infarction and to prevent coronary bypass graft occlusion. In combination with warfarin to prevent thromboembolism in patients with prosthetic heart valves.

Contraindications   Use with caution in patients with hypotension.

Untoward Reactions   *CNS:* Headaches, dizziness, weakness or syncope. *GI:* Nausea, GI distress. *Other:* Flushing, skin rashes. Rarely, aggravation of angina pectoris.

Drug Interaction   Anticoagulant effect is increased if given concomitantly with aspirin.

Dosage   **PO.** 50 mg t.i.d. 1 hr before meals with a full glass of fluid.

Note: Differences in bioavailability between products may occur.

Nursing Implications

1. *Assess*
   a. for aggravation of angina pectoris, which necessitates discontinuance of therapy.
   b. for positive clinical response demonstrated by increased exercise tolerance, reduced nitroglycerin requirement, and reduction or elimination of anginal attacks.
   c. for untoward reactions, because dosage adjustment may be necessary.
2. *Teach patient and/or family*
   a. to report subjective signs of hypotension, such as weakness, dizziness, and faintness, which may have been potentiated by medication and warrant a change in regimen.
   b. to continue drug compliance because patient may become discouraged by delayed clinical response (1–3 months).

NADOLOL   Corgard (Rx)

See Chapter 26, p. 336.

PROPRANOLOL HYDROCHLORIDE   Inderal (Rx)

See Chapter 26, p. 337.

Chapter Twenty-five

PERIPHERAL VASODILATORS

General Statement Many conditions, including arteriosclerosis, reduce blood flow to the limbs. The resulting peripheral vascular disease may have serious consequences, such as tissue hypoxia and gangrene. Treatment usually involves relaxation of the muscles surrounding the small arteries and capillaries. Many of the drugs that act on various components of the autonomic nervous system (see Part 6) are used for the treatment of peripheral vascular disease. The drugs that specifically act on the peripheral blood vessels are discussed here.

CYCLANDELATE   Cyclan, Cyclospasmol (Rx)

Classification Peripheral vasodilator, spasmolytic.

Action/Kinetics Direct papaverine-like action on smooth muscle of blood vessels, resulting in peripheral vasodilation. Drug has little effect on blood pressure and heart rate. Beneficial effects become noticeable gradually. **Onset:** 15 min. **Peak effect:** 1–1½ hr. **Duration:** 3–4 hr. Metabolic rate uncertain.

Uses Symptomatic therapy for occlusive vascular disease and vasospastic conditions including peripheral arteriosclerosis, intermittent claudication, thromboangiitis obliterans, acute thrombophlebitis, erythrocyanosis, Raynaud's disease, scleroderma, noctural leg cramps, diabetic ulcers of the leg, frostbite, and selected cases of occlusive cerebrovascular disease. Not intended as a substitute for other therapy.

Contraindications Should be used with extreme caution in patients with obliterative coronary artery or cerebrovascular disease. Safe use in pregnancy has not been established. Administer with caution to patients with glaucoma.

Untoward Reactions *GI:* Heartburn, GI distress. *CNS:* Headaches, dizziness, weakness. *CV:* Flushing, tachycardia. *Miscellaneous:* Tingling of extremities, sweating.

Dosage PO. **Initial,** 1,200–1,600 mg daily in divided doses before meals and at bedtime; **maintenance:** 100–200 mg q.i.d. Note: Beneficial effects may not be seen for several weeks.

Nursing Implications

Teach patient and/or family

    a. to take the drug with meals or with antacids when experiencing gastric distress.

(continued)

b. to continue taking medication, explaining that improvement with cyclandelate generally occurs gradually.

c. to report untoward symptoms; however, it is important to **stress** that flushing, headache, weakness, and tachycardia occur frequently during the first few weeks of therapy.

ETHAVERINE HYDROCHLORIDE Circubid, Ethaquin, Ethatab, Ethavex-100, Isovex (Rx)

Classification Peripheral vasodilator.

Action/Kinetics Closely resembles papaverine. Acts directly on heart muscle, depressing conduction and prolonging refractory period. Also acts as direct nonspecific relaxant on other smooth muscles.

Uses Various circulatory disorders accompanied by spasms of the blood vessels resulting in circulatory insufficiency. Spastic conditions of the genitourinary and gastrointestinal tracts. Efficacy is uncertain.

Contraindications Complete A-V block, serious arrhythmias, severe liver disease. Administer with extreme caution in presence of coronary insufficiency, pulmonary embolism, and glaucoma. Safe use during pregnancy and lactation not established.

Untoward Reactions *GI:* Nausea, anorexia, abdominal distress, dryness of throat. *CV:* Hypotension, cardiac depression, arrhythmias, flushing. *CNS:* Vertigo, headache, drowsiness, lassitude, dizziness, malaise. *Miscellaneous:* Skin rashes, sweating, respiratory depression.

Dosage **PO**: 100 mg t.i.d., up to 200 mg t.i.d. **Time-release capsule**: 150 mg q 12 hr, up to 300 mg q 12 hr.

Nursing Implications

1. Urge patient to report any untoward reactions, because they will necessitate reduction of dosage or discontinuance of drug.
2. Very carefully assess patients with coronary insufficiency, pulmonary embolus, or glaucoma who are receiving ethaverine hydrochloride.

ISOXSUPRINE HYDROCHLORIDE Vasodilan, Voxsuprine (Rx)

Classification Peripheral vasodilator.

Action/Kinetics Direct relaxation of vascular smooth muscle, increasing peripheral blood flow. Drug crosses placenta. **Peak serum levels (PO or IM)**: 1 hr, persisting for approximately 3 hr. t½: 1¼ hr. Mostly excreted in urine.

Uses Symptomatic treatment of cerebrovascular insufficiency. Improves peripheral blood circulation in arteriosclerosis obliterans, Buerger's disease, and Raynaud's disease. *Investigational:* Dysmenorrhea, threatened premature labor.

Contraindications Postpartum, arterial bleeding. Use with caution parenterally in patients with hypotension and tachycardia.

Untoward Reactions *CV:* Tachycardia, hypotension, chest pain. *GI:* Abdominal distress, nausea, vomiting. *CNS:* Lightheadedness, dizziness, nervousness, weakness. *Miscellaneous:* Severe rash.

Dosage **PO**: 10–20 mg t.i.d.–q.i.d. **IM**: 5–10 mg b.i.d. or t.i.d. Switch to PO as soon as possible.

Nursing Implication

Monitor frequency, intensity, and duration of contractions when given during premature labor to counteract threatened abortion.

NICOTINYL ALCOHOL Roniacol (Rx)

Classification Peripheral vasodilator.

Action/Kinetics Converted to niacin, which produces direct peripheral vasodilation, especially the cutaneous vessels of the face, neck, and chest. **Onset:** elixir, 5–10 min; tablet, 5–30 min. **Duration**: 10–60 min. Extended release: **Onset:** 30 min; **duration**: 6–12 hr.

Uses Intermittent claudication associated with peripheral arteriosclerosis and thromboangiitis obliterans, diabetic vascular disease, decubital and varicose ulcers, chilblains, Meniere's syndrome, vertigo.

Untoward Reactions *CV:* Flushing of face and neck, hypotension. *CNS:* Dizziness, syncope. *GI:* Heartburn, nausea, vomiting. *Miscellaneous:* Paresthesias, skin rashes, pruritus, allergic symptoms. Tolerance to drug may develop after prolonged use.

Dosage **PO**: 50–100 mg t.i.d. before meals. **Timed-release tablet:** 150–300 mg b.i.d. morning and night.

Nursing Implication

Advise patient to continue to maintain good skin care and to refrain from smoking and excessive standing, even though the drug offers symptomatic relief.

NYLIDRIN HYDROCHLORIDE Adrin, Arlidin, Arlidin Forte,* PMS Nylidrin* (Rx)

Classification Peripheral vasodilator.

Action/Kinetics Vasodilation, primarily of skeletal muscle, by beta-adrenergic receptor stimulation and by relaxation of vascular smooth muscle. **Onset:** 10 min; **maximum effect:** 30 min. **Duration:** 2 hr. Excreted in urine.

Uses Peripheral vascular disease, including Raynaud's disease, thromboangiitis obliterans, arteriosclerosis obliterans, diabetic vascular disease, frostbite, night leg cramps, ischemic ulcer, acrocyanosis, acroparesthesia, thrombophlebitis. Circulatory disturbances of inner ear. Not a drug of choice.

Contraindications Acute myocardial infarctions, angina pectoris, paroxysmal tachycardia, or thyrotoxicosis. Use with caution in all patients with cardiac disease.

Untoward Reactions *CV:* Palpitations, orthostatic hypotension. *CNS:* Tremors, weakness, dizziness, nervousness. *GI:* Nausea, vomiting.

Dosage **PO:** 3–12 mg t.i.d.–q.i.d.

Nursing Implications
Teach patient and/or family

a. that palpitations should subside as therapy continues.
b. that improvement might not be apparent for several weeks.

PAPAVERINE HYDROCHLORIDE Cerespan, Delapav, Dilart, Myobid, P-200, Papacon, Pavabid, Pavabid HP, Pavacap, Pavacen, Pavadur, Pavadyl, Pavagen, Pava-Par, Pavarine, Pava-Rx, Pavased, Pavasule, Pavatine, Pavatym, Paverolan, PT-300, Vasocap-150 and -300 Vasospan (Rx)

Classification Peripheral vasodilator.

Action/Kinetics Direct spasmolytic effect on smooth muscle, possibly by inhibiting oxidative phosphorylation and by interfering with role of calcium in muscle contraction. Absorbed fairly rapidly. Localized in fat tissues and liver. Steady plasma concentration maintained when drug is given q 6 hr.

Uses Various circulatory disorders accompanied by spasms of the blood vessels, resulting in circulatory insufficiency (myocardial, renal, cerebral, or peripheral). Ureteral or biliary spasm, GI colic. The drug is not considered very effective.

Contraindications Complete A-V block; administer with extreme caution in presence of coronary insufficiency and glaucoma. Safe use in pregnancy and lactation or for children not established.

Untoward Reactions *CV:* Flushing of face, hypertension. *GI:* Nausea, anorexia, abdominal distress, constipation or diarrhea, dry mouth and throat. *CNS:* Headache, drowsiness, sedation, vertigo. *Miscellaneous:* Sweating, pruritus, skin rashes, increase in depth of respiration, jaundice, eosinophilia.

Note: Both acute and chronic poisoning may result from use of papaverine. Symptoms are extensions of untoward effects. Also, acute poisoning symptoms include: Nystagmus, diplopia, coma, cyanosis, respiratory depression. Additional chronic poisoning symptoms include: Ataxia, blurred vision, erythematous macular eruptions, blood dyscrasias.

Drug Interaction Papaverine may ↓ effect of levodopa by blocking dopamine receptors.

Laboratory Test Interference ↑ SGOT, SGPT, and bilirubin.

Dosage **PO:** 100–300 mg 3 to 5 times/day; **time-release capsule:** 150 mg q 12 hr up to 150 or 300 mg q 8–12 hr for severe cases. **IM, IV:** 30–120 mg given slowly (over 1–2 min) q 3 hr. **Pediatric:** 6 mg/kg.

Administration
1. IV injections must be given by physician or under his immediate supervision.
2. Do not mix with Ringer's lactate solution because a precipitate will form.

Nursing Implications
1. Monitor pulse, respiration, and BP closely for at least a ½ hr after IV injection of papaverine.
2. Report untoward autonomic nervous system and GI symptoms to physician.

PHENOXYBENZAMINE HYDROCHLORIDE   Dibenzyline (Rx)

See *Adrenergic Blocking Agents* (Sympatholytic), p. 577.

TOLAZOLINE HYDROCHLORIDE   Priscoline HCl, Vasodil (Rx)

See *Adrenergic Blocking Agents* (Sympatholytic), p. 580.

Chapter Twenty-six

ANTIHYPERTENSIVE AGENTS

II. Peripherally Acting Agents

III. Beta-Adrenergic Blocking Agents

IV. Miscellaneous Agents

Monoamine Oxidse (MAO) Inhibitor

Agents That Act Directly on Vascular Smooth Muscle

General Statement Hypertension is a condition in which the mean arterial blood pressure is elevated. It is one of the most widespread chronic conditions for which medication is prescribed and taken on a regular basis. Most cases of hypertension are of unknown etiology and result from a generalized increase in resistance to flow in the peripheral vessels (arterioles). Such cases are known as primary or essential hypertension. Treatment of essential hypertension is aimed at reducing blood pressure to normal or near-normal levels, because this is believed to prevent or halt the slow, albeit permanent, damage caused by constant excess pressure.

Essential hypertension is commonly classified according to its severity as mild, moderate, or severe. Most early cases of hypertension are mild. Moderate or severe (malignant) hypertension can result in degenerative changes in the brain, heart, and kidneys and can be fatal.

Other types of hypertension (secondary hypertension) have a known etiology and can result from a complication of pregnancy (toxemic hypertension) or certain other diseases that cause impairment of kidney function. It can also be caused by a tumor of the adrenal gland (pheochromocytoma) or by blockage of certain arteries leading into the kidney (renal hypertension). The latter two cases can be corrected by surgery.

Most pharmacologic agents used to treat hypertension lower blood pressure by relaxing the constricted arterioles, thereby decreasing the resistance to peripheral blood flow. These drugs exert this effect by decreasing the influence of the sympathetic nervous system on smooth muscle of arterioles, by directly relaxing arteriolar smooth muscle, or by acting on the centers in the brain that control blood pressure.

Antihypertensive drug therapy is usually initiated when the diastolic blood pressure is greater than 90 mm Hg. Weight reduction, sodium restriction, stopping smoking, exercise, and behavior changes are all important components of antihypertensive treatment. Antihypertensive therapy is undertaken in a stepped care fashion. Stepped care therapy is initiated with a single drug. Additional agents may be added or substituted in gradually increasing doses until the desired effect is reached, maximal dosage has been reached, or side effects can not be tolerated. When additional drugs are added to the regimen, they should act by different mechanisms than the drugs already being used.

The following drugs are used for stepped care. Step 1: Thiazide diuretics (drugs of choice) and beta-adrenergic blocking agents. Step 2: Drugs that inhibit the activity of the adrenergic nervous system. Such drugs include those acting centrally (clonidine, guanabenz, methyldopa) and those acting peripherally (guanadrel, prazosin, reserpine). Beta-adrenergic blocking agents may also be considered Step 2 drugs. Step 3: Vasodilators, including hydralazine and minoxidil. Step 4: Guanethidine and captopril are reserved for Step 4 therapy due to the large number of side effects. However, captopril may be substituted in Steps 2 or 3 if side effects or ineffectiveness limit the use of other agents.

Note: The calcium channel blockers have also been used for hypertension (See Chapter 24, p. 305).

Other drugs used to treat hypertension include:

1. **Sedatives and antianxiety agents**. These are used for the management of mild hypertension especially if due to stress. See Chapter 31.
2. **Rauwolfia alkaloids**.
3. **Ganglionic blocking agents**. Used to treat moderate to severe hypertension.
4. **Monoamine oxidase inhibitors**.

Nursing Implications
1. Assess baseline blood pressure before initiating therapy with any antihypertensive medication.
2. Periodically reassess blood pressure as warranted by patient's condition and medication.
3. Report significant changes in blood pressure or lack of response to medication to physician.

RAUWOLFIA ALKALOIDS

General Statement   The rauwolfia alkaloids decrease elevated blood pressure that is accompanied by bradycardia but have no effect on renal blood flow. However, insufficient antihypertensive effects are manifested when reserpine is given alone at doses that produce a minimal incidence of side effects. Significant CNS effects produced by rauwolfia alkaloids resulted in their use in the treatment of psychoses.

Action/Kinetics   Reserpine is believed to exert its action by depleting nerve terminals of norepinephrine and serotonin. Thus less neurotransmitter is available to interact with receptors, resulting in relaxation of smooth muscle of blood vessels. Reserpine also acts directly to depress myocardial function, to increase gastric acid secretion, and to produce a variety of endocrine changes. It also produces antipsychotic effects. **PO:** Onset is slow, with maximum effects taking one or more weeks. **IM:** Onset, greater than 1 hr; duration: up to 10 hr. **IV:** Onset, 1 hr; maximum effect: 4 hr. Metabolized in liver and excreted in urine. t½: 50–100 hr.

Uses   In conjunction with a diuretic for primary hypertension of the mild or labile type, especially when associated with anxiety and emotional factors. Psychoses accompanied by agitation. *Investigational:* Adjunct in treatment of tachycardia, palpitations, and psychological disturbances in thyrotoxicosis; for vasospasms in Raynaud's disease.

Contraindications Pheochromocytoma, history of mental depression, in electroconvulsive therapy, colitis, or peptic ulcer. Use with caution in the presence of cardiac arrhythmias or asthma. Because the drugs have been reported to cause uterine contractions and to pass the placental barrier, they should be administered with caution during pregnancy. In nursing mothers, they may cause nasal congestion in the infant, which can result in serious respiratory problems during feeding.

Untoward Reactions *CNS:* Drowsiness, fatigue, lethargy, depression (may be severe and lead to suicide attempts). Headache, dizziness, nightmares, increased dreaming. *CV:* Bradycardia, severe hypotension, angina-like symptoms, arrhythmias. *GI:* Nausea, vomiting, diarrhea, anorexia, cramps, increased gastric acid secretion (may aggravate peptic ulcer), dry mouth. *Allergy:* Pruritus, rash, asthma symptoms in asthmatics. *Endocrine:* Impotence, decreased libido, breast engorgement, gynecomastia, galactorrhea. *Other:* Nasal congestion (common), flushing, sialorrhea, thrombocytopenic purpura, epistaxis, ecchymosis, increased bleeding time, muscle aches, blurred vision, ptosis.

Rauwolfia alkaloids may cause acute cardiovascular collapse in patients under sudden stress, and administration should be discontinued 2 weeks before surgery. Complications have been noted during the administration of anesthesia.

Rauwolfia alkaloids must be discontinued 1 week before electroshock therapy. Sodium and water retention may progress to congestive heart failure (CHF).

Overdosage is characterized by CNS depression, hypotension, miosis, and catatonia.

Drug Interactions

Interactant	Interaction
Anticholinergics	Rauwolfia alkaloids ↓ effect of anticholinergics due to ↑ gastric acid secretion
Anticonvulsant drugs	Reserpine ↓ convulsive threshold and shortens seizure latency. Anticonvulsant drug dose may have to be adjusted.
Antidepressants, tricyclic	↑ Stimulating effect in depressed patients
Beta-adrenergic blocking agents	Hypotension and bradycardia
Digitalis glycosides	↑ Possibility of cardiac arrhythmias
Ephedrine	↓ Effectiveness of ephedrine
General anesthetics	Hypotension, bradycardia
Mephentermine	↓ Effectiveness of mephentermine
Methotrimeprazine	Additive hypotensive effect
Monoamine oxidase	Reserpine-induced release of accumulated norepinephrine caused by monoamine oxidase inhibitors results in excitation and hypertension
Phenothiazines	Additive hypotensive effect
Procarbazine	Additive hypotensive effect
Quinidine	Additive hypotensive effect and ↑ chance of cardiac arrhythmias
Theophylline	↑ Chance of tachycardia
Thiazide diuretics	Additive hypotensive effect

Interactant	Interaction
Thioxanthines	Additive hypotensive effect
Vasodilator drugs, peripheral	Additive hypotensive effect

Laboratory Test Interference ↑ Serum glucose, urine glucose. ↓ Urine catecholamines, 17-hydroxycorticosteroids, and 17-ketosteroids.

Dosage **Usually PO.** See individual compounds, Table 10, below.

TABLE 10   RAUWOLFIA ALKALOIDS

Drug	Dosage	Remarks
Alseroxylon (Rauwiloid) Rx	**PO: initial,** 2–4 mg daily in single or divided doses; **maintenance:** 2 mg daily.	Reserpine preferred for institionalized patients. *Additional Drug Interactions* 1. Ethanol ↑ CNS depressant and hypotensive effects of alseroxylon. 2. Levodopa and methyldopa ↑ hypotensive effects of alseroxylon.
Deserpidine (Harmonyl) Rx	*Hypertension* **PO: initial,** 0.25 mg 3 to 4 times daily for up to 2 weeks; **maintenance:** 0.25 mg daily. *Psychiatry.* **PO, individualize, usual,** 0.5 mg/day. **Range:** 0.1–1 mg daily.	
Rauwolfia serpentina/ Whole root rauwolfia (Hiwolfia, Raudixin, Rauserpin, Rauval, Rauverid, Rawfola, Serfolia, Wolfina) Rx	**PO: initial,** 200–400 mg daily in AM and PM; **maintenance:** 50–300 mg/day in one or two doses.	A dosage of 200–300 mg of this preparation is equivalent to 0.5 mg reserpine.
Rescinnamine (Moderil) Rx	**PO. initial** 0.5 mg b.i.d. for 2 weeks; **maintenance:** 0.25–0.5 mg daily.	Causes less bradycardia than does reserpine. Reserpine preferred for institutionalized patients.
Reserpine (Releserp-5,Reserfia,* Sandril, Serpalan, Serpasil, Serpate, SK-Reserpine, Zepine) Rx	**PO.** *Hypertension:* **initial,** 0.5 mg/day for 1–2 weeks; **maintenance:** 0.1–0.25 mg daily. *Psychiatry:* 0.1–1 mg adjusted to response of patient.	Drug of choice for institutionalized patients. May cause postural hypotension and respiratory depression. Determine BP before each administration. 10 mg or more may cause delayed hypotensive reaction. When used alone, may not provide reliable control of hypertension. Most often used with thiazide diuretics or combined with hydralazine (e.g., Diupres, Hydropres, Regroton, Salutensin, Ser-Ap-Es). (See Appendix 3.)

Nursing Implications

1. *Assess*
   a. for personality changes, nightmares, or changes in sleep patterns, since these are early symptoms of depression that may lead to suicide attempts.
   b. BP under standard conditions and compare with baseline and other previous BP readings. Report significant changes (obtain significant guidelines for each patient from physician).
2. Weigh the patient at least twice weekly under standard conditions to monitor fluid retention and evaluate severity by pitting.
3. Evaluate for edema by measuring calf 5 cm above the medial malleolus and comparing measurements at least twice daily.
4. Have a sympathomimetic agent (ephedrine) available to treat overdose.
5. *Teach patient and/or family*
   a. signs that may precede depression, and stress the importance of medical supervision should these occur.
   b. possible side effects of rauwolfia alkaloids and how to check for edema; advise patients to report untoward effects.

Nursing Implications for Parenteral Rauwolfia

1. Observe the patient for respiratory depression.
2. Observe for postural hypotension.
3. Caution the patient not to get out of bed without assistance.
4. Monitor BP before each parenteral dose of reserpine.

GANGLIONIC BLOCKING AGENTS

Action/Kinetics   These drugs block transmission of nerve impulses at the ganglia of the autonomic nervous system. This action results in inhibition of nerve impulses, including those that constrict the vascular walls, thereby causing a reduction in blood pressure. Baroreceptor reflexes are also blocked, thus preventing an increase in heart rate due to the decreased blood pressure.

These drugs are of limited value in long-term management of chronic hypertension due to side effects including orthostatic hypotension, adynamic ileus, and urinary retention.

Untoward Reactions   Most untoward reactions are related to the blocking of parasympathetic and sympathetic nervous systems because the drugs block ganglia to all organs of the body—not just to the blood vessels. As with other powerful drugs that cause a major alteration of physiologic processes, it is often difficult to decide when an untoward reaction becomes excessive.

CV: Postural hypotension, interstitial pulmonary edema, and fibrosis. *GI:* Anorexia, diarrhea followed by constipation, paralytic ileus, dry mouth, nausea, vomiting, glossitis. *CNS:* Weakness, fatigue, dizziness, syncope, sedation. Rarely, seizures, chorieform movements, tremors, and mental disturbances especially with high doses. *GU:* Urinary retention, impotence, decreased libido. *Other:* Paresthesias.

Patients on low-sodium diets or those who have had sympathectomy and hypertensive encephalopathy are particularly sensitive to the ganglionic blocking agents.

Drug Interactions

Interactant	Interaction
Alcohol	↑ Hypotensive effect
Antihypertensive drugs	Additive hypotensive effects
General anesthetics	Additive hypothesic effects
Thiazide diuretics	↑ Additive hypotensive effects; concomitant use permits reduction of dosage of ganglionic blocking agents to about one-half

Dosage   Highly individualized. (See individual drug entries.) The required amount of drug depends on the time of day (higher doses are generally required at night), on the season (lower doses are required in warm weather), and on the position of the patient (higher doses are required for an ambulatory patient than for one confined to bed).

It is important always to measure blood pressure in patients taking ganglionic blocking agents in the standing position or as the physician orders.

Nursing Implications

1. *Assess*
   a. BP and pulse at the specific times ordered, and make sure that the patient is in position as ordered for all readings (either standing or sitting). If this is not possible, alterations in time and position should be indicated on the chart.
   b. the patient's weight daily and check for edema to determine whether weight gain is due to fluid or to increased appetite.
   c. intake and output, since oliguria may occur due to excessive hypotension.
   d. for constipation. Check with the physician regarding orders for laxatives, such as saline or other irritating cathartics, which could be administered if the patient fails to have regular bowel movements. Should constipation occur, the drug must be discontinued. Bulk-producing cathartics are ineffective.
   e. closely for additive hypotensive effect if other antihypertensives or diuretics are concomitantly administered, as adjustment in dosage may be required.
2. *Teach patient and/or family*
   a. that orthostatic hypotension is manifested by weakness, dizziness, and fainting and that these symptoms may occur when patients rapidly change from a supine to a standing position. To prevent this, they should slowly rise from the bed to a sitting position, dangle legs for a few minutes until they feel stable enough to stand up. A nurse or family member should assist as necessary.
   b. if weak, dizzy, or faint after standing or exercising for a long time, to lie down if possible or otherwise sit down and lower head between knees.
   c. how to prevent constipation and to report constipation if it occurs.

MECAMYLAMINE HYDROCHLORIDE   Inversine (Rx)

Classification   Ganglionic blocking agent, antihypertensive.

Action/Kinetics   The drug is less apt than other ganglionic blocking agents to induce tolerance. Withdraw or substitute mecamylamine slowly since sudden withdrawal or switching to other antihypertensive agents may result in severe hypertensive rebound. Since mecamylamine reduces peristalsis, it is a useful addition to a thiazide-guanethidine regimen in patients who experience persistent diarrhea with guanethidine.

Onset (gradual): ½–2 hr. **Duration:** 6–12 hr. May take 2–3 days to achieve full therapeutic potential.

Uses Moderate to severe hypertension including malignant hypertension.

Contraindications Coronary insufficiency, patients with recent myocardial infarction, uremia, chronic pyelonephritis being treated with antibiotics and sulfonamides, glaucoma, pyloric stenosis, uncooperative patients.

Abdominal distention, decreased bowel signs, and other symptoms of adynamic ileus are reasons for discontinuing the drug.

Dosage **PO: initial,** 2.5 mg b.i.d. Increase by increments of 2.5 mg every 2 or more days; **maintenance:** 25 mg daily in 3 divided doses.

Administration

1. For better control of hypertension, administer after meals.
2. The morning dose may be small or omitted; larger doses are given at noon and in the evening.

TRIMETHAPHAN CAMSYLATE Arfonad (Rx)

Classification Ganglionic blocking agent, antihypertensive.

Action/Kinetics In addition to acting as a ganglionic blockade, this agent directly dilates blood vessels as well as releases histamine. **Onset:** immediate. **Duration:** extremely short (10–30 min). BP increases 10 min after discontinuance of IV infusion.

Uses During surgery when controlled hypotension is desirable, as in the case of brain tumors, cerebral aneurysms, A-V fistula repair, aortic grafts and transplants, coarctation, anastomosis, and fenestration operations.

Trimethaphan is also indicated in hypertensive crises and in pulmonary edema resulting from hypertension. **Investigational:** Dissecting aortic aneurysm or ischemic heart disease when other drugs cannot be used.

Contraindications Anemia, shock, asphyxia, respiratory insufficiency, hypovolemia. Use with caution in arteriosclerosis, cardiac, hepatic, or renal disease, Addison's disease, diabetes, degenerative CNS disease, patients taking steroids.

Drug Interactions

Interactant	Interaction
Anesthetics, general	Additive hypotension
Antihypertensive drugs	Additive hypotension
Diuretics	↑ Effect of trimethaphan
Muscle relaxants, nondepolarizing	Additive muscle relaxation
Succinylcholine	↑ Muscle relaxation

Dosage **IV infusion: Adults, initial,** 1.0 mg/ml in 5% dextrose given at a rate of 3–4 ml/min (3–4 mg/min); **then,** individualize dosage. **Pediatric:** 50–150 μg/kg/min. Check BP frequently.

Administration
1. Administration should be stopped before wound closure to allow blood pressure to return to normal (usually within 10 min).
2. Patient should be placed to avoid cerebral anoxia.

Additional Nursing Implications
See also *Nursing Implications*, p. 321.

1. *Assess*
   a. BP closely. Systolic BP should be maintained above 60 mm Hg or at two-thirds the usual value in hypertensive patients.
   b. for peripheral vascular collapse as demonstrated by excessive hypotension, rapid pulse, cold clammy skin, and cyanosis.
2. Levarterenol, ephedrine, methoxamine, and phenylephrine should be on hand to correct undesirable low BP.
3. Teach patient who has a history of angina the importance of reporting any further anginal attacks, because medication may precipitate attack.

AGENTS THAT DEPRESS THE ACTIVITY OF THE SYMPATHETIC NERVOUS SYSTEM

Centrally Acting Drugs

CLONIDINE HYDROCHLORIDE   Catapres, Dixarit* (Rx)

Classification   Antihypertensive, centrally acting antiadrenergic.

Action/Kinetics   Stimulates alpha-adrenergic receptors of the CNS, which results in inhibition of the sympathetic vasomotor centers and decreased nerve impulses. Thus, bradycardia and a fall in both systolic and diastolic blood pressure occur. Plasma renin levels are decreased while peripheral venous pressure remains unchanged. The drug has few orthostatic effects. Although sodium chloride excretion is markedly decreased, potassium excretion remains unchanged. Tolerance to the drug may develop. **Onset:** 30–60 min. **Maximum effect:** 2–4 hr. **Duration:** 12–24 hr. **t½:** 12–16 hr. Excreted mainly in the urine.

Uses   Mild to moderate hypertension. A diuretic or other antihypertensive drugs, or both, are often used concomitantly. *Investigational:* Prophylaxis of migraine headaches, dysmenorrhea, and menopausal flushing. Treatment of Gilles de la Tourette syndrome. Detoxification of opiate dependence.

Contraindications   Use with caution in presence of severe coronary insufficiency, recent myocardial infarction, cerebrovascular disease, or chronic renal failure. Use in pregnancy only when benefits outweigh risks. Safe use in children not established.

Untoward Reactions   *CNS:* Drowsiness (common), sedation, dizziness, headache, fatigue, malaise, nightmares, nervousness, restlessness, anxiety, mental depression, increased dreaming, insomnia. *GI:* Dry mouth (common), constipation, anorexia, nausea, vomiting, weight gain. *CV:* Congestive heart failure, Raynaud's phenomenon, abnormalities in ECG. *Dermatologic:* Urticaria, skin rashes, angioneurotic edema, pruritus, thinning of hair. *Other:* Impotence, urinary retention, gynecomastia, increase in blood glucose (transient), increased sensitivity to alcohol, dryness of mucous membranes of nose, itching, burning, dryness of eyes, skin pallor.

Note: Rebound hypertension may be manifested if clonidine is abruptly withdrawn.

Drug Interactions

Interactant	Interaction
Alcohol	↑ Depressant effects
Beta-adrenergic blocking agents	Paradoxical hypertension; also, ↑ severity of rebound hypertension following clonidine withdrawal
CNS depressants	↑ Depressant effect
Levodopa	↓ Effect of levodopa
Tolazoline	Blocks antihypertensive effect
Tricyclic antidepressants	Blocks antihypertensive effect

Laboratory Test Interferences Transient ↑ of blood glucose and serum creatinine phosphokinase. Weakly + Coombs' test. Alteration of electrolyte balance.

Dosage *Hypertension.* **PO: initial,** 0.1 mg b.i.d.; **then,** increase by 0.1–0.2 mg/day until desired response attained; **maintenance:** 0.2–0.8 mg/day in divided doses (maximum: 2.4 mg/day). Tolerance necessitates increased dosage or concomitant administration of a diuretic. Gradual increase of dosage after initiation minimizes side effects. *Gilles de la Tourette syndrome:* 0.05–0.6 mg/day. *Withdrawal from opiate dependence:* 0.8 mg/day.

Administration Drug should be discontinued gradually over period of 2–4 days. Administer last dose of day at bedtime to ensure overnight blood pressure control.

Nursing Implications

1. Monitor BP closely during initiation of therapy, because a decrease occurs within 30 to 60 min after administration and may persist for 8 hr. Determine frequency of monitorings with medical supervision.
2. *Assess*
   a. closely for 3 to 4 days after initiation of therapy for weight gain (weigh daily in AM) and for edema, caused by sodium retention. Fluid retention should disappear after 3 to 4 days.
   b. for fluctuations in BP to determine whether it is preferable to use clonidine alone or concomitantly with a diuretic. A stable BP reduces orthostatic effects of postural changes.
   c. for further depressive episodes that may be precipitated by the drug in a patient who has a history of mental depression.
   d. for paradoxical hypertensive response, if patient is also receiving propranolol.
   e. for blocking of antihypertensive action if patient is concomitantly receiving tolazoline or a tricyclic antidepressant, as dosage adjustment would be indicated.
3. Report side effects, because dosage is based on patient's BP and tolerance. Side effects can be minimized by increasing dosage gradually.
4. Have on hand IV tolazoline (Priscoline) for treatment of acute toxicity caused by clonidine.

5. *Teach patient and/or family*
   a. not to engage in activities that require alertness, such as operative machinery or driving a car, because the drug may cause drowsiness.
   b. not to discontinue medication abruptly, but to consult with medical supervision before initiating any change in medication regimen. Rebound hypertension is prevented by gradual withdrawal of medication.
   c. **(in case of Parkinson's disease controlled with levodopa),** to report increase in signs and symptoms, as effect of levodopa may be reduced by clonidine.

GUANABENZ ACETATE   Wytensin (Rx)

Classification   Antihypertensive, centrally acting antiadrenergic.

Action/Kinetics   Guanabenz stimulates alpha-adrenergic receptors in the CNS resulting in a decrease in sympathetic impulses and a decrease in sympathetic tone. It also decreases pulse rate but postural hypotension has not been manifested.

Uses   Hypertension, alone or as adjunct with thiazide diuretics.

Contraindications   Pregnancy, lactation, children under 12 years of age. Use with caution in severe coronary insufficiency, cerebrovascular disease, recent myocardial infarction, hepatic or renal disease.

Untoward Reactions   *CNS:* Drowsiness and sedation (common), dizziness, weakness, headache, ataxia, depression, disturbances in sleep, excitement. *GI:* Dry mouth (common), nausea, vomiting, diarrhea, constipation, abdominal pain or discomfort. *CV:* Palpitations, chest pain, arrhythmias. *Miscellaneous:* Edema, blurred vision, muscle aches, dyspnea, rash, pruritus, nasal congestion, urinary frequency, gynecomastia, alterations in taste.

Drug Interaction   Use with CNS depressants may result in significant sedation.

Dosage   **PO. Adults: initial,** 4 mg b.i.d.; **then,** increase by 4–8 mg q 1–2 weeks until control achieved. Maximum recommended dose: 32 mg b.i.d.

Nursing Implications
1. Assess pulse rate for possible bradycardia.
2. *Teach patient and/or family*
   a. not to drive automobile or operate machinery until the sedative effect of this drug has been assessed.
   b. to be alert to disturbances in sleep, which may indicate a depressive episode.

METHYLDOPA   Aldomet, Apo-Methyldopa,* Dopamet,* Medimet-250,* Novomedopa* (Rx)

METHYLDOPATE HYDROCHLORIDE   Aldomet Hydrochloride (Rx)

Classification   Antihypertensive, centrally acting antiadrenergic.

Action/Kinetics Primary mechanism thought to be that the active metabolite, alpha-methyl-norepinephrine lowers BP by stimulating central inhibitory alpha-adrenergic receptors, false neurotransmission, and/or reduction of plasma renin. It causes little change in cardiac output. **PO: Onset:** 7–12 hr. **Duration:** 12–24 hr. All effects terminated within 48 hr. Absorption is variable. **IV: Onset,** 4–6 hr. **Duration:** 10–16 hr. 70% of drug excreted in urine. **Full therapeutic effect:** 1–4 days.

Note: Methyldopa is a component of Aldoril. (See Appendix 3.)

Uses Moderate to severe hypertension. Particularly useful for patients with impaired renal function, renal hypertension, resistant cases of hypertension complicated by stroke, coronary artery disease, or nitrogen retention, and for hypertensive crises (parenterally).

Contraindications Sensitivity to drug, labile and mild hypertension, pregnancy, active hepatic disease, or pheochromocytoma. Use with caution in patients with a history of liver or kidney disease.

Untoward Reactions *CNS:* Sedation (disappears with use), weakness, headache, asthenia, dizziness, paresthesias, Parkinson-like symptoms, psychic disturbances, choreoathetotic movements. *CV:* Bradycardia, orthostatic hypotension, hypersensitivity of carotid sinus, worsening of angina, hypertensive response (paradoxical), myocarditis. *GI:* Nausea, vomiting, abdominal distention, diarrhea or constipation, flatus, colitis, dry mouth, "black tongue," pancreatitis. *Hematologic:* Hemolytic anemia, leukopenia, granulocytopenia, thrombocytopenia. *Endocrine:* Gynecomastia, amenorrhea, galactorrhea, hyperprolactinemia. *Miscellaneous:* Edema, jaundice, hepatitis, rash, fever, lupus-like symptoms, impotence, failure to ejaculate, decreased libido, nasal stuffiness, joint pain, myalgia.

Drug Interactions

Interactant	Interaction
Anesthetics, general	Additive hypotension
Antidepressants, tricyclic	Tricyclic antidepressants may block hypotensive effect of methyldopa
Ephedrine	Action of ephedrine ↓ in methyldopa-treated patients
Fenfluramine	↑ Effect of methyldopa
Haloperidol	Methyldopa ↑ toxic effects of haloperidol
Levodopa	↑ Effect of levodopa
Lithium	↑ Possibility of lithium toxicity
Levodopa	↑ Effects of both drugs
Methotrimeprazine	Additive hypotensive effect
MAO inhibitors	May reverse hypotensive effect of methyldopa and cause headache and hallucinations
Norepinephrine	↑ Pressor response to norepinephrine
Phenoxybenzamine	Urinary incontinence
Phenylpropanolamine	↑ Pressor response to phenylpropanolamine
Propranolol	Paradoxical hypertension
Thiazide diuretics	Additive hypotensive effect
Tolbutamide	↑ Hypoglycemia due to ↓ breakdown by liver
Thioxanthines	Additive hypotensive effect
Tricyclic antidepressants	↓ Effect of methyldopa
Vasodilator drugs	Additive hypotensive effect
Verapamil	↑ Effect of methyldopa

Laboratory Test Interference   False + or ↑: Alkaline phosphatase, bilirubin, BUN, BSP, cephalin flocculation, creatinine, SGOT, SGPT, uric acid, Coombs' test, prothrombin time. Positive lupus erythematosis (LE) cell preparation and antinuclear antibodies.

Dosage   *Methyldopa*, **PO: initial:** 250 mg b.i.d.–t.i.d. for 2 days. Adjust dose every 2 days. If increased, start with evening dose. **Usual maintenance:** 0.5–2.0 gm daily in divided doses; **maximum:** 3 gm daily. Transfer to and from other antihypertensive agents should occur gradually, with initial dose of methyldopa not exceeding 500 mg. *Remarks*: Do not use combination medication to initiate therapy. **Pediatric: initial**, 10 mg/kg daily, adjusting maintenance to a maximum of 65 mg/kg. *Methyldopate Hydrochloride*: **IV infusion**, 250–500 mg q 6 hr; **maximum:** 1 gm q 6 hr for *hypertensive crisis*. Switch to oral methyldopa, at same dosage level, when blood pressure is brought under control. **Pediatric:** 20–40 mg/kg daily in divided doses q 6 hr; **maximum:** 65 mg/kg up to maximum of 3 gm daily.

Nursing Implications

1. Ascertain that hematologic, liver function, and Coombs' tests are done before initiation of therapy. Periodic tests should be performed throughout therapy.
2. If the patient needs a blood transfusion, ascertain that both direct and indirect Coombs' tests are done. If the indirect as well as the direct Coombs' tests are positive, anticipate consultation with a blood transfusion specialist.
3. *Assess*
   a. for signs of tolerance, which may occur during the second or third month of therapy.
   b. weight daily and observe carefully for edema.
   c. intake and output, observing particularly for reduced urine volume.
4. *Teach patient and/or family*
   a. that patient should rise from bed slowly and should dangle feet from edge of bed to prevent dizziness and fainting. Adjusting dosage may prevent morning hypotension.
   b. that sedation may occur when therapy is first started, but that it disappears once the maintenance dose is established.
   c. that in rare cases methyldopa may darken urine or turn it blue, but that this reaction is not harmful.
   d. to inform anesthesiologist that patient is on methyldopa, if surgery is required.
   e. to withhold drug and report to doctor tiredness, fever, or yellowing of skin and whites of eyes.
   f. to inform doctor that patient is on methyldopa if he requires a transfusion, because the drug induces a positive Coombs' test.

Peripherally Acting Drugs

GUANADREL SULFATE   Hylorel (Rx)

Classification   Antihypertensive, peripherally acting antiadrenergic

Action/Kinetics Similar to guanethidine. Inhibits vasoconstriction by blocking efferent, peripheral sympathetic pathways by depleting norepinephrine reserves and inhibiting norepinephrine release. Causes increased sensitivity to norepinephrine. **Peak plasma levels:** 1.5–2 hr. **t½:** approximately 10 hr.

Uses Hypertension (usually Step 2 therapy).

Contraindications Pheochromocytoma, congestive heart failure, within 1 week of monoamine oxidase drugs, within 2–3 days of elective surgery. Use with caution in bronchial asthma and peptic ulcer. Safety not established in pregnancy, lactation, and in children.

Untoward Effects *CNS:* Fainting, fatigue, headache, drowsiness, paresthesias, confusion, depression. *CV:* Exertional or resting shortness of breath, chest pain, orthostatic hypotension, palpitations. *GI:* Increase in number of bowel movements, constipation, anorexia, indigestion, flatus, glossitis, nausea and vomiting. *GU:* Difficulty in ejaculation, nocturia, urinary urgency or frequency. *Miscellaneous:* Cough, edema, leg cramps, changes in weight (gain or loss), backache, joint pain.

Drug Interactions

Interactant	Interaction
Beta-adrenergic blocking agents	Excessive hypotension, bradycardia
Ephedrine	↓ Effect of guanadrel
Norepinephrine	Guanadrel ↑ effect of norepinephrine
Phenothiazines	↓ Effect of guanadrel
Phenylpropanolamine	↓ Effect of guanadrel
Reserpine	Excessive hypotension, bradycardia
Tricyclic antidepressants	↓ Effect of guanadrel

Dosage PO. Individualized. **Initial:** 10 mg/day; **then,** increase dosage to maintenance of 20–75 mg/day in 2 divided doses.

Administration
1. Tolerance may occur with long-term therapy necessitating a dosage increase.
2. While adjusting dosage, both supine and standing blood pressure should be monitored.

Nursing Implications
1. *Assess* blood pressure in both sitting and standing positions at same times each day.
2. *Teach patient and/or family*
   a. that weakness, dizziness, and fainting may occur with rapid changes of position from supine to standing. Patient should rise from bed slowly and dangle feet from edge of bed before standing.
   b. that nonprescription drugs should not be taken without consultation with physician. Sympathomimetic amines in products used to treat asthma, colds, and allergies are specifically to be used with caution.

GUANETHIDINE SULFATE   Apo-Guanethidine,* Ismelin Sulfate (Rx)

Classification Antihypertensive, peripherally acting antiadrenergic.

Action/Kinetics Guanethidine produces selective adrenergic blockade of efferent, peripheral sympathetic pathways by depleting norepinephrine reserve and inhibiting norepinephrine release. It induces a gradual, prolonged drop in both systolic and diastolic blood pressure, usually associated with bradycardia, decreased pulse pressure, a decrease in peripheral resistance, and small changes in cardiac output. The drug is not a ganglionic blocking agent and does not produce central or parasympathetic blockade.

Incompletely and variably absorbed from the GI tract (3–50%) resulting in variable plasma levels. **Peak effect:** 6–8 hr. **Duration:** 24–48 hr. **Maximum effect:** 1–3 weeks. **Duration:** 7–10 days after discontinuation. **t½:** approximately 5 days.

Uses Moderate to severe hypertension—used alone or in combination. Renal hypertension.

Contraindications Mild, labile hypertension, pheochromocytoma, or CHF not due to hypertension.

Administer with caution and at a reduced rate to patients with impaired renal function, coronary disease, cardiovascular disease, especially when associated with encephalopathy, or to those who have suffered a recent myocardial infarction. During prolonged therapy, cardiac, renal, and blood tests should be performed. Used with caution in peptic ulcer.

Untoward Reactions *CNS:* Dizziness, weakness, lassitude. Rarely, dyspnea, fatigue, psychic depression. *CV:* Exertional or postural hypotension, bradycardia, edema with possible congestive heart failure. Rarely, angina. *GI:* Persistent diarrhea, increased frequency of bowel movements. Rarely, nausea, vomiting, parotid tenderness. *Miscellaneous:* Inhibition of ejaculation. Rarely, dyspnea, nocturia, urinary incontinence, dermatitis, alopecia, xerostomia, increased blood urea nitrogen, drooping of upper eye lid, blurred vision, myalgia, muscle tremors, chest paresthesia, nasal congestion.

Drug Interactions

Interactant	Interaction
Alcohol, ethyl	Additive orthostatic hypotension
Amphetamines	↓ Effect of guanethidine by ↓ uptake of the drug to its site of action
Anesthetics, general	Additive hypotension
Antidepressants, tricyclic	↓ Effect of guanethidine by ↓ uptake of the drug to its site of action
Cocaine	↓ Effect of guanethidine by ↓ uptake of the drug to its site of action
Ephedrine	↓ Effect of guanethidine by ↓ uptake of the drug to its site of action
Epinephrine	Guanethidine ↑ effect of epinephrine
Haloperidol	↓ Effect of guanethidine by ↓ uptake of the drug to its site of action
Levarterenol	See Norepinephrine
Metaraminol	Guanethidine ↑ effect of metaraminol
Methotrimeprazine	Additive hypotensive effect
Methoxamine	Guanethidine ↑ effect of methoxamine
Monoamine oxidase inhibitors	Reverse effect of guanethidine
Norepinephrine	↑ Effect of norepinephrine probably due to ↑ sensitivity of norepinephrine receptor and ↓

Interactant	Interaction
	uptake of norepinephrine by the neuron
Oral contraceptives	↓ Effect of guanethidine by ↓ uptake of the drug to its site of action
Phenothiazines	↓ Effect of guanethidine by ↓ uptake of the drug to its site of action
Phenylephrine	↑ Response to phenylephrine in guanethidine-treated patients
Phenylpropanolamine	↓ Effect of guanethidine by ↓ uptake of the drug to its site of action
Procainamide	Additive hypotensive effect
Procarbazine	Additive hypotensive effect
Propranolol	Additive hypotensive effect
Pseudoephedrine	↓ Effect of guanethidine by ↓ uptake of the drug to its site of action
Quinidine	Additive hypotensive effect
Reserpine	Excessive bradycardia, postural hypotension, and mental depression
Thiazide diuretics	Additive hypotensive effect
Thioxanthines	↓ Effect of guanethidine by ↓ uptake of the drug to its site of action
Vasodilator drugs, peripheral	Additive hypotensive effect
Vasopressor drugs	↑ Effect of vasopressor agents probably due to ↑ sensitivity of norepinephrine receptor and ↓ uptake of vasopressor agent by the neuron

Laboratory Test Interference ↑ BUN, SGOT, and SGPT. ↓ Prothrombin time, serum glucose, and urine catecholamines. Alteration of electrolyte balance.

Dosage **PO**. *Ambulatory patients*: **initial**, 10 mg daily; increase in 10 mg increments q 7 days; **maintenance**: 25–50 mg once daily. *Hospitalized patients*: **initial**, 25–50 mg; increase by 25 or 50 mg daily or every other day; **maintenance**: estimated to be approximately one-seventh of loading dose. **Pediatric: initial,** 0.2 mg/kg/day given in one dose; **then,** dose may be increased by 0.2 mg/kg/day q 7–10 days to maximum of 3 mg/kg/day.

Administration

1. Drug given daily or every other day.
2. Often used concomitantly with thiazide diuretics to reduce severity of sodium and water retention caused by guanethidine.
3. When control is achieved, dosage should be reduced to the minimal dose required to maintain lowest possible BP.
4. Guanethidine sulfate should be discontinued or dosage decreased at least 2 weeks before surgery.

Nursing Implications

1. Ascertain that cardiac, hepatic, and renal studies are completed before therapy is initiated.
2. *Assess*

a. BP, with patient in both the standing and supine positions, unless contraindicated by condition.

b. for bradycardia and diarrhea, and report to physician. An anticholinergic drug (atropine) may be given.

c. weight daily and observe for edema.

d. intake and output, particularly observing for reduced urine volume.

e. for stress, as this may precipitate cardiovascular collapse.

f. closely for drug interactions, as guanethidine interacts with many drugs, and dosage may require adjustment.

3. *Teach patient and/or family*

a. to limit alcohol intake; otherwise, orthostatic hypotension may be further precipitated.

b. to rise slowly from bed by sitting on the edge of the bed for a few minutes with feet dangling before standing. This is especially important in the morning when the patient should be assisted after lying flat all night, since hypotension may be more severe.

c. to lie down or sit down with head bent low, should he feel weak or dizzy.

d. to avoid sudden or prolonged standing or exercise.

PHENOXYBENZAMINE HYDROCHLORIDE   Dibenzyline (Rx)

Classification   Antihypertensive, adrenergic blocking agent. (See p. 577.)

PHENTOLAMINE MESYLATE   Regitine Mesylate (Rx)

Classification   Antihypertensive, adrenergic blocking agent. (See p. 578.)

PRAZOSIN HYDROCHLORIDE   Minipress (Rx)

Classification   Antihypertensive, peripherally acting antiadrenergic.

Action/Kinetics   Produces selective blockade of postsynaptic alpha-adrenergic receptors. Dilates arterioles and veins, thereby decreasing total peripheral resistance and decreasing diastolic more than systolic blood pressure. Cardiac output, heart rate, and renal blood flow are not affected. Can be used to initiate antihypertensive therapy and is most effective when used with other agents (e.g., diuretics, beta-adrenergic blocking agents).

Onset: 2 hr; **maximum effect**: 2–4 hr; **duration**: 6–12 hr. t½: 2–4 hr. Full therapeutic effect: 4–6 weeks. Metabolized extensively; excreted primarily in feces.

Uses   Mild to moderate hypertension. *Investigational:* Congestive heart failure refractory to other treatment. Raynaud's disease.

Contraindications   Safe use in pregnancy and during childhood has not been established.

Untoward Reactions   Syncope 30 to 90 minutes after administration of initial dose (usually 2 or more mg), increase of dosage, or addition of other antihypertensive agent. *CNS:* Dizziness, drowsiness, headache, fatigue, paresthesias, depression, vertigo, nervousness. *CV:* Palpitations, syncope, tachycardia, orthostatic hypotension, aggravation of angina. *GI:* Nausea, vomiting, diarrhea or constipation, dry mouth, abdominal pain. *Miscellaneous:* Sweating, symptoms of lupus, blurred vision, tinnitus, epistaxis, nasal congestion, reddening of sclera, rash, alopecia, pruritus.

Drug Interactions

Interactant	Interaction
Antihypertensives (other)	↑ Antihypertensive effect
Diuretics	↑ Antihypertensive effect
Propranolol	Especially pronounced additive hypotensive effect

Dosage   PO: *individualized*, always initiate with 1 mg b.i.d.–t.i.d.; **maintenance**: if necessary, increase gradually to 20 mg daily in 2 to 3 divided doses. If used with diuretics or other antihypertensives, reduce dose to 1–2 mg t.i.d.

Administration   Food may delay absorption and may minimize side effects of the drug.

Nursing Implications

1. In the event of syncope, place patient in a reclining position, and provide supportive care.
2. Place patient in a supine position should overdosage occur, and provide supportive measures. Treat for shock if necessary with plasma volume expanders and vasopressor drugs.
3. *Teach patient and/or family*
   a. to be drug compliant, since full effect of drug may not be evident for 4 to 6 weeks.
   b. report side effects to medical supervisor, because reduction in dosage may be indicated.
   c. not to discontinue medication unless so directed by medical supervision.
   d. to avoid any cold, cough, or allergy medication, unless he checks with medical supervision, because sympathomimetic component of such medication will interfere with action of prazosin.
   e. not to engage in activities requiring alertness, such as operating machinery or driving a car, as the drug may cause dizziness and drowsiness.
   f. to avoid rapid postural changes because these may precipitate weakness, dizziness, and syncope.
   g. if a very rapid heartbeat is felt, to lie down or sit down and put head below knees to avoid fainting.
   h. to avoid situations in which fainting would be dangerous.

Beta-Adrenergic Blocking Agents

Action/Kinetics   Beta-adrenergic blocking agents combine reversibly with beta-adrenergic receptors to block the response to sympathetic nerve impulses, circulating catecholamines, or adrenergic drugs. Beta-adrenergic receptors have been classified as beta-1 (predominately in the cardiac muscle) and beta-2 (mainly in the bronchi and vascular musculature). Blockade of beta-1 receptors decreases heart rate, myocardial contractility, and cardiac output; in addition, A-V conduction is slowed. These effects lead to a decrease in blood pressure as well as a reversal of cardiac arrhythmias. Blockade of beta-2 receptors increases airway resistance in the bronchioles and inhibits the vasodilating effects of catecholamines on peripheral blood vessels. The various beta-blocking agents differ in their ability to block beta-1 and beta-2 receptors; also, certain of these agents have intrinsic sympathomimetic action.

Uses   Depending on the drug, these agents may be used to treat hypertension, angina, cardiac arrhythmias, and myocardial infarction. Also, see individual agents.

Contraindications   Sinus bradycardia, partial or total heart block, cardiogenic shock, congestive heart failure, overt cardiac failure. Chronic bronchitis, asthma, bronchospasm, emphysema. Use with caution in diabetes, thyrotoxicosis, and impaired renal or kidney function. Safe use in pregnancy, lactation, and in children has not been established. Also, see individual agents.

Untoward Reactions   *CV:* Bradycardia, hypotension (especially following IV use), congestive heart failure, cold extremities, claudication, worsening of angina, strokes, edema, syncope, arrhythmias, increased heart rate, palpitations, precipitation or worsening of heart block, thrombosis of renal or mesenteric arteries, ischemic colitis, precipitation or worsening of Raynaud's phenomenon. Sudden withdrawal of large doses may cause angina, ventricular tachycardia, fatal myocardial infarction, or sudden death. *GI:* Nausea, vomiting, diarrhea, flatulence, dry mouth, constipation, anorexia, cramps, weight gain or loss, retroperitoneal fibrosis. *Respiratory:* Asthma-like symptoms, bronchospasms, worsening of chronic obstructive lung disease, dyspnea, cough, nasal stuffiness, rhinitis, pharyngitis, rales. *CNS:* Fatigue, lethargy, vivid dreams, depression, hallucinations, delirium, psychoses, paresthesias, insomnia, nervousness, nightmares, headache, vertigo. *Hematologic:* Agranulocytosis, thrombocytopenia. *Allergic:* Fever, sore throat, respiratory distress, rash. *Skin:* Pruritus, rashes, increased skin pigmentation, sweating, dry skin, alopecia, skin irritation. *Other:* Hyperglycemia or hypoglycemia, joint and muscle pain, arthralgia, back pain, lupus-like syndrome, Peyronie's disease, sexual dysfunction, dysuria, nocturia, visual disturbances, eye irritation or burning, conjunctivitis.

Drug Interactions

Interactant	Interaction
Anesthetics, general	Additive depression of myocardium
Anticholinergic agents	Anticholinergics counteract bradycardia produced by beta-adrenergic blockers
Antihypertensives	Additive hypotensive effect
Chlorpromazine	Additive beta-adrenergic blocking action
Cimetidine	↑ Effect beta-blockers due to ↓ breakdown by liver
Clonidine	Paradoxical hypertension; also, ↑ severity of rebound hypertension
Epinephrine	Beta-blockers prevent beta-adrenergic action of epinephrine but not alpha-adrenergic action → ↑ systolic and diastolic blood pressure and ↓ heart rate
Furosemide	↑ Beta-adrenergic blockade
Hydralazine	↑ Beta-adrenergic blockade

Interactant	Interaction
Insulin	Beta-blockers ↑ hypoglycemic effect of insulin
Indomethacin	↓ Effect of beta-blockers possibly due to inhibition of prostaglandin synthesis
Lidocaine	↑ Effect of lidocaine due to ↓ breakdown by liver
Methyldopa	Possible ↑ blood pressure to to alpha-adrenergic effect
Oral contraceptives	↑ Effect beta-blockers due to ↓ breakdown by liver
Phenformin	↑ Hypoglycemia
Phenobarbital	Phenobarbital ↓ effect of beta-blockers due to ↑ breakdown by liver
Phenothiazines	↑ Effect of both drugs
Phenytoin	Additive depression of myocardium; also phenytoin ↓ effect of beta-blockers due to ↑ breakdown by liver
Prazosin	↑ Effect of prazosin
Rifampin	Rifampin ↓ effect of beta-blockers due to ↑ breakdown by liver
Ritodrine	Beta-blockers ↓ effect of ritodrine
Salicylates	↓ Effect of beta-blockers possibly due to inhibition of prostaglandin synthesis
Succinylcholine	Beta-blockers ↑ effects of succinylcholine
Theophylline	Beta-blockers reverse the effect of theophylline; also, beta-blockers ↓ renal clearance of theophylline
Tubocurarine	Beta-blockers ↑ effects of tubocurarine

Laboratory Test Interference   ↓ Serum glucose

Dosage   See individual drugs.

Treatment of Overdosage   General supportive treatment such as inducing emesis or gastric lavage, artificial respiration, treatment of hypoglycemia or hypokalemia. *Excessive bradycardia:* **Atropine, 0.6 mg; if no response, give q 3 min for a total of 2–3 mg. Cautious administration of isoproterenol may be tried. Also, glucagon, 5–10 mg may reverse bradycardia.** *Cardiac failure:* Digitalis, diuretic, and oxygen; if failure is refractory, IV aminophylline or glucagon may be helpful. *Hypotension:* IV fluids; also vasopressors such as norepinephrine, dobutamine, dopamine. If refractory, glucagon may be helpful. *Premature ventricular contractions:* Lidocaine or phenytoin. *Bronchospasms:* Give a beta-2 adrenergic agonist or theophylline. *Heart block:* Isoproterenol or transvenous cardiac pacing.

Nursing Implications

1. *Assess*
   a. the pulse rate as these drugs may cause tachycardia or bradycardia.
   b. for symptoms of congestive heart failure, such as fatigue, increasing dyspnea and cough, and edema; these symptoms indicate that patient may require digitalization and diuretics and/or discontinuation of drug.

c. rate and quality of respirations as these drugs may cause dyspnea and bronchospasm.

d. diabetic patient for acute fatigue, restlessness, malaise, irritability, and weakness, which are symptoms indicative of hypoglycemia. (Most beta-adrenergic blockers mask signs of hypoglycemia such as tachycardia and hypotension.)

2. *Teach patient and/or family*

a. to take blood pressure at least twice a week and to take pulse rate immediately prior to first dose each day.

b. not to interrupt therapy without consulting physician, as abrupt withdrawal of most beta-adrenergic blocking agents may precipitate angina, myocardial infarction, or rebound hypertension.

ACEBUTOLOL HYDROCHLORIDE   Sectral (Rx)

Action/Kinetics Predominately beta-1 blocking activity. Acebutolol also has some intrinsic sympathomimetic activity. **t½:** 3–4 hr. Metabolized in liver and excreted in urine and bile.

Uses Hypertension (either alone or with other antihypertensive agents as thiazide diuretics). Premature ventricular contractions.

Dosage **PO.** *Hypertension:* **initial,** 400 mg 1–2 times/day. *Premature ventricular contractions:* **initial,** 200 mg b.i.d.; **then,** increase dose gradually to reach 600–1,200 mg/day. Dosage should be decreased in geriatric patients (should not exceed 800 mg daily) and in those with impaired kidney or liver function.

ATENOLOL   Tenormin (Rx)

Action/Kinetics Predominately beta-1 blocking activity. **Peak blood levels:** 2–4 hr. **t½:** 6–7 hr. Eliminated unchanged by the kidney.

Uses Hypertension (either alone or with other antihypertensives as thiazide diuretics). *Investigational:* Prophylaxis of migraine.

Dosage **PO. Initial:** 50 mg once daily either alone or with diuretics; if response inadequate, 100 mg once daily. Doses higher than 100 mg daily will not produce further beneficial effects. Adjust dosage in cases of renal failure.

METOPROLOL   Betaloc,* Lopressor (Rx)

Action/Kinetics Exerts mainly beta-1 adrenergic blocking activity. **Onset:** 15 min. **Peak plasma levels:** 90 min. **t½:** 3–4 hr. Effect of drug is cumulative. Food increases bioavailability. Exhibits significant first-pass effect. Metabolized in liver and excreted through urine.

Uses Hypertension (either alone or with other antihypertensive agents as thiazide diuretics). Acute myocardial infarction in stable patients. *Investigational:* IV to suppress atrial ectopy in chronic obstructive pulmonary disease.

Additional Contraindications   Myocardial infarction in patients with a heart rate less than 45 beats/min, in second-, or third-degree heart block, of if systolic blood pressure is less than 100 mg Hg. Cardiac failure.

Additional Drug Interactions   Methimazole or propylthiouracil may ↑ the effects of metoprolol.

Laboratory Test Interferences   ↑ Serum transaminase, LDH, alkaline phosphatase.

Dosage   PO. *Hypertension:* **initial,** 100 mg daily in single or divided doses; **then,** dose may be increased weekly to maintenance of 100–450 mg daily. A diuretic may also be used. *Myocardial infarction, early treatment:* 5 mg as an **IV** bolus q 2 min for a total of 3 doses (15 mg); **then,** if this dose is tolerated, give 50 mg PO q 6 hr for 48 hr, beginning 15 min after the last IV dose. **Maintenance:** 100 mg b.i.d. If patient can not tolerate full IV dose, begin PO dose at 25 or 50 mg q 6 hr. *Myocardial infarction, late treatment:* **PO,** 100 mg b.i.d. as soon as feasible; continue for 1–3 months.

NADOLOL   Corgard (Rx)

Action/Kinetics   Manifests both beta-1 and beta-2 adrenergic blocking activity. **Peak serum concentration:** 3–4 hr. **t½:** 20–24 hr (permits once daily dosage). **Duration:** 17–24 hr. Absorption variable, averaging 30%; steady plasma level achieved after 6–9 days administration. Excreted unchanged by the kidney.

Uses   Hypertension, either alone or with other drugs (e.g., thiazide diuretic). Angina pectoris. *Investigational:* Prophylaxis of migraine, treatment of lithium-induced tremors.

Dosage   PO. *Hypertension:* **initial,** 40 mg once daily; **then,** may be increased in 40–80 mg increments until optimum response obtained. **Maintenance:** 40–80 mg once daily although up to 320 mg once daily may be needed. *Angina:* **initial,** 40 mg once daily; **then,** increase dose in 40–80 mg increments q 3–7 days until optimum response obtained. **Maintenance:** 40–80 mg once daily although up to 240 mg once daily may be needed. Dosage for all uses should be decreased in patients with renal failure.

PINDOLOL   Visken (Rx)

Action/Kinetics   Manifests both beta-1 and beta-2 adrenergic blocking activity. Pindolol also has significant intrinsic sympathomimetic effects. **t½:** 3–4 hr. The drug is metabolized by the liver, and the metabolites and unchanged drug are excreted through the kidneys.

Uses   Hypertension (alone or in combination with other antihypertensive agents as thiazide diuretics).

Laboratory Test Interferences   ↑ SGOT and SGPT. Rarely, ↑ LDH, uric acid, alkaline phosphatase.

Dosage   PO. Initial: 5 mg b.i.d. (alone or with other antihypertensive drugs). If no response in 3–4 weeks, increase by 10 mg/day q 3–4 weeks to a maximum of 60 mg daily.

PROPRANOLOL HYDROCHLORIDE   Apo-Propranolol,* Detensol,* Inderal, Inderal LA, Novopranol,* PMS Propranolol* (Rx)

Action/Kinetics   Propranolol manifests both beta-1 and beta-2 adrenergic blocking activity. The antiarrhythmic action results from both beta-adrenergic receptor blockade and from a direct membrane stabilizing action on the cardiac cell. **PO: Onset,** 30 min. **Maximum effect:** 1–1½ hr. **Duration:** 3–6 hr. **t½:** 2–5 hr. Onset after IV administration is almost immediate. Completely metabolized by liver and excreted in urine. Although food increases bioavailability of the drug, absorption may be decreased.

Uses   Hypertension (alone or in combination with other antihypertensive agents). Angina pectoris, hypertrophic subaortic stenosis, prophylaxis of myocardial infarction, pheochromocytoma, prophylaxis of migraine. Cardiac arrhythmias including ventricular tachycardias, tachycardias due to digitalis intoxication, supraventricular arrhythmias. *Investigational:* Schizophrenia, tardive dyskinesia, acute panic symptoms, recurrent GI bleeding in cirrhosis, tremor (essential).

Additional Untoward Reactions   Psoriasis-like eruptions, skin necrosis, systemic lupus erythematosus (rare).

Additional Drug Interactions   Methimazole and propylthiouracil may ↑ the effects of propranolol.

Laboratory Test Interferences   ↑ Blood urea, serum transaminase, alkaline phosphatase, LDH. Interference with glaucoma screening test.

Dosage   PO. *Hypertension:* **initial,** 40 mg b.i.d. or 80 mg of sustained release/day; **then,** increase dose to maintenance of 120–240 mg daily given in 2–3 divided doses or 120–160 mg of sustained release once daily. Maximum daily dose should not exceed 640 mg. *Angina, prophylaxis:* **initial,** 10–20 mg t.i.d.–q.i.d. or 80 mg of sustained release once daily; **then,** increase dose gradually to maintenance of 160 mg/day. The maximum daily dose should not exceed 320 mg. *Arrhythmias:* 10–30 mg before meals and at bedtime. *Hypertrophic subaortic stenosis:* 20–40 mg t.i.d.–q.i.d. before meals and at bedtime or 80–160 mg of sustained release given once daily. *Myocardial infarction prophylaxis:* 180–240 mg daily given in 2–3 divided doses. *Pheochromocytoma, preoperatively:* 60 mg daily for 3 days before surgery given concomitantly with an alpha-adrenergic blocking agent; *inoperable tumors:* 30 mg/day in divided doses. *Migraine:* **initial,** 80 mg sustained release given once daily; **then,** increase dose gradually to maintenance of 160–240 mg daily.

IV. *Life-threatening arrhythmias:* 1–3 mg not to exceed 1 mg/min; a second dose may be given after 2 min with subsequent doses q 4 hr. Patients should begin PO therapy as soon as possible.

Administration

1. Do not administer for a minimum of 2 weeks after patient has received MAO inhibitor drugs.
2. If signs of serious myocardial depression occur following propranolol, isoproterenol (Isuprel) should be slowly infused IV.

Additional Nursing Implications

1. *Assess* for rash, fever, and/or purpura, indicative of hypersensitivity reaction. Withdrawal of drug may be necessary.

(continued)

2. Review list of drug interactions as there are extensive interactions requiring close assessment of patient and possible dose reduction.
3. To combat hypotension or circulatory collapse after IV administration, have available atropine for IV use.

TIMOLOL MALEATE   Blocadren, Timolide,* Timoptic (Rx)

Action/Kinetics   Timolol exerts both beta-1 and beta-2 adrenergic blocking activity. The mechanism of the protective effect in myocardial infarction is unknown. **Peak plasma levels:** 1–2 hr. **t½:** 4 hr. Metabolized in the liver, and metabolites and unchanged drug excreted through the kidney.

Uses   Hypertension (alone or in combination with other antihypertensives as thiazide diuretics). Within 1–4 weeks of myocardial infarction to reduce risk of reinfarction. Glaucoma (see Table 22, p. 588). *Investigational:* Prophylaxis of migraine.

Laboratory Test Interferences   ↑ BUN, serum potassium and uric acid. ↓ Hemoglobin and hematocrit.

Dosage   PO. *Hypertension:* **initial,** 10 mg b.i.d.; **maintenance:** 20–40 mg/day (up to 60 mg/day in 2 doses may be required). If dosage increase is necessary, wait 7 days. *Myocardial infarction prophylaxis:* 10 mg 2 times per week.

Additional Nursing Implications
Teach patient and/or family that when timolol is used for long-term prophylaxis against myocardial infarction, not to interrupt therapy without consulting with physician as abrupt withdrawal may precipitate reinfarction.

Miscellaneous Agents

CAPTOPRIL   Capoten (Rx)

Classification   Antihypertensive, inhibitor of angiotensin synthesis

Action/Kinetics   Mechanism not fully understood, but drug seems to inhibit biosynthesis of angiotensin II, which increases BP. Captopril also increases renin activity and decreases aldosterone secretion, leading to small increase in serum potassium. **Peak blood levels:** 1 hr; presence of food decreases absorption by 30–40%. **Plasma protein binding:** 25–30% **Duration:** 6–12 hr. **t½:** 2 hr; in 24 hr, 95% of absorbed dose excreted in urine (40–50% unchanged).

Uses   In combination with a thiazide diuretic in patients who have not responded to other antihypertensive drug regimens or in whom side effects have occurred with other regimens. (Concomitant use with diuretic therapy may, however, cause precipitous hypotension.)

In combination with diuretics and digitalis in treatment of heart failure not responding to conventional therapy.

Contraindications Use with caution in cases of impaired renal function. Use in pregnancy only if potential benefit outweighs risk. Use in children only if other antihypertensive therapy has proved ineffective in controlling BP. Lactation.

Untoward Reactions *Dermatologic*: Rash with pruritus, fever, eosinophilia. Angioedema of face, mucous membranes of mouth, or extremities. Flushing, pallor. *GI:* Gastric irritation, nausea, vomiting, anorexia, constipation or diarrhea, ulcers, dyspepsia, dry mouth. *CNS:* Headache, dizziness, insomnia, malaise, fatigue. *CV:* Hypotension, angina, congestive heart failure, myocardial infarction, Raynaud's phenomenon, chest pain, palpitations, tachycardia. *Renal:* Renal insufficiency or failure, proteinuria, urinary frequency, oliguria, polyuria. *Other:* Decrease or loss of taste perception with weight loss (reversible), neutropenia, paresthesias.

Drug Interactions

Interactant	Interaction
Antihypertensives, oral	↑ Effect of captopril if renin is released
Diuretics	Sudden ↓ BP within 3 hr
Potassium-sparing diuretics	↑ Serum potassium

Laboratory Test Interference False + urinary acetone. Transient ↑ BUN and creatinine. ↑ Serum potassium.

Dosage **PO.** *Hypertension:* **Adults:** 25 mg t.i.d. If unsatisfactory response after 1–2 weeks, increase to 50 mg t.i.d.; if still unsatisfactory after another 1–2 weeks, thiazide diuretic should be added (e.g., hydrochlorothiazide, 25 mg/day). Dosage may be increased to 100–150 mg t.i.d., not to exceed 450 mg daily. *Heart failure:* **initial,** 25 mg t.i.d.; **then,** increase dose to 50 mg t.i.d., and evaluate response. **Maintenance:** 50–100 mg t.i.d., not to exceed 450 mg daily.

For accelerated or malignant hypertension: **initial,** 25 mg t.i.d.; **then,** increase dose q 24 hr until satisfactory response obtained or maximum dose reached. For all uses, doses should be reduced in patients with renal impairment.

Administration

1. Since food decreases absorption, captopril should be taken 1 hr before meals.
2. In cases of overdosage, volume expansion with normal saline (IV) is the treatment of choice to restore BP.
3. Captopril should not be discontinued without the consent of a physician.

Nursing Implications

1. Ascertain that baseline hematologic, renal, and liver function tests are done before initiating therapy.
2. *Assess*
   a. for proteinuria periodically. Test urine and assess for edema.
   b. closely for a precipitous drop in BP within 3 hr after initial dose of captopril in a patient who has been on diuretic therapy and on a sodium-restricted diet. If BP falls precipitously, place patient in supine position and be prepared to assist with an infusion of saline (IV).
3. Withhold potassium-sparing diuretics and consult with doctor if patient is not hypokalemic because hyperkalemia may result.
4. Be alert to hyperkalemia occurring several months after spironolactone was administered and captopril initiated.

(continued)

5. *Teach patient and/or family*
   a. to take captopril 1 hr before meals on an empty stomach, as food interferes with absorption.
   b. to report fever, sore throat, mouth sores, irregular heart beat, or chest pain to doctor.
   c. to avoid sudden changes in posture to prevent dizziness and fainting.
   d. to report skin rash or interference with taste perception if these conditions continue.

LABETALOL HYDROCHLORIDE Normodyne, Trandate (Rx)

Classification   Alpha- and beta-adrenergic blocking agent.

Action/Kinetics   Labetalol decreases blood pressure by blocking both alpha- and beta-adrenergic receptors. Significant reflex tachycardia and bradycardia do not occur although AV conduction may be prolonged. **Onset: PO,** 2–4 hr; **IV,** 5 min. **Duration: PO,** 8–12 hr. **t½: PO,** 7 hr; **IV,** 5½ hr. Significant first-pass effect; metabolized in liver. Food increases bioavailability of the drug.

Uses   Alone or in combination with other drugs for hypertension.

Contraindications   Cardiogenic shock or failure, bronchial asthma, bradycardia, greater than first-degree heart block. Use with caution in pregnancy, lactation, impaired renal function, diabetes (may prevent premonitory signs of acute hypoglycemia). Safety and efficacy in children has not been established.

Untoward Reactions   *CV:* Postural hypotension, edema, flushing, ventricular arrhythmias. *GI:* Nausea, vomiting, diarrhea, altered taste, dyspepsia. *CNS:* Headache, drowsiness, fatigue, sleepiness, dizziness, vertigo. *GU:* Impotence, urinary bladder retention, difficulty in urination, failure to ejaculate. *Dermatologic:* Rashes, facial erythema, alopecia, urticaria, pruritus, psoriasis-like syndrome. *Other:* Bronchospasm, dyspnea, muscle cramps or weakness, toxic myopathy, jaundice, cholestasis, difficulties with vision, dry eyes, nasal stuffiness, numbness, wheezing, tingling of skin or scalp, sweating.
   There may be changes in laboratory values including increased serum transaminase, positive antinuclear factor, and increases in blood urea and creatinine.

Drug Interactions

Interactant	Interaction
Cimetidine	↑ Bioavailability of labetalol
Halothane	↑ Risk of severe hypotension
Nitroglycerin	Additive hypotension
Tricyclic antidepressants	↑ Risk of tremors

Dosage   **PO. Initial:** 100 mg b.i.d.; **maintenance:** 200–400 mg b.i.d. up to 1,200–2,400 mg daily for severe cases. **IV injections. Individualize. Initial:** 20 mg slowly over 2 min; **then,** 40–80 mg q 10 min until desired effect or a total of 300 mg has been given. **IV infusion. Initial:** 2 mg/min; **then,** adjust rate according to response. **Usual dose range:** 50–300 mg. *Transfer from IV to PO therapy:* **initial,** 200 mg;

then, 200–400 mg 6–12 hr later depending on response. Thereafter, dosage based on response.

Administration
1. When transferring to oral labetalol from other antihypertensive therapy, slowly reduce dosage of current therapy.
2. To transfer from IV to PO therapy in hospitalized patients, begin when supine blood pressure begins to increase.
3. Labetalol is not compatible with 5% sodium bicarbonate injection.

METYROSINE   Demser (Rx)

Classification   Tyrosine hydroxylase inhibitor.

Action/Kinetics   By inhibiting the enzyme tyrosine hydroxylase, which is the rate-limiting step in the biosynthesis of catecholamines, there is a decrease in both norepinephrine and epinephrine synthesis. **Peak effect:** over 6 hr. **Duration:** 2–3 days. **Absorption:** GI tract (70%); excreted unchanged in urine.

Use   Pheochromocytoma (preoperatively or for chronic therapy). Not used in the treatment of essential hypertension.

Contraindications   Hypersensitivity to drug. Safe use during pregnancy, lactation, and children under 12 yr not established.

Untoward Reactions   *CNS:* Sedation (100%), which decreases with usage; alteration in sleep patterns; insomnia and psychic stimulation upon drug removal; extrapyramidal symptoms (drooling, speech difficulties, tremors); anxiety, depression, hallucinations, disorientation, confusion, headaches. *GI:* Diarrhea (10%), nausea, vomiting, decreased salivation, dry mouth. *Other:* Galactorrhea, crystalluria, hematuria, transient dysuria, nasal stuffiness, impotence, swollen breasts. *Rarely:* Eosinophilia, peripheral edema, hypersensitivity. During anesthesia and surgery, life-threatening arrhythmias may result—treat with lidocaine or a beta-adrenergic blocking agent.

Drug Interactions

Interactant	Interaction
Alcohol	Additive CNS depression
Alpha-adrenergic blocking agents	Hypotension; ↓ perfusion of vital organs
CNS depressants	Additive CNS depression
Haloperidol	↑ Extrapyramidal side effects
Phenothiazines	↑ Extrapyramidal side effects

Laboratory Test Interferences   ↑ SGOT and urinary catecholamine levels.

Dosage   **Adults and children over 12 yr: Initial,** 250 mg q.i.d.; **then,** increase by 250–500 mg every day to maximum of 4 gm/day in divided doses. Usual optimum dosage: 2–3 gm/day. Dose must be individually determined by BP response and control of clinical symptoms. Phenoxybenzamine may be added if adequate control not achieved.

Nursing Implications

1. *Teach patient and/or family*
   a. that adequate fluid intake is essential to prevent low BP, crystals in urine, and poor circulation to vital organs.
   b. not to drive a car or operate hazardous machinery, as drowsiness may occur within the first 24 hr of therapy. Encourage patient that sedative effects usually do not occur after 1 week unless dosage is more than 2 gm or more per day.
   c. that he should report all symptoms noted in *Untoward Effects* to doctor.

MINOXIDIL   Loniten (Rx)

Classification   Antihypertensive, depresses sympathetic nervous system.

Action/Kinetics   Decreases elevated BP by decreasing peripheral resistance. Drug causes increase in renin secretion, increase in cardiac rate and output, and salt/water retention. It does not cause orthostatic hypotension. **Onset:** rapid. **Peak plasma level:** reached within 60 min; **plasma t½:** 4.2 hr. **Duration:** 75 hr. Absorbed from GI tract 90%; excretion: renal (90% metabolites). The time to maximum effect is inversely related to the dose.

Minoxidil can produce severe side effects; it should be reserved for resistant cases of hypertension. Use generally requires concomitant administration of beta-adrenergic blocking agents and diuretics. Close medical supervision required, including possible hospitalization during initial administration.

Use   Hypertension not controllable by use of a diuretic plus two other antihypertensive drugs.

Contraindications   Pheochromocytoma. Within 1 month after a myocardial infarction. Safe use during pregnancy and lactation not established. Use with caution and at reduced dosage in impaired renal function.

Untoward Reactions   *CV:* Edema, pericardial effusion, tamponade (acute compression of heart caused by fluid or blood in pericardium), CHF, angina pectoris, increased heart rate. *GI:* Nausea, vomiting. *CNS:* Headache, fatigue. *Other:* Hypertrichosis (enhanced growth, pigmentation and thickening of fine body hair 3–6 weeks after initiation of therapy) (80%), skin rashes (hypersensitivity), breast tenderness.

Drug Interactions   Concomitant use with guanethidine may result in severe hypotension.

Laboratory Test Interferences   Nonspecific changes in ECG. ↓ Hematocrit, erythrocyte count, and hemoglobin. ↑ Alkaline phosphatase, serum creatinine, and BUN.

Dosage   Usually taken with at least two other antihypertensive drugs, a diuretic, and a drug to minimize tachycardia (e.g., beta-adrenergic blocking agent). **Adults and children over 12 yr: Initial,** 5 mg once daily. For optimum control, dose can be increased to 10, 20, and then 40 mg in single or divided doses/day. Daily dosage should not exceed 100 mg. **Children under 12 yr: Initial,** 0.2 mg/kg once daily. Effective dose range: 0.25–1.0 mg/kg/day. Dosage must be titrated to individual response. Daily dosage should not exceed 50 mg.

Administration   Can be taken with fluids and without regard to meals.

Nursing Implications

1. Anticipate that minoxidil therapy will be initiated in the hospital, so that the patient can be rigorously monitored for rapid or large orthostatic decreases in BP. After medication, BP decreases within a ½ hr. Within 2–3 hr, the patient reaches minimum BP.

2. *Assess*
   a. patient for salt and water retention leading to CHF. Weigh every day and examine for edema.
   b. for tachycardia and report.
   c. for respiratory dysfunction and report.

3. Ensure that a patient on guanethidine discontinues its use before initiation of minoxidil, or that the patient is rigorously monitored for severe hypotensive effects that may be precipitated by drug interaction.

4. *Teach patient and/or family*
   a. the technique of monitoring pulse. Report pulse 20 beats above baseline to doctor.
   b. to weigh himself daily and to report rapid weight gain over 5 lb within 3 days.
   c. to report edema of extremities, face, and abdomen.
   d. to report any dyspnea that occurs when lying down.
   e. to report angina, dizziness, or fainting.
   f. that the medication might cause elongation, thickening, and increased pigmentation of body hair, but that there is a return to pretreatment norm with the discontinuance of drug.

MONOAMINE OXIDASE (MAO) INHIBITOR

PARGYLINE HYDROCHLORIDE   Eutonyl (Rx)

Classification   Antihypertensive, monoamine oxidase (MAO) inhibitor.

Action/Kinetics   Mechanism of antihypertensive effect not known. Hypotensive effect is primarily orthostatic (similar to ganglionic blocking agents). **Discontinue at least 2 weeks before elective surgery. Onset:** Slow. Full therapeutic effect may take several weeks. **Duration:** Residual effects persist 3 weeks after drug discontinued.

For *Untoward Reactions, Drug Interactions, Laboratory Test Interferences*, See Part 6, Chapter 33, Antidepressants.

Uses   Moderate to severe essential or secondary hypertension. Used in conjunction with thiazides or with other antihypertensive drugs, or both.

Contraindications   Labile and mild hypertension, advanced renal failure, pheochromocytoma, paranoid schizophrenia, or hyperthyroidism. Children under 12 years.

Dosage   **PO. Adult, initial:** 25 mg once daily for 1 week; increase at weekly intervals by 10 mg until desired therapeutic effect is attained. **Initial dose** *for elderly or sympathectomized patients*: 10–25 mg. **Maintenance:** 25–50 mg or higher daily but not to exceed 200 mg daily.

Nursing Implications

Teach patient and/or family

a. to avoid any other medication (particulary decongestants) unless they consult with their physician first.

b. to avoid aged or natural cheese (e.g. Cheddar, Camembert, and Stilton), as well as other foods that require the actions of molds or bacteria for their preparation, such as pickled herring. Alcoholic beverages in any form should not be consumed. Concomitant use of pargyline with such foods may lead to hypertensive crisis.

c. that he may feel dizzy or faint, particularly when changing position from supine to standing. Patient should rise slowly from bed. If he feels dizzy or faint, he should lie or sit down with head lowered.

d. to report headache or other unusual symptoms.

e. to avoid increase in physical activity while on medication, even though he might feel better. (This is particularly important for patients suffering from angina or coronary heart disease.)

f. to weigh himself daily, to check for edema, and to assess whether weight gain is due to fluid or to increased appetite.

g. to monitor intake and output.

h. to report constipation to physician, to determine whether laxative is needed.

i. to practice good mouth care, to counteract nausea and dry mouth.

AGENTS THAT ACT DIRECTLY ON VASCULAR SMOOTH MUSCLE

DIAZOXIDE Hyperstat IV (Rx)

Classification Antihypertensive, direct action on vascular smooth muscle.

Action/Kinetics Direct, prompt vasodilation of peripheral arterioles. **Onset:** 1–5 min. **Duration** (variable): usual 3–12 hr; extreme: 30 min to 72 hr.

Uses May be the drug of choice for hypertensive crisis (malignant hypertension). Often given concomitantly with a diuretic. Especially suitable for patients with impaired renal function, hypertensive encephalopathy, hypertension complicated by left ventricular failure and in eclampsia. Ineffective for hypertension due to pheochromocytoma.

Used orally for management of hyperinsulinism (see p. 696).

Contraindications Hypersensitivity to drug or thiazide diuretics.

Untoward Reactions *CV:* Hypotension (may be severe), sodium and water retention, arrhythmias, cerebral or myocardial ischemia, palpitations, bradycardia. *CNS:* Headache, dizziness, drowsiness, lightheadedness. Confusion, seizures, paralysis, unconsciousness, numbness (all due to cerebral ischemia). *Respiratory:* Tightness in chest, cough, dyspnea, sensation of choking. *GI:* Nausea, vomiting, diarrhea, anorexia, parotid swelling, change in sense of taste, salivation, dry mouth, ileus, constipation. *Other:* Hyperglycemia (may be serious enough to require treatment), sweating, flushing, sensation of warmth, tinnitus, hearing loss, retention of nitrogenous wastes, acute pancreatitis. Pain, cellulitis, phlebitis at injection site.

Drug Interactions

Interactant	Interaction
Anticoagulants, oral	↑ Effect of oral anticoagulants due to ↓ plasma protein binding
Nitrites	↑ Hypotensive effect
Phenytoin	Diazoxide ↓ anticonvulsant effect of phenytoin
Reserpine	↑ Hypotensive effect
Thiazide diuretics	↑ Hyperglycemic, hyperuricemic, and antihypertensive effect of diazoxide
Vasodilators, peripheral	↑ Hypotensive effect

Laboratory Test Interference False + or ↑ uric acid

Dosage **IV Push** (30 sec or less): **Adults,** 1–3 mg/kg up to a maximum of 150 mg; may be repeated at 5–15 min intervals until adequate blood presssure response obtained. Drug may then be repeated at 4- to 24-hr intervals for 4–5 days, or until oral antihypertensive therapy can be initiated.

A bolus of 300 mg may also be used but it is no more effective and increases the risk of severe hypotension.

Administration/Storage

1. Protect from light, heat, and freezing.
2. Inject rapidly (30 seconds) undiluted into a peripheral vein to maximize response.
3. Do not administer **IM** or **SC**.

Nursing Implications

1. Maintain patient in recumbent position during and for 30 minutes after injection.
2. Maintain patient in recumbent position for 8 to 10 hours if furosemide (Lasix) is administered as part of therapy.
3. Closely monitor BP after injection until it has stabilized and then every hour thereafter.
4. Assess final BP of patient on arising after injection.
5. Monitor urine for glycosuria while the patient is on therapy.
6. Assess for symptoms of hyperglycemia. See p. 680.

HYDRALAZINE HYDROCHLORIDE   Alazine, Apresoline (Rx)

Classification Antihypertensive, direct action on vascular smooth muscle.

Action/Kinetics Exerts a direct vasodilating effect on vascular smooth muscle. It also increases blood flow to the kidneys and brain and increases cardiac output by a reflex action. To minimize the cardiac effects, hydralazine is often given with drugs that decrease activity of sympathetic nerves. For example, it is found in Apresazide and Ser-Ap-Es. Food increases bioavilability of the drug.

PO: Onset, 20–30 min; **Peak plasma level:** 2 hr; **Duration:** 2–4 hr. **IM: Onset,**

10–30 min; **Peak plasma level**: 1 hr; **Duration**: 2–6 hr. **IV: Onset**, 5–10 min; **Maximum effect**: 10–80 min; **Duration**: 2–6 hr.

Uses   *PO:* In combination with other drugs for essential hypertension. *Parenteral:* Hypertensive emergencies. *Investigational:* To reduce afterload in congestive heart failure, severe aortic insufficiency after valve replacement.

Contraindications   Coronary artery disease, angina pectoris, advanced renal disease (as in chronic renal hypertension), and chronic glomerulonephritis. Use with caution in stroke patients.

Untoward Reactions   *CV:* Orthostatic hypotension, myocardial infarction, angina pectoris, palpitations, tachycardia. *CNS:* Headache, dizziness, psychoses, tremors, depression, anxiety, disorientation. *GI:* Nausea, vomiting, diarrhea, anorexia, constipation, paralytic ileus. *Allergic:* Rash, urticaria, fever, chills, arthralgia, pruritus, eosinophilia. Rarely, hepatitis, obstructive jaundice. *Hematologic:* Decrease in hemoglobin and red blood cells, purpura, agranulocytosis, leukopenia. *Other:* Peripheral neuritis, impotence, nasal congestion, edema, muscle cramps, lacrimation, conjunctivitis, difficulty in urination, lupus-like syndrome, lymphadenopathy, splenomegaly. Side effects are less severe when dosage is increased slowly.

Drug Interactions

Interactant	Interaction
Beta-adrenergic blocking agents	↑ Effect of both drugs
Methotrimeprazine	Additive hypotensive effect
Procainamide	Additive hypotensive effect
Quinidine	Additive hypotensive effect
Sympathomimetics	↑ Risk of tachycardia and angina

Dosage   **PO. Adult, initial**: 10 mg q.i.d for 2–4 days; **then**, increase to 25 mg q.i.d. for rest of first week. For second and following weeks, increase to 50 mg q.i.d. **Maintenance**: individualized to lowest effective dose; maximum daily dose should not exceed 300 mg. **Pediatric: initial**, 0.75 mg/kg/day in 4 divided doses; dosage may be increased gradually up to 7.5 mg/kg/day. Food increases the bioavailability of the drug.

   IV, IM. *Hypertensive crisis*: **adults, usual**, 20–40 mg, repeated as necessary. Blood pressure may fall within 5–10 min with maximum response in 10–80 min. Usually, switch to PO medication in 1–2 days. Dosage should be decreased in patients with renal damage. **Pediatric**: 0.1–0.2 mg/kg q 4–6 hr as required.

Administration   Parenteral injections should be made as quickly as possible after being drawn into the syringe.

Nursing Implications

1. *Assess*
   a. for an influenza-like syndrome early during therapy or for a rheumatoid syndrome, which may necessitate discontinuing hydralazine.
   b. BP several times a day under standardized conditions, either sitting or standing, as ordered by physician.
   c. BP within 5 min after the parenteral injection of the medication.
   d. weight daily.
   e. for edema.
   f. intake and output, observing particularly for a reduction in output.

2. *Teach patient and/or family*
   a. possible side effects of drug. After taking first dose, patient may experience headache, palpitations, and possibly mild postural hypotension. These symptoms may persist for 7 to 10 days with continued treatment.
   b. that patient may feel weak and dizzy. Should this occur, the patient should lie down or sit down with head low.
   c. to change slowly from supine to sitting position.

NITROPRUSSIDE SODIUM   Nipride, Nitropress (Rx)

Classification   Antihypertensive, direct action on vascular smooth muscle.

Action/Kinetics   Direct action on vascular smooth muscle, leading to peripheral vasodilation. **Onset** (drug must be given by IV infusion): 2 min; **Duration**: 3–5 min.

Uses   Hypertensive crisis to reduce BP immediately. To produce controlled hypotension during anesthesia to reduce bleeding. *Investigational:* Severe refractory congestive heart failure (may be combined with dopamine), in combination with dopamine for acute myocardial infarction, lactic acidosis due to impaired peripheral perfusion, to reduce the vasoconstrictor effects of norepinephrine and dopamine.

Contraindication   Compensatory hypertension. Use with caution in hypothyroidism, liver or kidney impairment, in pregnancy, and in lactation.

Untoward Reactions   Large doses may lead to cyanide toxicity. *Following rapid injection:* Dizziness, nausea, restlessness, headache, sweating, muscle twitching, palpitations, abdominal pain, apprehension. *Symptoms of thiocyanate toxicity:* Blurred vision, tinnitus, confusion, hyperreflexia, seizures. *CNS symptoms (transitory)*: Restlessness, agitation, and muscle twitching. Vomiting or skin rash.

Drug Interaction   Concomitant use of other antihypertensives, volatile liquid anesthetics, or certain depressants ↑ response to nitroprusside.

Dosage   **Adults and children, IV infusion only**: average 3 µg/kg/min. **Range**: 0.5–10 mg/kg/min. Smaller dose is required for patients receiving other antihypertensives.
   Monitor BP and use as guide to regulate rate of administration so as to maintain desired antihypertensive effect. Rate of administration should not exceed 10 µg/kg/minute.

Administration/Storage
1. Protect drug from heat, light, and moisture.
2. Protect dilute solutions during administration by wrapping flask with opaque material, such as aluminum foil.
3. Dilute with 5% D₅W injection or with sterile water **without preservative**.
4. Discard all unused dilute solutions after 4 hr.
5. Discard solutions that are any color but very light brown.
6. Do not add any other drug or preservative to solution.

Nursing Implications
1. Monitor BP closely to assist in regulating rate of administration and to check for excessive hypotensive effect.
2. Adjust the infusion pump or microdrip regulator to conform exactly to the rate of administration ordered.

Chapter Twenty-seven

ANTIARRHYTHMIC AGENTS

General Statement   The orderly sequence of contraction of the heart chambers, at an efficient rate, is necessary so that the heart can pump enough blood to the body organs. Normally the atria contract first, then the ventricles.

Altered patterns of contraction, or marked increases or decreases in the rate of the heart, reduce the ability of the heart to pump blood. Such altered patterns are called *cardiac arrhythmias*. Some examples of cardiac arrhythmias are:

1. *Premature ventricular beats* or beats that occasionally originate in the ventricles instead of in the sinus node region of the atrium. This causes the ventricles to contract before the atria and ultimately results in a decrease in the volume of blood pumped into the aorta.
2. *Ventricular tachycardia*. A rapid heartbeat with a succession of beats origi-nating in the ventricles.
3. *Atrial flutter*. Rapid contraction of the atria at a rate too fast to enable it to force blood into the ventricles efficiently.
4. *Atrial fibrillation*. The rate of atrial contraction is even faster than that noted during atrial flutter and more disorganized.
5. *Ventricular fibrillation*. Rapid, irregular, and uncoordinated ventricular con-tractions that are unable to pump any blood to the body. This condition will cause death if not corrected immediately.
6. *Atrioventricular heart block*. Slowing or failure of the transmission of the car-diac impulse from atria to ventricles, in the atrioventricular junction. This can result in atrial contraction *not* followed by ventricular contraction.

Antiarrhythmic drugs are used to correct disorders of the heart rate and rhythm. These drugs will either change the rate of the heart to more normal values or restore the origin of the heartbeat to the sinus nodes (pacemaker). The drugs regulate the heartbeat by depressing impulse formation in regions of the heart where the impulse should not arise. Some drugs normalize the time interval during which the heart cannot be stimulated to contract (refractory period).

Nursing Implications

1. *Assess*
   a. all patients receiving antiarrhythmic drugs by the IV route with a cardiac monitor.
   b. for variations in cardiac rhythm and report changes that may require alteration in drug administration.
   c. especially for depression of cardiac activity, such as the prolongation of the P-R interval, the QRS complex, or aggravation of the arrhythmia.
   d. blood pressure almost continuously during IV therapy, because antiarrhythmic patients are particularly susceptible to hypotension and cardiac collapse.
   e. cardiac rate. Bradycardia may be indicative of approaching cardiac collapse.
2. Should an adverse reaction occur, be prepared to assist in discontinuing the medication, to administer emergency drugs, and to use emergency resuscitative techniques.

BRETYLIUM TOSYLATE Bretylate Parenteral,* Bretylol (Rx)

Classification Antiarrhythmic, Type III.

Action/Kinetics The mechanism for the antiarrhythmic effect is not known but may involve a prolongation of repolarization. Bretylium also inhibits catecholamine release at nerve endings by decreasing excitability of nerve terminal. The drug may induce a small initial increase in heart rate and transient hypertension. **Peak plasma concentration**: Within 60 min after IM use. Antifibrillatory effect within a few minutes after IV use. Hypotensive effect within first hour; suppression of ventricular tachycardia and ventricular arrhythmias: 20 min to 2 hr; premature ventricular beats: 6–9 hr. **Plasma t½**: 5–10 hr. Excreted unchanged in urine (70–80%).

Uses Life-threatening ventricular arrhythmias, especially fibrillations and tachycardias failing to respond to other antiarrhythmics. For short-term use only.

Contraindications Severe aortic stenosis, severe pulmonary hypertension. Safe use in pregnancy and children not established.

Untoward Reactions *CV*: Hypotension, transient hypertension, increased frequency of premature ventricular contractions, bradycardia, precipitation of anginal attacks. *GI*: Nausea, vomiting especially after rapid administration, diarrhea, abdominal pain, hiccoughs. *CNS*: Vertigo, dizziness, lightheadedness, syncope, anxiety, paranoid psychosis, confusion, emotional ups and downs. *Other*: Renal dysfunction, flushing, hyperthermia, shortness of breath, nasal stuffiness, diaphoresis, conjunctivitis, erythematous macular rashes.

Drug Interactions

Interactant	Interaction
Digitalis glycosides	Bretylium may aggravate digitalis toxicity due to initial release of norepinephrine

Interactant	Interaction
Procainamide, Quinidine	Concomitant use with bretylium ↓ inotropic effect of bretylium and ↑ hypotension

Dosage *Ventricular fibrillation.* **IV**: 5 mg/kg of undiluted solution rapidly. Can increase to 10 mg/kg and repeat at 15–30 min. Dosage should not exceed 30 mg/kg. **Maintenance:** 1–2 mg/minute of diluted solution by continuous IV infusion or 5–10 mg/kg q 6 hr infused over 10–30 min. *Other ventricular arrhythmias.* **IV infusion:** 5–10 mg/kg of diluted solution over 10–30 min; **maintenance:** 5–10 mg/kg q 6 hr or continuous IV infusion of 1–2 mg/min. **IM**: 5–10 mg/kg of undiluted solution followed by a second dose in 1–2 hr; thereafter, same dosage q 6–8 hr. Usual course: 3–5 days.

Administration

1. *IV usual.* Dilute with four parts of dextrose or sodium chloride injection and administer slowly (over 10–30 min). For ventricular fibrillations, administer as rapidly as feasible, possibly without dilution.
2. *IM (use undiluted).* Avoid proximity of major nerve. Rotate injection site to avoid localized atrophy, fibrosis, degeneration, or inflammation. *Inject only 5 ml into any one site.*

Additional Nursing Implications

See also *Nursing Implications*, p. 349.

1. Keep patient supine during therapy and monitor for postural hypotension, until tolerance is developed. This may take several days. About 50% of patients are hypotensive in a supine position while receiving bretylium therapy.
2. Report and be prepared to administer dopamine or norepinephrine IV to raise BP below 75 mm Hg when patient is in a supine position.
3. Question concomitant use of digitalis preparations, because bretylium may aggravate digitalis toxicity.
4. Recognize that nausea and vomiting may be caused by too rapid IV infusion and report immediately.

DIGITALIS GLYCOSIDES

See *Cardiac Glycosides*, p. 291.

DILTIAZEM HYDROCHLORIDE Cardizem (Rx)

See *Calcium Channel Blocking Drugs*, p. 305.

DISOPYRAMIDE Norpace, Norpace CR, Rythmodan,* Rythmodan-LA* (Rx)

Classification Antiarrhythmic, Type I.

Action/Kinetics Disopyramide depresses the excitability of cardiac muscle to electrical stimulation and prolongs the refractory period. It manifests anticholinergic effects although it has fewer side effects than quinidine. The drug does not affect blood pressure significantly and it can be used in digitalized and nondigitalized patients. **Onset**: 30 min. **Peak plasma levels**: 2 hr. **Duration**: average of 6 hr (range 1.5–8 hr). t½: 5–8 hr. **Therapeutic serum levels**: 2–8 µg/ml. **Protein-binding**: 40–60%.

Uses   Prevention, recurrence, and control of unifocal, multifocal, and paired premature ventricular contractions. Arrhythmias in coronary artery disease. **Investigational**: Ventricular arrhythmias in emergency conditions, paroxysmal supraventricular tachycardia.

Contraindications   Hypersensitivity to drug. Cardiogenic shock, heart failure, heart block, especially preexisting second- and third-degree A-V block, glaucoma, urinary retention. Safe use during pregnancy, childhood, labor, and delivery has not been established.

Untoward Reactions   *Cardiovascular*: Hypotension, congestive heart failure, edema, weight gain, cardiac conduction disturbances, hypotension, shortness of breath, syncope, chest pain. *Anticholinergic*: Dry mouth, urinary retention, constipation, blurred vision, dry nose, eyes, and throat. *GU*: Urinary frequency and urgency. *GI*: Nausea, pain, flatulence, anorexia, diarrhea, vomiting. *CNS:* Headache, nervousness, dizziness, fatigue, depression, insomnia, psychoses. *Dermatologic*: Rash/dermatoses. *Other:* Fever, respiratory problems, gynecomastia, anaphylaxis, malaise, muscle weakness, numbness, tingling, angle-closure glaucoma.

Drug Interaction   Phenytoin and rifampin ↓ effect due to ↑ breakdown by liver.

Dosage   PO. *Individualized*. **Initial loading dose**: 300 mg (200 mg if patient weighs less than 110 lb); **maintenance**: 400–800 mg/day in 4 divided doses (usual: 150 mg q 6 hr). *For patients less than 110 lb*, **maintenance**: 100 mg q 6 hr. If controlled release form used, administer q 12 hr. *Severe refractory tachycardia*: up to 400 mg q 6 hr may be required. *Cardiomyopathy*: do not administer a loading dose; give 100 mg q 6 hr. For all uses, dosage must be decreased in patients with renal or hepatic insufficiency.

Administration
1. Administer drug only after ECG assessment.
2. Administer with caution to patients receiving (or who have recently received) other antiarrhythmic drugs.

Nursing Implications
1. *Assess*
   a. patients who are being transferred from another antiarrhythmic to disopyramide very carefully.
   b. BP b.i.d. for hypotensive effect.
   c. ECG for QRS widening and QT prolongation, indications for discontinuing disopyramide.
   d. patients with poor left ventricular function closely, because they are more susceptible to hypotension or worsened CHF manifested by cough, dyspnea, moist rales, and cyanosis.
   e. whether adequate serum potassium levels are present for effective response to disopyramide.
   f. for development of urinary retention, particularly in men with hypertrophy of the prostate.

(continued)

2. Report untoward reactions because dosage is based on patient's response and tolerance to the medication.
3. Do not administer if ECG shows a first-degree heart block. Check with medical supervision for reduced dosage.

LIDOCAINE HYDROCHLORIDE　IM: Lidopen Auto-Injector, Xylocaine HCl IM for Cardiac Arrhythmias (Rx). Direct IV or IV Admixtures: Lidocaine HCl without Preservatives, Xylocaine HCl IV for Cardiac Arrhythmias, Xylocard,* (Rx). IV Infusion: Lidocaine HCl in 5% Dextrose (Rx)

Classification　Antiarrhythmic, Type I.

Action/Kinetics　Lidocaine shortens the refractory period and suppresses the automaticity of ectopic foci without affecting conduction of impulses through cardiac tissue. It does not affect blood pressure, cardiac output, or myocardial contractility. **IV: Onset:** 45–90 sec. **Duration:** 10–20 min. **t½:** 1–2 hr. **Therapeutic serum levels:** 1.5–5 μg/ml. **Protein-binding:** 40–80%. Since lidocaine has little effect on conduction at normal antiarrhythmic doses, it should be used in acute situations (instead of procainamide) in instances in which heart block might occur.

Uses　**IV:** Treatment of acute ventricular arrhythmias such as those following myocardial infarctions or occuring during surgery. The drug is ineffective against atrial arrhythmias. **IM:** Certain emergency situations (e.g., ECG equipment not available; mobile coronary care unit, under advice of physician).

Contraindications　Hypersensitivity to amide-type local anesthetics, Adams-Stokes syndrome, or total or partial heart block. Use with caution in the presence of liver or severe kidney disease, CHF, marked hypoxia, severe respiratory depression, or shock. Use with caution in pregnancy, labor, delivery, and in children.

Untoward Reactions　*CV:* Precipitation or aggravation of arrhythmias (following IV use), hypotension, bradycardia (with possible cardiac arrest), cardiovascular collapse. *CNS:* Dizziness, restlessness, apprehension, euphoria, stupor, convulsions, unconsciousness. *Respiratory:* Difficulties in breathing or swallowing, respiratory depression. *Allergic:* Rash, urticaria, edema, anaphylaxis. *Other:* Tinnitus, blurred vision, vomiting, numbness, sensation of heat or cold, twitching, tremors.

　　During anesthesia, cardiovascular depression may be the first sign of lidocaine toxicity. During other usage, convulsions are the first sign of lidocaine toxicity.

Drug Interactions

Interactant	Interaction
Aminoglycosides	↑ Neuromuscular blockade
Cimetidine	↑ Effects of lidocaine
Metoprolol	↓ Lidocaine clearance
Phenytoin	IV phenytoin → excessive cardiac depression
Procainamide	Additive neurologic side effects
Propranolol	↓ Lidocaine clearance

Interactant	Interaction
Succinylcholine	↑ Action of succinylcholine by ↓ plasma protein binding
Tubocurarine	↑ Neuromuscular blockade

Dosage **IV Bolus:** 50–100 mg at rate of 25–50 mg/min. Repeat if necessary after 5-min interval. Onset of action is 10 sec. **Maximum dose/hr:** 200– 300 mg. **Infusion:** 1–4 mg/min (or 20–50 μg/kg/min for the average 70 kg adult). Onset of action is 10–20 min. **IM:** 300 mg. Switch to IV lidocaine or PO antiarrhythmics as soon as possible.

IV bolus dosage should be reduced in patients over 60 years of age or in those with CHF or liver disease.

Administration

1. **Do not add lidocaine to blood transfusion assembly.**
2. Lidocaine solutions that contain epinephrine should not be used to treat arrhythmias. Make certain vial states, "For Cardiac Arrhythmias."
3. Use 5% dextrose in water to prepare solution; this is stable for 24 hr.

Additional Nursing Implications

1. *Assess*
   a. for untoward CNS effects, such as twitching and tremors that may precede convulsions.
   b. for respiratory depression, characterized by shallow, slow respirations.
2. Have available a short-acting barbiturate, such as secobarbital (Seconal), for emergency use.

PHENYTOIN (DIPHENYLHYDANTION)   Dilantin, Novophenytoin* (Rx)

PHENYTOIN SODIUM (DIPHENYLHYDLANTOIN SODIUM)   Dilantin Sodium (Rx)

Classification   Antiarrhythmic (Type I), anticonvulsant (see p. 457).

Action/Kinetics   Phenytoin increases the electric stimulation threshold of heart muscle although it is less effective than quinidine, procainamide, or lidocaine. **Onset:** 30–60 min. **Duration:** 24 or more hr. t½: 22–36 hr. **Therapeutic serum level:** 10–20 μg/ml.

Uses   PO for certain premature ventricular contractions and IV for premature ventricular contractions and tachycardia. The drug is particularly useful for arrhythmias produced by digitalis overdosage.

For all details on this drug, including *Contraindications, Untoward Reactions, Drug Interactions,* and *Nursing Implications,* see Part 6, Chapter 36, *Anticonvulsants,* p. 457.

Laboratory Test Interference   False + or ↑ fasting glucose, Coombs' test.

Dosage   *Arrhythmias.* **PO:** 200–400 mg daily. **IV:** 100 mg q 5 min up to maximum of 1 gm.

PROCAINAMIDE HYDROCHLORIDE Procan SR, Promine, Pronestyl, Pronestyl-SR (Rx)

Classification Antiarrhythmic.

Action/Kinetics Prolongs refractory period of heart and depresses conduction of cardiac impulse. It has some anticholinergic and local anesthetic effects. **Onset: PO**, 30 min; **IV**, 1–5 min. **Duration**: 3 hr. t½: 2.5–4.5 hr. **Therapeutic serum level**: 4–8 µg/ml. **Protein binding**: 15%. 50–60% excreted unchanged.

Uses Ventricular tachycardia, atrial fibrillation, resistant paroxysmal atrial tachycardia. Emergency treatment of ventricular tachycardia, digitalis intoxication, prophylactic control of tachycardia for patients at risk during anesthesia or undergoing thoracic surgery.

Contraindications Hypersensitivity to drug, complete A-V heart block, second- or third-degree A-V heartblock, myasthenia gravis, or blood dyscrasias. Use with extreme caution in patients for whom a sudden drop in BP could be detrimental, in patients with liver or kidney dysfunction, and in those with bronchial asthma or other respiratory disorders. Safe use in pregnancy and lactation has not been established.

Untoward Reactions *CV:* Following IV use: hypotension, ventricular asystole or fibrillation, partial or complete heart block. *GI:* Nausea, vomiting, diarrhea, anorexia, bitter taste, abdominal pain. *Hematologic:* Thrombocytopenia, agranulocytosis. *Allergic:* Urticaria, pruritus, angioneurotic edema, maculopapular rash. *CNS:* Depression, giddiness, psychoses, hallucinations. *Other:* Lupus erythematosus-like syndrome especially in those on maintenance therapy. Also, granulomatous hepatitis, weakness, fever, chills.

Drug Interactions

Interactant	Interaction
Acetazolamide	↑ Effect of procainamide due to ↓ excretion by kidney
Anticholinergic agents, Atropine	Additive anticholinergic effects
Antihypertensive agents	Additive hypotensive effect
Cholinergic agents	Anticholinergic activity of procainamide antagonizes effect of cholinergic drugs
Cimetidine	↑ Effect of procainamide due to ↓ excretion by kidney
Ethanol	↓ Effect of procainamide due to ↑ rate of breakdown by liver
Kanamycin	Procainamide ↑ muscle relaxation produced by kanamycin
Lidocaine	Additive neurologic side effects
Magnesium salts	Procainamide ↑ muscle relaxation produced by magnesium salts
Neomycin	Procainamide ↑ muscle relaxation produced by neomycin
Succinylcholine	Procainamide ↑ muscle relaxation produced by succinylcholine
Sodium bicarbonate	↑ Effect of procainamide due to ↓ excretion by the kidney

Laboratory Test Interference May affect liver function tests. False + or ↑ serum alkaline phosphatase.

Dosage Individualized. **PO**. *Atrial arrhythmias*: **initial,** 1.25 gm followed in 1 hr by 0.75 gm; **then,** if no ECG changes, 0.5–1.0 gm q 2 hr until arrhythmia stopped. **Maintenance**: 0.5–1.0 gm q 4–6 hr. *Premature ventricular contractions*: 50 mg/kg daily in divided doses q 3 hr. *Ventricular tachycardia*: **initial,** 1.0 gm; **then,** 6 mg/kg q 3 hr. **Sustained release tablets**: not recommended for initial therapy; **maintenance**: 50 mg/kg/day in divided doses q 6 hr.

IM: 0.5–1.0 gm q 4–8 hr until PO therapy possible. *Arrhythmias associated with surgery or anesthesia*: 0.1–0.5 gm IM.

Direct IV use: 100 mg q 5 min by slow IV injection at a rate not to exceed 25–50 mg/min; give until arrhythmia stops or until 1 gm is administered; **maintenance**: IV infusion, 2–6 mg/min. **IV infusion**: initial, 500–600 mg over 25–30 min; **then,** 2–6 mg/min. Switch to PO therapy as soon as possible, but wait at least 3–4 hr after the last IV dose.

Administration/Storage

1. IV use should be reserved for emergency situations.
2. For IV initial therapy, the drug should be diluted with 5% dextrose and administered slowly to minimize side effects.
3. Discard solutions of drug that are darker than light amber or otherwise colored. Solutions that have turned slightly yellow on standing may be used.

Additional Nursing Implications

See also *Nursing Implications*, p. 349.

1. Monitor IV administration, checking that dose does not exceed 25–50 mg/min.
2. Assess patient in a supine position during IV infusion and monitor BP almost continuously.
3. Report and be prepared to discontinue infusion if diastolic BP falls 15 mm Hg or more during administration.
4. Have on hand phenylephrine hydrochloride injection (Neo-Synephrine) or lev-arterenol bitartrate (Levophed) injection to counteract excessive hypotensive response.
5. Assess patients on oral maintenance for symptoms of lupus erythematosus as manifested by polyarthralgia, arthritis, pleuritic pain, fever, myalgia, and skin lesions.

PROPRANOLOL HYDROCHLORIDE Apo-Propranolol,* Detensol,* Inderal, Inderal LA, Novopranol,* PMS Propranolol* (Rx)

Classification Antiarrhythmic (Type II), adrenergic blocking agent. See Antihypertensive Agents, p. 337 for all details on this drug.

QUINIDINE BISULFATE Bioquin Durules* (Rx)

QUINIDINE GLUCONATE Duraquin, Quinaglute, Quinatime, Quin-Release, (Rx)

QUINIDINE POLYGALACTURONATE   Cardioquin (Rx)

QUINIDINE SULFATE   Cin-Quin, Quinidex, Quinora, SK-Quinidine Sulfate (Rx)

Classification   Antiarrhythmic, Type I.

Action/Kinetics   Quinidine depresses the excitability of the heart and increases the refractory period by decreasing potassium efflux of cardiac fibers. It also decreases cardiac output and possesses anticholinergic, antimalarial, antipyretic, and oxytocic properties. **PO: Onset,** 0.5–3 hr. **Duration:** 6–8 hr. t½: 6–7 hr. **Therapeutic plasma levels:** 2–7 μg/ml. **Protein binding:** 60–80%. Metabolized by liver. Rate of urinary excretion (20% excreted unchanged) is affected by urinary pH.

Uses   Often the drug of choice for atrial fibrillation and atrial and ventricular arrhythmias. Not indicated for prophylaxis during surgery.

Contraindications   Hypersensitivity to drug or other cinchona drugs. Quinidine should be used with extreme caution for patients in whom a sudden change in blood pressure might be detrimental or those suffering from extensive myocardial damage, subacute endocarditis, bradycardia, coronary occlusion, disturbances in impulse conduction, chronic valvular disease, considerable cardiac enlargement, frank congestive failure, arrhythmias due to digitalis toxicity, renal disease.

Cautious use is also recommended in patients with acute infections, hyperthyroidism, myasthenia gravis, muscular weakness, respiratory distress, and bronchial asthma. Safety for use in pregnancy, lactation, and children has not been established.

Untoward Reactions   *CV:* Widening of QRS complex, hypotension, asystole, ectopic ventricular beats, ventricular tachycardia or fibrillation, arterial embolism, circulatory collapse, bradycardia, congestive heart failure, partial or total heart block. *GI:* Nausea, vomiting, abdominal pain, colic, anorexia, diarrhea, urge to defecate as well as urinate. *CNS:* Syncope, headache, confusion, excitement, vertigo, apprehension, tinnitus, decreased hearing acuity. *Dermatologic:* Skin eruptions, urticaria, exfoliative dermatitis, photosensitivity, flushing. *Allergic:* Acute asthma, angioneurotic edema, respiratory paralysis, dyspnea, fever, vascular collapse. *Hematologic:* Hypoprothrombinemia, acute hemolytic anemia, thrombocytopenic purpura, agranulocytosis. *Ophthalmologic:* Blurred vision, mydriasis, alterations in color perception, decreased field of vision, double vision, photophobia, optic neuritis, night blindness, scotomata. *Other:* Liver toxicity including hepatitis, lupus erythematosus (rare).

Drug Interactions

Interactant	Interaction
Acetazolamide ⎱ Antacids ⎰	↑ Effect of quinidine due to ↓ renal excretion
Anticholinergic agents, Atropine	Additive effect on blockade of vagus nerve action
Anticoagulants, oral	Additive hypoprothrombinemia
Barbiturates	↓ Effect of quinidine due to ↑ breakdown by liver
Cholinergic agents	Quinidine antagonizes effect of cholinergic drugs
Cimetidine	↑ Effect of quinidine due to ↓ breakdown by liver
Digoxin, Digitoxin	↑ Symptoms of digoxin toxicity

Interactant	Interaction
Guanethidine	Additive hypotensive effect
Methyldopa	Additive hypotensive effect
Neuromuscular blocking agents	↑ Respiratory depression
Phenobarbital ⎫ Phenytoin ⎬	↓ Effect of quinidine by ↑ rate of metabolism in liver
Phenothiazines	Additive cardiac depressant effect
Potassium	↑ Effect of quinidine
Propranolol	Both drugs produce a negative inotropic effect on the heart
Reserpine	Additive cardiac depressant effects
Rifampin	↓ Effect of quinidine due to ↑ breakdown by liver
Skeletal muscle relaxants	↑ Skeletal muscle relaxation
Sodium bicarbonate	↑ Effect of quinidine due to ↓ renal excretion
Thiazide diuretics	↑ Effect of quinidine due to ↓ renal excretion
Verapamil	Hypotension in patients with hypertrophic cardiomyopathy

Laboratory Test Interferences   False + or ↑ PSP, 17-ketosteroids, prothrombin time.

Dosage   *Individualized*. ECG monitoring recommended when large doses of quinidine are used. Administration of a test dose (single tablet or 200 mg IM) of quinidine is recommended to establish possibility of hypersensitivity reaction. **Plasma concentration:** 2–6 µg/ml; this can be achieved by giving 200–300 mg q.i.d. **PO.** *Paroxysmal supraventricular tachycardia*: 400–600 mg q 2–3 hr until beneficial effect obtained. *Premature atrial and ventricular contractions*: 200–300 mg t.i.d.–q.i.d. *Atrial fibrillation*: **initial**, 200 mg q 2–3 hr for 5 to 8 doses; **then**, increase daily dose until rhythm restored (or toxicity seen) to maximum of 3–4 gm daily. **Maintenance** for all uses: 200–300 mg t.i.d.–q.i.d. **Sustained release forms:** 300–600 mg q 8–12 hr. **IM.** *Acute tachycardia*: **initial**, 600 mg; **then**, 400 mg of gluconate repeated q 2 hr if necessary. **IV.** *Arrhythmias*: 330 mg (or less) of the gluconate; some patients may require 500–750 mg.

Administration/Storage

1. IV solution can be prepared by diluting 10 ml of quinidine gluconate injection to 50 ml with 5% glucose; this should be given at a rate of 1 ml/min.
2. Use only colorless clear solution for injection, because light may cause quinidine to crystallize, which turns solution brownish.
3. Administer with food to minimize GI effects.

Additional Nursing Implications

See also *Nursing Implications*, p. 349.

1. Anticipate that preliminary test dose will be given before instituting quinidine therapy. **Adult**: 200 mg quinidine sulfate or quinidine gluconate administered PO or IM. **Children**: test dose of 2 mg of quinidine sulfate per kilogram of body weight.

(continued)

2. *Assess*
   a. for hypersensitivity demonstrated by respiratory and integumentary symptoms.
   b. ECG and report prolongation of P-R intervals, absence of P waves, and cardiac rates above 120 beats/min, all of which are reasons for discontinuance of drug.
   c. patient on oral quinidine for signs of hypotension.
   d. BP of hospitalized patient on oral quinidine at least once daily.

TOCAINIDE HYDROCHLORIDE Tonocard (Rx)

Classification Antiarrhythmic (Type 1).

Action/Kinetics Tocainide, which is similar to lidocaine, decreases the excitability of cells in the myocardium. Tocainide produces increases in pulmonary and aortic arterial pressure and slight increases in peripheral resistance. Is effective in both digitalized and nondigitalized patients. **Peak plasma levels:** 0.5–2 hr. **t½:** 15 hr. **Therapeutic plasma level:** 4–10 μg/ml. Approximately 10% is bound to plasma protein. Forty percent is excreted unchanged in the urine.

Uses Ventricular arrhythmias including premature ventricular contractions, unifocal or multifocal, couplets, and ventricular tachycardia.

Contraindications Allergy to amide-type local anesthetics, second- or third-degree A-V block in the absence of artificial ventricular pacemaker. Safety in pregnancy, lactation, and children has not been established.

Untoward Reactions *CV:* Increased arrhythmias, increased ventricular rate, congestive heart failure, tachycardia, hypotension, conduction disturbances, bradycardia, chest pain, left ventricular failure. *CNS:* Lightheadedness, dizziness, vertigo, giddiness, headache, tremors, restlessness, confusion, disorientation, hallucinations, ataxia, paresthesias, numbness, nystagmus, drowsiness. *GI:* Nausea, vomiting, anorexia, diarrhea. *Hematologic:* Leukopenia, agranulocytosis, hypoplastic anemia, thrombocytopenia. *Other:* Pulmonary fibrosis, blurred vision, tinnitus, hearing loss, sweating, arthritis, myalgia, lupus-like syndrome.

Drug Interactions Use with metaprolol may result in additive effects.

Dosage **Individualized. PO. Adults: initial,** 400 mg q 8 hr up to a maximum of 2,400 mg/day. Total daily dose of 1,200 mg may be adequate in patients with liver or kidney disease.

Nursing Implications
Teach patient and/or family

   a. to report promptly any bruising, bleeding, or signs of infections such as fever, sore throat, or chills, which may indicate signs of blood dyscrasias.
   b. the importance of scheduled laboratory tests, especially during the first 6 months of therapy.
   c. to report promptly any pulmonary symptoms such as wheezing, coughing, or dyspnea, as this may indicate pulmonary fibrosis and drug must be discontinued.

VERAPAMIL   Calan, Isoptin (Rx)

See *Calcium Channel Blocking Drugs*, p. 305.

Chapter Twenty-eight

HYPOCHOLESTEROLEMIC AND ANTILIPEMIC AGENTS

General Statement   Atherosclerosis is characterized by a narrowing of the blood vessels by lipid deposits, as well as an increased incidence of stroke or myocardial infarction. The condition is associated with changes in the cholesterol, fat, and/or carbohydrate metabolism, although it is not known whether these changes are a cause or a consequence of the disease. Patients often manifest increased levels of plasma lipids, a complex mixture of triglycerides, phospholipids, free cholesterol, and cholesterol esters—all associated with protein. The lipoproteins are further subdivided into chylomicrons, very low density lipoproteins (VLDL),* low-density lipoproteins (LDL), and high-density lipoproteins (HDL). The latter are considered beneficial and protective. They occur in higher concentrations in women and are increased by exercise.

On the basis of their lipoprotein patterns and other characteristics, patients can be separated into five types (see Table 11).

A reduction of plasma lipids, especially cholesterol and LDL, to more normal levels is believed to be therapeutically useful in minimizing atherosclerosis and the closely related hyperlipoproteinemias (Table 11). Such a reduction is achieved primarily through diet (decreased intake of cholesterol, saturated fats, simple sugars, increased amounts of fiber), weight loss, and exercise. Antilipemic or hypocholesterolemic agents are sometimes prescribed, even though their long-term therapeutic effect has not been established. Their use, at present, is restricted to patients who have had one or more cardiovascular accidents, who are overweight, and who have a family history of atherosclerotic heart disease. The drugs will not

---

*VLDL are also called prebeta-lipoproteins, and LDL are also called beta-lipoproteins in classifications derived from electrophoresis.

TABLE 11 PRIMARY HYPERLIPOPROTEINEMIAS

Lipid Pattern	Characteristic Feature	Treatment
Type I (exogenous or "fat-induced")	High level of triglycerides. Normal levels of Cholesterol. This pattern occurs rarely and is related to dietary intake of fat. ↑ Chylomicrons	Low-fat diet. Treatment of underlying condition (diabetes, thyroid condition).
Type II (a and b) (familial hypercholesterolemia)	High plasma cholesterol level, normal or slightly elevated triglycerides. ↑ LDL	Substitution of unsaturated fats for saturated fats in diet. Most antilipemic drugs.
Type III (endogenous)	Increased LDL and VLDL, especially beta-lipoproteins. Hypercholesterolemia and hypertriglyceridemia	Weight reduction. Possible drug therapy (clofibrate).
Type IV (endogenous)	Carbohydrate-induced hyperlipoproteinemia, often associated with early onset of atherosclerosis. ↑ VLDL	Weight reduction, reduction in carbohydrate intake. Drug therapy (clofibrate and nicotinic acid).
Type V (mixed exogenous and endogenous)	Mixed I and IV caused both by dietary fat and abnormal carbohydrate metabolism. Hypertriglyceridemia. ↑ Chylomicrons and VLDL	Weight reduction. Reduced carbohydrate intake. Drug therapy (clofibrate and nicotinic acid).

remove existing intrarterial lipid plaques (atheromas) but may reduce the rate at which new ones are formed.

CHOLESTYRAMINE RESIN Questran (Rx)

Classification Resin, hypocholesterolemic agent.

Action/Kinetics Cholestyramine binds sodium cholate (bile salts) in the intestine; thus, the principal precursor of cholesterol is not absorbed due to formation of an insoluble complex. The drug decreases cholesterol, VLDL, and LDL. Also, there is relief of itching as a result of removing irritating bile salts. **Onset** (therapeutic): 1 week; **maximum effect**: 1–3 weeks. Return to pretreatment cholesterol levels 2–4 weeks after discontinuance.

Fat-soluble vitamins (A, D, K) and possibly folic acid may have to be administered IM during long-term therapy, since cholestyramine binds these vitamins in the intestine.

Uses Pruritus associated with obstructive jaundice, primary biliary cirrhosis and biliary obstruction, diarrhea for patients with ileac resections, and atherosclerosis. Hyperlipoproteinemia. *Investigational*: Treatment of poisoning by chlordecone (Kepone); antibiotic-induced *Pseudomonas* colitis.

Contraindications Complete obstruction or atresia of bile duct.

Untoward Reactions   *GI:* Nausea, vomiting, constipation, diarrhea, abdominal distention. Fecal impaction in elderly patients. Large doses may cause steatorrhea. *Other:* Osteoporosis, electrolyte imbalance, and CNS and musculoskeletal manifestations. Prolonged administration may interfere with absorption of fat-soluble vitamins.

Drug Interactions

Interactant	Interaction
Anticoagulants, oral	↓ Anticoagulant effect due to ↓ absorption from GI tract
Cephalexin	↓ Absorption of cephalexin from GI tract
Clindamycin	↓ Absorption of clindamycin from GI tract
Digitalis glycosides	Cholestyramine binds digitoxin in the intestine and ↓ its half-life
Iron preparations	↓ Effect of iron preparations due to ↓ absorption from GI tract
Phenobarbital	↓ Absorption of phenobarbital from GI tract
Phenylbutazone	Absorption of phenylbutazone delayed by cholestyramine—may ↓ effect
Thiazide diuretics	↓ Effect of thiazides due to ↓ absorption from GI tract
Thyroid hormones	↓ Effect of thyroid hormones due to ↓ absorption from GI tract

Dosage   **PO**: 4 gm of anhydrous resin t.i.d.–q.i.d. before or with meals, for 2 or more weeks. After relief of pruritus, dosage may be reduced. Doses greater than 24 gm daily result in an increased incidence of side effects.

Administration

1. Always mix with fluid before administering because resin may cause esophageal irritation or blockage.
2. Disguise unpalatable taste of drug by mixing it with fruit juice, soup, milk, water, applesauce, pureed fruits, or carbonated beverage.
3. After placing contents of one packet of resin on the surface of 4–6 oz of fluid, allow it to stand without stirring for 2 minutes, occasionally twirling the glass, and then stir slowly (to prevent foaming) to form a suspension.

Nursing Implications

1. Anticipate that vitamins A, D, K and folic acid may be administered in a water-miscible form when patient is receiving medication.
2. Assess for bleeding from any orifice or for purpura because bleeding tendencies are increased. Such symptoms are usually treated with parenteral administration of vitamin K.
3. Check that patient is scheduled for regular clinical laboratory evaluation, including serum cholesterol and triglyceride levels.
4. Anticipate that medication will be discontinued if it does not lower cholesterol levels.
5. *Teach patient and/or family*
   a. how to follow prescribed low-cholesterol diet.

(continued)

b. to take other prescribed medications at least 1 hr before or 4 hr after administration of antihyperlipidemic medication to minimize interference with their absorption.

c. the constipating effects of medication.

d. to drink extra fluids and to include roughage in diet. Check with physician whether laxatives should be ordered to overcome constipating effect of medication.

e. that relief of pruritus may become evident 1 to 3 weeks after initiation but may return after medication is discontinued.

CLOFIBRATE   Atromid-S, Claripex*, Novofibrate* (Rx)

Classification   Hypocholesterolemic agent.

Action/Kinetics   Clofibrate decreases triglycerides, VLDL, and, to a lesser extent, cholesterol and LDL. The mechanism is not known with certainty but may be due to increased catabolism of VLDL to LDL and decreased synthesis of VLDL by the liver. The higher the cholesterol level, the more effective the drug. **Peak plasma levels**: 2–6 hr. **t½**: 6–25 hr. **Therapeutic effect: Onset**, 2–5 days; **maximum effect**: 3 weeks. Triglycerides return to pretreatment levels 2–3 weeks after therapy is terminated. Active metabolite excreted in urine. The drug may concentrate in fetal blood. Liver function tests should be performed during therapy.

Uses   Hyperlipidemia—hypercholesterolemia, hypertriglyceridemia. Drug of choice for type III hyperlipidemia. Xanthoma (small, lumpy fat deposits in skin); therapy for this condition is limited to 1 year. The drug is ineffective in the presence of untreated hyperthyroidism.

Contraindications   Impaired hepatic or renal function, pregnancy or expectation thereof, lactation, children. Use with caution in patients with gout.

Untoward Reactions   *GI:* Nausea, dyspepsia, weight gain or loss, vomiting, flatulence, abdominal distress, stomatitis, loose stools. *CNS:* Headaches, dizziness, fatigue, weakness. *CV:* Changes in blood clotting time. *Skeletal muscle:* Myositis, asthenia, myalgia, weakness, muscle aches, cramps. *Enzyme changes:* Creatinine phosphokinase, increased serum transaminase (if levels continue to increase after maximum therapeutic response has been achieved, therapy should be discontinued). *Other:* Increased incidence of gallstones, leukopenia, skin rashes, urticaria, pruritus, dry and brittle hair (in women), dyspnea.

Drug Interactions

Interactant	Interaction
Anticoagulants	Clofibrate ↑ anticoagulant effect by ↓ plasma protein binding
Antidiabetics (sulfonylureas)	Clofibrate ↑ effect of antidiabetics
Furosemide	Concurrent use may ↑ effects of both drugs

Dosage   **PO**: 500 mg q.i.d. Therapeutic response may take several weeks to become apparent. Drug must be administered on a continuous basis, since lowered levels of cholesterol and other lipids will return to elevated state within several weeks after administration is stopped. Discontinue after 3 months if response is poor.

Nursing Implications

1. Ascertain that hematology, kidney and liver function tests, serum, lipid, and cholesterol levels, and electrolyte studies are completed before therapy is initiated.
2. *Teach patient and/or family*
   a. how to follow prescribed diet.
   b. to observe for bleeding from any orifice or for purpura if also on anticoagulant therapy. A reduction in anticoagulant drug dosage is usual if clofibrate therapy is instituted.
   c. to observe for symptoms of hypoglycemia (see p. 680), when taking oral antidiabetics because of possible drug interactions. Stress the importance of reporting such symptoms.
   d. to be alert to signs and symptoms associated with gallstones.
   e. that nausea usually decreases with continued therapy or reduced dosage.
   f. to use contraception if appropriate because clofibrate may be teratogenic.
   g. not to discontinue contraception for several months after discontinuing drug if pregnancy is planned.

COLESTIPOL HYDROCHLORIDE   Colestid (Rx)

Classification   Resin, hypocholesterolemic agent.

Action/Kinetics   Colestipol is an anion exchange resin that binds and removes bile acids, indirectly decreasing the concentration of cholesterol levels in the blood by stimulating its oxidation to bile acids. Colestipol also decreases LDL, but not triglycerides, and may increase VLDL. **Therapeutic onset:** 1–2 days; **maximum effect:** 1 month. Return to pretreatment cholesterol levels after discontinuance of therapy: 1 month.

Uses   Hypercholesterolemia, hyperlipoproteinemia (IIa).

Contraindications   Complete obstruction or atresia of bile duct. Use with caution in patients with preexisting constipation or hemorrhoids. Safe use during pregnancy and childhood not established.

Untoward Reactions   Constipation (10%), usually mild, but can result in fecal impaction; also, abdominal discomfort, GI irritation, muscle pain, headaches, dizziness, and hypersensitivity reactions.

Drug Interactions

Interactant	Interaction
Cephalexin Chlorothiazide Clindamycin Digitalis Phenobarbital Phenylbutazone	Colestipol may delay or ↓ absorption from the GI tract of the drugs listed

Interactant	Interaction
Tetracycline	
Trimethoprim	Colestipol may delay or ↓ absorption from the GI
Thyroid preparations	tract of the drugs listed
Warfarin sodium	

Dosage **PO**: 15–30 gm daily in 2 to 4 equally divided doses.

Administration

1. Always mix with fluid before administering, because resin may cause esophageal irritation or blockage.
2. Disguise unpalatable taste of drug by mixing it with fruit juice, soup, milk, water, applesauce, pureed fruit, breakfast cereals, carbonated beverages.
3. Take other drugs 1 hr before or 4 hr after colestipol to reduce interference with their absorption.

Nursing Implication
See *Cholestyramine Resin*, p. 361.

DEXTROTHYROXINE SODIUM Choloxin (Rx)

Classification Hypocholesterolemic agent.

Action/Kinetics Dextrothyroxine (the dextro isomer of thyroid hormone) increases the rate at which cholesterol is metabolized in the liver; excretion of cholesterol and metabolites is increased, leading to decreased serum levels of cholesterol and total serum lipids, including triglycerides, VLDL, and LDL. Dextrothyroxine has little effect on basal metabolic rate (BMR) but is otherwise physiologically similar to levothyroxine. The effectiveness increases as cholesterol levels increase. **t½**: 18 hr.

Uses Hypercholesterolemia in patients with no thyroid or heart disease. Occasionally used for hypothyroidism. Should be used mainly if dietary measures fail.

Contraindications Euthyroid patients with hypertensive organic heart disease, including angina pectoris, history of myocardial infarctions, cardiac arrhythmias or tachycardia, rheumatic disease, and CHF. Pregnancy, lactation, patients with advanced liver or kidney disease, or a history of hypersensitivity to iodine.

Untoward Reactions *CNS:* Insomnia, nervousness, fever, headache, changes in libido, dizziness, malaise, tiredness, psychic changes. *CV:* Palpitations, flushing, changes in cardiac activity in previously normal subjects, myocardial infarctions, angina pectoris, arrhythmias, ischemic myocardial changes, cerebrovascular accidents, thrombophlebitis. *GI:* Weight loss, bitter taste, GI hemorrhages. *Other:* Tremor, drooping eyelids, sweating, hair loss, diuresis, menstrual irregularities, hoarseness, tinnitus, peripheral edema, visual disturbances, paresthesia, muscle pain, gallstones, increases in blood sugar of diabetic patients.

Aggravation of existing cardiac disease is cause for discontinuation. Overdose is characterized by hyperthyroidism, diarrhea, cramps, vomiting, nervousness, twitching, tachycardia, and weight loss.

Drug Interactions

Interactant	Interaction
Anticoagulants, oral	↑ Effect of anticoagulants by ↑ hypoprothrombinemia
Antidiabetics, oral	↓ Diabetic control as dextrothyroxine ↑ blood sugar
Thyroid drugs	↑ Sensitivity of hypothyroid patients to thyroid drugs

Dosage   PO: *individualized*, **initial**, 1–2 mg daily. Daily dosage can be increased every 4 weeks by 1–2 mg; **maintenance**: 4–8 mg daily. **Maximum daily dosage**: 8 mg. It may take 2 to 4 weeks for the therapeutic response to become manifested. **Pediatric: initial**, 0.05 mg/kg daily. Increase by 0.05 mg/kg daily every month up to maximum of 4 mg daily, until satisfactory control is established. Withdraw drug 2 weeks before surgery.

Nursing Implications
1. Assist and encourage patient to follow prescribed diet.
2. Assess patients for attacks of angina.

GEMFIBROZIL   Lopid (Rx)

Classification   Antihyperlipidemic.

Action/Kinetics   Gemfibrozil, which resembles clofibrate, decreases VLDL and LDL fractions resulting in decreased serum triglycerides and possibly total serum cholesterol. The drug may be beneficial in inhibiting development of atherosclerosis. **Peak plasma levels**: 1–2 hr; **t½**: 1.3 hr. Nearly 70% is excreted unchanged.

Uses   Hypertriglyceridemia (type IV hyperlipidemia) unresponsive to dietary control or increased exercise. (Response variable; discontinue if significant improvement not observed within 3 months.)

Contraindications   To reduce elevated blood lipids for prophylaxis of coronary heart disease, primary biliary cirrhosis, gallbladder disease, and severe renal dysfunction. Use with caution in pregnancy and lactation.

Untoward Reactions   Cholelithiasis; increased chance of viral and bacterial infections. *GI*: Abdominal or epigastric pain, nausea, vomiting, diarrhea, flatulence. *CNS*: Dizziness, headache, blurred vision; possibly tinnitus, insomnia, vertigo, paresthesia. *Hematopoietic*: Anemia, leukopenia, eosinophilia. *Musculoskeletal*: Painful extremities; possibly arthralgia, muscle cramps, swollen joints, back pain, myalgia. *Miscellaneous*: Dermatitis, pruritus, urticaria; possibly fatigue, malaise, syncope.

Drug Interaction   Anticoagulant dosage should be ↓ if given with gemfibrozil.

Laboratory Test Interference   ↑ SGOT, SGPT, LDH, alkaline phosphatase.

Dosage   PO: 600 mg 30 min before the morning and evening meal (Range: 900–1,500 mg/day).

Nursing Implications

1. Ascertain that hematologic, kidney, liver function tests, serum cholesterol and triglyceride levels, and electrolyte studies are completed before therapy is initiated and then periodically thereafter.

2. *Teach patient and/or family*

   a. how to follow prescribed diet. Limit alcohol intake.

   b. to observe for bleeding from any orifice, or for purpura if patient is also on anticoagulant therapy. A reduction in anticoagulant drug dosage is indicated if gemfibrozil is instituted.

   c. to be alert for signs and symptoms associated with gallstones, such as abdominal pain and vomiting. Report persistent GI symptoms to physician.

   d. to use caution when driving or performing other dangerous tasks, since drug may cause dizziness or blurred vision.

NICOTINAMIDE   Niacinamide

NICOTINIC ACID   Diacin, Niac, Niacin, Nicobid, Nicocap, Nico-400, Nicolar, Nico-Span, Nicotinex, Nicotym, SK-Niacin, Span-Niacin, Tega-Span, Wampocap (Both Rx and OTC)

Classification   Hypocholesterolemic agent.

Action/Kinetics   By altering fat metabolism in adipose cells (increasing lipolysis, stimulating lipoprotein lipase), these drugs decrease serum cholesterol, triglycerides, chylomicrons, VLDL, and LDL. It stimulates the release of histamine from mast cells and increases gastric secretion. **Onset:** 30 min. **Peak serum concentration:** 45 min. **t½:** 45 min. **Therapeutic plasma concentration:** 0.5–1.0 $\mu g/ml$.

The drug has been effective in keeping the cholesterol and serum lipid level down for periods up to 5 years. When the drug is discontinued, the blood levels return to pretreatment levels within 2 to 6 weeks.

Uses   Hypercholesterolemia, hyperlipidemia.

Contraindications   Use with caution in patients with peptic ulcer or a history thereof, gallbladder disease, hepatic conditions, gout, diabetes, tuberculosis (active or arrested), asthma, allergic tendencies, or bronchial disease.

Untoward Reactions   *GI:* Nausea, dyspepsia, flatulence, anorexia, vomiting, epigastric pain, and diarrhea. These reactions can be severe but usually respond to dosage reduction. Concomitant administration of antacids helps. Activation of peptic ulcer. *Ophthalmologic:* Blurred vision, amblyopia, ocular edema. *CNS:* Panic reactions, nervousness. *Dermatologic:* Flushing, pruritus, urticaria, dry skin, dry mouth. *Alteration of glucose metabolism:* Hyperglycemia, glycosuria, precipitation of diabetes. *Other:* Tingling sensations, reactivation of tuberculosis, acanthosis nigricans (skin condition characterized by pigmented wartlike growths).

Prolonged therapy has resulted in a slight increase in uric acid levels (precipitation of gouty arthritis), as well as alteration of some blood and liver function tests.

Drug Interactions

Interactant	Interaction
Anticoagulants	Aluminum nicotinate ↑ effect
Antidiabetic agents	Change in sugar metabolism caused by aluminum nicotinate may require change in dosage of antidiabetic drugs
Tetracylines	Effect ↓ by aluminum nicotinate

Dosage   *Nicotinic acid*. **PO**: 1–2 gm t.i.d. with or following meals (to be taken with cold water). Dose is initiated slowly to minimize side effects. *Nicotinamide*. **PO or parenteral**: 50 mg, 3–10 times daily.

Nursing Implications

Teach patient and/or family

a. how to follow prescribed diet.

b. to limit alcohol intake.

c. to take drug in *divided* doses with meals. If GI side effects persist, report to physician, who may reduce dosage and/or order an antacid.

d. to avoid taking aluminum nicotinate on an empty stomach, because in addition to gastric side effects, the likelihood of flushing is increased.

e. that flushing, pruritis, and nausea may subside with continuing therapy.

f. that diabetic patients should be alert to symptoms of hyperglycemia (see p. 680) precipitated by nicotinic acid. Report symptoms of hyperglycemia to doctor as change in antidiabetic agent may be indicated.

g. that the patient on anticoagulant therapy should observe for purpura and/or bleeding from any orifice and to report to physician.

h. that the patient in whom acanthosis nigricans develops as an untoward reaction should expect warts to disappear 2 months after discontinuing drug.

PROBUCOL   Lorelco (Rx)

Classification   Hypocholesterolemic agent.

Action/Kinetics   Mechanism for alteration of cholesterol metabolism unknown. Decreases cholesterol with variable effects on triglycerides. After prolonged administration, the drug becomes deposited in the adipose tissues, and after discontinuation, persists in the body for up to 6 months. Absorption from the GI tract is variable. t½: (biphasic): **initial**, 24 hr; **final**: 20 days. **Therapeutic onset**: 2–4 weeks; maximum: 20–50 days. Poorly absorbed from GI tract.

Uses   Primary hypercholesterolemia, especially of type II and IIa. Not indicated when hypertriglyceridemia is the main finding.

Contraindication   Hypersensitivity. Safe use during pregnancy and in childhood has not been established.

Untoward Reactions   Mild and of short duration. *GI:* Most common. Diarrhea, flatulence, abdominal pain, nausea, vomiting. *Other:* Hyperhidrosis, fetid sweat, angioneurotic edema.

Dosage **Adults only, PO**: 500 mg b.i.d. with morning and evening meals.

Administration/ Storage

1. To be taken with morning and evening meal.
2. Store in dry place, in light-resistant containers away from excessive heat.

Nursing Implications

Teach patient and/or family

a. to follow prescribed low-cholesterol diet.
b. that if diarrhea occurs, it is usually transient. Roughage should, however, be eliminated until diarrhea stops.
c. to report GI symptoms to physician if they persist.

SITOSTEROLS   Cytellin (Rx)

Classification   Hypocholesterolemic agent.

Action/Kinetics   Sitosterols are a mixture of sterols obtained from vegetable oils. Sitosterols interfere with the absorption of dietary and endogenous cholesterol. Also, increased excretion of cholesterol and decreased levels of total lipid, including triglycerides. Effects are inconsistent, however. Absorption usually limited to 5%; cholesterol lowered by 12–16%.

Uses   Hypercholesterolemia and hyperbetalipoproteinemia. Sitosterols have been used successfully for patients who also suffer from diabetes, hypothyroidism, and idiopathic hypercholesterolemia. The higher the abnormal serum cholesterol level, the more effective the drug.

Contraindication   Administer with caution to patients with liver disease.

Untoward Reactions   GI effects: anorexia, diarrhea, and abdominal cramps.

Drug Interaction   Anticoagulants, oral: potentiated by sitosterols. Anticoagulant dosage must be reduced.

Dosage   **PO**: 3–6 gm (depending on quantity and fat content of meal) before meals, not to exceed 24–36 gm/day. If additional food ingested between meals, a partial or total dose should be taken. Effect of therapy becomes apparent during first month. Maximum effect usually becomes established during second or third month.

Administration   Improve palatability of drug by mixing with milk, coffee, tea, or fruit juice.

Nursing Implications

Teach patient and/or family

a. how to adjust dosage.
b. that stool will be bulky and light in color because of presence of sitosterols.
c. to restrict roughage in diet to minimize incidence of diarrhea.

Part Six

DRUGS AFFECTING THE CENTRAL NERVOUS SYSTEM

Chapter Twenty-nine

BARBITURATES

General Statement The barbiturates, especially their sodium salts, are readily absorbed after oral, rectal, or parenteral administration. They are distributed throughout all tissues, cross the placental barrier, and appear in breast milk. Toxic doses depress the activity of tissues in addition to the CNS, including the cardiovascular system. In some patients, barbiturates manifest an unusual action, including an excitatory response.

Action/Kinetics Barbiturates produce all levels of CNS depression, ranging from mild depression (sedation) following low doses to hypnotic (sleep-inducing) effects, and even coma and death, as dosage is increased. The depressant effects are thought to be manifested at the level of the reticular activating system by interfering with the transmission of nerve impulses to the cerebral cortex. The neurotransmitter gamma-aminobutryic acid (GABA) is thought to be associated with this action. Certain barbiturates also possess anticonvulsant activity; however, barbiturates are not analgesics and therefore should not be given to patients for the purpose of ameliorating pain.

The main difference between the various barbiturates is onset of action. *Ultrashort-acting*: **Onset: IV**, immediate; **duration**: up to 30 min. *Short-acting*: **Onset: PO**, 10–15 min; **peak effect**: 3–4 hr. *Intermediate-acting*: **Onset: PO**, 45–60 min; **peak effect**: 6–8 hr. *Long-acting*: **Onset: PO**, 60 or more minutes; **peak effect**: 10–12 hr. *Rectal administration*: Onset times are similar to PO. **Onset: IV**, immediate for short-acting up to 5 min for long-acting. **Duration of sedation**: 3–6 hr after IV; 6–8 hr, all other routes.

Note: It is currently believed that there is little difference in the duration of hypnosis after the use of any barbiturate; however there is a difference in the time of onset. Thus although widely used, the classification by duration of action may be outdated. Barbiturates are metabolized almost completely in the liver (except for barbital and phenobarbital) and are excreted in the urine. t½: See individual drugs, Table 12, p. 371.

Uses Preanesthetic medication, anesthesia (thiobarbiturates), sedation, hypnotic, and for the control of acute convulsive conditions (only phenobarbital, mephobarbital, metharbital) as in epilepsy, tetanus, and eclampsia. The benzodiazepines have replaced barbiturates for the treatment of many conditions.

TABLE 12 BARBITURATES

Drug	Use	Dosage	Remarks[a]
Amobarbital (Amobarbitone,* Amytal) C-II, Rx	Sedation, hypnotic, acute convulsive disorders, manic reactions	*Amobarbital.* **PO only.** *Sedation:* 30–50 mg 2–3 times daily. *Hypnotic:* 100–200 mg. *Amobarbital sodium.* **PO:** *Insomnia* 65–200 mg. *Preanesthetic:* 200 mg 1–2 hr before surgery. *Labor:* **Initial,** 200–400 mg; **then** 200–400 mg, if needed q 1–3 hr not to exceed total dose of 1 gm. **IM:** 65–200 mg. **IV:** Dose individualized	Intermediate-acting. *t½:* 8–42 hr. *Administration:* When dissolving drypacked ampules with accompanying sterile water for parenteral use, rotate ampule for mixing. Solutions that are not clear after 5 min should be discarded. Not more than 30 min should elapse between opening of ampule and usage. **IM:** Inject deeply, in large muscle, no more than 5 ml at one site. **IV:** Inject slowly at rates not exceeding 1 ml/min. Patients requiring IV administration should be closely monitored
Amobarbital sodium (Amytal) C-II, Rx			
Aprobarbital (Alurate) C-III, Rx	Daytime sedation, hypnotic	PO, *Sedation:* 40 mg t.i.d. *Hyponotic:* 80–160 mg. The preparation is supplied as an elixir. One teaspoon (5 ml) contains 40 mg.	Intermediate-acting. *t½:* 14–34 hr.
Butabarbital sodium (Butalan, Butatran, Buticaps, Butisol Sodium, Day-Barb,* Neobarb,* Sarisol No. 2, Soneryl) C-III, Rx	Hypnotic, mild sedation for anxiety	PO, *Sedation:* **Adult,** 15–30 mg t.i.d.–q.i.d.; **pediatric:** 7.5–30 mg (depending on age and degree of sedation desired). *Hypnotic:* **Adults** 50–100 mg; **pediatric:** depends on age and weight.	Intermediate-acting. *t½:* 34–42 hr. Most often used as sedative. Also found in Fiorinal Plain and with Codeine (see Appendix 3).
Mephobarbital (Mebaral) C-IV, Rx	Sedation, anticonvulsant for clonic-tonic or absence seizures	PO *Sedative:* **Adults** 32–100 mg t.i.d.–q.i.d.; **pediatric:** 16–32 mg	Long-acting. Anticonvulsant activity. Broken down in liver to phenobarbital, which is the active form. The hypnotic effects are mild

TABLE 12 (Continued)

Drug	Use	Dosage	Remarks[a]
		t.i.d.–q.i.d. *Epilepsy:* **Adults: usual,** 400–600 mg/day; **pediatric (over 5 years):** 32–64 mg t.i.d.–q.i.d.; **pediatric (under 5 years):** 16–32 mg t.i.d.–q.i.d. Administer at bedtime if seizures are likely to occur at night. Dosage should be increased gradually until optimum effects observed.	and compound causes little drowsiness or lassitude. For epilepsy, mephobarbital is often administered concurrently with phenytoin.
Metharbital (Gemonil) C-III, Rx	Anticonvulsant, suitable for treatment of petit mal, grand mal, myoclonic epilepsy and mixed types of seizures (not agent of first choice, however)	*Individualized, Usual,* **adult:** 100 mg 1–3 times daily, to be increased gradually until control is established; **pediatric:** 5–15 mg/kg daily.	Long-acting. Anticonvulsant with specific antiepileptic action. Often used with other anticonvulsant drugs.
Methohexital sodium (Brevital sodium, Brietal Sodium) C-IV, Rx	General anesthetic for brief procedures (oral surgery, gynecologic, and genitourinary examinations, reduction of fractures, prior to electroshock therapy)	**Induction:** 50–120 mg; **maintenance:** administer 20–40 mg as required usually q 4 to 7 min (as a 1% solution) or by continuous drip (0.2% solution-1 drop/min).	Ultrashort-acting; duration of anesthesia 5–8 min.
Pentobarbital (Nembutal) C-II Pentobarbital Sodium (Nembutal Sodium) C-II, Rx	Sedative, hypnotic, emergency use in convulsive states, preanesthetic medication	**PO.** *Sedation:* **Adults,** 30 mg t.i.d.–q.i.d.; **pediatric:** 8–30 mg. *Hypnotic:* **Adults,** 100 mg. **Rectal** (Suppositories): **Adults,** 120–200 mg; **pediatric, 2–12 months:** 30 mg; **1–4**	Short-acting; t½: 19–34 hr. Is 60–70% protein bound. *Administration:* Since pentobarbital is a potent CNS depressant that may cause adverse respiratory and circulatory response, the IV dose is given in fractions. Adults receive 100 mg initially; children and debilitated persons 50 mg. Subsequent fractions are administered after 1 minute observation pe-

| Phenobarbital (Barbita, Gardenal,* Luminal Ovoids, PBR/12, SK-Phenobarbital, Solfoton) C-IV, Rx

Phenobarbital sodium (Luminal Sodium) C-IV, Rx | Sedative, preanesthetic, postoperative sedation, hypnotic, anticonvulsant (tonic-clonic or cortical focal seizures); emergency control of acute convulsive disorders such as status epilepticus, meningitis, tetanus, eclampsia, toxicity of local anesthetics | years: 30–60 mg; **5–12 years:** 60 mg; **12–14 years:** 60–120 mg. IV **(slow): Adult (70 kg),** 100 mg *(See Remarks).* **IM, Adults:** 150–200 mg; **pediatric:** 25–80 mg (not to exceed 100 mg).

Phenobarbital. **PO.** *Sedation:* **Adults,** 30–120 mg/day in 2–3 divided doses. *Hypnotic:* **Adults,** 100–320 mg. *Anticonvulsant:* **Adults,** 50–100 mg b.i.d.–t.i.d.; **pediatric,** 4–6 mg/kg/day for 7–10 days (to achieve a blood level of 10–15 µg/ml) or 10–15 mg/kg/day. *Preanesthetic:* **Pediatric,** 1–3 mg/kg. **IM, IV.** *Sedation:* **Adults,** 100–130 mg. *Convulsions, eclampsia:* **Adults,** 200–300 mg (repeat in 6 hr if necessary). **IM only.** *Sedation:* **Infants, children,** 2 mg/kg. *Convulsions, eclampsia:* **Infants, children,** 3–5 mg/kg. *Preanesthetic:* **Adults,** 130–200 mg; **children,** | riods. Overdosage or too rapid administration may cause spasms of larynx or pharynx, or both. Pentobarbital solutions are highly alkaline. Administer no more than 5 ml at one site **IM** because of possible tissue irritation (pain, necrosis, gangrene).
Additional Nursing Implications (1) Observe closely for respiratory depression, which is the first sign of overdosage. (2) Observe for pain, delayed onset of hypnosis, pallor, cyanosis, and patchy discoloration of skin, signs of intra-arterial injection. (3) Stop IV injection if there is any pain in limb.

Long-acting. t½: 24–140 hr. **Anticonvulsant therapeutic serum levels:** 15–45 µg/ml. Is 50–60% protein bound. Long-acting barbiturate. A drug of choice for tonic-clonic seizures. Give major fraction of anticonvulsant dosage according to when seizures are likely to occur. On arising for daytime seizures, at bedtime when seizures occur at night. In most cases, when used for epilepsy, drug must be taken regularly to avoid seizures—even when no seizures are imminent. Aqueous solution for injection must be freshly prepared. Some ready-dissolved solutions for injection are available. The vehicle is propylene glycol, water, and alcohol. These solutions are stable. *IV administration:* Inject very slowly at rate of 50 mg/min. |

TABLE 12 (Continued)

Drug	Use	Dosage	Remarks[a]
Secobarbital (Seconal) C-II, Rx Secobarbital sodium (Seconal Sodium) C-II, Rx	Mild sedation, hypnotic, acute convulsive disorders due to local anesthetic reactions, tetanus, status epilepticus. Dentistry.	16–100 mg. *Postoperative sedation:* **Adults,** 32–100 mg; **children:** 8–30 mg. *Vomiting of pregnancy:* 100–130 mg q 6 hr. **PO.** *Sedation:* **Adult,** 30–50 mg t.i.d.; **pediatric:** 6 mg/kg/day in 3 divided doses. *Hypnotic:* **Adult,** 100 mg. *Preoperative sedation:* **Adult,** 200–300 mg 1–2 hr before surgery; **pediatric:** 50–100 mg 1–2 hr before surgery. **Rectal** (Dosage dependent on degree of sedation desired): **Adults:** 120–200 mg; **pediatric, up to 6 months:** 15–60 mg; **6 months-3 years:** 60 mg; **over 3 years:** 60–120 mg. **IM.** *Hypnotic:* **Adults,** 100–200 mg; **children,** 3–5 mg/kg up to a maximum total dose of 100 mg. *Dentistry:* **Adults, children,** 2.2 mg/kg	Short-acting. t½: 15–40 hr. Is 46–70% protein bound. Not effective for epilepsy. **Adults:** Aqueous solution preferred to polyethylene glycol-which may be irritating to kidneys, especially in patients with signs of renal insufficiency. *Administration* (1) Aqueous solutions for injection must be freshly prepared from dry-packed ampules. (2) Stable aqueous-polyethylene glycol solutions are available. These should be stored below 10°C.

Drug	Uses	Dosage	Remarks
(continued from previous page)		10–15 min before procedure. **Maximum dose**: 100 mg. **IV**. *Anesthetic procedures*: 50 mg/15 sec until desired degree of hypnosis reached. Total dose should not exceed 250 mg. *Convulsions in tetanus*: 5.5 mg/kg repeated q 3–4 hr if necessary. (Rate should not exceed 50 mg/15 sec).	
Talbutal (Lotusate) C-III, Rx	Hypnotic	**PO.** *Hypnotic*: 120 mg 15–30 min before bedtime.	Intermediate-acting
Thiamylal sodium (Surital Sodium) C-III, Rx		**IV**: 3–4 ml of a freshly prepared 2.5% solution; **maximum dose**: 1 gm (or 40 ml of 2.5% solution). Two-thirds of calculated dose may be sufficient for obstetric cases.	Ultrashort-acting. *Administration*: Solution should be administered slowly: 1 ml every 5 sec. Can also be administered by IV drip as 0.2% or 0.3% solution. *Additional Contraindication*: Porphyria.
Thiopental sodium (Pentothal Sodium) C-III, Rx	Preanesthetic or general anesthesia only	**IV only.** Dosage determined by anesthesiologist to fit needs of situation. **Rectal**: Dose determined by anesthesiologist	Ultrashort-acting. Administer cautiously to avoid severe respiratory depression. *Additional Drug Interaction*: Sulfisoxazole ↑ effects of thiopental by ↓ plasma protein binding.

[a]For Action/Kinetics, see p. 370.

Contraindications Hypersensitivity to barbiturates, severe trauma, pulmonary disease, edema, uncontrolled diabetes, history of porphyria, and for patients in whom they produce an excitatory response.

Barbiturates should be used with caution during pregnancy and lactation, and in patients with CNS depression, hypotension, marked asthenia (characteristic of Addison's disease, hypoadrenalism, and severe myxedema), porphyria, fever, anemia, hemorrhagic shock, cardiac, hepatic or renal damage, history of alcoholism, in suicidal patients, and in the elderly, especially those with senile psychosis.

Untoward Reactions Skin eruptions, blood dyscrasias, photosensitivity, muscle and joint pain, lassitude, vertigo, headache, nausea, diarrhea, and hangover. Also excitement, euphoria, and restlessness. Prolonged administration may produce jaundice and porphyria in susceptible people. Elderly patients usually have an increased sensitivity to barbiturates and sometimes respond with excitement.

Barbiturates can induce physical and psychological dependence if high doses are used regularly for long periods of time. Withdrawal symptoms usually begin after 12–16 hours of abstinence. Manifestations of withdrawal include anxiety, weakness, nausea, vomiting, muscle cramps, delirium, and even tonic-clonic seizures.

Drug Interactions

GENERAL CONSIDERATIONS

1. Barbiturates stimulate the activity of enzymes responsible for the metabolism of a large number of other drugs by a process known as enzyme induction. As a result, when barbiturates are given to patients receiving such drugs, their therapeutic effectiveness is markedly reduced or even abolished.
2. The CNS depressant effect of the barbiturates is potentiated by many drugs. Concomitant administration may result in coma or fatal CNS depression. Barbiturate dosage should either be reduced or eliminated when other CNS drugs are given.
3. Barbiturates also potentiate the toxic effects of many other agents.

Interactant	Interaction
Alcohol	Potentiation or addition of CNS depressant effects, concomitant use may lead to drowsiness, lethargy, stupor, respiratory collapse, coma, or death
Anesthetics, general	See *Alcohol*
Anorexiants	↓ Effect of anorexiants due to opposite activities
Antianxiety drugs	See *Alcohol*
Anticoagulants, oral	↓ Effect of anticoagulants due to ↓ absorption from GI tract and ↑ breakdown by liver
Antidepressants, tricyclic	↓ Effect of antidepressants due to ↑ breakdown by liver
Antidiabetic agents	Prolong the effects of barbiturates
Antihistamines	See *Alcohol*
Beta-Adrenergic agents	↓ Beta-blockade due to ↑ breakdown by the liver
Chloramphenicol	↑ Effect of barbiturates by ↓ breakdown by the liver and ↓ effect of chloramphenicol by ↑ breakdown by liver
CNS depressants	See *Alcohol*
Corticosteroids	↓ Effect of corticosteroids due to ↑ breakdown by liver

Interactant	Interaction
Digitoxin	↓ Effect of digitoxin due to ↑ breakdown by liver
Doxorubicin	↓ Effect of doxorubicin
Doxycycline	↓ Effect of doxycycline due to ↑ breakdown by liver
Estrogens	↓ Effect of estrogen due to ↑ breakdown by liver
Furosemide	↑ Risk or intensity of orthostatic hypotension
Griseofulvin	↓ Effect of griseofulvin due to ↓ absorption from GI tract
Haloperidol	↓ Effect of haloperidol due to ↑ breakdown by liver
Methoxyflurane	↑ Kidney toxicity due to ↑ breakdown of methoxyflurane by liver to toxic metabolites
Monoamine oxidase inhibitors	↑ Effect of barbiturates due to ↓ breakdown by liver
Narcotic analgesics	See *Alcohol*
Oral contraceptives	↓ Effect of contraceptives due to ↑ breakdown by liver
Phenothiazines	↓ Effect of phenothiazines due to ↑ breakdown by liver; also see *Alcohol*
Phenytoin	↓ Effect variable; monitor carefully
Procarbazine	↑ Effect of barbiturates
Quinidine	↓ Effect of quinidine due to ↑ breakdown by liver
Rifampin	↓ Effect of barbiturates due to ↑ breakdown by liver
Sedative-hypnotics, nonbarbiturate	*See Alcohol*
Theophyllines	↓ Effect of theophyllines due to ↑ breakdown by liver
Valproic acid	↑ Effect of barbiturates due to ↓ breakdown by liver

ACUTE TOXICITY Characterized by cortical and respiratory depression; anoxia; peripheral vascular collapse; feeble, rapid pulse; pulmonary edema; decreased body temperature; clammy, cyanotic skin; depressed reflexes; stupor; and coma. After initial constriction the pupils become dilated. Death results from respiratory failure or arrest followed by cardiac arrest.

CHRONIC TOXICITY Prolonged use of barbiturates at high doses may lead to physical and psychological dependence as well as tolerance. Doses of 600–800 mg daily for 8 weeks may lead to physical dependence. The addict usually ingests 1.5 gm a day. Addicts prefer short-acting barbiturates. Symptoms of dependence are similar to those associated with chronic alcoholism and withdrawal symptoms are as severe. Withdrawal symptoms usually last from 5 to 10 days and are terminated by a long sleep.

Treatment consists of a cautious withdrawal of the hospitalized addict over a 2- to 4-week period. A stabilizing dose of 200–300 mg of a short-acting barbiturate is administered every 6 hr. The dose is then reduced by 100 mg daily until the stabilizing dose is reduced by one half. The patient is then maintained on this dose for 2–3 days before further reduction. The same procedure is repeated when the initial stabilizing dose has been reduced by three quarters. If a mixed spike and slow activity appear on the ECG, or if insomnia, anxiety, tremor, or weakness is observed, the dosage is maintained at a constant level or increased slightly until symptoms disappear.

TREATMENT OF ACUTE TOXICITY   *This should consist of maintenance of an adequate airway, oxygen intake, and carbon dioxide removal*. Absorption following SC or IM administration of the drug may be delayed by the use of ice packs or tourniquets. After oral ingestion, gastric lavage or gastric aspiration may delay absorption. Emesis should not be induced once the symptoms of overdosage are manifested as the patient may aspirate the vomitus into the lungs. Also, if the dose of barbiturate is high enough, the vomiting center in the brain may be depressed. Maintenance of renal function and removal of the drug by peritoneal dialysis or artificial kidney should be carried out. Supportive physiologic methods have proven superior to analeptic methods.

Laboratory Test Interferences

1. **Interference with test method**: ↑ 17-Hydroxycorticosteroids.
2. **Caused by pharmacologic effects**: ↑ Creatinine phosphokinase, alkaline phosphatase, serum transaminase, serum testosterone (in certain women), urinary estriol, porphobilinogen, coproporphyrin, uroporphyrin. ↓ Prothrombin time in patients on coumarin. ↑ or ↓ Bilirubin. False + lupus erythematosus test.

Dosage   Aim for minimum effective dosage. As hypnotics, barbiturates should be administered intermittently because tolerance develops. Elderly patients should receive half dosage, children one-quarter to one-half of adult dose (see Table 12).

Administration/Storage

1. When used as hypnotics, barbiturates should not be given for more than 14–28 days.
2. Aqueous solutions of sodium salts are unstable and must be used within 30 min after preparation.
3. Discard parenteral solutions that contain precipitate.

Nursing Implications

1. Withhold drug and consult with a physician if symptoms of overdosage are observed.
2. Do not awaken a patient to administer a sleeping pill.
3. Note sleeping patterns of patients since these may influence the doctor in deciding what type of barbiturate the patient may need.
4. Anticipate that with some patients sedation is preceded by a period of transient elation, confusion, or euphoria and provide appropriate nursing measures to calm the patient and prevent injury.
5. Use safety measures, such as side rails and assistance when ambulatory, for patients receiving hypnotic doses, since they may be unsteady or confused.
6. Do not apply cuffs or other restraints at the first sign of excitement when a patient becomes confused by barbiturates. Attempt to calm the patient and orient him by switching on a light and talking quietly and calmly until he is calm and relaxed.
7. Use supportive nursing measures to enhance the effect of the drug (back rub, warm drink, quiet pleasant atmosphere, and empathetic attitude).
8. Use nursing judgment in deciding whether to administer a second PRN sleeping medication during the night. Try to find out why the patient cannot sleep, use comfort measures, and administer analgesics for pain if ordered, or consult with physician. The dazed, dizzy, lethargic hangover effect is sometimes caused by injudicious use of barbiturates during the night.

9. Observe that patient is actually taking the drug and not hoarding it when medication is given PO.

10. Assess patient for physical and psychological dependence and tolerance.

11. Be alert to the signs of developing porphyria characterized by nausea and vomiting, abdominal pain, and muscle spasm.

12. Anticipate that IV use of barbiturates will be limited to the treatment of acute convulsions and anesthesia.

13. Monitor IV administration of barbiturates closely for correct rate of flow; too rapid an injection may produce respiratory depression, dyspnea, and shock.

14. Monitor the site of the IV injection closely for extravasation, which may lead to pain, nerve damage, and necrosis.

15. Monitor the site of the IV injection for thrombophlebitis evidenced by redness and pain along site of vein.

16. Be familiar with the treatment of chronic and acute toxicity associated with barbiturates.

17. *Teach patient and/or family*

   a. that patient should avoid drinking alcohol because it potentiates barbiturates.

   b. not to drive a car or operate other hazardous machinery after taking medication.

   c. not to leave medication bottle on the bedside table. Patients have been known to forget how many pills they have taken and accidentally overdose as a result.

   d. that a patient who has been taking large doses of sedatives for 8 weeks or more should not discontinue medication suddenly, because withdrawal symptoms (e.g., weakness, anxiety, delirium, and tonic-clonic seizures) may occur. Dosage should not be reduced without checking with physician.

   e. to report immediately signs of infection, such as sore throat and fever; also report immediately symptoms of bleeding tendency, such as bruising easily or nosebleeds, all of which are signs of hematologic toxicity.

Chapter Thirty

BENZODIAZEPINE AND OTHER NONBARBITURATE SEDATIVE-HYPNOTICS

Action/Kinetics   The nonbarbiturate sedative-hypnotics act similarly to the barbiturates in that they interfere with transmission of nerve impulses in the reticular activating system. These drugs produce similar actions as the barbiturates (See Chapter 29, p. 370.

If an individual exceeds the recommended therapeutic dose, physical dependence and tolerance may result. Thus, the dose should never be increased without medical supervision. Treatment consists of a cautious and gradual withdrawal of the drug over a period of time under the care of a physician.

Drug Interactions   Concomitant use of nonbarbiturate sedative-hypnotics with alcohol, anesthetics, antianxiety drugs, antihistamines, barbiturates, narcotics, or phenothiazines may result in addition or potentiation of CNS depressant effects. Symptoms manifested are drowsiness, lethargy, stupor, respiratory collapse, coma, and possible death.

Nursing Implications

1. Avoid the use of alcohol with any of these drugs.
2. use caution in driving or operating machinery until daytime sedative effects are evaluated.
3. Assess for tolerance and psychological and physical dependence.
4. When suffering from simple insomnia, try warm baths, warm milk, and other interventions to induce sleep rather than becoming dependent on drugs.

ACETYLCARBROMAL   Paxarel (Rx)

Classification   Nonbarbiturate, nonbenzodiazepine sedative-hypnotic.

Action/Kinetics   Liberates bromide, which causes sedation. Since the active principle of acetylcarbromal is bromide, intoxiction (bromism) may result. If bromism develops, the drug should be discontinued and the excretion of bromide increased by administering sodium or ammonium chloride or a chloruretic diuretic. Hemodialysis is also effective. The drug is rarely used.

Uses   Anxiety, tension, insomnia. Premenstrual tension or menopausal syndrome. Preoperative, preprocedural, or postoperative sedative.

Contraindications   Sensitivity to bromides. Lactation.

Untoward Reactions   Large doses: Bromide intoxication characterized by dizziness, impaired thoughts, irritability, motor incoordination, skin rash, vomiting, profound stupor, and bromide psychosis.

Drug Interactions   Concomitant use with alcohol or other CNS depressants may lead to severe CNS depression.

Dosage   **Adults:** 250–500 mg b.i.d. - t.i.d. **Pediatric:** Dosage determined by age and weight.

Additional Nursing Implication

Teach patient and/or family to discontinue drug and report to doctor if symptoms of bromism as indicated in *Untoward Reactions* are observed.

CHLORAL HYDRATE   Aquachloral, Noctec, Novochlorhydrate,* SK-Chloral Hydrate (C-IV) (Rx)

Classification   Nonbarbiturate, nonbenzodiazepine sedative-hypnotic.

General Statement   Chloral hydrate only produces slight hangover effects and is said not to affect REM sleep. High doses lead to severe CNS depression, as well as depression of respiratory and vasomotor centers (hypotension). Both psychological and physical dependence develop.

Action/Kinetics   Chloral hydrate is metabolized to trichloroethanol, which is the active metabolite. **Onset:** 10–15 min. **Duration:** 4–8 hr. **t½:** 8–10 hr. The drug is readily absorbed from the GI tract and is distributed to all tissues; it passes the placental barrier and appears in breast milk as well. Metabolites excreted by kidney.

Uses   Hypnotic and sedative. Preoperative sedative and postoperative as adjunct to analgesics.

Contraindications   Marked hepatic or renal impairment, severe cardiac disease, or nursing mothers. Drugs should not be given orally to patients with gastritis or gastric ulcer.

Untoward Reactions   *CNS:* Paradoxical paranoid reactions. Sudden withdrawal in dependent patients may result in "chloral delirium." Sudden intolerance for the drug following prolonged use may result in respiratory depression, hypotension, cardiac effects, and possibly death. *GI:* Nausea, vomiting, diarrhea, bad taste in mouth, gastritis, increased peristalsis. *GU:* Renal damage, decrease urine flow and uric acid excretion. *Miscellaneous:* Skin reactions, hepatic damage, allergic reactions, leukopenia, eosinophilia.

  Chronic toxicity is treated by gradual withdrawal and rehabilitative measures as used in treatment of the chronic alcoholic. Poisoning by chloral hydrate resembles acute barbiturate intoxication; the same supportive treatment is indicated. (see p. 378).

Drug Interactions

Interactant	Interaction
Anticoagulants, oral	↑ Effect of anticoagulants by ↓ plasma protein binding
CNS depressants	Additive CNS depression. Concomitant use may lead to drowsiness, lethargy, stupor, respiratory collapse, coma, or death
Furosemide (IV)	Concomitant use results in diaphoresis, tachycardia, hypertension, flushing

Laboratory Test Interferences   ↑ 17-Hydroxycorticosteroids. Interference with fluoresence tests for catecholamines.

Dosage   **PO** (*capsules, elixir, and syrup*) and **rectally.** *Sedative*: 250 mg t.i.d; **pediatric:** one-half the hypnotic dose. *Hypnotic*: 0.5–1 gm 15–30 min before bedtime, not to exceed 2 gm daily; **pediatric:** 50 mg/kg not to exceed 1 gm daily.

Administration   PO: give capsules after meals with full glass of water or elixir with ½ glass of juice, water, or ginger ale.

Additional Nursing Implications

1. *Assess*
   a. for alertness of patient.
   b. for respiratory, cardiac, and vasomotor depression and dilation of cutaneous blood vessels.
   c. for reduced urine output and elevated BUN.
   d. for tolerance and psychological and physical dependence. Symptoms of dependence resemble those of acute alcoholism, but with more severe gastritis.
2. Have equipment ready for physiologic supportive treatment of acute poisoning: suction, respirator, oxygen, IV sets, and sodium bicarbonate and sodium lactate solutions.

ETCHLORVYNOL   Placidyl (C-IV) (Rx)

Classification   Nonbarbiturate, nonbenzodiazepine sedative-hypnotic.

Action/Kinetics   Manifests anticonvulsant and muscle relaxant properties as well as sedation and hypnotic effects. Said to depress REM sleep. Chronic use produces psychological and physical dependence. Produces less respiratory depression than occurs with barbiturates.

Onset: 15–30 min. **Peak blood levels:** 1–1.5 hr. **Duration:** 5 hr. t½: initial, 1–3 hr; final, 10–25 hr. Approximately 90% metabolized in liver and excreted in urine.

Uses   Insomnia (treatment not to exceed 1 week).

Contraindications   Porphyria, hypersensitivity.

Untoward Reactions   *CNS:* Initial excitement, giddiness, vertigo, mental confusion, headache, blurred vision, hangover, fatigue, ataxia. *GI:* Bad aftertaste, nausea, vomiting, gastric upset. *Cardiovascular:* Hypotension, fainting. *Miscellaneous:* Skin rash, thrombocytopenia, jaundice, pulmonary edema (following IV abuse). Overdose produces symptoms similar to barbiturate intoxication.

Drug Interactions

Interactant	Interaction
Anticoagulants, oral	↓ Effect of anticoagulants due to ↑ breakdown by liver
Antidepressants, tricyclic	Combination may result in transient delirium

Laboratory Test Interference   ↓ Prothrombin time (patients on coumadin).

Dosage   PO. Adult, usual: 500 mg at bedtime; up to 1,000 mg may be required if insomnia is severe. If patient awakens, a 100–200 mg supplemental dose can be given. Adjust dose carefully in geriatric or debilitated patients.

Administration   With food or milk to reduce or eliminate giddiness and ataxia.

Nursing Implications
See *Nursing Implications* for *Barbiturates*, p. 378.

ETHINAMATE   Valmid (C-IV) (Rx)

Classification   Nonbarbiturate, nonbenzodiazepine sedative-hypnotic.

Action/Kinetics   Drug may have some weak anticonvulsant and weak local anesthetic effects. Therapeutic doses produce quiet sleep with little or no hangover. Larger doses produce euphoria. *Overdosage:* respiratory depression. Ethinamate may cause psychological and physical dependence as well as tolerance. Withdrawal symptoms are similar to those of barbiturates.
   Onset: 20–30 min. **Duration:** 4 hr. A dose of 500 mg ethinamate is approximately equal to 100 mg secobarbital. Inactivated in liver and excreted in urine.

Uses   Insomnia (use should not exceed 1 week).

Contraindications   Hypersensitivty to drug. Safety in pregnancy, childhood, or during lactation has not been established. Not useful in patients suffering pain. *Not recommended* for routine daytime sedation because prolonged use may lead to psychological and physical dependence.

Untoward Reactions   Few. Thrombocytopenic purpura, mild GI symptoms, skin rashes, and paradoxical excitement in children. Abrupt withdrawal of large doses may be dangerous.

Drug Interactions   Concomitant use with alcohol or other CNS depressant may lead to severe CNS depression.

Laboratory Test Interference   Interferes with test by ↑ 17-hydroxycorticosteroids and 17-ketosteroids.

Dosage   PO: 500–1,000 mg 20 min before bedtime. Elderly or debilitated patients should receive a lower dosage.

Administration
   1. If insomnia persists after 1 week of therapy, a 1 week rest period should follow before a second course of therapy.

2. Due to possible drowsiness and dizziness, patients should be cautious while driving or operating machinery.

Nursing Implications
1. Assess patient receiving large dosages for symptoms of dependence.
2. See treatment for acute toxicity under *Barbiturates*, p. 378.
3. Be prepared to assist with gastric lavage for acute poisoning, because lavage must be done immediately as the drug is rapidly absorbed from the GI tract.
4. Caution the patient against abruptly discontinuing drug, since withdrawal symptoms may occur.

FLURAZEPAM HYDROCHLORIDE   Dalmane, Apo-Flurazepam,* Novoflupam,* Somnol*, Som-Pam* (C-IV) (Rx)

Classification   Benzodiazepine sedative-hypnotic.

Action/Kinetics   **Onset:** 15–45 min. The major active metabolite, N-desalkyl-flurazepam, is active and has a t½ of 47–100 hr. **Maximum effectiveness:** 2–3 days (due to slow accumulation of active metabolite).

Use   Insomnia (all types).

Contraindications   Hypersensitivity. Pregnancy or in women wishing to become pregnant. Depression, renal or hepatic disease, chronic pulmonary insufficiency, children under 15 years.

Untoward Reactions   *CNS:* Ataxia, dizziness, drowsiness/sedation, headache, disorientation. Symptoms of stimulation including nervousness, apprehension, irritability, and talkativeness. *GI:* Nausea, vomiting, diarrhea, gastric upset or pain, heartburn, constipation. *Miscellaneous:* Arthralgia, chest pains or palpitations. Rarely, symptoms of allergy, shortness of breath, jaundice, anorexia, blurred vision.

Drug Interactions

Interactant	Interaction
Cimetidine	↑ Effect flurazepam due to ↓ breakdown by liver
Disulfiram	↑ Effect flurazepam due to ↓ breakdown by liver
Ethanol	Additive depressant effects even the day following flurazepam
Isoniazid	↑ Effect flurazepam due to ↓ breakdown by liver
Oral contraceptives	Either ↑ or ↓ effect of benzodiazepines due to effect on breakdown by liver
Rifampin	↓ Effect of benzodiazepines due to ↑ breakdown by liver

Laboratory Test Interference   ↑ Alkaline phosphatase, bilirubin, serum transaminases.

Dosage   **PO. Adults:** 15–30 mg at bedtime; 15 mg for geriatric and/or debilitated patients.

GLUTETHIMIDE   Doriden (C-III) (Rx)

Classification   Nonbarbiturate, nonbenzodiazepine sedative-hypnotic.

Action/Kinetics   Glutethimide produces CNS depressant effects comparable to barbiturates, including suppression of REM sleep and REM rebound. Other effects include anticholinergic with mydriasis, inhibition of salivary secretion, and constipation. At comparable doses, glutethimide produces less respiratory depression but greater hypotension than occurs with barbiturates. Psychological and physical dependence may develop.

   Onset: 30 min. **Peak plasma concentration:** 1–6 hr (erratically absorbed from GI tract). **t½:** 10–12 hr. About 50% is bound to plasma protein. Metabolized in liver and excreted in urine.

Uses   Insomnia (use should not exceed 1 week).

Contraindications   Hypersensitivity to drug. Porphyria. Patients with a history of drug dependence, alcoholism, or emotional disorders. Use not recommended during pregnancy and in children.

   Do not give to patient with glaucoma or to patients with a history of drug dependence, alcoholism, or emotional disorders.

Untoward Reactions   *GI:* Nausea, vomiting, anorexia, xerostomia. *CNS:* Headache, dizziness, confusion, drowsiness. *Dermatologic:* Skin rash (cause for discontinuing drug), urticaria, purpura. *Miscellaneous:* Osteomalacia following long-term use.

   Rarely: Excitation, blurred vision, acute hypersensitivity, exfoliative dermatitis, intermittent porphyria, and blood dyscrasias including thrombocytopenia, aplastic anemia, and leukopenia.

   Abrupt withdrawal of large doses may be dangerous—withdrawal symptoms are similar to that of barbiturates. Occasionally, symptoms similar to withdrawal occur in patients who have been taking only moderate doses, even when there is no abstention (tremulousness, nausea, tachycardia, fever, tonic muscle spasms, generalized convulsions).

CHRONIC TOXICITY   Characterized by psychosis, confusion, delirium, hallucinations, ataxia, tremor, hyporeflexia, slurred speech, memory loss, irritability, fever, weight loss, mydriasis, xerostomia, nystagmus, headache, and convulsions. Treatment consists of careful, cautious withdrawal of drug over a period of several days or weeks.

ACUTE TOXICITY   Characterized by coma, hypotension, hypothermia, followed by fever, tachycardia, depression or absence of reflexes (including pupillary response), sudden apnea, cyanosis, tonic muscle spasms, convulsions, and hyperreflexia.

   Treatment of acute toxicity is supportive, starting with gastric lavage, CNS stimulants (used with caution), vasopressors, and maintenance of pulmonary ventilation. Parenteral fluids are administered cautiously, and hemodialysis may be necessary. Endotracheal intubation or tracheotomy may be indicated.

Drug Interactions

Interactant	Interaction
Anticoagulants, oral	↓ Effect of anticoagulants due to ↑ breakdown by liver
Antidepressants, tricyclic	Additive anticholinergic side effects

Laboratory Test Interference   Alters (↑ or ↓) 17-ketogenic steroids, 17-hydroxycorticosteroids.

Dosage   PO. Adults: Individualize to minimize chance of overdosage. **Usual:** 250–500 mg at bedtime. **Geriatric or debilitated patients:** Daily dose should not exceed 0.5 gm. **Not recommended for children.**

Additional Nursing Implications

1. Provide special mouth care, since the patient may have xerostomia.
2. Check that the patient is having regular bowel movements; glutethimide reduces intestinal motility. Provide extra fluids and roughage in diet. Consult with physician regarding need for a laxative.
3. Withhold drug from patients showing signs of depression or suicidal tendencies.
4. Warn patients receiving glutethimide not to drive a car or operate other machinery after taking medication because drug may cause drowsiness.

TREATMENT OF OVERDOSAGE

5. Be prepared to assist with gastric lavage for treatment of acute toxicity. Monitor vital signs.
6. In addition to providing an adequate airway, oxygen, fluids, electrolyte intake, and parenteral fluids, have on hand CNS stimulants and pressor agents.
7. Have on hand an endotracheal tube and tracheotomy setup.
8. Be prepared to handle request for hemodialysis.

METHYPRYLON   Noludar (C-III) (Rx)

Classification   Nonbarbiturate, nonbenzodiazepine sedative-hypnotic.

Action/Kinetics   The action of methyprylon is similar to that of the barbiturates in that it suppresses REM sleep and induces rebound when drug therapy is discontinued. **Onset:** 45 min. **Peak plasma level:** 1–2 hr; **duration:** 5–8 hr. **t½:** 4 hr. Both unchanged drug and liver metabolites are excreted in the urine.

Uses   Transient or intermittent insomnia. Especially useful for patients allergic to barbiturates.

Contraindications   Hypersensitivity to drug. Children under 12 years. Administer with caution in pregnancy and in the presence of renal and hepatic disease.

Untoward Reactions   Morning drowsiness, dizziness, mild to moderate gastric upset, headache, paradoxic excitement, skin rash. Overdosage is characterized by somnolence, confusion, coma, constricted pupils, respiratory depression, and hypotension.

Drug Interactions   Concomitant use with alcohol or other CNS depressant may lead to severe CNS depression.

Laboratory Test Interference   With test methods: ↑ 17-Hydroxycorticosteroids, 17-ketosteroids, 17-ketogenic steroids.

Dosage   PO. Adults: 200–400 mg before bedtime. **Pediatric over 12 years:** (effectiveness extremely variable), **initial,** 50 mg. If ineffective, may be increased to 200 mg at bedtime.

Nursing Implications

1. *Teach patient and/or family*
   a. not to engage in hazardous activities such as driving because drowsiness may develop.
   b. that when suffering from simple insomnia to try warm baths, warm milk, and so forth to induce sleep rather than becoming dependent on drugs.
2. Assist in treatment of toxicity by
   a. monitoring vital signs closely.
   b. assisting in evacuation of stomach contents by lavage.
   c. providing oxygen and assisting ventilation if necessary; have available caffeine and sodium benzoate to be used to stimulate respiration.
   d. monitoring IV fluids and electrolytes; have on hand Levophed or Aramine to be used for hypotension.
   e. monitoring urinary output; hemodialysis may be instituted if urinary output is too scant.
   f. providing supportive care for the comatose patient; turn patient on side to prevent aspiration of vomitus.
   g. providing safety measures such as side rails.

PARALDEHYDE   Paral (C-IV) (Rx)

Classification   Nonbarbiturate sedative-hypnotic.

Action/Kinetics   Paraldehyde is bitter tasting (liquid) and has a strong, unpleasant odor. In usual doses, it has little effect on either respiration or blood pressure. In the presence of pain, paraldehyde may induce excitement or delirium; it is not analgesic. (See *Chloral Hydrate*, p. 381.)

   Onset: 10–15 min. Approximately 70–80% is detoxified in the liver, with the remainder excreted unchanged by the lungs. **t½:** 3.4–9.8 hr.

Uses   Sedative and hypnotic. Delirium tremens and other excited states. Prior to EEG to induce artificial sleep. Emergency treatment of eclampsia, tetanus, status epilepticus, and overdose of stimulant or convulsant drug. (see p. 467).

Contraindications   Gastroenteritis, bronchopulmonary disease, hepatic insufficiency. Use with caution during labor.

Drug Interactions

Interactant	Interaction
Disulfiram (Antabuse)	Combination may produce an Antabuse-like reaction
Sulfonamides	↑ Chance of sulfonamide crystalluria

Laboratory Test Interference   17-Hydroxycorticosteroids, 17-ketogenic steroids.

Dosage   **PO.** *Hypnotic*: 4–8 ml. *Delirium tremens*: 10–35 ml. **Rectal**: 10–20 ml (see *Administration*). **IM. Adults:** *Sedation,* 2–5 ml; *Hypnosis:* 10 ml (no more than 5 ml per injection site). **Pediatric:** *Sedation,* 0.15 ml/kg; *Hypnosis,* 0.3 ml/kg. **IV. Adults:** *Hypnosis,* 10 ml; *Sedation,* 5 ml. Use Sterile paraldehyde for IM or IV.

Administration/ Storage

1. *PO.* Drug should be very cold to minimize odor and taste as well as gastric irritation. Mask the taste and odor by mixing drug with syrup, milk, fruit juice, or wine.
2. *Rectal.* Mix with a thin oil or isotonic sodium choride solution to minimize irritation—1 part medication to 2 parts diluent.
3. *IM.* A pure sterile preparation should be used. Prevent extravasation into subcutaneous tissue as drug is very irritating and may cause sterile abscesses.
4. *IV.* Only in an emergency, dilute with several volumes of physiologic saline and inject at a rate not to exceed 1 ml/minute since circulatory collapse or pulmonary edema may occur. Use glass syringe and metal needles because the drug may react with the plastic used in disposable syringes and needles.
5. Store in a tight, light-resistant container, well filled with a maximum of 120 gm in each container.

Nursing Implications

See *Nursing Implications* for *Chloral Hydrate*, for toxicity and treatment, p. 382.

1. Reassure patients disturbed by the odor that they will become accustomed to it.
2. Assess for dependence and toxicity.
3. Report coughing during IV administration, as this could indicate untoward effects on pulmonary capillaries.
4. Assess patient for symptoms of overdosage, such as rapid, labored breathing and a fast, feeble pulse, low BP, and the characteristic odor of paraldehyde on breath.

PROPIOMAZINE HYDROCHLORIDE   Largon (Rx)

Classification   Nonbarbiturate sedative, phenothiazine.

Action/Kinetics   At therapeutic dosages, this phenothiazine drug has sedative, antiemetic, antihistaminic, and anticholinergic effects. **Peak sedative effects: IV**, 15–30 min; **IM**, 40–60 min. **Duration:** 3–6 hr.

Uses   Preanesthetic to reduce anxiety and emesis during surgery and labor. Adjunct to narcotic analgesia during labor.

Contraindications   Intra-arterial injection. Use with caution in pregnancy.

Untoward Reactions   *GI:* Dry mouth, GI upset. *CNS:* Dizziness and confusion in the elderly. Transient restlessness. *CV:* Transient decrease in blood pressure after rapid IV administration, tachycardia. *Other:* Skin rashes, respiratory depression, altered respiratory pattern. Irritation and thrombophlebitis at injection site.

Dosage   IM and IV. Adults. *Preoperative sedation:* **usual**, 20 mg up to 40 mg with meperidine, 50 mg. *Obstetrics*: 20–40 mg with meperidine, 50 mg. *Sedation with local anesthesia*: 10–20 mg. **Pediatric.** *Pre- and postoperatively:* children weighing less than 27 kg: 0.55–1.1 mg/kg.

Administration/ Storage

1. Inject into large, undamaged vein.

2. Avoid extravasation.
3. Never administer subcutaneously or intra-arterially.
4. Do not use solutions that are cloudy or contain precipitate.
5. Aqueous solutions are incompatible with barbiturate salts or alkaline solutions.
6. Store at 15°–30°C and protect from light.

Nursing Implications
1. Anticipate that the dose of other sedatives administered with propiomazine will be reduced by one-fourth to one-half in strength.
2. Anticipate that should vasopressor drugs be administered with propiomazine, norepinephrine would be used rather than epinephrine.
3. Provide mouth care to relieve xerostomia except for patients scheduled for surgery, for whom a dry mouth is desirable.
4. Monitor BP for 5 hours after IM or IV administration because medication may have a hypotensive effect.
5. Assess patients for untoward reaction remembering that, although unlikely, the adverse reactions (blood dyscrasias, hepatotoxicity, extrapyramidal symptoms, reactivation of psychotic processes, cardiac arrest, endocrine disturbances, dermatologic disorders, ocular changes, and hypersensitivity reactions) associated with long-term use of phenothiazines may occur.
6. Provide a safe environment for geriatric patients experiencing dizziness, confusion, or amnesia after administration of the drug.
7. Consider that the antiemetic effect of propiomazine may be masking other pathology, such as toxicity to other drugs, intestinal obstruction, or brain lesions.

TEMAZEPAM Restoril (C-IV) (Rx)

Classification Benzodiazepine hypnotic.

Action/Kinetics Temazepam is a benzodiazepine derivative. Disturbed nocturnal sleep may occur the first one or two nights following discontinuance of the drug. Prolonged administration is not recommended, since physical dependence and tolerance may develop. See also *Flurazepam,* p. 384. **Peak blood levels:** 2–3 hr. t½, initial: 0.4–0.6 hr; **final:** 10 hr. **Steady-state plasma levels:** 382 ng/ml (2½ hr after 30 mg dose). The drug is metabolized in the liver to inactive metabolites.

Uses Insomnia in patients unable to fall asleep, with frequent awakenings during the night, and/or early morning awakenings.

Contraindications Pregnancy. Use with caution during lactation, in geriatric patients, and in severely depressed patients.

Untoward Reactions *CNS:* Drowsiness (after daytime use) and dizziness are common. Lethargy, confusion, euphoria, weakness, ataxia, lack of concentration, hallucinations. In some patients paradoxical excitement (less than 0.5%), including stimulation and hyperactivity, occurs. *GI:* Anorexia, diarrhea. *Other:* Tremor, horizontal nystagmus, falling, palpitations. Rarely, blood dyscrasias.

Dosage PO. **Adults: usual,** 30 mg at bedtime. **In elderly or debilitated: initial,** 15 mg; **then,** adjust dosage to response.

Nursing Implications
See *Antianxiety Agents, Benzodiazepines*, p. 393.

TRIAZOLAM   Halcion (C-IV) (Rx)

Classification   Benzodiazepine sedative-hypnotic.

Action/Kinetics   Triazolam decreases sleep latency, increases the duration of sleep, and decreases the number of awakenings. **t½:** 2.3 hr. Metabolized in liver and inactive metabolites excreted in the urine.

Uses   Insomnia (short-term management not to exceed 1 month).

Contraindications   Pregnancy, lactation. Safety and efficacy in children under 18 years of age not established.

Untoward Reactions   *CNS:* Rebound insomnia, anterograde amnesia, headache, ataxia, decreased coordination. Psychological and physical dependence.   *GI:* Nausea, vomiting.

Drug Interactions   Concomitant use with alcohol or other CNS depressants may lead to severe CNS depression.

Dosage   **Individualized. Adults: initial,** 0.125 mg; **then,** depending on response, 0.25–0.5 mg before retiring. In geriatric or debilitated patients, the dose should be reduced by one-half.

Chapter Thirty-one

ANTIANXIETY AGENTS

BENZODIAZEPINES

General Statement   The benzodiazepines exhibit a wide margin of safety between therapeutic and toxic doses. For example, ataxia and sedation are observed at doses higher than those required to achieve antianxiety effects. The major difference among benzodiazepines appears to be a function of duration of action and other pharmacokinetic properties.

All antianxiety agents have the ability to cause psychological and physical dependence. Withdrawal symptoms usually start within 12–48 hr after stopping the drug and last for 12–48 hr. When the patient has received large doses of these drugs for weeks or months, dosage should be reduced gradually over a period of 1–2 weeks. Alternatively, a short-acting barbiturate may be substituted and then withdrawn gradually. Abrupt withdrawal of high dosage may be accompanied by coma, convulsions, and even death.

Dosage and uses of the benzodiazepines are presented in Table 13. Meprobamate and the miscellaneous agents are presented individually.

Action/Kinetics   The major antianxiety agents include the benzodiazepines and meprobamate. The benzodiazepines are thought to affect the limbic system by reducing anxiety. This effect is believed to be mediated through the action of the benzodiazepines on the neurotransmitter GABA on its receptor. Meprobamate and the benzodiazepines also possess varying degrees of anticonvulsant activity, skeletal muscle relaxation, and the ability to alleviate tension. The benzodiazepines generally have long half-lives (1–8 days); thus cumulative effects can occur. Also, several of the benzodiazepines are metabolized to active metabolites in the liver, which prolongs their duration of action. Benzodiazepines are widely distributed throughout the body. Approximately 85–98% of an administered dose is bound to plasma protein. It is excreted through the kidneys.

Uses   Management of anxiety and tension occurring alone or as a side effect of other conditions including menopausal syndrome, premenstrual tension, asthma, and angina pectoris.

Neurologic conditions involving muscle spasm and tetanus. Adjunct in treatment of rheumatoid arthritis, osteoarthritis, trauma, low back pain, torticollis, and selected convulsive disorders including status epilepticus.

Premedication for surgery or electric cardioversion.

Rehabilitation of chronic alcoholics; delirium tremens; nocturnal enuresis in childhood; and to induce sleep.

Contraindications   Hypersensitivity, acute narrow-angle glaucoma, psychoses, pregnancy, lactation. Use with caution in impaired hepatic or renal function and in the geriatric or debilitated patient.

Untoward Reactions   *CNS:* Drowsiness, fatigue, confusion, ataxia, dizziness, vertigo, fainting, headache, weakness, dysarthria, hallucinations, suicide. Paradoxical excitement manifested by restlessness, talkativeness, acute rage reactions, muscle spasticity, increased reflexes, insomnia, euphoria, nightmares. *GI:* Increased appetite, constipation, hiccoughs, anorexia, weight gain or loss, dry mouth, bitter or metallic taste, increased salivation, swollen tongue. *Allergic:* Urticaria, rash, photosensitivity, pruritus, edema, nonthrombocytopenic purpura, hypotension. *Endocrine:* Increased or decreased libido, gynecomastia, galactorrhea, menstrual irregularities. *GU:* Difficulty in urination, urinary retention. *Ophthalmologic:* Diplopia, conjunctivitis, nystagmus, blurred vision. *Miscellaneous:* Joint pain, muscle cramps, paresthesia, lupus-like symptoms, tachycardia, sweating, shortness of breath, flushing.

SYMPTOMS OF OVERDOSE Severe drowsiness, confusion, tremors, slurred speech, staggering, coma, hypotension, shortness of breath, labored breathing, weakness, slow heart rate.

Note: Geriatric patients, debilitated patients, very young children, and patients with liver disease are more sensitive to the CNS effects of benzodiazepines.

TREATMENT OF OVERDOSE Supportive therapy. Gastric lavage provided an endotracheal tube with cuff inflated is used to prevent aspiration of vomitus. Emesis only if drug ingestion was recent and patient is fully conscious. Activated charcoal and saline cathartic may be given after emesis or lavage. Adequate respiratory function must be maintained. Hypotension may be reversed by IV fluids, norepinephrine, or metaraminol.

Drug Interactions (Benzodiazepines)

Interactant	Interaction
Alcohol	Potentiation or addition of CNS depressant effects. Concomitant use may lead to drowsiness, lethargy, stupor, respiratory collapse, coma, or death
Anesthetics, general	See *Alcohol*
Antidepressants, tricyclic	Concomitant use with benzodiazepines may cause additive sedative effect and/or atropine-like side effects
Antihistamines	See *Alcohol*
Barbiturates	See *Alcohol*
Cimetidine	Cimetidine ↑ effect of benzodiazepines by ↓ breakdown in liver
CNS depressants	See *Alcohol*
Disulfiram	Disulfiram ↑ effect of benzodiazepines by ↓ breakdown in liver
CNS depressants	See *Alcohol*
Isoniazid	↑ Effect of benzodiazepines due to ↓ breakdown in liver
Levodopa	↓ Effect of levodopa
Narcotics	See *Alcohol*
Oral Contraceptives	Possible ↑ or ↓ effect of benzodiazepines
Phenothiazines	See *Alcohol*
Phenytoin	Concomitant use with benzodiazepines may cause ↑ effect of phenytoin due to ↓ breakdown by liver
Rifampin	↓ Effect of benzodiazepines due to ↑ breakdown by liver
Sedative-hypnotics, non-barbiturate	See *Alcohol*
Valproic acid	↑ Effect of benzodiazepines due to ↓ breakdown by liver

Laboratory Test Interference   Altered liver function tests, including bilirubin values.

Dosage   See Table 13, p. 394. Persistent drowsiness, ataxia, or visual disturbances may require dosage adjustment.

Lower dosage is usually indicated for older patients. GI effects are decreased when drugs are given with meals or shortly after. Withdraw drugs gradually.

Nursing Implications

1. Assess for more frequent requests for the drugs or for ingestion of larger than recommended doses. Such patients may be developing physical and psychological dependence, which can lead to drug abuse.

2. Assess for manifestations of ataxia, slurred speech, and vertigo. Such symptoms are characteristic of chronic intoxication and are usually an indication that the patient is taking more than the recommended dose.

3. Carefully supervise the dose and amount prescribed, especially when prescription is for long-term treatment of alcoholics and other patients with a known predisposition to take excessive quantities of drugs.

4. Remain with patient until drug is swallowed when it is administered on the ward. This prevents omission of the drug or hoarding, which may result in a suicide attempt.

5. Be aware, and inform the patient, that sudden withdrawal of the drug after prolonged and excessive use may cause the recurrence of preexisting symptoms or precipitate a withdrawal syndrome manifested by anxiety, anorexia, insomnia, vomiting, ataxia, tremors, muscle twitching, confusion, hallucinations, and, rarely, convulsive seizures.

6. Anticipate that doses to the elderly or debilitated patient will be lowest effective dose.

7. Anticipate that the drug will be prescribed cautiously and in small doses to patients with suicidal tendencies, and observe such patients—indeed *all* patients—for signs of depression.

8. Provide side rails and assistance for patients affected by ataxia, weakness, or incoordination.

9. Monitor BP before and after the patient receives an antianxiety agent by IV route. Evaluate the presence and degree of hypotensive reaction. Preferably keep the patient in a recumbent position for 2–3 hr after IV administration of drug.

10. Assess for and report early symptoms of cholestatic jaundice, such as high fever, upper abdominal pain, nausea, diarrhea, and rash, which would necessitate liver function tests.

11. Withhold the drug and report to the physician should yellowing of skin, sclera, or mucous membranes occur. (These are late signs of cholestatic jaundice indicating biliary tract obstruction.)

12. Assess and report symptoms of blood dyscrasias, such as sore throat, fever, and weakness, which necessitate withholding the drug and reevaluation of blood tests.

13. Withhold the drug and consult with physician if the patient appears overly sleepy or confused or is comatose.

14. Be prepared to assist in the treatment of overdosage. This may involve respiratory assistance, gastric lavage, and general physiologic supportive measures. During such procedures, BP, respiration, and intake–output should be carefully monitored.

15. Be prepared to assist and have drugs on hand, such as epinephrine, antihistamines, and possibly corticosteroids, for treatment of hypersensitivity reactions.

16. *Teach patient and/or family*
    a. that these drugs may reduce ability to handle potentially dangerous equipment, such as cars and other machinery.

(*continued on page 398*)

TABLE 13   BENZODIAZEPINES USED AS ANTIANXIETY AGENTS

Drug	Main Use	Dosage	Remarks
Alprazolam (Xanax) C-IV, Rx	Anxiety associated with depression	**PO: Initial,** 0.25–0.5 mg t.i.d.; **then,** titrate to needs of patient with total daily dosage not to exceed 4 mg. **In elderly or debilitated: initial,** 0.25 mg b.i.d.–t.i.d.; **then** adjust dosage to needs.	**Peak plasma levels: PO,** 8–37 ng/ml after 1–2 hr. $t\frac{1}{2}$: 12–15 hr. 80% plasma protein bound. Metabolized to alpha-hydroxyalprazolam, an active metabolite. Excreted in urine.
Chlordiazepoxide (Apo-Chlordiazepoxide,* Libritabs, Librium, Lipoxide, Medilium,* Murcil, Novopoxide,* Reposans-10, Sereen, Solium,* SK-Lygen, Trilium) C-IV, Rx	Anxiety, acute withdrawal symptoms in chronic alcoholics. Preoperatively to reduce anxiety and tension	**PO. Adults:** *Anxiety and tension* 5–10 mg t.i.d.–q.i.d. (up to 20–25 mg t.i.d.–q.i.d. in severe cases). Reduce dose to 5 mg b.i.d.–q.i.d. in geriatric or debilitated patients. **Pediatric, over 6 years: initial,** 5 mg b.i.d.–q.i.d. May be increased to 10 mg b.i.d.–t.i.d. *Preoperatively:* 5–10 mg t.i.d.–q.i.d. on day before surgery. *Alcohol withdrawal:* 50–100 mg; may be increased to 300 mg per day; **then,** reduce to maintenance levels. **IM, IV (not recommended for children under 12 years.)** *Acute/severe agitation/anxiety:* **initial,** 50–100 mg; **then,** 25–50 mg t.i.d.–q.i.d. *Preoperatively:* **IM,** 50–100 mg 1 hr before surgery. *Alcohol withdrawal:* **IM, IV,** 50–100 mg; repeat in 2–4 hr if necessary. Dos-	PO absorption is more rapid than following IM administration. **Onset: PO,** 30–60 min; **IM,** 15–30 min; **IV,** 3–30 min. **Peak plasma levels (PO):** 1–4 hr. **Duration:** $t\frac{1}{2}$: 5–30 hr. Is metabolized to two active metabolites: desmethyldiazepam and oxazepam. Chlordiazepoxide has less anticonvulsant activity and is less potent than diazepam. *Additional Untoward Reactions* Jaundice, acute hepatic necrosis, hepatic dysfunction. *Laboratory Test Interferences* 1. *Interference with test methods:* ↑ 17-Hydroxycorticosteroids, 17-Ketosteroids. 2. *Caused by pharmacologic effects:* ↑ Alkaline phosphatase, bilirubin, serum transaminase, porpholbilinogen; ↓ prothrombin time (patients on coumarin). *Administration* **IM:** Prepare solution immediately before administration by adding diluent to ampule. Shake until dissolved. Discard any unused solution. Inject slowly into upper, outer quadrant of gluteal muscle. **IV:** Prepare immediately before administration. Inject directly into vein over 1-min period. Do not add to IV infusion because of instability of drug. Do not use IV solution for IM.

Clorazepate Dipotassium (Tranxene, Tranxene-SD, Tranxene-SD Half Strength) C-IV, Rx

Anxiety, tension. Acute alcohol withdrawal, as adjunct in treatment of seizures

age should not exceed 300 mg/day.
PO. *Anxiety,* **initial,** 30 mg/day in divided doses; **maintenance:** 15–60 mg/day in divided doses. **Elderly or debilitated: initial,** 7.5–15 mg/day. **Alternative: Single daily dosage: Adults, initial,** 15 mg; **then,** 11.25–22.5 mg once daily. *Acute alcohol withdrawal: Day 1,* **initial,** 30 mg; **then,** 30–60 mg in divided doses; *Day 2,* 45–90 mg/day; *Day 3,* 22.5–45 mg/day; *Day 4,* 15–30 mg/day. Thereafter, reduce to 7.5–15 mg/day, and discontinue as soon as possible. *Anticonvulsant:* **Adults, initial,** 7.5 mg t.i.d.; increase no more than 7.5 mg/week to maximum of 90 mg/day. **Children (9–12 years): initial,** 7.5 mg b.i.d.; increase no more than 7.5 mg/week to maximum of 60 mg/day.

Peak effect: 60 min. **t½:** 30–100 hr. Clorazepate is hydrolyzed in the stomach to desmethyldiazepam, the active metabolite. The drug is slowly excreted.
Additional Contraindications
Depressive patients, nursing mothers. Give cautiously to patients with impaired renal or hepatic function.

Diazepam (Apo-Diazepam,* E-Pam,* Meval,* Novodipam,* Neo-Calme,* Rival,* Stress-Pam,* Valium,* Valrelease, Vivol*) C-IV, Rx

Anxiety, tension (more effective than chlordiazepoxide), alcohol withdrawal, muscle relaxant, anticonvulsive agent.
Used prior to gastroscopy and esophagoscopy, preoperatively and prior to

PO, *Anxiety, anticonvulsant, muscle relaxant:* 2–10 mg b.i.d.–q.i.d. *Alcohol withdrawal:* **Initial,** 10 mg t.i.d.–q.i.d. Decrease gradually to 5 mg t.i.d.–q.i.d. **Elderly, debilitated patients:** 2–

Onset: PO, 30–60 min; **IM,** 15–30 min; **IV,** more rapid. **Peak plasma levels: PO,** 1–2 hr. **Duration:** 3 hr. **t½:** 20–50 hr. Diazepam is broken down in the liver to the active metabolites desmethyldiazepam and methyloxazepam.
Additional Contraindications
Narrow-angle glaucoma, children under 6

TABLE 13 (Continued)

Drug	Main Use	Dosage	Remarks
	cardioversion. Treatment of status epilepticus. Adjunct in cerebral palsy, paraplegia, or tetanus	2.5 mg 1–2 times daily. May be gradually increased to adult level. **Pediatric over 6 months: initial,** 1–2.5 mg t.i.d.–b.i.d. **IM, IV:** same as **PO** up to maximum of 30 mg in 8 hr. *Preop or diagnostic use,* **IM:** 5–15 mg 5 to 30 minutes before procedure. **IM, IV,** *Tetanus in children,* **over 1 month:** 1–2 mg; repeated q 3–4 hr as necessary; **age 5 years and over:** 5–10 mg q 3–4 hrs. **IV,** *Status epilepticus:* **Children over 1 month** 0.2–0.5 mg q 2–5 min up to maximum of 5 mg; **children, over 5 years:** 1 mg q 2–5 min up to maximum of 10 mg. Can be repeated in 2–4 hr. IV administration should not exceed 5 mg/min. **IV,** *Cardioversion:* 5–10 min before procedure. Elderly or debilitated patients should not receive more than 5 mg parenterally at any one time.	months, and parenterally under 12 years. *Additional Drug Interactions* 1. Diazepam potentiates antihypertensive effects of thiazides and other diuretics. 2. Diazepam potentiates muscle relaxant effects of *d*-tubocurarine and gallamine. 3. Ranitidine ↓ GI absorption of diazepam. 4. Isoniazid ↑ half-life of diazepam. *Laboratory Test Interferences* ↓ Urinary homovanilic acid, gastric acid; ↑ Porphobilinogen, coproporphyrin, uroporphyrin. *Administration/Storage* Be careful not to administer intra-arterially. Do not inject through small veins. Inject IM deep into muscle. Do not mix with other injectables. Have equipment available for respiratory assistance when administering IV to children. Store protected from light.
Halazepam (Paxipam) C-IV, Rx	Short-term relief of anxiety	**PO:** individualized. **Usual:** 20–40 mg t.i.d.–q.i.d. In debilitated patients: ini-	t½ 14 hr. Metabolized in liver to the *N*-desmethyldiazepam (**maximum plasma levels:** 3–6 hr), and to inactive conjugates.

Drug	Uses	Dosage	Remarks
Lorazepam (Ativan) C-IV, Rx	Anxiety, tension, anxiety with depression, insomnia, preanesthetic. *Investigational:* Status epilepticus.	tial, 20 mg 1–2 times daily. **PO.** *Anxiety:* 2–3 mg/day in 2–3 divided doses. *Hypnotic:* 2–4 mg at bedtime. **Geriatric/debilitated patients:** 1–2 mg/day in divided doses. **IM.** *Preoperatively:* 0.05 mg/kg up to maximum of 4 mg 2 hr before surgery. **IV.** *Anxiety:* initial, 0.044 mg/kg; up to 4 mg (0.05 mg/kg) may be required in some. Dosage not established in children under 18 years of age.	*Additional Contraindication* Acute narrow-angle glaucoma. Absorbed and eliminated faster than other benzodiazepines. **Peak plasma levels: PO,** 2.5 hrs. *t½:* 10–15 hrs. Is metabolized to inactive compounds. *Additional Contraindications* Narrow-angle glaucoma. Use cautiously in presence of renal and hepatic disease. *Additional Drug Interaction* With parenteral lorazepam, scopolamine → sedation, hallucination, and behavioral abnormalities.
Oxazepam (Apo-Oxazepam,* Ox-Pam,* Serax, Zapex*) C-IV, Rx	Anxiety, tension, anxiety with depression. Adjunct in acute alcohol withdrawal.	**PO.** *Anxiety:* 10–15 mg t.i.d.–q.i.d. (up to 30 mg t.i.d.–q.i.d. in severe states). **Geriatric and debilitated patients:** 10 mg t.i.d.; can be increased to 15 mg t.i.d.–q.i.d. *Alcohol withdrawal:* 15–30 mg t.i.d.–q.i.d.	**Peak plasma levels:** 2–4 hr. *t½:* 5–13 hr. Broken down in the liver to inactive metabolites. Drug is reputed to cause less drowsiness than chlordiazepoxide. Paradoxical reactions characterized by sleep disturbances, and hyperexcitement may occur during first weeks of therapy. Hypotension has occurred with parenteral administration. Dosage not established in children under 12 years of age.
Prazepam (Centrax) C-IV, Rx	Anxiety, psychoneurosis associated with various disease states	**PO.** *Usual:* 30 mg/day in divided doses (range: 20–60 mg/day, depending on patient response). **Geriatric and debilitated: initial,** 10–15 mg daily. Dosage may be administered to all patients in a single dose at night.	**Peak plasma levels:** 6 hr. *t½:* 30–100 hr. Significant first pass effect results in biotransformation to the active metabolite desmethyldiazepam.

b. not to drink alcohol while taking antianxiety agents because the depressant effect of both the alcohol and the antianxiety agents will be potentiated.

c. to rise slowly from a supine position and to dangle feet before standing.

d. to lie down immediately if feeling faint.

e. not to suddenly stop taking drug after prolonged and excessive use. (See *Nursing Implication* 5 above.)

MEPROBAMATE AND OTHER AGENTS

CHLORMEZANONE   Trancopal (Rx)

Classification   Antianxiety agent, meprobamate-type.

Action/Kinetics   Onset: 15–30 min. **Duration:** 4–6 hr. t ½: 24 hr.

Uses   Anxiety, tension.

Untoward Reactions   *CNS:* Dizziness, drowsiness, depression, excitement, tremors, headache, confusion, weakness. *GI:* Nausea, dry mouth. *Miscellaneous:* Rash, edema, flushing, inability to void, cholestatic jaundice (rare).

Drug Interactions   Additive effects when used with other CNS depressants.

Dosage   PO. Adults: 100–200 mg t.i.d.–q.i.d.; **pediatric, 5–12 years:** 50–100 mg t.i.d.–q.i.d.

Administration

1. Initial dosage should be the lowest possible, especially in children.
2. Can be taken on an empty stomach.
3. Patients should be warned about possible interference with driving or operating machinery.

HYDROXYZINE HYDROCHLORIDE   Atarax, Multipax,* Vistaril (Rx)

HYDROXYZINE PAMOATE   Vistaril (Rx)

Classification   Antianxiety agent, miscellaneous.

Action/Kinetics   The action of hydroxyzine may be due to a depression of activity in selected important regions of the subcortical areas of the CNS. Hydroxyzine manifests anticholinergic, antiemetic, antispasmodic, local anesthetic, antihistaminic, and skeletal relaxant effects. The drug also has mild antiarrhythmic activity and mild analgesic effects. **Onset:** 15–30 min. The pamoate salt is believed to be converted to the hydrochloride in the stomach.

Uses   Tranquilizer for psychoneurosis and tension states, anxiety and agitation. Adjunct in the treatment of chronic urticaria. Control of nausea and vomiting accompanying various diseases. Preanesthetic medication. When administered IM for the control of emesis, reduce narcotic requirement during surgery or delivery. Alcohol withdrawal. Postpartum adjunctive medication.

Contraindications Pregnancy; not recommended for the treatment of morning sickness during pregnancy or as sole agent for treatment of psychoses or depression. Hypersensitivity to drug. Not to be used IV, SC, or intra-arterially.

Untoward Reactions Low incidence at recommended dosages. Drowsiness, dryness of mouth, involuntary motor activity, dizziness, urticaria, or skin reactions.

Marked discomfort, induration, and even gangrene have been reported at site of IM injection.

Drug Interactions Additive effects when used with other CNS depressants. See *Drug Interactions* for *Benzodiazepines*, p. 392.

Laboratory Test Interference Hydroxycorticosteroids.

Dosage **PO. Hydroxyzine hydrochloride** and **hydroxyzine pamoate.** *Antianxiety:* **Adults,** 25–100 mg t.i.d.–q.i.d.; **pediatric under 6 years:** 50 mg daily; **over 6 years:** 50–100 mg daily in divided doses. *Pruritus:* **Adults,** 25 mg t.i.d.–q.i.d.; **children, under 6 years:** 50 mg daily in divided doses; **children, over 6 years:** 50–100 mg/day in divided doses. *Preoperatively:* **Adults,** 50–100 mg; **children:** 0.6 mg/kg.

IM. Hydroxyzine hydrochloride. *Acute anxiety, including alcohol withdrawal:* **Initial,** 50–100 mg repeated q 4–6 hr as needed. *Nausea, vomiting, pre- and postoperative, pre- and postpartum:* **Adults,** 25–100 mg; **pediatric,** 1.1 mg/kg. Switch to **PO** as soon as possible.

Administration Inject IM only. Injection should be made into the upper, outer quadrant of the buttock or the midlateral muscles of the thigh.

In children the drug should be injected into the midlateral muscles of the thigh.

Nursing Implications
See also *Nursing Implications* for *Benzodiazepines*, p. 393.
Encourage rinsing of mouth and increased fluid intake to relieve dryness of mouth.

MEPROBAMATE Apo-Meprobamate,* Equanil, Meditran,* Mepriam, Meprospan, Miltown, Neo-Tran,* Neuramate, Neurate-400, Novomepro,* Sedabamate, SK-Bamate, Tranmep (C-IV) (Rx)

Classification Antianxiety agent.

Action/Kinetics Meprobamate is a carbamate derivative that also possesses muscle relaxant and anticonvulsant effects. It acts in the limbic system and the thalamus as well as to inhibit polysynaptic spinal reflexes. **Onset:** 1 hr. **Blood levels, chronic therapy:** 5–20 μg/ml. **t½:** 6–24 hr. Extensively metabolized in liver. Mebrobamate is also found in *Equagesic.*

Uses Short-term relief of anxiety.

Contraindications Hypersensitivity to meprobamate or carisoprodol. Porphyria. Children under 6 years of age. Use with caution in pregnancy, lactation, epilepsy, liver and kidney disease.

Untoward Reactions *CNS:* Ataxia, dizziness, headache, excitement, slurred speech, vertigo. *GI:* Nausea, vomiting, diarrhea. *Miscellaneous:* Visual disturbances, allergic reactions including hematologic and dermatologic symptoms, paresthesias.

Drug Interactions Additive depressant effects when used with CNS depressants, MAO inhibitors, and tricyclic antidepressants.

Laboratory Test Interferences *With test methods:* ↑ 17-Hydroxycorticosteroids, 17-ketogenic steroids, and 17-ketosteroids. *Pharmacologic effects:* ↑ Alkaline phosphatase, bilirubin, serum transaminase, urinary estriol (colorimetric tests), porphobilinogen. ↓ Prothrombin time in patients on coumarin.

Dosage **PO. Adults, initial,** 400 mg t.i.d.–q.i.d. May be increased, if necessary, up to maximum of 2.4 gm daily. **Pediatric over 6 years:** 100–200 mg b.i.d.–t.i.d.

Nursing Implications
See *Nursing Implications* for *Benzodiazepines*, p. 393.

Chapter Thirty-two

ANTIPSYCHOTIC AGENTS

General Statement   The advent of antipsychotic drugs was responsible for a major change in the treatment of the mentally ill. Reserpine, an alkaloid derived from *Rauwolfia serpentina,* and chlorpromazine, both of which appeared during the early 1950s, almost singlehandedly revolutionized the care of the mentally ill both inside and outside the hospital. Patients who had not been helped for decades with electroshock, insulin therapy, and/or other forms of treatment could now often be discharged.

Antipsychotic drugs do not cure mental illness, but they calm the intractable patient, relieve the despondency of the severely depressed, activate the immobile and withdrawn, and make some patients more accessible to psychotherapy.

PHENOTHIAZINES

General Statement   Most phenothiazines induce some sedation, especially during the initial phase of the treatment. Medicated patients can, however, be easily roused. In this manner, the phenothiazines differ markedly from the narcotic analgesics and sedative hypnotics. However, phenothiazines potentiate the analgesic properties of opiates and prolong the action of CNS depressant drugs.

The drugs also decrease spontaneous motor activity, as in parkinsonism, and many lower blood pressure.

According to their detailed chemical structure, the phenothiazines belong to three subgroups:

1. Dimethylaminopropyl compounds
2. Piperazine compounds
3. Piperidine compounds

Drugs belonging to the *dimethylaminopropyl subgroup,* which includes chlorpromazine, are often the first choice for patients in acute excitatory states. Drugs belonging to this subgroup cause more sedation than other phenothiazines and are especially indicated for patients exhausted by lack of sleep.

Members of the *piperazine subgroup* act most selectively on the subcortical sites. This accounts for the fact that they can be administered in relatively small doses. This in turn results in minimal drowsiness and undesirable motor effects. The piperazines also have the greatest antiemetic effects because they specifically depress the chemoreceptor trigger zone (CTZ) of the vomiting center. Members of the *piperidyl subgroup* are less toxic in terms of extrapyramidal effects. Mellaril, a member of this group, has little effectiveness as an antiemetic drug.

Action/Kinetics   It has been postulated that excess amounts of dopamine in certain areas of the CNS cause psychoses. Phenothiazines are thought to act by blocking dopamine receptors postsynaptically, leading to a reduction in psychotic symptoms. Phenothiazines are also thought to depress various portions of the reticular activating system, which accounts for their effects on regulation of body temperature, as well as on emesis, hormonal balance, vasomotor tone, wakefulness, and basal metabolic rate. These drugs also act peripherally, exerting anticholinergic and alpha-adrenergic blocking properties. Kinetic information on the phenothiazines is scarce and often unreliable. Generally, peak plasma levels occur 2–4 hr after oral administration. Phenothiazines are widely distributed throughout the body. They have an average half-life of 10–20 hr. Most are metabolized in the liver and excreted by the kidney. Studies have shown that both oral dosage forms and suppositories from different manufacturers differ in their bioavailability. It is therefore not recommended that brands not be interchanged unless data indicating bioequivalance are available.

Uses Psychoses, especially if excessive psychomotor activity manifested. Involutional, toxic, or senile psychoses. Used in combination with monoamine oxidase inhibitors in depressed patients manifesting anxiety, agitation, or panic (use with caution). With lithium in acute manic phase of manic-depressive illness. As an adjunct in alcohol withdrawal to reduce anxiety, tension, depression, nausea, and/or vomiting. For severe behavioral problems in children manifested by hyperexcitable and/or combative behavior; also, for short-term use in hyperactive children who exhibit excess motor activity and conduct disorders.

Prophylaxis and control of severe nausea and vomiting due to cancer chemotherapy, radiation, postoperatively. Intractable hiccoughs, intermittent porphyria, tetanus (as adjunct). As preoperative and/or postoperative medications. Some phenothiazines are antipruritics.

Contraindications Severe CNS depression, in coma, patients with subcortical brain damage, bone marrow depression, lactation. In patients with a history of seizures and in patients on anticonvulsant drugs. Geriatric or debilitated patients, hepatic or renal disease, cardiovascular disorders, glaucoma, prostatic hypertrophy. Contraindicated in children with chickenpox, CNS infections, measles, gastroenteritis, dehydration due to increased risk of extrapyramidal symptoms in these patients.

Phenothiazines should be used with caution in patients exposed to extreme heat or cold, and in those with asthma, emphysema, or acute respiratory tract infections. Safe use in pregnancy not established; thus use only when benefits outweigh risks.

Untoward Reactions *CNS:* Depression, drowsiness, dizziness, lethargy, fatigue. Extrapyramidial effects, Parkinson-like symptoms including shuffling gait or tic-like movements of head and face, tardive dyskinesia (see below), akathisia, dystonia. Seizures, especially in patients with a history of such. *CV:* Orthostatic hypotension, increase or decrease in blood pressure, tachycardia, fainting. *GI:* Dry mouth, anorexia, constipation, paralytic ileus, diarrhea. *Endocrine:* Breast engorgement, galactorrhea, gynecomastia, increased appetite, weight gain, hyper- or hypoglycemia, glycosuria. Delayed ejaculation, increased or decreased libido. *GU:* Menstrual irregularities, loss of bladder control, urinary difficulty. *Dermatologic:* Photosensitivty, pruritus, erythema, eczema, exfoliative dermatitis, pigment changes in skin (long-term use of high doses). *Hematologic:* Aplastic anemia, leukopenia, agranulocytosis, eosinophilia, thrombocytopenia. *Ophthalmologic:* Deposition of fine particulate matter in lens and cornea leading to blurred vision, changes in vision. *Respiratory:* Laryngospasm, bronchospasm, laryngeal edema, breathing difficulties. *Miscellaneous:* Fever, muscle stiffness, decreased sweating, muscle spasm of face, neck, or back, obstructive jaundice, nasal congestion, pale skin, mydriasis, systemic lupus-like syndrome.

Tardive dyskinesia has been observed with all classes of antipsychotic drugs although the precise cause is not known. The syndrome is most commonly seen in older patients, especially women, and in individuals with organic brain syndrome. It is often aggravated or precipitated by the sudden discontinuance of antipsychotic drugs and may persist indefinitely after the drug is discontinued. Early signs of tardive dyskinesia include fine vermicular movements of the tongue and grimacing or tic-like movements of the head and neck. Although there is no known cure for the syndrome, it may not progress if the dosage of the drug is slowly reduced. Also, a few drug-free days for the patient may unmask the symptoms of tardive dyskinesia and help in early diagnosis.

Drug Interactions

Interactant	Interaction
Alcohol, ethyl	Potentiation or addition of CNS depressant effects. Concomitant use may lead to drowsiness, lethargy, stupor, respiratory collapse, coma, or death

Interactant	Interaction
Amphetamine	↓ Effect of amphetamine by ↓ uptake of drug to the site of action
Anesthetics, general	See *Alcohol*
Antacids, oral	↓ Effect of phenothiazines due to ↓ absorption from GI tract
Antianxiety drugs	See *Alcohol*
Anticholinergic drugs	Additive anticholinergic side effects and/or ↓ antipsychotic effect.
Antidepressants, tricyclic	Additive anticholinergic side effects
Antidiabetic agents	↓ Effect of antidiabetic agents, since phenothiazines ↑ blood sugar
Bacitracin	Additive respiratory depression
Barbiturates	See *Alcohol*
Barbiturate anesthetics	↑ Chance tremor, involuntary muscle activity, and hypotension
Capreomycin	Additive respiratory depression
CNS depressants	See *Alcohol*; also, ↓ effect of phenothiazines due to ↑ breakdown by liver
Colistimethate	Additive respiratory depression
Diazoxide	Additive hyperglycemic effect
Guanethidine	↓ Effect of guanethidine by ↓ uptake of drug at the site of action
Hydantoins	↑ Risk of hydantoin toxicity
Lithium carbonate	↓ Levels of phenothiazines
Meperidine	↑ Risk of meperidine toxicity
Metoprolol	Additive hypotensive effects
MAO inhibitors	↑ Effect of phenothiazines due to ↓ breakdown by liver
Narcotics	See *Alcohol*
Phenytoin	↑ Effect of phenytoin due to ↓ breakdown by liver
Polymyxin B	Additive respiratory depression
Propranolol	Additive hypotensive effects
Quinidine	Additive cardiac depressant effect
Sedative-hypnotics, nonbarbiturate	See *Alcohol*
Succinylcholine	↑ Muscle relaxation

Laboratory Test Interference   False +: Bile (urine dipstick), ferric chloride, pregnancy tests, urinary porphobilinogen, urinary steriods, urobilinogen (urine dipstick). False −: Inorganic phosphorus, urinary steroids. *Caused by pharmacologic effects*: ↑ Alkaline phosphatase, bilirubin, serum transaminases, serum cholesterol, urinary catecholamines. ↓ Glucose tolerance, serum uric acid, 5-hydroxyindoleacetic acid, FSH, growth hormone, luteinizing hormone, vanillylmandelic acid.

Dosage   The phenothiazines are effective over a wide dosage range. Dosage is usually increased gradually to minimize side effects over a period of 7 days until the minimal effective dose is attained. Dosage is increased more gradually in elderly or debilitated patients, since they are more susceptible to the effects and side effects of drugs. After symptoms are controlled, dosage is gradually reduced to maintenance levels. It is usually desirable to keep chronically ill patients on maintenance levels indefinitely.

Medication, especially in patients on high dosages, should not be discontinued abruptly.

Administration/Storage

1. Do not interchange brands of oral dosage forms or suppositories because they differ in bioavailability.
2. When preparing or administering parenteral solutions, both nurse and patient should avoid contact of drug with skin, eyes, and clothing.
3. Dilution of commercially available injectable solutions in saline or local anesthetic and massaging injection site after administration may reduce pain of administration.
4. Do not mix in syringe with other drug.
5. Discard pink or markedly discolored solutions.
6. Store solutions in a cool place in amber-colored containers.
7. A specific rate of flow should be ordered for parenteral doses. Rate of IV administration and blood pressure should be monitored carefully.
8. Prevent extravasation of IV solution.
9. Inject deeply and slowly IM.

Nursing Implications

Note: These *Nursing Implications* apply to all antipsychotic agents except lithium.

1. *Assess*
   a. for yellow-brown skin reaction that may turn to grayish purple (usually occurs in patients on long-term therapy).
   b. for hyperthermic or hypothermic reaction, as heat-regulating mechanism may be affected by the drug. Warmth for hypothermic reactions should be provided with blankets and *not* hot water bottles or heating appliances, since the patient's sensitivity to heat is blocked and burns may occur. Excessive hyperthermia may necessitate cooling baths, but care should be taken that the patient is not chilled.
   c. for symptoms of blood dyscrasias, such as sore throat, fever, and weakness, that necessitate withholding the drug and practicing reverse isolation until blood tests are reevaluated.
   d. signs of both physical and emotional depression or excessive stimulation, as well as extrapyramidal symptoms as a change in medication or additional medication may be required.
   e. neuromuscular reactions, particularly in children with acute infections or dehydration, as they are more susceptible to adverse effects.
   f. intake and output and observe for abdominal distention, as patient may fail to report urinary retention and constipation.
      (1) Report urinary retention, as this condition may require reduced dosage, antispasmodics, or change of drug.
      (2) Report constipation, as this condition may require increased roughage in diet, more fluids, and laxatives.
   g. for visual difficulties and check that periodic ocular examinations are completed.
   h. changes in carbohydrate metabolism, such as glycosuria, weight loss, po-

lyphagia, increased appetite, or excessive weight gain, that may necessitate dietary or medication changes.

i. menstrual irregularities, breast engorgement, lactation, increased libido in women, and decreased libido in men since these symptoms may be frightening to the patient and a change of medication may be necessitated. The patient should be reassured that these changes are drug induced and will be relieved by medication adjustment.

j. symptoms of hypersensitivity, such as fever, asthma, laryngeal edema, angioneurotic edema, and anaphylactoid reaction. Be prepared with epinephrine, steroids, antihistamines, and oxygen.

k. early symptoms of cholestatic juandice, such as high fever, upper abdominal pain, nausea, diarrhea, and rash, that would necessitate liver function tests.

2. Remain with patient until medication is swallowed, to prevent hoarding or omission of medication.

3. Take a base line reading of BP and pulse before IV administration.

4. Keep the patient recumbent for at least 1 hr after IV administration and monitor BP closely for hypotensive reaction. After 1 hr, slowly elevate the patient and observe for tachycardia, fainting, or dizziness. Side rails are an advisable precaution.

5. Withhold drug and report to physician should signs of cholestatic jaundice occur indicating bile tract obstruction, including yellowing of skin, sclera, or mucous membranes.

6. Anticipate that barbiturates (to relieve anxiety) will be reduced in dosage when given with phenothiazines but that barbiturates used as anticonvulsants will not be reduced in dosage.

7. Consider that the antiemetic effect of phenothiazines may be masking other pathology such as toxicity to other drugs, intestinal obstruction, or brain lesions.

8. *Teach patient and/or family*

a. that when dizzy or faint, to sit down or preferably lie down with feet elevated.

b. to prevent exposure to excessive sunlight.

c. not to drive a car or operate machinery requiring mental alertness for at least 2 weeks after therapy has begun, and then only after consulting physician, who will evaluate response to therapy.

d. to rinse mouth with water and to increase fluid intake to relieve excessive dryness of mouth.

e. not to stop high doses of phenothiazines abruptly, since this could cause nausea, vomiting, tremors, feelings of warmth and cold, sweating, tachycardia, headache, and insomnia.

f. to breathe deeply in presence of respiratory failure, because drug might depress cough reflex.

g. that drug may turn urine pink or reddish-brown.

h. the necessity to continue taking medication after discharge. Emphasize the need to return for follow-up care to avoid the revolving door syndrome.

ACETOPHENAZINE MALEATE   Tindal (Rx)

Classification   Antipsychotic, piperazine-type phenothiazine.

Action/Kinetics Acetophenazine manifests moderate sedation but a high incidence of extrapyramidal effects. It also produces a low incidence of orthostatic hypotension and anticholinergic effects.

Dosage **PO, adults, usual**: 20 mg t.i.d. (range: 40–80 mg daily in divided doses); 80–120 mg daily in divided doses for hospitalized schizophrenic patients (doses as high as 400–600 mg/day may be needed in severe schizophrenia).

Additional Nursing Implication

See also *Nursing Implications*, p. 404.
Administer 1 hr before bedtime to patient who has difficulty sleeping.

CHLORPROMAZINE   (Rx)

CHLORPROMAZINE HYDROCHLORIDE   Baychlor, Chlorazine, Chlorpromanyl,* Largactil,* Novochlorpromazine,* Ormazine, Promapar, Promaz, Thorazine, Thor-Prom (Rx)

Classification Antipsychotic, dimethylamino-type phenothiazine.

Action/Kinetics **Peak plasma levels**: 2–3 hr after both PO and IM administration. t½ (after IV, IM): **initial**, 4–5 hr; **final**: 3–40 hr. Chlorpromazine is extensively metabolized in the intestinal wall and liver; certain of the metabolites are active. **Steady-state plasma levels** (in psychotics): 10–1,300 ng/ml. After 2–3 weeks of therapy, plasma levels decline, possibly because of reduction in drug absorption and/or increase in drug metabolism.

Uses Acute and chronic psychoses, including schizophrenia; manic phase of manic-depressive illness. Acute intermittent porphyria. Preanesthetic, adjunct to treat tetanus, intractable hiccoughs, severe behavioral problems in children, neuroses, nausea and vomiting. Anesthetic.

Dosage **Adults.** *Psychiatry*: *Severe symptoms*, **IM**, 25 mg repeated in 1 hr. Then switch to **PO** therapy. **PO: initial**, 10 mg t.i.d.–q.i.d. or 25 mg b.i.d.–t.i.d.; **then**, may be increased by 20–50 mg twice weekly until improvement noted (dosage of 200–800 mg/day in some patients). *Nausea and vomiting*: **IM**, 25 mg **initially; then**, 25–50 mg q 3–4 hr if no hypotension occurs. **PO**, 10–25 mg q 4–6 hr. **Rectal**, 50–100 mg q 6–8 hr. *Preoperatively*: **PO**, 25–50 mg 2–3 hr before surgery or 12.5–25 mg **IM** 1–2 hr before surgery. *To control nausea/vomiting during surgery*: **IM**, 12.5 mg repeated in 30 min if necessary; **IV**, 2 mg at 2 min intervals not to exceed 25 mg (dilute with saline to 1 mg/ml). *Postoperative*: **PO**, 10–25 mg q 4–6 hr; **IM**, 12.5–25 mg q.i.d. *Hiccoughs*: **PO**, 25–50 mg t.i.d.–q.i.d.; if symptoms persist, after 2–3 days, **IM**, 25–50 mg; or, **slow IV infusion**, 25–50 mg in 500–1,000 ml saline. *Tetanus*: **IM**, 25–50 mg t.i.d.–q.i.d. with a barbiturate; **IV**, 25–50 mg (give 1 mg/ml at a rate of 1 mg/min). *Acute intermittent porphyria*: **PO**, 25–50 mg or **IM**, 25 mg both t.i.d.–q.i.d.

  Children. *Nausea, vomiting, psychiatry*: **PO, IM, rectal**, 0.55–1.1 mg/kg q 4–8 hr as needed; **maximum IM dose: up to 5 years**, 40 mg/day; **5–12 years**: 75 mg/day. **Not used in children less than 6 months of age.** *Preoperatively*: **PO**, 0.55 mg/kg 2–3 hr before surgery or **IM**, 0.55 mg/kg 1–2 hr before surgery. *To control nausea and vomiting during surgery*: **IM**, 0.25 mg/kg repeated in 30 min if necessary; **IV**, 1 mg administered at 2-min intervals. *Postoperatively*: **PO, IM**,

0.55 mg/kg. *Tetanus*: **IM, IV,** 0.55 mg/kg q 6–8 hr. **For IV,** dilute to 1 mg/ml and give at rate of 1 mg/2 min. Do not exceed 50 mg/day in children up to 50 lb; 75 mg/day in children 50–100 lb. *Schizophrenia, hospitalized patients:* **PO,** up to 50–100 mg daily (in some cases 500 mg/day); **IM, up to 5 years:** not to exceed 40 mg/day; **5–12 years:** not to exceed 75 mg/day.

FLUPHENAZINE DECANOATE   Prolixin Decanoate, Modecate* (Rx)

FLUPHENAZINE ENANTHATE   Prolixin Enanthate, Moditen Enanthate* (Rx)

FLUPHENAZINE HYDROCHLORIDE   Permitil, Prolixin, Moditen Hydrochloride* (Rx)

Classification   Antipsychotic, piperazine-type phenothiazine.

Action/Kinetics   Fluphenazine is accompanied by a high incidence of extrapyramidal symptoms and a low incidence of sedation, anticholinergic effects, and orthostatic hypotension. The enanthate and decanoate esters dramatically increase the duration of action. *Decanoate*: **Onset,** 24–72 hr; **peak plasma levels,** 12 hr; **t½** (approximate), 6.8–9.6 days; **duration:** up to 4 weeks. *Enanthate*: **Onset,** 24–72 hr; **peak plasma levels,** 48 hr; **t½** (approximate): 3.6 days; **duration:** 1–3 weeks.

Fluphenazine hydrochloride can be cautiously administered to patients with known hypersentivity to other phenothiazines. Fluphenazine enanthate may replace fluphenazine hydrochloride if desired response occurs with hypersensitivity reaction to fluphenazine.

Additional Uses   Chronic schizophrenia.

Dosage   *Individualized.* Fluphenazine hydrochloride is administered **PO and IM.** Fluphenazine enanthate or decanoate are administered **SC and IM.** *Hydrochloride.* **PO: initial,** 0.5–10 mg/day in divided doses q 6–8 hr; **then,** reduce gradually to maintenance of 1–5 mg/day (usually give as a single dose not to exceed 20 mg/day). *Geriatric patients:* **initial,** 1–2.5 mg/day; **then,** dosage determined by response. **IM: initial,** 1.25 mg; **then,** 2.5–10 mg/day in divided doses q 6–8 hr (do not exceed 10 mg/day). *Enanthate and decanoate.* **IM, SC, initial,** 12.5–25 mg. Subsequent doses determined by patient response, but should not exceed 100 mg.

Administration/Storage
1. Protect all forms of medication from light.
2. Store at room temperature and avoid freezing.
3. Color of parenteral solution may vary from colorless to light amber. Do not use solutions that are darker than light amber.

MESORIDAZINE BESYLATE   Serentil (Rx)

Classification   Antipsychotic, piperidine-type phenothiazine.

Action/Kinetics   Mesoridazine has pronounced sedative effects, moderate anticholinergic and orthostatic hypotensive effects, and a low incidence of extrapyramidal symptoms.

Uses Schizophrenia, acute and chronic alcoholism, behavior problems in patients with mental deficiency and chronic brain syndrome, psychoneurosis.

Dosage **PO**, *Schizophrenia*: **initial**, 50 mg t.i.d.; **optimum total dose**: 100–400 mg/day. *Alcoholism*: **initial**, 25 mg b.i.d.; **optimum total dose**: 50–200 mg/day. *Behavior problems*: **initial**, 25 mg t.i.d.; **optimum total dose**: 75–300 mg/day. *Psychoneurosis*: **initial**, 10 mg t.i.d.; **optimum total dose**: 30–150 mg. Total dosage is administered in 2 to 3 divided doses. **IM: initial**, 25 mg. Can be repeated, if necessary, after 30–60 min. **Optimum IM daily dose**: 25–200 mg.

Administration

1. Maintain patient supine for minimum of 30 minutes after parenteral administration to minimize orthostatic effect.
2. Acidified tap or distilled water, orange juice, or grape juice may be used to dilute the concentrate prior to use.

PERPHENAZINE   Apo-Perphenazine,* Phenazine,* Trilafon (Rx)

Classification Antipsychotic, antiemetic, piperazine-type phenothiazine.

Action/Kinetics Use accompanied by a high incidence of extrapyramidal effects, moderate anticholinergic effects, and a low incidence of orthostatic hypotension and sedation. Perphenazine is also found in Triavil (see Appendix 3).

Action/Kinetics Resembles chlorpromazine.

Dosage *Psychoses*: **PO, IM, IV**, 4–16 mg b.i.d.–q.i.d., depending on the severity of the condition. *Severe nausea and vomiting*: **PO**, 8–16 mg/day in divided doses; **IM**, 5 mg (up to 10 mg may be required in some). IV administration is seldom necessary and should be used with caution. Children over 12 years of age may receive the lowest adult dose.

Administration/Storage

1. Each 5.0 ml oral concentrate should be diluted with 60 ml diluent, such as water, milk, carbonated beverage, or orange juice.
2. Do not mix with tea, coffee, cola, grape juice, or apple juice.
3. Protect from light.
4. Store solutions in amber-colored containers.

PROCHLORPERAZINE   Compazine, Stemetil* (Rx)

PROCHLORPERAZINE EDISYLATE   Compazine Edisylate (Rx)

PROCHLORPERAZINE MALEATE   Chlorazine, Compazine Maleate (Rx)

Classification Antipsychotic, antiemetic, piperazine-type phenothiazine.

Action/Kinetics Prochlorperazine causes a high incidence of extrapyramidal effects, a moderate sedation, and a low incidence of anticholinergic effects and orthostatic hypotension. It also possesses significant antiemetic effects. Prochlorperazine is also a component of Combid (see Appendix 3).

Additional Uses Psychoneuroses. Severe nausea and vomiting.

Dosage **Adults.** *Severe nausea and vomiting*: **PO**: 5–10 mg t.i.d.–q.i.d. or 10 mg sustained release q 12 hr. **IM: initial**, 5–10 mg; repeat if necessary q 3–4 hr (total IM dose should not exceed 40 mg/day). **Rectal**: 25 mg suppository b.i.d. *To control nausea during surgery*: **IM**, 5–10 mg; **IV injection**, 5–10 mg 15–30 min before anesthesia; **IV infusion**, 20 mg/liter and add to infusion 15–30 min before anesthesia. *Excessive anxiety/psychoses*: **PO, initial**, 5–10 mg t.i.d.–q.i.d.; then, increase gradually to maintenance of 50–75 mg/day (up to 150 mg/day in some). **IM**: 10–20 mg q 2–4 hr until patient under control. For prolonged use, 10–20 mg q 4–6 hr.

    Children. *Nausea and vomiting*. **PO, Rectal: 20–29 lb**, 2.5 mg 1–2 times/day not to exceed 7.5 mg/day; **30–39 lb**, 2.5 mg b.i.d.–t.i.d. not to exceed 10 mg/day; **40–85 lb**: 2.5 mg t.i.d., not to exceed 15 mg/day. **IM**: 0.13 mg/kg. Therapy for more than 1 day not usually necessary. *Psychiatry*. **PO, rectal: 2–12 years**, 2.5 mg b.i.d.–t.i.d. (**ages 2–5**: not to exceed 20 mg/day; **ages 6–12**: not to exceed 25 mg/day). **IM, up to 12 years**: 0.13 mg/kg; switch to PO therapy after control reached. **Not recommended for children under 2 years of age or under 20 lb.**

Administration/Storage

1. Store all forms of drug in tight-closing amber-colored bottles, the suppositories below 37°C.
2. Add the desired dosage of concentrate to 60 ml of beverage (e.g., tomato or fruit juice, milk, soup) or semisolid food just before administration to disguise the taste.

Additional Nursing Implications

See also *Nursing Implications*, p. 404.

1. Advise parents not to exceed prescribed dose and to withhold drug if child reacts with signs of restlessness and excitement.
2. If the patient received spansule, continue treatment of overdosage until all signs of latter have worn off.
3. In treatment of overdosage, anticipate that saline cathartics may be used to hasten evacuation of pellets that have not already released their medication.

PROMAZINE HYDROCHLORIDE   Prozine, Sparine (Rx)

Classification Antipsychotic, dimethylaminopropyl-type phenothiazine.

Action/Kinetics The use of promazine is accompanied by significant anticholinergic side effects and moderate sedation, extrapyramidal symptoms, and orthostatic hypotension. This drug is ineffective in reducing destructive behavior in acutely agitated psychotic patients.

Uses See general information.

Dosage **PO, IV, IM**: Oral or IM route preferred. *Severe and moderate agitation*: **initial, IM**: 50–150 mg; **then, PO**: 10–200 mg q 4–6 hr. **Total daily dose should not exceed 1,000 mg. Children over 12 years**: 10–25 mg q 4–6 hr for chronic psychotic disorders.

Administration
1. Dilute concentrate as directed on bottle. Taste can be disguised with citrus fruit juice, milk, or flavored drinks.
2. IM injections should be given in the gluteal region.

THIORIDAZINE HYDROCHLORIDE Apo-Thioridazine,* Mellaril, Mellaril-S, Millazine, Novoridazine,* PMS Thioridazine* (Rx)

Classification Antipsychotic, piperidine-type phenothiazine.

Action/Kinetics The use of thioridazine is accompanied by a high incidence of anticholinergic, sedative, and orthostatic hypotensive effects and a low incidence of extrapyramidal effects. Thioridazine can often be used for patients intolerant to other phenothiazines. It has little or no antiemetic effects.

Peak plasma levels (after PO): 1–4 hr. Thioridazine may impair its own absorption at higher doses due to the strong anticholinergic effects. **t½:** 10 hr. Metabolized in the liver to both active and inactive metabolites.

Uses Acute and chronic schizophrenia; moderate to marked depression with anxiety; sleep disturbances. *In children*: treatment of hyperactivity in the retarded and behavior problems. Geriatric patients with organic brain syndrome. Alcohol withdrawal. Intractable pain.

Dosage **PO**. Highly individualized. *Neurosis, anxiety states, alcohol withdrawal, senility*, **range**: 20–200 mg daily; **initial**: 25 mg t.i.d. **Maintenance**, mild cases: 10 mg b.i.d.–q.i.d.; severe cases: 50 mg t.i.d.–q.i.d. *Psychotic, severely disturbed hospitalized patients* **initial**: 50–100 mg t.i.d. If necessary increase to maximum of 200 mg q.i.d. When control is achieved, reduce gradually to minimum effective dosage. **Pediatric above 2 years**: 0.5–3.0 mg/kg daily. *Hospitalized psychotic children*, **initial**: 25 mg b.i.d.–t.i.d. Increase gradually if necessary. **Not recommended for children under 2 years of age**.

Administration/Storage Dilute each dose just before administration with distilled water, acidified tap water, or suitable juices. Preparation and storage of bulk dilutions is not recommended.

TRIFLUOPERAZINE Apo-Trifluoperazine,* Novoflurazine,* Solazine,* Stelazine, Suprazine, Terfluzine* (Rx)

Classification Antipsychotic, antiemetic, piperazine-type phenothiazine.

Action/Kinetics Trifluoperazine is accompanied by a high incidence of extrapyramidal symptoms, and a low incidence of sedation, orthostatic hypotension, and anticholinergic side effects. It is an effective antiemetic. Recommended only for hospitalized or well-supervised patients. **Maximum therapeutic effect**: Usually 2–3 weeks after initiation of therapy.

Uses Schizophrenia. Suitable for patients with apathy or withdrawal. Anxiety, tension, agitation in neuroses.

Dosage *Hospitalized patients*, **PO: initial**, 2–5 mg b.i.d.–t.i.d.; **maintenance**: 15–20 mg daily in 2 or 3 divided doses. *Outpatients*, **PO**: 1–2 mg daily, up to 4 mg daily. *Severe symptoms,* **IM**: 1–2 mg q 4–6 hr. May be increased to 6–10 mg daily. **Pediatric 6–12 years: PO**: 1–2 mg daily. Increase gradually to maintenance levels, which rarely exceed 15 mg daily. IM (only if absolutely necessary): 1 mg 1–2 times/day. Dose may have to be reduced in elderly patients.

Administration/Storage
1. Dilute concentrate with 60 ml of suitable beverage (e.g., tomato or fruit juice, milk) or semisolid food.
2. Dilute just before administration.
3. Protect liquid forms from light.
4. Discard strongly colored solutions.
5. Avoid skin contact with liquid form to prevent contact dermatitis.

TRIFLUPROMAZINE HYDROCHLORIDE   Vesprin (Rx)

Classification   Antipsychotic, dimethylaminopropyl-type phenothiazine.

Action/Kinetics   This drug produces significant sedative and anticholinergic effects but minimal extrapyramidal symptoms and orthostatic hypotension.

Additional Uses   Severe nausea and vomiting. Should not be used for psychotic disorders with depression.

Dosage   *Psychoses*. **Adults, IM**: 60 mg up to maximum of 150 mg/day. **Pediatric: IM**, 0.2–0.25 mg/kg to maximum of 10 mg/day (not to be used in children under 2½ years of age). *Nausea and vomiting*. **Adults: IM**, 5–15 mg as single dose repeated q 4 hr to maximum of 60 mg/day (for elderly or debilitated: 2.5 mg up to maximum of 15 mg/day); **IV**, 1 mg up to maximum of 3 mg/day. **Children: IM**: 0.2–0.25 mg/kg up to maximum of 10 mg/day. IV use not recommended for children. **Not to be used in children less than 2½ years of age**.

Administration/Storage
1. Avoid excessive heat and freezing.
2. Store in amber-colored containers.
3. Do not use discolored (darker than light amber) solutions.
4. Avoid skin contact with liquid form to prevent contact dermatitis.

THIOXANTHENE AND BUTYROPHENONE DERIVATIVES

General Statement   Drugs belonging to two other chemical families—the thioxanthene derivatives and the butyrophenone derivatives—are used as antipsychotic agents. The thioxanthene derivatives, chlorprothixene and thiothixene, are closely related to the phenothiazines from a chemical, pharmacologic, and clinical point of view.

Although the butyrophenone derivatives (haloperidol and droperidol) differ chemically from the phenothiazines, they are closely related in their pharmacologic actions.

For all general information pertaining to these agents, see the Phenothiazines, p. 401.

THIOXANTHENE DERIVATIVES

CHLORPROTHIXENE   Taractan (Rx)

Classification   Antipsychotic, thioxanthine derivative.

Action/Kinetics   Chlorprothixene causes significant sedation and orthostatic hypotension, with moderate anticholinergic and extrapyramidal effects. It has antiemetic properties. It is a more potent inhibitor of postural reflexes and motor coordination than is chlorpromazine, but has less pronounced antihistaminic effects. **Onset: IM**, 30 min.

Uses   Neurosis, depression, schizophrenia, antiemesis, alcohol withdrawal. Adjunct in electroshock therapy. Drug may be effective in patients resistant to other psychotherapeutic drugs.

Untoward Reactions   Drowsiness, lethargy, orthostatic hypotension, tachycardia, dizziness, and dry mouth occur especially frequently.

Drug Interactions   May cause additive hypotensive effects with methyldopa or reserpine.

Dosage   **IM, adults and children over 12 years**: 25–50 mg t.i.d.–q.i.d. Doses exceeding 600 mg/day are rarely needed. Switch to oral when feasible. **PO** same as **IM. Pediatric, children 6–12 years: PO,** 10–25 mg t.i.d.–q.i.d. Dosage should be reduced in elderly patients.

Administration/Storage

1. Inject deeply into large muscle mass.
2. Patient should be supine during administration because of postural hypotension.
3. Protect from light.

THIOTHIXENE   Navane (Rx)

Classification   Antipsychotic, thioxanthine derivative.

Action/Kinetics   Thiothixene causes significant extrapyramidal symptoms, minimal sedation, orthostatic hypotension, and anticholinergic effects. It has antiemetic properties. Its actions closely resemble those of chlorprothixene with respect to postural reflexes and motor coordination. The margin between a therapeutically effective dose and one that causes extrapyramidal symptoms is narrow.

   Peak plasma levels, PO: 1–3 hr. t½: 34 hr. **Therapeutic plasma levels** (during chronic treatment): 10–150 ng/ml.

Uses   Symptomatic treatment of acute and chronic schizophrenia, especially when condition is accompanied by florid symptoms.

Contraindication   Children under 12 years of age.

Drug Interactions   See Chlorprothixene, above.

Dosage   **PO. Adults: initial,** 2 mg t.i.d.; can be increased gradually to usual maintenance of 20–30 mg/day, although some patients require 60 mg/day. **IM. Adults**: 4 mg b.i.d.–q.i.d.; **usual maintenance**: 16–20 mg/day, although up to 30 mg/day may be required in some cases. Switch to **PO** form as soon as possible. **Not recommended for children under 12 years of age.**

BUTYROPHENONE DERIVATIVES

DROPERIDOL   Inapsine (Rx)

Classification   Antipsychotic, butyrophenone; antianxiety agent.

Action/Kinetics   Droperidol causes sedation, alpha-adrenergic blockade, peripheral vascular dilation, and has antiemetic properties. For other details, see Haloperidol and Phenothiazines, below and p. 401, respectively. **Onset** (after IM, IV): 3–10 min. **Peak effect**: 30 min. **Duration**: 2–4 hr, although alteration of consciousness may last up to 12 hr.

Uses   Preoperatively; induction and maintenance of anesthesia. To relieve nausea and vomiting and reduce anxiety in diagnostic procedures or surgery. Antiemetic in cancer chemotherapy (used IV).

Drug Interactions

Interactant	Interaction
Anesthetics, conduction (e.g., spinal)	Peripheral vasodilation and hypotension
CNS depressants	Additive or potentiating effects
Narcotic analgesics	↑ Respiratory depressant effects

Dosage   *Preoperatively*. **Adults: IM**, 2.5–10 mg 30–60 min before surgery (modify dosage in elderly, debilitated); **pediatric, 2–12 years**, 88–165 µg/kg. *Adjunct to general anesthesia*: **Adults, IV**, 0.28 mg/kg with analgesic or anesthetic; **maintenance**: 1.25–2.5 mg (total dose). *Diagnostic procedures*: **Adults, IM**, 2.5–10 mg 30–60 min before procedure; **then**, if necessary, **IV**, 1.25–2.5 mg. *Adjunct to regional anesthesia*: **IM or IV (slow)**, 2.5–5 mg.

Additional Nursing Implications

1. See also *Nursing Implications* for *Phenothiazines*, p. 404.
2. Monitor BP and pulse closely during the immediate postoperative period until stabilized at satisfactory levels.

HALOPERIDOL   Apo-Haloperidol,* Haldol, Novoperidol,* Peridol* (Rx)

Classification   Antipsychotic, butyrophenone.

Action/Kinetics   Haloperidol causes significant extrapyramidal effects, as well as a low incidence of sedation, anticholinergic effects, and orthostatic hypotension. The margin between the therapeutically effective dose and that causing extrapyramidal symptoms is narrow. The drug also has antiemetic effects. **Peak plasma levels: PO**, 2–6 hr; **IM**, 20 min. **Therapeutic serum levels**: 3–10 ng/ml. **t½**: 12–38 hr. **Plasma protein binding**: 90%. Metabolized in liver, slowly excreted in urine and bile.

Uses   Tics and vocal utterances associated with Gilles de la Tourette's disease. Acute and chronic psychoses including schizophrenia, the manic phase of manic-depressive psychosis, and psychotic reactions in adults with brain damage and mental retardation. Severe behavioral problems in children. *Investigational*: Antiemetic in low dosage.

Contraindications Use with extreme caution, or not at all, in patients with parkinsonism.

Untoward Reactions Extrapyramidal symptoms, especially akathisia and dystonias, occur more frequently than with the phenothiazines. Overdosage is characterized by severe extrapyramidal reactions, hypotension or sedation. The drug does not elicit photosensitivity reactions like the phenothiazines.

Drug Interactions

Interactant	Interaction
Amphetamine	↓ Effect of amphetamine by ↓ uptake of drug at its site of action
Anticholinergics	↓ Effect of haloperidol
Antidepressants, tricyclic	↑ Effect antidepressant due to ↓ breakdown by liver
Barbiturates	↓ Effect of haloperidol due to ↑ breakdown by liver
Guanethidine	↓ Effect of guanethidine by ↓ uptake of drug at site of action
Lithium	Lithium increases toxicity of haloperidol
Methyldopa	Methyldopa increases toxicity of haloperidol
Phenytoin	↓ Effect of haloperidol due to ↑ breakdown by liver

Laboratory Test Interferences ↑Alkaline phosphatase, bilirubin, serum transaminase; ↓ prothrombin time (patients on coumarin), serum cholesterol.

Dosage **Adults: PO, Initial**: 0.5–2 mg b.i.d.–t.i.d. up to 3–5 mg b.i.d.–t.i.d. for severe symptoms; **maintenance**, reduce dosage to lowest effective level. Up to 100 mg/day may be required in some. Dosage should be reduced in geriatric or debilitated patients. **IM**: 2–5 mg (up to 10–30 mg may be required); may be repeated if necessary q 4–8 hr. Switch to **PO** therapy as soon as possible.

   Children, 3–12 years (or 15–40 kg): PO, initial, 0.5 mg/day; dose may be increased by 0.5 mg every 5 to 7 days until therapeutic response achieved. Total dose *for psychoses*, 0.05–0.15 mg/kg/day; *for nonpsychotic behavior or Tourette's disease*: 0.05–0.075 mg/kg/day. The total dose may be given in divided doses 2 to 3 times daily. The drug is not intended for children under 3 years, and doses higher than 6 mg/day do not enhance therapeutic effects.

MISCELLANEOUS ANTIPSYCHOTIC AGENTS

LITHIUM CARBONATE Eskalith, Lithane, Lithizine,* Lithobid, Lithonate, Lithotabs (Rx)

LITHIUM CITRATE Cibalith-S, Eskalith CR (Rx)

Classification Antipsychotic agent, miscellaneous.

General Statement To prevent toxic serum levels from occurring, blood levels should be determined 1 to 2 times per week during initiation of therapy, and monthly thereafter, on blood samples taken 8 to 12 hours after dosage. Full beneficial effects of lithium therapy may not be noted for 6 to 10 days after initiation. To reduce the danger of lithium intoxication, sodium intake must remain at normal levels.

Action/Kinetics Currently believed to normalize receptor site sensitivity in CNS of manic-depressive patients, reducing characteristic "highs" and "lows" of disease. **Peak serum levels** (regular release): 1–2 hr; (slow-release): 4–6 hr. **Therapeutic serum levels**: 0.6–1.4 mEq/liter (must be carefully monitored as toxic effects may occur at these levels and significant toxic reactions occur at serum lithium levels of 2 mEq/liter. **t½** (plasma): 24 hr (longer in presence of renal impairment and in the elderly).

Uses Control of manic episodes in manic-depressive patients. Prophylaxis. *Investigational*: To reverse neutropenia induced by cancer chemotherapy and in children with chronic neutropenia. Prophylaxis of cluster headaches and cyclic migraine headaches.

Contraindications Cardiovascular or renal disease. Brain damage. Patients receiving diuretics. Pregnancy, lactation.

Untoward Reactions These are related to the blood lithium level. *CNS:* Fainting, drowsiness, slurred speech, confusion, dizziness, tiredness, lethargy, ataxia, dysarthria, aphasia, vertigo, stupor, restlessness, coma, seizures. *GI:* Anorexia, nausea, vomiting, diarrhea, thirst, dry mouth, bloated stomach. *Muscular:* Tremors (especially of hand), muscle weakness, fasciculations, and/or twitching, clonic movements of limbs, increased deep tendon reflexes, choreoathetoid movements, cogwheel rigidity. *Renal:* Nephrogenic diabetes insipidus (polyuria, polydypsia). *Endocrine:* Hypothyroidism, goiter, hyperparathyroidism. *CV:* Changes in ECG, edema, hypotension, cardiovascular collapse, irregular pulse, tachycardia. *Dermatologic:* Acneform eruptions, pruritic-maculopapular rashes, drying and thinning of hair, alopecia, paresthesia, cutaneous ulcers, lupus-like symptoms. *Miscellaneous:* Hoarseness, swelling of feet, lower legs, or neck, cold sensitivity, leukemia, leukocytosis, dyspnea on exertion.

Drug Interactions

Interactant	Interaction
Acetazolamide	↓ Lithium effect by ↑ renal excretion
Aminophylline	↓ Lithium effect by ↑ renal excretion
Diazepam	↑ Risk of hypothermia
Bumetanide	
Ethacrynic acid }	↑ Lithium toxicity due to ↓ renal clearance
Furosemide	
Haloperidol	↑ Risk of neurologic toxicity
Indomethacin	↑ Chance of lithium toxicity due to ↓ renal clearance
Iodide salts	↑ Chance of hypothyroidism
Mannitol	↓ Lithium effect by ↑ renal excretion
Methyldopa	↑ Chance of lithium toxicity
Neuromuscular blocking agents	Lithium ↑ effect of these agents
Phenothiazines	↓ Levels of phenothiazines and ↑ neurotoxicity
Phenytoin	↑ Chance lithium toxicity
Piroxicam	↑ Chance of lithium toxicity due to ↓ renal clearance
Sodium bicarbonate	↓ Lithium effect by ↑ renal excretion
Sodium chloride	Excretion of lithium is proportional to amount of sodium chloride ingested; if patient on salt-free

Interactant	Interaction
	diet, may develop lithium toxicity since less lithium excreted
Succinylcholine	↑ Muscle relaxation
Theophyllines	↓ Effect of lithium due to ↑ renal excretion
Thiazide diuretics ⎫ Triamterene ⎬	↑ Chance of lithium toxicity due to ↓ renal clearance
Urea	↓ Lithium effect by ↑ renal excretion

Laboratory Test Interferences False + urinary glucose test (Benedict's), ↑ serum glucose, creatinine kinase. False − or ↓ serum protein bound iodine (PBI), uric acid; ↑ TSH; ↓ thyroxine.

Dosage **PO**. *Acute mania*: Individualized and according to lithium serum level (not to exceed 1.4 mEq/liter) and clinical response. *Usual*, **initial**: 600 mg t.i.d. or 900 mg b.i.d. of slow release form; **elderly and debilitated patients**: 0.6–1.2 gm daily in 3 doses. **Maintenance**: 300 mg t.i.d. - q.i.d.

Administration of drug is discontinued when lithium serum level exceeds 1.2 mEq/liter and resumed 24 hr after it has fallen below that level. *To reverse neutropenia*: 300–1,000 mg/day (to achieve serum levels between 0.5–1.0 mEq/liter) for 7–10 days. *Prophylaxis of cluster headaches*: 600–900 mg/day.

Administration

1. Due to drowsiness, patients should exercise caution when driving or operating machinery.
2. Advise patient to drink 10–12 glasses of water each day and to avoid dehydration (e.g., sunbathing, sauna).
3. The drug may be taken with food.

Nursing Implications

1. Be prepared to assist with gastric suction, parenteral administration of fluids and electrolytes to promote lithium excretion in case of toxicity.
2. *Teach patient and/or family*
   a. that blood tests to check lithium levels (therapeutic serum concentrations usually 0.6–1.2 mEq/liter) must be completed at least once weekly.
   b. that if diarrhea, vomiting, drowsiness, muscular weakness, and lack of coordination occur, lithium therapy must be immediately discontinued, and patient must report to medical supervision.
   c. not to engage in physical activities that require alertness or physical coordination because these may be impaired while on therapy.
   d. to eat a diet containing normal amounts of salt.
   e. to maintain a fluid intake of 2.5–3 liters a day.
   f. to report excessive sweating or diarrhea because this may indicate need for supplemental fluids or salt.

LOXAPINE SUCCINATE   Daxolin, Daxolin C, Loxapac,* Loxitane, Loxitane C, Loxitane IM (Rx)

Classification Antipsychotic, miscellaneous.

Action/Kinetics Loxapine belongs to a new subclass of tricyclic antipsychotic agents. It causes significant extrapyramidal symptoms, moderate sedative effects, and a low incidence of anticholinergic effects, as well as orthostatic hypotension. **Onset**: 20–30 min. **Peak effects**: 1.5–3 hr. **Duration**: about 12 hr. **t½**: 6–8 hr. Partially metabolized in the liver; excreted in urine, and unchanged in feces.

Use Schizophrenia.

Additional Contraindications History of convulsive disorders. Use with caution in patients with cardiovascular disease.

Additional Untoward Reactions Tachycardia, hypertension, hypotension, lightheadedness, and syncope.

Dosage **PO**, *individualized*: **initial**, 10 mg b.i.d. *Severe*: up to 50 mg daily. Increase dosage rapidly during 7 to 10 days until symptoms are controlled. **Range**: 60–100 mg up to 250 mg daily. **Maintenance**: If possible reduce dosage to 20–60 mg daily. Divide all daily dosages into 2 to 4 doses. **IM**: 12.5–50 mg q 4–6 hr; once adequate control has been established, switch to PO medication.

Administration

1. Measure the dosage of the concentrate *only* with the enclosed calibrated dropper.
2. Mix oral concentrate with orange or grapefruit juice immediately before administration, to disguise unpleasant taste.

MOLINDONE Moban (Rx)

Classification Antipsychotic, miscellaneous.

Action/Kinetics This drug is related chemically to serotonin. It produces moderate sedation, extrapyramidal symptoms, and anticholinergic effects and a low incidence of orthostatic hypotension.

Peak serum levels: 30–90 min. **t½**: 1.5 hr. A single oral dose may exert effects for 24–36 hr. Drug extensively metabolized in liver and metabolites and small amount unchanged drug eliminated through urine and feces.

Use Schizophrenia.

Contraindications Hypersensitivity to drug. Severe CNS depression caused by other agents.

Untoward Reactions *CNS:* Transient initial drowsiness, Parkinson-like reactions, akinesia, restlessness, insomnia, depression, hyperactivity, euphoria, headaches, increased libido. *GI:* Dry mouth, nausea. *Miscellaneous:* Postural hypotension, menstrual abnormalities, blurred vision.

Drug Interactions Calcium sulfate is found in these tablets; may interfere with absorption of tetracyclines or phenytoin.

Dosage Individualized and according to severity of symptoms. **Initial:** 50–75 mg/day increased to 100 mg within 3–4 days. **Maintenance:** *Mild schizophrenia*: 5–15 mg t.i.d.–q.i.d.; *moderate schizophrenia*: 10–25 mg t.i.d.–q.i.d.; *severe schizophrenia*: 225 mg daily, up to maximum of 400 mg/day. Can be given once daily.

Chapter Thirty-three

ANTIDEPRESSANTS

MONOAMINE OXIDASE (MAO) INHIBITORS

General Statement   Because of their relatively high toxicity, MAO inhibitors are prescribed only if tricyclic compounds are ineffective. MAO inhibitors may also interfere with detoxification mechanisms, and thus with biotransformation of certain drugs, which occurs in the liver. One MAO inhibitor—pargyline—is used as an antihypertensive (see p. 343).

Action/Kinetics   Monoamine oxidase is one of the enzymes that breaks down biogenic amines (norepinephrine, epinephrine, serotonin) in the body. Drugs classified as MAO inhibitors prevent the enzyme from metabolizing biogenic amines; these amines therefore accumulate in the presynaptic granules, increasing the concentration of neurotransmitters released upon nerve stimulation. This increase is thought to be responsible for the antidepressant effects of the monoamine oxiolase inhibitors. **Onset**: Few days to several months. Clinical effects of drug manifested for up to 2 weeks after termination of therapy.

Uses   Reactive or endogenous depression, depression of neuroses, involutional melancholia, depressive phases of manic-depressive psychoses. These drugs are rarely used as first drugs for therapy of depressive illness.

Contraindications   Hypersensitivity to MAO inhibitors. History of liver disease, abnormal liver function tests, pheochromocytoma (tumor of the adrenal medulla), impaired renal function, hyperthyroidism, paranoid schizophrenia, epilepsy, cerebrovascular disease, hypertension, cerebral or generalized arteriosclerosis, hypernatremia, atonic colitis, and cardiovascular disease. MAO inhibitors may aggravate glaucoma. They may also suppress anginal pain, which may serve as a warning sign for patients with angina pectoris. Use cautiously in elderly patients.

Untoward Reactions *CNS:* Restlessness, headache, dizziness, drowsiness, insomnia, hypomania, memory impairment, weakness, fatigue, euphoria, ataxia, coma, akathisia, neuritis. Rarely, convulsions, hallucinations, schizophrenic symptoms. Symptoms of excitation including agitation, anxiety, mania. *CV:* Orthostatic hypotension, changes in cardiac rate and rhythm. Rarely, palpitations. *GI:* Nausea, vomiting, abdominal pain, constipation or diarrhea, anorexia, dryness of mouth. *Neuromuscular:* Tremors, hyperreflexia, muscle twitching. *Genitourinary:* Urinary retention, dysuria, incontinence. Rarely, increased secretion of antidiuretic hormone. *Miscellaneous:* Edema, blurred vision, sweating, skin rashes, glaucoma, photosensitivity, sexual disturbances, hepatic complications, black tongue.

Drug Interactions MAO inhibitors potentiate both the pharmacologic actions and the toxic effects of a wide variety of drugs. Because of the long duration of action of MAO inhibitors, adverse drug reactions may also occur if any of the drugs listed below are given to patients within 2–3 weeks after the administration of MAO inhibitors has been terminated.

Interactant	Interaction
Alcohol, ethyl	Tyramine-containing beverages (e.g., Chianti wine) may result in hypertensive crisis
Amphetamine	See *Sympathomimetic drugs*
Anticholinergic agents, Atropine	MAO inhibitors ↑ effects of anticholinergic drugs
Antidepressants, tricyclics	Concomitant use may result in excitation, hyperpyrexia, delirium, tremors, convulsions although such combinations have been used successfully
Antidiabetic agents	MAO inhibitors ↑ and prolong hypoglycemic response to insulin and oral hypoglycemics
Antihypertensives	↑ Chance of hypotension
Barbiturates	↑ Effect of barbiturates due to ↓ breakdown by liver
Doxapram	MAO inhibitors ↑ adverse cardiovascular effects of doxapram (arrhythmias, increase in BP)
Ephedrine	See *Sympathomimetic drugs*
Guanethidine	Concomitant use may cause hypertensive crisis
Levodopa	Concomitant administration may result in ↑ effects of levodopa resulting in hypertension, lightheadedness, and flushing
Metaraminol	See *Sympathomimetic drugs*
Methylphenidate (Ritalin)	See *Sympathomimetic drugs*
Narcotic analgesics	Possible potentiation of either MAO inhibitor (excitation, hypertension), or narcotic (hypotension, coma) effects— death has resulted
Phenothiazines	↑ Effect of phenothiazines due to ↓ breakdown by liver; also ↑ chance of severe extrapyramidal effects and hypertensive crisis

Interactant	Interaction
Phenylephrine	See *Sympathomimetic drugs*
Phenylpropanolamine	See *Sympathomimetic drugs*
Reserpine	Concomitant use may cause hypertensive crisis
Succinylcholine	↑ Effect of succinylcholine due to ↓ breakdown of drug in plasma by pseudocholinesterase
Sympathomimetic drugs Amphetamine, ephedrine, metaraminol, methylphenidate, phenylephrine, phenylpropanolamine. (Many over-the-counter cold tablets and capsules, hayfever medications, and nasal decongestants contain one or more of these drugs)	All peripheral, metabolic, cardiac, and central effects are potentiated up to 2 weeks after termination of MAO inhibitor therapy (symptoms include acute hypertensive crisis with possible intracranial hemorrhage, hyperthermia, convulsions, coma—death may occur)
Tyramine-rich foods, such as beer, broad beans, cheeses (Brie, cheddar, Camembert, Stilton), Chianti wine, chicken livers, caffeine, cola beverages, figs, licorice, liver, pickled or kippered herring, tea, cream, yogurt, yeast extract, and chocolate	Severe headache, hypertension, intracranial hemorrhage, and even death have been reported if these foods are eaten by patient being treated with MAO inhibitor

Laboratory Test Interferences   ↑ Alkaline phosphatase, BUN, bilirubin, serum transaminase, urinary catecholamines, metanephrine, prothrombin time; ↓ urinary 5-HIAA.

Dosage   All agents are administered orally. The effectiveness of the MAO inhibitors is cumulative and it may take days or even months for the drugs to reach their full effectiveness. The effects of the drugs also take 2 to 3 weeks to wane. Therefore, if switching from one MAO inhibitor to another, the second drug should not be given for 2 weeks after the first drug has been discontinued. Also, all drug interactions between MAO inhibitors and other agents can occur up to 2 to 3 weeks after MAO inhibitor therapy has been discontinued. Rapid drug withdrawal in patients receiving high doses may cause a rebound effect characterized by headache, CNS excitability, and occasional hallucinations. (For specific dosages, see Table 14).

Nursing Implications
1. *Assess*
   a. BP and pulse when therapy is initiated and at regular intervals thereafter, so as to note hypertension, which would necessitate discontinuance of the drug.
   b. for peripheral edema, which may be an early symptom of impending CHF.
   c. for red-green vision impairment, as this may be the first indication of optic damage.
   d. diabetic patient for signs of hypoglycemia, because MAO inhibitors potentiate the effect of insulin and sulfonylurea compounds.

e. intake and output and for bladder distention to check on possible urinary retention, which may necessitate changes in medication.

f. for cues pointing to a possible suicide, because patients on antidepressants are more apt to make such an attempt when they emerge from the deepest phase of depression than they were before therapy.

2. Have on hand medication for treatment of overdosage. Agitation is treated with phenothiazine tranquilizers (IM). Excessive pressor response is treated with an alpha-adrenergic blocking agent (phentolamine) or a vasodilator-type drug.

3. *Teach patient and/or family*

a. not to ingest any other drug while on MAO inhibitor therapy and for 2 to 3 weeks after discontinuation before consulting the physician.

b. that foods rich in tyramine (see *Drug Interactions*) may be extremely harmful to patient and must be omitted from the diet. Give printed list of foods that are to be omitted.

c. to limit excessive drinking of coffee, tea, and cola beverages, because excessive caffeine with MAO inhibitors may cause hypertensive crisis, characterized by marked elevation of BP, occipital headaches, palpitation, stiffness and soreness of neck, nausea, vomiting, sweating, photophobia, dilated pupils, tachycardia or bradycardia, and constricting chest pain.

d. to rise slowly from supine position and to dangle feet before standing to minimize orthostatic hypotension.

e. to lie down immediately, if feeling faint.

f. not to overexert, because drugs suppress anginal pain, a warning sign of myocardial ischemia.

TABLE 14   ANTIDEPRESSANTS, MAO INHIBITOR TYPE

Drug	Dosage	Remarks
Isocarboxazid (Marplan), Rx	**PO: initial,** 30 mg daily as a single or divided dose. Reduce when clinical improvement is noted. **Maintenance:** 10-20 mg daily.	It may take 3 to 4 weeks for effect to become noticeable.
Phenelzine sulfate (Nardil), Rx	**PO: Initial,** 15 mg t.i.d.; increase dose rapidly to 60 mg/day (some may require 90 mg/day). **Maintenance** (after maximum beneficial effects noted): 15 mg/day or every other day.	Beneficial effects may not be noted until 60 mg/day have been given for 4 weeks or more.
Tranylcypromine (Parnate), Rx	**PO:** 10 mg b.i.d. for 2 to 3 weeks until beneficial effect is noted. If no response is noted, increase to 30 mg daily. **Maintenance:** Decrease dosage gradually to 10-20 mg daily. **Maximum daily dose:** 30 mg.	Onset of action more rapid than with other MAO inhibitors. More likely to cause hypertensive crisis. To be used for severely depressed, hospitalized patients. Reduce dosage gradually when withdrawing this drug.

TRICYCLIC ANTIDEPRESSANTS

General Statement Dosage levels vary greatly in effectiveness from one patient to another; therefore, dosage regimens must be carefully individualized. The tricyclic antidepressants are chemically related to the phenothiazines and, as such, they exhibit many of the same pharmacologic effects (e.g., anticholinergic, antiserotonin, sedative, antihistaminic, and hypotensive). The tricyclic antidepressants are less effective for depressed patients in the presence of organic brain damage or schizophrenia. Also, they can induce mania; this possibility should be kept in mind when given to patients with manic-depressive psychoses.

Leukocyte and differential counts and liver function tests are indicated in long-term therapy.

Action/Kinetics Tricyclic antidepressants prevent the reuptake of norepinephrine or serotonin, or both, into the storage granule of the presynaptic nerve. This results in increased concentrations of these neurotransmitters in the synapse, which alleviates depression. (Note: Endogenous depression is thought to be caused by low concentrations of norepinephrine and/or serotonin.) The tricyclic antidepressants are well absorbed from the GI tract. All these drugs have a long serum half-life. Up to 4 to 6 days may be required to reach steady plasma levels, and maximum therapeutic effects may not be noted for 2 to 4 weeks. Because of the long half-life, single daily dosage may suffice. The tricyclic antidepressants are more than 90% bound to plasma protein. They are partially metabolized in the liver and excreted primarily in the urine. (See Table 15 below.)

TABLE 15   TRICYCLIC ANTIDEPRESSANTS

Drug	Dosage	Kinetics/Remarks
Amitriptyline hydrochloride (Amitril, Apo-Amitriptyline,* Elavil, Emitrip, Endep, Enovil, Levate,* Meravil,* Novotriptyn,* SK-Amitriptyline), Rx	**PO. Adults (out-patients):** 75 mg/day in divided doses; may be increased to 150 mg/day. **Hospitalized patients: initial,** 100 mg/day; may be increased to 200–300 mg/day. **Maintenance: usual,** 40–100 mg/day (may be given as a single dose at bedtime). **Adolescent and geriatric:** 10 mg t.i.d. and 20 mg at bedtime. **IM only: initially,** 20–30 mg q.i.d.; switch to **PO** therapy as soon as possible.	Amitriptyline is metabolized to an active metabolite, nortriptyline. **Effective plasma levels of amitriptyline and nortriptyline:** approximately 125–250 ng/ml. t½: 17–40 hrs. Up to 1 month may be required for beneficial effects. *Additional Uses* Depression accompanied by anxiety and insomnia. Chronic pain due to cancer or other pain syndromes. Prophylaxis of cluster and migraine headaches. *Additional Nursing Implications* See also *Nursing Implications,* p. 428. Warn patient not to drive a car or operate hazardous machinery as drug causes high degree of sedation. Amitriptyline is also found in Limbitrol, and Triavil (see Appendix 3).

TABLE 15 (*Continued*)

Drug	Dosage	Remarks
Amoxapine (Asendin), Rx	**PO**: *individualized,* **initial**, 50 mg t.i.d. Can be ↑ to 100 mg t.i.d. during 1st week. **Maintenance**: 300 mg as a single dose at bedtime. **Hospitalized patients**: Up to 150 mg q.i.d. **Geriatric: initial**, 25 mg b.i.d.– t.i.d. If necessary, increase to 50 mg b.i.d.– t.i.d. after 1st week. **Maintenance**: Up to 300 mg once daily at bedtime.	**Peak blood levels**: 90 min. **Effective plasma levels**: 200–400 ng/ml. **t½**: 8 hr; t½ of major metabolite: 30 hr. Excreted in urine. Safe use in children under 16 years, pregnancy, lactation not established. Avoid high dose levels in patients with history of convulsive seizures. Do not use during acute recovery period after myocardial infarction. *Additional Use* Antianxiety agent.
Desipramine hydrochloride (Desmethylimipramine Hydrochloride, Norpramin, Pertofrane), Rx	**PO**, *individualized:* **initial**, 75–200 mg in single or divided doses. **Maximum daily dose**: 300 mg. **Maintenance**: 50–100 mg daily; **geriatric and adolescent patients**. 25–100 mg/day. **Not recommended for children**.	Effective plasma levels: 150–300 ng/ml. **t½**: 12– 76 hr. Patients who will respond to drug usually do so within the first week. *Additional Untoward Reactions* Bad taste in mouth.
Doxepin hydrochloride (Adapin, Sinequan), Rx	**PO**. *Individualized. Mild to moderate symptoms*: 25 mg t.i.d.; **then**, adjust dosage to individual response (usual optimum dosage: 75–150 mg/day). **Alternate dosage**: 150 mg at bedtime. *Severe symptoms*: 50 mg t.i.d.; **then**, gradually increase to 300 mg/day. **Not recommended for children under 12 years of age**.	Doxepin is metabolized to the active metabolite, desmethyldoxepin. **Minimum effective plasma level of both doxepin and desmethyldoxepin**: 150–250 ng/ml. **t½**: 8–36 hr. *Additional Uses* Antianxiety agent, depression accompanied by anxiety and insomnia, depression in patients with manic-depressive illness. *Administration* Oral concentrate is to be diluted with 4 oz of water, fruit juice, or milk just before ingestion. *Additional Contraindication* Glaucoma. *Additional Untoward Reactions* Drug has high incidence of side effects, including high degree of sedation, decreased libido, extrapyramidal symptoms, dermatitis, pruritus, fatigue, weight gain, edema, parasthesia, breast engorgement, in-

TABLE 15 TRICYCLIC ANTIDEPRESSANTS

Drug	Dosage	Kinetics/Remarks
		somnia, tremor, chills, tinnitus, and photophobia.
Imipramine hydrochloride (Apo-Imipramine,* Impril,* Janimine, Novopramine,* SK-Pramine, Tipramine, Tofranil), Rx Imipramine pamoate (Tofranil-PM), Rx	*Depression.* **PO, IM,** *individualized,* **hospitalized patients:** 50 mg b.i.d.–t.i.d. Can be increased by 25 mg every few days up to 200 mg daily. After 2 weeks, dosage may be increased gradually to maximum of 250–300 mg once daily at bedtime. **Outpatients:** 75–150 mg daily. Maximum dose for outpatients is 200 mg. Decrease when feasible to maintenance dosage: 50–150 mg once daily at bedtime. **Adolescent and geriatric patients** 30–40 mg/day **PO,** up to maximum of 100 mg/day. *Childhood enuresis:* **PO, ages 6 and over,** 25 mg/day 1 hr. before bedtime. Dose can be increased to 50 mg/day up to 12 years of age and 75 mg/day in children over 12 years of age.	Imipramine is biotransformed into its active metabolite, desmethylimipramine. **Effective plasma level of imipramine and desmethylimipramine:** 150–300 ng/ml. t½: 6–24 hr. High therapeutic dosage may increase frequency of seizures in epileptic patients and cause seizures in nonepileptic patients. Elderly and adolescent patients may have low tolerance to the drug. *Laboratory Test Interferences* ↑ Metanephrine (Pisano test); ↓ urinary 5-HIAA. *Storage* Protect from direct sunlight and strong artificial light. *Administration* Crystals that may be present in the injectable form can be dissolved by immersing closed ampuls into hot water for 1 minute. Total daily dose can be given once daily at bedtime. *Additional Nursing Implications* See also *Nursing Implications*, p. 428. Report increase in frequency of seizures in epileptics and occurrence of seizures in nonepileptics.
Maprotiline hydrochloride (Ludiomil), Rx	**Adults,** *mild to moderate depression,* **outpatients, initial:** 75 mg/day; can be increased to 150–225 mg/day, *if necessary.* **Adult,** *severe depression,* **hospitalized, initial:** 100–150 mg/day; can be increased to 225–300 mg, if necessary. Dosage should not exceed 300 mg/day. **Maintenance:** For all uses, 75–150 mg/day, adjusted depend-	**Effective plasma levels:** 200–300 ng/ml. t½: Approximately 25–60 hr. **Peak effect:** 12 hr. Beneficial effects may not be observed for 2–3 weeks. *Additional Uses* Depressive neuroses, depression in patients with manic-depressive illness, depression with anxiety. *Administration* 1. May be given in single or divided doses. 2. Should be discontinued

TABLE 15   TRICYCLIC ANTIDEPRESSANTS

Drug	Dosage	Kinetics/Remarks
	ing on therapeutic response. **Geriatric patients**: 50–75 mg/day. **Not recommended for patients under 18 years of age.**	as long as possible before elective surgery.
Nortriptyline hydrochloride (Aventyl Hydrochloride, Pamelor), Rx	**PO**: 25 mg t.i.d.–q.i.d. Dose individualized. **Doses above 100 mg not recommended. Elderly patients: 30–50 mg/day in divided doses. Not recommended for children.**	**Effective plasma levels**: 50–150 ng/ml. t½: 15–90 hr. *Administration* After meals and at bedtime *Laboratory Test Interference* ↓ Urinary 5-HIAA
Protriptyline hydrochloride (Triptil,* Vivactil), Rx	**PO**, *individualized*, **initial**, *severe depression*: 30–60 mg in 3 to 4 divided doses. After satisfactory response is obtained, decrease gradually to maintenance level of 15–40 mg daily in divided doses. **Elderly patients: initial**, 5 mg t.i.d., increase dose slowly. Monitor cardiovascular system closely if dose exceeds 20 mg/day in the elderly. **Not recommended for children.**	**Effective plasma levels**: 115–210 ng/ml. t½: Approximately 50–200 hr. *Additional Uses* Withdrawn and anergic patients. Obstructive sleep apnea. Protriptyline causes more cardiovascular side effects than the other tricyclic antidepressants. Administer with caution to patients with myocardial insufficiency and those in whom tachycardia or a drop in BP might lead to serious complications. Drug causes less sedation than other tricyclic antidepressants. *Administration* If drug causes insomnia give last dose no less than 8 hr before bedtime. *Nursing Implications* See also *Nursing Implications*, p. 428. Assess vital signs at least b.i.d. during initiation of therapy.
Trimipramine maleate (Surmontil), Rx	**Adults, outpatients: initial**, 75 mg/day in divided doses up to 150 mg/day. Daily dosage should not exceed 200 mg; **maintenance**: 50–150 mg/day. Total dosage can be given at bedtime. **Adults, hospitalized: initial**, 100 mg/day in divided doses up to 200 mg/day. If no improvement in 2–3 wk, increase to 250–300	**Effective plasma levels** 180 ng/ml. t½: 7–30 hr. Seems more effective in endogenous depression than in other types of depression. *Additional Uses* Peptic ulcer disease.

TABLE 15 (*Continued*)

Drug	Dosage	Kinetics/Remarks
	mg/day. **Adolescent/ geriatric patients: initial**, 50 mg/day up to 100 mg/day. Not recommended for children.	

Uses Endogenous and reactive depressions. Preferred over MAO inhibitors because they are less toxic. See individual drugs for special uses.

Contraindications Severely impaired liver function. Use with caution in patients with epilepsy, cardiovascular diseases, glaucoma, benign prostatic hypertrophy, suicidal tendencies, a history of urinary retention, and the elderly. Do not use together with MAO inhibitors.

Untoward Reactions Most frequent side effects are sedation and atropine-like reactions. *CNS:* Confusion, anxiety, restlessness, insomnia, nightmares, hallucinations, delusions, mania or hypomania, headache, dizziness, inability to concentrate, panic reaction, worsening of psychoses, fatigue, weakness. *Anticholinergic:* Dry mouth, blurred vision, mydriasis, constipation, paralytic ileus, urinary retention or difficulty in urination. *GI:* Nausea, vomiting, anorexia, gastric distress, unpleasant taste, stomatitis, glossitis, cramps, increased salivation, black tongue. *CV:* Fainting, tachycardia, hypo- or hypertension, arrhythmias, heart block, possibility of palpitation, myocardial infarction, stroke. *Neurologic:* Paresthesia, numbness, incoordination, neuropathies, extrapyramidal symptoms including tardive dyskinesia, dysarthria, seizures. *Dermatologic:* Skin rashes, urticaria, flushing, pruritus, petechiae, photosensitivity, edema. *Endocrine:* Testicular swelling and gynecomastia in males, increase or decrease in libido, impotence, menstrual irregularities and galactorrhea in females, hypo- or hyperglycemia, changes in secretion of antidiuretic hormone. *Miscellaneous:* Sweating, alopecia, nasal congestion, lacrimation, increase in body temperature, chills, urinary frequency including nocturia. Bone marrow depression including thrombocytopenia, leukopenia, agranulocytosis, eosinophilia.

High dosage increases the frequency of seizures in epileptic patients and may cause epileptiform attacks in normal subjects.

Drug Interactions

Interactant	Interaction
Acetazolamide	↑ Effect of tricyclics by ↑ renal tubular reabsorption of the drug
Alcohol, ethyl	Concomitant use may lead to ↑ GI complications and ↓ performance on motor skill tests—death has been reported
Ammonium chloride	↓ Effect of tricyclics by ↓ renal tubular reabsorption of the drug
Anticholinergic drugs	Additive anticholinergic side effects
Anticoagulants, oral	↑ Hypoprothrombinemia due to ↓ breakdown by liver
Anticonvulsants	Tricyclics may ↑ incidence of epileptic seizures
Antihistamines	Additive anticholinergic side effects
Ascorbic acid	↓ Effect of tricyclics by ↓ renal tubular reabsorption of the drug

Interactant	Interaction
Barbiturates	↑ Effect of barbiturates; also, barbiturates may ↑ breakdown of antidepressants by liver
Beta-adrenergic blocking agents	Tricyclic antidepressants ↓ effect of the blocking agents
Chlordiazepoxide	Concomitant use may cause additive sedative effects and/or additive atropine-like side effects
Cimetidine	↑ Effect of tricyclics due to ↓ breakdown by liver
Clonidine	Tricyclics ↓ effect of clonidine by preventing uptake at its site of action
Contraceptives, oral	Oral contraceptives may ↑ effect of tricyclic antidepressants
Diazepam	Concomitant use may cause additive sedative effects and/or additive atropine-like side effects
Ephedrine	Tricyclics ↓ effects of ephedrine by preventing uptake at its site of action
Estrogens	Depending on the dose, estrogens may ↑ or ↓ the effects of tricyclics
Ethchlorvynol	Combination may result in transient delirium
Furazolidone	Toxic psychoses possible
Glutethimide	Additive anticholinergic side effects
Guanethidine	Tricyclics ↓ effect of guanethidine by preventing uptake at its site of action
Haloperidol	↑ Effect of tricyclics due to ↓ breakdown by liver
Levodopa	↓ Effect of levodopa due to ↓ absorption
Meperidine	Tricyclics enhance narcotic-induced respiratory depression; also, additive anticholinergic side effects
Methyldopa	Tricyclics may block hypotensive effects of methyldopa
Methylphenidate	↑ Effect of tricyclics due to ↓ breakdown by liver
MAO inhibitors	Concomitant use may result in excitation, increase in body temperature, delirium, tremors, convulsions although combinations have been used successfully
Narcotic analgesics	Tricyclics enhance narcotic-induced respiratory depression; also, additive anticholinergic effects
Oxazepam	Concomitant use may cause additive sedative effects and/or atropine-like side effects
Phenothiazines	Additive anticholinergic side effects; also, phenothiazines ↑ effects of tricyclics due to ↓ breakdown by liver
Procainamide	Additive cardiac effects
Quinidine	Additive cardiac effects
Reserpine	Tricyclics ↓ hypotensive effect of reserpine

Interactant	Interaction
Sodium bicarbonate	↑ Effect of tricyclics by ↑ renal tubular reabsorption of the drug
Sympathomimetics	Potentiation of sympathomimetic effects → hypertension or cardiac arrhythmias
Thyroid preparations	Mutually potentiating effects observed
Vasodilators	Additive hypotensive effect

Laboratory Test Interferences   ↑ Alkaline phosphatase, bilirubin; ↑ or ↓ blood glucose. False + or ↑ urinary catecholamines.

Dosage   See individual agents, Table 15.

Overdosage

SYMPTOMS   Drowsiness, ataxia, tachycardia, ECG abnormalities, congestive heart failure, convulsions, mydriasis, severe hypotension, stupor, coma, agitation, hyperactive reflexes, muscle rigidity, diaphoresis, respiratory depression, cyanosis, shock, vomiting, hyperpyrexia.

TREATMENT OF OVERDOSAGE
1. Admit patient to hospital.
2. Empty stomach in alert patients by induced vomiting followed by gastric lavage and charcoal **after insertion of cuffed endotracheal tube**. Maintain respiration and avoid the use of respiratory stimulants.
3. Administer physostigmine salicylate to reverse CNS and cardiovascular effects. *Adults*: 1–3 mg; *pediatric*: 0.5 mg repeated q 5 min up to maximum of 2 mg, if necessary. For all patients, repeat, if needed, q 30–60 min.
4. Monitor ECG for at least 72 hr. Closely monitor cardiac function.
5. Control hyperpyrexia by external means (icepack, cool baths, spongings).
6. To reduce possibility of convulsions, minimize external stimulation. If necessary, use diazepam, short-acting barbiturates, paraldehyde, or methocarbamol to control convulsions. Avoid barbiturates, if MAO inhibitors have been used recently.
7. For life-threatening arrhythmias, lidocaine, propranolol, or phenytoin have been used. Monitor for myocardial depression caused by these agents.

Nursing Implications
1. Ascertain that baseline blood and liver function tests are done before onset of therapy and that a plan for periodic evaluations is implemented.
2. *Assess*
   a. for allergic response manifested by skin rash, alopecia, eosinophilia, or other allergic-type response.
   b. patient with a history of cardiovascular disorders for arrhythmia and tachycardia, which may lead to increased anginal attacks, myocardial infarction, and stroke. Ascertain that a plan for periodic ECG evaluations is implemented.
   c. and report symptoms of blood dyscrasias, such as sore throat, fever, weakness, and purpura, which necessitate withholding the drug and placing patient in reverse isolation until blood tests are reevaluated.
   d. for GI reactions manifested by nausea, vomiting, anorexia, epigastric distress, diarrhea, constipation, peculiar taste, abdominal cramps, and black tongue. These symptoms necessitate adjustment of dosage.
   e. for endocrine reactions, such as increased or decreased libido, gynecomastia,

testicular swelling, galactorrhea, interference with antidiuretic hormone secretion, and elevated or depressed blood sugar levels.

f. for behavior manifesting further psychological disturbances that may require either reduction in dosage or discontinuance of therapy.

g. patients with a history of closed-angle glaucoma for onset of an acute attack often characterized by severe headache, nausea, vomiting, eye pain, dilation of the pupil, and halos.

h. patient with hyperthyroidism, for cardiac arrhythmias precipitated by tricyclic compound.

i. for intake and output, abdominal distention, and bowel sounds that may indicate urinary retention, paralytic ileus, and constipation. These conditions may require reduction in dosage.

j. for symptoms of cholestatic jaundice (indicating biliary tract obstruction), such as high fever, upper abdominal pain, nausea, diarrhea, rash, yellowing of skin, sclera, or mucous membranes. Withhold drugs and report to medical supervision, should these signs and symptoms be present.

k. for other adverse reactions that may be manifestations of the tricyclic compounds described under *Untoward Reactions*.

3. Anticipate that dosage will be highly individualized according to patient's age, physical and mental condition, and response.

4. Anticipate that sedation and anticholinergic effects may be minimized by starting with small doses and then gradually increasing doses.

5. Closely supervise seriously depressed patients, particularly during the early therapy, because suicidal tendencies are increased when patients start recovering from depression. Also, ascertain that such patients are ingesting drugs and not hoarding them.

6. Check with medical supervision before administering tricyclic compounds to patients on electroshock therapy, because the combination may increase the hazard of therapy.

7. Be aware that patient may have epileptiform seizure precipitated by drug. Practice seizure precautions.

8. Ascertain that drug is discontinued several days before surgery, because tricyclic compounds may affect blood pressure during surgery.

9. Withdraw drug gradually to prevent withdrawal symptoms, such as nausea, headache, and malaise.

10. Be aware that although MAO inhibitors are usually contraindicated with tricyclic antidepressants, they may be used in small dosages, under close medical supervision, for patients refractory to more conservative therapy.

11. *Teach patient and/or family*

a. not to ingest any other drug while taking tricyclic antidepressants for 2 weeks after therapy has been completed without consulting medical supervision.

b. that 2 to 4 weeks may be needed to achieve maximum clinical response.

c. to rise gradually from a supine position and not to remain standing in one place for any length of time; if faint, lie down, to minimize orthostatic hypotension. Provide appropriate safety measures.

d. to rinse mouth with water. Encourage increased fluid intake to relieve excessive dryness of mouth, and assist in retention of false dentures if patient has these.

(continued)

e. that if therapy with tricyclic compound results in impotence, the doctor will adjust dosage to alleviate condition.

f. that diabetic patients are to monitor urine carefully, because drug may affect carbohydrate metabolism, and adjustment of hypoglycemic drugs and diet may be indicated.

g. that photosensitive patients are to remain out of the sun.

h. to use caution when performing hazardous tasks requiring mental alertness or physical coordination, because the drug causes drowsiness or ataxia.

MISCELLANEOUS AGENTS

TRAZODONE HYDROCHLORIDE   Desyrel (Rx)

Classification   Antidepressant, miscellaneous.

Action/Kinetics   Trazodone is a novel antidepressant that does not inhibit MAO and is also devoid of amphetamine-like effects. Response usually occurs after 2 weeks (75% of patients) with the remainder responding after 2–4 weeks. The drug may inhibit serotonin uptake by brain cells, therefore increasing serotonin concentrations in the synapse. **Peak plasma levels**: 1 hr (empty stomach). t½: initial, 3–6 hr; final, 5–9 hr.

Use   Depression with or without accompanying anxiety.

Contraindications   During the initial recovery period following myocardial infarction. Concurrently with electroshock therapy. Use with caution during pregnancy and lactation. Safety and efficacy in children less than 18 years of age have not been established.

Untoward Reactions   *General*: Dermatitis, edema, blurred vision, constipation, dry mouth, nasal congestion, skeletal muscle aches and pains. *CV*: Hypertension or hypotension, syncope, palpitations, tachycardia, shortness of breath, chest pain. *GI*: Diarrhea, nausea, vomiting, bad taste in mouth, flatulence. *GU*: Delayed urine flow, hematuria, increased urinary frequency. *CNS*: Nightmares, confusion, anger, excitement, decreased ability to concentrate, dizziness, disorientation, drowsiness, lightheadedness, fatigue, insomnia, nervousness, impaired memory. Rarely, hallucinations, impaired speech, hypomania. *Other*: Incoordination, tremors, paresthesia, decreased libido, appetite disturbances, red eyes, sweating or clamminess, tinnitus, weight gain or loss, anemia, hypersalivation. Rarely, akathisia, muscle twitching, increased libido, impotence, retrograde ejaculation, early menses, missed periods.

Drug Interactions

Interactant	Interaction
Antihypertensives	Additive hypotension
Clonidine	Trazodone ↓ effect of clonidine
CNS depressants	↑ CNS depression
Digoxin	Trazodone ↑ serum digoxin levels
Phenytoin	Trazodone ↑ serum phenytoin levels

Dosage PO. Initial, 150 mg/day; **then,** increase by 50 mg/day every 3–4 days to maximum of 400 mg/day in divided doses (outpatients). Inpatients may require up to but not exceeding 600 mg/day in divided doses. **Maintenance:** use lowest effective dose.

Administration

1. Take with food to enhance absorption and minimize dizziness and/or light-headedness.
2. To reduce side effects during day, take major portion of dose at bedtime.

Nursing Implications

1. *Assess*
   a. for untoward reactions and report to supervisor.
   b. for cues to suicide; patients on antidepressants are more prone to suicide when they emerge from the deepest phase of depression than they were before therapy.
2. *Teach patient and/or family*
   a. to use caution when driving or performing other hazardous tasks, since tra-zodone may cause drowsiness or dizziness.
   b. not to drink alcohol or take other depressant drugs.
   c. to share responsibility for drug therapy to optimize treatment and to prevent overdosage.
   d. to inform physician if elective surgery is planned so that therapy with tra-zodone may be adjusted to minimize interaction with anesthetic agent.

Chapter Thirty-four

ANTIPARKINSON AGENTS

Parkinson's disease is a progressive disorder of the nervous system, affecting mostly people over the age of 50.

Its main symptoms are slowness of motor movements (bradykinesia and akinesia), stiffness or resistance to passive movements (rigidity), muscle weakness, tremors, speech impairment, sialorrhea (salivation), and postural instability.

Parkinsonism is a frequent side effect of certain antipsychotic drugs, including prochlorperazine, chlorpromazine, and reserpine. Drug-induced symptoms usually disappear when the responsible agent is discontinued. Extrapyramidal Parkinson-like symptoms can accompany brain injuries (strokes, tumors) or other diseases of the nervous system.

The cause of Parkinson's disease is unknown; however, it is associated with a depletion of the neurotransmitter dopamine in the nervous system. Administration of levodopa—the precursor of dopamine—relieves symptoms in 75–80% of the patients. Anticholinergic agents also have a beneficial effect by reducing tremors and rigidity and improving mobility, muscular coordination, and motor performance. They are often administered together with levodopa. Certain antihistamines, notably diphenhydramine (Benadryl), are also useful in the treatment of Parkinsonism.

Patients suffering from Parkinson's disease need emotional support and encouragement because the debilitating nature of the disorder often causes depression. Comprehensive treatment includes physical therapy.

CHOLINERGIC BLOCKING AGENTS

General Statement   The administration of cholinergic blocking agents reduces tremors and rigidity seen with parkinsonism; in addition, improvement in mobility, muscular coordination, and motor performance is noted. Synthetic anticholinergics have largely replaced atropine and similar drugs for this disease.

Action/Kinetics   Parkinsonism is believed to result from a neurotransmitter imbalance in the corpus striatum of the CNS especially manifested by a deficiency of dopamine and an excess of acetylcholine. By blocking the action of acetylcholine on CNS neurons, the cholinergic blocking agents help balance cholinergic and dopaminergic activity, thus reversing the symptoms of Parkinsonism. There is also some evidence that the cholinergic blocking agents may inhibit the reuptake of dopamine into storage sites, thereby prolonging the effect of dopamine. Peripheral side effects of the cholinergic blocking agents (such as dry mouth, constipation, tachycardia, urinary retention) tend to limit their use for Parkinsonism.

Contraindications   Glaucoma, tachycardia, partial obstruction of the GI and biliary tract, and prostatic hypertrophy. The drugs are to be used with extreme caution for patients with hypertension, cardiac disease, especially those with a tendency to develop tachycardia, and in the elderly with atherosclerosis or evidence of mental impairment. Use with caution in patients on chronic phenothiazine therapy and in hot weather.

Untoward Reactions   *GI:* Constipation (frequent), nausea, vomiting, dry mouth (which may cause difficulty in swallowing), colon distention, paralytic ileus. *GU:* Urinary hesitantcy or retention, impotence. *Cardiovascular system*: Tachycardia, palpitations, hypotension. *Central nervous system*: Dizziness, drowsiness, lassitude, nervousness, disorientation; symptoms often may be mistaken for senility or mental deterioration. Excess dosage may cause agitation, psychotic reactions, and hallucinations. *Respiratory*: Decreased bronchial secretions, antihistamine effects. *Ocular*: Blurred vision, acute glaucoma, photophobia. *Miscellaneous*: Suppression of sweating, flushing, scarlatiniform rash, decreased glandular secretions, numbness of fingers, difficulty in achieving or maintaining an erection, suppression of perspiration, loss of libido.

Drug Interactions

Interactant	Interaction
Amantidine	Additive anticholinergic side effects, especially with trihexyphenidyl and benztropine
Antidepressants, tricyclic	Additive anticholinergic side effects
Antihistamines	↑ Risk of anticholinergic side effects
Haloperidol	↓ Effect of haloperidol
MAO inhibitors	MAO Inhibitors ↑ effects of anticholinergic drugs
Narcotic analgesics	↑ Risk of anticholinergic side effects
Phenothiazines	↑ Risk of GI side effects, including paralytic ileus; also, ↓ effect of phenothiazines
Procainamide	Additive anticholinergic side effects
Quinidine	Additive effect on blockade of vagus nerve action

Dosage See individual agents. The agents are usually initiated at low dosage and increased gradually, until optimum levels have been reached. Excessive untoward reactions can often be corrected by decrease in dosage. Agent should not be discontinued abruptly, but decreased gradually while another drug with the same effect is introduced slowly.

Administration

1. May be taken with food to minimize gastric upset.
2. Cholinergic blocking agents may increase risk of heat stroke if used in hot weather.
3. Due to drowsiness or dizziness, caution should be exercised when driving or performing other tasks requiring alertness.

Nursing Implications

1. Be alert to a history of asthma, glaucoma, or duodenal ulcer, which contraindicates the use of these drugs.
2. Check dosage and measure drug exactly because some of these antiparkinson agents are given in minute amounts, and overdosage results in toxicity.
3. *Teach patient and/or family*
   a. the side effects that may occur, and advise reporting these to physician who may reduce dose, or temporarily discontinue drug. The physician may encourage patient to tolerate certain side effects (e.g., dry mouth, blurred vision) because of overall beneficial effects.
   b. who improve with drug therapy to resume normal activity gradually, taking other medical problems he may have into consideration.
   c. that antiparkinson drugs should not be withdrawn abruptly. When changing medication, one drug should be withdrawn slowly and the other started in small doses.
   d. to relieve dry mouth by using cold beverages, hard candies, or gum if permitted.

BENZTROPINE MESYLATE   Apo-Benztropine,* Benzylate,* Cogentin, PMS Benztropine* (Rx)

Classification   Antiparkinson agent, synthetic anticholinergic.

Action/Kinetics   Benztropine is a synthetic anticholinergic possessing antihistamine and local anesthetic properties. Its effects are cumulative and it is long acting (24 hours). Full effects are manifested in 2 to 3 days. The drug produces a low incidence of side effects.

Uses   As adjunct in the treatment of parkinsonism (all types). Used to reduce severity of extrapyramidal effects in phenothiazine or other antipsychotic drug therapy (not effective in tardive dyskinesia).

Dosage   Patients can rarely tolerate full dosage. **PO (rarely by IV or IM).** *Parkinsonism*: 0.5–6 mg daily. *Drug-induced parkinsonism*: **initial**, 0.5 mg daily increased gradually to 1–4 mg 1 or 2 times daily.

Administration   When used as replacement for or supplement to other antiparkinsonism drugs, substitute or add gradually.

Additional Nursing Implications

See also *Nursing Implications*, p. 433.

1. Inform the patient that it takes 2 to 3 days for drug to show effects.
2. Advise patient to use caution while driving or operating dangerous machinery because drug has a sedative effect.
3. Assess for vomiting or excitement, which may require temporary withdrawal. Treatment may be resumed later at a lower dosage.

BIPERIDEN HYDROCHLORIDE   Akineton Hydrochloride (Rx)

BIPERIDEN LACTATE   Akineton Lactate (Rx)

Classification   Antiparkinson agent, synthetic anticholinergic.

Action/Kinetics   Tolerance may develop to this synthetic anticholinergic. Tremor may increase as spasticity is relieved.

Uses   Parkinsonism, especially of the postencephalitic, arteriosclerotic, and idiopathic type. Drug-induced (e.g., phenothiazines) extrapyramidal manifestations.

Additional Contraindications   Children under the age of 3 years; use with caution in older children.

Additional Untoward Effects   Muscle weakness, inability to move certain muscles.

Dosage   *Hydrochloride.* **PO**: *Parkinsonism*, 2 mg t.i.d.–q.i.d.; *Drug-induced extrapyramidal effects*: 2 mg 1–3 times/day. *Lactate.* **IM, IV**: 2 mg; repeat q 30 min until symptoms improve, but not more than 4 doses/day.

Administration   Administer with meals to reduce gastric irritation.

Additional Nursing Implications

See also *Nursing Implications*, p. 433.

1. Maintain patient recumbent during IV administration.
2. Dangle patients legs on edge of bed prior to walking after IV administration of drug to prevent transient hypotension, syncope, and falling.
3. Assist the patient in walking after IM or IV administration because of transient incoordination.

ETHOPROPAZINE HYDROCHLORIDE Parsidol Hydrochloride, Parsitan* (Rx)

Classification Antiparkinson agent, synthetic anticholinergic of the phenothiazine type.

Action/Kinetics This synthetic anticholinergic is considered by some to be a drug of choice for treatment of major tremors of parkinsonism. Ethopropazine also manifests antihistaminic, local anesthetic, and CNS depressant effects. **Onset**: 30 min. **Duration**: 4 hr. The drug produces a high incidence of side effects.

Uses To treat all types of parkinsonism and drug-induced extrapyramidal symptoms.

Additional Untoward Reactions Tachycardia, abnormal EEG, agranulocytosis, purpura, pancytopenia, endocrine disturbances, ocular disturbances, hallucinations, jaundice. Parkinsonian symptoms may become exacerbated.

Dosage **PO: initial**, 50 mg 1 or 2 times a day; increase by 10 mg per dose q 2 to 3 days until optimum effect or limit of tolerance. **Maintenance**: 100–600 mg daily. Most patients, especially the elderly, cannot tolerate full therapeutic dosage.

Additional Nursing Implications

See also *Nursing Implications*, p. 433.

1. Assess patients for high incidence of side effects.
2. Anticipate that dosage for elderly will be less than full therapeutic dosage.

ORPHENADRINE HYDROCHLORIDE Disipal (Rx)

Classification Antiparkinson agent, anticholinergic.

Action/Kinetics Orphenadrine improves rigidity but not the tremor of parkinsonism. **Peak effect**: 2 hr. **Duration**: 4–6 hr.

Uses Adjunct in the treatment of all types of parkinsonism. Drug-induced extrapyramidal reactions.

Additional Contraindications Glaucoma or myasthenia gravis. Use with caution for patients with tachycardia, signs of urinary retention, or in pregnancy.

Additional Untoward Reactions Adverse CNS manifestations (dizziness, drowsiness, increased tremor) may be present during initiation but will subside with continuation of usage or reduction in dose. Mild euphoria. Aplastic anemia occurs rarely.

Dosage PO: 50 mg t.i.d. Doses up to 250 mg daily have been used without ill effects.

Additional Nursing Implications
See also *Nursing Implications*, p. 433.

1. Assess closely for increased tremor or adverse CNS effects that may require decrease in dosage.
2. Report side effects, but encourage the patient to continue treatment since these may subside with continued treatment.

PROCYCLIDINE HYDROCHLORIDE   Kemadrin, PMS Procyclidine,* Procyclid* (Rx)

Classification Antiparkinson agent, synthetic anticholinergic.

Action/Kinetics Procyclidine, a synthetic anticholinergic, appears to be better tolerated by younger patients. **Onset:** 30–45 min. **Duration:** 4–6 hr. This drug is often more effective in relieving rigidity than tremor.

Uses Treatment of all types of parkinsonism. Drug-induced extrapyramidal symptoms. Control sialorrhea following neuroleptic drug use.

Dosage PO. *Parkinsonism (for patients on no other therapy):* **initial,** 2.5 mg t.i.d. after meals; dose may be increased slowly to 4–5 mg t.i.d. and, if necessary, before bedtime. *Parkinsonism (transferring from other therapy):* substitute 2.5 mg t.i.d.; slowly increase dose of procyclidine and decrease dose of other drug to appropriate maintenance levels. *Drug-induced extrapyramidal symptoms:* **initial,** 2.5 mg t.i.d.; increase to maintenance of 10–20 mg/day.

TRIHEXYPHENIDYL HYDROCHLORIDE   Aparkane,* Aphen, APO-Trihex,* Artane, Novohexidyl,* Trihexane, Trihexidyl, Trihexy-2 and -5 (Rx)

Classification Antiparkinson agent, anticholinergic.

Action/Kinetics Synthetic anticholinergic, which relieves rigidity but has little effect on tremor. Has a high incidence of side effects. **Onset:** 60 min. **Duration:** 6–12 hr.

Uses Adjunct in the treatment of all types of parkinsonism (often used as adjunct with levodopa). Drug-induced extrapyramidal symptoms. Sustained release is for maintenance dosage only.

Additional Contraindications Arteriosclerosis and hypersensitivity to drug.

Additional Untoward Reactions Serious CNS stimulation (restlessness, insomnia, delirium, agitation) and psychotic manifestations.

Dosage PO. *Parkinsonism:* **initial (day 1),** 1–2 mg; **then,** increase by 2 mg q 3–5 days until daily dose is 6–10 mg given in divided doses. Some patients may require l2–15 mg daily. *Adjunct with levodopa:* 3–6 mg/day in divided doses. *Drug-induced extrapyramidal reactions:* **initial,** 1 mg daily; **then,** increase as needed to total daily dose of 5–15 mg. **Maintenance:** Sustained release, 5–10 mg 1–2 times daily.

Additional Nursing Implications

See also *Nursing Implications*, p. 433.

1. Assess for high incidence of side effects and report to prevent overwhelming problems.
2. Assess for additional untoward reactions of CNS (i.e., restlessness, insomnia, delirium, agitation, and psychotic manifestations).

OTHER ANTIPARKINSON AGENTS

AMANTADINE HYDROCHLORIDE   Symmetrel (Rx)

Classification   Antiparkinson and antiviral agent.

General Statement   The drug decreases extrapyramidal symptoms, including akinesia, rigidity, tremors, excessive salivation, gait disturbances, and total functional disability. Favorable results have been obtained in about 50% of the patients. Improvements can last up to 30 months, although some patients report that the effect of the drug wears off in 1 to 3 months. A rest period or increased dosage may reestablish effectiveness. For parkinsonism, amantadine hydrochloride is usually used concomitantly with other agents, such as levodopa and anticholinergic agents.

Action/Kinetics   It is currently believed that amantadine either causes the release of dopamine from synaptosomes or blocks the reuptake of dopamine into presynaptic neurons. Either of these mechanisms would result in an increase in the levels of dopamine in dopaminergic synapses in the corpus striatum. **Onset:** 48 hrs. **Peak blood levels:** 1–4 hr after PO dosage. **Elimination t½:** 9–37 hr. The drug is excreted unchanged in the urine.

Amantadine is also used as an antiviral agent (see p. 193).

Uses   Symptomatic treatment of idiopathic parkinsonism and parkinsonian syndrome resulting from encephalitis, carbon monoxide intoxication, or cerebral arteriosclerosis. Prophylaxis or management of influenza A virus-induced respiratory illness.

Contraindications   Hypersensitivity to drug; history of epilepsy. Administer with caution to patients with liver and renal disease, CHF, peripheral edema, orthostatic hypotension, recurrent eczematoid dermatitis, or severe psychosis, to patients on CNS stimulant drugs, exposed to rubella, and nursing mothers. Safe use for those who may become pregnant not established.

Untoward Reactions   *CNS:* Depression (common), confusion, anxiety, irritability, psychoses, hallucinations, headache, fatigue, insomnia. *CV:* Congestive heart failure, orthostatic hypotension, edema. *GI:* Anorexia, nausea, constipation, vomiting, dry mouth. *Miscellaneous:* Urinary retention, dyspnea, weakness, skin rash, slurred speech, livedo reticularis (mottlng of skin of the extremities), impaired vision.

Drug Interactions

Interactant	Interaction
Anticholinergics	Additive anticholinergic effects (including hallucinations, confusion), especially with trihexyphenidyl and benztropine
CNS stimulants	May ↑ CNS and psychic effects of amantadine; use cautiously together
Levodopa	Potentiated by amantadine

Dosage   PO. *Parkinsonism*: When used as sole agent, usual, 100 mg b.i.d.; may be necessary to increase up to 400 mg/day in divided doses. When used with other antiparkinson drugs: 100 mg 1–2 times/day. *Drug-induced extrapyramidal symptoms*: 100 mg b.i.d. (up to 300 mg/day may be required in some). (*Antiviral*, see p. 194.) Dosage should be reduced in patients with impaired renal function.

Administration   Administer last daily dosage several hours before retiring to prevent insomnia.

Additional Nursing Implications

See also *Nursing Implications*, p. 433.

1. Anticipate that following loss of effectiveness of the drug, benefits may be regained by increasing the dosage or discontinuing the drug for several weeks and then reinstituting it.
2. *Teach patient and/or family*
   a. not to drive a car or operate other machinery after taking medication, since concentration and coordination may be affected.
   b. to report patchy discoloration of the skin, but also that discoloration lessens when legs are elevated and usually fades completely within weeks after discontinuing drug.
   c. to rise slowly from a prone position as orthostatic hypotension may occur.
   d. to lie down if dizzy or weak to relieve the orthostatic hypotension.

BROMOCRIPTINE MESYLATE   Parlodel (Rx)

Classification   Antiparkinson agent. Also, see p. 865

Remarks   Bromocriptine is also used for amenorrhea, galactorrhea, prevention of lactation, and female infertility. For uses, contraindications, untoward reactions, see p. 865.

Dosage   PO. *Parkinsonism:* 2.5 mg daily (one-half of the 2.5 mg tablet b.i.d. with meals). If necessary, the dosage may be increased by 2.5 mg/day every 2–4 weeks not to exceed 100 mg daily. Dosage should be assessed every 2 weeks to ensure the lowest effective dose is used.

Administration   In the event of untoward reactions, the dose should be reduced gradually in 2.5 mg increments.

CARBIDOPA   Lodosyn (Rx)

CARBIDOPA/LEVODOPA   Sinemet-10/100, -25/100, or -25/250 (Rx)

Classification   Antiparkinson agent.

Action/Kinetics   Carbidopa inhibits the peripheral decarboxylation of levodopa but not central decarboxylation, since it does not cross the blood–brain barrier. Since peripheral decarboxylation is inhibited, this allows more levodopa to be available for transport to the brain, where it will be converted to dopamine, thus relieving the symptoms of parkinsonism. It is recommended that both carbidopa and levodopa be given together (e.g., Sinemet). However, *the dosage of levodopa must be reduced by up to 80% when combined with carbidopa*. This decreases the incidence of levodopa-induced side effects.

Note: Pyridoxine will not reverse the action of carbidopa/levodopa.

Uses   All types of parkinsonism. *Investigational:* Postanoxic intention myoclonus.
See Levodopa, p. 440. **WARNING**: Levodopa must be discontinued at least 8 hr before carbidopa/levodopa therapy is initiated. Also, patients taking carbidopa/levodopa must not take levodopa concomitantly, because the former is a combination of carbidopa and levodopa.

Contraindications   See Levodopa, p. 440. History of melanoma. MAO inhibitors should be stopped 2 weeks before therapy.

Untoward Reactions   See Levodopa, p. 440. Also, because more levodopa reaches the brain, dyskinesias may occur at lower doses with carbidopa/levodopa than with levodopa alone.

Drug Interactions   Use with tricyclic antidepressants may cause hypertension and dyskinesia.

Dosage   Individualized. *Patients not receiving levodopa:* **initial,** 1 tablet of 10 mg carbidopa/100 mg levodopa or 25 mg carbidopa/100 mg levodopa t.i.d.; **then,** increase by 1 tablet every 1–2 days until a total of 6 tablets/day is taken. If additional levodopa is required, substitute 1 tablet of 25 mg carbidopa/250 mg levodopa t.i.d.–q.i.d. *Patients receiving levodopa:* **initial,** carbidopa/levodopa dosage should be about 25% of prior levodopa dosage (levodopa dosage is discontinued 8 hr before carbidopa/levodopa initiated); **then,** adjust dosage as required.
Carbidopa is available alone for patients requiring additional carbidopa, i.e. inadequate reduction in nausea and vomiting.

Additional Nursing Implications
See also *Nursing Implications*, p. 433.

1. Assess patient closely during the dose-adjustment period for involuntary movement, which may necessitate dosage reduction.
2. Assess for blepharospasm, which is an early sign of excessive dosage in some patients.
3. Do not administer with levodopa.
4. Facilitate patient's adjustment to change to medication by administering last dose of levodopa at bedtime and starting carbidopa/levodopa when patient arises in AM.

DIPHENHYDRAMINE HYDROCHLORIDE Allerdryl,* Bay Dryl, Belix, Bena-D and -D 50, Benadryl, Benahist 10 and 50, Benaphen, Bendylate, Benaject-10 and -50, Benylin, Diahist, Dihydrex, Diphen Cough, Diphenacen-10 and -50, Fenylhist, Fynex Cough, Hydril Cough, Hyrexin-50, Noradryl, Phen-Amin, Tusstat, Valdrene, Wehdryl-50 (Rx)

Classification Antihistamine.

Uses This antihistamine (see Chapter 51, p. 627) is useful for treating parkinsonism in geriatric patients unable to tolerate more potent drugs. Also for mild parkinsonism in other age groups. Drug-induced extrapyramidal symptoms.

Dosage **PO. Adults**: 25–50 mg t.i.d.–q.i.d.; **pediatric, over 20 lb**: 12.5–25 mg t.i.d.– q.i.d. (or 5 mg/kg/day). **IM, IV. Adults**: 10–50 mg (up to 100 mg may be necessary); maximum daily dose: 400 mg. **Pediatric**: 5 mg/kg/day divided into 4 doses; maximum daily dose: 300 mg.

LEVODOPA Dopar, Larodopa, L-Dopa (Rx)

Classification Antiparkinson agent.

General Statement Levodopa is effective in more than one-half the patients with parkinsonism. It, however, only provides symptomatic relief and does not alter the course of the disease. When effective it relieves rigidity, bradykinesia, tremors, dysphagia, seborrhea, sialorrhea, and postural instability.

Periodic hepatic, hematopoietic, cardiovascular and renal function tests should be performed on patients receiving long-term therapy. Levodopa is often administered together with an anticholinergic agent.

Action/Kinetics Levodopa, a dopamine precursor, is able to cross the blood–brain barrier. In the CNS it is converted to dopamine, thus replenishing depleted dopamine stores characteristic of parkinsonism. **Peak plasma levels**: 1–2 hr (may be delayed if ingested with food). Levodopa is extensively metabolized both in the GI tract and the liver and metabolites are excreted in the urine.

Uses Idiopathic, arteriosclerotic, or postencephalitic parkinsonism. Parkinsonism due to carbon monoxide or magnesium intoxication. *Investigational:* Pain from herpes zoster.

Contraindications Hypersensitivity to drug, narrow-angle glaucoma, blood dyscrasias, hypertension, coronary sclerosis. Use with extreme caution in patients with history of myocardial infarctions, convulsions, arrhythmias, bronchial asthma, emphysema, active peptic ulcer, psychosis or neurosis, wide-angle glaucoma.

Untoward Reactions The side effects of levodopa are numerous and usually dose related. Some may abate with usage.

GI effects include anorexia, nausea, vomiting, duodenal ulcer, GI bleeding, constipation, diarrhea, epigastric and abdominal distress, pain, flatulence, eructation, hiccups, sialorrhea, bitter taste, dry mouth, tightness of lips or tongue, difficulty in swallowing, burning sensation of the tongue.

Cardiac irregularities and orthostatic hypotension occur frequently. ECG abnormalities, palpitations, hypertension, flushing, and phlebitis occur more rarely, but their appearance necessitates discontinuation of drug.

Neurologic effects include grimacing, bruxism (grinding of teeth), twisting of tongue, waving of neck, hands, and feet, jerky and involuntary movements. Dizziness, sedation, dyskinesia, agitation, anxiety, confusion, depression, mental changes, antisocial behavior, ataxia, convulsions, torticollis and many other such neurologic and psychological effects. Less frequently, suicidal tendencies, increased libido, and possibly associated antisocial behavior.

Also respiratory side effects, such as cough, hoarseness, bizarre breathing patterns; increased urinary frequency, retention, incontinence, hematuria, dark urine, and nocturia. Blurred vision, diplopia, changes in blood cells, fever, hot flashes, and changes in many laboratory value parameters.

Levodopa interacts with many other drugs (see below) and must be administered cautiously.

Drug Interactions

Interactant	Interaction
Amphetamines	Levodopa potentiates the effect of indirectly acting sympathomimetics
Antacids	↑ Effect of levodopa due to ↑ absorption from GI tract
Anticholinergic drugs	Possible ↓ effect of levodopa due to ↑ breakdown of levodopa in stomach (due to delayed gastric emptying time)
Antidepressants, tricyclic	↓ Effect of levodopa due to ↓ absorption from GI tract; also, ↑ risk hypertension
Clonidine	↓ Effect of levodopa
Digoxin	↓ Effect of digoxin
Ephedrine	Levodopa potentiates the effect of indirectly acting sympathomimetics
Furazolidone	↑ Effect of levodopa due to ↓ breakdown
Guanethidine	↑ Hypotensive effect of guanethidine
Hypoglycemic drugs	Levodopa upsets diabetic control with hypoglycemic agents
Methyldopa	Additive effects including hypotension
MAO inhibitors	Concomitant administration may result in hypertension, lightheadedness, and flushing due to ↓ breakdown of dopamine and norepinephrine formed from levodopa
Papaverine	↓ Effect of levodopa
Phenothiazines	↓ Effect of levodopa due to ↓ uptake of dopamine into neurons
Phenytoin	Phenytoin antagonizes the effect of levodopa
Propranolol	Propranolol may antagonize the hypotensive and positive inotropic effect of levodopa
Pyridoxine	Pyridoxine reverses levodopa-induced improvement in Parkinson's disease.
Reserpine	Reserpine inhibits response to levodopa by ↓ dopamine in the brain
Thioxanthines	↓ Effect of levodopa in Parkinson patients

Laboratory Test Interferences   ↑ BUN, SGOT, LDH, SGPT, bilirubin, alkaline phosphatase, protein-bound iodine. False + Coombs' test. Interference with tests for urinary glucose and ketones.

Dosage **PO** (with meals). **Usual initial**: 0.5–1 gm/day divided in 2 doses; **then**, increase total daily dose by no more than 0.75 gm q 3–7 days until optimum dosage reached (should not exceed 8 gm/day). Up to 6 months may be required to achieve a significant therapeutic effect.

Administration

1. Administer to patients unable to swallow tablets or capsules by crushing tablets or emptying capsule into a small amount of fruit juice at time of administration.
2. The urine or sweat may darken; this is not harmful.

Additional Nursing Implications

See also *Nursing Implications*, p. 433.

1. Check with medical supervision whether drug is to be stopped 24 hours before surgery, and ascertain when the drug is to be reinstituted.
2. *Teach patient and/or family*
   a. that dosage of drug is not to exceed 8 gm daily.
   b. not to take multivitamin preparations containing 10–25 mg of vitamin B_6, which rapidly reverses the antiparkinson effect of levodopa.
   c. to continue drug even though effects may not yet be evident. Takes up to 6 months for significant effect.

Chapter Thirty-five

CENTRALLY ACTING SKELETAL MUSCLE RELAXANTS

Action/Kinetics　The centrally acting skeletal muscle relaxants decrease muscle tone and involuntary movement. Many relieve anxiety and tension as well. Although the precise mechanism of action is unknown, most of these agents depress spinal polysynaptic reflexes. Their beneficial effects may also be attributable to their antianxiety activity. Several of the drugs in this group also manifest analgesic properties.

Uses Musculoskeletal and neurologic disorders associated with muscle spasms, hyperreflexia, and hypertonia, including parkinsonism, tetanus, tension headaches, acute muscle spasms caused by trauma, and inflammation (e.g., low back syndrome, sprains, arthritis, bursitis). They also may be useful in the mangement of cerebral palsy and multiple sclerosis.

Untoward Reactions Untoward reactions often involve the central nervous system, gastrointestinal system, and urinary system. Symptoms of allergy may also be manifested. For specific untoward reactions, see individual drugs.

Drug Interactions Centrally acting muscle relaxants may increase the sedative and respiratory depressant effects of CNS depressants, for example, alcohol, barbiturates, sedatives and hypnotics, and antianxiety agents.

Dosage The drugs seem to be more effective when administered parenterally. For dosage, see individual agents.

Overdosage

SYMPTOMS Symptoms of overdosage are often extensions of the untoward reactions. Stupor, coma, shock-like syndrome, respiratory depression, loss of muscle tone, and impaired deep tendon reflexes may also occur.

TREATMENT Symptomatic. Emesis or gastric lavage (followed by activated charcoal). If necessary, artificial respiration, oxygen administration, pressor agents, and IV fluids may be used. It may be possible to increase the rate of excretion of selected drugs by diuretics (including mannitol), peritoneal dialysis, or hemodialysis.

> **Nursing Implication**
> Since these drugs cause drowsiness, patients should be instructed not to operate dangerous machinery or drive a car.

BACLOFEN   Lioresal, Lioresal DS (Rx)

Classification Centrally acting muscle relaxant.

Action/Kinetics The mechanism of action of baclofen is not fully known, but the drug is known to inhibit both mono- and polysynaptic spinal reflexes. It may also act at certain brain sites. **Peak serum levels**: 2 hr. t½: 3–4 hr. The drug is eliminated unchanged by the kidney.

Uses Multiple sclerosis (flexor spasms, pain, clonus, and muscular rigidity) and diseases and injuries of the spinal cord associated with spasticity. It is not effective for the treatment of cerebral palsy, stroke, parkinsonism, or rheumatic disorders.

Contraindications Hypersensitivity. Safe use in pregnancy or for children under 12 years of age not established. Rheumatic disorders, spasm resulting from Parkinson's disease, stroke, cerebral palsy.

Untoward Reactions *CNS*: Drowsiness, dizziness, weakness, fatigue, confusion, headaches, insomnia. Hallucinations following abrupt withdrawal. *Cardiovascular*: Hypotension. *GI*: Nausea, constipation. *GU*: Urinary frequency. *Other:* Rash, pruritus, ankle edema, increased perspiration, weight gain, fainting, nasal congestion.

Drug Interactions Concomitant use with CNS depressants → additive CNS depression.

Laboratory Test Interference ↑ SGOT, alkaline phosphatase, blood glucose.

Dosage PO. Initial, 5 mg t.i.d. for 3 days; **then,** increase by 5 mg t.i.d. q 3 days until optimum effective dosage is established. Maximum daily dosage should not exceed 20 mg q.i.d.

Administration If beneficial effects are not noted, the drug should be slowly withdrawn.

Nursing Implications
1. Report to medical supervision patients who use spasticity to stand upright, maintain balance when walking, or to increase their function. Baclofen may be contraindicated in these instances because it interferes with patients' coping mechanisms.
2. Assess epileptics for clinical signs and symptoms of disease, and arrange for EEG at regular intervals, because reduction in seizure control has been associated with baclofen.
3. Assist with lavage and maintain adequate respiratory exchange in treatment of overdosage. Do not use respiratory stimulants.
4. *Teach patient and/or family*
    a. not to operate an automobile or other dangerous machinery, because the major side effects of drug are drowsiness, dizziness, weakness, and fatigue.
    b. not to drink alcohol and/or take other CNS depressants, because effects may be additive.

CARISOPRODOL Rela, Soma, Sporodol (Rx)

Classification Centrally acting muscle relaxant.

Action/Kinetics Carisoprodol may produce skeletal muscle relaxation by inhibiting synaptic reflexes in the descending reticular formation and spinal cord. Its sedative effects may also be responsible for muscle relaxation. **Onset:** 30 min. **Duration:** 4–6 hr. **t½:** 8 hr.

Uses As an adjunct in skeletal muscle disorders including bursitis, low back disorders, contusions, fibrositis, spondylitis, sprains, muscle strains, and cerebral palsy.

Contraindications Porphyria. Hypersensitivity to carisoprodol or meprobamate. Children under 12 years of age. Use with caution in impaired liver or kidney function.

Untoward Reactions *CNS:* Ataxia, dizziness, drowsiness, excitement, tremor, syncope, vertigo, insomnia. *GI:* Nausea, vomiting, gastric upset, hiccoughs. *Cardiovascular:* Flushing of face, postural hypotension, tachycardia. *Allergic reactions:* Including dermatologic and hematologic symptoms.

Drug Interactions

Interactant	Interaction
Alcohol	Additive CNS depressant effects
Antidepressants, tricyclic	↑ Effect of carisoprodol
Barbiturates	Possible ↑ effect of carisoprodol, followed by inhibition of carisoprodol
Chlorcyclizine	↓ Effect of carisoprodol
CNS depressants	Additive CNS depression
MAO inhibitors	↑ Effect of carisoprodol by ↓ breakdown by liver
Phenobarbital	↓ Effect of carisoprodol by ↑ breakdown by liver
Phenothiazines	Additive depressant effects

Dosage   **PO**: 350 mg q.i.d. (take last dose at bedtime).

Administration   For patients unable to swallow tablets, mix with a flavoring agent such as jelly, syrup, or chocolate.

CHLORPHENESIN CARBAMATE   Maolate (Rx)

Classification   Centrally acting muscle relaxant.

Action/Kinetics   The action is thought to be due to depression of polysynaptic spinal reflexes as well as the sedative effects of the drug. **Peak serum concentration**: 1–3 hr. **t½**: 3.5 hr. Rapidly excreted in the urine as inactive metabolites.

Uses   As an adjunct for muscle spasms and muscle pain secondary to sprains, trauma, or inflammation.

Additional Contraindications   Hepatic dysfunction; hypersensitivity to drug.

Dosage   **PO**: **initial,** 800 mg t.i.d.; **maintenance,** 400 mg q.i.d. Safety for use longer than 8 weeks has not been established.

CHLORZOXAZONE   Paraflex (Rx)

Classification   Centrally acting muscle relaxant.

Action/Kinetics   Chlorzoxazone inhibits polysynaptic reflexes at both the spinal cord and subcortical areas of the brain. Its effect may also be due to the sedative properties of the drug. **Peak blood levels:** 3–4 hr. **Onset:** 1 hr. **Duration:** 3–4 hr. **t½:** 1 hr. The drug is metabolized in the liver and inactive metabolites excreted in the urine.

Note: Chlorzoxazone is also found in Parafon Forte. See Appendix 3.

Uses   Muscle spasms associated with low back pain, fibrositis, bursitis, myositis, spondylitis, sprains, muscle strain, torticollis, cervical root and disk syndrome.

Dosage   **PO. Adults:** 250–750 mg t.i.d.–q.i.d. with meals and at bedtime; **pediatric:** 125–500 mg t.i.d.–q.i.d.

Administration
1. Administer at mealtime to minimize gastric irritation.
2. May be mixed with food or beverages for administration to children.

Nursing Implications
1. Advise the patient that this drug may cause urine to appear orange or purple-red in color when it is exposed to air.
2. Since the drug causes drowsiness, patients should be instructed not to operate dangerous machinery or drive a car.

CYCLOBENZAPRINE HYDROCHLORIDE Flexeril (Rx)

Classification Centrally acting muscle relaxant.

Action/Kinetics Structurally and pharmacologically, cyclobenzaprine is related to the tricyclic antidepressants and possesses both sedative and anticholinergic properties. In contrast to many skeletal muscle relaxants, cyclobenzaprine hydrochloride is thought to act mainly at the level of the brainstem (as compared to spinal cord) to inhibit reflexes. **Peak plasma levels:** 4–6 hr. **Onset:** 1 hr. **Duration:** up to 24 hr. **t½:** 1–3 days. The drug is highly bound to plasma protein. Inactive metabolites are excreted in the urine.

Uses Adjunct to rest and physical therapy for relief of muscle spasms associated with acute and/or painful musculoskeletal conditions. It is not indicated for the treatment of spastic diseases or for cerebral palsy.

Contraindications Hypersensitivity. Arrhythmias, heart block, CHF, or soon after myocardial infarctions. Hyperthyroidism. Due to atropine-like effects, use with caution in situations where cholinergic blockade is not desired. Safe use in pregnancy, lactation, and in children under age 15 has not been established.

Untoward Reactions Symptoms of cholinergic blockade including dry mouth, dizziness, tachycardia, blurred vision, urinary retention. Also, drowsiness, weakness, dyspepsia, paresthesia, unpleasant taste, insomnia. Since cyclobenzaprine resembles tricyclic antidepressants, untoward reactions for these drugs should also be noted (p. 426).

Physostigmine salicylate, 1–3 mg, may be used to reverse symptoms of severe cholinergic blockade.

Drug Interactions

Interactant	Interaction
Anticholinergics	Additive anticholinergic side effects
CNS depressants	Additive depressant effects
Guanethidine	Cyclobenzaprine may block effect
MAO inhibitors	Hypertensive crisis, severe convulsions
Tricyclic antidepressants	Additive side effects

Dosage **PO:** *usual*; 10 mg t.i.d., up to 60 mg daily in divided doses.

Administration
1. Use cyclobenzaprine for 2–3 weeks only.

2. Do not administer for a minimum of 2 weeks after patient has received mono-amine oxidase inhibitor drugs.

Additional Nursing Implications
See *Nursing Implications* for *Tricyclic Antidepressants*, p. 428.

Teach patient not to extend course of medication beyond 2–3 weeks; longer therapy with this drug is contraindicated.

DANTROLENE SODIUM   Dantrium, Dantrium Intravenous (Rx)

Classification   Centrally acting muscle relaxant.

Action/Kinetics   Dantrolene is a hydantoin derivative and, as such, is chemically unrelated to other skeletal muscle relaxants. It acts directly on skeletal muscle probably by dissociating the excitation-contraction coupling mechanism. This action results in a decreased force of reflex muscle contraction and a reduction of hyperreflexia, spasticity, involuntary movements, and clonus. Absorption is slow and incomplete, but consistent. t½: **oral**, 8.7 hr; t½: **IV**, 5 hr. There is significant plasma protein binding of the drug.

Uses   Muscle spasticity associated with severe chronic disorders, such as multiple sclerosis, cerebral palsy, spinal cord injury, and stroke. Muscle pain due to exercise. Malignant hyperthermia due to hypermetabolism of skeletal muscle. *Investigational:* Exercise-induced muscle pain.

Contraindications   Rheumatic diseases, pregnancy, nursing mothers, or children under 5 years of age. Acute hepatitis and cirrhosis of the liver. Use with caution in impaired pulmonary function.

Untoward Reactions   Fatal and nonfatal hepatotoxicity. *CNS:* Drowsiness, dizziness, weakness, malaise, lightheadedness, headaches, insomnia, seizures, speech disturbances, fatigue, confusion, depression, nervousness. *GI:* Diarrhea (common), anorexia, gastric upset, cramps, GI bleeding. *Musculoskeletal:* Backache, myalgia. *Dermatologic:* Rashes, photosensitivity, pruritus, urticaria, hair growth, sweating. *Cardiovascular:* Blood pressure changes, phlebitis, tachycardia. *Genitourinary:* Urinary retention, hematuria, crystalluria, nocturia, impotence. *Miscellaneous:* Visual disturbances, chills, fever, tearing, feelings of suffocation, pleural effusion with pericarditis.

Untoward reactions are dose related and decrease with usage. Side effects listed are following oral use.

Dosage   PO. *Spastic conditions.* **Adults: initial**, 25 mg/day; **then**, increase to 25 mg b.i.d.–q.i.d.; dose may then be increased by 25-mg increments up to 100 mg b.i.d.–q.i.d. (doses in excess of 400 mg/day not recommended). **Pediatric: initial**, 0.5 mg/kg b.i.d.; **then**, increase to 0.5 mg/kg t.i.d.–q.i.d.; dose may then be increased by increments of 0.5 mg/kg to 3 mg/kg b.i.d.–q.i.d. (doses should not exceed 400 mg/day.). *Malignant hyperthermia, preoperatively.* **Adults and children:** 4–8 mg/kg daily in 3–4 divided doses 1–2 days before surgery. **IV. Malignant hyperthermia, crisis treatment: Adults and children, initial**, 1 mg/kg rapidly; dose may be repeated to cumulative dose of 10 mg/kg; **then,** to prevent recurrence, 4–8 mg/kg/day orally in divided doses.

Administration

1. Can be given in fruit juice or other liquid vehicle.
2. Beneficial effects may not be seen for 1 week for spasticity and the drug should be discontinued after 6 weeks if beneficial effects not evident.
3. Due to potential hepatotoxicity, long-term benefits must be evaluated for each patient.
4. Reconstituted solution should be protected from light and used within 6 hr.

Nursing Implications

1. Encourage the patient by telling him that the effect of drug may become apparent after 1 week and that side effects decrease with usage.
2. Since this drug causes drowsiness, patients should be instructed not to operate dangerous machinery or drive a car.

DIAZEPAM   Valium (Rx)

Antianxiety agent and muscle relaxant. For details, see Table 13, p. 395.

METAXALONE   Skelaxin (Rx)

Classification   Centrally acting muscle relaxant.

Action/Kinetics   The beneficial effects of metaxalone may be due to its sedative effects. The drug resembles meprobamate. **Onset:** 1 hr. **Duration:** 4–6 hr. **t½:** 2–3 hr.

Uses   As an adjunct for acute skeletal muscle spasm associated with sprains, strains, dislocation, and other trauma.

Contraindications   Liver disease, epilepsy, impaired renal function, history of drug-induced hemolytic or other anemias, pregnancy, children under 12 years.

Untoward Reactions   *CNS:* Drowsiness, dizziness, headache, nervousness, irritability. *GI:* Nausea, vomiting, gastric upset. *Miscellaneous:* Allergic reactions, jaundice, leukopenia, hemolytic anemia.

Dosage   **PO. Adults and children over 12 yr of age:** 800 mg t.i.d.–q.i.d.

Nursing Implications

1. *Assess*
   a. for abdominal pain, high fever, nausea, and diarrhea (early symptoms of hepatotoxicity).
   b. for sore throat, fever, and lassitude (symptoms of blood dyscrasias).
   c. patient with history of grand mal for accentuation of seizures precipitated by metaxalone.

2. Encourage rinsing of mouth and intake of more fluids in diet to relieve dryness of mouth.
3. Since drug causes drowsiness, patients should be instructed not to operate dangerous machinery or drive a car.

METHOCARBAMOL   Delaxin, Marbaxin-750, Robaxin, Robaxin-750 (Rx)

Classification   Centrally acting muscle relaxant.

Action/Kinetics   The beneficial action of methocarbamol may be related to the sedative properties of the drug. Of limited usefulness. The drug may be given IM or IV in polyethylene glycol 300 (50% solution). PO therapy should be initiated as soon as possible. **Onset**: 30 min. **t½**: 1–2 hr.

Uses   Muscle spasms associated with sprains and/or trauma, acute back pain due to nerve irritation or discogenic disease, postoperative orthopedic procedures, bursitis, and torticollis. Acute phase muscle spasms. Adjunct in tetanus.

Contraindications   Hypersensitivity, when muscle spasticity is required to maintain upright position, pregnancy, lactation, children under 12 years. Renal disease (parenteral dosage form only). Use with caution in epilepsy.

Untoward Reactions   *Following PO use. CNS:* Dizziness, drowsiness, lightheadedness, vertigo, lassitude, headache. *GI:* Nausea. *Miscellaneous:* Allergic symptoms including rash, urticaria, pruritus, conjunctivitis, blurred vision, fever. *Following IV use (in addition to above). Cardiovascular:* Fainting, hypotension, bradycardia. *Miscellaneous:* Metallic taste, nasal congestion, flushing, nystagmus, double vision, thromboplebitis, pain at injection site, anaphylaxis.

Drug Interaction   CNS depressants (including alcohol) may increase the effect of methocarbamol.

Laboratory Test Interference   Color interference for 5-hydroxyindoleacetic acid (5-HIAA) and vanillylmandelic acid (VMA).

Dosage   **PO. Adults, initial**: 1.5 gm q.i.d.; **maintenance**: 1 gm q.i.d.
   (*Note*:   for the first 48–72 hrs, 6 gm/day recommended).
   IM, IV: usual initial, 1 gm; in severe cases, up to 2–3 gm may be necessary. **IV administration should not exceed 3 days.** *Tetanus*: **IV**, 1–3 gm given into tube of previously inserted indwelling needle. May be given q 6 hr until **PO** administration is feasible.

Administration
1. Rate of IV not to exceed 3 ml/min.
2. For IV drip, one ampule may be added to not more than 250 ml of sodium chloride or 5% dextrose injection.
3. Clamp off tubing before removing IV, to prevent extravasation of hypertonic solution which may cause thrombophlebitis.
4. For IM use, inject no more than 5 ml into each gluteal region.

Nursing Implications

1. Position the patient in recumbent position during IV administration and have him maintain this position for 10 to 15 minutes after injection to minimize postural hypotensive side effects.
2. Advise the patient to lie down immediately if he feels faint.
3. Check IV for infiltration frequently because extravasation of fluid may cause thrombophlebitis or sloughing.
4. Have side rails in place unless the patient is attended during IV administration. Use seizure precautions.
5. Have the patient rise slowly from a recumbent position and dangle feet before standing up.
6. Since drug causes drowsiness, patients should be instructed not to operate dangerous machinery or drive a car.

ORPHENADRINE CITRATE   Banflex, Flexoject, Flexon, K-Flex, Myolin, Neocyten, Norflex, O-Flex, Orflagen, Orphenate, X-Otag, X-Otag S.R. (Rx)

Classification   Centrally acting muscle relaxant.

Action/Kinetics   Action may be related, in part, to its analgesic effects. It also possesses anticholinergic activity. **Peak effect:** 2 hr. **Duration:** 4–6 hr. **t½:** 14 hr.

Uses   Adjunct to the treatment of acute musculoskeletal disorders.

Contraindications   Angle-closure glaucoma, stenosing peptic ulcers, prostatic hypertrophy, pyloric or duodenal obstruction, cardiospasm, and myasthenia gravis. Use in pregnancy, children. Use with caution in cardiac disease.

Untoward Reactions   Anticholinergic effects, including dryness of mouth, tachycardia, urinary retention, blurred vision, constipation. Also, symptoms of allergy, gastric irritation, tremor, headache, dizziness.

Drug Interactions

Interactant	Interaction
Anticholinergics	↑ Effect of anticholinergic drugs
Contraceptives, oral	Orphenadrine ↑ breakdown by liver
Griseofulvin	Orphenadrine ↑ breakdown by liver
Propoxyphene	Concomitant use may result in anxiety, tremors, and confusion

Dosage   PO: 100 mg b.i.d. **IV or IM:** 60 mg. May be repeated q 12 hr.

Administration   IV injections should be given over a period of 5 min with the patient in a supine position; IV administration should be followed by a 5–10 min rest period.

Nursing Implications

1. Observe the patient for dryness of mouth, which indicates need for reduction of dosage.

2. Encourage rinsing of mouth and more fluids in diet to relieve dryness of mouth.
3. Since drug causes drowsiness, patients should be instructed not to operate dangerous machinery or drive a car.

Chapter Thirty-six

ANTICONVULSANTS

General Statement Anticonvulsant agents are used for the control of the chronic seizures and involuntary muscle spasms or movements characteristic of certain neurologic diseases. They are most frequently used in the therapy of epilepsy, which results from disorders of nerve impulse transmission in the brain.

Therapeutic agents cannot cure these convulsive disorders, but they attempt to suppress their manifestations without impairing the normal functions of the CNS. This is often accomplished by selective depression of hyperactive areas of the brain responsible for the convulsions. Therefore, these drugs are taken at all times (prophylactically) to prevent the occurrence of the seizures.

There are several different types of epileptic disorders, including tonic-clonic (grand mal), absence seizures (petit mal), and psychomotor epilepsy. All the drugs listed under this group of anticonvulsants are not effective against all types of epilepsy; only certain ones can be used for each type of disorder (see individual drugs). Drugs effective against one type of epilepsy may not be effective against another.

Barbiturates, especially phenobarbital, mephobarbital, and metharbital, are effective anticonvulsant drugs. They were discussed in Chapter 29, p. 370.

Anticonvulsant therapy must be individualized. Therapy begins with a small dose of the drug, which is continuously increased until either the seizures disappear or drug toxicity occurs. If a certain drug decreases the frequency of seizures but does not completely prevent them, another drug can be added to the dosage regimen and administered concomitantly with the first. Often a drug is ineffective and then another agent must be given. Failure of therapy most often results from the administration of doses too small to have a therapeutic effect and from failure to use two or more drugs together.

If for any reason drug therapy is discontinued, the anticonvulsant drugs must be withdrawn gradually over a period of days or weeks to avoid severe, prolonged convulsions. This rule also applies when one anticonvulsant is substituted for another. The dosage of the second drug is built up at the same time the first drug is being reduced.

With modern drugs, four out of five cases of epilepsy can be controlled adequately, but it may take the physician some time to find the best drug or combination of drugs with which to treat the patient. Anticonvulsants may cause postpartum hemorrhages, as well as birth and coagulation defects in neonates of patients on these drugs.

Dosage   Dosage is highly individualized. However, trauma or emotional stress may necessitate an increase in drug dosage requirements (e.g., if the patient requires surgery and starts having seizures). For details see individual agents.

Administration

1. Anticonvulsants may be taken with food to decrease GI upset.
2. Medication should not be discontinued abruptly without physician advice.
3. Many anticonvulsants interfere with driving or performing tasks requiring alertness.
4. Individuals on anticonvulsant therapy should carry identification indicating epilepsy and the drug therapy being taken.

Nursing Implications

1. Check whether the patient has a history of hypersensitivity to a particular type of anticonvulsant; if so, derivatives of that type should not be administered (e.g., if the patient has shown hypersensitivity to any of the hydantoins, he should not be administered any other drug of this type).
2. Check whether the physician wishes the patient to have folic acid supplementation to prevent megaloblastic anemia.
3. Check whether the physician wishes the patient to have vitamin D supplementation to prevent hypocalcemia (4,000 units of vitamin D per week is the usual dose).
4. Anticipate that vitamin K will be administered to pregnant women 1 month before parturition to prevent bleeding in the newborn.
5. Monitor patient closely after IV administration of anticonvulsants for respiratory depression and cardiovascular collapse. Be prepared, in case of acute toxicity, to assist with inducing emesis (provided the patient is not comatose) and with gastric lavage along with other supportive measures such as administration of fluids and oxygen.
6. Anticipate that peritoneal dialysis or hemodialysis may be instituted in the treat-

ment of acute toxicity for barbiturates and hydantoins and hemodialysis for succinimides.

7. *Teach patient and/or family*

a. the need for close medical supervision during anticonvulsant therapy.

b. to take the prescribed doses of the drug.

c. that anticonvulsant drugs are not to be increased, decreased, or discontinued without medical supervision because convulsions may result.

d. that excessive use of alcohol may interfere with the action of anticonvulsants.

e. during initiation of therapy not to perform hazardous tasks requiring mental alertness and coordination, because the anticonvulsants often cause drowsiness, vertigo, headache, and ataxia. CNS symptoms are often dose related and may disappear with a change of dosage or continued therapy.

f. that GI distress may be minimized by taking medication with large amounts of fluid or with food.

g. to report rash, fever, severe headache, stomatitis, rhinitis, urethritis, or balanitis (inflammation of the glans penis), which are early signs of hypersensitivity syndromes.

h. how to avoid fever, low blood sugar, and low salt, since these lower the seizure threshold.

i. to report sore throat, easy bruising, petechiae, or nosebleeds, which are signs of hematologic toxicity. Hematologic studies should be performed before initiation of therapy and at periodic intervals during therapy.

j. to report jaundice, dark urine, anorexia, and abdominal pain, which are signs of hepatotoxicity. Liver function tests should be performed before initiation of therapy and at periodic intervals during therapy.

k. to discuss with doctor the effects of medication on pregnancy, if conception were to occur.

l. to observe a nursing infant whose mother is on anticonvulsant therapy for signs of drug toxicity and report.

m. to inform doctor of unusual events in the patient's life, since dosage requirements may change when the patient is undergoing trauma or emotional stress.

HYDANTOINS

General Statement   The hydantoins currently used for the treatment of epilepsy and other convulsive disorders are phenytoin, ethotoin, and mephenytoin. Of these, phenytoin (Dilantin) is the most widely used. However, patients refractory to phenytoin may respond to one of the other hydantoins.

Action/Kinetics   The hydantoins act in the motor cortex of the brain to reduce the spread of electrical discharges from the rapidly firing epileptic foci in this area. This is accomplished by stabilizing hyperexcitable cells possibly by affecting sodium efflux. Also, the hydantoins decrease activity of centers in the brain stem responsible for the tonic phase of grand mal seizures. These drugs have few sedative effects.

Uses   Chronic epilepsy, especially of the tonic-clonic, psychomotor type. Not effective against petit mal and may even increase the frequency of seizures in this disorder. Parenteral phenytoin is sometimes used to treat status epilepticus, to control seizures during neurosurgery, and in cardiac arrhythmias.

Contraindications Hypersensitivity to hydantoins or exfoliative dermatitis. Administer with extreme caution to patients with a history of asthma or other allergies, impaired renal or hepatic function, and heart disease. Should not be administered to nursing mothers. Use with caution in porphyria.

Untoward Reactions *CNS:* Drowsiness, incoordination, ataxia, slurred speech, dizziness, extrapyramidal reactions, paradoxical increase in motor activity, psychotomimetic effects including hallucinations and delusions, fatigue, insomnia, and apathy. *GI:* Nausea, vomiting, either diarrhea or constipation. *Dermatologic:* Various dermatoses including a measles-like rash (common), scarlatiniform, maculopapular, and urticarial rashes. Rarely, drug-induced lupus erythematosus, Stevens-Johnson syndrome, exfoliative or purpuric dermatitis, and toxic epidermal necrolysis. Skin reactions may necessitate withdrawal of therapy. *Hematopoietic:* Megaloblastic anemia, lymph node hyperplasia, thrombocytopenia, leukopenia, agranulocytosis, pancytopenia, anemias including hemolytic and aplastic. *Hepatic:* Hepatitis, jaundice, toxic hepatitis. *Miscellaneous:* Hyperglycemia, osteomalacia, gingival hyperplasia (with phenytoin), hirsutism, pulmonary fibrosis, alopecia, edema, photophobia.

Rapid parenteral administration may cause serious cardiovascular effects, including hypotension, arrhythmias, cardiovascular collapse, and heart block, as well as CNS depression.

Overdosage is characterized by nystagmus, ataxia, dysarthria, coma, unresponsive pupils, hypotension, as well as by some of the CNS effects described above.

Many patients have a partial deficiency in the ability of the liver to degrade phenytoin, and as a result toxicity may develop after a small oral dose. Liver and kidney function tests and hematopoietic studies are indicated prior to and periodically during drug therapy.

Drug Interactions (Phenytoin)

Interactant	Interaction
Alcohol, ethyl	In alcoholics, ↓ effect of phenytoin due to ↑ breakdown by liver
Allopurinol	↑ Effect of phenytoin due to ↓ breakdown by liver
Antacids	↓ Effect of phenytoin due to ↓ GI absorption
Anticoagulants, oral	↑ Effect of phenytoin due to ↓ breakdown in liver. Also, possible ↑ in anticoagulant effect by ↓ plasma protein binding
Antidepressants, tricyclic	May ↑ incidence of epileptic seizures or ↑ effect of phenytoin
Barbiturates	Effect of phenytoin may be ↑, ↓, or not changed; possible ↑ effect of barbiturates
Benzodiazepines	↑ Effect of phenytoin due to ↓ breakdown by liver
Carbamazepine	↓ Effect of phenytoin due to ↑ breakdown by liver
Chloral hydrate	↓ Effect of phenytoin due to ↑ breakdown by liver
Chloramphenicol	↑ Effect of phenytoin due to ↓ breakdown by liver
Cimetidine	↑ Effect of phenytoin due to ↓ breakdown by liver
Contraceptives, oral	Estrogen-induced fluid retention may precipitate seizures; also, ↓ effect of contraceptives due to ↑ breakdown by liver

Interactant	Interaction
Corticosteroids	Effect of corticosteroids ↓ due to ↑ breakdown by liver
Cyclosporine	↓ Effect of cyclosporine due to ↑ breakdown by liver
Diazoxide	↓ Effect of phenytoin due to ↑ breakdown by liver
Dicoumarol	Phenytoin ↓ effect of dicoumarol
Digitalis glycosides	↓ Effect of digitalis glycosides by ↑ breakdown by liver
Disulfiram (Antabuse)	↑ Effect of phenytoin due to ↓ breakdown by liver
Dopamine	IV phenytoin results in hypotension and bradycardia
Doxycycline	↓ Effect of doxycycline due to ↑ breakdown by liver
Estrogens	See *Contraceptives, oral*
Folic acid	↓ Phenytoin blood levels due to ↑ breakdown by liver
Furosemide	↓ Effect of furosemide due to ↓ absorption
Haloperidol	↓ Effect of haloperidol due to ↑ breakdown by liver
Isoniazid	↑ Effect of phenytoin due to ↓ breakdown by liver
Levodopa	Phenytoin ↓ effect of levodopa
Meperidine	↓ Effect of meperidine due to ↑ breakdown by liver
Methadone	↓ Effect of methadone due to ↑ breakdown by liver
Methotrexate	↓ Effect of phenytoin due to ↓ absorption from GI tract
Metyrapone	↓ Effect of metyrapone due to ↑ breakdown by liver
Phenacemide	↑ Effect of phenytoin due to ↓ breakdown by liver
Phenothiazines	↑ Effect of phenytoin due to ↓ breakdown by liver
Phenylbutazone	↑ Effect of phenytoin due to ↓ breakdown by liver and ↓ plasma protein binding
Primidone	Possible ↑ effect of primidone
Quinidine	↓ Effect of quinidine due to ↑ breakdown by liver
Salicylates	↑ Effect of phenytoin by ↓ plasma protein binding
Sulfonamides	↑ Effect of phenytoin due to ↓ breakdown in liver
Sulfonylureas	↓ Effect of sulfonylureas
Theophylline	↓ Effect of both drugs due to ↑ breakdown by liver
Trimethoprim	↑ Effect of phenytoin due to ↓ breakdown by liver
Valproic acid	↑ Chance of phenytoin toxicity
Vinblastine	↑ Effect of phenytoin due to ↓ breakdown by liver

Laboratory Test Interferences Alters liver function tests, ↑ blood glucose values, and ↓ PBI values. ↑ Gammaglobulins. Phenytoin ↓ Immunoglobulins A and G.

Dosage See individual drugs. Full effectiveness of orally administered hydantoins is delayed and may take 6 to 9 days to be fully established. A similar period of time will elapse before effects disappear completely.

When hydantoins are substituted for or added to other anticonvulsant medication, their dosage is gradually increased, while dosage of the other drug is decreased proportionally.

Additional Nursing Implications

See also *Nursing Implications* for *Anticonvulsants*, p. 452.
Teach patient and/or family

a. not to take any other medication without medical supervision, because hydantoins interact with many other medications and the addition of other drugs may require adjustment of the anticonvulsant dose.

b. in cases of diabetes, to report any changes in fractional urine tests because hydantoins may affect blood sugar levels.

c. that hydantoin may cause urine to appear pink, red, or brown.

d. to practice good oral hygiene, including brushing, flossing, and gum massage, to minimize bleeding from gums.

e. to report excessive hair growth on face and trunk to physician.

f. the need for good skin care, because the androgenic effect of hydantoin on the hair follicle may cause acne.

ETHOTOIN   Peganone (Rx)

Classification   Anticonvulsant, hydantoin type.

General Statement   Ethotoin is said to be less toxic, but also less effective, than phenytoin. Serum level monitoring is necessary because serum concentrations may increase disproportionately with increasing doses. May be used with other anticonvulsant drugs (except phenacemide) for combined seizure disorders. Contraindicated in hepatic or hematologic disorders.

Action/Kinetics   The kinetics of ethotoin have not been widely studied. **Therapeutic plasma levels**: 15–50 μg/ml.

Dosage   PO: initial, individualized, 1 gm daily in 4 – 6 divided doses. Dosage is increased until control has been established. Usual **maintenance**: 2–3 gm daily; **pediatric: initial**, not to exceed 0.75 gm/day; **maintenance**: 0.5–1 gm/day (up to 2 or even 3 gm may be required in some patients).

MEPHENYTOIN   Mesantoin (Rx)

Classification   Anticonvulsant, hydantoin type.

General Statement   Mephenytoin is a potentially dangerous drug since it is more toxic than the other hydantoins and is to be used only for patients refractory to other anticonvulsants. Blood dycrasias, skin and mucous membrane manifestations, and central effects are more common than with other hydantoins. Also mephenytoin has a sedative effect, which phenytoin does not have. Liver function tests are indicated before initiating therapy.

Action/Kinetics   Rapidly absorbed from GI tract. Metabolized in liver to active metabolites.

Additional Uses   Focal and Jacksonian seizures and patients refractory to other drugs.

Dosage   PO, adults and children: initial, 50–100 mg daily to be increased gradually over a period of 8 to 10 weeks until symptoms are under control. Dosage should be taken at least one week before it is increased. Usual **maintenance, adults**: 200–600 mg in 3 to 4 divided doses; **pediatric maintenance**: 100–400 mg in 3 to 4 divided doses.

Additional Nursing Implications

See also *Nursing Implications*, p. 452.
Advise patients against running machinery since drowsiness occurs more frequently with this drug than with other hydantoins.

PHENYTOIN (DIPHENYLHYDANTOIN)   Dilantin Infatab, Dilantin-30 Pediatric, Dilantin-125, Novophenytoin* (Rx)

PHENYTOIN SODIUM, EXTENDED   Dilantin Kapseals (Rx)

PHENYTOIN SODIUM, PARENTERAL   Dilantin (Rx)

PHENYTOIN SODIUM PROMPT (DIPHENYLHYDANTOIN SODIUM) Diphenylan Sodium (Rx)

Classification   Anticonvulsant, hydantoin type.

Action/Kinetics   Serum levels must be monitored because the serum concentrations of phenytoin increase disproportionately as the dosage is increased. Phenytoin extended is designed for once a day dosage. It has a slow dissolution rate—no more than 35% in 30 min, 30–70% in 60 min, and less than 85% in 120 min. Absorption is variable following oral dosage. **Peak serum levels: PO**, 4–8 hr. Since the rate and extent of absorption depend on the particular preparation, the same product should be used for a particular patient. **Peak serum levels (following IM)**: 24 hr (wide variation). **Therapeutic serum levels**: 10–20 µg/ml. t½: 8–60 hr (average: 20–30 hr). Steady state attained 7–10 days after initiation. Phenytoin is biotransformed in the liver. Both inactive metabolites and unchanged drug are excreted in the urine.

Dosage   PO. Adults: 100 mg t.i.d. initially; adjust dosage until seizures are controlled (**usual, maintenance**: 300–400 mg/day, although 600 mg/day may be required in some). **Pediatric: initial**, 5 mg/kg/day in 2–3 divided doses; **maintenance**, 4–8 mg/kg (up to maximum of 300 mg/day). Children over 6 years may require up to 300 mg/day. Once dosage level has been established, the extended capsules may be used for once a day dosage. **IV**. *Status epilepticus*: 150–250 mg administered slowly; **then,** 100–150 mg after 30 min, if necessary. **Pediatric**: Dosage may be calculated on the basis of 250 mg/m². **IM**. If IM dosage is required in a patient stabilized on PO therapy, the IM dose should be 50% greater than the PO dose. *Neurosurgery*: 100–200 mg IM q 4 hr during and after surgery (during first 24 hr, no more than 1,000 mg should be administered; after first day, give maintenance dosage). *Phenytoin extended*: **PO: Maintenance only**, 300–400 mg as a single dose each day.

Administration (Parenteral)

1. Dilute with special diluent supplied by manufacturer. Vials must be shaken until solution is clear. The drug takes about 10 minutes to dissolve. The process can be hastened by warming the vial in warm water after the addition of the diluent. Drug is incompatible with acid solutions. Only a clear solution may be used.
2. Avoid subcutaneous or perivascular injection, as pain, inflammation, and necrosis may be caused by the highly alkaline solution.
3. Administer sodium chloride injection through the same needle or IV catheter after IV administration of the drug to avoid local irritation of the vein due to alkalinity of solution.
4. *Do not* add phenytoin to a running IV solution.
5. Inject IV slowly for treatment of status epilepticus, at a rate not exceeding 50 mg/min. If necessary, dose may be repeated 30 minutes after initial administration.

Additional Nursing Implications

See also *Nursing Implications* for *Anticonvulsants*, p. 452, and for *Hydantoins*, p. 456.

1. Ascertain that total serum phenytoin levels are done periodically, particularly for patients receiving drugs that interact with hydantoins or for patients with impaired renal function (10–20 μg/ml is the clinically effective serum range). Seven to 10 days may be required to achieve recommended serum levels.
2. Do not substitute phenytoin products or exchange brands, as bioavailability of phenytoin may vary. There may be a loss of seizure control or toxic blood levels if a substitution is made.
3. *Teach patient and/or family on phenytoin extended*
   a. not to substitute chewable tablets for capsules, as the strength of medication (phenytoin) is not equal.
   b. to check that label on bottle indicates that capsule is *extended*.
   c. to take only a single dose a day.
   d. to take only brand or dosage form prescribed by doctor.

OXAZOLIDINEDIONES

Action/Kinetics   Two oxazolidinediones (paramethadione and trimethadione) are currently used for the treatment of absence seizures only. The drugs may depress rapid activity of neurons in the epileptogenic focus or depress the spread of seizure from focus by depressing synaptic transmission during rapid activity. The drugs are well absorbed from the GI tract.

Uses   Absence seizures (petit mal). Because of its toxicity, it is not the drug of choice; reserved for refractory cases.

Contraindications   Anemia, leukopenia, thrombocytopenia, renal and hepatic disease, disease of the optic nerve. Pregnancy (may be teratogenic).

Untoward Reactions   *CNS:* May increase frequency of tonic-clonic seizures. Myasthenia-gravis-like syndrome, drowsiness, irritability, insomnia, fatigue, headache, malaise, personality changes. *Hematologic:* Pancytopenia, leukopenia, thrombocytopenia, eosinophilia, agranulocytosis, neutropenia, anemia (aplastic or hypoplastic). Also, petechiae, retinal hemorrhage, bleeding from gums, nose, or vagina. *Dermatologic:* Skin rash, exfoliative dermatitis, erythema multiforme. Alopecia, pruritus. *GI:* Nausea, vomiting, abdominal distress and pain, anorexia, weight loss, hiccoughs. *Other:* Lupus erythematosus, pseudolymphomas, nephrotic symptoms (nephrosis, proteinuria), hepatitis (rare), photophobia, double vision, blood pressure changes.

Complete blood counts should be undertaken before therapy begins and at monthly intervals thereafter. Periodic ophthalmologic examinations are necessary.

Drug Interactions

Interactant	Interaction
Aminosalicylic acid (PAS)	PAS ↑ CNS depressant effects of the oxazolidinediones
Anticoagulants, oral	↑ CNS depressant effects of oxazolidinediones
Narcotic analgesics	Concomitant administration may cause severe respiratory depression, coma, and death

Additional Nursing Implications
See also *Nursing Implications* for *Anticonvulsants*, p. 452.

1. *Assess*
   a. for history of visual problems before initiating therapy.
   b. for increased frequency of grand mal seizures.
   c. for unusual vaginal bleeding.
   d. for excessive hair loss.
2. *Teach patient and/or family*
   a. to report signs of renal damage demonstrated by edema, frequency of urination, burning on urination, and albuminuria (cloudy urine). Stress the importance of periodic urine analysis.
   b. that drowsiness occurs frequently with these anticonvulsants and that activities should be planned to minimize hazard caused by lack of alertness and coordination.
   c. that day blindness should be reported and that it may be relieved by wearing dark glasses.

PARAMETHADIONE   Paradione (Rx)

Classification   Anticonvulsant, oxazolidinedione type.

Action/Kinetics   Has greater sedative effects but is said to be less toxic and less effective than trimethadione. Toxic doses may lead to unconsciousness and respiratory depression. Is converted in the liver to the active metabolite dimethadione.

Dosage   PO. *Individualized.* **Adults: initial**, 900 mg/day; increase 300 mg at weekly intervals until seizures controlled or toxicity appears. **Maintenance**: 300–600 mg t.i.d.–q.i.d. **Pediatric**: 300–900 mg/day in 3–4 divided doses.

Administration   Available in capsules and alcoholic solution that must be diluted with milk, juice, or other diluent before administration.

TRIMETHADIONE   Tridione (Rx)

Classification   Anticonvulsant, oxazolidinedione type.

Action/Kinetics   **Peak plasma levels**: $1/2$ - 2 hr. Biotransformed by the liver to the active metabolite dimethadione. t$1/2$(trimethadione): 12–24 hr; t$1/2$(dimethadione): 6–13 days. **Therapeutic serum levels of dimethadione**: 700 μg/ml (approximate). Dimethadione is excreted unchanged by the kidney. Trimethadione does not bind significantly to plasma protein.

Dosage   See Paramethadione, above.

SUCCINIMIDES

General Statement   Three succinimide derivatives are currently used primarily for the treatment of absence seizures (petit mal): ethosuximide, methsuximide, and phensuximide. Ethosuximide is currently the drug of choice in the treatment of absence seizures. Methsuximide should be used only when the patient is refractory to other drugs. These drugs may be given concomitantly with other anticonvulsants if other types of epilepsy are manifested with absence seizures.

Action/Kinetics   The succinimide derivatives suppress the abnormal brain wave patterns associated with lapses of consciousness in absence seizures. They apparently do so by depressing the motor cortex and by raising the threshold of the CNS to convulsive stimuli.

Uses   Primarily absence seizures (petit mal).

Contraindications   Hypersensitivity to succinimides. Safe use in pregnancy has not been established. Must be used with caution in patients with abnormal liver and kidney function.

Untoward Reactions   *CNS:* Drowsiness, ataxia, dizziness, headaches, euphoria, lethargy, fatigue, insomnia, hyperactivity. Psychiatric or psychological aberrations such as mental slowing, hypochondriasis, sleep disturbances, inability to concentrate, depression, confusion, aggressiveness. *GI:* Nausea, vomiting, hiccoughs, anorexia, diarrhea, gastric distress and pain, cramps, constipation. *Hematologic:* Leukopenia, granulocytopenia, eosinophilia, agranulocytosis, pancytopenia, aplastic anemia, monocytosis. *Dermatologic:* Pruritus, urticaria, erythema multiforme, lupus erythematosus, Stevens-Johnson syndrome, photophobia. *Miscellaneous:* Blurred vision, alopecia, muscle weakness, hirsutism, hyperemia, hypertrophy of gums, swollen tongue, myopia, vaginal bleeding.

Drug Interactions   Succinimides may increase the effects of hydantoins by decreasing breakdown by the liver.

Dosage   *Individualized*. See individual agents. Succinimides may be given in combination with other anticonvulsants if two or more seizure types are present.

Additional Nursing Implications

See also *Nursing Implications*, for *Anticonvulsants*, p. 452.

1. Report increase in frequency of tonic-clonic (grand mal) seizures.
2. Alert the family to the possibility of transient personality changes, hypochondriacal behavior, and aggressiveness. Stress reporting these personality changes.

ETHOSUXIMIDE   Zarontin (Rx)

Classification   Anticonvulsant, succinimide type.

Note: See information on Succinimides, p. 460, and Anticonvulsants, p. 451.

Action/Kinetics   Peak serum levels: 3–7 hr. **t¹/₂: adults**, 60 hr; **t¹/₂: children**, 30 hr. Steady serum levels reached in 7–10 days. **Therapeutic serum levels**: 40–100 μg/ml. The drug is metabolized in the liver. Both inactive metabolites and unchanged drug are excreted in the urine.

Additional Drug Interactions   Both isoniazid and valproic acid may ↑ the effects of ethosuximide.

Dosage   PO: *individualized*. **Usual initial; adults and children over 6 years**: 250 mg b.i.d.; **pediatric, children under 6 years**: 250 mg daily.
   Dosage may be increased gradually (increments of 250 mg every 4 to 7 days) until control is established. This may require 1–1.5 gm or more daily. Doses exceeding 1 gm daily are seldom more effective than smaller amounts.
   May be used with other anticonvulsants in the presence of other forms of epilepsy.

METHSUXIMIDE   Celontin (Rx)

Classification   Anticonvulsant, succinimide type.

Note: See information on Succinimides, p. 460 and Anticonvulsants, p. 451.

Uses   Methsuximide is used for absence seizures refractory to other drugs.

Additional Untoward Reactions   Most common are ataxia, dizziness, and drowsiness.

Additional Drug Interaction   Methsuximide may ↑ the effect of primidone.

Dosage   PO. *Individualized*. **Adults and children: initial**, 300 mg daily for first week; **then**, increase dosage by 300 mg at weekly intervals until control established. **Maximum daily dose**: 1.2 gm in divided doses.

PHENSUXIMIDE   Milontin (Rx)

Classification   Anticonvulsant, succinimide type.

Note: Phensuximide is said to be less effective as well as less toxic than other succinimides. May color the urine pink, red, or red-brown. See information on Succinimides, p. 460, and Anticonvulsants, p. 451.

Additional Untoward Reactions   Kidney damage, hematuria, urinary frequency.

Dosage   PO. *Individualized*. **Adults**: 0.5–1.0 gm b.i.d.–t.i.d. **Pediatric**: 0.6–1.2 gm b.i.d.–t.i.d. Total daily dosage, regardless of age, varies between 1 and 3 gm. May be used with other anticonvulsants in the presence of multiple types of epilepsy.

MISCELLANEOUS ANTICONVULSANTS

ACETAZOLAMIDE   AK-Zol, Dazamide, Diamox (Rx)

Classification   Anticonvulsant (miscellaneous), diuretic.

Action/Kinetics Carbonic anhydrase inhibitor—a sulfonamide derivative—that appears to retard abnormal, paroxysmal discharges from CNS neurons. Beneficial effects may be due to either inhibition of carbonic anhydrase or resultant acidosis. Absorbed from the GI tract and widely distributed throughout the body, including the CNS. Excreted unchanged in the urine.

Uses Adjunct in clonic-tonic, myoclonic seizures, absence seizures (petit mal), mixed seizures. Also used as a diuretic and for glaucoma. *Investigational:* Prophylaxis of acute mountain sickness.

Contraindications Low serum levels of sodium and potassium. Renal and hepatic dysfunction. Hyperchloremic acidosis, adrenal insufficiency, hypersensitivity to thiazide diuretics. Not to be used chronically in presence of noncongestive angle-closure glaucoma.

Untoward Reactions *Short-term therapy* (minimal adverse reactions): Anorexia, polyuria, drowsiness, confusion, paresthesia. *Long-term therapy:* Acidosis, transient myopia. *Rarely:* Urticaria, glycosuria, hepatic insufficiency, melena, flaccid paralysis, convulsions. Also, side-effects similar to those produced by sulfonamides (see p. 140).

Drug Interactions See Diuretics, p. 793.

Dosage **PO. Adults/children:** 8–30 mg/kg/day in divided doses. Optimum daily dosage: 375–1,000 mg (doses higher than 1,000 mg do not increase therapeutic effect). *If used as adjunct to other anticonvulsants:* **initial,** 250 mg once daily; dose can be increased up to 1,000 mg/day if necessary.

Administration/Storage

1. Change from other anticonvulsant therapy to acetazolamide should be gradual.
2. Use parenteral solutions within 24 hr after reconstitution.
3. IV administration is preferred; IM administration is painful.
4. Reconstitute with at least 5 ml of sterile water for injection.

Nursing Implications

See also *Nursing Implications* for *Diuretics*, p. 791 and *Sulfonamides*, p. 141.
    Teach patient to report symptoms of acidosis, such as weakness, headache, malaise, abdominal pain, nausea, and vomiting, to doctor, who might prescribe bicarbonate or other antacid to neutralize excessive acidity.

CARBAMAZEPINE Apo-Carbamazepine,* Mazepine,* Tegretol (Rx)

Classification Anticonvulsant, miscellaneous.

Action/Kinetics Carbamazepine is chemically similar to the cyclic antidepressants; it also manifests analgesic, anticholinergic, and sedative effects. Due to the potentially serious blood dyscrasias, a benefit-to-risk evaluation should be undertaken before the drug is instituted.
    The mechanism of action of carbamazepine is unknown, but its anticonvulsant properties are similar to those of the hydantoins. **Peak plasma levels:** 2–6 hr. **t½** (serum): 12–17 hr with repeated doses. **Therapeutic serum levels:** 5–12 μg/ml. Carbamazepine is metabolized in the liver to an active metabolite (epoxide derivative) with a half-life of 5–8 hr.

Uses   Carbamazepine is not the drug of choice for seizure disorders but is reserved for seizures unresponsive to other agents. Epilepsy, especially partial seizures with complex symptomatology. Grand mal, psychomotor epilepsy, and disease with mixed seizure patterns. To treat pain associated with tic douloureux (trigeminal neuralgia) and glossopharyngeal neuralgia. *Investigational:* Neurogenic diabetes insipidus, alcohol withdrawal, selected psychiatric disorders such as resistant schizophrenia.

Contraindications   History of bone marrow depression. Hypersensitivity to drug or tricyclic antidepressants. In patients taking MAO inhibitors. Use with caution in glaucoma and in hepatic, renal, and cardiovascular disease. Safe use in pregnancy or lactation not established. Do not use when other antiepileptic agents are effective.

Untoward Reactions   *GI:* Nausea, vomiting, diarrhea, abdominal pain or upset, anorexia, glossitis, stomatitis, dryness of mouth and pharynx. *Hematologic:* Aplastic anemia, leukopenia, eosinophilia, thrombocytopenia, purpura, agranulocytosis, leukocytosis. *CNS:* Fatigue, drowsiness, ataxia, incoordination, vertigo, confusion, headache, nystagmus, hallucinations, involuntary movements, speech disturbances, depression. *CV:* Congestive heart failure, hypertension, hypotension, syncope, thrombophlebitis, worsening of angina, arrhythmias, myocardial infarction. *GU:* Urinary frequency or retention, oliguria, impotence. *Dermatologic:* Pruritus, urticaria, photosensitivity, exfoliative dermatitis, Stevens-Johnson syndrome, aggravation of systemic lupus erythematosus, alopecia, erythema nodosum. *Ophthalmologic:* Nystagmus, double vision, blurred vision, oculomotor disturbances, conjunctivitis. *Other:* Peripheral neuritis, paresthesias, tinnitus, sweating, fever, chills, joint and muscle aches and cramps, adenopathy or lymphadenopathy.

Drug Interactions

Interactant	Interaction
Anticoagulants, oral	↓ Effect of anticoagulant due to ↑ breakdown by liver
Cimetidine	↑ Effect of carbamazepine due to ↓ breakdown by liver
Contraceptives, oral	↓ Effect of contraceptives due to ↑ breakdown by liver
Doxycycline	↓ Effect of doxycycline due to ↑ breakdown by liver
Erythromycin	↑ Effect of carbamazepine due to ↓ breakdown by liver
Ethosuximide	↓ Effect of ethosuximide due to ↑ breakdown by liver
Isoniazid	↑ Effect of carbamazepine due to ↓ breakdown by liver
Lithium	↑ CNS toxicity
MAO inhibitors	Exaggerated side effects of carbamazepine
Phenobarbital	↓ Effect of carbamazepine due to ↑ breakdown by liver
Phenytoin	↓ Effect of carbamazepine due to ↑ breakdown by liver
Posterior pituitary hormones	Carbamazepine ↑ effect of posterior pituitary hormones
Primidone	↓ Effect of carbamazepine due to ↑ breakdown by liver
Propoxyphene	↑ Effect of carbamazepine due to ↓ breakdown by liver
Theophyllines	↓ Effect theophyllines due to ↑ breakdown by liver
Troleandomycin	↑ Effect of carbamazepine due to ↓ breakdown by liver
Valproic acid	↓ Effect of valproic acid due to ↑ breakdown by liver

Dosage   **PO**, *individualized, epilepsy*, **adults and children over 12 years: initial**, 200 mg b.i.d. Increase by 200 mg/day until best response is attained. Divide total dose and administer q 6 to 8 hours. **Maximum dose, children 12–15 years**: 1,000 mg daily; **adults and children over 15 years**: 1,200 mg daily. **Maintenance**: decrease dose gradually to 800–1,200 mg daily. **Children, 6–12 years: initial,** 100 mg b.i.d.; **then,** increase slowly by 100 mg/day; dose is divided and given q 6–8 hr. Daily dose should not exceed 1,000 mg. **Maintenance:** 400–800 mg daily. *Trigeminal neuralgia*: **initial,** 100 mg b.i.d. on day 1. Increase by no more than 200 mg/day using increments of 100 mg q 12 hr as needed, up to maximum of 1,200 mg daily. **Maintenance**: *usual*, 400–800 mg daily. Attempt discontinuation of medicine at least 1 time q 3 months.

Administration/ Storage

1. Do not administer for a minimum of 2 weeks after patient has received MAO inhibitor drugs.
2. Protect tablets from moisture.
3. The drug should be taken with meals.

Nursing Implications

1. Ascertain that baseline hematologic, liver function, and renal function tests are completed before initiation of therapy. Do not initiate therapy until significant abnormalities have been ruled out.
2. Ascertain that above tests are done periodically (hematologic tests are to be done every week during first 3 months of therapy and monthly thereafter for 2 to 3 years). Withhold drug and report to medical supervision if the test results indicate abnormalities.
3. Use the following guide to assess for bone marrow depression:

    Erythrocyte count less than 4 million/mm^3; hematocrit less than 32%; hemoglobin less than 11 gram%; leukocytes less than 4,000/mm^3; reticulocytes less than 0.3% of erythrocytes (20,000/mm^3); serum iron greater than 150 μg%.
4. Ascertain that baseline periodic eye examination for opacities and intraocular pressure is completed.
5. Anticipate that therapy will start gradually with low doses to minimize adverse reactions, such as dizziness, drowsiness, nausea, and vomiting.
6. Assess patients with history of psychosis for activation of symptoms.
7. Assess elderly patients for confusion and agitation and provide protective measures for them.
8. Anticipate that when carbamazepine is added to an antiepilepsy regimen the drug will be gradually added while the other antiepilepsy agents are maintained or gradually decreased.
9. Unless bone marrow depression or other life-threatening side effects occur, the drug should be withdrawn slowly to avoid precipitating status epilepticus.
10. Practice seizure precautions for patients who may have seizures precipitated by abrupt withdrawal of drug.
11. *Teach patient and/or family*
    a. to withhold drug and check with medical supervision should the following symptoms occur:
       (1) *Early signs of bone marrow depression*. Fever, sore throat, mouth ulcer, easy bruising, petechial and purpuric hemorrhages.
       (2) *Early signs of GU dysfunction*. Frequency, acute retention, oliguria, and impotence.
       (3) *Cardiovascular side effects*. Symptoms of CHF, syncope, collapse, edema, thrombophlebitis or cyanosis.

b. to use caution in operating an automobile or other dangerous machinery because drug interferes with vision and coordination.

c. to report skin eruptions, which may necessitate withdrawal of drug.

CLONAZEPAM Clonopin, Rivotril* (C-IV) (Rx)

Classification Anticonvulsant, miscellaneous.

Action/Kinetics Benzodiazepine derivative. Clonazepam depresses frequency of discharge in absence seizures and decreases the frequency, amplitude, spread, and duration of discharge in minor motor seizures. **Peak plasma levels**: 1–2 hr. **t½**: 18–50 hr. **Peak serum levels**: 20–80 ng/ml. The drug is more than 80% bound to plasma protein; it is metabolized almost completely in the liver to inactive metabolites, which are excreted in the urine.

Even though a benzodiazepine, clonazepam is used only as an anticonvulsant. However, contraindications, untoward reactions, and so forth are similar to those for diazepam (see p. 391).

Uses Absence seizures (petit mal) including Lennox-Gastant syndrome, akinetic and myoclonic seizures.

Contraindications Sensitivity to benzodiazepines. Severe liver disease, acute narrow angle glaucoma. Safe use in pregnancy and childhood not established.

Untoward Reactions In patients in whom different types of seizure disorders exist, clonazepam may elicit or precipitate grand mal seizures.

Drug Interactions

Interactant	Interaction
CNS depressants	Potentiation of CNS depressant effect of clonazepam
Phenobarbital	↓ Effect of clonazepam due to ↑ breakdown by liver
Phenytoin	↓ Effect of clonazepam due to ↑ breakdown by liver
Valproic acid	↑ Chance of absence seizures

Dosage **PO, adults**: *individualized*, **initial**, 0.5 mg t.i.d. Increase by 0.5–1 mg daily q 3 days until seizures are under control or side effects become excessive; **maximum**: 20 mg/day. **Pediatric up to 10 years or 30 kg**: 0.01–0.03 mg/kg/day in 2 to 3 divided doses to maximum of 0.05 mg/kg/day. Increase by increments of 0.25–0.5 mg q 3 days until seizures are under control or maintenance of 0.1–0.2 mg/kg is attained.

Nursing Implications

See *Nursing Implications* for *Benzodiazepines*, *Antianxiety Agents*, p. 393 and for *Anticonvulsants*, p. 452.

CLORAZEPATE DIPOTASSIUM Tranxene, Tranxene-SD, Tranxene-SD Half Strength (Rx)

Classification Benzodiazepine, anticonvulsant.

Action/Kinetics For information in action, uses, contraindications, untoward re-actions, and drug interactions, see Chapter 31, p. 391.

Uses Adjunct for treating partial seizures.

Dosage PO. Adults and children over 12 years, initial: 7.5 mg t.i.d.; **then,** dose may be increased by 7.5 mg weekly to a maximum of 90 mg/day. **Pediatric, 9–12 years, initial:** 7.5 mg b.i.d.; **then,** dose may be increased by 7.5 mg weekly to a maximum of 60 mg/day. Not recommended for children under 9 years of age.

DIAZEPAM   Valium (C-IV) (Rx)

See Chapter 31, Table 13, p. 395.

MAGNESIUM SULFATE (Rx)

Classification Anticonvulsant, electrolyte, cathartic.

Action/Kinetics Magnesium depresses the CNS and controls convulsions by block-ing neuromuscular transmission. **Effective serum levels**: 2.5–7.5 mEq/liter (nor-mal Mg levels: 1.5–3.0 mEq/liter). **Onset: IM**, 1 hr; **IV**, immediate. **Duration: IM**, 3–4 hr; **IV**, 30 min. Mg is excreted by kidney.

Uses Seizures associated with toxemia of pregnancy, epilepsy, or when abnormally low levels of magnesium may be a contributing factor in convulsions such as in hypothyroidism or glomerulonephritis. Acute nephritis in children.

Contraindications Renal impairment, myocardial damage, heart block.

Untoward Reactions Symptoms of high plasma levels of magnesium including CNS depression, sweating, hypotension, circulatory collapse, flushing, and cardiovas-cular depression. Suppression of knee jerk reflex can be used to determine toxicity. Respiratory failure may occur if given beyond disappearance of knee jerk.

Drug Interactions

Interactant	Interaction
CNS depressants (general anesthetics, sedative hypnotics, narcotics)	Additive CNS depression
Digitalis	Heart block when Mg intoxication is treated with calcium in digitalized patients
Neuromusclear blocking agents (succinylcho-line, tubocurarine, de-camethonium)	Possible additive neuromuscular blocking activity

Dosage *Anticonvulsant.* **IM**: 1–5 gm of a 25–50% solution up to 6 times daily. **Pediatric:** 20–40 mg/kg using the 20% solution (may be repeated if necessary). **IV**: 1–4 gm using 10–20% solution not to exceed 1.5 ml/min of the 10% solution. **IV infusion:** 4 gm in 250 ml 5% dextrose at a rate not to exceed 3 ml/min. *Magnesium deficiency.* **IM, IV**: 1–2 gm or until desired response achieved.

Administration

1. For IV injections, administer only 1.5 ml of 10% solution per minute. Discontinue administration when convulsions cease.
2. For IV infusion, administration should not exceed 3 ml/min.

Nursing Implications

1. Assess for symptoms of toxicity as noted in *Untoward Reactions*.
2. Assess the presence of knee-jerk reflexes before administering drug. If knee jerk is absent, withhold drug and report to physician as further administration may result in respiratory failure requiring artificial respiration or administration of calcium.
3. Have available calcium gluconate or calcium gluceptate IV to be used as an antidote.
4. Anticipate that the dose of CNS depressants administered to patients receiving magnesium sulfate will be adjusted.
5. Monitor especially closely any patient receiving digitalis preparations *and* magnesium sulfate, because if toxicity occurs treatment with calcium is extremely dangerous and may result in heart block.

PARALDEHYDE   Paral (Rx)

Classification   Hypnotic, anticonvulsant.

Action/Kinetics   Paraldehyde is a rapidly acting hypnotic devoid of analgesic activity. It is colorless, with an unpleasant odor and bitter taste. Onset of hypnosis: 10–15 min. Metabolized in liver.

Uses   Emergency treatment of convulsive disorders arising from status epilepticus, tetanus, eclampsia, poisoning by convulsive drugs including anesthetics. Frequently used in treatment of delirium tremens. Also used as a sedative-hypnotic (see p. 387).

Contraindications   Hepatic insufficiency, occasionally in bronchopulmonary disease. May cause GI irritation in presence of gastroenteritis. Can be habit forming.

Untoward Reactions   *IV only*: Massive pulmonary hemorrhage, edema, dilation and failure of right heart, constriction of pulmonary capillaries, coughing. Metabolic acidosis with overdosage.

Drug Interactions

Interactant	Interaction
CNS depressants	Additive CNS depression
Disulfiram (Antabuse)	Antabuse-like reaction

Dosage   **IM**: 5 ml. **IV infusion**: 3–5 ml (diluted with sodium chloride injection). See p. 387 for dosage of other uses.

Administration

1. Do not infuse at a rate more than 1 ml/minute.
2. Do not use liquid medication with brownish tinge and/or sharp penetrating odor—indicative of presence of acetic acid.

3. Do not use paraldehyde from container that has been open for more than 24 hr.
4. Use glass equipment to administer, as drug interacts with plastics.
5. If parenteral administration is necessary, IM is the route of choice, even though the injection is painful until the drug takes effect.
6. Use great care to avoid nerve trunks during IM injection, because the drug may cause nerve injury and paralysis.

Nursing Implications
1. Reassure patients disturbed by the odor that they will become accustomed to it.
2. Do not administer concomitantly with disulfuram, as an Antabuse-like reaction may occur.
3. Report coughing during IV administration, as this may indicate untoward effects on pulmonary capillaries.
4. Assess patient for symptoms of overdosage, such as rapid labored breathing and a rapid, feeble pulse, low blood pressure, and the characteristic odor of paraldehyde on breath.
5. Have equipment ready for physiologic supportive treatment of acute poisoning: suction, respirator, oxygen, IV sets, and sodium bicarbonate and sodium lactate solutions.
6. Anticipate use of hemodialysis or peritoneal dialysis to correct metabolic acidosis.

PHENACEMIDE   Phenurone (Rx)

Classification   Anticonvulsant, miscellaneous.

Action/Kinetics   Phenacemide reduces focal seizures of the psychomotor type; the drug also increases the anticonvulsant effect of mephenytoin, phenobarbital, and trimethadione. It is absorbed well following oral administration. **Duration:** 5 hr. It is metabolized in the liver to inactive metabolites, which are excreted in the urine.

Uses   Mixed types of psychomotor seizures refractory to other drugs. Not the drug of choice for any disorder because of its *severe toxic effects*.

Contraindications   Hypersensitivity to drug or impaired liver function. Use with caution in patients with history of psychoneurosis and allergy.

Untoward Reactions   Phenacemide is more toxic than most other anticonvulsants and its administration requires close supervision of patient. *CNS:* Psychic changes, toxic psychoses, dizziness, fatigue, fever, sedation, drowsiness, insomnia, headache. *GI:* Anorexia, nausea, weight loss. *Hematologic:* Aplastic anemia, leukopenia. *Other:* Dermatologic manifestations, hepatitis, liver damage, nephritis, muscle pain, palpitations.
   Liver function tests and complete blood counts are indicated before and periodically after therapy has been initiated.

Drug Interactions

Interactant	Interaction
Hydantoins	↑ Effect of hydantoins due to ↓ breakdown by liver
Mephenytoin Oxazolidinediones Succinimides }	Since these anticonvulsants have similar toxic effects as phenacemide, they should not be used concomitantly

Dosage   **PO**: *highly individualized*. Aim at minimum effective dosage. **Adult, initial**, 250–500 mg t.i.d. Dose may be increased at weekly intervals by 500 mg and up to a maximum of 3 gm daily; **pediatric 5–10 years**: half of adult dose.

Additional Nursing Implications

See also *Nursing Implications* for *Anticonvulsants*, p. 452.

1. Check as to whether there is any history of allergy and/or personality disorder before administering phenacemide.
2. Assess and report changes in mental attitude, such as loss of interest or depression, since such changes may indicate severe personality change leading to toxic psychoses.
3. *Teach patient and/or family*
   a. to discontinue drug and check with physician at the first sign of a rash or other allergic manifestation.
   b. to report signs of renal damage demonstrated by edema, frequency, burning on urination, and albuminuria (cloudy urine). Stress the importance of periodic urine analysis.

PRIMIDONE   Apo-Primidone,* Myidone, Mysoline, Sertan* (Rx)

Classification   Anticonvulsant, miscellaneous.

Action/Kinetics   Primidone is closely related to the barbiturates; however, the mechanism for its anticonvulsant effects is unknown. Primidone produces a greater sedative effect than barbiturates when used for seizure treatment. Side effects usually subside with use. **Peak plasma levels**: 3 hr. Primidone is converted in the liver to two active metabolites, phenobarbital and phenylethylmalonamide (PEMA). **Peak plasma levels (PEMA)**: 7–8 hr. t½ **(primidone)**: 8 hr; t½ **(PEMA)**: 24–48 hr; t½ **(phenobarbital)**: 48–120 hr. The appearance of phenobarbital in the plasma may be delayed several days after initiation of therapy. **Therapeutic plasma levels, primadone**: 5–12 μg/ml; **phenobarbital**, 10–30 μg/ml.

Uses   Psychomotor seizures, focal seizures, or refractory tonic-clonic seizures. May be used alone or with other drugs. Often reserved for patient refractory to barbiturate–hydantoin regimen. *Investigational:* Benign familial tremor.

Contraindications   Porphyria. Hypersensitivity to phenobarbital. Lactation.

Untoward Reactions   *CNS:* Drowsiness, ataxia, vertigo, irritability, general malaise, headache, emotional disturbances. GI: Nausea, vomiting, anorexia, painful gums. *Miscellaneous:* Skin rash, edema of eyelids and legs, megaloblastic anemia, diplopia, nystagmus, alopecia, or impotence. Occasionally has caused hyperexcitability, especially in children. Postpartum hemorrhage and hemorrhagic disease of the newborn. Symptoms of systemic lupus erythematosus.

Drug Interactions   See also Barbiturates, p. 376.

Interactant	Interaction
Carbamazepine	↑ Plasma levels of phenobarbital
Isoniazid	↑ Effect of primidone due to ↓ breakdown by liver
Phenytoin	↑ Effect of primidone due to ↓ breakdown by liver

Dosage   **PO. Adults and children over 8 years: initial**, *in patients on no other anticonvulsant medication*: Days 1–3, 100–125 mg at bedtime; Days 4–6, 100–125 mg b.i.d.; Days 7–9, 100–125 mg t.i.d.; **maintenance**: 250 mg t.i.d.–q.i.d. (may be increased to 250 mg 5–6 times per day; daily dosage should not exceed 500 mg q.i.d.). **Children under 8 years: initial**, Days 1–3, 50 mg at bedtime; Days 4–6, 50 mg b.i.d.; Days 7–9, 100 mg b.i.d.; **maintenance**: 125 mg b.i.d.–250 mg t.i.d.

If patient receiving other anticonvulsants: **initial**, 100–125 mg at bedtime; **then**, increase to maintenance levels as other drug is slowly withdrawn (transition should take at least 2 weeks).

Additional Nursing Implications

See also *Nursing Implications* for *Anticonvulsants*, p. 452.

1. *Assess*
   a. for and report hyperexcitability in children.
   b. for excessive loss of hair.
   c. for edema of eyelids and legs.
   d. for impotence.
2. Check whether the physician wishes a pregnant patient to be administered vitamin K during the last month of pregnancy to prevent postpartum hemorrhage and hemorrhagic disease of the newborn.

VALPROIC ACID   Depakene, Depakote (Rx)

Classification   Anticonvulsant, miscellaneous.

Action/Kinetics   The precise anticonvulsant action is unknown, but activity is believed to be caused by increased brain levels of the neurotransmitter GABA. Absorption from the GI tract is more rapid following administration of the syrup (sodium salt) than capsules. **Peak serum levels**: 1–4 hr (delayed if the drug is taken with food). t½: 6–16 hr. **Therapeutic serum levels**: 50–100 μg/ml. The drug is approximately 90% bound to plasma protein. It is metabolized in the liver and inactive metabolites are excreted in the urine; small amounts of valproic acid are excreted in the feces.

Uses   Alone or in combination with other anticonvulsants for treatment of epilepsy characterized by simple and multiple absence seizures (petit mal).

Contraindications   Safe use in pregnancy and during lactation has not been established. Use with caution in presence of liver disease.

Untoward Reactions   *GI*: (most frequent): Nausea, vomiting, indigestion. *CNS*: Sedation. *Hematologic:* Thrombocytopenia, leukopenia, eosinophilia, anemia, bone marrow suppression. *Miscellaneous:* **Hepatotoxicity.** Also transient alopecia, emotional disturbances, changes in behavior, weakness, skin rashes, petechiae, menstrual irregularities, acute pancreatitis, increase in SGOT and serum alkaline phosphatase values.

Drug Interactions

Interactant	Interaction
Alcohol	↑ Incidence of CNS depression
Aspirin	↑ Effect of valproic acid due to ↓ plasma protein binding
Benzodiazepines	↑ Effect of benzodiazepines due to ↓ breakdown by liver.
Clonazepam	↑ Chance of absence seizures (petit mal)
CNS depressants	↑ Incidence of CNS depression
Ethosuximide	↑ Effect ethosuximide
Phenobarbital	↑ Effect of phenobarbital due to ↓ breakdown by liver
Phenytoin	↑ Effect of phenytoin due to ↓ breakdown by liver
Warfarin sodium	Inhibition of platelet aggregation

Laboratory Test Interference False + for ketonuria.

Dosage PO: initial, 15 mg/kg/day. Increase at 1-week intervals by 5–10 mg/kg/day; **maximum:** 60 mg/kg/day. If the total daily dose exceeds 250 mg, the dosage should be divided.

Administration

1. Divide daily dosage if it exceeds 250 mg/day.
2. Initiate at lower dosage or give with food to patients who suffer from GI irritation.
3. Capsules should be swallowed whole to avoid local irritation.

Nursing Implications

1. Advise diabetic patients on valproic acid therapy that the drug may cause a false + urine test for acetone. Review symptoms of ketoacidosis (dry mouth, thirst, dry flushed skin) so that patients can evaluate whether they are acidotic.
2. Do not administer valproic acid syrup to patients whose *sodium* intake must be restricted. Consult doctor if a sodium restricted patient is unable to swallow capsules.

Chapter Thirty-seven

NARCOTIC ANALGESICS AND ANTAGONISTS

NARCOTIC ANALGESICS

General Statement The narcotic analgesics include opium, morphine, codeine, various opium derivatives, and totally synthetic substances with similar pharmacologic properties. Of these, meperidine (Demerol) is the best known. The relative strength of all narcotic analgesics is measured against morphine.

Opium itself is a mixture of alkaloids obtained since ancient times from the poppy plant. Morphine and codeine are two of the pure chemical substances isolated from opium. Certain drugs (pentazocine, butorphanol, nalbuphine) have both narcotic agonist and antagonist properties. Such drugs may precipitate a withdrawal syndrome if given to patients dependent on narcotics.

DEPENDENCE AND TOLERANCE It is important to remember that all drugs of this group are addictive. Psychological and physical dependence and tolerance develop even when using clinical doses. Tolerance is characterized by the fact that the patient requires shorter periods of time between doses or larger doses for relief of pain. Tolerance usually develops faster when the narcotic analgesic is administered regularly and when the dose is large.

EFFECTS OF NARCOTIC ANALGESICS The most important effect of the narcotic analgesics is on the CNS. In addition to an alteration of pain perception (analgesia), the drugs, especially at higher doses, induce euphoria, drowsiness, changes in mood, mental clouding, and deep sleep.

The narcotic analgesics also depress respiration. The effect is noticeable at small doses. Death, by overdosage, is almost always the result of respiratory arrest.

The narcotic analgesics have a nauseant and emetic effect (direct stimulation of the chemoreceptor trigger zone). They depress the cough reflex, and small doses of narcotic analgesics (codeine) are part of several antitussive preparations.

The narcotic analgesics have little effect on blood pressure when the patient is in a supine position. However, most narcotics decrease the capacity of the patient to respond to stress. Morphine and other narcotic analgesics induce peripheral vasodilation, which may result in hypotension.

Many narcotic analgesics constrict the pupil. With such drugs, pupillary constriction is the most obvious sign of dependence.

The narcotic analgesics also decrease peristaltic motility. The constipating effects of these agents (Paregoric) are sometimes used therapeutically in severe diarrhea. The narcotic analgesics also increase the pressure within the biliary tract.

ACUTE TOXICITY   This state is characterized by profound respiratory depression, deep sleep, stupor or coma, and pinpoint pupils. The respiratory rate may be as low as 2–4 breaths/min. The patient may be cyanotic. The blood pressure falls gradually. Urine output is decreased, the skin feels clammy, and there is a decrease in body temperature. Death almost always results from respiratory depression.

TREATMENT OF ACUTE OVERDOSAGE   Gastric lavage and induced emesis are indicated in case of PO poisoning. Treatment, however, is aimed at combating the progressive respiratory depression (usually artificial respiration). Although respiratory stimulants (caffeine, pentylenetetrazole, nikethamide) have been used, severe depression follows the stimulatory effects. Such depression adds to the depression from the narcotic overdosage.

Narcotic antagonists: levallorphan (Lorfan), 0.5–1.0 mg IV, or naloxone (Narcan), 0.4 mg IV, is effective in the treatment of acute overdosage. Naloxone is currently the drug of choice.

CHRONIC TOXICITY   The problem of chronic dependence is well known and does not need to be detailed here. Suffice to say that dependence is not only a problem of "the street" but is often found among those who have easy access to narcotics (physicians, nurses, pharmacists). All the principal narcotic analgesics (morphine, opium, heroin, codeine, and meperidine) are at times used for nontherapeutic purposes.

The nurse must be aware of the problem and be able to recognize signs of chronic dependence. These are constricted pupils, GI effects (constipation), skin infections, needle scars, abscesses, and itching, especially on the anterior surfaces of the body, where patient may inject drug.

Withdrawal signs appear after drug is withheld 4 – 12 hr. They are characterized by intense craving for the drug, insomnia, yawning, sneezing, vomiting, diarrhea, tremors, sweating, mental depression, muscular aches and pains, chilliness, and anxiety. Although the symptoms of narcotic withdrawal are uncomfortable, they are rarely life-threatening. This is to be contrasted with the withdrawal syndrome from depressants where the life of the individual may be endangered because of the possibility of tonic-clonic seizures.

Action/Kinetics   The narcotic analgesics attach to specific receptors located in the CNS (cortex, brainstem, and spinal cord), resulting in analgesia. Although details are unknown, mechanism is believed to involve decreased permeability of the cell membrane to sodium, which results in diminished transmission of pain impulses. For kinetics, see individual agents.

Uses   Severe pain, especially of coronary, pulmonary, or peripheral origin. Hepatic and renal colic. Preanesthetic medication and adjuncts to anesthesia. Postsurgical pain. Acute vascular occlusion, especially of coronary, pulmonary, and peripheral origin. Diarrhea and dysentery. Pain from myocardial infarction, carcinoma, burns. Postpartum pain. Some members of this group are primarily used as antitussives. Methadone is used for heroin withdrawal and maintenance (details for this use are not discussed in this book).

Contraindications Asthmatic conditions, emphysema, kyphoscoliosis, severe obesity, convulsive states as in epilepsy, delirium tremens, tetanus and strychnine poisoning, diabetic acidosis, myxedema, Addison's disease, hepatic cirrhosis, and children under 6 months. To be used cautiously in patients with head injury or after head surgery because of morphine's capacity to elevate intracranial pressure.

To be used with caution in the elderly, the debilitated, in young children, in cases of increased intracranial pressure, in obstetrics, and with patients in shock or during acute alcoholic intoxication.

Morphine should be used with extreme caution in patients with pulmonary heart disease (cor pulmonale). Deaths following ordinary therapeutic doses have been reported. Use cautiously in patients with prostatic hypertrophy, since it may precipitate acute urinary retention.

To be used cautiously in patients with reduced blood volume such as in hemorrhaging patients who are more susceptible to the hypotensive effects of morphine.

Since the drugs depress the respiratory center, they should be given early in labor, at least 2 hr before delivery, so as to reduce the danger of respiratory depression to the newborn. When given before surgery, the narcotic analgesics should be given at least 1 to 2 hr preoperatively so that the danger of maximum depression of the respiratory function will have passed before anesthesia is initiated.

These drugs should sometimes be withheld prior to diagnostic procedures so that physician can use pain to locate dysfunction.

Untoward Reactions *Respiratory:* Respiratory depression, apnea. *CNS:* Dizziness, lightheadedness, sedation, lethargy, headache, euphoria, mental clouding, fainting. Idiosyncratic effects including excitement, restlessness, tremors, delirium, insomnia. *GI:* Nausea, vomiting, constipation, increased pressure in biliary tract, dry mouth, anorexia. *Cardiovascular:* Flushing, changes in heart rate and blood pressure, circulatory collapse. *Allergic:* Skin rashes including pruritus and urticaria. Sweating, laryngospasm, edema. *Miscellaneous:* Urinary retention, oliguria, reduced libido, changes in body temperature. Narcotics cross the placental barrier and depress respiration of the fetus or newborn.

Drug Interactions

Interactant	Interaction
Alcohol, ethyl	Potentiation or addition of CNS depressant effects; concomitant use may lead to drowsiness, lethargy, stupor, respiratory collapse, coma, or death
Anesthetics, general	See *Alcohol*
Antianxiety drugs	See *Alcohol*
Antidepressants, tricyclic	↑ Narcotic-induced respiratory depression
Antihistamines	See *Alcohol*
Barbiturates	See *Alcohol*
Cimetidine	↑ CNS toxicity from narcotics
CNS depressants	See *Alcohol*
Methotrimeprazine	Potentiation of CNS depression
Monoamine oxidase inhibitors	Possible potentiation of either monoamine oxidase inhibitor (excitation, hypertension) or narcotic (hypotension, coma) effects; death has resulted

Interactant	Interaction
Phenothiazines	See *Alcohol*
Sedative-hypnotics, nonbarbiturate	See *Alcohol*
Skeletal muscle relaxants (surgical)	↑ Respiratory depression and ↑ muscle relaxation

Laboratory Test Interference Altered liver function tests. False + or ↑ urinary glucose test (Benedict's). ↑ Plasma amylase or lipase.

Dosage (See individual drugs.) The dosage of narcotics and the reaction of a patient to the dosage depend on the amount of pain. Two to four times the usual dose may be tolerated for relief of excruciating pain. However, the nurse should be aware that, if for some reason the pain disappears, severe respiratory depression may result. This respiratory depression is not apparent while the pain is still present.

Nursing Implications

1. Account for narcotics (given or wasted) in a written record as required by the provisions of the Controlled Substances Act of 1970 and state law.
2. Request that the physician rewrite order at time intervals required for continued administration.
3. Use discrimination and judgment in evaluating the needs of a patient complaining of pain.
   a. Preferably use supportive nursing care measures, such as repositioning patient and reassurance, to relieve pain.
   b. If there is a choice, preferably administer a nonaddictive type of analgesic.
   c. Do not make the patient wait for resumption of full pain before administering medication, for then effect of drug will be reduced.
   d. Do not withhold medication when it is needed.
4. *Assess*
   a. for growing dependence and tolerance. However, dependence is not considered a problem in treating the terminally ill cancer patient.
   b. for allergic or idiosyncratic effects.
   c. for early signs of toxicity, such as depressed respiration (10–12 breaths/min), deep sleep, and constricted pupils. Withhold drug when any of these symptoms appear, and consult physician. Have naloxone hydrochloride (Narcan) available to treat toxicity.
   d. food intake and provide meals that patient can tolerate.
   e. for abdominal distention, gas, and constipation; report such signs to the physician, who may order laxatives. Encourage more roughage and fluids in diet.
   f. for bladder distention, because drug may inhibit stimulus to void. This may cause urinary retention. Offer fluids and urge the patient to attempt to empty bladder at least every 3 to 4 hours.
5. Use safety measures (particularly side rails) for the bedridden patient who has been medicated with narcotics.
6. Adequately supervise and assist the ambulatory patient, who is more likely to experience dizziness, nausea, and vomiting after medication. Have the patient gradually rise to a sitting position to minimize hypotension.

(continued)

7. Be prepared to dry patient and change linens more frequently, because the patient perspires when receiving drug.
8. Reassure the patient that flushing and feeling of warmth are sometimes caused by therapeutic doses of narcotics.
9. Provide nursing care to a dependent patient in a friendly but firm manner.
10. Warn ambulatory patient not to drive a car or operate hazardous machinery, because dizziness and sedation may occur.

ALPHAPRODINE HYDROCHLORIDE   Nisentil (C-II) (Rx)

Classification   Narcotic analgesic, morphine type

Action/Kinetics   **Onset: IV,** 1–2 min; **SC,** 2–30 min. **Duration:** 0.5–2 hr. **t½:** 2 hr.

Additional Uses   Cystoscopy. Rapid analgesia in minor surgery. Use in children restricted to dental procedures.

Dosage   *Analgesic:* **Adults: IV,** 0.4–0.6 mg/kg, not to exceed 30 mg initially; **SC,** 0.4–1.2 mg/kg, not to exceed 60 mg initially. Total daily dose, either IV or SC, should not exceed 240 mg. *Obstetrics:* **SC,** 40–60 mg q 2 hr as needed (often combined with scopolamine or atropine). *Dentistry.* **Pediatric: submucosally only,** 0.3–0.6 mg/kg.

BROMPTON'S COCKTAIL (BROMPTON'S MIXTURE) (Rx)

Classification   Narcotic analgesic mixture.

General Statement   Brompton's Cocktail is a complex variable mixture of a narcotic analgesic (usually morphine or methadone), a CNS stimulant (cocaine or *d*-amphetamine), alcohol (ethanol, gin, brandy, or vermouth), and flavoring agents (honey, syrups). Little tolerance to this combination occurs.

Action/Kinetics   The stimulant is believed to increase and potentiate endorphins or to provide sensory overload, which decreases sensation of pain. The alcohol increases palatability, improves mood, and enhances sedation. The stimulant and/or alcohol enhances activity of narcotic analgesic. **Duration:** morphine, 3–4 hr; methadone, 6–8 hr.

Uses   Pain relief, especially in terminal cancer patients when use of narcotic analgesic alone has proved ineffective.

Dosage   The range of doses is as follows: morphine or methadone, 5–15 mg; cocaine or *d*-amphetamine, 5–15 mg; ethanol (90–98%), 1.25–2.5 ml. Frequency of administration must be titrated for each patient and should be on a regular schedule.

Administration

1. The mixture should be discarded after 2 weeks if unused and if stability is unknown.
2. If excessive stimulation is manifested, a phenothiazine can be added to the regimen.

3. Dosage adjustments should be made every 48–72 hr and only one drug dosage varied at any given time.
4. If cocaine is used, the mixture should be swished around in the mouth before swallowing (to increase absorption through oral mucosa).
5. Never mix with soft drinks or fruit juices; the cocktail may be served on ice.

Nursing Implications
1. Assist health team in assessing patient's need for Brompton's cocktail by evaluating severity of pain, fear, anxiety, and depression.
2. Administer on schedule as ordered to maintain continuous analgesia and euphoric state. The patient is then relaxed and does not fear the return of pain.
3. Assess and report to physician excessive sedation, respiratory depression, and nausea. These assessment data are essential for titrating dosage.
4. Teach patient and/or family
   a. Brompton's cocktail should be administered on a regular schedule around the clock as ordered so that pain is always controlled and patient neither fears its return nor associates medication with pain or dependence.
   b. how to monitor for excessive sedation, respiratory depression, and nausea. Emphasize that these assessment data are essential for the physician to adjust dosage to the needs of the individual patient.
   c. accurate measurement of dose and appropriate method of administration.
   d. consult with physician if dose is ineffective, rather than to increase dosage themselves.
   e. that tolerance usually does not develop and that dependence is not considered a problem in treating the terminally ill cancer patient.

BUTORPHANOL TARTRATE   Stadol (Rx)

Classification   Narcotic analgesic—agonist-antagonist.

Action/Kinetics   Butorphanol has both narcotic agonist and antagonist properties. Its analgesic potency is said to be up to 7 times that of morphine and 30–40 times that of meperidine. Overdosage responds to naloxone. **Onset: IM**; 10 min; **IV**; rapid. **Duration**: 3–4 hr. **Peak analgesia**: 30–60 min following IM and more rapidly following IV. **t½**: 2½–3½ hr. Butorphanol is metabolized in the liver and excreted by the kidney.

Additional Uses   Moderate to severe pain especially after surgery. Also as preoperative medication (as part of balanced anesthesia). Postpartum pain.

Additional Contraindications   Use with extreme caution in patients with acute myocardial infarction, ventricular dysfunction, and coronary insufficiency (morphine or meperidine are preferred). Safe use in pregnancy, during labor or in children under 18 years of age not yet established.

Additional Drug Interactions   Butorphanol may precipitate withdrawal in patients physically dependent on narcotics.

Dosage   IM: usual; 2 mg q 3–4 hr, as necessary; **range**: 1–4 mg q 3 to 4 hr. **IV**: **usual**: 1 mg q 3 to 4 hr; **range**: 0.5–2 mg q 3 to 4 hr. **Not recommended for use in children**.

CODEINE PHOSPHATE   Paveral* (C-II) (Rx)

CODEINE SULFATE   (C-II) (Rx)

Classification   Narcotic analgesic, morphine type.

Action/Kinetics   Codeine resembles morphine pharmacologically but produces less respiratory depression, nausea, and vomiting than morphine. It is moderately habit-forming and constipating. Dosages over 60 mg often cause restlessness and excitement and irritate the cough center. However, in lower doses, it is a potent antitussive and is an ingredient in many cough syrups. **Onset**: 15–30 min. **Peak effect**: 60–90 min. **Duration**: 4–6 hr. t½: 3–4 hr.

It is often used to supplement the effect of nonnarcotic analgesics such as aspirin and acetaminophen; see Appendix 3, p. 898. Codeine is also found in combination cough/cold products; see Appendix 3.

Uses   Analgesic, antitussive. Analgesia for severe pain and pre- and postoperative medication.

Additional Drug Interaction   Combination with chlordiazepoxide may induce coma.

Dosage   *Adults. Analgesia,* **IV, IM, SC, PO:** 15–60 mg q 4–6 hr. *Antitussive,* **PO:** 10–20 mg q 4–6 hr up to maximum of 120 mg/day. **Pediatric.** *Analgesia,* **1 year and older, IM, SC, PO:** 0.15 mg/kg q 4–6 hr. *Antitussive,* **PO: 2–6 years:** 2.5–5 mg q 4–6 hr not to exceed 30 mg/day; **6–12 years:** 5–10 mg q 4–6 hr not to exceed 60 mg/day.

FENTANYL CITRATE   Sublimaze (C-II) (Rx)

Classification   Narcotic analgesic, morphine type.

Action/Kinetics   Similar to morphine and meperidine. **Onset**: 5–15 min. **Peak effect**: approximately 30 min. **Duration**: 1–2 hr. t½: 1.5–6 hr. The drug is faster-acting and of shorter duration than morphine or meperidine.

Uses   Analgesia for severe pain, pre- and postoperative medication; especially suitable for minor surgery in outpatients. Tachypnea and postoperative emergence delirium. Combined with droperidol for preanesthetic medication, induction of anesthesia, and adjunct in maintenance of anesthesia. Combined with oxygen in open heart surgery or complicated neurologic or orthopedic procedures in high-risk patients.

Additional Contraindications   Myasthenia gravis and other conditions in which muscle relaxants should not be used. Patients particularly sensitive to respiratory depression. Use with caution and at reduced dosage in poor-risk patients, children, the elderly, and when other CNS depressants are used.

Additional Untoward Reaction   Skeletal and thoracic muscle rigidity, especially after rapid IV administration.

Additional Drug Interaction   ↑ Risk of cardiovascular depression when high doses of fentanyl are combined with nitrous oxide or diazepam.

Dosage   *Preoperatively*: **IM**, 50–100 μg 30–60 min before surgery. *Adjunct to anesthesia: induction*, **IV**, 0.002–0.05 mg/kg, depending on length and depth of anesthesia desired; *maintenance*: **IV, IM**, 0.025–0.1 mg/kg when indicated. *Adjunct to regional anesthesia*: **IM, IV**, 50–100 μg over 1–2 min when indicated. *Postop-*

eratively: **IM**, 50–100 µg q 1–2 hr for control of pain. **Pediatric, 2–12 years of age:** *Induction and maintenance*: 1.7–2.6 µg/kg.

Storage   Protect from light.

HYDROCHLORIDES OF OPIUM ALKALOIDS   Pantopon (C-II) (Rx)

Classification   Narcotic analgesic, morphine type.

Action/Kinetics   This preparation is a mixture of alkaloids obtained from opium. It is rapidly absorbed from the GI tract and has a low incidence of side effects.

Uses   Analgesia for severe pain and pre- and postoperative medication. Antidiarrheal.

Dosage   IM or SC only: 5–20 mg q 4–5 hr. Each 20 mg of pantopon is equivalent to 15 mg of morphine.

HYDROMORPHONE HYDROCHLORIDE (DIHYDROMORPHINONE HYDROCHLORIDE)   Dilaudid Hydrocholoride, Dilaudid-HP* (C-II) (Rx)

Classification   Narcotic analgesic, morphine type.

Action/Kinetics   Hydromorphine is 7 to 10 times more analgesic than morphine, with a shorter duration of action. It manifests less sedation, less vomiting and less nausea than morphine although it induces pronounced respiratory depression. **Onset**: 15–30 min. **Peak effect**: 30–90 min. **Duration**: 4–5 hr. t½: 4 hr. The drug can be given rectally for prolonged activity.

Uses   Analgesia for severe pain (e.g., surgery, cancer, biliary colic, burns, renal colic, myocardial infarction, bone trauma).

Additional Contraindication   Migraine headaches. Use in children.

Dosage   *Analgesic* **PO, IM, IV, SC**: 2–4 mg q 4–6 hr as necessary. **Rectally**: 3 mg (suppository), q 6–8 hr.

Additional Nursing Implications
See also *Nursing Implications*, p. 475.

1. Administer slowly by IV to minimize hypotensive effects and respiratory depression.
2. Assess closely for respiratory depression, as it is more profound with hydromorphone.

LEVORPHANOL TARTRATE   Levo-Dromoran (C-II) (Rx)

Classification   Narcotic analgesic, morphine type.

Action/Kinetics   Levorphanol is 5 times more potent than morphine as an analgesic; respiratory depression, smooth muscle contraction, and dependence liability are increased proportionally. Levorphanol may be used safely with a wide range of anesthetics, including nitrous oxide. **Onset**: approximately 60 min. **Peak effect**: 60–90 min. **Duration**: 4–5 hr. t½: approximately 80 min.

Dosage **PO, SC** 2–3 mg. Give slow IV for special conditions.

MEPERIDINE HYDROCHLORIDE (PETHIDINE HYDROCHLORIDE)
Demerol Hydrochloride, Pethadol (C-II) (Rx)

Classification Narcotic, synthetic.

General Statement The pharmacologic activity of meperidine is similar to that of the opiates; however, it is only one-tenth as potent an analgesic as morphine. Its analgesic effect is only one-half when given orally rather than parenterally. Meperidine has no antitussive effects and does not produce miosis. The duration of action of meperidine is less than that of most opiates and this must be kept in mind when a dosing schedule is being established.

Meperidine will produce both psychological and physical dependence; overdosage is manifested by severe respiratory depression (see morphine overdosage).

Action/Kinetics Unrelated chemically to morphine. **Onset**: 10–15 min. **Peak effect**: 30–60 min. **Duration**: 2–4 hr. t½: 3–8 hr. Meperidine also possesses moderate spasmogenic effects on smooth muscle.

Uses Any situation that requires a narcotic analgesic: severe pain, hepatic and renal colic, obstetrics, preanesthetic medication, adjunct to anesthesia. These drugs are particularly useful for minor surgery as in orthopedics, ophthalmology, rhinology, laryngology, and dentistry, and for diagnostic procedures such as cystoscopy, retrograde pyelography and gastroscopy. Spasms of GI tract, uterus, urinary bladder. Anginal syndrome and distress of CHF.

Additional Contraindications Hypersensitivity to drug, convulsive states as in epilepsy, tetanus and strychnine poisoning, children under 6 months, diabetic acidosis, head injuries, shock, liver disease, respiratory depression, increased cranial pressure, and pregnancy before labor. To be used with caution in obstetrics, lactating mothers, and in older or debilitated patients. Use with extreme caution in patients with asthma. Meperidine has atropine-like effects that may aggravate glaucoma especially when given with other drugs, which should be used with caution in glaucoma.

Additional Untoward Reactions Transient hallucinations, transient hypotension (high doses), visual disturbances.

Additional Drug Interactions

Interactant	Interaction
Antidepressants, tricyclic	Additive anticholinergic side effects
Hydantoins	↓ Effect meperidine due to ↑ breakdown by liver
Monoamine oxidase inhibitors	↑ Risk of severe symptoms including hyperpyrexia, restlessness, hyper- or hypotension, convulsions, or coma

Dosage **PO, IM, SC**: *Analgesic.* **Adults**: 50–100 mg q 3–4 hr as needed; **pediatric**: 1.1–1.8 mg/kg, up to adult dosage, q 3–4 hr as needed. *Preoperatively*: **Adults, IM, SC**, 50–100 mg 30–90 min before anesthesia; **pediatric: IM, SC**, 1.1–2.2 mg/kg 30–90 min before anesthesia. *Support of anesthesia*: **IV infusion** (1 mg/ml) or **slow IV injection** (10 mg/ml) until patient needs met. *Obstetrics*: **IM, SC**: 50–100 mg q 1–3 hr.

METHADONE HYDROCHLORIDE   Dolophine Hydrochloride (C-II) (Rx)

Classification   Narcotic analgesic, morphine type.

General Statement   Methadone produces only mild euphoria, which is the reason it is used as a heroin withdrawal substitute and for maintenance programs. Methadone produces physical dependence but the abstinence syndrome develops more slowly upon termination of therapy; also, withdrawal symptoms are less intense but more prolonged than for morphine. Methadone does not produce sedation or narcosis.

Methadone is not effective for preoperative or obstetric anesthesia. When administered orally, it is only one-half as potent as when given parenterally.

Action/Kinetics   Morphine-type analgesic. **Onset:** 10–15 min. **Peak effects:** 1–2 hr. **Duration:** 4–6 hr. t½: 22–25 hr (increased with repeated use due to cumulative effects).

Uses   Analgesic; drug withdrawal and maintenance of narcotic dependence.

Additional Contraindications   IV use, liver disease; give rarely if at all during pregnancy.

Additional Untoward Reactions   Marked constipation, excessive sweating, or pulmonary edema.

Drug Interactions   Rifampin and phenytoin ↓ plasma methadone levels by ↑ breakdown by liver; thus, possible symptoms of narcotic withdrawal may develop.

Laboratory Test Interference   ↑ Immunoglobulin G.

Dosage   *Analgesia*: **IM, SC, PO,** 2.5–10 mg q 3–4 hr. *Narcotic withdrawal*: **PO, initial,** 15–20 mg/day (some may require 40 mg/day); **then,** depending on need of the patient, slowly decrease dosage. *Maintenance (individualized)*: **PO,** 60–120 mg/day, once stabilized.

Additional Nursing Implications
See also *Nursing Implications*, p. 475.

1. Inspect injection site for irritation.
2. Anticipate that side effects are more prominent in ambulatory patients and in those who are not suffering acute pain.
3. Anticipate that relief of nausea and vomiting may be achieved by lowering the dosage and by administering medication only when needed to control pain.
4. Caution patients on withdrawal therapy to store medication out of the reach of children.

MORPHINE SULFATE   Epimorph,* MS Contin, RMS Uniserts, Roxanol, Roxanol SR, Statex* (C-II) (Rx)

Classification   Narcotic analgesic, morphine type.

General Statement   In low doses, morphine is more effective against dull, continuous pain than against intermittent, sharp pain. Large doses, however, will dull almost any kind of pain. Morphine should not be used with papaverine for analgesia in biliary spasms but may be used with papaverine in acute vascular occlusions. Morphine is least effective by the oral route.

Action/Kinetics Morphine is the prototype for opiate analgesics. **Onset:** approximately 20 min. **Peak effect:** 30–90 min. **Duration:** up to 7 hr. t½: 2–3 hr.

Additional Uses Acute left ventricular failure (for dyspneic seizures) and pulmonary edema. Intrathecally, epidurally, or by continuous IV infusion for acute or chronic pain.

Dosage **PO, sustained release:** 30 mg q 8 hr depending on patient needs and response. **IM, SC: Adults,** 5–20 mg q 4 hr as needed; **pediatric:** 100–200 μg/kg up to a maximum of 15 mg. **IV: Adults,** 4–10 mg in 4–5 ml of water for injection (should be administered slowly over 4–5 min). **Rectal:** 10–20 mg q 4 hr. **PO (not recommended):** 10–20 mg q 4 hr. Dose may be lower in geriatric patients or those with respiratory disease.

NALBUPHINE HYDROCHLORIDE Nubain (Rx)

Classification Narcotic analgesic—agonist-antagonist.

Action/Kinetics Nalbuphine, a synthetic compound resembling oxymorphone and naloxone, is a potent analgesic with both narcotic agonist and antagonist actions. Its analgesic potency is approximately equal to morphine while its antagonistic potency is approximately one-fourth that of nalorphine.

Onset: **IV,** 2–3 min; **SC or IM,** less than 15 min. **Peak effect:** 30–60 min. **Duration:** 3–6 hr; t½: 5 hr.

Uses Moderate to severe pain, preoperative analgesia, anesthesia adjunct, obstetric analgesia.

Contraindications Hypersensitivity to drug. Safe use during pregnancy (except for delivery) and lactation not established. Children under 18 years. Use with caution in presence of head injuries and asthma, myocardial infarction (if patient is nauseous or vomiting), biliary tract surgery (may induce spasms of sphincter of Oddi), renal insufficiency.

Additional Untoward Reactions Even though nalbuphine is an agonist/antagonist, it may cause dependence and may precipitate withdrawal symptoms in an individual physically dependent on narcotics. *CNS:* Sedation is common. Crying, feelings of unreality, and other psychic feelings. *GI:* Cramps, dry mouth, bitter taste, dyspepsia. *Skin:* Itching, burning, urticaria, sweaty, clammy skin. *Other:* Blurred vision, difficulty with speech, urinary frequency.

Drug Interactions Concomitant use with CNS depressants, other narcotics, phenothiazines, may result in additive depressant effects.

Dosage **Adult: SC, IM, IV,** 10 mg for 70-kg patient (single dose should not exceed 20 mg q 3–6 hr; total daily dose should not exceed 160 mg).

Overdosage See p. 473 and *Narcotic Antagonists,* p. 485.

Additional Nursing Implications

1. See also *Nursing Implications,* p. 475.
2. *Assess*
   a. for history of dependency on narcotics, as nalbuphine may precipitate withdrawal symptoms in such a patient.

b. for withdrawal symptoms, such as restlessness, lacrimation, rhinorrhea, yawning, perspiration, and pupil dilation, which are indicative of narcotic dependence. Report symptoms as dosage adjustment is indicated.

OXYCODONE HYDROCHLORIDE   Oxycodan* (C-II) (Rx)

OXYCODONE TEREPHTHALATE   (C-II) (Rx)

Classification   Narcotic analgesic, morphine type.

Action/Kinetics   A semisynthethic opiate, oxycodone produces mild sedation with little or no antitussive effect. It is most effective in relieving acute pain. **Duration:** 4–5 hr. Dependence liability is moderate. Oxycodone is only available in combination with aspirin (e.g., Percodan) or acetaminophen.

Uses   Moderately acute pain, such as bursitis, injuries, dislocations, simple fractures, pleurisy, and neuralgia. Also for obstetric, postoperative, postextractional, and postpartum pain.

Additional Drug Interactions   Patients with gastric distress, such as colitis or gastric or duodenal ulcer, and patients who have glaucoma should not receive Percodan, which also contains aspirin.

Dosage   **PO. Adults:** 5 mg q 6 hr. Use in children not recommended.

OXYMORPHONE HYDROCHLORIDE   Numorphan Hydrochloride (C-II) (Rx)

Classification   Narcotic analgesic, morphine type.

Action/Kinetics   Oxymorphone, on a weight basis, is said to be 2 to 10 times more potent as an analgesic than morphine although potency depends on the route of administration. It produces mild sedation and moderate depression of the cough reflex. **Onset:** 5–10 min. **Peak effect:** 30–90 min. **Duration:** 4–5 hr.

Additional Uses   Dyspnea associated with pulmonary edema or acute left ventricular failure.

Dosage   **SC, IM. Initial:** 1–1.5 mg q 4–6 hr; dose can be increased carefully until analgesic response obtained. *Obstetrics*: **IM,** 0.5–1.0 mg. **IV: initial,** 0.5 mg. **Rectal (suppositories):** 5 mg q 4–6 hr. **Not recommended for children under 12 years of age.**

Administration   Suppositories should be stored in the refrigerator.

PAREGORIC   Camphorated Tincture of Opium (C-III) (Rx)

Classification   Narcotic analgesic, morphine type.

Note: Paregoric contains 2 mg of morphine equivalent per 5 ml. For all details, consult morphine, general statement on narcotic analgesics, and paregoric, anti-diarrheal, p. 659.

Uses   Moderate to severe pain, diarrhea.

Dosage   Adults: 5–10 ml (2–4 mg morphine) 1–4 times/day. **Pediatric:** 0.25–0.5 ml/kg 1–4 times/day.

Additional Nursing Implications

See *Nursing Implications* for *Narcotic Analgesics*, p. 475 and *Antidiarrheal Agents*, p. 656.

PENTAZOCINE HYDROCHLORIDE WITH NALOXONE   Talwin NX (C-IV) (Rx)

PENTAZOCINE LACTATE   Talwin (C-IV) (Rx)

Classification   Narcotic analgesic—agonist-antagonist.

General Statement   When administered preoperatively for pain, pentazocine is approximately one-third as potent as morphine. It is a weak antagonist of the analgesic effects of meperidine, morphine, and other narcotic analgesics. It also manifests sedative effects.

Pentazocine has been abused by combining it with the antihistamine tripelennamine (combination known as T's and Blues). This combination has been injected intravenously as a substitute for heroin. To reduce this possibility, the oral dosage form of pentazocine has been combined with naloxone (Talwin NX), which will prevent the effects of intravenously administered pentazocine but will not affect the efficacy of pentazocine when taken orally.

Action/Kinetics   Pentazocine manifests both narcotic agonist and antagonist properties. **Onset: IM,** 15–20 min; **PO,** 15–30 min; **IV,** 2–3 min. **Duration:** 3 hr. However, onset, duration, and degree of relief depend on both dose and severity of pain. t½: 2–3 hr.

Uses   Obstetrics. Preoperative analgesic and sedative. Moderate to severe pain.

Additional Contraindications   Increased intracranial pressure or head injury. Use with caution in impaired renal or hepatic function as well as after myocardial infarction when nausea and vomiting are present. Not recommended for use in children under 12 years of age.

Note: The narcotic antagonist levallorphan is *ineffective* in reversing respiratory depression or overdosage of pentazocine. Naloxone, however, can be used for such purposes. Avoid using methadone or other narcotics for pentazocine withdrawal.

Additional Untoward Reactions   Edema of the face, syncope, dysphoria, nightmares, and hallucinations. Also, decreased white blood cells, paresthesia, chills. Both psychological and physical dependence are possible, although the addiction liability is thought to be no greater than for codeine.

Dosage   *Pentazocine hydrochloride with naloxone.* **PO: Adults,** 50 mg q 3–4 hr, up to 100 mg. Daily dose should not exceed 600 mg. *Pentazocine lactate.* **IM, SC, IV:** 30 mg q 3–4 hr; doses exceeding 30 mg IV or 60 mg IM not recommended. Total daily dosage should not exceed 360 mg. *Obstetric analgesia*: **IM,** 30 mg; **IV,** 20 mg. Dosage may be repeated 2–3 times at 2–3-hr intervals.

Administration   Do not mix soluble barbiturate in the same syringe with pentazocine, because a precipitate will form.

NARCOTIC ANTAGONISTS

General Statement   The narcotic antagonists are able to prevent or reverse many of the pharmacologic actions of morphine-type analgesics and meperidine. For example, respiratory depression induced by these drugs is reversed within minutes.

Naloxone is considered a pure antagonist in that it does not produce any morphine-like effects. However, levallorphan, when administered alone, may cause respiratory depression and even some analgesic effects.

The narcotic antagonists are not effective in reversing the respiratory depression induced by barbiturates, anesthetics, or other nonnarcotic agents.

Narcotic antagonists almost immediately induce withdrawal symptoms in narcotic addicts and are sometimes used to unmask dependence.

Action/Kinetics   Narcotic antagonists block the action of narcotic analgesics by attaching to the opiate receptors, thereby preventing access by the analgesic (competitive inhibition).

Nursing Implications

1. Try to obtain a history about cause of respiratory depression from the patient or a friend because narcotic antagonists will not relieve the toxicity of nonnarcotic CNS depressants.
2. *Assess*
   a. vital signs before and after administration of narcotic antagonist to evaluate response to therapy.
   b. respiration closely when duration of action of narcotic antagonist is over as additional doses may be necessary.
   c. the appearance of withdrawal symptoms after administration of antagonist. Withdrawal symptoms are characterized by restlessness, lacrimation, rhinorrhea, yawning, perspiration, and pupil dilation.
3. Be prepared to assist in the use of other resuscitative measures for the narcoticized patient, such as gastric lavage, maintenance of a patent airway, artificial ventilation, provision of oxygen, cardiac massage, and vasopressor agents.
4. Provide supportive care to the comatose patient by turning him on his side to prevent aspiration and by providing side rails, and so forth.
5. Assess for initial dilation followed by constriction of the pupil when the narcotic antagonists are used to diagnose narcotic use or dependence.

LEVALLORPHAN TARTRATE   Lorfan (Rx)

Classification   Narcotic antagonist.

Action/Kinetics   Levallorphan will reverse respiratory depression increasing both rate and depth of respiration. **Onset:** rapid (1 min). **Duration:** 2–5 hr.

Uses To overcome narcotic-induced respiratory depression. Diagnosis of narcotic dependence.

Contraindications Mild respiratory depression. Respiratory depression induced by barbiturates and anesthetics (unless levallorphan used in a test dose to determine whether toxicity is due to a narcotic analgesic). Drug may induce severe withdrawal symptoms in narcotic addicts.

Untoward Reactions Respiratory depression when used alone. Also dysphoria, miosis, lethargy, dizziness, drowsiness, GI upsets, and sweating. At high dosages the drug may induce psychotomimetic manifestations.

Dosage **IV.** *Narcotic overdosage*: **initial**, 1 mg; then, if necessary, 1–2 additional doses of 0.5 mg at 10–15 min intervals up to maximum of 3 mg. **Neonates** (respiratory depression as a result of narcotic administration to the mother): 0.05–0.1 mg with 2–3 ml of sodium chloride injection into the umbilical vein after delivery. Can also be given IM or SC if umbilical vein cannot be used.

NALOXONE HYDROCHLORIDE   Narcan (Rx)

Classification Narcotic antagonist.

Action/Kinetics The drug can reverse the respiratory depression induced by narcotic analgesics and that induced by pentazocine (Talwin), propoxyphene (Darvon), and cyclazocine. Since the action of naloxone is shorter than that of the narcotic analgesics, the respiratory depression may return when the narcotic antagonist has worn off. **Onset: IV**, 2 min; **SC, IM**: less than 5 min. **Duration**: Usually 1–4 hr but is dependent on dose and route of administration. **t½:** 1 hr.

Uses Respiratory depression induced by natural and synthetic narcotics. Drug of choice when nature of depressant drug is not known. Diagnosis of acute opiate overdosage. Not effective when respiratory depression is induced by hypnotics, sedatives, or anesthetics, and other nonnarcotic CNS depressants.

Contraindications Sensitivity to drug. Narcotic addicts (drug may cause severe withdrawal symptoms). Not recommended for use in neonates. Safe use in children is not established.

Untoward Reactions Nausea, vomiting, sweating, hypertension, tremors, sweating. If used postoperatively, tachycardia, fibrillation, hypo- or hypertension, pulmonary edema.

Dosage *Narcotic overdosage*: **IV, IM, SC, initial**, 0.4–2 mg; if necessary, additional IV doses may be repeated at 2–3-min intervals. If no response after 10 mg, reevaluate diagnosis. *To reverse postoperative narcotic depression*: **IV, initial**, 0.1–0.2-mg increments at 2–3-min intervals; **then,** repeat at 1–2-hr intervals if necessary. Supplemental IM dosage increases the duration of reversal. **Pediatric.** *Narcotic overdosage*: **IV, IM, SC**, initial, 0.01 mg/kg; may be repeated if necessary. **Neonates.** *To reverse narcotic depression*: **IV, IM, SC**, initial 0.01 mg/kg; may be repeated if necessary.

NALTREXONE   Trexan (Rx)

Classification Narcotic antagonist.

Action/Kinetics Naltrexone binds to opiate receptors thereby reversing or preventing the effects of narcotics. This is an example of competitive inhibition. **Peak**

plasma levels: 1 hr. **Duration:** 24–72 hr. Metabolized in the liver; a major metabolite—6-β-naltrexol—is active. t½: **naltrexone,** approximately 4 hr; **6-β-naltrexol,** 13 hr.

Uses To prevent narcotic use in former narcotic addicts.

Contraindications Patients taking narcotic analgesics, those dependent on narcotics, those in acute withdrawal from narcotics. Liver disease, acute hepatitis. Safety in pregnancy, lactation, and in children under 18 years of age has not been established.

Untoward Reactions *CNS:* Headache, anxiety, nervousness, sleep disorders, dizziness, change in energy level, depression, confusion, restlessness, disorientation, hallucinations, nightmares. *GI:* Nausea, vomiting, diarrhea, constipation, anorexia, abdominal pain or cramps, flatulence, ulcers, increased appetite, weight gain or loss, increased thirst, xerostomia. *CV:* Phlebitis, edema, increased blood pressure, changes in ECG, palpitations, epistaxis, tachycardia. *GU:* Delayed ejaculation, increased urinary frequency or urinary discomfort, changes in interest in sex. *Respiratory:* Cough, sore throat, nasal congestion, rhinorrhea, sneezing, excess secretions, hoarseness, shortness of breath. *Dermatologic:* Rash, oily skin, pruritus, acne, cold sores, alopecia. *Other:* Hepatoxicity, joint/muscle pain, muscle twitches, blurred vision, tinnitus, painful ears, aching or strained eyes, chills, swollen glands, inguinal pain.

A severe narcotic withdrawal syndrome may be precipitated if naltrexone is administered to a dependent individual. The syndrome may begin within 5 min and last for up to 2 days.

Dosage **PO.** *To produce blockade of opiate actions:* 50 mg daily. **Range:** 50 mg weekdays and 100 mg on weekends; 100 mg q other day; 150 mg q third day.

Administration

1. Naltrexone therapy should **never** be initiated until it has been determined that the individual is not dependent on narcotics.
2. The patient should be opiate-free for at least 7–10 days before beginning naltrexone therapy.
3. When initiating naltrexone therapy, begin with 25 mg and observe for 1 hr for any signs of narcotic withdrawal.
4. The blockade produced by naltrexone may be overcome by taking large doses of narcotics. Such doses may be fatal.
5. Patients taking naltrexone may not respond to preparations containing narcotics for use in coughs, diarrhea, or pain.

Nursing Implications

1. Be aware that physician will order a naloxone challenge prior to administration of this drug because patient must be opiate-free 7–10 days prior to administration.
2. Inform patient/family that self-administration of large doses of narcotics during treatment can result in serious illness or fatality.

Chapter Thirty-eight

NONNARCOTIC ANALGESICS AND ANTIPYRETICS

General Statement   Drugs such as aspirin and acetaminophen are available without a prescription and are thus consumed in large quantities for the relief of pain and fever. However, if used improperly, their administration may cause serious side effects. Aspirin is often responsible for accidental poisonings in small children.

In addition to their analgesic and antipyretic effects, many of the drugs of this group have specific anti-inflammatory effects and are the drug for choice for rheumatic diseases. For these conditions the drugs are, however, prescribed at much higher dosage levels than for fever or simple analgesia.

The nonnarcotic analgesics include the salicylates, acetaminophen, nonsteroidal anti-inflammatory agents, and various miscellaneous drugs.

SALICYLATES

Classification   Analgesic, antipyretic, and anti-inflammatory.

Action/Kinetics   Salicylates manifest antipyretic, anti-inflammatory, and analgesic effects. Their antipyretic effect is due to an action on the hypothalamus that results in heat loss by vasodilation of peripheral blood vessels and promoting sweating. The anti-inflammatory effects are probably mediated through inhibition of prostaglandin synthetase, which results in a decrease in prostaglandin synthesis. Prostaglandins have been implicated in the inflammatory process as well as in mediation of pain. Thus, if levels are decreased, the inflammatory reaction may subside. The mechanism of action for the analgesic effects of aspirin is not known fully but is partly attributable to improvement of the inflammatory condition. Aspirin also produces inhibition of platelet aggregation by decreasing the synthesis of endoperoxides and thromboxanes—substances which mediate platelet aggregation.

Large doses of aspirin (5 gm/day or more) increase uric acid secretion, while low doses (2 gm/day or less) decrease uric acid secretion. However, aspirin antagonizes drugs used to treat gout.

Salicylates are rapidly absorbed after PO administration. Aspirin is hydrolyzed to the active salicylic acid, which is 70–90% protein bound. **Therapeutic salicylic acid serum levels**: 150–300 μg/ml, although tinnitus occurs at serum levels above 200 μg/ml and serious toxicity above 400 μg/ml. t½: aspirin, 15 min; salicylic acid, 2–20 hr, depending on dose. Salicylic acid and metabolites are excreted by the kidney.

The bioavailability of enteric-coated salicylate products may be poor.

The salicylates are listed in Table 16.

Uses Pain arising from integumental structures, myalgias, neuralgias, arthralgias, headache, dysmenorrhea, and similar types of pain. Antipyretic. Anti-inflammatory agents in conditions such as arthritis, systemic lupus erythematosus, acute rheumatic fever, and many other conditions. Aspirin is also used to reduce the risk of recurrent transient ischemic attacks and strokes in men. Gout. May be effective in less severe postoperative and postpartum pain; pain secondary to trauma and cancer. *Topical*: salicylic acid is used for its keratolytic activity. Methylsalicylate (oil of wintergreen) is used as a counterirritant.

Contraindications Hypersensitivity to salicylates. Patients with asthma, hay fever, or nasal polyps have a higher incidence of hypersensitivity reactions. Salicylates are to be used with caution in the presence of peptic ulcers, in conjunction with anticoagulant therapy, and in patients with cardiac disease. Salicylates can cause congestive failure in the large doses used for rheumatic diseases. Vitamin K deficiency, one week before and after surgery. Use with caution in liver or kidney disease.

In children with chickenpox or flu due to possibility of development of Reye's syndrome.

Untoward Reactions The toxic effects of the salicylates are dose related. *GI:* Dyspepsia, heartburn, anorexia, nausea, occult blood loss. *Allergic:* Bronchospasm, asthma-like symptoms, anaphylaxis, skin rashes, urticaria, rhinitis, nasal polyps.

Salicylism—mild toxicity. Seen at serum levels between 150–200 μg/ml. *GI:* Nausea, vomiting, diarrhea, thirst. *CNS:* Tinnitus (most common), dizziness, difficulty in hearing, mental confusion, lassitude. *Miscellaneous:* Flushing, sweating, tachycardia. Symptoms of salicylism may be observed with doses used for inflammatory disease or rheumatic fever.

Severe salicylate poisoning. Seen at serum levels over 400 μg/ml. *CNS:* Excitement, confusion, high fever, coma, seizures. *Metabolic:* Respiratory alkalosis (initially), respiratory acidosis and metabolic acidosis, dehydration. *Miscellaneous:* Hemorrhage, pulmonary edema, cardiovascular collapse, renal and respiratory failure, tetany.

For treatment, see Nursing Implications, p. 493.

Drug Interactions

Interactant	Interaction
Acetazolamide	↑ CNS toxicity of salicylates
Alcohol, ethyl	↑ Chance of GI bleeding caused by salicylates
Aminosalicylic acid (PAS)	Possible ↑ effect of PAS due to ↓ excretion by kidney or ↓ plasma protein binding
Ammonium chloride	↑ Effect of salicylates by ↑ renal tubular reabsorption
Antacids	↓ Salicylate levels in plasma due to ↑ rate of renal excretion
Anticoagulants, oral	↑ Effect of anticoagulant by ↓ plasma protein binding and plasma prothrombin

TABLE 16 SALICYLATES

Drug	Uses	Dosage	Remarks
Acetylsalicylic acid (Apo-Asen,* Arthritis Bayer, A.S.A., Aspirin, Aspergum, Bayer, Bayer Children's, Coryphen,* Cosprin 650, Easprin, Ecotrin, Ecotrin Maximum Strength, Empirin, Measurin, Norwich Aspirin, Norwich Extra Strength Aspirin, Nova-sen,* Riphen-10,* Su-pasa,* Triaphen-10,* Zorprin), OTC (Easprin and Zorprin are Rx)	Analgesic, anti-inflammatory, antipyretic, rheumatic fever, myocardial infarction pro-phylaxis	**PO. Adults:** *Analgesic,* 325–650 mg q 4hr. *Arthritis/rheumatic diseases:* 2.6–5.2 gm/day in divided doses. *Transient ischemic attacks in men:* 650 mg b.i.d. or 325 mg q.i.d. **Pediatric:** *Analgesic, antipyretic;* 65 mg/kg/day in divided doses q 6 hr not to exceed 3.6 gm/day.	Aspirin is commonly found in many combination products including Darvon Compound, Empirin Compound Plain and with Codeine, Equagesic, Fiorinal Plain and with Codeine, Norgesic and Norgesic Forte, and Synalgos DC. See Appendix 3.
Acetylsalicylic acid, buff-ered (Alka-Seltzer, Arthritis Pain Formula, Asadrin C-200,* Ascriptin, Ascriptin A/D, Asperbuf, Buff-A, Buffaprin, Buffered Aspirin, Bufferin, Bufferin Arthritis Strength, Bufferin Extra Strength, Buffex, Buffinol, Buf-Tabs, Cama Arthritis Strength, Wesprin Buffered), OTC			
Choline salicylate (Arthro-pan), OTC	Analgesic, antipyretic, anti-inflammatory	**PO:** *Analgesic, antipyretic:* **Adults and children over 12 years,** 870 mg q 4 hr but no more than 6 times daily. *Anti-inflammatory:* 870–1,740 mg up to q.i.d.	May be preferred to sodium salicylate when sodium restriction is necessary. Administer syrup in ½ glass water to reduce aftertaste. Do not give antacids at the same time that choline salicylate is administered. If antacids are required, give choline salicylate before meals and antacid 2 hours after meal. Fewer GI effects than aspirin.

490

Drug	Use	Dosage	Remarks
Magnesium salicylate (Doan's Pills, Durasal, Efficin, Magan, Mobidin, MS-650), Rx (Doan's Pills and Efficin are OTC)	Analgesic, antipyretic, anti-inflammatory	PO: *Analgesic, antipyretic,* 500–600 mg t.i.d.–q.i.d. up to 3.6–4.8 gm daily. *Anti-inflammatory/rheumatic fever:* up to 9.6 gm daily.	A sodium-free salicylate derivative. Not recommended for children under 12 years of age. Fewer GI side effects than aspirin.
Salicylamide (Uromide), OTC	Analgesic	PO: *Analgesic,* **adults:** 325–650 mg t.i.d.	Compound less effective than aspirin. Overdosage does not produce metabolic acidosis, but does produce CNS symptoms, respiratory depression, and convulsions. Patients allergic to aspirin may be able to tolerate salicylamide. Administer after meals or with fluids to minimize gastric irritation.
Salsalate (Artha-G, Disalcid, Mono-Gesic, Salicylsalicylic Acid), Rx	Analgesic, antipyretic	PO: **Adults:** 325–1,000 mg b.i.d.–t.i.d.	Insoluble in stomach. Slowly releases two molecules of salicylic acid in small intestine. Take last dose at bedtime.
Sodium salicylate (Uracel 5), OTC (tablets); Rx (injection)	Antipyretic, analgesic, acute rheumatic fever	*Antipyretic, analgesic,* **PO and IV:** 325–650 mg q 4–6 hr. *Acute rheumatic fever:* 10–15 gm daily in divided doses q 4–5 hr.	Do not give to patients on low-sodium diet. One gram of menadione (vitamin K) should be given per gram of sodium salicylate during long-term therapy. Some physicians order concurrent administration of ½ gm sodium biocarbonate/gm sodium salicylate. This will reduce rate of elimination of drug. Do not infuse rapidly. Check frequently to avoid extravasation, as sloughing may occur.
Sodium thiosalicylate (Arthrolate, Asproject, Rexolate, Thiocyl, Thiosal, Thiosul, Tusal), Rx	Rheumatic fever, gout, analgesic for muscle pain	IM: *analgesic,* 50–100 mg/day or on alternate days. *Acute gout:* 100 mg q 3–4 hr for 2 days; **then** 100 mg/day. *Rheumatic fever:* 100–150 mg q 4–6 hr for 3 days; **then** 100 mg b.i.d. until no symptoms are present.	

Interactant	Interaction
Antirheumatics	Both are ulcerogenic and may cause ↑ GI bleeding
Ascorbic acid	↑ Effect of salicylates by ↑ renal tubular reabsorption
Corticosteriods	Both are ulcerogenic; also, corticosteroids may ↓ blood salicylate levels by ↑ breakdown by liver and ↑ excretion
Dipyridamole	Additive anticoagulant effects
Furosemide	↑ Chance salicylate toxicity due to ↓ renal excretion
Heparin	Inhibition of platelet adhesiveness by aspirin may result in bleeding tendencies
Hypoglycemics, oral	↑ Hypoglycemia due to ↓ plasma protein binding and ↓ excretion
Indomethacin	Both are ulcerogenic and may cause ↑ GI bleeding
Insulin	↑ Hypoglycemic effect of insulin
Methotrexate	↑ Effect of methotrexate by ↓ plasma protein binding; also, salicylates block renal excretion of methotrexate
Nonsteroidal anti-inflammatories	Additive ulcerogenic effects
Phenylbutazone	Combination may produce hyperuricemia
Phenytoin	↑ Effect of phenytoin by ↓ plasma protein binding
Probenecid	Salicylates inhibit uricosuric activity of probenecid
Sodium bicarconate	↓ Effect of salicylates by ↑ rate of excretion
Spironolactone	Aspirin ↓ effect of spironolactone
Sulfinpyrazone	Salicylates inhibit uricosuric activity of sulfinpyrazone
Sulfonamides	↑ Effect of sulfonamides by ↑ blood levels of salicylates
Valproic acid	↑ Effect of valproic acid due to ↓ plasma protein binding

Laboratory Test Interferences False + or ↑: Amylase, SGOT, SGPT, uric acid, catecholamines, urinary glucose (Benedict's, Clinitest), and urinary uric acid (at high doses) values. False − or ↓: CO_2 content, glucose (fasting), potassium and thrombocyte values.

Dosage See Table 16, p. 490.

Administration

1. Administer with meals or with milk or crackers to reduce gastric irritation.
2. If ordered by the doctor, sodium bicarbonate may be given concurrently to lessen irritation.
3. Enteric-coated tablets or buffered tablets are better tolerated by some patients.

Nursing Implications

1. Assess for a history of hypersensitivity to salicylates before administration. Patients who have tolerated salicylates well for a long period of time may suddenly have an allergic or anaphylactoid reaction. Have on hand epinephrine for emergency treatment. Asthma caused by hypersensitive reaction to salicylates may

be refractory to epinephrine so that antihistamines should also be available for parenteral and oral use.

2. For hospitalized patients only, administer salicylates at the order of a physician and at the time scheduled. Advise patients against the indiscriminate use of aspirin at home.

3. Administer salicylates for antipyretic effect only at the TPR ordered by the physician. After administering aspirin for antipyretic effect, monitor the patient's temperature at least once an hour and check the patient for marked diaphoresis. Use supportive nursing care measures, such as drying patient, changing linen, giving fluids, and preventing chilling after marked diaphoresis.

4. Assess patient on anticoagulant therapy for bruises, bleeding of the mucous membranes, or bleeding from any orifice, because large doses of drugs may increase the prothrombin time.

5. Assess for gastric irritation and pain.

6. *Teach patient and/or family*
    a. that sodium bicarbonate should only be taken with the knowledge of the physician, as it may decrease serum level of aspirin sooner and thus reduce its effectiveness.
    b. the therapeutic and toxic effects of the drug (noted in *Untoward Reactions*).
    c. that in diabetic patients symptoms of hypoglycemia may occur, because salicylates potentiate antidiabetic drugs. Check with physician for possible dosage adjustment.
    d. that cardiac patients on large doses should be alert to symptoms of CHF.
    e. that if a child refuses to take aspirin or vomits the medication, check with the doctor as to whether aspirin suppositories or acetaminophen may be used.
    f. to consult physician if patient is taking aspirin because aspirin is usually discontinued one week before surgery because of the possibility of postoperative bleeding.

7. For salicylate toxicity
    a. after repeated administration of large doses of salicylate, assess patient for symptoms of salicylism characterized by hyperventilation, auditory and visual disturbances and report promptly to physician.
    b. anticipate that severe salicylate poisoning, whether due to overdose or cumulation, will also have an exaggerated effect on the CNS and metabolic system. The patient sometimes develops a salicylate jag characterized by garrulous behavior as though inebriated. Convulsions and coma may follow.
    c. be aware that even topically applied salicylates, such as salicylic acid and methylsalicylate, are rapidly absorbed from intact skin, especially when applied in lanolin, and may cause systemic poisoning.
    d. maintain adequate fluid intake in febrile children treated with aspirin as they are more susceptible to salicylate intoxication if they are dehydrated.
    e. emergency supplies for treatment of acute salicylate toxicity should include
        (1) apomorphine.
        (2) emetics; also, equipment for gastric lavage (lavage for toxicity due to methylsalicylate should continue until all odor of the drug is gone from the washings).
        (3) IV equipment and solution of dextrose, saline, potassium, and sodium bicarbonate; vitamin K.

(continued)

    (4) oxygen and respirator.
    (5) short-acting barbiturates (for convulsions), such as pentobarbital or se-
        cobarbital.
  f. *Teach parents and those caring for children*
    (1) that salicylates must be kept out of child's reach (4 ml of oil of wintergreen
        may be fatal for a child, 30 ml for an adult).
    (2) that aspirin should not be given routinely to children without consultation
        with a physician.
    (3) that children with fever and dehydration are particularly susceptible to
        intoxication from relatively small amounts of aspirin.
    (4) to report gastric irritation and pain to the doctor and to be alert for
        symptoms of hypersensitivity or toxicity.

ACETAMINOPHEN

ACETAMINOPHEN (PARACETAMOL)   A'cenol, A'Cenol D.S.,
Acephen, Aceta, Actamin, Actamin Extra, Anacin-3, Anacin-3 Maximum
Strength, Anuphen, Apap, Apo-Acetaminophen,* Atasol,* Banesin,
Campain,* Children's Anacin-3, Children's Bayapap, Children's
Genapap, Children's Halenol, Children's Tylenol, Conacetol, Dapa,
Datril Extra Strength, Dolanex, Dorcol Children's Fever and Pain
Reliever, Exdol,* Exdol Strong,* Genebs, Genebs Extra Strength,
Halenol, Halenol Extra Strength, Infants' Anacin-3 Drops, Infants'
Bayapap Drops, Infants' Genapap Drops, Infants' Tylenol Drops,
Liquiprin Drops, Meda Cap, Meda Tab, Mejoralito, Mejoralito w/o
Aspirin, Neopap, Oraphen-PD, Pain Relief w/o Aspirin, Panadol, Panex,
Panex 500, Pedric, Peedee Dose Aspirin Alternative, Phenaphen,
Robigesic,* Rounox,* St. Joseph Aspirin-Free For Children,
Suppap-120 and - 650 Tapanol Extra Strength, Tapar, Tempra, Tenol,
Tylenol Extra Strength, Tylenol Junior Strength, Tylenol Regular
Strength, TY-Tabs, TY-Tabs Extra Strength, Valadol, Valorin (All OTC
except for Neopap Suppositories)

ACETAMINOPHEN, BUFFERED   Bromo Seltzer (OTC)

Classification   Nonnarcotic analgesic, para-aminophenol type.

Action/Kinetics   The only para-aminophenol derivative currently used is acetaminophen. It resembles the salicylates in the manner in which it produces analgesia
and antipyresis. The magnitude of its effect is comparable to that of aspirin. Acetaminophen is devoid of anti-inflammatory, uricosuric, and has minimal, if any,
anticoagulant effects. It does not cause GI ulceration and irritation and does not
antagonize antigout agents.
   Peak plasma levels: 30–120 min. **t½:** ¾–3 hr. **Therapeutic serum levels** (an-

algesia): 5–20 μg/ml. **Plasma protein binding**: Approximately 25%. Acetaminophen is metabolized in the liver and is excreted in the urine as glucuronide and sulfate conjugates. However, an intermediate hydroxylated metabolite is hepatotoxic following large doses of acetaminophen.

Acetaminophen is often combined with other drugs as in Darvocet-N, Parafon Forte, Phenaphen with Codeine, and Tylenol with Codeine. See Appendix 3.

The buffered product is a mixture of acetaminophen, sodium bicarbonate, and citric acid that effervesces when placed in water. This product has a high sodium content (0.76 gm per ¾ capful).

Uses   Control of pain due to headache, dysmenorrhea, arthralgia, myalgia, musculoskeletal pain, immunizations, teething, tonsillectomy. To reduce fever in bacterial or viral infections. As a substitute for aspirin in upper GI disease, aspirin allergy, bleeding disorders, patients on anticoagulant therapy, and gouty arthritis.

Contraindications   Renal insufficiency, anemia. Patients with cardiac or pulmonary disease are more susceptible to toxic effects of acetaminophen. Evidence indicates acetaminophen may have to be used with caution in pregnancy.

Untoward Reactions   Few when taken in usual therapeutic doses. Chronic and even acute toxicity can develop after long symptom-free usage. *Hematologic:* Methemoglobinemia, hemolytic anemia, neutropenia, thrombocytopenia, pancytopenia, leukopenia. *Allergic:* Skin rashes, fever. *Miscellaneous:* CNS stimulation, hypoglycemia, jaundice, drowsiness, glossitis.

SYMPTOMS OF OVERDOSAGE   There may be few initial symptoms. *Hepatic toxicity. CNS:* CNS stimulation, general malaise, delirium followed by depression, seizures, coma, death. *GI:* Nausea, vomiting, diarrhea, gastric upset. *Miscellaneous:* Sweating, chills, fever, vascular collapse.

TREATMENT OF OVERDOSAGE   Initially, induction of emesis, gastric lavage, activated charcoal. Oral *N*-acetylcysteine is said to reduce or prevent hepatic damage by inactivating acetaminophen metabolites, which cause liver effects.

Drug Interactions

Interactant	Interaction
Carbamazepine	↓ Effect of acetaminophen by ↑ breakdown by liver
Oral contraceptives	↑ Breakdown of acetaminophen by liver
Phenobarbital	↓ Effect of acetaminophen by ↑ breakdown by liver
Phenytoin	↓ Effect of acetaminophen by ↑ breakdown by liver

Dosage   **PO. Adults**, 300–650 mg q 4 hr; doses up to 1 gm q.i.d. may be used for short-term therapy; for long-term therapy daily dosage should not exceed 2.6 gm/day. **Pediatric.** Doses given 4–5 times/day. **Up to three months:** 40 mg/dose; **4–12 months:** 80 mg/dose; **1–2 years:** 120 mg/dose; **2–3 years:** 160 mg/dose; **4–5 years:** 240 mg/dose; **6–8 years:** 320 mg/dose; **9–10 years:** 400 mg/dose; **11–12 years:** 480 mg/dose.

Buffered. **Adult, usual:** 1 or 2, ¾ capfuls are placed into an empty glass; add ½ glass cool water. May be taken while fizzing or after settling. Can be repeated every 4 hr as required or directed by physician.

Nursing Implications

1. *Assess for*
   a. methemoglobinemia (bluish color of mucosa and fingernails, dyspnea, vertigo, weakness, and headache) caused by anoxia.

(continued)

   b. hemolytic anemia (pallor, weakness, and heart palpitations).

   c. nephritis (hematuria and albuminuria).

   d. chronic poisoning (dyspnea, rapid weak pulse, cold extremities, clammy sweat, subnormal temperatures, and collapse with confusion).

   e. toxicity (CNS stimulation, excitement, and delirium).

   f. psychic disturbances accompanying withdrawal of the drug.

2. *Teach patient and/or family that*

   a. phenacetin may color urine dark brown or wine.

   b. the long-term ingestion of headache remedies containing acetaminophen can result in toxic reactions.

   c. so-called headache and minor pain relievers containing combinations of salicylates, acetaminophen, and caffeine may be no more beneficial than aspirin alone and that such combinations may be more dangerous.

MISCELLANEOUS AGENTS

METHOTRIMEPRAZINE   Levoprome, Nozinan* (Rx)

Classification   Analgesic, nonnarcotic, miscellaneous.

Action/Kinetics   Methotrimeprazine is a phenothiazine derivative with many pharmacologic effects, including sedation, analgesic, amnesic, antipruritic, local anesthetic, and anticholinergic effects. The effects on the CNS are thought to be due to depression of subcortical areas of the brain including the thalamus, limbic and reticular systems, and the hypothalamus all of which result in a decrease in sensory impulses, reduction of locomotor activity and subsequent sedation, and an antiemetic effect. **Peak effect:** 20–40 min after IM use. **Duration:** about 4 hr. **Therapeutic blood level:** 1 mg/ml. The drug is metabolized in the liver and the metabolites (which possess minimal pharmacologic activity) are excreted in the urine and feces.

Uses   Analgesic in nonambulatory patients. Obstetric analgesia where respiratory depression is to be avoided. As preanesthetic for producing sedation and relief of anxiety and tension.

Contraindications   This drug should be used with caution in geriatric patients or in individuals with heart disease. It should not be administered to patients in premature labor or with an antihypertensive agent as well as in severe myocardial, renal, or hepatic disease.

Untoward Reactions   *CV:* Orthostatic hypotension accompanied by fainting or weakness. *CNS:* Dizziness, speech problems, excess sedation, disorientation. *GI:* Nausea, vomiting, dry mouth, discomfort. *Miscellaneous:* Urinary difficulties, allergic symptoms, jaundice, agranulocytosis, chills, nasal congestion, pain at injection site.

Drug Interactions

Interactant	Interaction
Alcohol, ethyl	Potentiation or addition of CNS depressant effects; concomitant use may lead to drowsiness, leth-

Interactant	Interaction
	argy, stupor, respiratory depression, coma, and possibly death
Anticholinergic agents	Tachycardia and possibility of extrapyramidal symptoms with concomitant use
Antihypertensives	Additive hypotensive effect
CNS depressants	See *Alcohol, ethyl*
Antianxiety agents, barbiturates, narcotics, phenothiazines, sedative-hypnotics	
Guanethidine	Additive hypotensive effect
Methyldopa	Additive hypotensive effect
Phenothiazines	See *Alcohol, ethyl*; also, additive extrapyramidal effects
Reserpine	Additive hypotensive effect
Skeletal muscle relaxants, surgical	↑ Muscle relaxation

Dosage **IM. Adults**: 10–20 mg q 4–6 hr as needed for analgesia. Dose should be reduced in geriatric patients: **initial,** 5–10 mg; **then,** increase gradually, if necessary. *Obstetric analgesia*: **initial,** 15–20 mg; may be repeated if necessary. *Preanesthetic medication*: 2–20 mg given 45 min to 3 hr before surgery. *Postoperative analgesia*: **initial,** 2.5–7.5 mg (due to residual effects of anesthetic); **then,** give additional dosage, as required, q 4–6 hr. **Do not administer SC or IV.**

Administration

1. Administer by deep IM injection into a large muscle mass. Rotation of sites is advisable.
2. Do not administer SC, as irritation may occur.
3. Should only be mixed with either atropine or scopolamine in the same syringe.

Nursing Implications

Avoid ambulation for at least 6 hours following the initial dose as orthostatic hypotension, fainting, and dizziness may occur. Tolerance to these effects occurs with repeated administration.

PROPOXYPHENE HYDROCHLORIDE 642 Tablets,* 692 Tablets,* Darvon, Dolene, Doxaphene, Novopropoxyn,* Profene 65, SK-65 (C-IV) (Rx)

PROPOXYPHENE NAPSYLATE Darvon-N (C-IV) (Rx)

Classification Analgesic, nonnarcotic, miscellaneous.

General Statement When taken in excessive doses for long periods, psychological dependence, and occasionally physical dependence and tolerance, will be manifested.

Propoxyphene is often prescribed in combination with salicylates. In such instances, the information on salicylates should also be consulted. Propoxyphene hydrochloride is found in Darvon Compound, and Wygesic, while propoxyphene napsylate is found in Darvocet-N. See Appendix 3.

Action/Kinetics Propoxyphene resembles the narcotics with respect to its mechanism and analgesic effect; it is 1/2–2/3 as potent as codeine.

It is devoid of antitussive, anti-inflammatory or antipyretic activity. **Peak plasma levels:** *Hydrochloride:* 2–2½ hr; *napsylate:* 3–4 hr. **Analgesic onset:** up to 1 hr. **Duration:** 3½–4 hr. **Therapeutic serum levels:** 0.05–0.12 µg/ml. Extensive first-pass effect; metabolites are excreted in the urine.

Uses To relieve mild to moderate pain. Propoxyphene napsylate has been used experimentally to suppress the withdrawal syndrome from narcotics.

Contraindications Hypersensitivity to drug.

Untoward Reactions *GI:* Nausea, vomiting, constipation, abdominal pain. *CNS:* Sedation, dizziness, lightheadedness, headache, weakness, euphoria, dysphoria. *Other:* Skin rashes, visual disturbances.

Propoxyphene can produce psychological dependence as well as physical dependence and tolerance.

Symptoms of overdosage are similar to those of narcotics and include respiratory depression, coma, pupillary constriction, and circulatory collapse. Treatment of overdosage consists of maintaining an adequate airway, artificial respiration, and the use of a narcotic antagonist (naloxone, levallorphan) to combat respiratory depression. Gastric lavage or administration of activated charcoal may be helpful.

Drug Interactions

Interactant	Interaction
Carbamazepine	↑ Effect of carbamazepine due to ↓ breakdown by liver
CNS depressants	Additive CNS depression
Alcohol Antianxiety agents Antipsychotic agents Narcotics Sedative-hypnotics	Concomitant use may lead to drowsiness, lethargy, stupor, respiratory, depression, and coma
Orphenadrine	Concomitant use may lead to confusion, anxiety, and tremors
Phenobarbital	↑ Effect of phenobarbital due to ↓ breakdown by liver
Skeletal muscle relaxants	Additive respiratory depression
Warfarin	↑ Hypoprothrombinemic effects of warfarin

Dosage *Hydrochloride.* **PO:** 65 mg q 4 hr, not to exceed 390 mg/day. *Napsylate.* **PO:** 100 mg q 4 hr, not to exceed 600 mg/day. **Not recommended for use in children.**

Nursing Implications
1. *Assess*
   a. for growing dependence and tolerance.

b. for early signs of toxicity, as manifested by depressed respiration or constricted pupils.
2. *Teach patient and/or family*
   a. to use caution when operating potentially hazardous machinery or while driving, because drug may cause dizziness and sedation.
   b. to lie down if dizziness, nausea, or vomiting occur.

Chapter Thirty-nine

ANTIRHEUMATIC AND ANTI-INFLAMMATORY AGENTS

General Statement Arthritis, which means inflammation of the joints, refers to about 80 different conditions also called rheumatic, collagen, or connective tissue diseases. The most prominent symptoms of these conditions are painful, inflamed joints, but the cause for this joint inflammation varies from disease to disease.

The joint pain of gout, for example, results from sodium urate crystals that are formed as a consequence of the overproduction or underelimination of uric acid. Osteoarthritis is caused by the degeneration of the joint; rheumatoid arthritis and systemic lupus erythematosus (SLE) are autoimmune diseases. Immune factors trigger the release of corrosive enzymes in the joints in a complex manner. Infectious arthritis is the result of rapid joint destruction by microorganisms like gonococci that invade the joint cavity. Treatment must obviously be aimed at the cause of the particular form of arthritis, and a thorough diagnostic evaluation must therefore precede the initiation of therapy. Gout is treated with urocosuric agents, which alter uric acid metabolism (Chapter 40); infectious arthritis responds to antibiotics (Chapter 9); osteoarthritis is treated with analgesics and anti-inflammatories; rheumatoid arthritis, SLE, and ankylosing spondylitis respond to anti-inflammatories. Rheumatoid arthritis is also treated with two remitting agents: gold and penicillamine. Aspirin (Chapter 38) is an important agent in the treatment of all rheumatic diseases. Corticosteroids are used, preferably for short-term therapy only, for some of the more recalcitrant cases of rheumatoid arthritis and SLE (Chapter 61). Corticosteroids also are used for intra-articular injection. Antimalarials, especially hydroxychloroquine sulfate (Plaquenil Sulfate), are sometimes used for rheumatoid arthritis and SLE (Chapter 14).

Drug therapy of the arthritides must be supplemented by a physical therapy program, as well as proper rest and diet. Total joint replacement is also becoming an increasingly important mode of therapy to correct the ravages of arthritis.

PROPIONIC ACID DERIVATIVES AND RELATED COMPOUNDS

Action/Kinetics Over the past decade, a growing number of nonsteroidal anti-inflammatory agents have been developed. Chemically, these drugs are related to indene, indole, or propionic acid. As in the case of aspirin, the therapeutic actions of these agents are believed to result from the inhibition of prostaglandin synthesis. The agents are effective in reducing joint swelling, pain, and morning stiffness, as well as increasing mobility in arthritic patients. They do not alter the course of the disease, however. Their anti-inflammatory activity is comparable to that of aspirin. They also have analgesic activity; most have some antipyretic action.

The nonsteroidal anti-inflammatory agents have an irritating effect on the GI tract. They differ from one another slightly with respect to their rate of absorption, length of action, anti-inflammatory activity and effect on the gastrointestinal mucosa.

Uses Rheumatoid arthritis (acute flares and long-term management), osteoarthritis, anklyosing spondylitis, gout, and other musculoskeletal diseases. Mild to moderate pain. Primary dysmenorrhea, episiotomy pain, strains and sprains, postextraction dental pain.

Contraindications Most for children under 14 years of age. Hypersensitivity to any of these agents or to aspirin. Acute asthma, rhinitis, or urticaria. Use with caution in patients with a history of GI disease, reduced renal function.

Untoward Reactions *GI (most common)*: Peptic ulceration and GI bleeding, reactivation of preexisting ulcers. Heartburn, dyspepsia, nausea, vomiting, anorexia, diarrhea, constipation, indigestion, stomatitis. *CNS*: Dizziness, drowsiness, vertigo, headaches. *Skin*: Pruritus, skin eruptions, sweating, ecchymoses, rashes, urticaria, purpura. *Other*: Tinnitus, blurred and other vision disturbances. *Blood dyscrasias*: Anemia, alteration of platelet function, increased bleeding time. *Cardiovascular*: Edema, palpitations, tachycardia.

Drug Interactions

Interactant	Interaction
Anticoagulants (Coumarin)	Concomitant use results in ↑ prothrombin time
Aspirin	↓ Effect of nonsteroidal agents
Phenobarbital	↓ Effect of fenoprofen to ↑ breakdown by liver
Phenytoin	↑ Effect of phenytoin due to ↓ plasma protein binding
Probenecid	↑ Effect of nonsteroidal agents due to ↑ plasma levels
Sulfonamides	↑ Effect of sulfonamides due to ↓ plasma protein binding
Sulfonylureas (oral hypoglycemics)	↑ Effect of sulfonylureas due to ↓ plasma protein binding

Nursing Implications

Teach patient and/or family

a. to take anti-inflammatory agents with meals, with milk, or with an antacid prescribed by their doctor to minimize gastric irritation.

b. drug compliance, because regular intake of medications is necessary for anti-inflammatory effect.

c. the need for regular medical supervision for adjustment of dosage on the basis of patient's age, condition, and changes in disease activity.

d. to report to the doctor signs and symptoms of GI irritation or bleeding, blurred vision or other eye symptoms, tinnitus, skin rashes, purpura, weight gain or edema.

e. to use caution in operating machinery or operating a car because medication may cause dizziness or drowsiness.

FENOPROFEN CALCIUM   Nalfon (Rx)

Classification   Nonsteroidal, anti-inflammatory analgesic.

Action/Kinetics   **Peak serum levels**: 1–2 hr; t½: 3 hr. Ninety-nine percent protein bound. Food (but not antacids) delays absorption and decreases the total amount absorbed. When used for arthritis, 2 to 3 weeks may be necessary to assess full therapeutic effects. Safety and efficacy in children has not been established.

Additional Untoward Reactions   *GU:* Dysuria, hematuria, nephrotic syndrome.

Additional Drug Interaction   Phenobarbital ↓ effect of fenoprofen due to ↑ breakdown by liver.

Dosage   *Rheumatoid and osteoarthritis.* **PO**: 300–600 mg t.i.d.–q.i.d. Adjust dose according to response of patient. *Mild to moderate pain*: 200 mg q 4–6 hr. Maximum daily dose for all uses: 3,200 mg.

Administration   Give drug 30 min before or 2 hr after meals, because food decreases the rate and extent of absorption of fenoprofen.

IBUPROFEN   Advil, Amersol,* Motrin, Nuprin, Rufen (Rx: Motrin, Rufen; OTC: Advil, Nuprin)

Classification   Anti-inflammatory, nonsteroidal analgesic.

Action/Kinetics   **Peak serum levels**: 1–2 hr. **t½**: 2 hr. Food delays absorption rate but not total amount of drug absorbed.
   Advil and Nuprin each contain 200 mg of ibuprofen and are available without a prescription.

Dosage   **PO**. *Arthritis*: 300–600 mg t.i.d.–q.i.d.; adjust dosage according to patient response. Full therapeutic response may not be noted for 2 or more weeks. *Mild to moderate pain*: 200–400 mg q 4–6 hr. *Dysmenorrhea:* 400 mg q 4 hrs. Maximum daily dose for all uses: 2,400 mg.

INDOMETHACIN   Indocid,* Indocin, Indocin SR, Novomethacin* (Rx)

INDOMETHACIN SODIUM TRIHYDRATE   Indocin I.V. (Rx)

Classification   Anti-inflammatory, analgesic, antipyretic.

Action/Kinetics   **PO. Onset**: 1–2 hr. **Peak plasma levels**: 30–120 min. **Duration**: 4–6 hr. **Therapeutic plasma levels**: 10–18 µg/ml. **t½**: Approximately 5 hr. **Plasma t½ following IV in infants**: 12–20 hr depending on age and dose. Approximately 90% plasma protein bound. The drug is metabolized in the liver and excreted in both the urine and feces.

Additional Uses   Bursitis, tendinitis. *IV:* Pharmacologic closure of persistent patent ductus arteriosus in premature infants.

Additional Contraindications   GI lesions. To be used with caution in patients with history of epilepsy, psychiatric illness, parkinsonism, and in the elderly. Indomethacin should be used with extreme caution in the presence of existing, controlled infections. IV use: GI or intracranial bleeding, thrombocytopenia, renal disease, defects of coagulation, necrotizing enterocolitis.

Additional Untoward Reactions   Reactivation of latent infections. More marked CNS manifestations than for other drugs of this group.

Drug Interactions

Interactant	Interaction
Antacids	↓ Effect of indomethacin due to ↓ absorption from GI tract
Anticoagulants, oral	↑ Effect of anticoagulants by ↓ plasma protein binding; also indomethacin is ulcerogenic and may inhibit platelet function, leading to hemorrhage

Interactant	Interaction
Beta-adrenergic blocking agents	Indomethacin ↓ antihypertensive effects of these drugs
Bumetanide	↓ Effect of diuretic possibly due to inhibition of prostaglandin
Captopril	↓ Effect of captopril possibly due to inhibition of prostaglandin
Corticosteroids	Increased chance of GI ulceration
Ethacrynic acid	*See* Bumetanide
Furosemide	*See* Bumetanide
Lithium	↑ Lithium toxicity due to ↓ renal excretion
Probenecid	↑ Effect of indomethacin by ↓ renal excretion
Salicylates	Both are ulcerogenic and cause ↑ GI bleeding
Sulfonamides	↑ Effect of sulfonamides by ↑ blood levels
Sympathomimetic amines	Possibility of hypertension
Thiazides	*See* Bumetanide
Triamterene	↑ Risk of nephrotoxicity

Dosage **PO.** *Arthritis:* **initial**, 25 mg b.i.d.–t.i.d.; may be increased by 25 mg at weekly intervals according to condition, until satisfactory response is obtained. **Maximum daily dosage**: 150–200 mg. *Gouty arthritis*: 50 mg t.i.d. for 3 to 5 days. Reduce dosage rapidly until drug is withdrawn. *Bursitis/tendinitis:* 75–150 mg/day in 3–4 divided doses for 1–2 weeks. A sustained release formulation (75 mg, of which 25 mg is released immediately) is available for use 1–2 times daily.

   IV. *Patent ductus arteriosus:* 3 IV doses, depending on age of the infant, are given at 12–24 hr intervals. **Infants, less than 2 days:** first dose, 0.2 mg/kg followed by 2 doses of 0.1 mg/kg each; **infants 2–7 days of age:** 3 doses of 0.2 mg/kg each; **infants greater than 7 days of age:** first dose, 0.2 mg/kg followed by 2 doses of 0.25 mg/kg each. If ductus arteriosus reopens, a second course of 1–3 doses may be given. Surgery may be required if there is no response after 2 courses of therapy.

Administration/Storage

1. Store in amber-colored containers.
2. The IV solution should be prepared with sodium chloride injection or water for injection. Diluent should not contain preservatives.
3. IV solutions should be freshly prepared prior to use.
4. The IV solution should be given over 5–10 seconds.

Additional Nursing Implications

See also *Nursing Implications*, p. 501.

1. Make every effort by assessing, teaching, and reporting to help the physician establish the smallest effective dose for the individual patient, because adverse reactions are dose related.
2. Withhold drug and report untoward reaction to physician, because any one reaction may necessitate withdrawal of the drug.
3. Assess the patient for concurrent infection or reactivation of old infection because infectious symptoms may have been masked by indomethacin.

(continued)

4. *Teach patient and/or family*
   a. that medical supervision is essential during therapy with indomethacin. Ophthalmologic examinations and total blood counts are usually indicated during long-term therapy.
   b. to use caution operating potentially hazardous equipment because of possible lightheadedness and decreased alertness.

MECLOFENAMATE SODIUM   Meclomen (Rx)

Classification   Anti-inflammatory, nonsteroidal, analgesic.

Remarks   Not indicated as the initial drug for rheumatoid arthritis due to GI side effects. Has been used in combination with gold salts or corticosteroids.

Action/Kinetics   Peak plasma levels: 30–60 min. t½: 2–3.3 hr. Excreted through urine and feces.

Additional Contraindications   Not recommended for use in pregnancy. Safe use in lactation and children under 14 years not established.

Additional Untoward Reactions   Abdominal pain, pyrosis, flatulence, malaise, fatigue, paresthesia, insomnia, depression, taste disturbances, nocturia, blood loss (through feces: 2 ml/day).

Drug Interactions

Interactant	Interaction
Aspirin	↓ Plasma levels of meclofenamate
Warfarin	↑ Effect warfarin

Laboratory Test Interferences   ↑ Serum transaminase, alkaline phosphatase; rarely, ↑ serum creatinine or BUN.

Dosage   PO: 200–400 mg/day in 3 to 4 equal doses. Initiate at lower dose, and increase to 400 mg daily if necessary. After initial satisfactory response, lower dosage to decrease severity of side effects.

NAPROXEN   Apo-Naproxen,* Naprosyn, Naxen,* Novonaprox* (Rx)

NAPROXEN SODIUM   Anaprox (Rx)

Classification   Nonsteroidal, anti-inflammatory, analgesic.

Action/Kinetics   Peak serum levels of naproxen: 2–4 hr; **for sodium salt**: 1–2 hr. t½: 13 hr. Naproxen is more than 90% bound to plasma protein. Food delays the rate but not the amount of drug absorbed. Clinical improvement may not be observed for 2 weeks.

Additional Uses   Mild to moderate pain. Musculoskeletal and soft tissue inflammation including rheumatoid arthritis, osteoarthritis, bursitis, tendinitis, ankylosing spondylitis. Dysmenorrhea, acute gout.

Drug Interactions   Probenecid ↓ plasma clearance of naproxen.

Laboratory Test Interferences   Naproxen may increase urinary 17-ketosteroid values. Both forms may interfere with urinary assays for 5-hyroxyindoleacetic acid.

Dosage   **PO.** *Arthritis (rheumatoid, osteoarthritis, ankylosing spondylitis)*: **individualized. Usual:** 250–375 mg naproxen (sodium salt: 275 mg) b.i.d. Improvement should be observed within 2 weeks. *Acute gout:* **initial,** 750 mg naproxen (sodium salt: 825 mg); **then,** 250 mg naproxen (sodium salt: 275 mg) q 8 hr until symptoms subside. *Pain, dysmenorrhea, bursitis, tendinitis:* **initial,** 500 mg (550 mg sodium salt); **then,** 250 mg (275 mg sodium salt) q 6–8 hr. Total daily dosage should not exceed 1,250 mg (1,375 mg of sodium salt).

Administration   A morning and evening dose is recommended.

PIROXICAM   Feldene (Rx)

Classification   Nonsteroidal anti-inflammatory, analgesic, antipyretic.

Action/Kinetics   Piroxicam may inhibit prostaglandin synthesis. **Peak plasma levels**: 1.5–2 μg/ml after 3–5 hr (single dose). **Steady state plasma levels** (after 7–12 days): 3–8 μg/ml. **t½**: 50 hr. Metabolites and unchanged drug excreted in urine and feces.

The effect of piroxicam is comparable to aspirin but with fewer GI side effects and tinnitus. May be used with gold, corticosteroids, and antacids.

Laboratory Test Interference   Reversible ↑ BUN

Dosage   **PO**: 20 mg once daily. Effect of therapy should not be assessed for 2 weeks. Safety and efficacy have not been established in children.

Additional Nursing Implications

Teach patient and/or family

a. that effects of therapy cannot be fully evaluated until 2 weeks after onset of therapy with piroxicam.
b. not to take aspirin during therapy with piroxicam because effectiveness of piroxicam will be decreased and the possibility of adverse reactions may be increased.

SULINDAC   Clinoril (Rx)

Classification   Antirheumatic, analgesic.

Action/Kinetics   Sulindac is biotransformed in the liver to a sulfide, the active metabolite. **Peak plasma levels of sulfide**: after fasting, 2 hr; after food, 3–4 hr. **t½**, of sulindac: 7.8 hr; of metabolite: 16.4 hr. Excreted in both urine and feces.

Additional Use   Acute, painful shoulder.

Additional Drug Interactions   Sulindac ↑ effect of warfarin due to ↓ plasma protein binding.

Dosage   *Osteoarthritis, rheumatoid arthritis, ankylosing spondylitis*: 150 mg b.i.d. up to 400 mg daily. *Acute painful shoulder, acute gouty arthritis*: 200 mg b.i.d. for 7 to 14 days. For acute conditions, reduce dosage when satisfactory response is attained. Safety and efficacy have not been established for children.

Additional Nursing Implications

See also *Nursing Implications*, p. 501.

1. Assess intake and output closely of patient with impaired renal function because the drug is excreted by the kidneys.
2. Anticipate reduction of dosage to prevent excessive drug accumulation, should intake and output indicate renal dysfunction.
3. Teach patients not to take aspirin while they are on sulindac, as plasma levels of sulindac would be reduced.

TOLMETIN SODIUM   Tolectin, Tolectin DS (Rx)

Classification   Nonsteroidal, anti-inflammatory, analgesic.

Action/Kinetics   **Peak plasma levels**: 30–60 min. t½: 1 hr. **Therapeutic plasma levels**: 40 µg/ml. Inactivated in liver and excreted in urine.

Additional Use   Juvenile rheumatoid arthritis.

Laboratory Test Interference   Tolmetin metabolites give a false + test for proteinuria using sulfosalicylic acid.

Dosage   **PO. Adults**: 400 mg t.i.d. (one dose on arising and one at bedtime); adjust dosage according to patient response. Doses larger than 2,000 mg/day for rheumatoid arthritis and 1,600 mg/day for osteoarthritis are not recommended. **Pediatric, 2 years and older**: 20 mg/kg/day in 3–4 divided doses to start; **then**, 15–30 mg/kg/day. Beneficial effects may not be observed for several days to a week.

Administration

1. One dose should be taken on arising, one during the day, and one dose at bedtime.
2. Administer with meals, milk, or antacids (other than sodium bicarbonate) if GI symptoms occur.

PYRAZOLONE DERIVATIVE

PHENYLBUTAZONE   Algoverine,* Alkabutazolidin,* Alkabutazone,* Alka-Phenylbutazone,* Apo-Phenylbutazone,* Azolid, Butazolidin, Intrabutazone,* Neo-Zoline,* Novobutazone* (Rx)

Classification   Anti-inflammatory, pyrazolone derivative.

General Statement   Phenylbutazone is potentially dangerous for a number of patients. The most serious toxic reactions are blood dyscrasias, including agranulocytosis, leukopenia, and thrombocytopenia. The untoward reactions are of a hypersensitivity nature and are not necessarily dose related. The effects can be developed by persons who have taken these drugs without ill effects for a number of years. Aim for the lowest dosage.

Action/Kinetics Phenylbutazone possess antipyretic, analgesic, anti-inflammatory, and weak uricosuric effects. The anti-inflammatory effects are believed to result from a combination of the inhibition of prostaglandin synthesis, leukocyte migration, and release of lysosomal enzymes. **Onset**: 30–60 min, **peak plasma levels**: 2 hr; **duration**: 3–5 days. t½: 72 hr. **Plasma protein binding**: 98%. Phenylbutazone is metabolized to oxyphenbutazone, which is active.

Uses Acute gouty arthritis, active rheumatoid arthritis, degenerative joint disease of the hips and knees. Due to the possibility of severe toxic effects, phenylbutazone should be used only as a last resort when other therapy has proven unsuccessful.

Contraindications History of peptic ulcer disease, cardiac failure, pancreatitis, senility, children under 14 years of age, hypertension, thyroid disease, blood dyscrasias, edema, arteritis, drug allergy, stomatitis, parotiditis. Severe cardiac, renal, or hepatic disease. Concomitantly with drugs causing similar untoward reactions. Pregnancy and lactation.

Untoward Reactions Phenylbutazone is associated with a large number of side effects. Patients should be monitored carefully. *GI:* GI upset, nausea, indigestion, heartburn, vomiting, flatulence, diarrhea or constipation, gastritis, stomatitis, GI ulceration, hematemesis. *CNS:* Headache, weakness, drowsiness, confusion, numbness, lethargy, agitation. *Hematologic:* Thrombocytopenia, pancytopenia, agranulocytosis, aplastic anemia, generalized bone marrow depression, hemolytic anemia, leukopenia. *CV:* Edema, congestive heart failure, hypertension, myocarditis, pericarditis. *Allergic:* Urticaria, rashes, fever, polyarteritis, vasculitis, Stevens-Johnson syndrome, anaphylaxis, exfoliative dermatitis, exacerbation of lupus erythematosus. *Renal:* Glomerulonephritis, necrosis, obstruction, nephrotic syndrome, hematuria, proteinuria, anuria, oliguria, renal stones, azotemia with renal failure. *Ophthalmologic:* Blurred vision, double vision, detached retina, optic neuritis, corneal ulceration, hemorrhage of retina. *Other:* Hepatitis, hyperglycemia, thyroid disorders, hearing loss, tinnitus, lymphadenopathy.

Drug Interactions

Interactant	Interaction
Alcohol	Impairment of psychomotor skills
Anabolic steroids	Certain androgens ↑ effect of phenylbutazone
Anticoagulants, oral	↑ Effect of anticoagulants by ↓ plasma protein binding and ↓ breakdown by the liver; phenylbutazone may also produce GI ulceration and therefore ↑ chance of bleeding
Antidiabetic agents	↑ Hypoglycemic response due to ↓ breakdown by liver and ↓ plasma protein binding
Digitalis glycosides	↓ Effect of digitalis glycosides due to ↑ breakdown by liver
Phenytoin	↑ Effect of phenytoin due to ↓ breakdown by liver
Salicylates	Phenylbutazone inhibits uricosuric activity of salicylates

Laboratory Test Interferences May alter liver function tests. False + Coombs, test. ↑ Prothrombin time.

Dosage PO. *Rheumatoid arthritis, degenerative joint disease*: **Adults**, 300–600 mg/day in 3 to 4 doses; maintenance: 100–200 mg/day, not to exceed 400 mg/day. To determine effectiveness, a 1-week trial period is adequate. *Acute gouty arthritis*: **initial**, 400 mg; **then**, 100 mg q 4 hr for 4–7 days.

Administration

1. Administer before or after meals with a glass of milk to minimize gastric irritation.
2. The dose should be discontinued in patients over 60 years of age as soon as possible after 7 days of therapy due to increased risk of severe untoward reactions.
3. Hemogram tests and urinalysis should be done prior to and at 1–2 week intervals during therapy.

Nursing Implications

1. Discontinue drug and notify the physician should the patient demonstrate any allergic manifestations to the drug such as rash, edema, or wheezing.
2. Be prepared for treatment of toxicity with equipment for gastric lavage, oxygen, and blankets for warmth.
3. Practice reverse isolation technique in caring for patient, if agranulocytosis is severe.
4. Weigh patient daily and report weight gain.
5. Anticipate positive results of treatment by third to fourth day. Trial therapy is not usually continued beyond 1 week in the absence of favorable results.
6. *Teach patient and/or family*
   a. that drug must be discontinued immediately and the physician notified, should skin reactions, fever, malaise, sore throat, and ulcerated mucous membranes develop—symptoms of possible irreversible agranulocytosis.
   b. the need for regular and frequent blood tests.
   c. to take only the dose ordered, and not to increase the dose.
   d. to weigh each morning before breakfast under standard conditons and to record on chart. Report progressive weight gain.
   e. how to assess for edema daily and to report edema if present.
   f. to keep a written report of intake and output and to report a decrease in urinary excretion.
   g. how to follow a low-sodium or low-salt diet, if ordered, to minimize edema.

REMITTING AGENTS

AURANOFIN Ridaura (Rx)

Classification Oral gold compound for arthritis.

Action/Kinetics Auranofin is a gold-containing (29%) compound that was developed for oral administration. The oral drug has fewer side effects than injectable gold products. Although the mechanism is not known, auranofin will improve symptoms of rheumatoid arthritis; it is most effective in the early stages of active synovitis. Gold will not reverse damage to joints caused by disease. Approximately 25% of an oral dose is absorbed. **Plasma t½ of auranofin gold:** 26 days. Approximately 3 months are required for steady state blood levels to be achieved. The drug is metabolized and excreted in both the urine and feces.

Uses   Adults with rheumatoid arthritis that has not responded to other drugs. Up to 6 months may be required for beneficial effects to occur. Auranofin should be a part of a total treatment regimen for rheumatoid arthritis including nondrug treatments.

Contraindications   History of gold-induced disorders including necrotizing enterocolitis, pulmonary fibrosis, exfoliative dermatitis, bone marrow aplasia, or other hematologic disorders. Use in pregnancy, lactation, and children. Use with caution in renal or hepatic disease, skin rashes, or history of bone marrow depression.

Untoward Reactions   *GI:* Nausea, vomiting, diarrhea (common), abdominal pain, metallic taste, stomatitis, glossitis, gingivitis, anorexia, constipation, flatulence, dyspepsia, dysgeusia. Rarely, melena, GI bleeding, dysphagia, ulcerative enterocolitis. *Dermatologic:* Skin rashes, pruritus, alopecia, urticaria, angioedema. *Hematologic:* Leukopenia, anemia, thrombocytopenia, hematuria, neutropenia, agranulocytosis. *Renal:* Proteinuria, hematuria. *Other:* Conjunctivitis, cholestatic jaundice, fever, interstitial pneumonia and fibrosis, peripheral neuropathy.

Laboratory Test Interference   ↑ Liver enzymes.

Dosage   **PO. Adults: initial,** either 6 mg once daily or 3 mg b.i.d. If response is unsatisfactory after 6 months, increase to 3 mg t.i.d. If response is still inadequate after 3 additional months, the drug should be discontinued. Dosages greater than 9 mg daily are not recommended. *Transfer from injectable gold:* Discontinue injectable gold and begin auranofin at a dose of 6 mg daily.

Nursing Implications

Teach patient and/or family

 a. the numerous signs of toxicity and which ones need to be reported to the physician immediately.
 b. the importance of complying with schedule of laboratory testing (usually monthly) to detect early signs of toxicity.

AUROTHIOGLUCOSE   Gold Thioglucose, Solganal (Rx)

GOLD SODIUM THIOMALATE   (Sodium Aurothioglucose)
Myochrysin (Rx)

Classification   Antirheumatic.

Action/Kinetics   Although the exact mechanism is not known, gold salts inhibit lysosomal enzyme activity in macrophages and decrease macrophage phagocytic activity. Gold salts suppress, but do not cure, arthritis and synovitis. The beneficial effects may not be seen for 3–12 months. Most patients experience transient side effects although serious effects may be manifested in some. **Peak blood levels (IM):** 4–6 hr. **t½:** increases with continued therapy. Gold may accumulate in tissues and persist for years. Gold is not metabolized and is excreted in both urine and feces.

Uses   Adjunct to the treatment of rheumatoid arthritis (active and progressive stages) in children and adults. It is most effective in the early stages of the disease.

Contraindications Hepatic disease, cardiovascular problems such as hypertension or congestive heart failure, severe diabetes, debilitated patients, renal disease, blood dyscrasias, agranulocytosis, hemorrhagic diathesis, patients receiving radiation treatments, colitis, lupus erythematosus, pregnancy, lactation, children under 6 years of age. Patients with eczema or urticaria.

Untoward Reactions *Skin:* Dermatitis (most common), pruritus, erythema, dermatoses, gray to blue pigmentation of tissues, alopecia, loss of nails. *GI:* Stomatitis (second most common), metallic taste, gastritis, colitis, gingivitis, glossitis, nausea, vomiting, diarrhea, colic, anorexia, cramps, enterocolitis. *Hematologic:* Anemia, thrombocytopenia, granulocytopenia, leukopenia, eosinophilia, hemorrhagic diathesis. *Allergic:* Flushing, fainting, sweating, dizziness, anaphylaxis, syncope, bradycardia, angioneurotic edema, respiratory difficulties. *Other:* Interstitial pneumonitis, pulmonary fibrosis, nephrotic syndrome, glomerulitis (with hematuria), hepatitis, fever, headache, arthralgia, opthalmologic problems including corneal ulcers, iritis, gold deposits, EEG abnormalities, peripheral neuritis.

Corticosteroids may be used to treat symptoms such as stomatitis, dermatitis, GI, renal, hematologic, or pulmonary problems. Also, if symptoms are severe and do not respond to corticosteroids a chelating agent such as dimercaprol may be used. Patients should be monitored carefully.

Drug Interactions Concomitant use contraindicated with drugs known to cause blood dyscrasias (e.g. antimalarials, cytotoxic drugs, pyrazolone derivatives).

Laboratory Test Interference Alters liver function tests. Urinary protein and RBCs, altered blood counts (indicative of toxic effect of drug).

Dosage *Gold sodium thiomalate, aurothioglucose—rheumatoid arthritis,* **adults, IM**, week 1: 10 mg/week; weeks 2 and 3: 25 mg/week. Thereafter, 50 mg/week until 0.8–1 gm total has been given. Thereafter according to individual response. *Usual*: 25 mg/week or 50 mg q 3–4 weeks. **Pediatric, IM:** *Gold sodium thiomalate:* **initial**, 10 mg; **then**, usual is 1 mg/kg not to exceed 50 mg/injection. *Aurothioglucose*: one-fourth of adult dose (use body weight as guide).

Administration

1. Shake vial well to insure uniform suspension before withdrawing medication.
2. Inject into gluteus maximus.
3. Gold therapy may be reinstituted following mild toxic symptoms but not after severe symptoms.

Nursing Implications

1. Have the patient recumbent for at least 20 minutes after injection to prevent falling caused by transient giddiness or vertigo that may occur.
2. Have on hand dimercaprol (BAL) to use as an antidote in case of severe toxicity.
3. *Teach patient and/or family*
   a. that close medical supervision is required during gold therapy.
   b. that beneficial effects are slow to appear but that therapy may be continued up to 12 months in anticipation of relief.

PENICILLAMINE Cuprimine, Depen (Rx)

Classification Antirheumatic, heavy metal antagonist, to treat cystinuria.

Action/Kinetics   Penicillamine, a degradation product of penicillin, is a chelating agent also used as a heavy metal antagonist and an antirheumatic. The anti-inflammatory activity (rheumatoid arthritis) of penicillamine may be due to its effect on the altered immune response (depression of IgM rheumatoid factor). Penicillamine chelates excess copper and therefore reduces the toxic concentration of copper characteristic of Wilson's disease. In cystinuria, penicillamine is able to reduce excess cystine excretion probably by disulfide interchange between penicillamine and cystine. This results in penicillamine-cysteine disulfide, which is a complex that is more soluble than cystine and is thus readily excreted. Penicillamine is well absorbed from GI tract and is excreted in urine. **Peak plasma levels:** 1 hr. t½: Approximately 2 hr. **It may take 2–3 months for positive responses to become apparent when treating rheumatoid arthritis.**

Uses   Wilson's disease, cystinuria, and rheumatoid arthritis—severe active disease that does not respond to conventional therapy. Heavy metal antagonist. *Investigational:* Primary biliary cirrhosis.

Contraindications   Pregnancy, penicillinase-related aplastic anemia or agranulocytosis, hypersensitivity to drug. Patients allergic to penicillin may cross-react with penicillamine. Renal insufficiency or history thereof.

Untoward Reactions   This drug manifests a high number of potentially serious side effects. Patients should be carefully monitored. *GI:* Altered taste perception (common), nausea, vomiting, diarrhea, anorexia, GI pain, stomatitis, oral ulcerations, reactivation of peptic ulcer, glossitis, cheilosis. *Hematologic:* Thrombocytopenia, leukopenia, agranulocytosis, aplastic anemia, eosinophilia, monocytosis, red cell aplasia. *Renal:* Proteinuria, hematuria, nephrotic syndrome, Goodpasture's syndrome (a severe and ultimately fatal glomerulonephritis). *Allergic:* Rashes (common), lupus-like syndrome, pruritus, pemphigoid-type symptoms (e.g., bullous lesions), drug fever, arthralgia, lymphadenopathy, dermatoses, urticaria, obliterative bronchiolitis. *Other:* Tinnitus, optic neuritis, neuropathy, thrombophlebitis, alopecia, precipitation of myasthenia gravis, increased body temperature, pulmonary fibrosis, pneumonitis, bronchial asthma, renal vasculitis (may be fatal), hot flashes, increased skin friability.

Drug Interactions

Interactant	Interaction
Antacids	↓ Effect of penicillamine due to ↓ absorption from GI tract
Digoxin	Penicillamine ↓ effect of digoxin
Iron salts	↓ Effect of penicillamine due to ↓ absorption from GI tract
Antimalarials Cytotoxic drugs Gold therapy Pyrazolone derivatives	↑ Risk of blood dyscrasias and adverse renal effects

Dosage   **PO.** *Wilson's disease:* Dosage is usually calculated on the basis of the urinary excretion of copper. One gram penicillamine promotes excretion of 2 mg copper. **PO, adults and children:** *usual, initial,* 250 mg q.i.d. Dosage may have to be increased to 2 gm daily. A further increase does not produce additional excretion. *Cystinuria:* individualized and based on excretion rate of cystine (100–200 mg/day in patients with no history of stones, below 100 mg with patients with history of stones or pain). Initiate at low dosage (250 mg/day) and increase gradually to minimum effective dosage. **Adult:** *usual,* 2 gm/day (range: 1–4 gm); **children:** 30 mg/kg/day in 4 divided doses. If divided in less than 4 doses, give larger dose at night. *Rheumatoid arthritis,* **PO,** *individualized:* **initial,** 125–250 mg/day. Dosage may be increased at 1–3 month intervals by 125–250 mg increments until adequate response is attained. **Maximum**: 500–750 mg/day. Up to 500 mg/day can be given as a single dose; higher dosages should be divided.

Administration

1. Give penicillamine on an empty stomach 1 hr before or 2 hr after meals. Also wait 1 hr after any other food, milk, or drug.
2. If patient cannot tolerate dosage for cystinuria, the bedtime dosage should be larger and should be continued.
3. For treatment of cystinuria, the patient should be advised to consume large amounts of fluid (e.g., 1 pint at bedtime and another pint during the night, since the urine is more concentrated and more acidic during the night).
4. Administer the contents of the capsule in 15–30 ml of chilled juice or pureed fruit if patient is unable to swallow capsules or tablets.

Nursing Implications

1. Ascertain that urinalysis and hematology tests are performed every 2 weeks for first 6 months of therapy and monthly thereafter.
2. Withhold penicillamine if WBC falls below 3,500 per mm³ and report platelet count below 100,000 per mm³. If there is a progressive fall in WBC and platelet count during 3 successive laboratory tests, a temporary interruption of therapy is indicated.
3. Ascertain that liver function tests are done before initiation of therapy and q 6 months during first 1 1/2 yr of therapy.
4. Rule out infection, if white papules appear at site of venipuncture and at surgical sites. Do not assume papules are due to penicillamine.
5. Anticipate reduction in dose to 250 mg/day before surgery and until wound healing is completed.
6. Note that a positive antinuclear antibody (ANA) test does not mandate discontinuance of drug, but suggests that a lupus-like syndrome may occur in the future.
7. Anticipate that pyridoxine will be ordered as a supplement, because penicillamine increases that body's need for this vitamin.
8. *Teach patient and/or family*
   a. to report fever, sore throat, chills, bruising, or bleeding—all early signs of granulocytopenia.
   b. to take temperature nightly during first few months of therapy, because fever may be an indicator of hypersensitivity reaction.
   c. oral care for stomatitis, which must be reported, as it usually requires discontinuance of drug.
   d. that a blurring of taste perception may last 2 or more months but that it is usually self-limiting, and adequate nutrition should be maintained.
   e. the necessity for a period of at least 2 hours to elapse between ingestion of penicillamine and therapeutic iron, because iron decreases cupruretic effects of penicillamine.
   f. that especially the elderly, should avoid excessive pressure on shoulders, elbows, knees, toes, and buttocks, because skin becomes more friable with penicillamine.
   g. to observe urine for proteinuria (cloudy in appearance) and for hematuria (smoky brown in early state, slightly blood tinged later, and then grossly bloody). Report positive findings.

h. that for a woman of childbearing age, use of penicillamine during pregnancy is contraindicated, because drug can cause fetal damage.

i. that a woman should report to medical supervision, if a menstrual period is missed or other symptoms of pregnancy are noted.

j. for a patient with Wilson's disease to

(1) continue on low-copper diet by excluding chocolate, nuts, shellfish, mushrooms, liver, molasses, broccoli, and cereals enriched with copper.

(2) use distilled or demineralized water if drinking water contains more than 0.1 mg of copper/liter.

(3) ingest sulfurated potash or Carbo-Resin with meals to minimize absorption of copper except when patient is also receiving supplemental iron.

(4) continue therapy because it may take 1–3 months until neurologic symptoms show improvement.

(5) check that any vitamin preparations ingested are copper free.

k. for a patient with cystinuria

(1) to drink large amounts of fluid to prevent formation of renal calculi. Patients should drink 1 pint at bedtime and another pint during the night when urine tends to be the most concentrated and most acidic. Urine should have a specific gravity less than 1.010 and a pH of 7.5–8.

(2) to have yearly x-ray films of kidneys performed to determine whether renal calculi are present.

(3) to continue on diet low in methionine, a major precursor of cystine, by excluding rich meat soups and broths, milk, eggs, cheeses, and peas.

(4) that diet low in methionine is contraindicated for children and during pregnancy because of its low-protein content.

l. for a patient with rheumatoid arthritis to continue using other modalities to achieve relief of symptoms, because the therapeutic response to penicillamine may take up to 6 months.

MISCELLANEOUS AGENTS

DIFLUNISAL   Dolobid (Rx)

Classification   Nonsteroidal analgesic, anti-inflammatory, antipyretic.

Action/Kinetics   Diflunisal is a salicylic acid derivative although it is not metabolized to salicylcic acid. Its mechanism is not known although it is thought to be an inhibitor of prostaglandin synthetase. **Peak plasma levels:** 2–3 hr. **Peak effect:** 2–3 hr. **t½:** 8–12 hr. Ninety-nine percent protein bound. Metabolites excreted in urine.

Uses   Analgesic, osteoarthritis, musculoskeletal pain.

Contraindications   Hypersensitivity to drug, aspirin, or other anti-inflammatory drugs. Acute asthmatic attacks, urticaria, or rhinitis precipitated by aspirin. Use with caution in presence of ulcers or history thereof and in patients with hypertension, compromised cardiac function, or in conditions leading to fluid retention. Lactation and children less than 12 years of age. Use with caution in only first two trimesters of pregnancy.

Untoward Reactions *GI:* Nausea, dyspepsia, GI pain, diarrhea, vomiting, constipation, flatulence, peptic ulcer, GI bleeding, eructation, anorexia. *CNS:* Headache, fatigue, fever, malaise, dizziness, somnolence, insomnia, nervousness, vertigo, depression, paresthesias. *Dermatologic:* Rashes, pruritus, sweating, Stevens-Johnson syndrome, dry mucous membranes, erythemia multiforme. *CV:* Palpitations, syncope, edema. *Other:* Tinnitus, asthenia, chest pain, hypersensitivity reactions, anaphylaxis, dyspnea, dysuria, muscle cramps, thrombocytopenia.

Drug Interactions

Interactant	Interaction
Acetaminophen	↑ Plasma levels of acetaminophen
Antacids	↓ Plasma levels of diflunisal
Anticoagulants	↑ Prothrombin time
Furosemide	↓ Hyperuricemic effect of furosemide
Hydrochlorothiazide	↑ Plasma levels and ↓ hyperuricemic effect of hydrochlorothiazide
Indomethacin	↓ Renal clearance of indomethacin → ↑ plasma levels
Naproxen	↓ Urinary excretion of naproxen and metabolite

Dosage   PO. *Mild to moderate pain:* **initial,** 1,000 mg; **then,** 250–500 mg q 8–12 hr. *Osteoarthritis:* 250–500 mg b.i.d. Doses in excess of 1,500 mg/day are not recommended.

Administration

1. May be given with water, milk, or meals to decrease gastric upset.
2. Acetaminophen or aspirin should not be taken with diflunisal.

Additional Nursing Implications

See also *Nursing Implications,* p. 501.

1. *Assess*
   a. for bleeding in patient on high doses of diflunisal, since drug may inhibit platelet aggregation.
   b. for bleeding in patient on oral anticoagulant therapy because of increased prothrombin time due to drug interaction.
2. Teach patient and/or family to consult with physician before using antacids as they may lower plasma levels and thus reduce effectiveness of diflunisal.

HYDROXYCHLOROQUINE SULFATE   Plaquenil Sulfate (Rx)

Classification   Antimalarial.

General Statement   Antimalarial sometimes used for treatment of rheumatoid arthritis, discoid and systemic lupus erythematosus.

For most details, see *4-Aminoquinoline Antimalarials,* p. 168, and drug entry for that section, p. 170.

Hydroxychloroquine is not a drug of choice for rheumatoid arthritis and should be discontinued after 6 months if no beneficial effects are noted. Patients on long-term therapy should be examined thoroughly at regular intervals for knee and ankle reflexes and hematopoietic studies. *Drug may cause retinopathy;* thus baseline ophthalmologic examinations, repeated at 3-month intervals, must be performed, and drug discontinued in the event of ophthalmic damage, impaired reflexes, and blood dyscrasias.

Treatment of toxic symptoms: Administration of 8 gm ammonium chloride in divided doses 3 to 4 times week for several months to improve residual excretion of drug.

Dosage   See p. 170.

Nursing Implications

See *Nursing Implications* for *Antimalarials*, p. 169.

1. When the drug is given for rheumatoid arthritis
   a. reassure patient and indicate that benefits may not occur until 6 to 12 months after therapy has been initiated.
   b. anticipate that side effects may necessitate a reduction of therapy. After 5 to 10 days of reduced dosage, it may gradually again be increased to the desired level.
   c. anticipate that dosage will be reduced when the desired response is attained. Drug again will be effective in case of flare-up.
   d. reduce GI irritation by administering drug with meal or glass of milk.
2. When drug is given for lupus erythematosus, administer with evening meal.

MEFENAMIC ACID   Ponstan,* Ponstel (Rx)

Classification   Mild analgesic, antipyretic, nonnarcotic, miscellaneous.

Action/Kinetics   Mefenamic acid manifests anti-inflammatory, analgesic, and antipyretic effects. Like aspirin, it inhibits prostaglandin synthesis. **Peak plasma levels**: 2–4 hr; **duration**: 4–6 hr. The drug is absorbed slowly from the GI tract, metabolized by the liver, and excreted in urine and feces.

Uses   Short-term relief of mild to moderate pain such as that associated with toothache, tooth extraction, and musculoskeletal disorders. Dysmenorrhea.

Contraindications   Ulceration or chronic inflammation of the GI tract, pregnancy or possibility thereof, children under 14, and hypersensitivity to drug.

To be used with caution in patients with impaired renal or hepatic function, asthma, or patients on anticoagulant therapy.

Untoward Reactions   Neurologic and GI effects, including headache, drowsiness, dizziness, GI cramps, diarrhea, GI hemorrhage, and blood dyscrasias.

Drug Interactions

Interactant	Interaction
Anticoagulants	↑ Hypoprothrombinemia due to ↓ plasma protein binding
Insulin	↑ Insulin requirement

Laboratory Test Interference   False + test for urinary bile using diazo tablets.

Dosage   **PO.** *Analgesic.* **Adults and children over 14: initial,** 500 mg, followed by 250 mg q 6 hr. Length of therapy should not exceed 1 week. *Dysmenorrhea:* **initial,** 500 mg; **then,** 250 mg q 6 hr for 2–3 days.

Administration   With food.

Nursing Implications
1. Withhold drug and report rash or diarrhea.
2. Assess the patient for any signs of bleeding, as drug lowers the prothrombin time.
3. Advise patient to use caution when operating potentially hazardous machinery as in driving because drug may cause dizziness, lightheadedness, or confusion.

Chapter Forty

ANTIGOUT AGENTS

General Statement   Gout or gouty arthritis is characterized by an excess of uric acid in the body. This excess results either from an overproduction of uric acid or from a defect in its breakdown or elimination.

When the concentration of sodium urate in the blood exceeds a certain level (6 mg in 100 ml), it may start to form fine, needlelike crystals that can become deposited in the joints and cause an acute inflammatory response in the synovial membrane. Hyperuricemia may also accompany other diseases such as leukemia or lymphomas. High levels of uric acid may also accompany treatment with certain antineoplastic agents or thiazide diuretics. High uric acid levels in the kidney may lead to precipitation of uric acid crystals, which can cause kidney damage.

Therapy is aimed at reducing the uric acid level of the body to normal or near-normal levels. Drugs used for the treatment of gout or hyperuricemia either promote the excretion of uric acid by the kidney or reduce the amount of uric acid formed. These drugs, however, have no analgesic or anti-inflammatory properties although colchicine will decrease urate crystal-induced inflammation.

Previously, gout was often treated by dietary measures—reduced intake of purine-rich foods such as meat. Dietary restrictions are seldom prescribed today, except for organ meats, which have a high purine content.

Acute gout. As opposed to other forms of arthritis, acute gout has a dramatic onset. Maximum pain, joint swelling, and joint tenderness are reached within hours. An acute attack of gout is often accompanied by a low-grade fever and an increase in the WBC count.

In between attacks the patient with hyperuricemia is usually symptom free; however, since acute attacks usually recur in patients with hyperuricemia, patients are often kept on a maintenance dose of a uricosuric agent.

ALLOPURINOL   Alloprin,* Apo-Allopurinol,* Lopurin, Novopurol,* Purinol,* Roucol,* Zyloprim (Rx)

Classification   Antigout agent.

Remarks   Allopurinol is not useful for the treatment of *acute* attacks of gout, but is the drug of choice for *chronic* gouty arthritis. Allopurinol reduces uric acid without disrupting the biosynthesis of essential purines.

Action/Kinetics   Allopurinol and its major metabolite, oxypurinol, are potent inhibitors of xanthine oxidase, an enzyme involved in the synthesis of uric acid without disrupting the biosynthesis of essential purine. This results in decreased levels of uric acid. **Peak plasma levels**: 2–6 hr. **t½** (allopurinol); 2–3 hr; **t½** (oxypurinol): 18–30 hr. **Maximum therapeutic effect**: 1–3 weeks. Well absorbed from GI tract, metabolized in liver, excreted in urine.

Uses   Not useful for the treatment of *acute* gout, but is the drug of choice for *chronic* gouty arthritis. Gout, hyperuricemia associated with polycythemia vera, myeloid metaplasia or other blood dyscrasias, and certain cases of primary and secondary renal disease. Prophylaxis in hyperuricemia and as an adjunct in some antineoplastic therapy.

Allopurinol is sometimes administered concomitantly with uricosuric agents in patients with severe tophaceous gout. (A tophus is a deposit of sodium urate).

Contraindications   Hypersensitivity to drug. Patients with idiopathic hemochromatosis or relatives of patients suffering from this condition. Children except as an adjunct in treatment of neoplastic disease. Severe skin reactions on previous exposure. Use with caution in patients with liver or renal disease.

Untoward Reactions   *Dermatologic* (most frequent): Pruritic maculopapular skin rash (may be accompanied by fever and malaise). Exfoliative urticarial, purpura-type dermatitis and alopecia. Stevens Johnson syndrome. Skin rash has been accompanied by hypertension and cataract development. *Allergy:* Fever, chills, leukopenia, eosinophilia, arthralgia, skin rash, pruritus, nausea, vomiting, nephritis.

Drug Interactions

Interactant	Interaction
Ampicillin	Concomitant use may result in skin rashes
Anticoagulants, oral	↑ Effect of anticoagulant due to ↓ breakdown by liver
Azathioprine	↑ Effect of azathioprine due to ↓ breakdown by liver
Iron preparations	Allopurinol ↑ hepatic iron concentrations
Mercaptopurine	↑ Effect of mercaptopurine due to ↓ breakdown by liver
Theophylline	Allopurinol ↑ plasma theophylline levels

Laboratory Test Interferences   Alters liver function test. ↑ Serum cholesterol. ↓ Serum glucose levels.

Dosage   **PO**. *Gout/hyperuricemia*: 200–600 mg/day, depending on severity. *Prevention of uric acid nephropathy during treatment of neoplasms*: 600–800 mg/day for 2–3 days (with high fluid intake); minimum effective dose: 100–200 mg/day. *Prophylaxis of acute gout*: **initial**, 100 mg/day; increase by 100 mg at weekly intervals until serum uric acid level of 6 mg/100 ml or less is reached. **Pediatric**, *Hyperuricemia associated with malignancy*, **6–10 years of age**: 300 mg per day; **under 6 years of age**: 150 mg/day. Transfer from colchicine: uricosuric agents and/or anti-inflammatory agents to allopurinol should be made gradually by decreasing the dosage of the above agents and increasing the dosage of allopurinol.

Dosage should be decreased in renal impairment.

Administration

1. May be taken with food to decrease GI upset.
2. At least 10–12 eight-ounce glasses of fluid should be taken each day.
3. To prevent uric acid stone formation, the urine should be kept slightly alkaline.

Nursing Implications

1. Anticipate that during transfer of patient from uricosuric drug to allopurinol the dosage of the uricosuric agent is gradually decreased as the allopurinol dosage is gradually increased.
2. *Teach patient and/or family*
   a. to report a skin rash that may start months after initiation of drug therapy, because it may be caused by allopurinol and be an indication for discontinuing drug.
   b. to maintain a fluid intake that will result in a minimum excretion of 2 liters of urine daily (unless other medical condition contraindicates this) so as to prevent kidney damage.
   c. not to take iron salts while under treatment with allopurinol, because high iron concentrations in liver may occur.
   d. to use caution driving a car or carrying out other mechanical tasks requiring mental alertness, because allopurinol may cause drowsiness.
   e. to avoid excessive intake of vitamin C, which might lead to increased potential of kidney stone formation.
   f. to avoid use of alcohol, which would decrease effect of allopurinol.

COLCHICINE   Colsalide (Rx)

Classification   Antigout agent.

Action/Kinetics   Colchicine, an alkaloid, does not increase the excretion of uric acid (not uricosuric), but is is believed to reduce the crystal-induced inflammation by reducing lactic acid production by leukocytes (resulting in a decreased deposition of sodium urate), by inhibiting leukocyte migration, and by reducing phagocytosis. $t\frac{1}{2}$ (IV) (biphasic) initial: 20 min; final (in leukocytes): 60 hr. Colchicine is metabolized in liver and mostly excreted in the feces.

Uses   Agent of choice in acute attacks of gout, either spontaneous or induced by allopurinol or uricosuric agents; diagnosis of gout. Prophylaxis of recurrent gouty arthritis.

Contraindications   Use with extreme caution for elderly, debilitated patients, especially in the presence of chronic renal, hepatic, GI or cardiovascular disease.

Untoward Reactions   The drug is toxic; thus patients must be carefully monitored. Nausea, vomiting, diarrhea, abdominal cramping (discontinue drug at once and wait at least 48 hours before reinstating drug therapy). Prolonged administration can cause bone marrow depression, thrombocytopenia and aplastic anemia, peripheral neuritis, and liver dysfunction.

Acute colchicine intoxication is characterized at first by violent GI tract symptoms, such as nausea, vomiting, abdominal pain, and diarrhea. The latter may be profuse, watery, bloody, and associated with severe fluid and electrolyte loss. Also, burning of throat and skin, hematuria and oliguria, rapid and weak pulse, general exhaustion, muscular depression, and CNS involvement. Death is usually caused by respiratory paralysis. Treatment of acute poisoning involves gastric lavage, symptomatic support, including atropine and morphine, artificial respiration, hemodialysis, peritoneal dialysis, and treatment of shock.

Drug Interactions

Interactant	Interaction
Acidifying agents	Inhibit the action of colchicine
Alkalinizing agents	Potentiate the action of colchicine
CNS depressants	Patients on colchicine may be more sensitive to CNS depressant effect of these drugs
Sympathomimetic agents	Enhanced by colchicine
Vitamin B_{12}	Colchicine may interfere with absorption from the gut

Laboratory Test Interferences   Alters liver function tests. ↑ Alkaline phosphatase. False positive for hemoglobin or red blood cells in urine.

Dosage   *Acute attack of gout,* **PO**: 1–1.2 mg followed by 0.5–0.6 mg q hr (or 1–1.2 mg q 2 hr) until pain is relieved or diarrhea occurs. **Total amount required**: 4–8 mg. **IV: initial**, 1–2 mg; **subsequently**, 0.5 mg q 3–6 hr until pain is relieved; give up to 4 mg. *Prophylaxis*: **PO**: 0.5–0.6 mg/day for 3–4 days/week. Usually, oral route is used exclusively.

Administration/Storage

1. Store in tight light-resistant containers.
2. Parenteral administration is only to be by IV route. Drug would cause severe local irritation if given SC or IM.

Nursing Implications

1. Withhold drug if GI effects occur, and check with physician.
2. Anticipate that Paregoric may be ordered for treatment of severe diarrhea due to colchicine.
3. *Teach patient and/or family*
   a. to always have colchicine available if physician has prescribed its use for an acute attack of gout.
   b. to start or increase dosage of colchicine as ordered at first sign of joint pain or symptom of impending attack.

PROBENECID   Benemid, Benuryl,* Probalan, SK-Probenecid (Rx)

Classification   Antigout agent, uricosuric agent.

Action/Kinetics   Probenecid, a uricosuric agent, increases the excretion of uric acid by inhibiting the tubular reabsorption of uric acid; this action results in a decreased serum level of uric acid. Probenecid also inhibits the renal secretion of penicillins and cephalosporins; this effect is often taken advantage of in the treatment of infections, since concomitant administration of probenecid will increase plasma levels of antibiotics. **Peak plasma levels**: 2–4 hr. **Therapeutic plasma levels for inhibition of antibiotic secretion**: 40–60 μg/ml; **therapeutic plasma levels for uricosuric effect**: 100–200 μg/ml. t½: 8–10 hr. Probenecid is metabolized in the liver and is excreted in urine.

Uses   Hyperuricemia in chronic gout and gouty arthritis. Adjunct in therapy with penicillins or cephalosporins to elevate and prolong plasma antibiotic levels.

Contraindications   Hypersensitivity to drug, blood dyscrasias, uric acid, and kidney stones. Administer with caution to patients with renal disease, and children below 2 years of age. Use with caution in porphyria, glucose 6-phosphate dehydrogenase deficiency, and peptic ulcer.

Untoward Reactions   *CNS*: Headaches, dizziness. *GI*: Anorexia, nausea, vomiting, diarrhea, constipation, and abdominal discomfort. *Allergic:* Skin rash or drug fever, and very rarely anaphylactoid reactions. *Miscellaneous:* Flushing, hemolytic anemia, nephrotic syndrome, sore gums.

Initially, the drug may increase frequency of acute gout attacks due to mobilization of uric acid.

Drug Interactions

Interactant	Interaction
Acyclovir	Probenecid ↓ renal excretion of acyclovir
Aminosalicyclic acid (PAS)	↑ Effects of PAS due to ↓ excretion by kidney
Captopril	↑ Effect of captopril due to ↓ excretion by kidney
Cephalosporin	↑ Effect of cephalosporins due to ↓ excretion by kidney
Clofibrate	↑ Effect of clofibrate due to ↓ excretion and ↓ plasma protein binding
Dyphylline	↑ Effect dyphylline due to ↓ excretion by kidney
Indomethacin	↑ Effect of indomethacin due to ↓ excretion by kidney
Methotrexate	↑ Effect of methotrexate due to ↓ excretion by kidney
Naproxen	↑ Effect of naproxen due to ↓ excretion by kidney
Penicillins	↑ Effect of penicillins due to ↓ excretion by kidney
Pyrazinamide	Probenecid inhibits hyperuricemia produced by pyrazinamide
Rifampin	↑ Effect of rifampin due to ↓ excretion by kidney
Salicylates	Salicylates inhibit uricosuric activity of probenecid
Sulfinpyrazone (Anturane)	↑ Effect of sulfinpyrazone due to ↓ excretion by kidney
Sulfonamides	↑ Effect of sulfonamides due to ↓ plasma protein binding
Sulfonylureas, oral	↑ Action of sulfonylureas →hypoglycemia
Thiopental	↑ Effect of thiopental

Dosage   *Gout*, **PO: initial**, 250 mg b.i.d. for 1 week. **Maintenance**: 500 mg b.i.d. Dosage may have to be increased further (by 500 mg daily q 4 weeks to maximum of 2 gm) until urate excretion is less than 700 mg in 24 hr. *Adjunct to penicillin or cephalosporin therapy*: 500 mg q.i.d. Dosage is decreased for elderly patients with renal damage. **Pediatric, 2–14 years: initial**, 25 mg/kg; **maintenance**, 40 mg/kg/day in divided doses. **For children 50 kg or more**: give adult dosage. **Not recommended for use in children under 2 years of age**. Colbenemid, a combination tablet containing colchicine (0.5 mg) and probenecid (500 mg), is available.

Nursing Implications

1. Anticipate that urine may be alkalinized by sodium bicarbonate to prevent urates from crystallizing out of acid urine and forming kidney stones.
2. Be alert to the possibility that medication may cause a false Benedict test.
3. Report gastric intolerance promptly so that dosage may be corrected without loss of therapeutic effect.
4. Be alert to hypersensitivity reactions that occur more frequently with intermittent therapy.
5. Assess patient receiving medication whose excretion is inhibited by probenecid, as plasma levels may be toxic. Appropriate dosage adjustments should be made.
6. *Teach patient and/or family*
   a. that a liberal intake of fluids is essential to help prevent the formation of sodium urate stones.
   b. to note carefully whether there has been an increase in the number of attacks at the initiation of therapy, because physician may decide to add colchicine to regimen.
   c. to continue taking probenecid during acute attacks with colchicine as ordered unless specifically told by physician to discontinue use.
   d. not to take salicylates during uriscosuric therapy. Acetaminophen preparations may be used for analgesia instead of salicylates.

SULFINPYRAZONE   Antazone,* Anturane, Apo-Sulfinpyrazone,* Novopyrazone,* Zynol* (Rx)

Classification   Antigout agent, uricosuric.

General Statement   Sulfinpyrazone is not effective during acute attacks of gout and may even increase the frequency of acute episodes during the initiation of therapy. However, drug should not be discontinued during acute attacks. Concomitant administration of colchicine during initiation of therapy is recommended.

Action/Kinetics   Sulfinpyrazone inhibits the tubular reabsorption of uric acid thereby increasing the excretion of uric acid. Sulfinpyrazone also manifests antithrombotic and platelet inhibitory actions. **Peak plasma levels**: 1–2 hr. **Therapeutic plasma levels**: 10 μg/ml (for uricosuria). **Duration**: 4–6 hr (up to 10 hr in some). **t½**: 3–8 hr. Sulfinpyrazone is metabolized in the liver. Approximately 45% of the drug is excreted unchanged by the kidney, and a small amount is excreted in the feces.

Uses   Chronic gouty arthritis to reduce frequency and intensity of acute attacks of gout. *Investigational*: To decrease sudden death during first year after myocardial infarction.

Contraindications   Active peptic ulcer. Use with extreme caution in patients with impaired renal function and those with a history of peptic ulcers. Blood dyscrasias. Sensitivity to phenylbutazone. Use with caution in pregnant women.

Untoward Reactions   *GI*: Nausea, vomiting, abdominal discomfort. May reactivate peptic ulcer. *Hematologic*: Leukopenia, agranulocytosis, anemia, thrombocytopenia. *Miscellaneous*: Skin rash, which usually disappears with usage.

Acute attacks of gout may become more frequent during initial therapy. Give concomitantly with colchicine at this time.

Drug Interactions

Interactant	Interaction
Anticoagulants	↑ Effect of anticoagulant due ↓ plasma protein binding
Insulin	Potentiation of hypoglycemic effect
Probenecid	↑ Effect of sulfinpyrazone due to ↓ excretion by kidney.
Salicylates	Salicylates inhibit uricosuric effect of sulfinpyrazone
Sulfonamides	↑ Effect of sulfonamides by ↓ plasma protein binding
Sulfonylureas, oral	Potentiation of hypoglycemic effect

Dosage   **PO. Intitial**: 200–400 mg/day in 2 divided doses with meals. Patients who are transferred from other uricosuric agents can receive full dose at once. **Maintenance**: 400 mg/day in 2 divided doses up to 800 mg/day, if necessary. Maintain full dosage without interruption even during acute attacks of gout. *Following myocardial infarction*: 200 mg q.i.d.

Administration

1. Take with meals or antacids to minimize gastric upset.
2. At least 10–12 eight-ounce glasses of fluid should be taken daily.
3. Acidification of the urine may cause formation of uric acid stones.

Nursing Implications

1. Encourage liberal fluid intake to help prevent the formation of uric acid stones.
2. Anticipate the urine may be alkalinized by sodium bicarbonate to help prevent urates from crystallizing out of acid urine and forming kidney stones.
3. Administer with meals or with an antacid to minimize gastric distress.

Chapter Forty-one

ANOREXIANTS, ANALEPTICS, AND AGENTS FOR ATTENTION DEFICIT DISORDERS

General Statement   It is difficult to separate the central nervous system (CNS) stimulants into rigid pharmacologic classes because their effect is dose dependent. For example, any agent with primarily cerebral action will stimulate respiration, because respiratory control centers are located in the brainstem. Moreover, they can induce paradoxical reactions that are taken advantage of pharmacologically. For example, certain CNS stimulants have a quietening effect on children who suffer from hyperkinesia or other behavior problems of neurologic rather than psychological origin. (These conditions are called attention deficit disorders.) These agents and other CNS stimulants can be beneficial for patients suffering from extrapyramidal motor symptoms and spasticity.

The effect of these drugs is often not limited to the CNS. For example, the cardiovascular and autonomic nervous systems may also be affected; such effects are unwanted when the primary goal is stimulation of the CNS.

Even though there is a great deal of overlap among the indications for the various CNS stimulants, they have been divided according to their main clinical uses or pharmacologic action, into *Anorexiants, Analeptics,* and *Agents for Attention Deficit Disorders.* Spinal cord stimulants cause convulsions and are not used clinically; thus, they are not discussed.

ANOREXIANTS, AMPHETAMINES, AND DERIVATIVES

General Statement   Response to amphetamines is individualized. Psychic stimulation is often followed by a rebound effect manifested as fatigue. Tolerance will develop to all drugs of this class. The slight differences in the pharmacologic and untoward reactions of the different anorexiants (appetite suppression, respiratory stimulation, length of action) dictates their principal use.

Action/Kinetics   These drugs are thought to act on the cerebral cortex and reticular activating system (including the medullary respiratory and vasomotor centers) by releasing norepinephrine from adrenergic neurons. There is also some evidence that amphetamine might exert direct effects on adrenergic receptors. The stimulatory effect on the CNS causes an increase in motor activity and mental alertness, a mood-elevating effect, a slight euphoric effect, and an anorexigenic effect. The anorexigenic effect is thought to be produced by direct stimulation of the satiety center in the limbic and hypothalamic areas of the brain. Amphetamines are readily absorbed from the GI tract and are distributed throughout most tissues, with highest concentrations in the brain and CSF. Duration of anorexia (PO): 3–6 hr. Metabolized in liver and excreted by kidneys.

Uses   Appetite control (short term), narcolepsy, to counteract overdoses of depressants, to treat the depressive phase of manic-depressive psychoses. Also to treat hyperkinetic children and other abnormal behavior patterns in children.

Note: Many physicians recommend that amphetamines be used *only* for narcolepsy or hyperactive syndrome in children.

Contraindications   Hyperthyroidism, nephritis, diabetes mellitus, hypertension, narrow-angle glaucoma, angina pectoris, cardiovascular disease, and patients with hypersensitivity to drug. To be used with caution in patients suffering from hyperexcitability states; in elderly, debilitated, or asthenic patients; in patients with psychopathic personality traits or a history of homicidal or suicidal tendencies. Contraindicated in emotionally unstable persons susceptible to drug abuse.

Untoward Reactions   *CNS:* Nervousness, dizziness, depression, headache, insomnia, euphora, symptoms of excitation. Rarely, psychoses. *GI:* Nausea, vomiting, cramps, diarrhea, dry mouth, constipation, metallic taste, anorexia. *CV:* Arrhythmias, palpitations, dyspnea, pulmonary hypertension, peripheral hyper- or hypotension, precordial pain, fainting. *Dermatologic:* Symptoms of allergy including rash, urticaria, erythema, burning. Pallor. *GU:* Urinary frequency, dysuria. *Ophthalmologic:* Blurred vision, mydriasis. *Hematologic:* Agranulocytosis, leukopenia. *Endocrine:* Menstrual irregularities, gynecomastia, impotence and changes in libido. *Miscellaneous:* Alopecia, increased motor activity, fever, sweating, chills, muscle pain, chest pain.

Long-term use results in psychic dependence as well as a high degree of tolerance.

TOXIC REACTIONS   There is a relatively wide margin of safety between the therapeutic and toxic doses of amphetamines. However, amphetamines can cause both acute and chronic toxicity. Amphetamines are excreted very slowly (5 to 7 days) and cumulative effects may occur with continued administration.

Acute toxicity (overdosage) is characterized by cardiovascular symptoms (flushing, pallor, palpitations, labile pulse, changes in BP, heart block, or chest pains), hyperpyrexia, mental disturbances (confusion, delirium, acute psychoses, disorientation, delusions and hallucinations, panic states, paranoid ideation).

Death usually results from cardiovascular collapse or convulsions.

Chronic toxicity due to abuse is characterized by emotional lability, loss of appetite, somnolence, mental impairment, occupational deterioration, a tendency to withdraw from social contact, teeth grinding, continuous chewing, and ulcers of the tongue and lips.

Prolonged use of high doses can elicit symptoms of paranoid schizophrenia, including auditory and visual hallucinations and paranoid ideation.

Treatment of Acute Toxicity (Overdosage)   Symptomatic treatment. After oral ingestion, induce emesis or perform gastric lavage followed by activated charcoal. Adequate circulation and respiration should be maintained. Hyperpyrexia and other CNS symptoms may be treated with chlorpromazine. Diazepam or a barbiturate may be given for sedation. Phentolamine maybe used for hypertension while hypotension may be reversed by IV fluids and possibly vasopressors (used with caution). Stimuli should be reduced so that the patient is maintained in a quiet, dim environment. Patients who have ingested an overdosage of long-acting products should be treated for toxicity until all symptoms of overdosage have disappeared.

Drug Interactions

Interactant	Interaction
Acetazolamide	↑ Effect of amphetamine by ↑ renal tubular reabsorption
Ammonium chloride	↓ Effect of amphetamine by ↓ renal tubular reabsorption
Anesthetics, general	↑ Risk of cardiac arrhythmias
Antihypertensives	Amphetamines ↓ effect of antihypertensives
Ascorbic acid	↓ Effect of amphetamine by ↓ renal tubular reabsorption
Furazolidone	↑ Toxicity of anorexiants
Guanethidine	↓ Effect of guanethidine by displacement from its site of action
Haloperidol	↓ Effect of amphetamine by ↓ uptake of drug at its site of action
Insulin	Amphetamines alter insulin requirements
Methyldopa	↓ Hypotensive effect of methyldopa by ↑ sympathomimetic activity
MAO inhibitors	All peripheral, metabolic, cardiac, and central effects of amphetamine are potentiated up to 2 weeks after termination of MAO inhibitor therapy (symptoms include hypertensive crisis with possible intracranial hemorrhage, hyperthermia, convulsions, coma)—death may occur ↓ Effect of amphetamine by ↓ uptake of drug into its site of action
Phenothiazines	↓ Effect of amphetamine by ↓ uptake of drug into its site of action
Sodium bicarbonate	↑ Effect of amphetamine by ↑ renal tubular reabsorption
Thiazide diuretics	↑ Effect of amphetamine by ↑ renal tubular reabsorption

Laboratory Test Interference   ↑ Urinary catecholamines.

Dosage   Individualized (see Table 17). Many compounds are timed-release preparations.

TABLE 17 ANOREXIANTS, AMPHETAMINES AND DERIVATIVES

Drug	Dosage	Remarks
Amphetamine complex (Biphetamine 12½ and 20) C-II, Rx	**PO.** *Anorectic:* 12.5 mg daily (1 capsule). *Hyperkinesis.* Maintenance only: dosage variable.	Resin complex of amphetamine and dextroamphetamine. *Kinetics* See Amphetamine sulfate. *Administration* 10 to 14 hours before bedtime.
Amphetamine sulfate (Benzedrine *) C-II, Rx	**PO** *Narcolepsy:* **adult:** 5–60 mg/day. **Pediatric 12 years or older:** 10 mg daily; **6–12 years:** 5 mg daily. *Hyperkinetic behavior in children:* **3–5 years of age, initial,** 2.5 mg/day; increase by 2.5 mg weekly until optimum dosage achieved; **6 years and older, initial,** 5 mg 1–2 times/day; increase by 5 mg weekly until optimum level reached (rarely over 40 mg/day). *Anorectic:* **adult,** 5–30 mg daily in divided doses 30–60 min before meals (long-acting: 10 or 15 mg in AM).	*Administration* Give last dose 6 hr before bedtime. Should only be used for short-term therapy as an anorexiant. *Kinetics* After PO administration, completely absorbed in 3 hr. **Duration: PO,** 4–24 hr; t½: 5 hr. Excreted in urine. Acidification will increase excretion, while alkalinization will decrease excretion.
Benzphetamine hydrochloride (Didrex) C-III, Rx	**PO:** 25–50 mg 1 to 3 times daily 1 hour before meals.	Long-term use of large doses may result in psychic dependence. Contraindicated in pregnancy. *Administration* A single daily dose is preferably given in midmorning or midafternoon, depending on eating habits of patient.
Dextroamphetamine sulfate (Dexampex, Dexedrine, Ferndex, Oxydess, Spancap No. 1) C-II, Rx	Same dosage as Amphetamine sulfate (see above)	Has stronger central action and weaker peripheral action than does amphetamine, hence fewer undesirable cardiovascular effects. *Kinetics* See Amphetamine sulfate.
Diethylpropion hydrochloride (Depletite-25, Nobesine-75,* Propion,* Regibon,* Tenuate, Tepanil) C-IV, Rx	**PO:** 25 mg t.i.d. 1 hr before meals or as a single, 75-mg extended-release tablet at midmorning.	*Kinetics* **Duration: PO,** 4 hr. *Additional Untoward Reaction* May cause ↑ risk of seizures in epileptics. *Administration* Give timed-release in midmorning. The drug may also be given in mideven-

TABLE 17 (*Continued*)

Drug	Dosage	Remarks
		ing to reduce night hunger.
Fenfluramine hydrochloride (Ponderal,* Pondimin) C-IV, Rx	**PO:** 20 mg t.i.d. before meals. May be increased weekly to a maximum of 40 mg t.i.d. If initial dose is not well tolerated, reduce to 40 mg daily, and increase very gradually. Total daily dose should not exced 120 mg.	*Kinetics* **Onset:** 1–2 hr; **Duration:** 4–6 hr. t½: 20 hr. Excreted in urine. This drug produces more CNS depression and less stimulation than does standard amphetamine. *Additional Use* To treat autistic children with high serotonin levels. *Additional Contraindication* Do not use in alcoholics. *Additional Untoward Reactions* Hypoglycemia, CNS depression, impotence, drowsiness. *Additional Drug Interactions* Fenfluramine may ↑ effect of alcohol, CNS depressants, guanethidine, methyldopa, reserpine, thiazide diuretics, and tricyclic antidepressants.
Mazindol (Mazanor, Sanorex) C-III, Rx	**PO:** 1 mg t.i.d. 1 hr before meals or 2 mg once daily 1 hr before lunch.	*Kinetics* **Onset:** 30–60 min; **Duration:** 8–15 hr. **Therapeutic blood levels:** 0.003–0.012 µg/ml. Excreted in urine partially unchanged. *Administration* In event of GI distress, take with meals.
Methamphetamine hydrochloride(Desoxyn, Desoxyephedrine, Methampex) C-II, Rx	*Anorectic.* **PO, adult:** 5 mg 30 min before meals or long-acting, 10–15 mg in AM. Not to be used as an anorectic in children under 12 yrs. *Hyperkinesis.* **Pediatric over 5 years: initial,** 5 mg 1–2 times/day; **then,** increase by 5 mg/week to total of 20–25 mg/day.	When used to facilitate verbalization during psychotherapeutic interview, only give second dose if the first has proved effective. When used to treat hyperkinesis, evaluate therapy periodically to determine need for continued therapy. *Kinetics* See Amphetamine sulfate.
Phendimetrazine tartrate (Adipost, Adphen, Anorex, Bacarate, Bontril PDM and Slow-Release, Di-Ap-Trol, Dyrexan-OD, Hyrex 105, Melfiat, Mel-	**PO:** 35 mg 2 to 3 times daily 1 hr before meals or one sustained release capsule (105 mg) in AM.	**Duration:** 4 hr for regular tablet. t½: 5.5 hr (average).

527

TABLE 17 (*Continued*)

Drug	Dosage	Remarks
fiat-105, Metra, Obalan, Obeval, Obezine, PDM, Phenzine, Plegine, Prelu-2, Slyn-LL, Sprx-1, -3, and -105, Statobex, Statobex-G, Trimcaps, Trimstat, Trimtabs, Weightrol, Weh-Less, Wehless 105) C-III, Rx		
Phenmetrazine hydrochloride (Preludin) C-II, Rx	**PO:** *individualized:* 25 mg 2 to 3 times daily 1 hr before meals or as a single sustained release tablet (75 mg) in the AM.	**Duration:** 4 hr for regular tablet.
Phentermine hydrochloride (Adipex-P, Dapex-37.5, Fastin, Obe-Nix, Obephen, Obermine, Obestin-30, Parmine, Phentermine, Phentrol, Phentrol 2, 4, and 5, Tora, Unifast, Wilpowr) C-IV, Rx	**PO.** 8 mg t.i.d. ½ hr before meals. Or, 15–37.5 mg once daily before breakfast.	**Duration:** 4 hr for hydrochloride.
Phentermine resin (Ionamin) C-IV, Rx		
Phenylpropanolamine HCl (Acutrim Maximum Strength, Control, Dex-A-Diet, Dexatrim-15, Diadax, Prolamine, Resolution I Maximum Strength and II Half-Strength, Unitrol), OTC	**PO.** *Immediate release:* 25 mg t.i.d. 30 min before meals. *Timed/Precision release:* 75 mg in the morning.	**Peak plasma levels:** 1–2 hr. t½: 3–4 hr. This drug is available without a prescription. For other uses, side effects, etc., see Chapter 44, p 568.

Administration

1. Initial doses should be small and then increased gradually as necessary on an individual basis.
2. Administer last daily dose at least 6 hours before patient retires unless specified otherwise by physician.
3. As an appetite depressant, administer one-half hour before meals.

Nursing Implications

1. *Assess*
   a. for hypertensive crisis characterized by fever, marked sweating, excitation, delirium, tremor, twitching, convulsions, coma, and circulatory collapse. (Patient is susceptible to hypertensive crisis if he is concurrently receiving a MAO inhibitor or has received them 7–14 days before amphetamine therapy was initiated.)
   b. for acute toxicity as demonstrated by cardiovascular symptoms followed by psychotic syndrome. Be prepared to assist in treatment for overdosage as noted above in treatment of acute toxicity.
   c. for chronic toxicity manifested by emotional lability, loss of appetite, som-

nolence, mental impairment, and occupational deterioration. Drug should be discontinued.

d. for marked psychological dependence and tolerance. Drug should be discontinued.

e. for dryness of mouth and constipation.

f. for weight at least once a week, as anorexic effect may occur in patients being treated for other problems. Note insomnia or restlessness in these patients.

2. Follow agency policy in handling amphetamines. They are regulated by the Controlled Substances Act; availability and use are restricted to prevent drug abuse.

3. *Teach patient and/or family*

a. that when anorexiants are used for weight reduction, they are only a short-term crutch, that their effect lasts only 4 to 6 weeks, and that tolerance develops rapidly.

b. to stress curtailing of food intake. Assist with selection of appropriate diet.

c. that if tolerance develops, not to increase medication, but rather to decrease it.

d. that amphetamines may mask extreme fatigue, which can impair ability to perform potentially hazardous tasks, such as operating a machine or an automobile.

e. to seek medical supervision for management of extreme fatigue and depression when drug is discontinued.

f. that diabetic patients should be alert to untoward symptoms of diabetes, as amphetamines may alter insulin and dietary requirements.

MISCELLANEOUS AGENTS

CAFFEINE Caffedrine, Dexitac, No Doz, Quick Pep, Tirend, Vivarin (OTC)

CAFFEINE AND SODIUM BENZOATE (Rx)

CAFFEINE, CITRATED (OTC)

Classification CNS stimulant, miscellaneous.

Note: Caffeine is found in a number of widely used combination drugs, including Fiorinal Plain and with Codeine, and Synalgos DC (see Appendix 3).

Action/Kinetics Caffeine stimulates all levels of the CNS (cerebral cortex, medulla, and spinal cord). It also possesses other pharmacologic activity, including dilation of coronary and peripheral blood vessels, constriction of cerebral blood vessels, increase in heart rate, stimulation of skeletal muscle, increased gastric acid secretion, and diuresis. **Peak plasma levels**: 50–75 min. **Therapeutic plasma levels**: 6–13 μg/ml. Levels above 20 μg/ml produce toxic effects. t½: 3–4 hr. Approximately 17% bound to plasma protein. Metabolized primarily in liver and excreted by the kidneys. Both citric acid and sodium benzoate increase water solubility of caffeine.

Uses *Orally:* Adjunct with nonnarcotic and narcotic analgesics, increased wakefulness by increasing mental alertness, adjunct in migraine headache therapy. *Parenteral:* Analeptic in poisonings, acute circulatory failure, diuretic, headaches following spinal puncture, comatose alcoholic.

Although caffeine has been used to overcome hangover effects occuring during arousal from drug-induced coma such as that from intoxication with morphine, barbiturates, alcohol, and other CNS depressants, the use of caffeine for this purpose is neither advisable nor logical.

Contraindications Use with caution in cardiovascular, renal, ulcer disease, depression. Safety not established during pregnancy.

Untoward Reactions *CNS:* Symptoms of overexcitation including insomnia, nervousness, restlessness, headaches. *GI:* Nausea, vomiting, diarrhea, gastric upset. *GU:* Diuresis.

Note: Large doses may cause anxiety neurosis with sensory disturbances, palpitations, tremors, arrhythmias, flushing, and other symptoms mentioned above.

Drug Interactions

Interactant	Interaction
Cimetidine	Cimetidine ↓ excretion of caffeine
MAO inhibitors	Excessive caffeine may cause hypertensive crisis; reduce intake of caffeine-containing medication
Oral contraceptives	Oral contraceptives ↓ excretion of caffeine
Propoxyphene (Darvon)	Caffeine given to patients taking large doses of propoxyphene may cause convulsions

Laboratory Test Interference ↑ Urinary catecholamines.

Dosage *Caffeine sodium benzoate*: **IM, IV, or SC**. *Usual route*: **IM**: 0.2–0.5 gm. *Caffeine citrate*: **PO**, 100–200 mg q 4 hr. **Long-acting**: 200–250 mg q 4–6 hr. **Pediatric**: 8 mg/kg not to exceed 500 mg. PO form not recommended for children.

Nursing Implication
Assess for high caffeine intake, manifested by insomnia, irritability, tremors, cardiac irregularities, and gastritis.

ANALEPTICS

General Statement Analeptic drugs act directly on the medulla, located in the brainstem. At therapeutic doses, these agents are supposed to stimulate respiration. At higher doses, the analeptics stimulate the hindbrain and spinal cord. The drugs do not stimulate the myocardium. The analeptic agents are no longer considered drugs of choice in the treatment of CNS depression caused by an overdosage of sedatives and hypnotics. Current therapy for overdose of sedative-hypnotics relies largely on supportive therapy, such as establishing a patent airway, administering oxygen, assisting or controlling respiration when necessary, and maintaining blood pressure and blood volume. See also *Agents for Attention Deficit Disorders*.

DOXAPRAM HYDROCHLORIDE   Dopram (Rx)

Classification   CNS stimulant, analeptic.

Action/Kinetics   Doxapram increases the rate and depth of respiration directly by stimulating respiratory centers in the medulla as well as indirectly through reflex activation of carotid and aortic peripheral chemoreceptors. An increase in blood pressure may also occur due to increased cardiac output. The drug will antagonize respiratory depression, but not analgesia, induced by narcotics. An increased salivation and release of both gastric acid and catecholamines may be seen. As dosage is increased, other CNS centers are stimulated and doses may be given that cause tonic–clonic convulsions. **Onset** (after IV): 20–40 sec. **Peak effect**: 1–2 min. **Duration**: 5–12 min. Doxapram is metabolized in the liver and is excreted in the urine.

Uses   Adjunct in treatment of postanesthetic respiratory depression induced by narcotic analgesics or anesthetics. However, artificial respiration is more effective and use of this drug for this purpose is neither advisable nor logical. Temporary use (2 hr) in chronic pulmonary disease with acute hypercapnia in hospitalized patients.

Contraindications   Epilepsy, convulsive states, respiratory incompetence due to muscle paresis, pneumothorax, airway obstruction and extreme dyspnea, severe hypertension, and cerebrovascular accidents. Hypersensitivity. Use with caution in patients with cerebral edema, asthma, severe cardiovascular disease, hyperthyroidism and pheochromocytoma (cancer of adrenals), peptic ulcer, or gastric surgery.

Untoward Reactions   *CNS:* Excess stimulation including hyperactivity, clonus, convulsions. Headache, apprehension, dizziness. *GI:* Nausea, vomiting, diarrhea, urge to defecate. *Respiratory:* Bronchospasm, dyspnea, cough, hiccoughs, hypoventilation, laryngospasm. *CV:* Arrhythmias, abnormal ECG, tightness in chest or chest pain, phlebitis, flushing. *GU:* Spontaneous micturition, urinary retention. Burning or sensation of heat in genitalia and perineum areas. *Miscellaneous:* Mydriasis, muscle spasms, involuntary movements, sweating, pruritus.

OVERDOSAGE   Characterized by respiratory alkalosis and by hypocapnia (too little CO_2 in blood) with tetany and apnea. Also excessive stimulation of CNS, which may result in convulsions.

Drug Interactions

Interactant	Interaction
Anesthetics, general	Since doxapram increases epinephrine release, do not give until 10 min after anesthetic discontinued if halothane, cyclopropane, or enflurane used in order to minimize cardiac arrhythmias
MAO inhibitors	Additive pressor effects
Sympathomimetic amines	Additive pressor effects

Laboratory Test Interferences   ↓ Hemoglobin, hematocrit, RBCs. ↑ BUN, proteinuria.

Dosage   *After anesthesia*: **IV**, 0.5–1.0 mg/kg, not to exceed 1.5–2.0 mg/kg; may be given in several injections at 5-min intervals. *Chronic obstructive lung disease with acute hypercapnia*: **IV infusion**, 1–2 mg/min up to maximum of 3 mg/min. *Drug-induced CNS depression*: **IV, initial**, 2 mg/kg; repeat in 5 min and every 1–2 hr until patient is conscious.

Administration Allow minimum of 10 minutes between the discontinuation of anesthetic administration and administration of doxapram. Doxapram can also be administered by IV drip (dextrose, isotonic saline) at an initial rate of 5 mg of doxapram/minute.

Nursing Implications

1. Assess BP, heart rate, and deep tendon reflexes after administration of doxapram to prevent overdosage and to provide a guide for adjustment of rate of infusion.
2. After administration, assess the patient for at least ½ to 1 hour after he is alert, for possible poststimulation respiratory depression.
3. Administer oxygen along with the drug to patients suffering from chronic pulmonary insufficiency.
4. Have on hand short-acting barbiturates, oxygen, and resuscitative equipment to manage overdosage.
5. Use seizure precautions after administration of drug.

NIKETHAMIDE Coramine (Rx)

Classification CNS stimulant, analeptic.

Action/Kinetics The mechanism of action of nikethamide is similar to that of doxapram (see above). Nikethamide is rapidly absorbed after PO, IM, or SC administration and is converted to nicotinamide. Metabolized in liver and excreted in urine.

This drug is not widely used, as it has a narrow margin of safety and is not as effective as doxapram.

Uses Respiratory depression, CNS depression, circulatory failure.

Contraindications Intra-arterial injection (arterial spasm or thrombosis may occur).

Untoward Reactions *CNS:* Excess stimulation including convulsions. *CV:* Flushing, feeling of warmth, tachycardia, hypertension. *GI:* Nausea, vomiting. *Respiratory:* Burning or itching at back of nose, cough, sneezing, increased rate and depth of respiration (often the desired effect). *Miscellaneous:* Sweating, feeling of fear, facial muscle twitching.

Dosage **IV**: *narcotic depressant overdose, carbon monoxide poisoning*, 5–10 ml followed by 5 ml q 5 min for first hour, **then** 5 ml q 30–60 min if necessary. *Acute alcoholism*: 5–20 ml to overcome CNS depression. *Cardiac decompensation/coronary occlusion*: 5–10 ml **IM or IV**. *Electroshock therapy*: 5 ml with 5 ml sterile water in antecubital vein. Apply electrical stimulus when face of patient is flushed and respiratory rate increases noticeably. *Shock (as an adjunct)*: **IV, IM**, 10–15 ml. *Anesthetic overdosage*: **IM, IV**, 2–10 ml, depending on reason for use. **PO**: Maintenance, 3–5 ml of oral solution q 4–6 hrs.

Nursing Implication
Have barbiturates on hand to treat overdosage.

AGENTS FOR ATTENTION DEFICIT DISORDERS

General Statement   Several CNS stimulants are currently used for the treatment of children suffering from hyperkinesia and other behavior problems, stemming from neurologic and not psychologic causes. To treat decline in mental capacity in geriatric patients.

Before drug therapy of this ill-defined condition is undertaken in children, the child must undergo extensive evaluation including medical and psychological tests.

The mode of action of the agents used for attention deficit disorders is not fully understood. It is possible that the agents increase the concentration of choline, acetylcholine, and dopamine in the brain.

ERGOLOID MESYLATES (DIHYDROGENATED ERGOT ALKALOIDS)
Circanol, Deapril-ST, Gerimal, H.E.A., Hydergine, Trigot (Rx)

Classification   Agent for attention deficit disorders.

Action/Kinetics   This combination of equal proportions of the mesylate salts of dihydroergocornine, dihydroergocristine, and dihydroergocryptine is thought to act by increasing cerebral blood flow. **Peak plasma levels**: 1 hr. **t½**: 3.5 hr. Oral tablets are rapidly but incompletely absorbed from the GI tract; significant first-pass effect after oral use.

Uses   Primary progressive dementia, Alzheimer's dementia.

Contraindications   Any type of acute or chronic psychosis. Patients with tartrazine sensitivity. Use with caution in porphyria.

Untoward Reactions   Acute intermittent porphyria in susceptible patients. Sublingual use: irritation, nausea, heartburn

Dosage   **PO, sublingual: initial**, 1 mg t.i.d. Beneficial effects may not be seen for 3 to 4 weeks.

Administration   Patient should be sure the sublingual tablet dissolves completely under the tongue.

METHYLPHENIDATE HYDROCHLORIDE   Ritalin, Ritalin-SR Hydrochloride (C-II) (Rx)

Classification   CNS stimulant.

Action/Kinetics   The mechanism of action of methylphenidate is not known, but it manifests pharmacologic effects similar to amphetamine. **Peak blood levels**: 1–3 hr. **Duration**: 4–6 hr. **t½**: **PO**, 2–7 hr; **t½**: **IV**, 1–2 hr. The drug is metabolized by the liver and excreted by the kidney.

Uses   Attention deficit disorders in children as part of overall treatment regimen. Narcolepsy. Mild depression. Senility.

Contraindications   Marked anxiety, tension and agitation, glaucoma. Use with great caution in patients with history of hypertension or convulsive disease. Tourette's syndrome, motor tics.

Untoward Reactions *CNS:* Nervousness, insomnia, headaches, dizziness, drowsiness, chorea. Toxic psychoses. Psychological dependence. *CV:* Palpitations, tachycardia, angina, arrhythmias, hyper- or hypotension. *GI:* Nausea, anorexia, abdominal pain. *Allergy:* Skin rashes, fever, arthralgia, dermatoses, erythema.

OVERDOSAGE Characterized by cardiovascular symptoms (hypertension, cardiac arrhythmias, tachycardia), mental disturbances, agitation, headaches, vomiting, hyperreflexia, hyperpyrexia, convulsions, and coma.

TREATMENT OF OVERDOSAGE Symptomatic. Excess CNS stimulation may be treated by keeping the patient in quiet, dim surroundings. A short-acting barbiturate may be used. Emesis or gastric lavage if the patient is conscious. Adequate circulatory and respiratory function must be maintained. Hyperpyrexia may be treated by cooling the patient (e.g. cool bath).

Drug Interactions

Interactant	Interaction
Anticoagulants, oral	↑ Effect of anticoagulants due to ↓ breakdown by liver
Anticonvulsants (phenobarbital, phenytoin, primidone)	↑ Effect of anticonvulsants due to ↓ breakdown by liver
Guanethidine	↓ Effect of guanethidine by displacement from its site of action
MAO inhibitors	Possibility of hypertensive crisis, hyperthermia, convulsions, coma
Phenylbutazone	↑ Effect of phenylbutazone due to ↓ breakdown by liver
Tricyclic antidepressants	↑ Effect of antidepressants due to ↓ breakdown by liver

Laboratory Test Interference ↑ Urinary excretion of epinephrine.

Dosage PO. **Individualized, adults**: 20–60 mg/day in divided doses before meals. *Attention deficit disorders,* **6 years and older: initial**, 5 mg b.i.d. before breakfast and lunch; **then** increase 5–10 mg/week to a maximum of 60 mg daily.

Administration
1. Give before breakfast and lunch to avoid interference with sleep.
2. For attention deficit disorders, discontinue if no improvement in one month or if stimulation occurs.

Nursing Implications
1. Monitor BP and pulse b.i.d., as changes may occur.
2. Weigh 2 times/week since patients tend to lose weight on drug.
3. Provide cooling procedures in event of hyperpyrexia associated with drug overdosage.
4. Be prepared to provide supportive measures for maintenance of adequate circulation and respiratory exchange in case of overdosage. Protect patient against self-injury and reduce possible external stimuli.
5. Teach patient and/or family that caution must be used when driving or operating hazardous machinery when medicated with methylphenidate because drug may mask fatigue and/or cause physical incoordination, dizziness, or drowsiness.

PEMOLINE   Cylert (C-IV) (Rx)

Classification   CNS stimulant.

Action/Kinetics   Although pemoline resembles amphetamine and methylphenidate pharmacologically, its mechanism of action is not fully known. Pemoline is believed to act by dopaminergic mechanisms. **Peak serum levels**: 2–4 hr. **t½**: 12 hr. Steady state reached in 2–3 days, and beneficial effects may not be noted for 3–4 weeks. Approximately 50% is bound to plasma protein. Pemoline is metabolized by the liver, but more than 40% is excreted unchanged by the kidneys.

Uses   Attention deficit disorders, hyperkinetic syndrome. *Investigational*: Excessive daytime sleepiness, narcolepsy.

Contraindications   Hypersensitivity to drug. Tourette's syndrome. Children under 6 years of age.

Untoward Reactions   *CNS:* Insomnia (most common). Dyskinesia of the face and extremities, precipitation of Tourette's syndrome. Mild depression, headache, nystagmus, dizziness, hallucinations. *GI:* Transient weight loss, gastric upset, nausea. *Miscellaneous:* Skin rash.

For treatment of overdosage, see methylphenidate.

Dosage   PO: initial, 37.5 mg/day; increase at 1-week intervals by 18.75 mg until desired response is attained up to maximum of 112.5 mg/day. **Usual maintenance**: 56.25–75 mg daily. *Narcolepsy, daytime sleepiness*: 50–200 mg/day in 2 divided doses.

Administration

1. Administer as a single dose each AM.
2. Interrupt treatment 1 or 2 times annually to determine whether behavioral symptoms still necessitate therapy.

Nursing Implications

1. *Teach parents*
   a. to measure height of child every month, to weigh him twice a week, to record all measurements on a chart, and to bring chart to medical supervisor for evaluation of growth pattern.
   b. to report weight loss or failure to grow to medical supervision.
   c. to administer drug early in AM to minimize insomnia caused by drug.
   d. to continue with therapy, because behavioral changes take 3 to 4 weeks to occur.
   e. to interrupt drug administration, as recommended by medical supervision; then observe behavior to help doctor decide whether therapy should be resumed.
   f. to bring child in periodically for liver function tests in order to detect adverse reactions that would necessitate withdrawal of drug.
   g. to note signs of overdosage, such as agitation, restlessness, hallucinations, and tachycardia. Should these symptoms occur, instruct parents to withhold drug, to give supportive care, and to report to medical supervision.

Chapter Forty-two

LOCAL AND GENERAL ANESTHETICS

General Statement Since local and general anesthetics are often administered to patients, they are reviewed here briefly in tabular form. Note their duration of action and other characteristics, since they interfere with the other drugs a patient is receiving.

LOCAL ANESTHETICS

General Statement Local anesthetics stabilize the nerve membrane and thus prevent the initiation and transmission of impulses; this leads to the anesthetic action. The use of epinephrine in conjunction with local anesthetics decreases systemic absorption and prolongs the duration of action.

Use See Table 18, p. 537.

TABLE 18 LOCAL ANESTHETICS

Generic Name (Trade name)	Duration of Action (hr)	Indications
Benzocaine (*Topical:* Americaine Anesthetic, Benzocaine Topical, Benzocol, Bicozene, Chigger-Tox, Col-Vi-Nol, Dermoplast, Foille, Soft 'N Soothe, Solarcaine, Unguentine), OTC. *Mucous membrane:* Americaine Anesthetic Lubricant, Hurricaine), Rx	0.5–1	*Topical:* Anesthetic for skin disorders (0.5–20% as aerosol solution, cream, liquid, lotion, ointment, spray). *Mucous membrane anesthesia:* dental procedure (22%); Anesthetic for pharyngeal and nasal catheters and airways, nasogastric or endoscopic tubes, urinary catheters, laryngoscopes, proctoscopes, sigmoidscopes, vaginal specula (20% gel).
Bupivacaine HCl (Marcaine HCl, Sensorcaine), Rx	4–5	Local infiltration, dental block, caudal block, peripheral block, sympathetic block (all 0.25% or 0.5%); lumbar or epidural block (0.25–0.75%); retrobulbar block (0.75%).
Butamben picrate (Butesin Picrate), OTC		*Topical:* Anesthetic for skin disorders (1% ointment).
Chlorprocaine HCl (Nescaine, Nescaine-CE), Rx	1	Infiltration and nerve block (1–2%); caudal and epidural block (2–3%, preservative free).
Cocaine, Rx	0.5–2	*Mucous membrane anesthesia:* nose, throat, ear, bronchoscopy (all 1–4% solution).
Cyclomethycaine sulfate (Surfacaine), OTC and Rx		*Topical:* Anesthetic for skin disorders (0.5 % cream or 1% ointmen). *Mucous membrane anesthesia:* Mouth, respiratory tract, or urethra prior to examination or instrumentation (0.75% jelly).
Dibuciane HCl (Nupercaine HCl, Nupercainal), OTC and Rx	2–4	*Topical:* For skin disorders (0.5% cream, 1% ointment). Isobaric spinal anesthesia (1:200); hypobaric spinal anesthesia (1:1,500); low spinal anesthesia (2.5 mg with 5% dextrose).
Dyclonine HCl (Dyclone), Rx	Less then 1	*Mucous membrane anesthesia:* mouth, respiratory tract or urethra prior to endoscopy (all 0.5–1% solution); pain associated with oral or anogenital lesions (0.5% solution).
Etidocaine HCl (Duranest HCl), Rx	5–10 hr	Percutaneous infiltration (0.5%); peripheral nerve block (0.5–1%); central nerve block (0.5–1.5%), caudal block (0.5–1%).
Hexylcaine HCl (Cyclaine), Rx	0.5	*Mucous membrane anesthesia:* respiratory, upper GI, or urinary tracts (5% solution).
Lidocaine HCl (*Topical:* Lida-Mantle Creme, Xylocaine. *Mu-*	0.5–1	*Topical:* anesthetic for skin disorders (2.5–5% as cream or oint-

TABLE 18 (*Continued*)

Generic Name (Trade name)	Duration of Action (hr)	Indications
cous Membrane: Anestacon, Baylocaine 2% and 4%, Lida-Mangle, Xylocaine, Xylocaine 10% Oral, Xylocaine Viscous. *Injectables:* Bay Caine-1 and -2, Dalcaine, Dilocaine, Dolicaine 2%, Duo-Trach Kit, L-Caine, Li-doject-1 and -2, Nervocaine 1% and 2%, Nulicaine, Ultracaine 1% and 2%, Xylocaine HCl. *Injectables with Epinephrine:* Bay Caine-E-1 and -E-2, Octocaine, Xylocaine HC1.), OTC and Rx		ment). *Mucous membrane anesthesia:* oral and nasal cavities, endotracheal intubation, ureth-ritis, for urethral procedures (all 2–10% as cream, jelly, ointment, solution). Infiltration (0.5–2%); peripheral nerve block (1–2%); sympathetic nerve block (cervical or lumbar, 1%); central nerve block, epidural: thoracic (1%) or lumbar (1–2%); caudal block (1–1.5%); spinal anesthesia (5% with glucose); low spinal anesthesia (1.5% with dextrose); retrobulbar or transtracheal (4%).
Mepivacaine HCl (Carbocaine HCl, Carbocaine with Neo-Cob-efrin, Isocaine HCl), Rx	2–2½	Nerve block (1–2%); transvaginal block (1%); paracervical block (obstetrics, 1%); caudal and epidural (1–2%); infiltration (1%); management of pain (1–2%); dental (infiltration or nerve block 3% or 2% with levonorde-frin)
Pramoxine HCl (Prax Anti-Itch, Proxine, Tronothane HCl), OTC		*Topical:* anesthetic for skin disorders (1% cream, jelly, or lotion).
Prilocaine HCl (Citanest HC1), Rx	2–2½	Infiltration (1–2%); peripheral nerve block: intercostal or par-avertebral (1–2%), brachial plexus or sciatic/femoral (2–3%); central nerve block: epidural or caudal (1–3%); dental (4%).
Procaine HCl (Novocain), Rx	1	Infiltration (0.25–0.5%); peripheral nerve block (0.5–2%); spinal anesthesia (10%).
Proparacaine HCl (AK-Taine, Alcaine, Ophthaine, Ophthetic), Rx		*Ophthalmology:* anesthesia for cataract removal, removal of foreign bodies or sutures, tonometry (all 0.5% solution).
Tetracaine HCl (Pontocaine, Pontocaine Eye), Rx	0.5–1	*Topical:* For skin disorders (0.5% ointment or 1% cream). *Mucous membrane anesthesia:* nose or throat in preparation for bronchoscopy or other procedures (2% solution). *Spinal anesthesia:* High, medium, low, and saddle block (0.2–0.3% solution); prolonged (1% solution). *Ophthalmology:* Anesthesia, removal of foreign bodies, tonometry (all: 0.5% ointment or solution).

Contraindications Hypersensitivity. Large doses should not be used in patients with heart block. **Preparations containing preservatives should not be used for spinal or epidural anesthesia.**

Untoward Reactions Swelling and paresthesia of lips and oral tissue. Systemic reactions occur when plasma levels are high, and in rare cases such reactions can be fatal. Systemic symptoms include CNS excitation with tremors, shivering, and convulsions; cardiovascular effects, including hypotension, intraventricular conduction defect, or A-V block, which may lead to cardiac and respiratory arrest; eczematoid dermatitis.

Epinephrine in local anesthetic preparations may result in anginal pain, tachycardia, tremors, headache, restlessness, palpitations, dizziness, and hypertension.

Drug Interactions

Interactants	Interaction
Local anesthetics containing vasoconstrictors with MAO inhibitors, tricyclic antidepressants, phenothiazines	Severe hypo- or hypertension
Local anesthetics containing vasoconstrictors and oxytocic drugs	Excess hypertensive response
Local anesthetics containing vasoconstrictors and chloroform, halothane, cyclopropane, trichloroethylene	↑ Chance of cardiac arrhythmias

Administration/ Storage

1. Do not use preparations of local anesthetics containing preservatives for spinal or epidural anesthesia.
2. Store local anesthetics containing *epinephrine* separately from those that do not.
3. Store local anesthetics containing *preservatives* separately from those that do not.
4. Clearly mark each container indicating exactly which local anesthetics are stored in the compartment.
5. Autoclave vials of anesthetics that are not destroyed by heat for sterile handling.
6. Use antiseptic or detergent with dye as a solution in which to store anesthetics that cannot be autoclaved, but that must be sterile and ready for use. The dye will indicate if there is a crack in the vial and if the sterilizing solution is seeping into the anesthetic.
7. Read label three times to ascertain that the correct local anesthetic is being prepared or provided to the doctor for administration.
8. Discard remainder of preparations without preservatives following initial use.
9. *Do not use epinephrine* in nerve block of digits, because blood supply can be compromised and tissue damage can result.

Nursing Implications

1. Have resuscitative equipment and drugs available whenever local anesthetics are used.
2. Remember patient is awake when local anesthesia is used. Minimize anxiety provoking noise and conversation.

(continued)

3. Assess patient for CNS excitation symptoms, such as nervousness, dizziness, blurred vision, and tremors and for depression symptoms, such as drowsiness, respiratory distress, convulsions, and unconsciousness. The initial symptoms may be depressive.

4. Have available for treatment of patient with convulsions ultrashort-acting barbiturates (i.e., thiopental, thiamylal) or short-acting barbiturates (i.e., secobarbital, pentobarbital). Since CNS depressants should not be administered when cardiac or respiratory depression is present, have available a short-acting muscle relaxant (succinylcholine) to administer IV.

5. Assess patient for depressant cardiovascular reactions characterized by hypotension (monitor BP), myocardial depression, bradycardia (monitor pulse), and possibly cardiac arrest (assess BP, pulse rate, ECG, and appearance of patient).

6. Have available for treatment of patient with cardiovascular reaction vasopressors (i.e., ephedrine, metaraminol) and IV fluids. *Do not administer epinephrine* when patient is anoxic, because ventricular fibrillation may occur.

7. Support respiratory efforts by maintaining a patent airway and supplying oxygen by assisted or controlled ventilation methods.

8. Assess patient for allergic reactions characterized by cutaneous lesions, urticaria, edema, or anaphylaxis.

9. Have available for treatment of patient with allergic reaction oxygen, epinephrine, corticosteroids, and antihistamines.

10. Assess for local reactions characterized by burning, tenderness, swelling, tissue irritation, sloughing, and tissue necrosis. Report immediately and implement appropriate therapy ordered.

ANESTHESIA FOR EYE

1. Administer as noted on p. 29 (Chapter 6).

2. Do not allow dropper to come into contact with eyelid and surrounding tissue during administration.

3. Administer precisely the number of drops ordered since excess dosage causes serious side effects and retards wound healing in surgical conditions of the eye.

4. Rinse tonometer (instrument used for measuring intraocular pressure) with sterile distilled water prior to use to avoid introducing foreign bodies into the anesthetized eye.

5. Protect eye from irritating chemicals, foreign bodies, and rubbing of eye while eye is anesthetized. Cover eye with a patch following procedure because blink reflex is temporarily absent.

6. *Teach patient and/or family* not to touch or rub anesthetized eye.

ANESTHESIA FOR NASOPHARYNX   Advise patient not to eat food or drink fluids for at least 1 hour following use of topical anesthetic, as the second stage (pharyngeal) of swallowing is interfered with and aspiration may occur.

ANESTHESIA FOR RECTUM AND ANUS

1. Teach patient to use the lowest possible dose to minimize systemic toxicity.

2. Examine anal area for break in skin if patient complains of burning on administration.

ANESTHESIA BY NERVE BLOCK

ORAL CAVITY BLOCK   (1) Advise patient not to eat food for at least 1 hour after injection, because swallowing reflex is depressed. Aspiration and loss of sensation in tongue may result in injury during chewing. (2) Observe for swelling of lips and oral tissue, which may necessitate use of cold compresses.

PUDENDAL BLOCK   (1) Assess for increase in patient's apprehension, anxiety, and fear, which may indicate ineffectiveness of block. (2) Assess for hematoma formation or rectal puncture (blood flow through rectum) following block, which would indicate complications.

EPIDURAL BLOCK   (1) Assess for diminished cardiac and respiratory function, which may result inadvertently from the anesthesia itself. (2) Monitor pulse, BP, and skin color. If hypotension develops, summon assistance, elevate patient's legs, turn patient on left side, administer oxygen, and increase IV flow rate. (3) Constantly monitor the progress of labor because patient will have diminished sensation of contractions. (4) Palpate bladder for urinary retention. Catheterization may be indicated. (5) Check for fecal incontinence and cleanse perineal area as necessary while patient is in labor.

CAUDAL BLOCK   (1) Assess for diminished cardiac and respiratory function indicative of excessively high level of anesthesia. If hypotension develops, summon assistance, elevate patient's legs, turn patient on left side, and administer oxygen and increase IV flow rate. (2) Assess for marked restlessness, anxiety, tremor or twitching, early signs of impending convulsions due to absorption of local anesthetic into bloodstream. Use seizure precautions. (3) Assess for cessation of sweating and in lower extremities a pronounced vasodilatation, early signs of effective anesthesia. Consult physician before changing patient's position during the early stages of anesthesia. (4) Constantly monitor the progress of labor because patient will have diminished sensation of contractions. (5) Palpate bladder for urinary retention. Catheterization may be indicated. (6) Check for fecal incontinence and cleanse perineal area as necessary while patient is in labor.

PARACERVICAL BLOCK   Monitor fetal heart closely, preferably with a fetal monitor because local anesthesia by paracervical block may cause fetal bradycardia and acidosis.

SPINAL ANESTHESIA   (1) Maintain patient supine 8–12 hr after anesthesia to reduce occurrence of headache. (2) Apply ice bag to head if headache occurs. (3) Protect patient from burns because patient's bodily sensations are absent. (4) Chart when motion and sensation are recovered. When patient can move toes, sensation is completely recovered. (5) Provide analgesics and sedatives ordered as needed. (6) Hydrate adequately to prevent hypotension. (7) Assist in exercising lower limbs to prevent thrombophlebitis.

GENERAL ANESTHETICS

The objectives of general anesthesia are to produce (1) a state of unconsciousness and amnesia, (2) analgesia, (3) hyporeflexia, and (4) skeletal muscle relaxation.

There are two types of general anesthetics: inhalation anesthetics that include gases, such as nitrous oxide and cyclopropane, and highly volatile liquids, such as halothane and related drugs; and intravenous, or fixed-dose, anesthetics. This group includes the ultrashort-acting barbiturates, such as methohexital and thiopental.

Since general anesthetics should be used only by those with specialized training and experience, only general information on special uses, advantages, and disadvantages of general anesthetics currently in use will be presented. Since the nurse is largely responsible for patient care after anesthesia, extensive nursing implications have been included.

Action/Kinetics Most general anesthetics are excreted unchanged through the lungs. However, agents such as halothane, enflurane, methoxyflurane, and isoflurane are metabolized by the liver. Biotransformation of enflurane, methoxyflurane, and isoflurane releases flouride ion, which may cause renal toxicity (see Table 19).

Nursing Implications

1. Obtain a complete report (diagnosis, surgery, or procedure done, anesthetic administered, and time of administration, response to surgery anesthetic, current condition, and level of consciousness) before accepting responsibility for patient from the anesthetist.
2. Assess for adequate airway. Attach a ventilator, with the assistance of the anesthetist, if the endotracheal tube is still in place and adjust it as ordered to maintain adequate ventilation.
3. Keep patient on side at least until conscious, unless contraindicated, to prevent aspiration of vomitus.
4. Note excessive mucus in nasopharynx and oral cavity and suction as needed.
5. Monitor BP, pulse rate, respiratory rate, and patient's appearance as ordered. Assessments usually may be decreased in frequency as vital signs are stabilized.
6. Note which anesthetic the patient received and whether a short or long recovery to consciousness is anticipated. Plan care accordingly.
7. Monitor parameters by CVP, arterial pressures, cardiac monitor, and urinary drainage as ordered.
8. Remember that the first sense to return is hearing and that anxiety-provoking noise or conversation should be minimized. Orientation and positive encouragement should be provided by the nurse.
9. Help patient reestablish normal physiologic balance with the least anxiety possible.
10. Administer analgesic ordered if patient complains of pain after exhalation of anesthetic.
11. Assess patient experiencing hypotension and pain, because the pain may, in fact, cause the hypotension. Report assessment to doctor and determine with him whether analgesia should be administered even though patient is hypotensive.
12. Cover patient adequately to prevent vasodilation and subsequent heat loss, which tend to occur after administration of anesthetic agents.
13. Note that temperature is not a reliable vital sign for 1 to 2 hours after surgery, because the patient is adjusting to different environmental conditions.
14. Refer to medical-surgical nursing text for complete care of the postoperative patient.
15. *Prevent fire and explosive hazards.* Follow the protocols for preventing fire and explosive hazard associated with general anesthesia in the institution in which it is administered.
    a. Learn which gases are explosive.
    b. Avoid using explosive gases when electrocautery and electric dessication are to be used.

(continued on page 547)

TABLE 19　GENERAL ANESTHETICS

Generic/Trade Name	Uses	Advantages	Disadvantages	Additional Nursing Implications
		Volatile Liquids		
Enflurane (Ethrane), Rx	Induction and maintenance of general anesthesia (widely used). Analgesic for obstetrics.	Induction and recovery are rapid. No significant stimulation of salivation, bronchial secretions, or bronchomotor tone. Usually provides sufficient muscle relaxation for abdominal surgery. No significant bradycardia.	As depth of anesthesia increases, hypotension increases. High concentrations may cause uterine relaxation and increased uterine bleeding. Less chance to cause renal problems due to release of free flouride ion. High levels accompanied by hypercapnia may cause seizures.	Monitor cardiac function more closely if epinephrine is administered, because arrhythmias are more likely to occur.
Halothane (Fluothane, Somnothane*), Rx	Induction and maintenance of general anesthesia.	Rapid, pleasant induction and recovery. Little nausea/vomiting. Nonexplosive. Not an irritant to respiratory tract thus no increase in secretions. Hepatic toxicity does not appear to occur in children.	Hypoxia, acidosis, or apnea may occur during deep anesthesia. Sensitizes heart to epinephrine with possible serious arrhythmias. Bradycardia. Has been said to cause hepatic damage with repeated doses. Produces only moderate muscle relaxation. Assisted or controlled ventilation may be required. May produce hypotension or malignant hyperthermia.	
Isoflurane (Forane), Rx	Induction and maintenance of general anesthesia.	Induction and recovery are rapid. Less toxicity due to fluoride ion. Does not sensitize the myocardium to epinephrine.	Causes significant respiratory depression. Pungent odor. Less smooth induction than halothane. Profound peripheral di-	

543

TABLE 19 (Continued)

Generic/Trade Name	Uses	Advantages	Disadvantages	Additional Nursing Implications
		Good skeletal muscle relaxation when used alone.	lation may cause a decrease in blood pressure and increase in heart rate. May cause malignant hyperthermia.	
Methoxyflurane (Penthrane), Rx	Induction and maintenance of general anesthesia. May be combined with nitrous oxide and oxygen for surgery expected to last 4 hr or less. Also may be used alone or in combination with nitrous oxide for analgesia in obstetrics or minor surgery.	Analgesia and drowsiness persist so need for narcotics during immediate postop period reduced. Nonexplosive. Less incidence of laryngeal spasm or bronchoconstriction. Excellent skeletal muscle relaxation. No significant sensitization of myocardium to catecholamines. Pleasant odor with minimal respiratory tract irritation.	Induction and recovery are slow. Metabolized to free fluoride ion, which may cause renal damage or failure. May cause malignant hyperthermia.	
		Gases		
Trichloroethylene (Trilene), Rx	Analgesia and light anesthesia—used in childbirth.	Rapid induction and recovery. No liver or kidney damage.	Possibility of cardiac arrhythmias. Causes rapid, shallow respiration.	
Cyclopropane, Rx	Analgesia. Induction and maintenance of anesthesia.	Induction is rapid. Skeletal muscle relaxation in full anesthetic doses. Stimulates sympathetic nervous system thus maintaining blood pressure.	Sensitizes heart to epinephrine leading to arrhythmias. Difficult to detect planes of anesthesia. May produce laryngospasms and arrhythmias. Postanesthetic nausea, vomiting, and headache are frequent. Cyclopropane/oxygen mixtures	

544

Drug	Use	Effects / Remarks	Nursing Implications
Ethylene, **Rx**		Rapid onset and recovery. Few bronchospasms and laryngospasms; little postanesthetic vomiting. Nontoxic.	are explosive. May cause malignant hyperthermia. Adequate analgesia but poor muscle relaxant properties. Must be administered in high concentrations (80%) with oxygen (20%). Hypoxia can occur. Ethylene/oxygen mixtures are explosive. High concentrations may cause vomiting, hypoxia, respiratory depression.
Nitrous oxide, **Rx**	Adjunct with other anesthetics, antianxiety agents, narcotics, or muscle relaxants. Dentistry. Analgesic. In combination with halothane to reach equilibrium of halothane more rapidly.	Rapid, pleasant induction and recovery. Nonexplosive gas. No significant effects on hepatic, renal, or autonomic nervous systems.	With 100% gas, which is necessary for anesthesia, hypoxia and anoxia occur; with 80% gas + 20% oxygen, get good analgesia but poor anesthesia. Does not cause skeletal muscle relaxation. May cause malignant hyperthermia.

Miscellaneous

Drug	Use	Effects / Remarks	Nursing Implications
Etomidate (Amidate), **Rx**	IV for induction of general anesthesia. Adjunct with nitrous oxide for short surgical procedures.	Is considered a hypnotic. No effect on the cardiovascular system. Rapid onset.	No analgesic activity. Should not be used in pregnancy, lactation, or in children less than 10 years of age.
Innovar, **Rx**	A combination of a narcotic analesic (fentanyl)	Produces general quiescence, reduced motor	1. Be aware that post-operative nausea and vomiting are likely to occur. 2. Be aware that during the immediate post-operative period, both hypotension and hypertension and tachycardia and bradycardia can occur.

TABLE 19 *(Continued)*

Generic/Trade Name	Uses	Advantages	Disadvantages	Additional Nursing Implications
	and an antipsychotic (droperidol)—combined effect referred to as neuroleptanalgesia. Used to produce tranquilization and analgesia for surgical or diagnostic procedures or for anesthetic premedication. Adjunct in maintenance of general and regional anesthesia.	activity, and excellent analgesia; complete loss of consciousness usually does not occur.		
Ketamine (Ketalar), Rx	For procedures in which skeletal muscle relaxation not required. Induction of anesthesia.	Rapid acting; produces good analgesia. No effect on pharyngeal-laryngeal reflexes. Used to supplement low-potency agents as nitrous oxide.	Cardiovascular and respiratory stimulation. Inadequate skeletal muscle relaxation. In adults—vivid, unpleasant dreams during recovery.	To prevent dreams likely to occur with ketamine, place patient in a quiet area after anesthesia. Do not disturb as patient emerges from anesthesia. Take vital signs gently. Avoid making noises, bumping bed, or vigorously rousing patient. Anticipate that a low dose of a barbiturate sedative may be required if patient sively active during recovery phase.
Sufentanil (Sufenta), Rx	Narcotic analgesic used as an adjunct to maintain balanced general anesthesia. Anesthetic blood concenration: 8–30 μg/kg.	Will allow appropriate oxygenation of the heart and brain during prolonged surgical procedures. May be used in children.	Dosage must be decreased in the obese, elderly, or debilitated patient. Extended postoperative respiratory depression.	

c. Wear conductive shoes or boots.

d. Do not wear nylon uniforms where anesthetic gases may be used.

e. Do not use wool blankets in area.

f. Ascertain that all electrical equipment used is adequately grounded.

g. Check with anesthesiologist before activating any electrical equipment in the operating room.

h. Matches are not to be used in the operating room.

Part Seven

DRUGS AFFECTING THE AUTONOMIC NERVOUS SYSTEM

Chapter Forty-three

INTRODUCTION TO THE AUTONOMIC NERVOUS SYSTEM

The system that automatically regulates the basic physiologic functions of the body is called the involuntary, visceral, or autonomic nervous system (ANS).

Among the important functions regulated by the ANS are respiration, perspiration, body temperature, carbohydrate metabolism, digestion, bowel motility, pupil size, blood pressure, heart rate, and glandular secretions such as salivation.

The ANS is a composite of two opposing subsystems—the sympathetic and the parasympathetic divisions—that interact with one another to maintain the body in physiologic equilibrium. Even though it is difficult to separate the precise functions of the sympathetic and the parasympathetic systems, since both play a role in all major physiologic processes, the sympathetic system is more closely associated with the quick regulation of the expenditure of energy during emergencies (fight or flight response), whereas the parasympathetic system is more directly involved in the storage and conservation of energy (e.g., digestion and absorption of food).

The manner in which the two divisions of the ANS work together can best be illustrated by looking at a major organ like the heart. Impulses transmitted via the *sympathetic* division will have a tendency to *increase* the heart rate, the contractibility of the muscle, and the speed at which the impulse is transmitted. The *parasympathetic* system will *decrease* the rate of contractibility and conduction.

Normally the two divisions of the ANS are in balance. In an emergency situation, however, when there is an increased need for rapidly circulating blood, the sympathetic system dominates. Impulses are sent that increase the rate of the heart. Blood pressure rises. The small arterioles that supply the skin and outlying parts of the body constrict, and blood supply to the GI tract decreases. When the situation returns to normal the parasympathetic division returns the body to more normal housekeeping functions.

Each nerve pathway in the ANS is composed of two nerve cells. The preganglionic cell is located in the spinal cord, and the axon of this cell (preganglionic fiber) travels to a nerve cell outside the cord where there is a neurojunction or synapse. This nerve cell outside the cord is in a nerve ganglion and the neurojunction is the ganglionic synapse. Most of the sympathetic ganglia are located in the paravertebral ganglionic chain. The parasympathetic ganglia are located near the effector organ. The axon of the ganglionic cell (postganglionic fiber) then travels to the effector organ, where there is a second synapse at the organ or effector structure.

When a nerve impulse reaches any of these synapses, it releases the chemical mediator, a neurohormone, from special storage sites in the nerve terminal. The chemical mediator flows across the synapse and combines with a part of the cell called a receptor site. This then initiates a specific response of the effector organ. Once this is accomplished (the entire sequence of events is almost instantaneous), the remaining hormone is either destroyed by a specific enzyme or taken back up into the special storage sites of the cell. Also, a small amount of the hormone is carried away in the blood. Then the entire system is ready to respond again.

Three neurohormones are known to transmit the nerve impulse at the synapses of the ANS: *acetylcholine, epinephrine* (also known as Adrenalin, which is also found in the adrenal gland) and *norepinephrine* (Levarterenol).

Acetylcholine is found at both *synapses* (preganglionic and postganglionic) of the *parasympathetic* nervous system as well as in the ganglionic synapses of the sympathetic nervous system. Drugs whose actions reinforce or mimic acetylcholine are called cholinergic, or parasympathomimetic. Furthermore, drugs that act at the junction of the postganglionic fiber and effector organ are called muscarinic, while drugs that act at the ganglia are called nicotinic.

Norepinephrine and/or epinephrine (Adrenalin) are the chemical mediators at the postganglionic sympathetic nerve endings (junction at the effector organ). Norepinephrine combines with sites called alpha receptors. Epinephrine combines with *alpha* and *beta* receptors. In the heart both norepinephrine and epinephrine combine with beta receptor sites. Drugs whose actions reinforce or mimic these chemical mediators are called adrenergic or sympathomimetic.

Drugs that interfere with the enzymes that destroy the excess neurohormone after it is released from its storage vessels also increase the effectiveness of the neurohormones. Such drugs are also called *cholinergic* or *adrenergic*.

The other types of drugs that act on the ANS interfere with or block ANS nerve transmission. They are referred to as cholinergic blocking agents (*parasympatholytic*) and adrenergic blocking agents (*sympatholytic*).

From an anatomic point of view, the sweat glands and some of the salivary glands belong to the sympathetic system. However, since acetylcholine is found at both their neurojunctions, they respond to some of the drugs effective for the parasympathetic system.

Chapter Forty-four

SYMPATHOMIMETIC (ADRENERGIC) DRUGS

Sympathomimetics

Theophylline Derivatives

Nasal Decongestants

General Statement The adrenergic drugs supplement, mimic, and reinforce the messages transmitted by the natural neurohormones—norepinephrine and epinephrine. These hormones are responsible for transmitting nerve impulses at the postganglionic neurojunctions of the sympathetic nervous system. The physiologic effects of adrenergic drugs are listed in Table 20.

The adrenergic drugs work in two ways: (1) by mimicking the action of norepinephrine or epinephrine (directly acting sympathomimetics), or (2) by causing the release of the natural neurohormones from their storage sites at the nerve terminals (indirectly acting sympathomimetics). Some drugs exhibit a combination of effects 1 and 2.

The myoneural junction is equipped with special receptors for the neurohormones. These receptors have been classified into two types: alpha (α) and beta (β), according to whether they respond to norepinephrine, epinephrine, or isoproterenol and to certain blocking agents. Alpha-adrenergic receptors are blocked by phenoxybenzamine and phentolamine, whereas beta-adrenergic receptors are blocked by propranolol and similar drugs.

TABLE 20   OVERVIEW OF EFFECTS OF ADRENERGIC DRUGS[a]

Action	Therapeutic Use
Heart Excitation resulting in increase in heart rate and force of contraction. Dilation or constriction of coronary vessels. Results in increase in stroke volume and cardiac output, strengthening of pulse.	Cardiogenic shock, heart block, Stokes-Adams disease, cardiac slowing (bradycardia), resuscitation.
Blood vessels, systemic vasoconstriction Blood supply to abdominal viscera, cerebrum, skin, and mucosa sharply reduced (vasoconstriction of peripheral blood circulation). BP in large vessels increased (pressor effect) and regulated.	Increase in BP in drug-induced acute hypotension during anesthesia or after myocardial infarction or hemorrhage. Isoproterenol causes vasodilation of vessels in skeletal muscle accompanied by increase in cardiac output. Increased blood flow. Nasal decongestion, certain dermatoses, nosebleeds, migraine headaches, all types allergic reactions, anaphylactic reaction.
GI and GU tracts Inhibition of glandular secretion. Constriction of sphincters. Decrease of muscle tone and motility in GI tract, urinary bladder. Increase of muscle tone and motility in ureter.	To relieve spasms during ureteral and biliary colic, dysmenorrhea, and labor. Enuresis.
Lungs Relaxes muscles of bronchial tree.	Acute and chronic asthma, pulmonary emphysema and fibrosis, chronic bronchitis.
Eyes Dilates iris, increases ocular pressure, relaxes ciliary muscle.	
CNS stimulation Excitatory action, respiratory stimulation, wakefulness.	Appetite control, overdosage with CNS depressant drugs, narcolepsy.
Metabolism Increase in glycogenesis (sugar metabolism). Increase in lipolysis (release of free fatty acids).	
Miscellaneous Stimulates salivary glands.	
Sex organs Ejaculation.	

[a]Not all drugs are useful under all circumstances.

Both alpha and beta receptors have been subdivided into subtypes. Thus adrenergic stimulation of receptors will manifest the following general effects:

alpha-Adrenergic:	Vasoconstriction, decongestion. There is evidence of more than one subtype of alpha receptors.
beta$_1$-Adrenergic:	Myocardial (inotropic) contraction, regulation of heartbeat (chronotropic), improved impulse conduction
beta$_2$-Adrenergic:	Peripheral vasodilation, bronchial dilation

In addition, adrenergic agents affect the gut, the sphincter of the genitourinary (GU) tract, the exocrine glands, the salivary glands, the ocular musculature, and the CNS.

The adrenergic stimulants discussed in this section act preferentially on one or more of the above receptor subtypes; their pharmacologic effect must be carefully monitored and balanced.

Uses Sympathomimetic agents are mainly used for the treatment of shock induced by sudden cardiac arrest, decompensation, myocardial infarction, trauma, bronchodilation, acute renal failure, drug reactions, anaphylaxis. Adrenergic drugs are also used to reverse bronchospasm caused by bronchial asthma, emphysema, chronic bronchitis, and other respiratory disorders. Sympathomimetic drugs having predominately an alpha-receptor activity are used for the relief of nasal and nasopharyngeal congestion due to rhinitis, sinusitis, head colds. Also, see individual drugs.

Before considering the specific effects of each drug, examine Table 20, p. 552, to get an overview of the general physiologic effects of the adrenergic drugs.

Contraindications Tachycardia due to arrhythmias or digitalis toxicity. Use with caution in hyperthyroidism, diabetes, prostatic hypertrophy, seizures, degenerative heart disease especially in geriatric patients or patients with asthma, emphysema, or psychoneuroses. Also, use with caution in coronary insufficiency, coronary artery disease, hypertension, or history of stroke.

Untoward Reactions *CV:* Tachycardia, arrhythmias, palpitations, blood pressure changes, anginal pain, precordial pain, pallor, cerebral hemorrhage. *GI:* Nausea, vomiting, heartburn, anorexia, altered taste. *CNS:* Restlessness, anxiety, tension, insomnia, hyperkinesis, drowsiness, vertigo, irritability, dizziness, headache, tremors. *Other:* Pulmonary edema, respiratory difficulties, muscle cramps, coughing, bronchospasms, irritation of oropharynx.

Drug Interactions

Interactant	Interaction
beta-Adrenergic blocking agents	Inhibit adrenergic stimulation of the heart and bronchial tree; cause bronchial constriction; hypertension, asthma, not relieved by adrenergic agents
Ammonium chloride	↓ Effect of sympathomimetics due to ↑ excretion by kidney
Anesthetics	Halogenated anesthetics sensitize heart to adrenergics—causes cardiac arrhythmias
Anticholinergics	Concomitant use aggravates glaucoma
Antidiabetics	Hyperglycemic effect of epinephrine may necessitate ↑ in dosage of insulin or oral hypoglycemic agents

Interactant	Interaction
Corticosteroids	Used chronically with sympathomimetics may result in or aggravate glaucoma; aerosols containing sympathomimetics and corticosteroids may be lethal in asthmatic children
Digitalis glycosides	Combination may cause cardiac arrhythmias
Furazolidone	Furazolidone ↑ alpha-adrenergic effects of sympathomimetics
Guanethidine	Direct-acting sympathomimetics ↑ effects of guanethidine while indirect-acting sympathomimetics ↓ effects of guanethidine
MAO inhibitors	All effects of sympathomimetics are potentiated; symptoms include hypertensive crisis with possible intracranial hemorrhage, hyperthermia, convulsions, coma; death may occur
Methyldopa	↑ Effects of sympathomimetics
Methylphenidate	Potentiates pressor effect of sympathomimetics; combination hazardous in glaucoma
Oxytocics	↑ Chance of severe hypertension
Phenothiazines	↑ Risk of cardiac arrhythmias
Reserpine	↑ Risk of hypertension following direct-acting sympathimimetics and ↓ effect of indirect-acting sympathomimetics
Sodium bicarbonate	↑ Effect of sympathomimetics due to ↓ excretion by kidney
Thyroxine	Potentiation of pressor response of sympathomimetics
Tricyclic antidepressants	↑ Effect of direct-acting sympathomimetics and ↓ effect of indirect-acting sympathomimetics

Administration/Storage   Discard colored solutions.

Nursing Implications
1. Plan to have patients receiving IV administration of adrenergic drugs constantly attended and closely monitored for BP and pulse.
2. Do not administer maintenance doses of these drugs at bedtime, because they may cause insomnia.
3. *Teach patient and/or family*
   a. untoward side effects of drugs and the need to report these to physician should they occur when on maintenance doses.
   b. not to increase or administer the medication more frequently when on maintenance doses. If symptoms become more severe, consult the physician.

Special Nursing Implications for Adrenergic Bronchodilators
See *Administration by Inhalation*, Chapter 6, p. 26.
1. Monitor BP before and after patient uses bronchodilator for the first time to evaluate cardiac response.
2. Continue to provide oxygen mixture and ventilating assistance for patients with

status asthmaticus and abnormal blood gases, even though symptoms appear relieved by bronchodilator.

3. Use the method and the amount of oxygen per minute ordered, on the basis of evaluation of clinical symptomatology and blood gases of the individual patient, geared to preventing depression of respiratory effort.

4. Further treatment with the same agent is inadvisable if 3–5 aerosol treatments within the last 6 to 12 hours have only produced minimal relief.

5. Be prepared to assist with alternative therapy, if patient's dyspnea worsens after repeated excessive use of inhalator, as paradoxical airways resistance may occur.

6. *Teach patient and/or family*
   a. that a single aerosol treatment is usually enough to control an asthma attack.
   b. to contact medical supervision if the patient requires more than 3 aerosol treatments within a 24-hour period.
   c. that overuse of adrenergic bronchodilators may result in reduced effectiveness, possible paradoxical reaction, and cardiac arrest.
   d. to consult a doctor if bronchodilator causes dizziness, chest pain, or lack of therapeutic response to usual dose.
   e. to initiate inhalation therapy on arising in the morning and before meals, to improve lung ventilation and to reduce fatigue that accompanies eating.
   f. that increased fluid intake is an aid in the liquefaction of secretions.
   g. to accomplish postural drainage, to cough productively, and to clap and vibrate to promote good respiratory hygiene.
   h. that other adrenergic medications are not to be taken by patient, unless expressly prescribed by medical supervision.
   i. that regular consistent use of drug as ordered is essential for maximum benefit.

SYMPATHOMIMETICS

ALBUTEROL   Proventil, Ventolin (Rx)

Classification   Direct-acting adrenergic (sympathomimetic) agent.

Action/Kinetics   Albuterol stimulates beta$_2$-receptors of the bronchi, leading to bronchodilation. Causes less tachycardia and is longer-acting than isoproterenol. **Onset, PO**: within 30 min.; **inhalation,** within 15 min. **Peak effect, PO**: 30–60 min. **Duration, PO**: 4–6 hr.; **inhalation,** 3–4 hr. Metabolites and unchanged drug excreted in urine. **Not to be used in children less than 12 years of age.**

Use   Bronchial asthma; bronchospasm due to bronchitis or emphysema; exercise-induced asthma.

Dosage   **Inhalation. Adults and children over 12 years**: 2 inhalations (90 μg/inhalation) q 4–6 hr. (some patients require only 1 inhalation every 4 hr). *Exercise-induced asthma.* **Adults and children over 12 years:** 2 inhalations 15 min before exercising. **PO. Adults and children over 12 years: initial,** 2–4 mg t.i.d.–q.i.d.; **then,** adjust dosage depending on response, not to exeed 32 mg/day. Geriatric patients should receive an initial dose of 2 mg t.i.d.–q.i.d.

Administration

1. The recommended dose should not be exceeded.
2. Since the contents of the container are under pressure, do not store near heat or open flame and do not puncture.
3. When using albuterol inhalers, other inhalation medication should be used only if prescribed by a physician.
4. If previously effective dosage no longer provides relief, the physician should be contacted immediately.

DOBUTAMINE HYDROCHLORIDE   Dobutrex (Rx)

Classification   Direct-acting adrenergic (sympathomimetic) agent.

Action/Kinetics   Stimulates beta$_1$-receptors (in the heart) increasing cardiac function, cardiac output, and stroke volume with minor effects on heart rate. Has slight effects on alpha-adrenergic receptors (vasoconstriction). **Onset:** 1–2 min. **Peak effect:** 10 min. **t½:** 2 min. **Therapeutic plasma levels:** 40–190 ng/ml. Metabolized by the liver and excreted in urine.

Uses   Short-term treatment of cardiac decompensation. Atrial fibrillation with rapid ventricular rate (only after digitalis). *Investigational:* To increase heart function in children with congenital heart disease requiring cardiac catheterization.

Contraindications   Idiopathic hypertrophic subaortic stenosis. Safe use during pregnancy, childhood, or after acute myocardial infarctions not established.

Untoward Reactions   *CV:* Marked increase in heart rate, BP, and ventricular ectopic activity. Anginal and nonspecific chest pain, palpitations. *Other:* Nausea, headache, and shortness of breath.

Additional Drug Interactions   Concomitant use with nitroprusside causes ↑ cardiac output and ↓ pulmonary wedge pressure.

Dosage   **IV infusion:** *individualized*, **usual,** 2.5–10 µg/kg/min (up to 40 µg/kg/min). Rate of administration and duration of therapy are determined by response of patient as determined by heart rate, presence of ectopic activity, BP, and urine flow.

Administration/Storage

1. Reconstitute solution according to direction provided by manufacturer. Dilution process takes place in two stages.
2. The more concentrated solution may be stored in refrigerator for 48 hours and at room temperature for 6 hours.
3. Before administration, the solution is diluted further according to the fluid needs of patient. This more dilute solution should be used within 24 hours.
4. Dilute solutions of dobutamine may darken. This does not affect the potency of the drug when used within the time spans detailed above.
5. The drug is incompatible with alkaline solutions.

Nursing Implications

1. Have IV equipment readily available to infuse volume expanders before therapy with dobutamine hydrochloride is initiated.
2. Be prepared to monitor central venous pressure to assess vascular volume and

efficiency of cardiac pumping of the right side of the heart. The normal range is 5 to 8 mm H_2O. An elevated CVP is indicative of disruption in cardiac output as in pump failure or pulmonary edema. A low CVP is indicative of hypovolemia.

3. Be prepared to monitor pulmonary artery wedge pressure to determine the pressure in the left atrium and left ventricle and measure efficiency of cardiac output. The mean pressure range is 4–12 mm Hg.

4. Monitor ECG and BP continuously during administration.

5. Report overdosage as evidenced by excessive alteration of BP or tachycardia and be prepared to reduce rate of administration or temporarily discontinue.

6. Monitor intake and output.

DOPAMINE HYDROCHLORIDE   Dopastat, Intropin, Revimine* (Rx)

Classification   Direct- and indirect-acting adrenergic (sympathomimetic) agent.

Action/Kinetics   Dopamine is the immediate precursor to epinephrine in the body. Exogenously administered, dopamine produces direct stimulation of $beta_1$-receptors and variable (dose-dependent) stimulation of alpha receptors (peripheral vasoconstriction). Also, dopamine will cause a release of norepinephrine from its storage sites. These actions result in increased myocardial contraction, cardiac output, and stroke volume, as well as increased renal blood flow and sodium excretion. Exerts little effect on diastolic BP and induces fewer arrhythmias than seen with isoproterenol. **Onset:** 5 min. **Duration:** 10 min. t½: 2 min. Metabolized in liver and excreted in urine.

Uses   Cardiogenic shock, especially in myocardial infarctions associated with severe CHF. Also shock associated with trauma, septicemia, open heart surgery, renal failure and congestive heart failure. Especially suitable for patients who react adversely to isoproterenol. Poor perfusion of vital organs; hypotension due to poor cardiac output.

Additional Contraindications   Pheochromocytoma, uncorrected tachycardia or arrhythmias. Pediatric patients.

Additional Untoward Reactions   *CV:* Ectopic heartbeats, tachycardia, anginal pain, palpitations, vasoconstriction, hypotension, hypertension. *Other:* Dyspnea, headache, mydriasis.

Additional Drug Interactions

Interactant	Interaction
Diuretics	Additive or potentiating effect
Phenytoin	Hypotension and bradycardia
Propranolol	↓ Effect of dopamine

Dosage   IV infusion: Initial, 2–5 µg/kg/min; **then,** increase up to 20–50 µg/kg/min (depending on severity of illness) in increments of 5–10 µg/kg/min.

Administration/Storage

1. Drug must be diluted before use—see package insert.

2. Dilute solution is stable for 24 hr. Protect from light.

3. In order not to overload system with excess fluid, patients receiving high doses of dopamine may receive more concentrated solutions than average.

Additional Nursing Implications

See also *Nursing Implications*, p. 554.

1. Monitor BP, ECG, cup and pulmonary wedge pressure, and urine flow of patients receiving dopamine very closely. Report changes to physician.
2. Be prepared to adjust rate of flow of infusion frequently.
3. Check infusion frequently for extravasation because sloughing and necrosis may occur.

EPHEDRINE   (Rx)

EPHEDRINE HYDROCHLORIDE   Efedron Nasal (OTC)

EPHEDRINE SULFATE   Vatronol (Rx: Injection; OTC: Oral and nasal dosage forms)

Classification   Direct- and indirect-acting adrenergic agent.

Action/Kinetics   Releases norepinephrine from synaptic storage sites. Has slight direct effects on alpha, beta$_1$-, and beta$_2$-receptors, causing increased blood pressure due to arteriolar constriction and cardiac stimulation, bronchodilation, relaxation of GI tract smooth muscle, mydriasis, and increased tone of the bladder trigone and vesicle sphincter. It may also increase skeletal muscle strength especially in myasthenia patients. Ephedrine is more stable and longer lasting than epinephrine. **Onset, IM:** 10–20 min; **PO,** 15-60 min. **Duration, IM, SC, IV,:** 30-60 min; **PO,** 3–5 hr.

Uses   Acute hypotensive states (e.g., due to spinal anesthesia), Stokes-Adams syndrome. Asthmatic conditions, acute bronchospasm, narcolepsy, angioneurotic edema, hay fever. Nasal decongestion (also used topically).

Additional Untoward Reactions   Precordial pain, urinary retention, painful urination, decrease in urine formation, pallor, respiratory difficulty.

Drug Interactions

Interactant	Interaction
Dexamethasone	Ephedrine ↓ effect of dexamethasone
Diuretics	Diuretics ↓ response to sympathomimetics
Guanethidine	↓ Effect of guanethidine by displacement from its site of action
Methyldopa	Effect of ephedrine ↓ in methyldopa-treated patients

Dosage   *Bronchodilator*: **Adults, PO:** 25–50 mg q 3–4 hr. **SC, IM, slow IV: Adult,** 25–50 mg. **Pediatric (all routes):** 3 mg/kg/day divided into 4 to 6 doses. *Vasopressor*: **Adults, SC, IM, IV:** 25–50 mg (maximum dose should not exceed 150 mg/24 hr). **Pediatric, IM, SC:** 25–100 mg/m^2 in 4–6 divided doses. **Topical** (drops, jelly): **Adults and children over 6 years:** 2–3 drops of solution or small amount of jelly in each nostril q 3–4 hr. Should not be used topically for more than 3 or 4 consecutive days.

Additional Nursing Implications

See also *Nursing Implications*, p. 554.

1. Take baseline BP and pulse before initiating therapy and monitor frequently until stabilized when drug is given for hypotension.
2. After prolonged usage of ephedrine, observe the patient for resistance to the drug. This may necessitate a rest period of 3 to 4 days. Patient usually will again respond to drug after a rest period.
3. *Teach patient and/or family*
   a. to count radial pulse and to report elevated or irregular pulse.
   b. in the case of a male patient, report difficulty in voiding, which may be caused by drug-induced urinary retention.

EPINEPHRINE   Adrenalin Chloride Solution, Bronkaid Mist, Primatene Mist Solution, Sus-Phrine (Both Rx and OTC)

EPINEPHRINE BITARTRATE   Asthmahaler, Bronitin Mist, Bronkaid Mist Suspension, Medihaler-Epi, Epitrate, Primatene Mist Suspension (OTC)

EPINEPHRINE BORATE   Epinal Ophthalmic, EPPY/N 1/2%, 1%, 2% Ophthalmic Solutions (Rx)

EPINEPHRINE HYDROCHLORIDE   Adrenalin,* Adrenaline Chloride, Asthma Nefrin, Dey-Dose Epinephrine, Micronephrine, Dysne-Inhal,* Epifrin, Glaucon, Vaponefrin (Both Rx and OTC)

Classification   Direct-acting adrenergic agent.

Action/Kinetics   Epinephrine, a natural hormone produced by the adrenal medulla, induces marked stimulation of alpha, beta$_1$, and beta$_2$ receptors causing sympathomimetic stimulation, pressor effects, cardiac stimulation, bronchodilation, and decongestion. For all effects, see p. 552. **Extreme caution must be taken never to inject 1:100 solution intended for inhalation—injection of this concentration has caused death. Onset: IV, IM, SC, topical,** 3–10 min; **inhalation:** 1 min. **Peak (inhalation):** 3–5 min. **Duration:** 20 min. Epinephrine is ineffective when given orally.

Uses   Cardiac arrest, Stokes-Adams syndrome, to prolong the action of local anesthetics, hemostatic agent. Acute bronchial asthma, bronchospasms due to emphysema, chronic bronchitis, or other pulmonary disease. To treat hypersensitivity reactions to drugs, allergens, etc. As an adjunct in the treatment of open-angle glaucoma. To produce mydriasis, to treat conjunctivitis, to control bleeding in eye surgery.

Additional Contraindications   Administer parenteral epinephrine to children with caution.

Additional Untoward Reactions *CV:* Fatal ventricular fibrillation, cerebral or sub-arachnoid hemorrhage, obstruction of central retinal artery. *GU:* Decreased urine formation, urinary retention, painful urination. *At injection site:* Bleeding, urticaria, wheal formation.

Laboratory Test Interferences False + or ↑ BUN, fasting glucose, lactic acid, urinary catecholamines, glucose (Benedict's), ↓ in coagulation time. The drug may affect electrolyte balance.

Dosage *Cardiac arrest:* **IV,** 0.5–1 mg q 5 min (use 1:10,000 solution). **Intracardiac (only by trained personnel):** 0.3–0.5 mg (3–5 ml of 1:10,000 solution). *Intraspinal use:* 0.2–0.4 ml of 1:1,000 solution added to anesthetic fluid mixture. *Use with local anesthetic:* 1:100,000 to 1:20,000.

   Bronchial asthma. **Solution (1:1,000): Adults, SC, IM,** 0.3–0.5 mg q 20 min– 4 hr. **Infants and children, SC:** 0.01 mg/kg q 20 min–4 hr (single dose should not exceed 0.5 mg). **Suspension (1:200): Adults, SC only,** 0.5–1.5 mg; **infants and children, SC only:** 0.025 mg/kg. At least 6 hr should elapse between doses. *Inhalation:* Aqueous solution is administered from nebulizer with least number of inhalations that will produce relief.

   Glaucoma: 1 drop of 0.25%–2% solution in eye(s) 1–2 times/day (response determined by tonometry). *Conjunctivitis, rapid pupillary dilation:* 1–2 drops of 0.1% solution in eye(s); may be repeated once if required.

Administration/Storage

1. *Never administer* 1:100 solution IV. Use 1:1,000 solution for IV administration.
2. Preferably use a tuberculin syringe to measure epinephrine, as the parenteral doses are very small and the drug is very potent. An error in measurement may be disastrous.
3. Administer epinephrine IV by a double bottle setup so that rate of administration may be easily adjusted.
4. For IV administration to adults the drug must be well diluted as a 1:1,000 solution and quantities of 0.05 to 0.1 ml of solution should be injected cautiously and very slowly, taking about a minute for each injection, noting the response of the patient (BP and pulse). Dose may be repeated several times if necessary.
5. Briskly massage site of SC or IM injection to hasten the action of the drug. Do not expose epinephrine to heat, light, or air as this causes deterioration of the drug.
6. Discard if solution is reddish-brown color and after expiration date.

Additional Nursing Implications

See also *Nursing Implications*, p. 554.

1. Constantly attend patient on IV epinephrine.
2. *Assess*
   a. BP and pulse. Take baseline reading of BP and pulse rate before initiation of therapy and then monitor closely, every minute, until desired effect is achieved; then every 2 to 5 minutes until patient has stabilized and then monitor BP every 15 to 30 minutes. Report the rate and character (regularity and force) of pulse.
   b. for signs of shock such as cold, clammy skin; cyanosis; and loss of consciousness.

3. Be prepared to assist with the administration of IV fluids and blood to patients in hypovolemic shock.
4. Check where epinephrine and syringes are stored on the unit, so that in the event of an emergency you will be able to administer the drug without delay.

ETHYLNOREPINEPHRINE HYDROCHLORIDE   Bronkephrine (Rx)

Classification   Direct-acting adrenergic agent.

Action/Kinetics   Ethylnorepinephrine stimulates beta receptors similarly to epinephrine. Has little effect on BP and may be safer than epinephrine. Especially suitable for children, for diabetic asthmatics, and for patients refactory to isoproterenol or epinephrine. **Onset:** 6–12 min. **Duration:** 1–2 hr.

Use   Bronchial asthma, bronchospasms due to emphysema or bronchitis.

Dosage   IM, SC. Adults: 1–2 mg (0.5–1 ml of 0.2% solution); **pediatric**: 0.2–1 mg (0.1–0.5 ml of 0.2% solution).

HYDROXYAMPHETAMINE HYDROBROMIDE   Paredrine 1% Ophthalmic (Rx)

Classification   Direct-acting adrenergic agent.

Action/Kinetics   Used only topically to dilate the pupil. **Duration**: Few hours.

Use   Pupillary dilation.

Additional Contraindications   Hypersensitivity to drug, narrow-angle glaucoma.

Additional Untoward Reactions   Transitory stinging on initial instillation. Conjunctival allergy.

Dosage   *Pupillary dilatation*: 1–2 drops of 1% solution in each eye.

ISOETHARINE HYDROCHLORIDE   Arm-a-Med, Beta-2, Bronkosol, Dey-Dose Isoetharine HCl, Dey-Lute Isoetharine HCl, Dispos-a-Med (Rx)

ISOETHARINE MESYLATE   Bronkometer (Rx)

Classification   Adrenergic agent, bronchodilator.

Action/Kinetics   Isoetharine has a greater stimulating activity on beta$_2$ receptors of the bronchi than on beta$_1$ receptors of the heart. Causes relief of bronchospasms. **Inhalation: Onset**, 1 min; **peak effect**: 15–60 min; **duration**: 1–3 hr. Partially metabolized; excreted in urine.

Uses   Bronchial asthma, bronchospasms due to chronic bronchitis or emphysema.

Dosage **Inhalation.** *Hand nebulizer*: 3-7 inhalations (use undiluted).
   Aerosol nebulizer: 1-2 inhalations (wait at least 1 min after initial dose to ensure that a second dose is necessary).
   IPPB or oxygen aerosolization: 0.25-1 ml of 1% solution diluted with saline (1:3) or other diluent. Also, **0.5% solution:** 0.5 ml; **0.25% solution:** 1.25-5 ml; **0.125% solution:** 2-8 ml; **0.1% solution:** 2.5-10 ml.

Administration

1. One or two inhalations are usually sufficient. Wait 1 min after initial dose to ensure necessity of another dose.
2. Treatment usually needs not be repeated more than q 4 hours.
3. Do not use if solution contains a precipitate or is brown.

Nursing Implications

See *Nursing Implications* for *Adrenergic Bronchodilators*, p. 554 and *Administration by Inhalation*, p. 26.

ISOPROTERENOL HYDROCHLORIDE Aerolone, Dispos-a-Med, Dey-Dose, Isuprel, Isuprel Mistometer (Rx)

ISOPROTERENOL SULFATE Medihaler-Iso, Norisodrine Sulfate (Rx)

Classification Direct-acting sympathomimetic agent.

Action/Kinetics Isoproterenol produces pronounced stimulation of both beta$_1$ and beta$_2$ receptors of the heart, bronchi, skeletal muscle vasculature, and the GI tract. In contrast with other sympathomimetics, isoproterenol produces a drop in BP. It also causes less hyperglycemia than occurs with epinephrine, but produces bronchodilation and the same degree of CNS excitation. **Inhalation: Onset**, 2-5 min; **peak effect**: 3-5 min; **duration**: 30-120 min. **IV: Onset**, immediate; **duration**: less than 1 hr. **Sublingual: Onset**, 15-30 min; **duration**: 1-2 hr. **Rectal: Onset**, 30 min; **duration**: 4 hr. Partially metabolized; excreted in urine.

Uses Bronchodilator in asthma, chronic pulmonary emphysema, bronchitis, and other conditions involving bronchospasms. Adjunct in cardiogenic and other types of shock. Adams-Stokes and carotid sinus syndrome, adjunct in anesthesia. Certain cardiac arrhythmias. A-V heart block, ventricular tachycardia, and ventricular arrhythmias.

Additional Contraindications Use with caution in the presence of tuberculosis and in pregnancy.

Additional Untoward Reactions Flushing, sweating, swelling of the parotid gland. Excessive inhalation causes refractory bronchial obstruction. Sublingual administration may cause buccal ulceration. Side effects of drug are less severe after inhalation.

Drug Interaction Beta-adrenergic blocking agents reverse the effects of isoproterenol.

Dosage *Isoproterenol hydrochloride. Shock*: **IV Infusion**, 0.5-5 µg/min (0.25-2.5 ml of 1: 500,000 diluted solution). *Cardiac standstill and cardiac arrhythmias*:

Adults, IM, SC: 1 ml (0.2 mg) of 1:5,000 solution (range: 0.02–1 mg); **IV**: 1–3 ml (0.02–0.06 mg) of 1:50,000 solution (range: 0.01–0.2 mg); **IV infusion**: 5 μg/min (1.25 ml of 1:250,000 solution/min); **Intracardiac (in extreme emergencies)**: 0.1 ml of 1:5,000 solution. *Heart block*. **IV, SC, IM:** as above. **Sublingual, adults, initial:** 10 mg; **maintenance:** 5–50 mg. **Rectal, adults, initial:** 5 mg; **maintenance:** 5–15 mg.

Acute bronchial asthma: **Hand bulb nebulizer**: 5–15 deep inhalations of 1:200 solution (or, in adults, 3–7 inhalations of the 1:100 solution); repeat once more if relief not obtained after 5–10 min. **Metered dose inhaler: Usual**, one inhalation; if relief not obtained after 2–5 min, administer again. **Maintenance**: 1–2 inhalations 4–6 times/day (**Note**: No more than 2 inhalations should be taken at once and no more than 6 in one hour). *Chronic obstructive lung disease (bronchospasm)*: **Hand bulb nebulizer**: 5–15 deep inhalations of 1:200 solution (or 3–7 inhalations of 1:100 solution) q 3–4 hrs. **Nebulization by IPPE**: Dilute 0.5 ml of 1:200 solution in 2–2.5 ml diluent (to achieve concentration of 1:800–1:1,000) and deliver over 10–20 min. Can be repeated 5 times/day. **Metered dose inhaler**: 1–2 inhalations q 3–4 hr. **Sublingual: Adults**, 10–20 mg depending on response (not to exceed 60 mg daily). **Pediatric:** 5–10 mg up to a maximum of 30 mg daily. Dosage should not be more than t.i.d. *Bronchospasms during anesthesia:* **IV**, 0.01–0.02 mg as required (1 ml of a 1:5,000 solution diluted to 10 ml with sodium chloride or dextrose injection.

Isoproterenol sulfate. Dispensed from metered aerosol for bronchospasms. See dosage above for Hydrochloride.

Administration Administration to children, except where noted, is the same as that for adults, because a child's smaller ventilatory exchange capacity will permit a proportionally smaller aerosol intake.

Nursing Implications

See also *Nursing Implications* for *Adrenergic Bronchodilators*, p. 554.

1. Assess and report if respiratory problems seem worse after administration of drug. Refractory reaction may occur and necessitate withdrawal of the drug.
2. *Teach patient and/or family*
   a. to rinse mouth with water to minimize dryness after inhalation therapy.
   b. that sputum or saliva may appear pink after inhalation therapy, due to the drug.
   c. not to use inhalation therapy more frequently than prescribed, because severe cardiac and respiratory problems have occurred due to excessive use.
   d. to withhold drug and report parotid gland enlargement that may occur after prolonged use, which would necessitate stopping the drug.

LEVARTERENOL BITARTRATE (NOREPINEPHRINE) Levophed Bitartrate (Rx)

Classification Direct-acting adrenergic agent.

Action/Kinetics Levarterenol produces vasoconstriction (increase in BP) by stimulating alpha-adrenergic receptors. Also causes a moderate increase in contraction of heart by stimulating beta$_1$ receptors. Minimal hyperglycemic effect. **Onset**: immediate; **duration**: 1–2 min. Metabolized in liver; excreted in urine.

Uses Hypotensive states caused by trauma, septicemia, blood transfusions, drug reactions, spinal anesthesia, poliomyelitis, central vasomotor depression, and myocardial infarctions. Adjunct to treatment of cardiac arrest.

Additional Contraindications Hypotension due to blood volume deficiency (except in emergencies), mesenteric or perpheral vascular thrombosis, in halothane or cyclopropane anesthesia (due to possibilities of fatal arrhythmias).

Additional Untoward Reaction Drug may cause bradycardia that can be abolished by atropine.

Dosage **IV infusion only** (effect on BP determines dosage): **average**, 2–4 μg/min or 0.5–1 ml of a 0.004 mg/ml solution/min.

Administration/Storage

1. Discard solutions that are brown or that have a precipitate.
2. Do not administer through same tube as blood products.

Additional Nursing Implications

See also *Nursing Implications*, p. 554.

1. Take baseline reading of BP and pulse before initiation of therapy.
2. *Assess*
   a. patient constantly when he is receiving levarterenol.
   b. BP every 2 minutes from start of drug until desired level is obtained, and then every 5 minutes during administration of drug. After administration, check BP frequently to ascertain that desired level is being maintained.
   c. rate of flow constantly.
   d. pulse frequently for bradycardia. Have atropine on hand for treatment of bradycardia, should this occur.
   e. frequently for extravasation, as ischemia and sloughing may occur.
   f. for blanching along the course of the vein, an indication of permeability of the vein wall, which would permit leakage to occur. This effect would necessitate changing site of IV.
3. Administer levarterenol IV, using a double-bottle setup, to permit simple adjustment of the rate of administration.
4. Anticipate that IV administration will be via a large vein, preferably the antecubital, and not a limb demonstrating poor circulation.
5. Have on hand phentolamine (Regitine), which may be used at site of extravasation to dilate local blood vessels.

MEPHENTERMINE SULFATE   Wyamine Sulfate (Rx)

Classification Indirect-acting adrenergic agent.

Action/Kinetics Slight effects on alpha and beta₁ receptors and moderate effects on beta₂ receptors mediating vasodilation. The drug causes increased cardiac output; also elicits slight CNS effects. **IV: Onset**, immediate; **duration**: 15–30 min. **IM: Onset**, 5–15 min; **duration**: 1–4 hr. **SC: Duration**, 30–60 min. Metabolized in liver. Excreted in urine within 24 hr (rate increased in acidic urine).

Uses Hypotension due to anesthesia, ganglionic blockade, or hemorrhage (only as emergency treatment until blood or blood substitutes can be given).

Additional Contraindications Hypotension due to phenothiazines; in combination with MAO inhibitors.

Additional Drug Interactions Mephentermine will potentiate hypotensive effects of phenothiazines.

Dosage *Hypotension during spinal anesthesia*: **IV**, 30–45 mg; 30-mg doses may be repeated as required; or, **IV infusion**: 0.1% mephentermine in D₅W. *Prophylaxis of hypotension in spinal anesthesia*: **IM**, 30–45 mg 10–20 min before anesthesia. *Shock following hemorrhage*: Not recommended, but IV infusion of 0.1% in D₅W may maintain BP until blood volume is replaced.

Additional Nursing Implications

See also *Nursing Implications*, p. 554.

Take an initial reading of BP and pulse before initiating therapy; then, every 5 minutes until stable, and then every 15 to 30 minutes beyond the duration of the drug's action to check that BP is stabilized at a satisfactory level.

METAPROTERENOL SULFATE (ORCIPRENALINE SULFATE*)
Alupent, Metaprel (Rx)

Classification Direct-acting adrenergic agent, bronchodilator.

Action/Kinetics Metaproterenol markedly stimulates beta₂ receptors, resulting in relaxation of smooth muscles of the bronchial tree, as well as peripheral vasodilation. It is similar to isoproterenol, but it has a longer duration of action and fewer side effects. **Onset: Inhalation**, 1–5 min. **Peak effect**: 10 min. **PO: Onset**, 15 min; **Peak effect**: 1 hr. **Duration**: 3–4 hr. Oral administration produces a marked first-pass effect.

Uses Bronchodilator in asthma, bronchitis, emphysema, and other conditions associated with reversible bronchospasms.

Contraindications Inhalation for children under the age of 12 years. Safe use in pregnancy not established.

Drug Interactions Possible potentiation of adrenergic effects if used before or after other sympathomimetic bronchodilators.

Dosage **PO. Adults and children over 60 lb**: 20 mg t.i.d.–q.i.d.; **children under 60 lb**: 10 mg t.i.d.–q.i.d.; **children under 6 years**: 1.3–2.6 mg/kg/day in divided doses. **Inhalation. Hand nebulizer**: single dose, 10 inhalations of undiluted 5% solution. **IPPB**: 0.3 ml of 5% solution diluted in saline or other diluent. **Metered dose inhaler**: 2–3 inhalations (1.30–1.95 mg). Total daily dose should not exceed 12 inhalations (7.8 mg). **Inhalation not recommended for children under 12 years of age**. For acute bronchospasms administer metaproterenol every 4 hr. For chronic bronchospasms (pulmonary disease), administer 3–4 times/day.

Administration

1. Instruct patient to shake the container.
2. See *Nursing Implications* for *Administration by Inhalation*, p. 26.

Nursing Implications
See *Nursing Implications* for *Adrenergic Bronchodilators*, p. 554.

METARAMINOL BITARTRATE Aramine Bitartrate (Rx)

Classification Directly acting adrenergic agent.

Action/Kinetics Metaraminol directly stimulates primarily alpha receptors and to a slight extent beta$_1$ receptors, resulting in marked increases in BP due primarily to vasoconstriction and to a slight increase in cardiac output. Reflex bradycardia is also manifested. **Onset: IV**: 1–2 min; **IM**: 10 min; **SC**: 5–20 min. **Duration**: 20–60 min.

Uses Hypotension associated with surgery, anesthesia, hemorrhage, trauma, infections, and adverse drug reactions. Adjunct to the treatment of either septicemia or cardiogenic shock.

Additional Contraindications As a substitute for blood or fluid replacement. Use with caution in cirrhosis and malaria.

Dosage *Prophylaxis of hypotension*: **IM, SC**, 2–10 mg; **pediatric**: 0.01 mg/kg. *Treatment of hypotension*: **IV infusion** (only sodium chloride injection or 5% dextrose injection should be used as a diluent), 15–100 mg in 500 ml fluid (up to 500 mg/500 ml have been used). *Severe shock*: **Direct IV**, 0.5–5.0 mg followed by **IV infusion** of 15–100 mg in 500 ml fluid.

Administration Do not inject IM in areas that seem to have poor circulation, as sloughing has occurred with extravasation.

Additional Nursing Implications
See also *Nursing Implications*, p. 554.
   Assess

   a. BP before administering drug and at frequent intervals thereafter for at least 2 hours until BP is stabilized at satisfactory level.
   b. site of IV administration frequently, as extravasation followed by sloughing may occur.

NYLIDRIN HYDROCHLORIDE   Adrin, Arlidin (Rx)

See *Peripheral Vasodilators,* Chapter 25, p. 311.

PHENYLEPHRINE HYDROCHLORIDE   AK-Dilate Ophthalmic, AK-Nefrin Ophthalmic, Alconefrin 12, 25, and 50, Allerest Nasal, Coricidin Nasal Mist, Doktors Nose Drops, Duration Mild, Efricel 1/8% Ophthalmic, Efricel 2.5% and 10%, Eye Cool Ophthalmic, Isopto Frin, 2.5% Mydfrin Ophthalmic, Neo-Synephrine, Neo-Synephrine 2.5% Ophthalmic, Neo-Synephrine 10% Plain Ophthalmic, Neo-Synephrine Viscous Ophthalmic, Nostril, Rhinall, Rhinall 10, Sinarest Nasal, Sinex, Sinophen, Tear-Efrin Eye Drops, Vacon (Rx: Injection and Ophthalmic Solutions greater than 2.5%; OTC: Nasal products and ophthalmic solutions 0.12% and less)

Classification   Adrenergic agent.

Action/Kinetics   Phenylephrine stimulates alpha-adrenergic receptors, producing pronounced vasocontriction, hence an increase in BP. The drug is also a potent decongestant. It resembles epinephrine, but it has more prolonged action and few cardiac effects. **IV: Onset,** immediate; **duration:** 15–20 min. **IM: Onset,** 10–15 min; **duration:** ½–2 hr. *Nasal decongestion* (topical): **Onset:** 15–20 min; **duration:** 3–4 hr. Excreted in urine.

Phenylephrine is also found in Chlor-Trimetron Expectorant, Naldecon, Dimetane, and Dimetapp. See Appendix 3.

Uses   Acute hypotensive states caused by peripheral circulatory collapse. Maintain blood pressure during spinal anesthesia; to prolong spinal anesthesia. Paroxysmal supraventricular tachycardia. Nasal congestion, to decrease congestion around the middle ear. Ophthalmologic: Decongestant in hay fever, colds, or minor eye irritations. Decongestant and vasoconstrictor in uveitis, wide-angle glaucoma, surgery. Refraction, prior to intraocular surgery, diagnostic procedures.

Additional Contraindications   Use with caution in geriatric patients, severe arteriosclerosis, pregnancy, lactation.

Additional Untoward Reactions   Reflex bradycardia. Overdosage may cause ventricular extrasystoles and short paroxysm or ventricular tachycardia, tingling of the extremities and a sensation of heavy head.

Dosage   *Mild to moderate hypotension*: **SC, IM, usual:** 2–5 mg (range: 1–10 mg); initial dose should not exceed 5 mg. **IV, usual:** 0.2 mg (range: 0.1–0.5 mg); initial does should not exceed 0.5 mg. *Severe hypotension, shock*: **IV Infusion, initial,** 100–180 drops/min of 1:50,000 solution (or 10 mg per 500 ml); **maintenance:** 40–60 drops/min of 1:50,000 solution. *Prolongation of spinal anesthesia*: 2–5 mg added to anesthetic solution. *Vasoconstrictor in anesthesia:* 1 mg/20 ml anesthetic solution. *Hypotension during spinal anesthesia:* **IM, SC,** 2–3 mg 3–4 min prior to anesthetic. *For hypotensive emergencies:* **IV, Adults, initial,** 0.2 mg; **then,** increase by increments of 0.1–0.2 mg, if necessary, not to exceed 0.5 mg/dose. **Pediatric: IM, SC,** 0.5–1 mg/25 pounds. *Paroxysmal supraventricular tachycardia*: **Rapid IV,** initial dose not to exceed 0.5 mg; **then,** depending on response, can increase by no more than 0.1–0.2 mg increments, never to exceed a total of 1 mg.

Nasal decongestion: **Adults,** 1–2 sprays of 0.25–0.5% solution or small amount of 0.5% jelly in each nostril q 3–4 hr; **children, over 6 years of age**: 1–2 sprays of 0.25% solution in each nostril q 3–4 hr; **infants**: 1 drop of 0.125–0.2% solution in each nostril q 2–4 hr.

Glaucoma: 1 gtt of 10% solution in upper surface of cornea as often as necessary. *Refraction of eye,* **adults:** Use cycloplegic first followed in 5 min by 1 gtt of 2.5% solution and in 10 min with cycloplegic. **Pediatric:** 1 drop of 1% atropine sulfate followed by 1 drop phenylephrine 2.5% in 10–15 min and finally with 1 drop of atropine sulfate 1%. *Vasoconstriction and pupil dilation*: Local anesthetic followed by 1 gtt of 2.5% or 10% solution in upper limbus; may be necessary to repeat in 1 hr. *Uveitis and posterior synechiae*: Prophylaxis of synechiae: 2.5% or 10% ophthalmic solution with atropine; to free posterior synechiae: 1 gtt of 2.5% or 10% solution; continue on second day. (Also, hot compresses for 5–10 min t.i.d. with 1 gtt of 1% or 2% atropine sulfate before and after each series of compresses.) *Surgery*: wide dilatation of pupil before intraocular surgery: apply the 2.5% or 10% solution topically 30–60 min before surgery. *Ophthalmologic examination:* 1 drop of 2.5% solution in each eye; exam may be performed in 15–30 min (duration of mydriasis: 1–3 hr). *Eye irritation:* 2 drops in eye(s) b.i.d.–t.i.d. as required.

Administration/Storage

1. Store drug away from light in a brown bottle.
2. Anticipate that before administering Neosynephrine Ophthalmic Solution, a drop of local anesthetic will be necessary.
3. Tell the patient to blow nose before administration, when drug is used as a nasal decongestant.

Nursing Implications
See *Nursing Implications*, p. 554.

PHENYLPROPANOLAMINE HYDROCHLORIDE   Acutrim Maximum Strength, Control, Dex-a-Diet Caffeine Free, Dexatrim Caffeine Free, Diadax, Dietac Maximum Strength, Diet Gard, Propagest, Resolution II Half-Strength and I Maximum Strength, Rhindecon, Sucrets Cold Decongestant Formula, Unitrol, Westrim, Westrim LA 75 (OTC except Rhindecon)

Classification   Direct- and indirect-acting adrenergic agent.

Action/Kinetics   Phenylpropanolamine is thought to stimulate both alpha and beta receptors as well as indirectly through release of norepinephrine from storage sites. Increases in blood presssure are due mainly to increased cardiac output rather than vasoconstriction; has minimal CNS effects. **Onset:** 15–30 min; **duration:** 3 hr. Extended release: 12 hr. **Peak plasma levels:** 100 ng. t½: 3–4 hr. Excreted in urine.

Uses   Nasal congestion due to colds, hay fever, allergies. Often used in OTC products as an anorexiant (See Table 17).

Additional Contraindications   Arteriosclerosis, depression, glaucoma, kidney disease. Safety and efficacy in pregnancy, lactation, and children not established.

Additional Untoward Reactions   Renal failure, dysphoria, hallucinations, seizures, dry mouth, dysuria.

Dosage   *Decongestion*: **PO. Adults**: 25 mg q 4 hr or 50 mg q 6–8 hr (not to exceed 150 mg/day). **Children, 2–6 years**: 6.25 mg q 4 hr or 12.5 mg q 8 hr. **Children, 6–12 years**: 12.5 mg q 4 hr or 25 mg q 8 hr. *Anorexiant*: **PO**, 25 mg t.i.d.; timed release: 75 mg in the a.m. Dosage should not exceed 75 mg/day.

Additional Nursing Implications
See also *Nursing Implications*, p. 554.
    Caution older men to report difficulties in voiding, because they are more susceptible to drug-induced urinary retention.

PSEUDOEPHEDRINE HYDROCHLORIDE   Cenafed, Decofed, Dorcol Pediatric Formula, Eltor 120,* Halofed, Halofed Adult Strength, Neofed, Novafed, Neo-Synephrinol Day Relief, Peedee Dose Decongestant, Pseudofrin,*, Robidrine,* Sudafed, Sudafed S.A., Sudagest Decongestant, Sudrin (OTC)

PSEUDOEPHEDRINE SULFATE   Afrinol (OTC)

Classification   Direct- and indirect-acting sympathomimetic.

Action/Kinetics   Pseudoephedrine produces direct stimulation of both alpha- (pronounced) and beta-adrenergic receptors, as well as indirect stimulation through release of norepinephrine from storage sites. These actions produce a decongestant effect on the nasal mucosa. Systemic administration eliminates possible damage to the nasal mucosa. **Onset**: 30 min. **Duration**: 4–8 hr. **Extended release: Duration**, 12 hr. Urinary excretion slowed by alkalinization, causing reabsorption of drug.
    Pseudoephedrine is also found in Actifed, Chlor-Trimeton, and Drixoral. See Appendix 3.

Uses   Nasal congestion associated with sinus conditions, otitis, allergies.

Dosage   *Hydrochloride*. **Adults**: 60 mg q.i.d. or sustained release, 120 mg q 12 hr. Total daily dosage should not exceed 240 mg. **Children, 2–5 years**: 15 mg q 6 hr not to exceed 60 mg/day.; **Children, 6–12 years**: 30 mg q 6 hr not to exceed 120 mg/day. *Sulfate*. **Adults and children over 12 years**: 120 mg q 12 hr.

Nursing Implications
See also *Nursing Implications*, p. 554.
1. Avoid taking drug at bedtime, because it causes stimulation that may result in insomnia.
2. Assess patient with hypertension for symptoms due to elevation of BP, such as headache or dizziness. Alert the patient that these symptoms should be reported because they may be drug related.

TERBUTALINE SULFATE   Brethaire, Brethine, Bricanyl Sulfate (Rx)

Classification   Direct-acting adrenergic agent, bronchodilator.

Action/Kinetics   Terbutaline is specific for stimulating beta$_2$ receptors, resulting in bronchodilation and relaxation of peripheral vasculature. Drug action resembles that of isoproterenol. **PO: Onset**: 30 min; **maximum effect**: 2–3 hr; **duration**: 4–8 hr. **SC: Onset**, 6–15 min; **maximum effect**: 1/2–1 hr; **duration**: 1 1/2–4 hr. **Inhalation: Onset**: 5–30 min; **duration**: 3–6 hr.

Uses   Bronchodilator in asthma, bronchitis, emphysema, and other conditions associated with reversible bronchospasms. *Investigational*: To decrease premature labor.

Additional Contraindications   Safe use during pregnancy or childhood not established.

Dosage   **PO, adult**: 5 mg t.i.d. q 6 hr during waking hours, not to exceed 15 mg/24 hr. If disturbing side effects are observed, dose can be reduced to 2.5 mg t.i.d. without loss of beneficial effects. Anticipate use of other therapeutic measures, if patient fails to respond after second dose. **Children 12–15 years**: 2.5 mg t.i.d., not to exceed 7.5 mg/24 hr. **SC**: 250 µg. May be repeated 1 time after 15 to 30 minutes, if no significant clinical improvement was noted. Dose should not exceed 0.5 mg over 4 hr. *Premature labor:* **Initial, IV**, 10 µg/min up to a maximum of 80 µg/min maintained for up to 4 hr; **then, PO**, 2.5 mg q 4–6 hr until term.

Nursing Implications
See *Nursing Implications* for *Adrenergic Bronchodilators*, p. 554.

THEOPHYLLINE DERIVATIVES

Theophylline derivatives are used for the treatment of asthma. Thus, they are discussed in Chapter 49, *Antiasthmatic Drugs*, p. 612.

NASAL DECONGESTANTS

Action/Kinetics   The most commonly used agents for relief of nasal congestion are the adrenergic drugs. They act by stimulating alpha-adrenergic receptors thereby constricting the arterioles in the nasal mucosa; this reduces blood flow to the area reducing congestion. Both topical (sprays, drops) and systemic agents may be used. For topical, See Table 21.

Uses   Symptomatic relief of acute rhinitis associated with colds or other respiratory infections, allergic rhinitis, acute and chronic sinusitis, and hay fever.

Contraindications   Hyperthyroidism, arteriosclerosis, increased intraocular pressure, prostatic hypertrophy, angina, diabetes, ischemic heart disease, hypertension. Also, patients receiving MAO inhibitors may manifest hypertensive crisis following the use of oral nasal decongestants. Use with caution in geriatric patients and in pregnancy and lactation.

Untoward Reactions   *Topical use:* Stinging and burning, mucosal dryness, rebound congestion. Systemic use may produce the following symptoms. *CV:* Hypotension,

TABLE 21 TOPICAL NASAL DECONGESTANTS

Drug	Dosage	Remarks
Ephedrine hydrochloride (Efedron Nasal), OTC Ephedrine sulfate (Vatronol Nose Drops), OTC	**Adults and children over 6 years:** 2–3 gtt or small amount of jelly in each nostril 2–3 times daily. Not to be used for more than 3–4 consecutive days.	Available as 0.5% drops and 0.5% jelly.
Epinephrine hydrochloride (Adrenalin Chloride), OTC	**Adults and children over 6 years:** 1–2 gtt in each nostril q 4–6 hr.	1. Available as a 0.1% aqueous solution. 2. Because of presence of sodium bisulfite as a preservative, there may be a slight stinging after administration. 3. Not to be used in children under 6 years of age.
Naphazoline hydrochloride (Albalon Liquifilm,* Degest-2,* Naphcon-Forte,* Opcon,* Privine), OTC	**Adults and children over 6 years:** 2 gtt or sprays in each nostril no more than q 3 hr.	Available as 0.05% drops and spray.
Oxymetazoline hydrochloride (4-Way Long-Acting Nasal, Afrin, Afrin Pediatric, Dristan Long Lasting, Duramist Plus, Duration, Nafrine,* Neo-Synephrine 12 Hour, Nostrilla, NTZ Long Acting Nasal, Ocu-clear,* Sinex Long-Lasting), OTC	**Adults and children over 6 yr:** 2–3 gtt or sprays of 0.05% solution in each nostril in AM and PM. **Pediatric, 2–5 yr:** 2–3 gtt of 0.025% solution in each nostril in AM and PM.	Available as 0.05% drops or spray and as 0.025% drops.
Phenylephrine hydrochloride (Alconefrin 12, 25, and 50, Allerest Nasal, Coricidin Nasal Mist, Duration Mild, Doktors Nose Drops, Neo-Synephrine, Nostril, Rhinall, Rhinall-10, Sinarest Nasal, Sinex, Sinophen, Vacon), OTC	**Adults:** 1–2 sprays or several drops of the 0.25% solution in each nostril q 3–4 hr. (In severe cases, use 0.5–1% solution.) **Children over 6 yr:** 1–2 sprays of 0.25% solution in each nostril q 3–4 hr. **Infants:** 1 drop of 0.125–0.2% solution in each nostril q 2–4 hr. Nasal spray or small amount of the jelly may be placed into each nostril and inhaled.	1. Available as a 0.125%, 0.16%, or 1% solution; as a 0.2%, 0.25%, or 0.5% solution or spray; and, as a 0.5% jelly. 2. For infants the 0.125% or 0.16% solution should be used.
Propylhexedrine (Benzedrex, Vicks Inhaler), OTC	Used as an inhaler.	Inhale vapor through each nostril while blocking other nostril.
Tetrahydrozoline hydrochloride (Tyzine, Tyzine Pediatric), Rx	**Adults and children over 6 yr:** 2–4 gtt of 0.1% solution in each	1. Available as 0.05% pediatric solution, 0.1% solution and as 0.1% spray.

TABLE 21   *(Continued)*

Drug	Dosage	Remarks
	nostril no more than q 3 hr. **2–6 yr**: 2–3 gtt of 0.05% solution in each nostril no more than q 3 hr.	2. Not recommended for children less than 2 yr of age.
Xylometazolone hydrochloride (Chlorohist LA, Neo-Spray Long Acting, Neo-Synephrine II Long Acting, Otrivin Pediatric Nasal Drops, Sinutab Sinus Spray,* Sustaire*), OTC	**Adults and children over 12 yr**: 2–3 gtt of 0.1% solution in each nostril or 1–2 inhalations of 0.1% spray q 8–10 hr; **pediatric under 12 years**: 2–3 gtt of 0.05% solution in each nostril or 1 inhalation of 0.05% spray q 8-10 hr.	1. Available as a 0.1% solution and spray and as a 0.05% pediatric solution. 2. Should not be used in atomizers made of aluminum.

arrhythmias, palpitations, precordial pain, tachycardia. *CNS:* Anxiety, dizziness, headache, restlessness, tremors, insomnia, psychoses, hallucinations, seizures, depression. *GI:* Nausea, vomiting. *Opthalmologic:* Irritation, photophobia, tearing, blurred vision. *Other:* Dysuria, sweating, pallor, breathing difficulties, orofacial dystonia.

Note: Ephedrine may also produce anorexia and urinary retention in males with prostatic hypertrophy.

Dosage   See Table 21, p. 571.

Administration

1. Most nasal decongestants are used topically in the form of sprays, drops, or solutions.
2. See *Nursing Implications* for *Administration by Nasal Application*, p. 28.
3. Solutions of topical nasal decongestants may become contaminated with use and result in the growth of bacteria and fungi. Thus, the dropper or spray tip should be rinsed in hot water after each use.

Chapter Forty-five

ADRENERGIC BLOCKING (SYMPATHOLYTIC) DRUGS

General Statement As their name implies, the adrenergic blocking agents (sympatholytics) reduce or prevent the action of the sympathomimetic agents discussed in Chapter 44. They do this by competing with norepinephrine or epinephrine (the neurotransmitters) for either the alpha-adrenergic or beta-adrenergic receptor sites. For example, alpha-adrenergic blocking agents prevent the smooth muscles surrounding the arterioles from contracting, while beta-adrenergic blocking agents prevent the excitatory effect of the neurotransmitters on the heart. It should also be noted that several of the antihypertensive agents described in Chapter 26 involve blockade of alpha or beta receptors.

Some of the adrenergic blocking agents also have a direct systemic cardiac effect in addition to their peripheral vasodilating effect. The fall in blood pressure that accompanies their administration may trigger a compensatory tachycardia (reflex stimulation). The cardiac blood vessels of a patient with arteriosclerosis may be unable to dilate rapidly enough to accommodate these changes in blood volume and the patient may experience an acute attack of angina pectoris or even cardiac failure.

Adrenergic blocking agents have many undesirable effects which, although not toxic, limit their use. Treatment should always be started at low doses, to be increased gradually.

ALPHA-ADRENERGIC BLOCKING AGENTS These drugs reduce the tone of muscles surrounding peripheral blood vessels and consequently increase peripheral blood circulation and decrease blood pressure.

BETA-ADRENERGIC BLOCKING AGENTS These drugs block the nerve impulse transmission to the beta-type receptors of the sympathetic division of the ANS. These receptors are particularly numerous at the postjunctional terminals of the nerve fibers that control the heart muscle and reduce muscle tone. These drugs are discussed in Chapter 26, *Antihypertensives*.

ACEBUTOLOL Sectral (Rx)

See *Antihypertensives*, Chapter 26, p. 335.

ATENOLOL   Tenormin (Rx)

See *Antihypertensives*, Chapter 26, p. 335.

DIHYDROERGOTAMINE MESYLATE   D.H.E. 45 (Rx)

Classification   Alpha-adrenergic blocking agent.

Action/Kinetics   Dihydroergotamine manifests alpha-adrenergic receptor blocking activity as well as a direct stimulatory action on vascular smooth muscle of peripheral and cranial blood vessels, resulting in vasoconstriction thus preventing the onset of a migraine attack. Dihydroergotamine manifests greater adrenergic blocking activity, less pronounced vasoconstriction, and less nausea and vomiting than does ergotamine although it has no oxytocic effect. It is more effective when given early in the course of a migraine attack. **Onset: IM**, 15–30 min; **IV**, minutes. **Duration**: 3–4 hr. t½ initial: 1.4 hr; final: 18–22 hr. Metabolized in liver and excreted in urine.

Uses   Migraine, migraine variant, and cluster headaches. Especially useful when rapid effect is desired.

Contraindications   See *Ergotamine*, p. 575.

Untoward Reactions   See *Ergotamine*, p. 575. Side effects of Dihydroergotamine are milder than those of Ergotamine.

Drug Interactions   Oral nitroglycerin ↑ bioavailability of dihyroergotamine.

Dosage   IM: initial, 1 mg repeated every 1 to 2 hr to a total of 3 mg, if necessary. **IV**: similar to IM but to a maximum of 2 mg. **Total weekly dose should not exceed 6 mg**.

Nursing Implication

Encourage patient to take drug at onset of migraine headache, because this drug is most effective when administered early in an attack.

ERGOTAMINE TARTRATE   Ergomar, Ergostat, Medihaler Ergotamine, Wigrettes (Rx)

Classification   Alpha-adrenergic blocking agent.

Action/Kinetics   Ergot alkaloid with alpha-adrenergic blocking activity as well as direct stimulatory activity on vascular smooth muscle, causing vasoconstriction. The result is a decrease in pulsations responsible for migraine and other symptoms of vascular headaches. Ergotamine also has oxytocic and emetic effects. **Onset**: variable. **Peak plasma levels**: 0.5–3 hr. t½: Initial, 1.8–3.6 hr; final, 17–25 hr. Metabolized by the liver and excreted in the bile.

Uses   Drug of choice for acute attacks of migraine, although it is most effective when administered before the onset of an acute attack. Cluster headache.

ADRENERGIC BLOCKING (SYMPATHOLYTIC) DRUGS   575

Contraindications   Pregnancy and lactation. Peripheral vascular disease, coronary heart disease, hypertension, impaired hepatic or renal function, sepsis, hypersensitivity, or malnutrition, severe pruritus, presence of infection.

Untoward Reactions   *CV:* Precordial pain, transient tachycardia or bradycardia. Large doses may cause increased blood presssure, vasoconstriction of coronary arteries, and bradycardia. *GI:* Nausea, vomiting, diarrhea. *Other:* Numbness and tingling of fingers and toes, muscle pain in extremities, weakness in legs, localized edema, and itching. *Prolonged use:* Gangrene, ergotism.

Drug Interactions

Interactant	Interaction
Caffeine	Caffeine ↑ rate of absorption of ergotamine
Troleandomycin	↑ Effect of ergotamine due to ↓ breakdown by liver
Vasoconstrictors	Significant hypertension

Dosage   **Sublingual**: 2 mg at start of migraine attack followed by 2 mg every 30 min if necessary, but not more than 6 mg in 24 hr and 10 mg in 1 week. **Oral**: Same as sublingual, **IM, SC**: 0.25 mg initially, but not more than 0.5 mg in 24 hr, and 10 mg/week. **Inhalation**: 0.36 mg in a single inhalation at start of attack. Can take up to 6 doses in 24 hr or 15 doses/week. *Combination with caffeine:* 100 mg caffeine for every 1 mg ergotamine.

Nursing Implications
Teach patient and/or family

a. to check for coldness of extremities or tingling of fingers when on long-term therapy. These symptoms appear before onset of gangrene.
b. that female patients of childbearing age should not take ergotamine when suspecting pregnancy, because drug has an oxytocic effect.

METHYSERGIDE MALEATE   Sansert (Rx)

Classification   Serotonin antagonist.

Action/Kinetics   Methysergide is an ergot alkaloid derivative structurally related to LSD. The drug blocks the effects of serotonin, a powerful vasodilator believed to play a role in vascular headaches; it also inhibits release of histamine from mast cells and prevents the release of serotonin from platelets. It has weak vasoconstrictor, emetic, and oxytocic activity. **Peak plasma levels**: 60 ng/ml. **Therapeutic effect**: minimum of 1–2 days, but may take 3–4 wk. **t½**: long.

Uses   Prophylaxis of migraine or other vascular headache. Use should be limited to 6 months or less and for patients with severe headaches or who are refractory to other therapy. Patients should remain under supervision.

Contraindications   Severe renal or hepatic disease, severe hypertension, coronary artery disease, peripheral vascular disease, or tendency toward thromboembolic disease, cachexia (profound ill health or malnutrition), infectious disease, or peptic ulcer. Pregnancy, lactation, use in children.

Untoward Reactions   The drug is associated with a high incidence of side effects.

Fibrosis: Retroperitoneal fibrosis, cardiac fibrosis, pleuropulmonary fibrosis, Peyronie's-like disease. The fibrotic condition may result in vascular insufficiency in the lower legs. *CV:* Vasoconstriction of arteries leading to paresthesia, chest pain, abdominal pain, or extremities that are cold, numb, or painful. Tachycardia, postural hypotension. *CNS:* Dizziness, ataxia, drowsiness, vertigo, insomnia, euphoria, lightheadedness, and psychic reactions such as depersonalization, depression, and hallucinations. *GI:* Nausea, vomiting, diarrhea, heartburn, abdominal pain. *Hematologic:* Eosinophilia, neutropenia. *Other:* Peripheral edema, flushing of face, skin rashes, transient alopecia, myalgia, arthralgia, weakness, weight gain.

Drug Interactions   Narcotic analgesics are inhibited by methysergide.

Dosage   PO. Administer 4–8 mg daily, in divided doses. Continuous administration should not exceed 6 months. Drug may be readministered after a 3–4-week rest period.

Administration

1. Administer drug with meals or milk to minimize irritation due to increased hydrochloric acid production.
2. The drug must be discontinued gradually to avoid migraine headache rebound.

Nursing Implications

1. Assess the patient's behavior and use interviewing techniques to check whether hallucinatory experiences or other untoward CNS symptoms are occurring.
2. *Teach patient and/or family*
   a. to remain under medical supervision and that blood tests must be done at periodic intervals to check for complications.
   b. to weigh daily, keep a record of weight, and report unusually rapid weight gain.
   c. how to check extremities for edema.
   d. how to maintain a low-salt diet if ordered.
   e. to adjust caloric intake if weight gain is excessive.
   f. to immediately report chest girdle or flank pain and dyspnea.
   g. not to drive a car or engage in other hazardous tasks, as drug may cause drowsiness.
   h. to be alert to psychic changes.
   i. to be alert to circulatory disturbances.
   j. to rise slowly from a supine position and to dangle feet for a few minutes before standing erect.
   k. to lie down with legs elevated, if feeling faint.
   l. not to discontinue medication abruptly, because migraine headache rebound may occur. Medication must be discontinued gradually.

METOPROLOL TARTRATE   Lopressor (Rx)

See *Antihypertensives*, Chapter 26, p. 335.

NADOLOL   Corgard (Rx)

See *Antihypertensives*, Chapter 26, p. 336.

PHENOXYBENZAMINE HYDROCHLORIDE   Dibenzyline (Rx)

Classification   Alpha-adrenergic blocking agent.

Action/Kinetics   Phenoxybenzamine is an irreversible alpha-adrenergic blocking agent. The drug increases blood flow to the skin, mucosa, and abdominal viscera as well as lowers blood pressure. Beneficial effects may not be noted for 2–4 weeks. **Onset**: gradual. **Peak effect**: 4–6 hr. Metabolized slowly and excreted in urine.

Uses   Pheochromocytoma, peripheral vascular disease, Raynaud's disease, acrocyanosis, chronic ulceration of the extremities, frostbite sequelae.

Contraindications   Conditions in which a decrease in blood pressure is not desired. Use with caution in coronary or cerebral arteriosclerosis, respiratory infections, and renal disease.

Untoward Reactions   Due to adrenergic blockade and include: miosis, postural hypotension, tachycardia, nasal congestion, and inhibition of ejaculation.

Dosage   PO: initial, 10 mg daily; may be increased by 10 mg daily q 4 days, up to maximum of 60 mg daily.

Nursing Implications

1. *Assess*
   a. BP every 4 hours to check for excessive hypotension both in supine and erect position.
   b. BP, pulse, quality of peripheral pulses, and extremities for increased warmth for 4 days after a change in dosage to assist in evaluating as to whether patient needs an adjustment in dosage.
2. Anticipate that the symptoms of respiratory infections may be aggravated by the drug. The patient will then require more supportive care.
3. Have levarterenol (Levophed) on hand to treat overdosage. Epinephrine is ineffective and may increase heart rate as well as cause further peripheral dilatation.
4. Keep the patient flat for 24 hours after overdosage and apply Ace bandages to legs as well as an abdominal binder, unless contraindicated.
5. *Teach patient and/or family*
   a. to rise slowly from a supine position and to dangle feet for a few minutes before standing erect.
   b. to lie down immediately and elevate legs if feeling faint.
   c. how to monitor radial pulse and to report tachycardia, because it is a sign of autonomic blockade.

PHENTOLAMINE MESYLATE Regitine Mesylate, Rogitine* (Rx)

Classification Alpha-adrenergic blocking agent.

Action/Kinetics Phentolamine is an alpha-adrenergic blocking agent that produces vasodilation and cardiac stimulation. It is also said to exert mild stimulatory effects on beta$_2$ receptors. **Onset** (parenteral): immediate. **Duration**: short. Poorly absorbed from th GI tract.

Uses Treatment of hypertension caused by pheochromocytoma. Dermal necrosis and sloughing following IV use or extravasation of norepinephrine or serotonin. *Investigational*: Mesylate has been used to treat hypertensive crises due to MAO inhibitors or sympathomimetic drug use. Also, rebound hypertension due to withdrawal of antihypertensive agents such as clonidine or propranolol.

Contraindications Coronary artery disease including angina, myocardial infarction, or coronary insufficiency. Use with great caution in the presence of gastritis, ulcers, and history thereof. Safety in pregnancy and lactation has not been established.

Untoward Reactions *CV:* Acute and prolonged hypotension, tachycardia, and arrhythmias especially after parenteral administration. Orthostatic hypotension, flushing. *GI:* Nausea, vomiting, diarrhea. *Other:* Dizziness, weakness, nasal stuffiness.

Drug Interactions

Interactant	Interaction
Epinephrine	Not to be used to treat overdosage of phentolamine as concomitant use leads to severe tachycardia and hypotension
Norepinephrine	Suitable antagonist to treat overdosage induced by phentolamine.
Propranolol	Concomitant use during surgery for pheochromocytoma is indicated

Dosage *To treat hypertension preoperatively*: **IV, IM, adults**: 5 mg 1–2 hr before surgery; **children**: 1 mg 1–2 hr before surgery. *Dermal necrosis/sloughing following IV or extravasation of norepinephrine*: *Prevention*, 10 mg/1,000 ml norepinephrine solution; *treatment*: 5–10 mg/10 ml saline injected into area of extravasation within 12 hr. *Diagnosis of pheochromocytoma*: **IV, adults**, 5 mg; **children**, 1 mg. **IM, adults**: 5 mg; **children**: 3 mg.

Nursing Implications

1. Monitor BP and pulse before and after parenteral administration, until stabilized at satisfactory level.
2. Avoid postural hypotension after parenteral administration by keeping the patient supine for at least 30 minutes after injection. Then have patient rise slowly and dangle feet before standing to avoid orthostatic hypotension.
3. Treat overdosage by placing the patient in Trendelenburg position, assisting with administration of parenteral fluids, and having levarterenol available for use to minimize hypotension. *Do not use epinephrine*.

PINDOLOL Visken (Rx)

See *Antihypertensives*, Chapter 26, p. 336.

PROPRANOLOL HYDROCHLORIDE   Inderal (Rx)

See *Antihypertensives*, Chapter 26, p. 337.

TIMOLOL MALEATE   Blocadren, Timoptic (Rx)

See *Antihypertensives*, Chapter 26, p. 338.

Classification   Ophthalmic agent, beta-adrenergic blocking agent.

Remarks   Timolol has minimal sympathomimetic effects, direct myocardial depressant effects, and local anesthetic action. It does not cause pupillary constriction or nightblindness.

Action/Kinetics   Timolol exerts both beta$_1$- and beta$_2$-adrenergic receptor blockade. It reduces both elevated and normal intraocular pressure whether or not glaucoma is present; it is thought to act by reducing aqueous humor formation and/or slightly increasing outflow of aqueous humor. For use in eye: **Onset**: 30 min. **Maximum effect**: 2 hr. **Duration**: 24 hr. For systemic use, see p. 338.

Uses   Chronic open-angle glaucoma, selected cases of secondary glaucoma, ocular hypertension, aphakic (no lens) patients with glaucoma. Hypertension and to reduce mortality and rate of reinfarction in patients surviving acute myocardial infarction.

Contraindications   Hypersensitivity to drug. Use with caution in patients for whom systemic beta-adrenergic blocking agents are contraindicated. Safe use in pregnancy and in children not established.

Untoward Reactions   Few. Occasionally, ocular irritation, local hypersensitivity reactions, slight decrease in resting heart rate.

Drug Interactions   Possible potentiation with systemically administered beta-adrenergic blocking agents.

Dosage   *Glaucoma*: One drop of 0.25–0.50% solution in each eye, b.i.d. When patient is transferred from other antiglaucoma agent, continue old medication on day 1 of timolol therapy (one drop of 0.25%). Thereafter, discontinue former therapy. Initiate with 0.25% solution. Increase to 0.50% solution if response is insufficient. Further increases in dosage are ineffectual. For prophylaxis of myocardial infarction and hypertension see p. 338.

Administration   Teach patient to apply finger lightly on lacrymal sac for 1 minute following administration.

Nursing Implications
Teach importance of continued regular intraocular measurements by an ophthamologist, because ocular hypertension may recur and/or progress without overt signs or symptoms.

TOLAZOLINE HYDROCHLORIDE   Priscoline Hydrochloride (Rx)

Classification   Alpha-adrenergic blocking agent.

Action/Kinetics   Tolazoline is a peripheral vasodilator but with incomplete and transient effects as an alpha-adrenergic blocking agent. The vasodilation is due to a direct effect on the smooth muscle of blood vessels. Other effects produced include cardiac and GI stimulation, increased cutaneous blood flow, and histamine-like effects. Excreted unchanged in the urine.

Uses   Spastic peripheral vascular disease, endarteritis, diabetic arteriosclerosis, gangrene, postthrombotic conditions, scleroderma, Raynaud's disease, Buerger's disease, frostbite sequelae, acrocyanosis, acroparesthesia, and arteriosclerosis obliterans. *Investigational:* In infants as a pulmonary vasodilator. Intraarterially to increase blood flow to an injured limb.

Contraindications   Following cerebrovascular accidents and in patients with coronary artery disease. Use with caution in patients with gastritis, peptic ulcer, or mitral stenosis. Safety in pregnancy and lactation not established.

Untoward Reactions   *CV:* Increase or decrease in blood pressure, tachycardia, arrhythmias, angina, flushing. Possible cause of myocardial infarction. *CNS:* Confusion, hallucinations. *GI:* Nausea, vomiting, diarrhea, aggravation of peptic ulcer, abdominal discomfort, perforation of duodenum. *Other:* Thrombocytopenia, leukopenia, oliguria, hematuria, edema, hepatitis, rashes, tingling or chilliness, increased pilomotor activity.

Intra-arterial: Warm or burning sensation at injected area, transient weakness or postural vertigo, apprehension, palpitations.

Drug Interactions

Interactant	Interaction
Alcohol	Antabuse reaction when alcohol is ingested with tolazoline
Clonidine	Tolazoline ↓ effect of clonidine
Epinephrine	↓ Blood pressure with rebound (epinephrine reversal)

Dosage   *Individualized.* **SC, IM, IV:** 10–50 mg q.i.d. **Intra-arterial: initial,** 25 mg test dose then 50–75 mg 1 or 2 times daily. **Maintenance:** usual, 2-3 injections per week.

Administration
1. Administer parenteral drugs only to hospitalized patients.
2. Position patient supine for intra-arterial injection.

Nursing Implications
1. *Assess*
   a. BP and pulse at least b.i.d., as patients are subject to either hypertensive or hypotensive reactions.
   b. that the patient is experiencing a feeling of warmth in the affected limb and not a feeling of increased cold due to a paradoxic reaction.
   c. affected extremity for flushing and piloerection (hair erected) after drug is administered, because these indicate optimal dosage.
2. Keep the patient warm to increase effectiveness of drug.
3. Avoid postural hypotension after injection by keeping patient supine for at least 30 minutes after administration. Then have patient rise slowly and dangle feet before standing.

4. Warn the patient not to ingest alcohol before or after administration of drug, as an Antabuse-like reaction may occur.
5. Treat overdosage by placing patient in Trendelenburg position, assisting with administration of parenteral fluids, and having ephedrine available for use to minimize hypotension. (*Do not use epinephrine or norepinephrine.*)

Chapter Forty-six

PARASYMPATHOMIMETIC (CHOLINERGIC) DRUGS

PARASYMPATHOMIMETICS

The neurohormone acetylcholine is necessary for nerve impulse transmission in the parasympathetic (cholinergic) portion of the autonomic nervous system (ANS).

Acetylcholine is stored at the neurojunction; after appropriate stimulation, the neurohormone is released, crosses the synapse, and interacts with receptors located on the postsynaptic membrane.

Although all postjunctional cholinergic receptors of the parasympathetic ANS share certain characteristics, they vary with respect to the intensity with which they respond to stimulation by acetylcholine and drugs that either mimic the effects of acetylcholine or block its action. This difference in response was first identified in studies on receptors involving the alkaloids muscarine and nicotine. The receptors were classified into a muscarinic type and a nicotinic type, some of which were recently further subdivided.

Cholinergic drugs can be divided into two classes: directly acting drugs that mimic the action of acetylcholine and indirectly acting drugs that increase the concentration of acetylcholine, usually by inhibiting acetylcholinesterase, the enzyme that degrades acetylcholine. The direct-acting drugs include bethanecol and guanidine while the indirect-acting drugs include ambenonium, edrophonium, neostigmine, physostigmine, and pyridostigmine.

Cholinergic drugs have the following pharmacologic effects on various structures:

GI TRACT   Enhance secretion by gastric and other glands (may cause belching, heartburn, nausea, and vomiting). Increase smooth muscle tone and stimulate bowel movement.

GENITOURINARY SYSTEM   Stimulation of ureter and relaxation of urinary bladder, resulting in micturition.

CARDIAC MUSCLE   Slowing of heart rate (bradycardia), decrease in atrial contractility, impulse formation, and conductivity.

BLOOD VESSELS   Vasodilation, resulting in increased skin temperature and local flushing.

RESPIRATION   Increased mucus secretion and bronchial constriction, which causes coughing, choking, and wheezing, especially in patients with history of asthma.

EYES   Contraction of radial and sphincter muscles of iris (pupillary constriction or miosis). Contraction of the ciliary body producing spasm of accommodation of the lens, which then no longer adjusts to see at various distances. Reduction of intraocular pressure.

SKIN   Sweat and salivary glands: Activation, increased pilomotor response.

Note that some of these effects are more pronounced with some drugs than with others. Also, the cholinergic drugs are rather nonspecific because they affect so many different parts of the body and thus have many side effects.

Directly Acting Cholinergic Drug

BETHANECHOL CHLORIDE   Duvoid, Myotonachol, Urecholine (Rx)

Classification   Cholinergic (parasympathomimetic), direct acting.

Action/Kinetics   Directly stimulates cholinergic receptors, primarily muscarinic type. This results in stimulation of gastric motility, increases gastric tone, and stimulates the detrusor muscle of the urinary bladder. Bethanecol produces a slight transient fall of diastolic BP, accompanied by minor reflex tachycardia. The drug is resistant to hydrolysis by acetylcholinesterase, which increases its duration of action. **PO: Onset**, 30 min; **maximum**: 60–90 min; **duration**: up to 6 hr. **SC: Onset**, 5–15 min; **maximum**: 15–30 min.; **duration**: 2 hr.

Uses   Postpartum or postoperative urinary retention, atony of the bladder with urinary retention. *Investigational:* Reflux esophagitis.

Contraindications   Pregnancy. Hypertension, hypotension, coronary artery disease, coronary occlusion, AV conduction defects, bradycardia. Also, peptic ulcer, asthma, hyperthyroidism, parkinsonism, epilepsy, obstruction of the bladder, peritonitis, GI spastic disease, vagotonia.

Untoward Reactions   Serious side effects are uncommon with oral dosage; symptoms observed are those of overdosage. *GI:* Nausea, vomiting, diarrhea, salivation, GI upset, involuntary defecation, cramps, colic, belching. *CV:* Heart block, orthostatic hypotension, syncope with cardiac arrest, atrial fibrillation (in hyperthyroid patients). *CNS:* Headache, malaise. *Other:* Flushing, urinary urgency, attacks of asthma, dyspnea, chest pain or pressure.

Drug Interactions

Interactant	Interaction
Cholinergic inhibitors	Additive cholinergic effects
Ganglionic blocking agents	Critical hypotensive response
Procainamide	Antagonism of cholinergic effects
Quinidine	Antagonism of cholinergic effects

Dosage   **PO** (preferred): **Adults, usual**, 10–50 mg b.i.d.–q.i.d. to a maximum of 120 mg/day. **SC: usual**, 5 mg. Repeated after 15 to 30 minutes if necessary up to maximum of 10 mg. Never give **IM** or **IV**.

Administration   Bethanecol should be taken 1 hr before or 2 hr after meals to avoid nausea and vomiting.

Nursing Implication
See *Nursing Implications*, p. 584.
   Have on hand a syringe containing 0.6 mg of atropine whenever drug is given SC.

Indirectly Acting Cholinergic Drugs (Cholinesterase Inhibitors)

Action/Kinetics   By inhibiting the enzyme acetylcholinesterase, these drugs cause an increase in the concentration of acetylcholine at the myoneural junction.

Uses See individual drugs.

Contraindications Hypersensitivity, mechanical obstruction of GI or urinary tract, bradycardia, hypotension, vagotonia, peptic ulcer, asthma, hyperthyroidism, coronary occlusion, vesical neck obstruction of urinary bladder. Safety during pregnancy and lactation not established.

Untoward Reactions *GI:* Nausea, vomiting, diarrhea, abdominal cramps, involuntary defecation, salivation, dysphagia. *CV:* Bradycardia, hypotension, A-V block, substernal pain. *CNS:* Headache, seizures, malaise, dysphonia. *Respiratory:* Increased secretions, bronchoconstriction, skeletal muscle paralysis, laryngospasm. *Ophthalmologic:* Miosis, double vision, lacrimation, accomodation difficulties, hyperemia of conjunctiva. *Other:* Urinary frequency and incontinence, sweating, flushing, muscle weakness or cramps. These effects can usually be reversed by parenteral administration of 0.6 mg of atropine sulfate, which should be readily available.

Cholinergic crisis, due to overdosage, must be distinguished from myasthenic crisis (worsening of the disease) since cholinergic crisis involves removal of drug therapy while myasthenic crisis involves an increase in anticholinesterase therapy.

Drug Interactions

Interactant	Interaction
Aminoglycoside antibiotics	↑ Neuromuscular blockade
Atropine	Atropine suppresses symptoms of excess GI stimulation caused by cholinergic drugs
Magnesium salts	Antagonize the effects of anticholinesterases
Mecamylamine	Intense hypotensive response
Organophosphate-type insecticides/pesticides	Added systemic effects with cholinesterase inhibitors

Dosage See individual drugs.

Nursing Implications

1. Assess for toxic reaction demonstrated by generalized cholinergic stimulation.
2. Have atropine and epinephrine available for treatment of cholinergic overdose. Epinephrine is also valuable in overcoming severe cardiovascular or bronchoconstrictor reactions to cholinomimetic drugs.

AMBENONIUM CHLORIDE Mytelase (Rx)

Classification Indirectly acting cholinergic-acetylcholinesterase inhibitor.

Action/Kinetics **Onset:** 20–30 min. **Duration:** 3–8 hr. Observe closely for toxicity when daily dose is greater than 200 mg.

Uses Myasthenia gravis.

Dosage **PO: initial,** 5 mg, increased gradually as required; **maintenance,** usual, 5–25 mg t.i.d.–q.i.d. (range 5–75 mg/dose). Dosage should be adjusted q 1–2 days to prevent toxicity. Doses as high as 200 mg/day have been used, but the patient must be carefully observed for cumulative effects.

Additional Nursing Implications

See also *Nursing Implications*, p. 584.

1. *Assess*
   a. closely for side effects, as they are an indication of overdosage with this drug.
   b. for reactions peculiar to this cholinergic drug, such as nervousness, dizziness, headache, and mental confusion.
   c. response to initial and subsequent doses as dosage is highly individualized and based on patient's response.
2. Have on hand 0.5–1 mg of atropine sulfate as an antidote to be administered slowly IV, and be prepared to administer supportive therapy such as artificial respiration and oxygen inhalation.

EDROPHONIUM CHLORIDE   Tensilon (Rx)

Classification   Indirectly acting cholinergic-acetylcholinesterase inhibtor.

Action/Kinetics   Edrophonium is a short-acting agent mostly used for diagnosis and not for maintenance therapy. **Onset: IM**, 2–10 min; **IV**, less than 1 min. **Duration: IM**, 12–40 min; **IV**, 6–25 min.

Uses   Diagnosis of myasthenia gravis, adjunct to treat respiratory depression due to curare and curare-like drugs.

Dosage   *Diagnosis of myasthenia gravis*. **IV: Adults**, 2 mg initially; with needle in place, wait 45 sec; if no response occurs after 45 seconds inject an additional 8 mg. If a reaction is obtained following 2 mg, test is discontinued and atropine, 0.4–0.5 mg, is given IV. **Pediatric, up to 75 lb: IV**, 1 mg; if no response after 45 sec, can give up to 5 mg. **Infants**: 0.5 mg. If IV injection is not feasible, IM can be used. **IM: Adults**, 10 mg; if hyperreactivity occurs, retest after 30 min with 2 mg IM to rule out false negatives. **Pediatric, up to 75 lb**: 2 mg; **more than 75 lb**: 5 mg. (There is a 2–10 min delay in reaction with IM route.)

   To evaluate treatment needs in myasthenic patients: 1 hr after PO administration of drug used to treat myasthenia, give edrophonium **IV**, 1–2 mg (Note: response will be myasthenic in undertreated patients, adequate in controlled patients, and cholinergic in overtreated patients). *Curare antagonist*: **Slow IV**, 10 mg over 30–45 seconds; repeat if necessary to maximum of 40 mg.

Additional Nursing Implications

See also *Nursing Implications*, p. 584.

1. *Assess*
   a. for side effects such as increased salivation, bronchiolar spasm, bradycardia, and cardiac dysrhythmia in older patients.
   b. the effect of each dose of drug when it is used as antidote for curare before next dose is given.
2. Evaluate respiratory effort. Provide assisted ventilation when needed.

NEOSTIGMINE BROMIDE   Prostigmin Bromide (Rx)

NEOSTIGMINE METHYLSULFATE   Prostigmin Methylsulfate (Rx)

Classification   Indirectly acting cholinergic-acetylcholinesterase inhibitor.

Action/Kinetics   Shorter acting than ambenonium chloride and pyridostigmine. Atropine is often given concomitantly to control side effects. **Onset: PO**, 45–75 min; **IM**, 20 min; **IV**, 4–8 min. **Duration**: All routes, 2–4 hr.

Uses   Myasthenia gravis—diagnosis and management. Postoperative distention and urinary retention. Antidote for *d*-tubocurarine and similar drugs following surgery.

Additional Untoward Reactions   Skin rashes, thrombophlebitis after IV use.

Dosage   *Neostigmine bromide for myasthenia gravis*, **PO. Adults**: 15–375 mg/day; **usual**, 150 mg/day. **Pediatric**: 7.5–15 mg t.i.d.–q.i.d. *Neostigmine methylsulfate for myasthenia gravis*, **IM, SC. Adults**: 0.5 mg (use 1 ml of 1:2,000 solution). **Pediatric**: 0.01–0.04 mg/kg q 2–3 hr. *Diagnosis of myasthenia gravis*, **IM: Adults**, 0.022 mg/kg; **pediatric**: 0.04 mg/kg. *Antidote for tubocurarine*, **IV: Adults**, 0.5–2 mg slowly with 0.6–1.2 mg atropine sulfate. Can repeat if necessary up to total dose of 5 mg. **Pediatric**: 0.07–0.08 mg/kg with 0.008–0.025 mg/kg atropine sulfate.
   Postoperative distention and urinary retention. Prophylaxis, **SC, IM**: 0.25 mg (1 ml of 1:4,000 solution) as soon as possible after surgery; **then**, repeat q 4–6 hr for 48–72 hr. *Treatment:* **SC, IM**: 0.5 mg (1 ml of 1: 2,000 solution); may be repeated q 3 hr for a total of 5 doses.

Additional Nursing Implications

See also *Nursing Implications*, p. 584.

1. *Assess*
   a. for toxic reaction demonstrated by generalized cholinergic stimulation.
   b. for vaginal bleeding when medication is used for treatment of functional amenorrhea.
2. Assist in ventilation of the patient and maintenance of a patent airway when medication is used as an antidote for tubocurarine.
3. Have atropine available to be used with neostigmine when it is used as an antidote.
4. Anticipate the use of atropine before the administration of neostigmine if there is bradycardia. Pulse rate should be increased to 80 beats/min before giving neostigmine.

PHYSOSTIGMINE SALICYLATE   Antilirium (Rx)

Classification   Indirectly acting cholinergic-acetylcholinesterase inhibitor.

Action/Kinetics   Physostigmine is a reversible acetylcholinesterase inhibitor. **Onset** (parenteral): 3–5 min. **Duration**: 45–60 min. **t½:** 1–2 hr.

Uses   Belladonna (atropine) and tricyclic antidepressant overdosage. Reversal of CNS depressant effects of diazepam. Decrease respiratory depression and drowsiness due to morphine but without loss of analgesia. Glaucoma (see p. 591 and Table 22). *Investigational:* Delirium tremens, Alzheimer's disease.

Dosage *Anticholinergic drug overdosage:* **Adults, IV, IM,** 2 mg at a rate of 1 mg/min; may be repeated if necessary. *Following anesthesia:* **IM, IV,** 0.5–1 mg at a rate of 1 mg/min; may be repeated q 10–30 min if necessary. **Pediatric** *(life-threatening conditions only)*: no more than 0.5 mg by very slow IV injection; the dose may be repeated at 5–10 min intervals up to a maximum of 2 mg if no toxic effects are manifested. *Glaucoma*: See Table 22, p. 590.

PYRIDOSTIGMINE BROMIDE   Mestinon Bromide, Regonol (Rx)

Classification Indirectly acting cholinergic-acetylcholinesterase inhibitor.

Action/Kinetics Longer acting acetylcholinesterase inhibitor with fewer side effects than neostigmine. **Onset, PO:** 20–30 min; **IM:** 15 min; **IV:** 2–5 min. **Duration, PO:** 3–6 hr; **IM, IV:** 2- 4 hr. Poorly absorbed from the GI tract; excreted in urine up to 72 hr after administration.

Uses Myasthenia gravis. Antidote for nondepolarizing muscle relaxants (e.g., curare).

Dosage *Myasthenia gravis.* **PO: Usual,** 600 mg daily (in severe cases up to 1,500 mg may be required; *Sustained-release tablets*: 1–3 180-mg tablets 1–2 times/day, with an interval of at least 6 hr between doses. **Pediatric:** 7 mg/kg/day divided into 5–6 doses. *During myasthenic crisis, pre- and postoperatively, during labor and postpartum*: **IV (slow), IM,** 1/30 the oral dose. *Antidote for nondepolarizing muscle relaxants*: **IV,** 10–20 mg together with atropine sulfate, 0.6–1.2 mg.

Additional Nursing Implications

See also *Nursing Implications*, p. 584.

1. *Assess*
   a. for toxic reaction demonstrated by generalized cholinergic stimulation.
   b. for muscular weakness, which may be a sign of impending myasthenic crisis and cholinergic overdose.
2. *Teach patient and/or family*
   a. how extended-release tablets work, and caution them not to take these tablets more often than q 6 hr.
   b. that conventional tablets may be taken with extended-release tablets if ordered.
   c. to recognize symptoms of toxic reaction and myasthenic crisis.

OPHTHALMIC CHOLINERGIC (MIOTIC) AGENTS

General Statement Cholinergic agents are commonly used for the treatment of glaucoma and less frequently for the correction of accommodative (nonparalytic) convergent strabismus and ocular myasthenia gravis.
   The drugs are instilled directly into the conjunctival sac of the eye.

TABLE 22 OPHTHALMIC CHOLINERGIC DRUGS (MIOTICS)

Drug	Uses	Dosage	Remarks
Acetylcholine chloride, intra-ocular (Miochol Intraocular), Rx	Rapid, intense miosis during eye surgery	0.5–2 ml of 1% solution.	Irrigate slowly to avoid atrophy of iris. Rapid acting, short duration. (10–20 min). Since aqueous solutions of acetylcholine are unstable, prepare immediately before use.
Carbachol, intraocular (Miostat Intraocular), Rx	Miosis during surgery	0.5 ml of 0.01% solution placed in anterior chamber.	Administered together with wetting agent. **Maximum effect:** Within 2–5 min. **Duration:** 8 hr.
Carbachol, topical (Carbacel Ophthalmic, Isopto Carbachol), Rx	Glaucoma especially those resistant to pilocarpine	1–2 gtt of 0.75–3% solution b.i.d.–q.i.d.	*Side Effects* Slight hyperemia during first few days, aching of eyes and head which usually passes after third day of treatment. *Nursing Implications* After instillation of gtts, absorption may be improved by gentle massage of the lids.
Demecarium bromide (Humorsol Ophthalmic), Rx	Chronic simple and selected cases of secondary glaucoma, accommodative esotropia	*Glaucoma:* Preferred dosage: 1–2 drops of 0.125% solution b.i.d. (some may require dosage only twice/week). *Esotropia therapy:* **Initial,** 1 drop q day for 2–3 weeks; **then,** 1 drop q 2 days to 1 drop twice a week. Evaluate condition every 4 to 12 weeks.	Effect may last several days. *Nursing Implications* Initial instillation should be made by a physician after it has been confirmed that the angle of the eye is open. Available as 0.125% and 0.25% solution.
Dipivefrin hydrochloride (Propine), Rx	Chronic open-angle glaucoma	**Initial:** 1 drop q 12 hr. *Transfer from other glaucoma drugs (except epinephrine):*	Dipiverin slowly releases epinephrine (enzymatic liberation) from inactive compound into anterior

588

For first day, continue old medication together with dipivefrin as above. If transferring from epinephrine, discontinue and begin dipivefrin. *Concomitant therapy* (with pilocarpine, carbachol, echothiophate, acetazolamide): 1 drop dipivefrin q 12 hr..

chamber. This reduces production of aqueous humor and improves its outflow from eye. Dipivefrin is 17 times as potent as epinephrine. Smaller dosage reduces side effects and frequency of administration. *Kinetics:* **Onset:** 30 min; **peak:** 1 hr. **Duration:** 12 hr. Available as a 0.1% solution.

Untoward Reactions: Slight stinging on instillation. Tachycardia, arrhythmia, hypertension.

Additional Nursing Implications: Can be used concomitantly with other anti-glaucoma drugs. Teach patient to report rapid, irregular heartbeat or headache.

Echothiophate iodide (Phospholine Iodide), Rx

Early and advanced simple glaucoma; glaucoma following cataract surgery; accomodative esotropia.

Glaucoma: 1 drop of 0.03–0.06% solution every 12 to 48 hr. *Accommodative Esotropia:* **Initial,** 1 drop of 0.125% solution/day before bedtime in both eyes for 2 to 3 weeks, **then,** 1 drop of 0.125% solution every other day or 0.06% solution daily.

Duration: Several days. Available as 0.06%, 0.125%, and 0.25% solution. Miotic effect reversible by atropine. Enhanced by concomitant administration of Diamox.

Isoflurophate (DFP, Diisopropyl-flurophosphate, Floropryl Ophthalmic), Rx

Glaucoma, accommodative esotropia

Glaucoma: ¼-inch strip of ointment (0.025%) in eye q 8-72 hr. *Esotropia therapy:* **Initial:** ¼-inch strip in both eyes q night for 2 weeks; **then,** ¼-inch strip q other day to ¼-inch strip once a week for 2 months. Then reevaluate therapy.

Duration: Several days. Drug should be refrigerated. Accidental systemic ingestion treated with atropine; if severe also with magnesium sulfate.

TABLE 22 (*Continued*)

Drug	Uses	Dosage	Remarks
Physostigmine salicylate (Isopto Eserine), Rx Physostigmine sulfate (Eserine Sulfate), Rx	Glaucoma, especially after cataract extrusion	*Solution:* (0.25% and 0.5% as the salicylate): 2 gtt in eye up to q.i.d. *Ointment* (0.25% as the sulfate): Place a small quantity in the eye up to t.i.d.	**Onset:** 2 min. **Duration:** 12–26 hr.
Pilocarpine hydrochloride (Adsorbocarpine, Akarpine, Almocarpine, Isopto Carpine, Miocarpine HC1,* Pilocar, Pilocel, Pilomiotin, Piloptic), Rx	Acute or chronic simple glaucoma; secondary glaucoma; to reverse effect of cycloplegics and mydriatics following eye examination	*Usual:* 1–2 drops of 0.5%–4% solution 1 to 6 times/day.	**Onset of action:** 15 min, **Duration:** 4–6 hr. Available as 0.25%, 0.5%, 1%, 1.5%, 2%, 3%, 4%, 5%, 6%, 8%, and 10% solutions.
Pilocarpine nitrate (P.V. Carpine Liquifilm), Rx	See Pilocarpine hydrochloride		Available as 0.5%, 1%, 2%, 3%, 4%, and 6% solution.
Pilocarpine ocular therapeutic system (Ocusert Pilo-20 and -40), Rx	Glaucoma responsive to pilocarpine	A unit designed to be placed in cul-de-sac of eye for release of pilocarpine at rate of 20 or 40 µg/hr for 1 week.	Patient should check for presence of unit before bed and upon arising. Myopia may be observed during the first several hours of therapy.
Timolol maleate (Timoptic), Rx	Chronic open-angle and selected cases of secondary glaucoma and ocular hypertension	**Initial:** 1 drop of 0.25% solution in each eye b.i.d. If response inadequate, instill 1 drop of 0.5% solution b.i.d. Dose may be decreased to 1 drop/day if intra-ocular pressure remains low.	The drug does not affect pupil size or visual acuity. **Onset:** 30 min. **Maximum effect:** 1–2 hr. **Duration:** 24 hr. This beta-adrenergic blocking agent is also used in the treatment of hypertension, see p. 338.

The ophthalmic cholinergic drugs fall into two classes: Direct-acting (carbachol, pilocarpine) and indirect-acting (demecarium, echothiophate, isoflurophate, neostigmine, physostigmine), which inhibit the enzyme cholinesterase. In the treatment of glaucoma, the drugs lead to an accumulation of acetylcholine, which stimulates the ciliary muscles and increases contraction of iris sphincter muscle. This opens the angle of the eye and results in increased outflow of aqueous humor and consequently in a decrease of intraocular pressure. This effect is of particular importance in narrow-angle glaucoma. Hourly tonometric measurements are recommended during initiation of therapy. The drugs also cause spasms of accommodation. (For individual agents and dosages, see Table 22, p. 588.)

Uses Glaucoma: primary acute narrow angle glaucoma (acute therapy) and primary chronic wide angle glaucoma (chronic therapy). Selected cases of secondary glaucoma. Accommodative (nonparalytic) convergent strabismus (squint). Ocular myasthenia gravis. Antidote against harmful effects of atropine-like drugs in patients suffering from glaucoma. Alternately with a mydriatic drug to break adhesions between lens and iris.

Contraindications *Direct-acting drugs*: Inflammatory eye disease (iritis), asthma, hypertension.

Indirect-acting drugs: Same as *Direct-acting drugs* as well as acute-angle glaucoma, history of retinal detachment, ocular hypotension accompanied by intraocular inflammatory processes, intestinal or urinary obstruction, peptic ulcer, epilepsy, parkinsonism, spastic GI conditions, vasomotor instability, severe bradycardia or hypotension, and recent myocardial infarctions.

Untoward Reactions *Local*: Painful contraction of ciliary muscle, pain in eye, blurred vision, spasms of accommodation, darkened vision, failure to accommodate to darkness, twitching, headaches, painful brow. Most of these symptoms lessen with prolonged usage. Iris cysts and retinal detachment (indirect-acting drugs only).

Systemic: Systemic absorption of drug may cause nausea, GI discomfort, diarrhea, hypotension, bronchial constriction, and increased salivation.

Dosage *Individualized*, see Table 22, p. 588.

Nursing Implications
1. Side effects can be minimized by administering at least one dose at bedtime.
2. Prevent overflow of solution into nasopharynx after topical instillation of gtts by exerting pressure on the nasolacrimal duct for 1 to 2 minutes before allowing lid to close.
3. Have epinephrine and atropine available for emergency treatment of increased intraocular pressure.
4. Report redness around the cornea, as epinephrine or phenylephrine hydrochloride (10%) may be ordered with demecarium bromide, echothiophate iodide, and isoflurophate to minimize this type of reaction
5. *Teach patient and/or family*
   a. not to drive for 1 to 2 hours after administration of drugs.
   b. that pain and blurred vision usually diminish with prolonged usage.
   c. the need for regular medical supervision while on drug therapy.
   d. that painful eye spasms may be relieved by application of cold compresses.

Chapter Forty-seven

CHOLINERGIC BLOCKING (PARASYMPATHOLYTIC) DRUGS

PARASYMPATHOLYTICS

Action/Kinetics   The cholinergic blocking agents prevent the neurotransmitter acetylcholine from combining with receptors on the postganglionic parasympathetic nerve terminal (muscarinic site). In therapeutic doses these drugs have little effect on transmission of nerve impulses across ganglia (nicotinic sites) or at the neuromuscular junction.

The main effects of cholinergic blocking agents are

1. to reduce spasms of smooth muscles like those controlling the urinary bladder or spasms of bronchial and intestinal smooth muscle.
2. to block vagal impulses to the heart, resulting in an increase in the rate and speed of impulse conduction through the atrioventricular conducting system.
3. to suppress or decrease gastric secretions, perspiration, salivation, and secretion of bronchial mucus.
4. relax the sphincter muscles of the iris and cause pupillary dilation (mydriasis) and loss of accommodation for near vision (cycloplegia).
5. to act in diverse ways on the CNS, such as depression (scopolamine) or stimulation (toxic doses of atropine). Many of the anticholinergic drugs also have

antiparkinsonism effects. They abolish or reduce the signs and symptoms of Parkinson's disease, such as tremors and rigidity and result in some improvement in mobility, muscular coordination, and motor performance. These effects may be due to blockade of the effects of acetylcholine in the CNS. This section also discusses miscellaneous synthetic antispasmodics related to anticholinergic drugs. Agents used primarily for Parkinson's disease are presented in Chapter 34.

The anticholinergics that are related to atropine are quickly absorbed following oral ingestion. These agents cross the blood brain barrier and may exert significant CNS effects. Examples of these drugs are scopolamine, *l*-hyoscyamine, and belladonna alkaloids. The drugs classified as quaternary ammonium anticholinergic drugs are erratically absorbed from the GI tract and exert minimal CNS effects since they do not cross the blood-brain barrier. Examples of these drugs are glycopyrrolate, methantheline, propantheline, tridihexethyl chloride, clidinium bromide, isopropamide, and others.

Uses   See individual drugs.

Contraindications   Glaucoma, tachycardia, partial obstruction of the GI and biliary tracts, and prostatic hypertrophy, renal disease, myasthenia gravis, hepatic disease, paralytic ileus, intestinal atony, ulcerative colitis, obstructive uropathy. Cardiac patients, especially when there is danger of tachycardia; older persons suffering from atherosclerosis or mental impairment. Use with caution in pregnancy and lactation. Use with caution in hyperthyroidism, congestive heart failure, cardiac arrhythmias, hypertension, Down's syndrome, asthma, allergies, and chronic lung disease. Safety and efficacy have not been shown in children.

Untoward Reactions   These are desirable in some conditions and undesirable in others. Thus, the anticholinergics have an antisalivary effect that is useful in parkinsonism. This same effect is unpleasant when the drug is used for spastic conditions of the GI tract.

Most untoward reactions are dose related and decrease when dosage decreases. Sometimes it helps to discontinue the medication for several days. With this in mind, anticholinergic drugs have the following untoward reactions. *GI:* Nausea, vomiting, dry mouth, dysphagia, constipation, heartburn, change in taste perception, paralytic ileus. *CNS:* Dizziness, drowsiness, nervousness, disorientation, headache, weakness, insomnia, fever. Large doses may produce CNS stimulation including tremor and restlessness. *GU:* Urinary retention or hesitancy, impotence. *Ophthalmologic:* Blurred vision, dilated pupils, photophobia, cyloplegia, precipitation of acute glaucoma. *Allergic:* Urticaria, skin rashes, anaphylaxis. *Other:* Flushing, decreased sweating, nasal congestion, suppression of glandular secretions including lactation.

Drug Interactions

Interactant	Interaction
Amantadine	Additive anticholinergic side effects
Antacids	↓ Absorption of anticholinergics from GI tract
Antidepressants, tricyclic	Additive anticholinergic side effects
Antihistamines	Additive anticholinergic side effects
Benzodiazepines	Additive anticholinergic side effects
Corticosteroids	Additive increase in intraocular pressure
Cyclopropane	↑ Chance of ventricular arrhythmias
Digoxin	↑ Effect of digoxin due to ↑ absorption from GI tract
Disopyramide	Potentiation of anticholinergic side effects

Interactant	Interaction
Guanethidine	Reversal of inhibition of gastric acid secretion caused by anticholinergics
Haloperidol	Additive increase in intraocular pressure
Histamine	Reversal of inhibition of gastric acid secretion caused by anticholinergics
Levodopa	Possible ↓ effect of levodopa due to ↑ breakdown of levodopa in stomach (due to delayed gastric emptying time)
Meperidine	Additive anticholinergic side effects
Methylphenidate	Potentiation of anticholinergic side effects
Metoclopramide	Anticholinergics block action of metoclopramide
Monoamine oxidase inhibitors	↑ Effects of anticholinergics due to ↓ breakdown by liver
Nitrates, nitrites	Potentiation of anticholinergic side effects
Nitrofurantoin	↑ Bioavailability of nitrofurantoin
Orphenadrine	Additive anticholinergic side effects
Phenothiazines	Additive anticholinergic side effects
Primidone	Potentiation of anticholinergic side effects
Procainamide	Additive anticholinergic side effects
Quinidine	Additive anticholinergic side effects
Reserpine	Reversal of inhibition of gastric acid secretion caused by anticholinergics
Sympathomimetics	↑ Bronchial relaxation
Thiazide diuretics	↑ Bioavailability of thiazide diuretics
Thioxanthines	Potentiation of anticholinergic side effects

Dosage   See individual agents and Table 23, p. 596.

Nursing Implications
1. Assess for history of asthma, glaucoma, or duodenal ulcer, which contraindicates use of these drugs.
2. Check dosage and measure drug exactly, because some drugs are given in minute amounts and overdosage leads to toxicity.
3. Relieve dry mouth by providing cold drinks (particularly postoperatively) or sugarless hard candies and chewing gum if permitted.
4. Be alert to drug interactions that may necessitate reduction in dosage of either drug.
5. *Teach patient and/or family*
   a. that certain side effects are to be expected and advise to report these to the physician, who may alleviate symptoms by reducing the dose or temporarily stopping the drug. Sometimes patient will be expected to tolerate certain side effects (e.g., dry mouth, blurred vision) for other beneficial effects.
   b. the importance of maintaining the dietary regimen prescribed by the physician. Help the patient to understand and plan diet.

c. that antiparkinsonism drugs are not to be withdrawn abruptly. If there is to be a change in medication, one drug should be withdrawn slowly and the other started in small doses.

Additional Nursing Implications Related to Pathologic Condition for Which Drug is Administered

CARDIOVASCULAR   Assess for alterations in pulse rate and palpitations.

OCULAR

1. Assist hospitalized patient who is dizzy or who has blurred vision, and advise safety precautions.
2. *Teach patient and/or family*
   a. how long vision will be affected by medication, so that activities can be planned to include safety measures.
   b. that photophobia, which may occur, is relieved by wearing dark glasses.
   c. to report marked visual changes.

GASTROINTESTINAL

1. Administer medication for treatment of GI pathology early enough before a meal so that medication will be effective when needed (at least 20 min).
2. Teach patients with GI pathology how to maintain their prescribed diets and to continue taking other medication as ordered.

GENITOURINARY

1. Assess, particularly middle-aged male patient, for infrequent voiding, which may indicate retention.
2. Teach male patient that if impotence occurs it may be drug related and that he should consult with doctor.

Belladonna Poisoning

Infants and children are especially susceptible to the toxic effects of atropine and scopolamine. Poisoning (dose dependent) is characterized by the following symptoms: dry mouth, burning sensation of the mouth, difficulties in swallowing and speaking, blurred vision, photophobia, rash, tachycardia, increased respiration, increased body temperature [fever up to 109°F (42.7°C)], restlessness, irritability, confusion, muscle incoordination, dilated pupils, hot dry skin, respiratory depression and paralysis, tremors, seizures, hallucinations, and death.

TREATMENT OF BELLADONNA POISONING   *After PO intake*: gastric lavage or induction of vomiting followed by activated charcoal.

   Systemic antidote: physostigmine (Eserine), 1–3 mg IV (effectiveness uncertain; thus use other agents if possible). Neostigmine methylsulfate, 0.5–2 mg IV, repeated as necessary. If there is excitation, diazepam or a short-acting barbiturate may be given. For fever, cool baths may be used. Keep patient in a darkened room if photophobia is manifested.

TABLE 23 CHOLINERGIC BLOCKING AGENTS

Drug	Main Use	Dosage	Remarks
Anisotropine methylbromide (Valpin 50), Rx	Adjunct in peptic ulcer therapy.	**PO:** 50 mg t.i.d. before meals.	Quaternary ammonium compound. **Onset:** 1 hr; **duration:** 4–6 hr.
Atropine sulfate (S.M.P. Atropine*), Rx	Adjunct in peptic ulcer treatment; during anesthesia to control salivation and bronchial secretions; treatment of anticholinesterase poisoning or mushroom (e.g., Amanita) poisoning. Pylorospasms; in hypotonic radiography to relax upper GI tract and colon. With morphine for biliary and uretal colic. Inhalation for prophylaxis and treatment of bronchospasm due to asthma, chronic obstructive pulmonary disease or bronchitis. For mydriasis/cycloplegia (see Table 24).	**PO. Adults:** 0.4–0.6 mg; **pediatric, over 90 lb:** Same as adult; **65–90 lb:** 0.4 mg; **40–65 lb:** 0.3 mg; **24–40 lb:** 0.2 mg; **16–24 lb:** 0.15 mg; **7–16 lb:** 0.1 mg. *Surgery.* **SC, IM, IV: Adults:** 0.4–0.6 mg; **pediatric:** 0.1–0.6 mg, depending on age. *Anticholinesterase poisoning.* **SC, IM:** 2–3 mg repeated until signs of atropine toxicity occur. *Hypertonic radiography.* **IM,** 1 mg.	Atropine sulfate is found in a large number of combination products including Donnagel, Donnagel PG, Donnatal, and Lomotil. See Appendix 3.
Belladonna extract, Rx Belladonna tincture, Rx Belladonna, levorotatory alkaloids (Bellafoline), Rx	*Extract.* **GI:** Adjunct for peptic ulcer treatment; spastic, mucous, or ulcerative colitis; diarrhea, diverticulitis. *Tincture.* Pancreatitis. **CNS:** Parkinsonism, motion sickness. **GU:** Dysmenorrhea, nocturnal enuresis. *Levorotatory alkaloids.* **GI:** Peptic ulcer treatment, pylorospasms, colic, spastic colitis. **CNS:** Parkinsonism, motion sickness. **GU:** Renal	**PO.** *Extract:* 15 mg t.i.d.–q.i.d. *Tincture:* 0.6–1.0 ml t.i.d.–q.i.d.; **pediatric:** 0.03 ml/kg t.i.d. *Levorotatory alkaloids:* **PO: Adults,** 0.25–0.5 mg t.i.d.; **pediatric, over 6 years:** 0.125–0.25 mg t.i.d. **SC: Adults,** 0.25–0.5 mg 1–2 times/day; **pediatric:** Not recommended.	Often prescribed in fixed combination with phenobarbital.

Clidinium bromide (Quarzan), Rx

colic, dysmenorrhea, nocturnal eneursis. **Respiratory:** Bronchial asthma, excess secretions.
Adjunct in peptic ulcer therapy.

PO. **Adults,** 2.5–5.0 mg t.i.d. before meals and at bedtime. **Geriatric or debilitated patients:** 2.5 mg t.i.d. before meals.

Synthetic anticholinergic. Also found in Librax (Appendix 3).

Dicyclomine hyrochloride (Antispas, A-Spas, Baycyclomine, Bentyl, Bentylol,* Cyclocen, Dicen, Di-Cyclonex, Dibent, Dilomine, DiSpaz, Formulex,* Neoques, Protylol,* Spasmoban,* Spasmoban-PH,* Spasmoject, Viscerol*), Rx

Hypermotility and spasms of GI tract associated with irritable colon and spastic colitis, ulcerative colitis, diverticulitis, and peptic ulcers. Infant colic.

PO. **Adults:** 10–20 mg t.i.d.–q.i.d.; **children:** 10 mg t.i.d.–q.i.d.; **Infants** (use syrup): 5 mg t.i.d.–q.i.d. diluted with an equal volume of water. **IM (adults only):** 20 mg q 4–6 hr. **Not for IV use.**

Additional Untoward Reactions: Brief euphoria, slight dizziness, feeling of abdominal distention. Not contraindicated in glaucoma.

Glycopyrrolate (Robinul, Robinul Forte), Rx

Adjunct in treatment of peptic ulcer. To reduce salivation, tracheobronchial and pharyngeal secretions during surgery. To block cardiac vagal inhibitory reflexes during anesthesia. Adjunct with neostigmine or pyridostigmine to reverse neuromuscular blockade due to nondepolarizing muscle relaxants.

Peptic ulcer. **PO:** 1 mg t.i.d. or 2 mg b.i.d.–t.i.d.; **maintenance:** 1 mg b.i.d. **IM, IV:** 0.1 - 0.2 mg t.i.d.–q.i.d. *Preanesthetic medication.* **IM: Adults,** 0.004 mg/kg 30–60 min prior to anesthesia; **pediatric,** less than 12 yr: 0.004–0.008 mg/kg. *Reversal of neuro-muscular blockade.* **IV: Adults and children:** 0.2 mg/each 1 mg neostigmine or 5 mg pyridostigmine.

Onset: PO, 1 hr; **IV,** 10 min. **Duration: PO,** 6 hr. Not to be used for peptic ulcer in children under 12 years of age. Do not add to IV solution containing sodium chloride or bicarbonate.
Parenteral use may slow stomach emptying and cause pain at the injection site.

Hexocyclium methylsulfate (Tral), Rx

Adjunct in therapy of peptic ulcer.

PO. **Adults:** 25 mg q.i.d. before meals and at bedtime. *Timed release:* 50 mg b.i.d. (before lunch and at bedtime).

Synthetic anticholinergic. Quaternary ammonium compound. **Onset:** 1 hr. **Duration:** 3–4 hr. Not for use in children.

Hyoscyamine sulfate (Anaspaz, Bellaspaz, Cystospaz, Cysto-

GI: Peptic ulcer therapy. Gastric hypersecretion, intes-

PO. **Adults:** 0.125–0.25 mg t.i.d–q.i.d. or 0.375 mg sus-

Synthetic anticholinergic. Quaternary ammonium compound. **Onset:** 1 hr. **Duration:** 3–4 hr. Not for use in children.

Principal alkaloid of belladonna, which is also found in Donnagel

TABLE 23 (Continued)

Drug	Main Use	Dosage	Remarks
spaz-M, Levsin, Levsinex, Neoquess), Rx	tinal hypermotility (with cramps), mild dysenteries and diverticulitis, colitis. Biliary and infant colic. Pancreatitis. **Respiratory**: Preanesthetic to dry secretions. **CNS**: Poisoning by anticholinesterase agents. Parkinsonism. **GU**: Cystitis, renal colic.	tained release q 12 hr; **pediatric, 2–10 yr**: ½ adult dose; **pediatric, up to 2 yr**: ¼ adult dose. **IM, IV, SC**: 0.25–0.6 mg t.i.d.–q.i.d.	and Donnagel PG and in Donnatal. See Appendix 3.
Isopropamide iodide (Darbid), Rx	Adjunct in peptic ulcer therapy.	**PO. Adults**: 5 mg q 12 hr up to 10 mg q 12 hr. Not for use in children under 12 years.	Synthetic anticholinergic, antispasmodic. Quaternary ammonium compound. **Duration**: 12 hr. Sedatives and antacids can be given concurrently. Also found in Combid, Ornade, and Tuss-Ornade. See Appendix 3.
Mepenzolate bromide (Cantil), Rx	Adjunct in peptic ulcer therapy.	**PO: Initial**: 25 mg q.i.d. before meals and at bedtime. Increase gradually to 50 mg q.i.d. until therapeutic response is attained or side effects appear.	Synthetic anticholinergic, antispasmodic, quaternary ammonium salt. Safety and efficacy in children have not been established. *Additional Nursing Implication* See also *Nursing Implications*, p. 594. Observe carefully for side-effects and onset of therapeutic response to determine maintenance dosage.
Methantheline bromide (Banthine), Rx	Adjunct in peptic ulcer therapy.	**PO: Adults**: 50–100 mg q.i.d. **Pediatric**; over 1 yr: 12.5–50 mg q.i.d. **Infants, 1-12 months**: 12.5 up to 25 mg q.i.d. **Newborns**: 12.5 mg b.i.d.; then, 12.5 mg t.i.d.	Synthetic anticholinergic, antispasmodic (quarternary ammonium compound). *Kinetics* **PO: Onset**: 30 min. **Duration**: 6 hr. **IM: Duration**: 2-4 hr. Drug has some ganglionic blocking effects. *Additional Untoward Reactions* Postural hypotension, impotence.

598

Respiratory paralysis and tachycardia (overdosage).

Additional Nursing Implications
See also *Nursing Implications*, p. 594.

1. Initiate therapy for duodenal ulcer while patient is on liquid diet.
2. Assess ulcer patient for abdominal distention, epigastric distress, and vomiting, because drug reduces gastric motility.
3. *Teach patient and/or family*
   a. to rise slowly from supine position, to prevent hypotension.
   b. the possibility of drug-induced impotence, which should be reported to doctor.

Drug	Uses	Dosage	Remarks
Methscopolamine bromide (Hyoscine Methylbromide, Pamine Bromide, Scopolamine Methylbromide), Rx	Adjunct in peptic ulcer therapy.	PO: 2.5 mg ½ hr before meals and 2.5–5 mg at bedtime.	Quaternary ammonium derivative of belladonna. **Onset:** 1 hr. **Duration:** 4–6 hr. Dose-related side effects may be relieved by decreasing dose for 5 to 7 days.
Oxyphencyclimine hydrochloride (Daricon), Rx	Peptic ulcer, pylorospasms, spastic and inflammatory conditions of GI, urinary, and biliary tracts.	PO: **Adults:** 10 mg b.i.d. (in the AM and at bedtime) Not recommended for children under 12 years.	Anticholinergic, antispasmodic of the tertiary amine type. Can be given with antacids and sedatives. High doses may cause CNS stimulation. Neostigmine may be used to treat overdosage.
Oxyphenonium bromide (Antrenyl), Rx	Adjunct in peptic ulcer therapy.	PO. **Adults:** 10 mg q.i.d. before meals and at bedtime for several days; **then,** adjust dosage according to response. Not for use in children.	Anticholinergic, antispasmodic of the tertiary amine type. **Onset:** ½ hr. **Duration:** 6 hr. High incidence of side effects. Neostigmine should be used to treat overdosage.
Propantheline bromide (Norpanth, Pro–Banthine, Pro–	Adjunct in peptic ulcer therapy. Spastic and inflamma-	PO. **Adults:** 15 mg ½ hr before meals and 30 mg at bedtime.	Anticholinergic, antispasmodic quaternary ammonium compound.

TABLE 23 (*Continued*)

Drug	Main Use	Dosage	Remarks
panthel,* SK–Propantheline Bromide), Rx	tory disease of GI and urinary tracts. Control of salivation and enuresis.	Reduce dose to 7.5 mg t.i.d. for mild symptoms, geriatric patients or patients with small stature. **Pediatric:** *Anti-secretory:* 1.5 mg/kg/day in 3–4 doses. *Antispasmodic:* 2–3 mg/kg/day in divided doses q 4–6 hr and at bedtime.	Mix just prior to parenteral administration. *Additional Nursing Implication:* See also *Nursing Implications,* p. 594. A liquid diet is recommended during initiation of therapy for patients with edematous duodenal ulcer.
Scopolamine hydrobromide (Hyoscine Hydrobromide), Rx	**PO:** Motion sickness. **Parenteral:** Pre-anesthetic sedation and obstetrical amnesia. Mydriatic/cycloplegic (see Table 24).	**PO:** 0.25–0.8 mg 1 hr before travel. **SC, IM, IV** (only if diluted with water): **Adults,** 0.3–0.6 mg; **pediatric, 6 mo–3 yr:** 0.1–0.15 mg; **3 to 6 yr:** 0.15–0.2 mg; **6–12 yr:** 0.2–0.3 mg.	Anticholinergic with CNS depressant effects. Produces amnesia when given with morphine or meperidine. Tolerance may develop if given alone. In the presence of pain, may produce delirium. Also present in Donnagel and Donnagel PG, and Donnatal. See Appendix 3. *Additional Untoward Reactions* Disorientation, delirium, increased heart rate, decreased respiratory rate. *Additional Nursing Implications* See also *Nursing Implications,* p. 594.

Drug	Uses	Dosage	Remarks
Scopolamine transdermal therapeutic system (Transderm-Scop), Rx	Prophylaxis of nausea and vomiting associated with motion sickness.	One system is applied to post-auricular skin several hours before effect needed. System should be replaced q 3 days if continuous therapy required.	1. Assess a. for additional side effects. b. for tolerance after a long course of therapy. 2. Do not administer drug alone for pain, as it is likely to cause delirium. 3. Orient and reassure patient who experienced amnesia after receiving drug. *Kinetics* The system contains 1.5 mg scopolamine, which is slowly released from a mineral oil/polyisobutylene matrix. Approximately 0.5 mg is released per day. *Contraindications* Children, lactating women. *Additional Nursing Implications* Warn patient not to drive a car or operate dangerous machinery, as drug may cause drowsiness, confusion, and disorientation.
Tridihexethyl chloride (Pathilon), Rx	Adjunct in peptic ulcer therapy.	**PO:** 25–50 mg t.i.d.–q.i.d. before meals and at bedtime.	Neostigmine should be used to treat toxic reactions.

MYDRIATICS AND CYCLOPLEGICS

Action/Kinetics   These agents dilate the pupil (mydriasis) and paralyze the muscles required to accommodate for close vision (cycloplegia). This enables the physician to examine the inner structure of the eye including the retina. Also permits examination of refractive errors of the lens without the patient automatically accomodating.

Uses   Diagnostic ophthalmoscopic examination, refraction in children, pre- and postoperative mydriasis during eye surgery, and anterior uveitis.

Contraindications   Glaucoma, infants less than three months of age. Use with caution in infants, children, geriatric patients, diabetes, hypo- or hyperthyroidism, narrow anterior chamber angle.

TABLE 24   MYDRIATICS AND CYCLOPLEICS

Drug	Dosage	Remarks
Atropine sulfate (Atropisol Ophthalmic, Atropine–Care Ophthalmic, Isopto Atropine Ophthalmic), Rx	*Refraction,* **adults:** 1–2 gtt in eye 1 hr before examination; **children:** 1–2 gtt, 0.5% solution in eyes b.i.d. for 1 to 3 days before examination and 1 hr before examination. *Uveitis,* **adults:** 1–2 gtt in eye up to t.i.d.; **children:** 1–2 gtt of 0.5% solution in eye up to t.i.d.	**Peak effect:** *Mydriasis,* 30–40 min; *cycloplegia,* 1–3 hr. **Recovery:** Up to 12 days. Drug particularly prone to have systemic effects such as contact dermatitis, allergic conjunctivitis. Available in 0.5-3% solutions or 1.0% ointment.
Cyclopentolate hydrochloride (AK–Pentolage Ophthalmic, Cyclogel Ophthalmic), Rx	*Refraction,* **adults:** 1 gtt of 0.5% solution followed by 1 gtt in 5 min; **children:** 1 gtt of 0.5, 1, or 2% solution in each eye followed in 10 min by 1 gtt of 0.5 or 1% solution.	**Onset:** 25–75 min. **Duration:** 24 hr. Recovery time can be reduced by using 1–2 gtt pilocarpine, 1 or 2%. To reduce absorption, pressure should be applied over the nasolacrimal sac for 2–3 min.
Homatropine hydrobromide (Homatrocel Ophthlamic, Isopto Homatropine Ophthalmic), Rx	*Refraction:* 1–2 gtt; repeat in 5 to 10 minutes if necessary. *Uveitis:* 1–2 gtt q 3–4 hr.	Short acting. **Onset:** 60 min. **Duration:** 24–72 hr. Available as 2% or 5% solution.
Scopolamine hydrobromide (Isopto Hyoscine Ophthalmic), Rx	*Refraction:* 1–2 gtt of 0.25% solution 1 hr before examination. *Uveitis:* 1–2 gtt in eyes up to t.i.d.	**Onset:** 20–60 min. **Duration:** Up to 7 days. Fewer side effecs than atropine. Also used for iridocyclitis either pre- or postoperatively.
Tropicamide (Mydriacyl Ophthalmic), Rx	*Refraction:* 1–2 drops of 1% solution repeated after 5 min. Maximum cycloplegia occurs in 20 to 35 minutes when a second drop is given 5 minutes after first. *Examination of fundus:* 1–2 drops of 0.5% solution 15–20 min before exam.	**Rapid onset:** 20–40 min; **Duration:** 2–6 hr. Drug particularly likely to cause systemic side effects.

Untoward Reactions   *Ophthalmologic:* Blurred vision, stinging, increased intraocular pressure. Long-term use may cause irritation, photophobia, conjunctivitis, hyperemia, or edema. For systemic side effects, see p. 593.

Dosage   See individual agents, Table 24.

Administration

1. Drops are instilled in conjunctival sac.
2. Patients should not drive or operate machinery when eyes are dilated.

Nursing Implications

1. Before administering, check whether the patient has a history of angle-closure glaucoma because the drug may precipitate an acute crisis.
2. Warn the patient that these drugs will temporarily impair vision and that he should not do close work, operate machinery, or drive a car until the effects have worn off.

Chapter Forty-eight

NEUROMUSCULAR BLOCKING AGENTS

General Statement   The drugs considered in this section interfere with nerve impulse transmission between the motor endplate and the receptors of skeletal muscle (i.e., peripheral action). Upon stimulation, these muscles normally contract when acetylcholine is released from storage sites embedded in the motor endplate.

The drugs fall into two groups: competitive (nondepolarizing agents) and depolarizing agents. Competitive agents—atracurium, gallamine, metocurine, pancuronium, tubocurarine, vercuronium—compete with acetylcholine for the receptor site in the muscle cells. These agents are also called curariform because their mode of action is similar to that of the poison curare in which ancient hunters dipped their arrows to paralyze their prey. The depolarizing agent—succinylcholine—initially excites skeletal muscle and then prevents the muscle from contracting by prolonging the time during which the receptors at the endplate cannot respond to acetylcholine (depolarization).

The muscle paralysis caused by the neuromuscular blocking agents is sequential.

Therapeutic doses produce muscle depression in the following order: heaviness of eyelids, difficulty in swallowing and talking, diplopia, progressive weakening of the extremities and neck, followed by relaxation of the trunk and spine. The diaphragm (respiratory paralysis) is affected last. The drugs do not affect consciousness, and their use, in the absence of adequate levels of general anesthesia, may be frightening to the patient.

There is a narrow margin of safety between a therapeutically effective dose causing muscle relaxation and a toxic dose causing respiratory paralysis. **The neuromuscular blocking agents are always administered by a physician**. However, the nurse must be prepared to maintain and monitor a patient's respiration until the drug wears off.

Uses See individual agents.

Contraindications The neuromuscular blocking agents should be used with caution in patients with myasthenia gravis; renal, hepatic, or pulmonary impairment; respiratory depression; and in elderly or debilitated patients.

Depolarizing agents should be used with caution for patients with electrolyte imbalance, especially hyperkalemia, and in patients on digitalis.

Untoward Reactions *Respiratory paralysis. Severe and prolonged muscle relaxation.* Some neuromuscular blocking agents cause hypotension, bronchospasms, cardiac disturbances, hyperthermia. Also see individual agents.

Drug Interactions The following drug interactions are for nondepolarizing skeletal muscle relaxants. For succinylcholine, see individual entry.

Interactant	Interaction
Aminoglycoside antibiotics	Additive muscle relaxation
Amphotericin B	↑ Muscle relaxation
Anesthetics, inhalation	Additive muscle relaxation
Clindamycin	Additive muscle relaxation
Colistin	↑ Muscle relaxation
Furosemide	Furosemide ↑ effect of skeletal muscle relaxants
Lincomycin	↑ Muscle relaxation
Magnesium salts	↑ Muscle relaxation
Methotrimeprazine	↑ Muscle relaxation
Narcotic analgesics	↑ Respiratory depression and ↑ muscle relaxation
Phenothiazines	↑ Muscle relaxation
Polymyxin B	↑ Muscle relaxation
Procainamide	↑ Muscle relaxation
Procaine	↑ Muscle relaxation by ↓ plasma protein binding
Quinidine	↑ Muscle relaxation
Thiazide diuretics	↑ Muscle relaxation due to hypokalemia

Nursing Implications

1. *Assess*
   a. respiration, BP, and pulse very closely for the duration of action of the drug, and report untoward signs.
   b. for signs of respiratory embarrassment or apnea and be prepared to assist with artificial respiration and provision of oxygen.

c. for excessive bronchial secretions or respiratory wheezing.
2. Have oxygen, a respirator, neostigmine, atropine, and epinephrine available for emergency use.
3. Be aware that the respiratory depression caused by nondepolarizing type may be relieved by anticholinesterase drugs, such as neostigmine, which increase the body's production of acetylcholine, but that the antidote for depolarizing drugs is oxygen under pressure followed by whole blood or plasma if apnea is prolonged.
4. Be especially alert to drug interactions because potentiation of muscle relaxation may be fatal.

ATRACURIUM BESYLATE   Tracrium Injection (Rx)

Classification   Nondepolarizing skeletal muscle relaxant.

Action/Kinetics   Atracurium prevents the action of acetylcholine by competing for the cholinergic receptor at the neuromuscular junction. It may also release histamine leading to hypotension. **Peak effect:** 2–3 min. **Duration:** 20–40 min. Recovery occurs more quickly than with other nondepolarizing agents (e.g., *d*-tubocurarine). **t½:** 20 min. Drug is metabolized in the plasma.

Uses   Skeletal muscle relaxant during surgery; adjunct to general anesthesia; assist in endotracheal intubation.

Contraindications   Use with caution in pregnancy and during labor and delivery. Also, in patients with myasthenia gravis, Eaton-Lambert syndrome, electrolyte disorders, bronchial asthma. Safety and efficacy has not been determined in lactation and in children under 2 years of age.

Additional Untoward Reactions   *CV:*Bradycardia. Other untoward reactions may be due to histamine release and include: flushing, erythema, wheezing, urticaria, bronchial secretions, blood pressure and heart rate changes.

Dosage   **IV only. Adults and children over 2 years, initial:** 0.4–0.5 mg/kg as IV bolus; **maintenance:** 0.08–0.1 mg/kg. The first maintenance dose can be given after 20–45 min and repeated at 15–25 min intervals under balanced anesthesia or longer intervals using inhalation anesthetics. *Following use of succinylcholine for intubation:* **initial,** 0.3–0.4 mg/kg using balanced anesthesia. *Use in cardiovascular disease or patients with history of asthma or anaphylaxis:* **initial,** 0.3–0.4 mg/kg given slowly over 1 min.

Administration
1. Initial dosage should be reduced if being used with inhalation anesthetics.
2. Dosage should be reduced in patients with myasthenia gravis or other neuromuscular diseases, electrolyte disorders, or carcinomatosis.
3. Atracurium should not be mixed with alkaline solutions.

GALLAMINE TRIETHIODIDE   Flaxedil I.V. (Rx)

Classification   Nondepolarizing neuromuscular blocking agent.

Action/Kinetics Similar to tubocurarine. Does not release histamine or produce bronchospasms. Has no effect on GI tract. **Onset**: immediate. **Duration**: 20 min. Excreted unchanged by kidney.

Uses Muscle relaxant during surgery; adjunct to manage patients requiring mechanical ventilation.

Additional Contraindications Myasthenia gravis. Cardiac disease, especially for patients in whom tachycardia may be dangerous. Also in presence of hypertension, hyperthyroidism, impaired renal function or respiratory depression, and hypersensitivity to iodine.

Additional Untoward Reactions Anaphylaxis.

Dosage **IV, after general anesthesia has been introduced:** *highly individualized*. **Initial**, 1 mg/kg body weight up to maximum of 100 mg; an additional dose of 0.5–1 mg/kg body weight may be given at 30–40 min intervals.
    Dose should be reduced if used with cyclopropane, ether, halothane, or methoxyflurane.

Administration A precipitate will form if gallamine is mixed with anesthetic agents.

HEXAFLUORENIUM BROMIDE Mylaxen (Rx)

Classification Cholinesterase inhibitor.

Action/Kinetics Only used in conjunction with succinylcholine to prolong action. Permits reduction of dosage of succinylcholine and thus decreases side effects of the latter. Has no muscle relaxing effect by itself. **Duration**: 20–30 min.

Use Adjunct with succinylcholine to prolong muscle relaxation.

Contraindictions Use with caution in renal, hepatic, cardiovascular, or pulmonary disease. Also, in patients with glaucoma, neuromuscular diseases, fractures, severe burns, digitalized patients. Safety in pregnancy has not been established.

Untoward Reactions Untoward reactions are due to inhibition of cholinesterase and include the following. *CV:* Blood pressure changes, arrhythmias, tachycardia, bradycardia, cardiac arrest. *Skeletal muscle:* Paralysis, respiratory depression, bronchospasm, apnea. *Other:* Fever, allergic reactions, salivation, increased intraocular pressure.

Dosage **IV, after general anesthesia has been induced**: 0.4 mg/kg followed in 3 min by 0.2 mg/kg succinylcholine. Subsequent doses may be administered depending on the response of the patient and the length of the surgical procedure.

Administration Drug is administered after anesthetization and prior to surgery.

METOCURINE IODIDE Metubine Iodide Injection (Rx)

Classification Nondepolarizing neuromuscular blocking agent.

Action/Kinetics Metocurine is two times as potent as tubocurarine and does not cause ganglionic blockade. Histamine may be released. Effects are cumulative. **Onset**: few minutes; maximal effects persist for 35–60 min; **Duration**: 25–90 min. t½: 3.6 hr. About 50% excreted unchanged in urine.

Uses Muscle relaxation during surgery; to decrease muscle contractions during seizures; as adjunct in patients requiring mechanical ventilation; adjunct in electroshock therapy.

Contraindications Patients sensitive to iodide.

Additional Untoward Reactions Allergic reactions to drug or iodine. *Symptoms due to histamine release: CV:* Hypotension, erythema, tachycardia, flushing, circulatory collapse. *Other:* Edema, bronchospasm.

Additional Drug Interactions Succinylcholine chloride ↑ relaxant effect of both drugs.

Dosage IV. *Surgery:* Dose depends on type of anesthetic and nature of surgery. *For endotracheal intubation:* 0.2–0.4 mg/kg. *Supplemental doses:* 0.5–1 mg. *When used with halothane, enflurane, methoxyflurane, ether:* Reduce incremental doses by one-third to one-half. *Electroshock therapy:* 1.75–5.5 mg (usual: 2–3 mg). **IM use is not recommended.**

Administration Metocurine is incompatibile with alkaline solutions.

Additional Nursing Implications

See also *Nursing Implications*, p. 604.

1. Have neostigmine methylsulfate on hand during IV administration to combat respiratory depression.
2. Do not give neostigmine when respiratory depression is associated with fall in blood pressure as it may aggravate shock.

PANCURONIUM BROMIDE   Pavulon (Rx)

Classification Nondepolarizing neuromuscular blocking agent.

Action/Kinetics Effects similar to *d*-tubocurarine although pancuronium is 5 times as potent. Kinetics are dose-dependent. **Onset, after 0.04 mg/kg:** 45 sec; **peak effect:** 4.5 min; **duration:** 1 hr.

Use Muscle relaxation during anesthesia and for endotracheal intubation.

Additional Contraindications Hypersentivity to bromide, tachycardia, children under 10 years of age, and patients in whom increase in heart rate is undesirable.

Additional Untoward Reactions Salivation, skin rashes, increased pulse rate.

Additional Drug Interactions

Interactant	Interaction
Acetylcholine	Acetylcholine ↓ effect of pancuronium
Cardiac glycosides	Additive toxic effects on heart
Potassium	Antagonizes action of pancuronium
Succinylcholine	Succinylcholine ↑ intensity and duration of action of pancuronium

Dosage **IV: initial**, 40–100 μg/kg. Additional doses of 10 μg/kg may be administered at 25–60 min intervals. Dosage requirements for children are the same as adults. **Neonates**: A test dose of 20 $\mu g/kg$ should be administered first to determine responsiveness. *Endotracheal intubation*: 60–100 $\mu g/kg$.

SUCCINYLCHOLINE CHLORIDE   Anectine, Quelicin, Succinylcholine Chloride Min-I-Mix, Sucostrin (Rx)

Classification   Depolarizing neuromuscular blocking agent.

Action/Kinetics   Succinylcholine initially excites skeletal muscle and then prevents the muscle from contracting by prolonging the time during which the receptors at the neuromuscular junction cannot respond to acetylcholine. Short acting. **IV: Onset**, 1 min; **duration**: 4–6 min. **Recovery**: 8–10 min. **IM: Onset**, 3 min. Metabolized by plasma pseudocholinesterase.

Uses   Muscle relaxant during surgery, endotracheal intubation, endoscopy and short manipulative procedures; electroshock therapy.

Additional Contraindications   Use with caution in patients with severe liver disease, severe anemia, malnutrition, impaired cholinesterase activity, acute narrow angle glaucoma, history of malignant hyperthermia, penetrating eye injuries, in fractures. Also, in cardiovascular, pulmonary, renal, or metabolic diseases. Safe use in pregnancy not established.

Untoward Reactions   *Skeletal muscle:* May cause severe, persistent respiratory depression or apnea. Muscle fasciculation, postoperative muscle pain. *CV:* Bradycardia or tachycardia, blood pressure changes, arrhythmias, cardiac arrest. *Respiratory:* Apnea, respiratory depression. *Other:* Fever, malignant hyperthermia, salivation, hyperkalemia, anaphylaxis, myoglobinemia, skin rashes, increased intraocular pressure.

Drug Interactions

Interactant	Interaction
Aminoglycoside antibiotics	Additive skeletal muscle blockade
Antibiotics, nonpenicillin	Additive skeletal muscle blockade
Anticholinesterases	Additive effects
Beta-adrenergic blocking agents	Additive skeletal muscle blockade
Chloroquine	Additive skeletal muscle blockade
Clindamycin	Additive skeletal muscle blockade
Cyclophosphamide	↑ Effect of succinylcholine by ↓ breakdown of drug in plasma by pseudocholinesterase
Diazepam	↓ Effect of succinylcholine
Digitalis glycosides	↑ Chance of cardiac arrhythmias
Echothiophate Iodide	↑ Effect of succinylcholine by ↓ breakdown of drug in plasma by pseudocholinesterase
Furosemide	↑ Action of succinylcholine
Isoflurane	Additive skeletal muscle blockade
Lidocaine	↑ Effect of succinylcholine
Lincomycin	Additive skeletal muscle blockade

Interactant	Interaction
Lithium	↑ Effect of succinylcholine
Magnesium salts	Additive skeletal muscle blockade
Phenothiazines	↑ Effect of succinylcholine
Polymyxin	Additive skeletal muscle blockade
Procaine	↑ Effect of succinylcholine by inhibiting plasma pseudocholinesterase activity
Procainamide	↑ Effect of succinylcholine
Quinidine	Additive skeletal muscle blockade
Quinine	Additive skeletal muscle blockade
Trimethaphan	↑ Effect of succinylcholine by inhibiting plasma pseudocholinesterase activity
Thiotepa	↑ Effect of succinylcholine by ↓ breakdown of drug in plasma by pseudocholinesterase

Dosage **IV: Usual**, an initial test dose of 0.1 mg/kg should be given to assess sensitivity and recovery time. *Surgical procedures:* **Adults, 0.6 mg/kg (range: 0.3–1.1 mg/kg). Older children**: 1 mg/kg; **infants and younger children**: 1–2 mg/kg. For prolonged procedures, use **intermittent IV injections: Adults: initial**, 0.3–1.1 mg/kg; **then**, 0.04–0.07 mg/kg as required. **IM**: 3.3 mg/kg not to exceed a total dose of 150 mg.

Administration/Storage

1. For IV infusion, use 1 or 2 mg/ml solution of drug in 5% dextrose injection, 0.9% sodium chloride, or other suitable IV solution. Succinylcholine is not compatible with alkaline solutions.
2. Alter degree of relaxation by altering rate of flow.
3. Store in refrigerator.
4. Do not mix with anesthetic.

TUBOCURARINE CHLORIDE   Tubarine,* D-Tubocurarine Chloride (Rx)

Classification Nondepolarizing neuromuscular blocking agent.

Action/Kinetics Cumulative effects may occur. Narrow margin between therapeutic dose and toxic dose. Overdosage chiefly treated by artificial respiration, although neostigmine, atropine, and edrophonium chloride should be on hand. **Onset**: few minutes; maximal effects persist for 35–60 min; **Duration**: 25–90 min. t½: 1–3 hr. About 43% excreted unchanged in urine.

Uses Muscle relaxant during abdominal surgery, setting of fractures and dislocations; spasticity caused by injury to or disease of CNS; electroshock therapy; diagnosis of myasthenia gravis.

Additional Contraindications Use with extreme caution in patients with renal dysfunction, liver disease, or obstructive states. Drug may cause excessive secretion and circulatory collapse. Patients in whom release of histamine is hazardous. Use with caution in pregnancy, lactation, and in children.

Additional Untoward Reactions Allergic reactions.

Additional Drug Interactions

Interactant	Interaction
Acetylcholine	Acetylcholine antagonizes effect of tubocurarine
Anticholinesterases	Anticholinesterases antagonize effect of tubocurarine
Calcium salts	↑ Effect of tubocurarine
Diazepam	Diazepam may cause malignant hyperthermia with tubocurarine
Potassium	Antagonizes effect of tubocurarine
Propranolol	↑ Effect of tubocurarine
Quinine	↑ Effect of tubocurarine
Succinylcholine chloride	↑ Relaxant effect of both drugs
Trimethophan	↑ Effect of tubocurarine

Dosage **IV, IM**: initial dose should be 20 units *less* than the calculated amount. *Surgery*, **IV**: usually 1.1 unit/kg (40-60 units at time of incision followed by 20–30 units in 3–5 min, if necessary). *Electroshock therapy*: 1.1 units/kg **IV** over 60–90 sec. *Diagnosis of myasthenia gravis*, **IV**: 0.07–0.22 units/kg.

Administration Tubocurarine is incompatible with alkaline solutions.

VERCURONIUM BROMIDE   Norcuron (Rx)

Classification Nondepolarizing neuromuscular blocking agent.

Action/Kinetics Vercuronium acts by blocking receptors at the neuromuscular junction in a fashion similar to tubocurarine. **Onset:** 2.5–3 min; **peak effect:** 3–5 min; **duration:** 25–40 min. Metabolized in liver and excreted through the kidney. Is bound to plasma protein.

Uses To induce skeletal muscle relaxation during surgery or to assist in endotracheal intubation. As an adjunct to general anesthesia.

Additional Untoward Reactions Moderate to severe skeletal muscle weakness, which may require artificial respiration.

Additional Drug Interactions Succinylcholine ↑ effect of vercuronium.

Dosage **IV only. Individualized. Adults and children 10–17 years of age: initial,** 0.08–0.1 mg/kg as IV bolus; **maintenance:** 0.01–0.015 mg/kg given within 25–40 min after initial dose. Subsequent doses may be given q 12–15 min when using balanced anesthesia. *When succinylcholine used first for intubation:* 0.04–0.06 mg/kg with inhalation anesthesia and 0.05–0.06 mg/kg with balanced anesthesia. **Pediatric, 1–10 years:** May require somewhat higher initial dosage and supplementation more often than adults. **Pediatric, 7 weeks–1 year:** More sensitive to the drug than adults (monitor carefully).

Administration Dosage must be individualized and depends on prior or concomitant use of anesthetics or succinylcholine.

Part Eight

DRUGS AFFECTING THE RESPIRATORY SYSTEM

Chapter Forty-nine

ANTIASTHMATIC DRUGS

Theophylline Derivatives

Miscellaneous Antiasthmatics

General Statement   Asthma is a disease characterized by difficulty in breathing. Breathing difficulties may result from smooth muscle contraction of the bronchi and bronchioles, edema of the mucosa of the respiratory tract, or mucus secretions that adhere to the walls of the bronchi and bronchioles. The cause of asthma is not known with certainty but in some patients allergy is the underlying reason.

   The overall objectives of drug therapy for asthma are to open blocked airways and to alter the characteristics of respiratory tract fluid. The drugs and drug classes that are used to treat asthma are bronchodilators such as theophyllines and sympathomimetic amines (see Chapter 44), mucolytics (see Chapter 50), corticosteroids (see Chapter 61), and cromolyn sodium. Theophyllines and cromolyn sodium are discussed in this chapter.

THEOPHYLLINE DERIVATIVES

Action/Kinetics The theophylline derivatives are plant alkaloids, which, like caffeine, belong to the xanthine family. They are CNS stimulants, relax the smooth muscles of the bronchi and pulmonary blood vessels (relieve bronchospasms), produce diuresis, stimulate gastric acid secretion, and increase the rate and force of contraction of the heart. Theophylline and its derivatives competitively inhibit phosphodiesterase, which is the enzyme responsible for metabolizing cyclic AMP to 5-AMP. The resultant increase in cyclic AMP increases the release of endogenous epinephrine, which can cause bronchodilation. There is also evidence that the increase in cyclic AMP inhibits the release of slow reacting substance of anaphylaxis (SRS-A) and histamine. Response to the drugs is highly individualized.

Theophylline salts: **Onset**: 1–5 hr, depending on route and formulation. **Therapeutic plasma levels**: 10–20 μg/ml t½: 7–9 hr in nonsmoking adults, 4–5 hr in adult heavy smokers, and 3–5 hr in children. Because of great variations in absorption as well as extremely narrow therapeutic range, theophylline therapy is best monitored by determination of the serum levels. If these determinations cannot be obtained, saliva (which contains 60% of corresponding theophylline serum levels) determinations can be used. Metabolized in liver to the active 3-methylxanthine; excretion is through the kidneys.

Dyphylline: Less potent than theophylline, with a half-life of 2 hr. All drugs metabolized in liver, excreted in urine.

Uses Relief of acute bronchial asthma, reversible bronchospasms associated with chronic bronchitis, and emphysema.

Contraindications Hypersensitivity to drug, hypotension, coronary artery disease, angina pectoris. Safe use in pregnancy has not been established. Xanthines are not usually tolerated by small children because of excessive CNS stimulation. Use with caution in the presence of gastritis, peptic ulcer, alcoholism, acute cardiac diseases, hypoxemia, severe renal and hepatic disease, severe hypertension, severe myocardial damage, hyperthyroidism, glaucoma, the elderly, and neonates.

Untoward Reactions *GI:* Nausea, vomiting, diarrhea, anorexia, epigastric pain, hematemesis, dyspepsia, rectal irritation (following use of suppositories). *CNS:* Headache, insomnia, irritability, fever, dizziness, lightheadedness, vertigo, reflex hyperexcitability, seizures, depression, speech abnormalities, alternating periods of mutism and hyperactivity, brain damage, death. *CV:* Hypotension, arrhythmias, palpitations, tachycardia, peripheral vascular collapse, extrasystoles. *Renal:* Proteinuria, excretion of erythrocytes and renal tubular cells, dehydration due to diuresis, urinary retention (males with prostatic hypertrophy). *Other:* Tachypnea, respiratory arrest, fever, flushing, hyperglycemia, antidiuretic hormone syndrome, leukocytosis.

Note: Aminophylline given by rapid IV may produce: hypotension, flushing, palpitations, precordial pain, headache, dizziness, or hyperventilation. Also, the ethylenediamine in aminophylline may cause allergic reactions including urticaria and skin rashes.

Overdosage   Early signs of toxicity include anorexia, nausea, vomiting, wakefulness, restlessness, irritability. Later symptoms include agitated, manic behavior, frequent vomiting, extreme thirst, delirium, convulsions, hyperthermia, vasomotor collapse. Serious toxicity can develop without earlier signs of toxicity. Toxicity is usually associated with parenteral administration but can be observed after oral administration, especially in children.

Drug Interactions

Interactant	Interaction
β-adrenergic blocking agents	↓ Effect of theophylline
Cimetidine	↑ Theophylline toxicity due to ↓ breakdown by liver
Digitalis	Theophylline ↑ toxicity of digitalis
Ephedrine and other sympathomimetics	↑ CNS stimulation
Erythromycin	↑ Effect of theophylline due to ↓ breakdown by liver
Furosemide	↑ Effect of theophylline
Halothane	↑ Risk of cardiac arrhythmias
Lithium	↓ Effect of lithium due to ↑ rate of excretion
Muscle relaxants, nondepolarizing	Theophylline ↓ effect of these drugs
Oral contraceptives	↑ Effect of theophyllines due to ↓ breakdown by liver
Phenytoin	↓ Effect of both drugs due to ↑ breakdown by liver
Reserpine	Concomitant use → tachycardia
Tobacco smoking	↓ Effect of theophylline due to ↑ breakdown by liver
Troleandomycin	↑ Effect of theophylline due to ↓ breakdown by liver
Verapamil	↑ Effect of theophyllines

Laboratory Test Interference   ↑ Plasma free fatty acids, bilirubin, urinary catecholamines, RBC sedimentation rate. Interference with uric acid tests and tests for furosemide, probenecid, theobromine, and phenylbutazone.

Dosage   See Table 25. Individualized. Initially, dosage should be adjusted according to plasma level of drug. Usual: 10–20 μg theophylline /ml plasma.

Administration   Diet influences the excretion of theophylline in that it is increased by a high protein and/or low carbohydrate diet and decreased by a low protein and/or high carbohydrate diet.

Nursing Implications

1. *Assess*
   a. closely for clinical response and signs of toxicity.
   b. that serum levels of theophylline are in the 10–20-μg/ml range. Levels above 20 μg/ml require dosage adjustments.
   c. small children particularly for excessive CNS stimulation, because they are unable to report side effects.
2. Dilute drugs properly and maintain proper infusion rates to minimize problems of overdosage. Preferably, use an infusion pump to regulate IV flow rate.

(continued on page 615)

TABLE 25 THEOPHYLLINE DERIVATIVES USED FOR ACUTE BRONCHOSPASMS

Drug	Dosage	Remarks
Aminophylline (Amoline, Corophylline,* Palaron,* Phyllocontin, Phyllocontin-350,* Somophyllin, Somophyllin-DF, Theophylline Ethylenediamine, Truphylline), Rx	**PO**: *Acute asthmatic attacks*, **adults**: 500 mg **STAT; pediatric**: 7.5 mg/kg **STAT. Maintenance, adults**: 200–315 mg q 6–8 hr; **pediatric**: 3–6 mg/kg q 6–8 hr. **Rectal solution, adults**: 300 mg 1 to 3 times/day or 450 mg b.i.d.; **pediatric**: 5 mg/kg no more than q 6 hr. **Rectal suppositories: Adults**: 500 mg 1–2 times/day not to exceed 1 gm/day; **pediatric**: 7 mg/kg. **IM**: 500 mg as required (painful). **IV**: Use only 25 mg/ml preparations. **Loading dose**: 6 mg/kg at a rate not to exceed 25 mg/min. **Maintenance**: Up to 0.9 mg/kg/hr by infusion.	Drug of choice when one cannot differentiate between bronchospasms and pulmonary edema. Contains 79–86% theophylline. *Administration* Dilute in 10–20 ml diluent and inject slowly over period of 5–10 min to avoid severe hypotension. *Additional Nursing Implications* See also *Nursing Implications*, p. 613 1. Monitor BP closely during IV administration because drug may cause a transitory lowering of BP that requires immediate dosage and flow rate adjustment. 2. Encourage administration by other than IM injection, because this route is painful.
Dyphylline (Asminyl, Dilin, Dilor, Dyflex, Dyflex-400, Dy-Phyllin, Lufyllin, Lufyllin-400, Oxystat, Neothylline, Protophylline*), Rx	**PO. Adults**: 15 mg/kg q.i.d.; **pediatric (PO only)**: 4.5–5.8 mg/kg b.i.d.–t.i.d. **IM. Adults**: 250–500 mg (injected slowly); dose should not exceed 15 mg/kg q 6 hr; **pediatric**: 4.4–6.6 mg/kg/day in divided doses.	**Not to be used IV**. *Additional Drug Interaction* Probenecid ↓excretion of dyphylline. Less irritating than theophylline or aminophylline. Equivalent to 70% theophylline. *Note*: Serum theophylline levels do not measure dyphylline.
Oxtriphylline (Apo-Oxtriphylline*, Choledyl, Choledyl SA, Choline Theophyllinate, Novotriphyl*), Rx	**PO. Adults**: 200 mg q.i.d.; **pediatric, 2–12 years**: 3.7 mg/kg q.i.d. **Sustained release**: 400–600 mg q 12 hr.	Choline salt of theophylline containing 64% theophylline. Less irritating than aminophylline. Preferentially give after meals and at bedtime.
Theophylline (*Immediate release*: Accurbron, Aerolate, Asmalix, Bronkodyl, Elixicon, Elixomin, Elixophyllin, Lanophyllin, Lixolin, PMS Theophylline,* Quibron-T, Slo-Phyllin, Somophyllin-T, Theoclear-80, Theolair, Theolixir, Theon, Theophyl, Theophyl-225, Theostat 80. *Timed Release*:	**PO. Adults**, 200–250 mg q 6 hr; **pediatric**: 100 mg q 6 hr. Timed release: Dosage depends on preparation.	

TABLE 25   *(Continued)*

Drug	Dosage	Remarks
Aerolate, Bronkodyl S–R, Constant–T, Dur-aphyl, Elixophyllin SR, LaBID, Lodrane, Quibron–T/SR, Respbid, Slo-bid, Slo-Phyllin, Somophyllin-12,* Somophyllin–CRT, Sustaire, Theo–24, Theobid, Theo-clear L.A., Theo–Dur, Theo–Dur Sprinkle, Theolair–SR, Theo-phyl–SR, Theophylline SR, Theospan–SR), Rx		
Theophylline sodium glycinate (Acet–Am,* Synophylate), Rx	**PO. Adults:** 330–660 mg q 6–8 hr after meals; **pediatric, under 6 years:** 55–165 mg q 6–8 hr after meals; **pediatric, 6–12 years:** 220–330 mg q 6–8 hr after meals.	Contains 44.5–47.3% theophyl-line.

3. Wait to initiate oral therapy at least 4 to 6 hours after switching from IV therapy.
4. Have available a respirator, oxygen, diazepam (Valium), and IV fluids for treatment of overdosage.
5. Teach patient and/or family, to notify doctor if nausea, vomiting, GI pain, or restlessness occur.

MISCELLANEOUS ANTIASTHMATICS

BITOLTEROL MESYLATE Tornalate Aerosol (Rx)

Classification   Bronchodilator.

Action/Kinetics   Bitolterol is considered a prodrug in that it is converted by esterases in the body to the active colterol. Colterol is said to combine with β-2 adrenergic receptors producing dilation of bronchioles. **Onset following inhalation:** 3–4 min. **Duration:** 6–7 hr.

Uses   Prophylaxis and treatment of bronchial asthma. May be used with theophylline and/or steroids.

Contraindications   Use with caution in ischemic heart disease, hypertension, hyperthyroidism, diabetes mellitus, cardiac arrhythmias, seizure disorders, or in those who respond unusually to β-adenergic agonists. Safety has not been established for use in pregnancy, lactation, and in children less than 12 years of age.

Untoward Reactions   *CNS:* Tremors, dizziness, lightheadedness, nervousness, headache, insomnia. *CV:* Palpitations, tachycardia, premature ventricular contractions, flushing. *Respiratory:* Cough, dyspnea, tightness in chest, bronchospasm. *Other:* Nausea, throat irritation.

Drug Interactions   Additive effects with other β-adrenergic bronchodilators.

Laboratory Test Interference   ↑ SGOT. ↓ Platelets, white blood cells. Proteinuria.

Dosage   **Inhalation: Adults and children over 12 years,** 2 inhalations at an interval of 1–3 minutes q 8 hr (if necessary, a third inhalation may be taken). The dose should not exceed 3 inhalations q 6 hr or 2 inhalations q 4 hr.

Administration

1. Bitolterol is available in a metered dose inhaler. With the inhaler in an upright position the patient should breathe out completely in a normal fashion. As the patient is breathing in slowly and deeply, the cannister and mouthpiece should be squeezed between the thumb and forefinger, which activates the medication. The breath should be held for 10 seconds and then slowly exhaled.
2. The medication should not be stored above 120° F.

CROMOLYN SODIUM   Intal, Nalcrom,* Nasalcrom, Opticrom,* Rynacrom* (Rx)

Classification   Respiratory inhalant for bronchial asthma.

Action/Kinetics   Cromolyn sodium appears to act locally on the lung mucosa, preventing the release of histamine and slow-reacting substance of anaphylaxis. The drug has no antihistaminic, anti-inflammatory, or bronchodilator effects and has no role in terminating an acute attack of asthma. After inhalation some of the drug is absorbed systemically. It is excreted about equally in urine and bile (feces). t½: 81 min; from lungs: 60 min.

When effective, cromolyn reduces the number of asthmatic attacks and the intensity of the disease. Improvement is usually seen within 4 weeks.

Uses   Prophylactic and adjunct in the management of severe bronchial asthma in selected patients. Prophylaxis of exercise-induced bronchospasms, allergic rhinitis. *Investigational*: Orally to treat food allergies.

Contraindications   Hypersensitivity. Children under 5 years of age. Safe use in pregnancy not established. Acute attacks and status asthmaticus. Use with caution for long periods of time or in the presence of renal or hepatic disease.

Untoward Reactions   *Respiratory:* Bronchospasm, cough, laryngeal edema (rare), eosinophilic pneumonia. *CNS:* Dizziness, drowsiness, headache. *Allergic:* Urticaria, rash, angioedema, serum sickness, anaphylaxis. *Other:* Nausea, urinary frequency, dysuria, joint swelling and pain, lacrimation, swollen parotid gland.

Following nebulization: Sneezing, wheezing, itching, nose bleeds, burning, nasal congestion. **Following nasal solution:** Burning, stinging, irritation of nose; sneezing, nose bleeds, headache, bad taste in mouth, postnasal drip.

Dosage   *Asthma.* **Capsules for nebulization: Adults and children over 5 years: initial,** 20 mg q.i.d. at regular intervals, **Solution for nebulization: Adults and**

children over 2 years: same dosage as capsules. *Prophylaxis of exercise-induced bronchospasm:* inhalation of 20 mg (1 capsule) 1 hr before exercise. *Rhinitis:* **Nasal solution: Adults and children over 6 years:** 1 spray in each nostril 3–6 times/day.

Administration/Storage

1. Institute only after acute episode is over when airway is clear and patient can inhale adequately.
2. Teach patient to use special inhaler and not to swallow capsule.
3. Corticosteroid dosage should be continued when initiating cromolyn therapy; however, if improvement occurs, the steroid dosage may be tapered slowly. Steroid therapy may have to be reinstituted if cromolyn inhalation is impaired, in times of stress, or in adrenocortical insufficiency.

Nursing Implications

Teach patient and/or family

a. to load capsule into inhaler.
b. to inhale fully and introduce mouthpiece between lips.
c. to tilt head back and inhale deeply and rapidly through inhaler to cause propeller to turn rapidly and supply more medication in one breath.
d. to remove inhaler, hold breath a few seconds, and exhale slowly.
e. to repeat procedure until powder is completely administered.
f. to not to wet powder with breath while exhaling.
g. to continue self-administration of medication as ordered, because it may take up to 4 weeks for frequency of asthmatic attacks to decrease.
h. to consult with medical supervision if he/she wishes to discontinue medication because discontinuation may precipitate an asthmatic attack, and concomitant corticosteroid therapy may require adjustment.

Chapter Fifty

ANTITUSSIVES, EXPECTORANTS, AND MUCOLYTICS

ANTITUSSIVES

General Statement   The cough is a useful protective reflex mechanism through which the body attempts to clear the respiratory tract of excess mucus or foreign particles. Coughing may accompany upper respiratory tract infections and as such will usually clear up by itself within a few days. It may also indicate an underlying organic disease whose cause should be ascertained.

There are two common types of cough: productive (cough accompanied by expectoration of mucus and phlegm) and nonproductive (dry cough). When a cough becomes excessive and interferes with normal activities or sleep, it should be treated symptomatically.

Antitussive agents can be divided into narcotic and nonnarcotic products. Such agents depress a cough either by depressing the activity of the cough center in the brain or by a local action.

NARCOTIC ANTITUSSIVE

CODEINE

See *Narcotic Analgesics,* p. 478.

NONNARCOTIC ANTITUSSIVES

General Statement The drugs belonging to this category depress the cough reflex by a variety of mechanisms. All of them are more effective in the treatment of nonproductive cough than in cough associated with copious sputum. Many of the agents have local anesthetic properties. Unlike narcotics, they do not produce dependence.

Contraindication Antitussive medication should be avoided during the first trimester of pregnancy unless otherwise decided by a physician.

Nursing Implications

1. Report if the patient continues to sound congested or is unable to bring up secretions.
2. Provide supportive nursing care measures, such as offering and encouraging increased fluid intake, positioning the patient in a sitting position, splinting an incision during coughing, and providing soothing warm liquids to reduce mucosal irritation.
3. *Teach patient and/or family*
   a. to take antitussive as prescribed and to discard remaining medication after course of therapy because medication for cough should be taken under medical supervision.
   b. when a woman is of childbearing age, that antitussives are, for the most part, contraindicated in pregnancy.
   c. not to eat or drink fluids for at least 15 minutes after taking a cough syrup that has a demulcent effect.

BENZONATATE Tessalon (Rx)

Classification Nonnarcotic antitussive.

Action/Kinetics Antitussive action is due to local anesthetic effect on stretch receptors in respiratory tract thus depressing cough reflex at its source. It is as effective as codeine. **Onset:** 30 min. **Duration:** 2–8 hr.

Uses Respiratory conditions including pneumonia and bronchitis; chronic conditions including emphysema, tuberculosis, and pulmonary tumors; bronchial asthma. Adjunct in surgery when cough should be suppressed. Nonproductive cough.

Contraindications Use with caution in pregnancy and lactation.

Untoward Reactions *GI:* Nausea, gastric upset, constipation. *CNS:* Drowsiness, dizziness, headache. *Other:* Skin rash, pruritus, nasal congestion, chills, burning of the eyes, hypersensitivity.

Dosage **PO. Adults and children over 10:** 100 mg t.i.d. up to maximum of 600 mg/day.

Administration/ Storage Swallow perles without chewing to avoid local anesthetic effect on oral mucosa.

DEXTROMETHORPHAN HYDROBROMIDE Balminil D.M. Syrup,* Benylin DM, Broncho-Grippol-DM,* Congespirin For Children, Cremacoat 1, Delsym, DM Cough, DM Syrup,* Extend 12, Hold, Koffex,* Mediquell, Neo-DM,* Pedia Care 1, Pertussin 8 Hour, Robidex,* Romilar CF, Romilar Children's, St. Joseph For Children, Sedatuss,* Sucrets Cough Control Formula (OTC)

Classification Nonnarcotic antitussive.

Action/Kinetics Dextromethorphan selectively depresses the cough center in the medulla and its antitussive activity is about equal to that of codeine. It is a common ingredient of nonprescription cough medications; does not produce physical dependence or respiratory depression. Well absorbed from GI tract. **Onset:** 15–30 min. **Duration:** 3–6 hr.

Use Symptomatic relief of nonproductive chronic cough.

Contraindications Persistent or chronic cough. Use with caution in patients with nausea, vomiting, high fever, rash, or persistent headache.

Drug Interaction Contraindicated with monoamine oxidase inhibitors.

Dosage Syrup, lozenges. **Adults and children over 12:** 10–30 mg q 4–8 hr not to exceed 60–120 mg/day; **pediatric, 6–12 years:** either 5–10 mg q 4 hr or 15 mg q 6–8 hr, not to exceed 40–60 mg/day; **pediatric, 2–6 years:** either 2.5–5 mg q 4 hr or 7.5 mg q 6–8 hr not to exceed 30 mg/day. **Controlled release liquid. Adults:** 60 mg b.i.d.; **pediatric, 6–12 years:** 30 mg b.i.d.; **pediatric, 2–5 years:** 15 mg b.i.d.

Administration Increasing the dose of dextromethorphan will not increase the effectiveness but will increase the duration of action.

DIPHENHYDRAMINE HCl Benylin Cough, Diphen, Noradryl Cough, Tusstat, Valdrene (Rx)

See *Antihistamines,* p. 629

Dosage **PO. Adults: 25 mg q 4 hr, not to exceed 100 mg/day; pediatric, 6–12 years:** 12.5 mg q. 4 hr, not to exceed 50 mg/day; **pediatric, 2–6 years:** 6.25 mg q 4 hr, not to exceed 25 mg/day.

EXPECTORANTS

GUAIFENESIN (GLYCERYL GUAIACOLATE) 2G, Anti-Tuss, Balminil Expectorant,* Baytussin, Breonesin, Colrex Expectorant, Cremacoat 2 Liquid, Gee-Gee, Gg-CEN, Glyate, Glycotuss, Glytuss, Guiamid, Halotussin, Hytuss, Hytuss-2X, Malotuss, Neo-Spec,* Nortussin, Peedee Dose Expectorant, Resyl,* Robafet, Robitussin, S-T Expectorant SF & DF (OTC)

Classification Expectorant.

Action/Kinetics Guaifenesin increases the fluid of the respiratory tract. This reduces the viscosity of respiratory secretions and facilitates their expectoration. Data for efficacy are lacking; however, guaifenesin is an ingredient of many nonprescription cough preparations.

Uses   To loosen and expel accumulated mucus in the respiratory tract. Dry, non-productive cough.

Note: Also found in Chlor-Trimeton Expectorant. See Appendix 3, p. 899.

Contraindications   Chronic cough, cough accompanied by excess secretions.

Untoward Reactions   *GI:* Nausea, vomiting, GI upset. *CNS:* drowsiness.

Drug Interaction   Inhibition of platelet adhesiveness by guaifenesin may result in bleeding tendencies.

Dosage   PO. Adults and children over 12 years: 100–400 mg q 4–6 hr, not to exceed 2.4 gm/day; **pediatric, 6–12 years:** 50–100 mg q 4–6 hr, not to exceed 600 mg/day; **pediatric, 2–6 years:** 50 mg q 4 hr, not to exceed 300 mg/day.

TERPIN HYDRATE ELIXIR   (OTC)

TERPIN HYDRATE AND CODEINE ELIXIR   (Rx or OTC)

Classification   Expectorant.

General Statement   Terpin hydrate is alleged to increase respiratory tract fluid secretion, liquefy sputum, and facilitate expectoration; however, the recommended doses probably do not cause this effect. Terpin hydrate is often combined with codeine, a narcotic, which specifically depresses the cough reflex. Terpin hydrate elixir contains 43% alcohol, while terpin hydrate and codeine elixir contains 40% alcohol, 85 mg terpin hydrate, and 10 mg codeine per 5 ml and is subject to federal narcotic regulations.

Use   Symptomatic treatment of cough.

Contraindications   Peptic ulcer and severe diabetes mellitus. Use in children. See also *Codeine*, p. 478.

Untoward Reactions   See *Codeine*, p. 478.

Dosage   *Terpin hydrate elixir*, **PO**: 5–10 ml every 3 to 4 hr as needed. *Terpin hydrate and codeine elixir*, **PO**: 5 ml 3 to 4 times daily.

> **Nursing Implications**
> Warn the patient that excessive use of drug may lead to oversedation and prolonged use may lead to dependence.

MUCOLYTICS

ACETYLCYSTEINE   Airbron,* Mucomyst (Rx)

Classification   Mucolytic.

General Statement   Acetylcysteine reduces the viscosity of purulent and nonpurulent pulmonary secretions by splitting disulfide bonds.This permits expectoration, or removal by mechanical means. Action increases with increasing pH (peak: pH 7–9).

Uses   Adjunct in the treatment of acute and chronic bronchitis, emphysema, tuberculosis, pneumonia, bronchiectasis, atelectasis. Routine care of patients with tracheostomy, pulmonary complications after thoracic or cardiovascular surgery, or in post-traumatic chest conditions. Pulmonary complications of cystic fibrosis. Diagnostic bronchial studies. *Investigational:* Antidote in acetaminophen poisoning to reduce hepatotoxicity, as an ophthalmic solution for dry eye.

Contraindications Sensitivity to drug. Use with caution in patients with asthma and in the elderly.

Untoward Reactions *Respiratory:* Acetylcysteine increases the incidence of bronchospasm in patients with asthma. The drug may also increase the amount of liquefied bronchial secretions, which must be removed by suction if cough is inadequate. Bronchial and tracheal irritation, tightness in chest, bronchoconstriction . *GI:* Nausea, vomiting, stomatitis. *Other:* Rashes, fever, drowsiness, rhinorrhea.

Drug Interactions Acetylcysteine is incompatible with antibiotics and should be administered separately.

Dosage Administer 10% or 20% solution by nebulization, direct application, or direct intratracheal instillation.
Nebulization into face mask: 1–10 ml of 20% solution or 2–10 ml of 10% solution 3 to 4 times daily. *Closed tent or croupette*: 300 ml of 10% or 20% solution per treatment. *Direct instillation into tracheostomy*: 1–2 ml of 10–20% solution every 1 to 4 hr. *Percutaneous intratracheal catheter:* 1–2 ml of 20% solution or 2–4 ml of 10% solution q 1–4 hr by syringe attached to catheter. *Diagnostic procedures*: 2 to 3 doses of 1–2 ml of 20% or 2–4 ml of 10% solution by nebulization or intratracheal instillation. *Acetaminophen overdosage:* **PO, initial,** 140 mg/kg; **then,** 70 mg/kg q 4 hr for a total of 17 doses.

Administration/ Storage
1. Use nonreactive plastic, glass, or stainless steel equipment for administration.
2. Administer via face mask, face tent, oxygen tent, head tent, or by positive pressure breathing machine as indicated.
3. Administer with compressed air for nebulization. Hand nebulizers are contraindicated.
4. After prolonged nebulization, dilute the last fourth of the medication with sterile water for injection to prevent concentration of medication.
5. Note that the solution may develop a light purple color which does not affect the action of the medication.
6. Closed bottles are stable for 2 years when stored at 20°C. Open bottles should be stored at 2°–8°C and should be used within 96 hours.

Nursing Implications
1. Assess asthmatic patient particularly for onset of bronchial spasm demonstrated by wheezing and increased congestion.
2. Have available bronchodilators such as isoproterenol for aerosol inhalation should bronchospasm occur.
3. Provide mechanical suction to remove secretions if patient is unable to cough up secretions and have endotracheal tube available.
4. Advise the patient that the nauseous odor that may be perceived on the initiation of treatment will soon not be noticeable.
5. Wash the patient's face after nebulization, as medication may cause stickiness.

Chapter Fifty-one

HISTAMINE AND ANTIHISTAMINES

HISTAMINE

General Statement Histamine is stored in almost every type of tissue in the body; to date, however, the pharmacologic importance of histamine rests primarily on the suppression of its action by various histamine receptor blockers (antihistamines). Appropriate stimuli, including tissue injury, antigen–antibody (allergic) reactions, and extreme cold trigger the release of histamine from its storage sites into the vascular system, where it induces the following responses.

1. Dilation and increased permeability of the small arterioles, capillaries, and precapillaries, which result in increased permeability to fluid. This causes a fall of blood pressure in humans. The outflow of fluid into the subcutaneous spaces results in edema. The local edema in the nasal mucosa caused by histamine is responsible for the nasal congestion associated with allergies. It may also cause laryngeal edema.
2. Contraction of some smooth muscles such as those in the bronchioles; the resulting bronchoconstriction is believed to account for the role histamine plays in bronchial asthma. Histamine also causes the uterus to contract.
3. Stimulation of acid secretion in the stomach. It is used diagnostically to stimulate the gastric glands to test gastric function. It also increases bronchial, intestinal, and mild salivary secretions.
4. Dilation of cerebral vessels, and small doses can cause an intense headache.
5. Pain and itch, because it stimulates the sensory nerve endings.

Action   Upon release, histamine interacts with specific histamine receptors currently subdivided into H_1 receptors and H_2 receptors. Bronchoconstriction and intestinal motility are controlled by H_1 receptors, whereas gastric secretion involves H_2 receptors. Other processes in which histamine has a role, such as hypotension resulting from vascular dilation, involve both H_1 and H_2 receptors. *Histamine phosphate* is used for the diagnosis of pheochromocytoma and achlorhydria.

ANTIHISTAMINES (H_1 BLOCKERS)

Action/Kinetics   The effects of histamine may be reversed either by drugs that block histamine receptors (antihistamines) or by drugs that have effects opposite to histamine (i.e., epinephrine). Antihistamines used for the treatment of allergic conditions are referred to as H_1-receptor blockers while antihistamines used for the treatment of GI disorders (e.g., peptic ulcer) are referred to as H_2-receptor blockers (see Chapter 53).

Antihistamines do not prevent the release of histamine; rather, they compete with histamine for histamine receptors (competitive inhibition) thus preventing or reversing the effects of histamine. Antihistamines prevent or reduce increased capillary permeability (i.e., decrease edema, itching) and bronchospasms. Allergic reactions unrelated to histamine release are not affected by antihistamines.

The H_1-blockers manifest varying degrees of CNS depression, anticholinergic, antiemetic, and antiserotonin effects.

From a chemical point of view the antihistamines can be divided into the following five classes.

1. **Ethylenediamine Derivatives.** This group manifests weak sedative effects and almost no anticholinergic or antiemetic activity. They frequently cause GI distress. Available agents: Pyrilamine, Tripelennamine.
2. **Ethanolamine Derivatives.** Group most likely to cause CNS depression (drowsiness). Low incidence of GI side effects. Significant anticholinergic and antiemetic effects. Available agents: Carbinoxamine, Clemastine, Diphenhydramine.
3. **Alkylamines.** Members of this group are among the most potent antihistamines. They are effective at relatively low dosage and are most suitable agents for daytime use. This group manifests minimal sedation, moderate anticholinergic effects, and no antiemetic effects. Paradoxical excitation may also occur. Individual response to agents is variable. Available agents: Brompheniramine, Chlorpheniramine, Dexchlorpheniramine, Triprolidine.
4. **Phenothiazines** (see also *Phenothiazines,* Chapter 32). The agents used possess significant antihistaminic action, varying degrees of sedation, and a high degree of both anticholinergic and antiemetic effects. Available agents: Methdilazine, Promethazine, Trimeprazine.
5. **Piperidines.** Members of this group have prolonged antihistaminic activity, with a comparatively low incidence of drowsiness, moderate anticholinergic activity, and no antiemetic effects. Available agents: Azatadine, Cyproheptadine, Diphenylpyraline, Phenindamine.

The kinetics of most antihistamines is similar. **Onset:** 30–60 min; **peak: 1–2 hr; duration:** 4–6 hr (piperidines have a longer duration). Many antihistamines are available as timed-release preparations. Most antihistamines are metabolized by the liver and excreted in the urine.

Uses   Symptomatic relief of allergic symptoms caused by histamine release including urticaria, angioedema, dermatographism, anaphylaxis (used as adjunct), and blood or plasma reactions. Also, reactions due to drug-induced skin reactions, atopic dermatitis, contact dermatitis, pruritus ani, vulvae, and insect bites (topical products may also be used for these conditions). Nasal congestion accompanying allergic rhinitis, hay fever, and the common cold.

The CNS-depressant and anticholinergic effects of certain of the drugs has proven helpful in the treatment of parkinsonism and drug-induced extrapyramidal reactions. They decrease rigidity and improve speech and voluntary movements.

Certain antihistamines have been used as antimotion drugs and as nighttime sleep aids.

Contraindications   Hypersensitivity to the drug, narrow-angle glaucoma, prostatic hypertrophy, stenosing peptic ulcer, and pyloroduodenal or bladder neck obstruction.

Pregnancy, or possibility thereof (some agents), lactation, premature and newborn infants. Administer with caution to patients with convulsive disorders, in geriatric patients, in respiratory disease, and in infants and children (may cause hallucinations, convulsions, and death).

The phenothiazine-type antihistamines are contraindicated in CNS depression from any cause, bone marrow depression, jaundice, dehydrated or acutely ill children, and in comatose patients.

Untoward Reactions   *CNS*: Sedation ranging from mild drowsiness to deep sleep. Dizziness, lassitude, disturbed coordination, muscular weakness. Paradoxical excitation (especially in children) including: restlessness, insomnia, tremors, euphoria, nervousness, delirium, palpitations, and even convulsions. Antihistamines can precipitate epileptiform seizures in patients with focal lesions. *GI*: Epigastric distress, dryness of mouth, anorexia or increased appetite, nausea, vomiting, and diarrhea or constipation. *CV:* Palpitations, increased heart rate, hypotension, extrasystoles. *GU:* Urinary frequency, retention, or difficulty. Impotence, decreased libido, menstrual irregularities. *Respiratory:* Dryness of nose, mouth, throat; nasal stuffiness, respiratory depression, wheezing and tightness of chest. *Hematologic:* Anemias (hemolytic, hypoplastic), leukopenia, pancytopenia, agranulocytosis, thrombocytopenia. *Allergic:* Anaphylaxis, rash, photosensitivity, urticaria. *Miscellaneous:* Hands become heavy and weak, tingling, excess sweating, chills.

Topical use: Prolonged use may result in local irritation and allergic contact dermatitis.

Acute Toxicity   Antihistamines have a wide therapeutic range. Overdosage can nevertheless be fatal. Children are particularly susceptible. Overdosage can cause both CNS overstimulation and depression. The overstimulation is characterized by hallucinations, incoordination, and tonic–clonic convulsions. Fixed, dilated pupils, flushing, and fever are common in children. Cerebral edema, deepening coma, and respiratory collapse occur usually within 2 to 18 hours.

Overdosage in adults usually starts with severe CNS depression. Treatment of overdosage is symptomatic and supportive. Induction of vomiting with syrup of ipecac (do not use for phenothiazine overdosage) followed by activated charcoal and a cathartic. If vomiting has not been induced within 3 hours of ingestion, gastric lavage can be undertaken. Hypotension can be treated with a vasopressor such as norepinephrine, dopamine, or phenylephrine (do not use epinephrine). For convulsions, IV phenytoin is indicated; **do not use CNS depressants, including diazepam.**

Drug Interactions

Interactant	Interaction
Alcohol, ethyl	See *CNS depressants*
Antidepressants, tricyclic	Additive anticholinergic side effects
CNS depressants	Potentiation or addition of CNS depressant effects.
Antianxiety agents	Concomitant use may lead to drowsiness, leth-

Interactant	Interaction
Barbiturates	argy, stupor, respiratory depression, coma, and possibly death
Narcotics	
Phenothiazines	
Sedative-hypnotics	
MAO inhibitors	Intensification and prolongation of anticholinergic side effects.

Note: Also see Drug Interactions for phenothiazines, p. 402.

Laboratory Test Interference Discontinue antihistamines 4 days before skin testing to avoid false negatives.

Dosage **Usually PO.** See Table 26, p. 627. Parenteral administration is seldom used because of irritating nature of drugs.

Topical usage is also limited because antihistamines often cause hypersensitivity reactions. When given for motion sickness, antihistamines are usually given 30 to 60 minutes before anticipated travel.

Administration

1. Inject IM preparations deep into the muscle because preparations tend to be irritating to tissue.
2. Decrease GI side effects by administering with meals or with milk.
3. Topical preparations should not be applied to raw, blistered, or oozing areas of the skin, around the genitalia, eyes, or mucous membranes.

Nursing Implications

1. Use side rails for patients sedated with antihistamines.
2. Assist patients experiencing dizziness, lassitude, or weakness.
3. *Teach patient and/or family*
   a. caution against driving a car or operating other machinery until response to medication (drowsiness) has worn off. Sedative effect may disappear spontaneously after several days' administration.
   b. to report side effects to physician, who may change dose or order another antihistamine, which may have less side effects for this particular patient. The patient should not discontinue medication without consulting physician.
   c. to consult with physician before taking any depressants because antihistamines tend to potentiate other CNS depressants.
   d. to store antihistamines out of the reach of children, because large doses may be fatal.

TABLE 26 ANTIHISTAMINES

Drug	Type[a]	Dosage	Remarks
Azatadine maleate (Optimine), Rx	5	**PO:** 1–2 mg b.i.d. Use lower dosage in elderly.	Has prolonged action. Used for allergic rhinitis and chronic urticaria. Should not be used in children under 12 years of age.
Brompheniramine maleate (Bromphen, Brombay, Codimal–A, Diamine, Dimetane, Dimetane–Ten, Veltane), Rx (Dimetane and Dimetane Extend tabs are OTC)	3	**PO. Adults and children over 12:** 4 mg q 4–6 hr, or 8–12 mg sustained release b.i.d.–t.i.d. not to exceed 24 mg/day. **Pediatric, 6–12 years:** 2 mg q 4–6 hr or 8–12 mg sustained release q 12 hr; **2–6 years:** 1 mg q 4–6 hr not to exceed 6 mg/day. **IM, IV, SC. Adults: usual,** 10 mg (range 5–20 mg) b.i.d (maximum daily dose: 40 mg); **pediatric, under 12 years:** 0.5 mg/kg/day divided in 3 to 4 doses.	Can be given parenterally. Causes mild drowsiness. Do not use solution containing preservatives for IV injection. Also found in Dimetane Expectorant and Dimetapp (Appendix 3).
Buclizine Hydrochloride (Bucladin–S Softabs), Rx		**PO. Adults: usual,** 50 mg b.i.d.–t.i.d. with first dose 30 min before travel.	Used for motion sickness. Tablets may be placed in the mouth to dissolve, be chewed, or swallowed whole.
Carbinoxamine maleate (Clistin), Rx	2	**PO. Adults:** 4–8 mg t.i.d.–q.i.d **Pediatric: 1–3 years,** 2 mg t.i.d.–q.i.d.; **3–6 years:** 2–4 mg t.i.d.–q.i.d.: **over 6 years:** 4–6 mg t.i.d.–q.i.d.	Low incidence of side effects; drowsiness. The drug can be administered parenterally as prophylaxis to drug reactions or blood transfusion. Only preparation *without* preservative may be given IV. If drugs are compatible, chlorpheniramine may be administered in same syringe. Chlorpheniramine for injection *without* preservative may be added directly to blood transfusion. Not recommended for children under 6 years of age. Also found in Naldecon, Ornade, and Tuss–Ornade. See Appendix 3.
Chlorpheniramine maleate (Alermine, Aller–Chlor, Allerid–O.D.–8 and –12, Chlor–100, Chlo–Amine, Chlorate, Chlor–Niramine, Chlorphen,* Chlor–Pro, Chlorspan–12, Chlortab 4 and 8, Chlor–Trimeton, Hal–Chlor, Histrey, Novopheniram,* Phenetron, T.D. Alermine, Telachlor S.R., Teldrin), OTC and Rx	3	**PO. Adults and children over 12:** 4 mg q 4–6 hr or 8–12 mg sustained release q 8–12 hr or at bedtime not to exceed 24 mg/day. **Pediatric, 6–12 years:** 2 mg q 4–6 hr not to exceed 112 mg/day. **Do not use sustained release in children. IM, IV, SC.** *Allergic reactions to blood or plasma:* 10–20 mg as single dose up to 40 mg/day. *Other allergic reactions:* 5–20 mg as single dose. *Anaphylaxis:* **IV,** 10–20 mg as a single dose.	Low incidence of side effects; drowsiness. The drug can be administered parenterally as prophylaxis to drug reactions or blood transfusion. Only preparation *without* preservative may be given IV. If drugs are compatible, chlorpheniramine may be administered in same syringe. Chlorpheniramine for injection *without* preservative may be added directly to blood transfusion. Not recommended for children under 6 years of age. Also found in Naldecon, Ornade, and Tuss–Ornade. See Appendix 3.

627

TABLE 26 *(Continued)*

Drug	Type[a]	Dosage	Remarks
Clemastine fumarate (Tavist, Tavist 1), Rx	2	**PO. Adults and children over 12 years:** 1.34 mg b.i.d. to 2.68 mg t.i.d. not to exceed 8.04 mg daily. *Dermatoses:* Use 2.68 mg tablet only.	Do not use in children under 12 years of age. Frequently causes drowsiness.
Cyclizine hydrochloride (Marezine), OTC / Cyclizine lactate (Marezine), Rx	5	**PO:** 50 mg t.i.d.–q.i.d. up to maximum of 200 mg daily; **pediatric 6–12 years:** ½ adult dose (24 hr). **IM:** 50 mg t.i.d.–q.i.d. or as required	Contraindicated in pregnancy. Used widely as an antiemetic and for vertigo.
Cyproheptadine hydrochloride (Vimicon*, Periactin), Rx	5	**PO:** 4–20 mg daily. Not to exceed 0.5 mg/kg daily; **pediatric (use for maximum of 6 months) 2–6 years:** 2 mg t.i.d. not to exceed 12 mg daily; **6-14 years:** 4 mg t.i.d. Not to exceed 16 mg daily.	Contraindicated in glaucoma and urinary retention. Also used for treatment of pruritic dermatoses, angioedema, cluster headaches, and as an appetite stimulant in under-weight patients in anorexia nervosa.
Dexchlorpheniramine maleate (Dexchlor, Poladex–T.D., Polaramine), Rx	3	**PO: Adults:** 2 mg q 4–6 hr or 4–6 mg sustained release q 8–10 hr and at bedtime. **Pediatric, 6–11 years:** 1 mg q 4–6 hr or 4 mg sustained release once daily (usually at bedtime); **2–5 years:** 0.5 mg q 4–6 hr. **Do not use sustained release form.**	May cause mild drowsiness.
Dimenhydrinate (Apo–Dimenhydrinate,* Calm X, Dimentabs, Dinate, Dommanate, Dramamine, Dramaban, Dramamine, Dramilin, Dramocen, Dramoject, Dymenate, Gravol,* Marmine, Motion–Aid, Nauseatol,* Novodimenate,* PMS–Dimenhydrinate,* Travamine,* Wehamine), OTC and Rx	2	**PO. Adults:** 50–100 mg q 4–6 hr not to exceed 400 mg/day. **Pediatric, 6–12 years:** 25–50 mg q 6–8 hr not to exceed 150 mg/day; **2–6 years:** Up to 25 mg q 6–8 hr not to exceed 75 mg/day. **IM. Adults:** 50 mg. **IV. Adults:** 50 mg in 10 mg sodium chloride injection given over 2 min. **Pediatric, under 2 years, IM:** 1.25 mg/kg q.i.d. not to exceed 300 mg/day.	Contains diphenhydramine and chlorotheophylline. Widely used against motion sickness; may cause drowsiness. May mask ototoxicity due to aminoglycoside antibiotics (Gentamicin, Kanamycin, Neomycin, Streptomycin)
Diphenhydramine hydrochloride (Allerdyl,* Bay Dryl, Belix, Bena–D	2	**PO: Adults,** 25–50 mg t.i.d.–q.i.d.; **pediatric, over 20 lb:** 12.5–25 mg	Also used for motion sickness, antiemetic, as a sleep-aid, for parkinson-

Drug		Dosage	Remarks
and –D 50, Benadryl, Benahist 10 and 50, Benaphen, Bendylate, Benaject–10 and –50, Fenylhist, Fynex Cough, Hydril Cough, Hyrexin–50, Noradryl, Tusstat, Valdrene, Wehdryl–50), Rx		t.i.d.–q.i.d. (or 5 mg/kg/day not to exceed 300 mg daily). *Sleep aid:* **Adults,** 50 mg at bedtime. **IV, deep IM: Adults,** 10–50 mg up to 100 mg (not to exceed 400 mg daily); **pediatric:** 5 mg/kg/day not to exceed 300 mg daily.	ism, in geriatric patients unable to tolerate more potent drugs. For motion sickness, the full prophylactic dose should be given 30 min prior to travel with similar doses with meals and at bedtime.
Diphenylpyraline hydrochloride (Hispril), Rx	5	**PO. Adults,** 5 mg q 12 hr. **Pediatric, 6–12 years:** 5 mg/day. **Not for children under 6 years.**	Low incidence of side effects: drowsiness, headaches, dizziness, dry mouth.
Meclizine hydrochloride (Antivert, Antivert/25, Bonine, Dizmiss, Motion Cure, Wehvert), OTC and Rx	5	**PO.** *Motion sickness:* 25–50 mg 1 hr before travel. *Vertigo:* 25–100 mg daily in divided doses.	Mostly used for motion sickness or vertigo. May cause drowsiness, dry mouth, blurred vision.
Methdilazine hydrochloride (Dilosyn,* Tacaryl), Rx	4	**PO. Adults:** 8 mg b.i.d.–q.i.d.; **pediatric, over 3 years:** 4 mg b.i.d.–q.i.d.	Indicated for allergic and nonallergic pruritus. Tablet must be chewed properly. May cause drowsiness. See also *Phenothiazines.*
Phenindamine tartrate (Nolahist), OTC	5	**PO. Adults:** 25 mg q 4–6 hr not to exceed 150 mg/day. **Pediatric, 6–12 years:** 12.5 mg q 4–6 hr not to exceed 75 mg/day.	For children under 6 years, physician should be consulted.
Promethazine hydrochloride (Anergan 25 and 50, Baymeth, Baymethazine, Ganphen, Histanil,* K–Phen, Mallergan, Pentazine, Phenameth, Phenazine 25 and 50, Phencen–50, Phenergan, Phenoject–50, PMS Promethazine,* Prometh 25 and 50, Prorex–25 and –50, Prothazine, Provigan, V–Gan–25 and –50), Rx	4	**PO, Rectal.** *Allergy:* **Adults,** 25 mg at bedtime or 12.5 mg before meals and at bedtime; **pediatric:** 25 mg at bedtime or 6.25–12.5 mg t.i.d. *Motion sickness:* **Adults,** 25 mg b.i.d. with 1st dose 30–60 min before travel; **pediatric:** 12.5–25 mg b.i.d. *Preoperatively on night before surgery:* **Adults,** 50 mg; **pediatric:** 12.5–25 mg. Given in combination with meperidine and an anticholinergic. *Sedation including postoperatively or as adjunct to analgesics:* **Adults:** 25–50 mg; **pediatric:** 12.5–25 mg. **IM (usual), IV.** *Allergy:* 25 mg repeated in 2 hr, if necessary. *Nausea/vomiting:* 12.5–25 mg repeated q 4 hr or longer. *Pre- and postoperatively:* **Adults,** 25–50 mg combined with analgesic	Very potent antihistamine with prolonged action. Also used as sedative and for motion sickness. Severe drowsiness. See also *Phenothiazines.* Because of high incidence of side effects, use cautiously in ambulatory patients. If used IV, the concentration should be 25 mg/ml or less with a rate not to exceed 25 mg/minute. Also found in Phenergan Expectorant and Synalgos DC(see Appendix 3).

TABLE 26 *(Continued)*

Drug	Type[a]	Dosage	Remarks
		and anticholinergic; **pediatric**, under 12 years: 1 mg/kg. *Nighttime sedation*: **Adults**, 25–50 mg. *Labor*: 50 mg in early labor with 25–75 mg given with a narcotic when labor is established, up to 100 mg/day.	
Pyrilamine maleate	1	**PO. Adults:** 25–50 mg t.i.d.	
Terfenadine (Seldane), Rx	5	**PO. Adults and children over 12 years:** 60 mg b.i.d.	Is said to manifest significantly less drowsiness than other antihistamines. Safety and effectiveness in children less than 12 years of age have not been established.
Trimeprazine tartrate (Panectyl,* Temaril), Rx	4	**PO. Adults:** 2.5 mg q.i.d. or 5 mg sustained release q 12 hr. **Pediatric, 6 months to 3 years:** 1.25 mg t.i.d. or at bedtime (use syrup); **over 3 years:** 2.5 mg t.i.d. or at bedtime; **over 6 years:** 5 mg/day of sustained release.	Symptomatic relief of acute and chronic pruritus. Also see *Phenothiazines*. May cause drowsiness (decreasing with usage), dizziness, dry mouth.
Tripelennamine hydrochloride (PBZ, PBZ-SR, Pelamine), Rx	1	**PO. Adults: usual,** 25–50 mg q 4–6 hr or 100 mg b.i.d.–t.i.d. of sustained release; **pediatric:** 5 mg/kg/day divided into 4 to 6 doses up to maximum of 300 mg/day. Do not use sustained release form in children.	Low incidence of side effects: moderate sedation, mild GI distress, paradoxical excitation, hyperirritability.
Triprolidine hydrochloride (Actidil, Bayidyl), OTC and Rx	3	**PO. Adults:** 2.5 mg t.i.d.–q.i.d. **Pediatric: 4 months to 2 years:** 0.3 mg t.i.d.–q.i.d; **2–4 years:** 0.6 mg t.i.d.–q.i.d.; **4–6 years:** 0.9 mg t.i.d.–q.i.d.; **6 to 12 years:** ½ adult dose. Use syrup only up to 6 years of age.	Rapid onset; low incidence of side effects. May cause drowsiness, dizziness, GI distress, paradoxical excitation, hyperirritability. Also found in Actifed and Actifed-C (see Appendix 3).

[a]Type 1: Ethylenediamine derivatives. Type 2: Ethanolamine derivatives. Type 3: Alkylamines. Type 4: Phenothiazines. Type 5: Piperidines.

Chapter Fifty-two

ANTACIDS

General Statement   Hydrochloric acid maintains the stomach at a pH (1–2) necessary for optimum activity of the digestive enzyme pepsin. Under certain circumstances, however, people suffer adverse reactions due to gastric acid ranging from heartburn to life-threatening peptic or duodenal ulcers. It is believed that peptic ulcers are caused by a decrease in the resistance of stomach tissue to hydrochloric acid, whereas duodenal ulcers are associated with an increase in the secretion of acid by the parietal cells. Acute and chronic GI disturbances are among the most common medical conditions requiring treatment.

Various drugs and dietary measures are used for the treatment of hyperacidity states and ulcers, and use of antacids is an important part of such regimens.

Action/Kinetics   Antacids act by neutralizing or reducing gastric acidity thus increasing the pH of the stomach. If the pH is increased to 4, the activity of pepsin is inhibited. The ability of a specific antacid to neutralize acid is termed *acid neutralizing capacity* and antacids are selected on this basis. Ideally, antacids should not be absorbed systemically although substances such as sodium bicarbonate or calcium carbonate may produce significant systemic effects. The most effective dosage form for antacids is suspensions. Antacids also promote healing of peptic ulcer.

Antacids containing magnesium have a laxative effect while those containing aluminum or calcium have a constipating effect. This is why patients are often given alternating doses of laxative and constipating antacids. **Duration of antacids:** 30 min, if fasting; up to 3 hr if taken after meals.

Uses   Peptic ulcer, hyperacidity conditions, hiatal hernia, esophagitis, gastritis.

Drug Interactions

Interactant	Interaction
Amphetamine	Systemic antacids ↓ excretion → ↑ effect
Anticholinergics	↓ Effect of anticholinergic due to ↓ absorption
Indomethacin	↓ Effect of indomethacin due to ↓ absorption
Iron, oral	↓ Effect of iron due to ↓ absorption
Phenothiazines	↓ Effect of phenothiazines due to ↓ absorption
Quinidine	Systemic antacids ↓ excretion → ↑ effect
Salicylates	Systemic antacids ↑ excretion → ↓ effect
Tetracyclines	↓ Effect of tetracyclines due to ↓ absorption

Administration/Storage

1. Administer laxative or cathartic dose at bedtime as medication takes about 8 hours to be effective and the effect should not interfere with the patient's rest.
2. Tablets should be thoroughly chewed before swallowing and followed by a glass of milk or water.
3. The absorption of many drugs may be affected by antacids; thus, oral drugs should not be taken within 1–2 hours of antacid ingestion.
4. For active peptic ulcer disease, antacids should be given every hour for the first 2 weeks during waking hours.

Nursing Implications

1. *Assess*
   a. patient on antacid therapy for constipation if on medication containing calcium or aluminum. Encourage extra fluids unless contraindicated and consult with

physician when laxatives or enemas seem indicated.
  b. patient on antacid therapy for diarrhea if on medication containing magnesium. Report diarrhea to physician because change of medication or alternation with an aluminum- or calcium-containing antacid may be indicated.
2. Teach patient on antacid therapy to take medication with the amount of water or milk prescribed because liquid acts as a vehicle transporting the medication to the stomach where the action is desired.

ALUMINUM HYDROXIDE GEL   Alagel, Alternagel, Amphojel (OTC)

ALUMINUM HYDROXIDE GEL, DRIED   Alu-Cap, Alu-Tab, Amphojel Tablets, Dialume (OTC)

Classification   Antacid.

Action/Kinetics   Aluminum hydroxide is nonsystemic, has demulcent activity, and is constipating. Aluminum hydroxide and phosphorus form insoluble phosphates that are eliminated in the feces. This yields a relatively phosphorus-free urine and prevents phosphate stone formation in susceptible patients. Acid neutralizing capacity: 6.5–18 mEq/tablet, capsule, or 5 ml.

Uses   Adjunct in the treatment of gastric and duodenal ulcer. Hyperphosphatemia, chronic renal failure.

Contraindications   Sensitivity to aluminum. Peptic ulcer associated with pancreatic deficiency, diarrhea, or low-phosphorus diet. Aluminum hydroxide preparations contain sodium and thus should not be administered to patients on a low-sodium diet.

Untoward Reactions   Chronic use may lead to bone pain, muscle weakness, or malaise due to chronic phosphate deficiency and osteomalacia. Constipation, intestinal obstruction. Decreased absorption of fluoride.

Additional Drug Interactions   Aluminum hydroxide gel inhibits the absorption of barbiturates, digoxin, phenytoin, corticosteroids, quinidine, warfarin, and isoniazid, thereby decreasing their effect.

Dosage   *Suspension, tablets, capsules.* **Usual:** 600 mg 3–6 times/day after meals, between meals, and at bedtime.
   Hyperphosphatemia. **Children:** 50–150 mg/kg/day in divided doses q 4–6 hr; adjust dosage until normal serum phosphate levels achieved.

Administration
1. Administer gel in a one-half glass of water.
2. Teach the patient to chew tablets before swallowing them and to take them with milk or water.
3. For administration by stomach tube, dilute commercial solution 2 or 3 times with water. Administer this at a rate of 15–20 gtt/min. Total daily dose is approximately 1.5 liters of the diluted suspension.

Additional Nursing Implications

See also *Nursing Implications*, p. 632

1. Check that urine specimen is collected at least once a month to determine urinary phosphate when drug is given in management of phosphatic urinary calculi.
2. Check that patient is on a low-phosphorus diet of 1.3 gm of phosphorus, 700 mg of calcium, 13 gm of nitrogen, and 2,500 cal when patient is being treated for phosphatic urinary calculi.

ALUMINUM PHOSPHATE GEL   Phosphaljel (OTC)

Classification   Antacid.

Action/Kinetics   Aluminum phosphate has antacid, astringent, and demulcent properties similar to those of aluminum hydroxide gel but with only half the neutralizing power. The drug does not interfere with phosphate metabolism and is therefore preferred for patients who cannot maintain a high-phosphorus diet. Acid neutralizing capacity: 1.5 mEq/5 ml.

Note: See Aluminum hydroxide gel for uses, contraindications, untoward reactions, and additional drug interactions.

Dosage   PO: 15–30 ml undiluted q 2 hr between meals and at bedtime, alone or with milk or water.

BASIC ALUMINUM CARBONATE GEL   Basaljel (OTC)

Classification   Antacid.

Action/Kinetics   Acid neutralizing capacity: 11–14 mEq/capsule, tablet, or 5 ml.

Uses   Hyperacidity. With low phosphorus diet to prevent phosphate urinary stones by reducing urinary phosphate levels.

Note: See Aluminum hydroxide gel for contraindications, untoward reactions, and additional drug interactions.

Dosage   *Antacid:* 1–2 tablets or capsules or 1–2 teaspoons of suspension. *Extra strength suspension:* 1/2–1 teaspoon. *Urinary calculi:* 2–6 capsules or tablets or 1–2 tablespoons suspension 1 hr after meals and at bedtime. *Extra strength suspension:* 1–3 teaspoons.

Administration

1. Dilute liquid form in water or juice. Give after meals and at bedtime.
2. It may be necessary to give the antacid dose up to 12 times daily.

CALCIUM CARBONATE PRECIPITATED   Amitone, Alka-2, Chooz, Dicarbosil, Equilet, Mallamint, Tums, Tums E-X (OTC)

Classification   Antacid.

Remarks Nonsystemic antacid regarded by some as the antacid of choice. Since calcium carbonate is constipating, it is often alternated or even mixed with magnesium salts. Acid neutralizing capacity: 8.25–10 mEq/tablet.

Action/Kinetics Excellent acid-neutralizing capacity (8.25–10 mEq/tablet) although chronic use may lead to systemic effects. Rapid onset of action and a relatively prolonged activity.

Uses Antacid; peptic ulcer.

Untoward Reactions *GI:* Constipation, rebound hyperacidity, flatulence, eructation, intestinal obstruction. *Milk-alkali syndrome:* Hypercalcemia, metabolic alkalosis, renal dysfunction.

Dosage **PO**: *individualized usual dose.* 0.5–2 gm 4 or more times daily with water. *Severe symptoms*: 2–4 gm q hr. Tablets should be chewed before swallowing.

DIHYDROXYALUMINUM SODIUM CARBONATE   Rolaids (OTC)

Classification Antacid.

Action/Kinetics Nonsystemic antacid with adsorbent and protective properties similar to aluminum hydroxide but reported to act more rapidly. Acid neutralizing capacity: 7 mEq/tablet.
Note: See Aluminum hydroxide gel for uses, contraindications, untoward reactions, and additional drug interactions.

Dosage **PO**: 1–2 tablets chewed after meals and at bedtime; 1–2 tablets chewed q 2–4 hr may be required to alleviate severe discomfort.

MAGALDRATE (HYDROXYMAGNESIUM ALUMINATE)   Lowsium, Riopan (OTC)

Classification Antacid.

Remarks Chemical combination of aluminum hydroxide and magnesium hydroxide. This compound is an effective nonsystemic antacid. It buffers (pH 3.0–5.5) without causing alkalosis. Acid neutralizing capacity: 13.5 mEq/tablet or 5 ml.

Use Antacid.

Contraindication Sensitivity to aluminum. Use with caution in patients with impaired renal function.

Untoward Reactions Mild constipation and hypermagnesemia.

Dosage **PO: tablets or suspension**, 480–960 mg q.i.d. between meals and at bedtime. Frequency of administration may have to be increased initially to every hour to control severe symptoms.

MAGNESIUM HYDROXIDE (MAGNESIA)   Milk of Magnesia, M.O.M (OTC)

Classification Antacid, laxative.

Action/Kinetics Depending on dosage, drug acts as an antacid or as a laxative. Neutralizes hydrochloric acid. Does not produce alkalosis and has a demulcent effect. One milliliter neutralizes 2.7 mEq of acid. As an antacid, often alternated with aluminum hydroxide to counteract laxative effect.

Uses Antacid, laxative.

Contraindications Poor renal function.

Untoward Reactions Diarrhea, abdominal pain, nausea, vomiting. Hypermagnesemia and CNS depression (especially in patients with renal failure).

Additional Drug Interactions

Interactant	Interaction
Procainamide	Procainamide ↑ muscle relaxation produced by Mg salts
Skeletal muscle relaxants (surgical) Succinylcholine Tubocurarine	↑ Muscle relaxation

Dosage **PO. Adults and children over 12 yrs:** *antacid*, 5–10 ml liquid or 600 mg tablets q.i.d.; *laxative*, 15–30 ml liquid once daily with water. **Children, 6–12 yr:** *antacid*, 2.5–5 ml liquid with water; *laxative*, 15–30 ml (depending on age) once daily with water. **Children, 2–6 yr:** *laxative*, 5–15 ml liquid once daily with water.

Administration

1. Give suspension with water. Administer combined magnesia magma and aluminum hydroxide gel with one-half glass of water.
2. Provide a slice of orange or orange juice after administration as a laxative to minimize the unpleasant aftertaste.
3. Administer laxative dose at bedtime as medication takes about 8 hours to be effective and therefore will not interfere with patient's rest.

MAGNESIUM OXIDE Maox, Mag-Ox 400, Par-Mag, Uro-Mag (OTC)

Classification Antacid, laxative.

Action/Kinetics Magnesium oxide is a nonsystemic antacid with a laxative effect. The compound has a rather high neutralizing capacity (1.0 gm neutralizes 50 mEq acid). Magnesium oxide is slower acting than sodium bicarbonate, but has a more prolonged activity.

Uses Antacid, laxative.

Contraindication Poor renal function.

Untoward Reactions Abdominal pain, nausea, diarrhea. Hypermagnesemia and CNS depression in patients with poor renal function.

Additional Drug Interactions See Magnesium hydroxide.

Dosage **PO,** *antacid*: 0.25–1.5 gm with water or milk as required. *Cathartic*: 4 gm.

Administration Administer antacid with water or milk.

Additional Nursing Implications

See also *Nursing Implications*, p. 632.

Explain to patients why Sippy Powder No. 1 and 2 are alternated to reduce cathartic effect.

MAGNESIUM TRISILICATE (OTC)

Classification   Antacid.

Action/Kinetics   Nonsystemic antacid with marked adsorbent and protective properties and a relatively long action (1.0 gm neutralizes 50 mEq acid). Mild laxative effect; thus, used with aluminum antacids. The drug protects the crater of the ulcer.

Use   Antacid.

Contraindication   Use with caution in patients with renal disease.

Untoward Reactions   Abdominal pain, nausea, diarrhea, and magnesium intoxication.

Additional Drug Interactions   See Magnesium hydroxide.

Dosage   PO: 1–4 gm q.i.d. Tablets should be chewed before swallowing. Combined with aluminum hydroxide: 5–30 ml in one-half glass of water every 2–4 hr.

Administration

1. Instruct the patient to chew tablets before swallowing and then drink 60 ml of water.
2. Administer combination of magnesium trisilicate with aluminum hydroxide in 120 ml of water.

SODIUM BICARBONATE   Bell/Ans, Soda Mint (OTC)

Classification   Antacid, systemic alkalizer.

Action/Kinetics   Systemic antacid that neutralizes hydrochloric acid by forming sodium chloride and carbon dioxide (1 gm of sodium bicarbonate neutralizes 12 mEq of acid). Provides temporary relief of peptic ulcer pain and of discomfort associated with indigestion. Although widely used by the public, sodium bicarbonate is rarely prescribed as an antacid because of its high sodium content, short duration of action, and ability to cause alkalosis. Also, see Chapter 69 for details on sodium bicarbonate as an electrolyte.

Uses   Antacid. As an alkalinizing agent for the treatment of acidosis or to alkalinize the urine to increase or decrease excretion of drugs.

Contraindications   Renal disease, congestive heart failure, patients on restricted sodium diet, pyloric obstruction. Use with caution in patients with edema and cirrhosis. Do not use as an antidote for strong mineral acids because carbon dioxide is formed, which may cause discomfort and even perforation.

Untoward Reactions *GI:* Acid rebound, gastric distention. *Milk-alkali syndrome:* Hypercalcemia, metabolic alkalosis (dizziness, cramps, thirst, anorexia, nausea, vomiting, diminished breathing, seizures), renal dysfunction.

Drug Interactions See Chapter 69, Drug Interactions for Sodium Bicarbonate, p. 830.

Dosage *Antacid*: **PO**, 0.3–2 gm, 1–4 times/day. *Urinary or systemic alkalinization*: **PO**, 0.325–2 gm up to q.i.d. (not to exceed 16 gm/day). *As systemic electrolyte*, see p. 830.

Administration

1. Hypertonic solutions must be administered by the physician.
2. Isotonic solution should be administered slowly as ordered as too rapid administration may result in death due to cellular acidity. Check rate of flow frequently.

Nursing Implications

1. *Assess*
   a. acidotic patient being treated with sodium bicarbonate for relief of dyspnea and hyperpnea and report as the drug must be discontinued when these conditions are relieved.
   b. acidotic patients being treated with sodium bicarbonate for edema, which may necessitate a change to potassium bicarbonate.
2. Caution the general public not to take sodium bicarbonate routinely for gastric distress but rather to consult a physician instead. Excessive use of the drug may cause rebound effect with increased acid secretion or systemic alkalosis and formation of phosphate crystals in the kidney.

Chapter Fifty-three

ANTIULCER AND OTHER GASTROINTESTINAL DRUGS

CIMETIDINE   Apo-Cimetidine,* Novocimetidine,* Peptol,* Tagamet (Rx)

Classification   Histamine H$_2$-receptor blocking agent.

Action/Kinetics   Cimetidine decreases the acidity of the stomach by blocking the action of histamine, a substance involved in triggering gastric acid secretion. Cimetidine blocks the action of histamine by competitively occupying the histamine (H$_2$) receptors in the gastric mucosa. This, in turn, inhibits the release of gastric (hydrochloric) acid. Cimetidine reduces postprandial daytime and nighttime gastric acid secretion by about 50–80%. It is well absorbed from GI tract. **Peak plasma level**: 1 hr. t½: 2 hr, longer in presence of renal impairment. After PO use, most metabolized in liver; after parenteral use, about 75% of drug excreted unchanged in the urine.

Uses   Short-term (up to 8 weeks) treatment of active duodenal or benign gastric ulcers, prophylaxis in duodenal ulcers. Management of gastric acid hypersecretory states (Zollinger-Ellison syndrome, systemic mastocytosis). *Investigational:* Prior to surgery to prevent aspiration pneumonitis, primary or secondary hyperparathyroidism in chronic hemodialysis patients, prophylaxis of stress-induced ulcers, upper GI bleeding, gastroesophageal reflux, herpes virus infections, tinea capitis.

Contraindications   Pregnancy, children under 16, nursing mothers.

Untoward Reactions   *GI:* Diarrhea, pancreatitis, hepatitis, hepatic fibrosis. *CNS:* Dizziness, sleepiness, headache, confusion, delirium, hallucinations, double vision, dysarthria, ataxia. *CV:* Hypotension and arrhythmias following rapid IV administration. *Hematologic:* Agranulocytosis, thrombocytopenia, hemolytic or aplastic anemia, granulocytopenia. *GU:* Impotence (high doses for prolonged periods of time), gynecomastia (long-term treatment). *Other:* Arthralgia, myalgia, rash, vasculitis, galactorrhea, alopecia, bronchoconstriction.

Drug Interactions

Interactant	Interaction
Antacids	↓ Effect of cimetidine due to ↓ absorption from GI tract

Interactant	Interaction
Anticholinergics	↓ Effect of cimetidine due to ↓ absorption from GI tract
Anticoagulants, oral	↑ Effect of anticoagulant due to ↓ breakdown by liver
Barbiturates	↓ Effect of cimetidine due to ↓ absorption from GI tract and ↑ breakdown by liver
Benzodiazepines	↑ Effect of benzodiazepines due to ↓ breakdown by liver
Beta-adrenergic blocking drugs	↑ Effect of beta-blockers due to ↓ breakdown by liver
Caffeine	↑ Effect of caffeine due to ↓ breakdown by liver
Carbamazepine	Cimetidine ↑ effect of carbamazepine
Carmustine	Additive bone marrow depression
Chlorpromazine	↓ Effect chlorpromazine due to ↓ absorption from GI tract
Iron salts	↓ Effect of iron due to ↓ absorption from GI tract
Ketoconazole	↓ Effect of ketoconazole due to ↓ absorption from GI tract
Lidocaine	↑ Effect of lidocaine due to ↓ breakdown by liver
Metoclopramide	↓ Effect cimetidine due to ↓ absorption from GI tract
Metronidazole	↑ Effect metronidazole due to ↓ breakdown by liver
Narcotics	Possible ↑ toxic effects of narcotics
Phenytoin	↑ Effect of phenytoin due to ↓ breakdown by liver
Procainamide	↑ Effect of procainamide due to ↓ excretion by kidney
Quinidine	↑ Effect of quinidine due to ↓ breakdown by liver
Tetracyclines	↓ Effect of tetracyclines due to ↓ absorption from GI tract
Theophylline	↑ Effect of theophyllines due to ↓ breakdown by liver

Dosage **PO.** *Duodenal ulcers*: 300 mg q.i.d. with meals and at bedtime for 4 to 6 weeks (administer with antacids). *Prophylaxis of recurrent ulcers*: 400 mg at bedtime. *Active benign peptic ulcers:* 300 mg q.i.d. with meals and at bedtime for no more than 8 weeks. *Hypersecretory conditions*: 300 mg q.i.d. with meals and at bedtime up to a maximum of 2,400 mg daily. *Hospitalized patients with hypersecretory conditions or intractable ulcers*: **IM, IV**, 300 mg q 6 hr up to maximum of 2,400 mg/day. *Impaired renal function*: **PO, IV**, 300 mg q 12 hr.

Administration

1. For IV injection or infusion: dilute as specified by manufacturer and inject over period of 1–2 minutes, or infuse intermittently.
2. Administer oral medication with meals and at bedtime.
3. If antacids are to be used, the dose should be staggered with that of cimetidine.

Nursing Implication
Teach patient to continue taking medication as ordered even though he may feel asymptomatic.

DEXPANTHENOL   Ilopan, Panol (Rx)

Classification   Gastrointestinal stimulant.

Action/Kinetics   Dexpanthenol (*d*-pentothenyl alcohol), a precursor of coenzyme A, stimulates the smooth muscles of the GI tract, probably by increasing the synthesis of acetylcholine. Satisfactory response is unlikely in the presence of hypokalemia.

Uses   Prophylactic after major abdominal surgery to minimize development of paralytic ileus or abdominal distention. To treat retention of flatus or delay in resumption of normal intestinal motility after surgery or parturition. Paralytic ileus.

Contraindications   Hemophilia. Within one hour of succinylcholine. Safety and effectiveness in pregnancy, lactation, and in children has not been established.

Untoward Reactions   *GI*: Intestinal colic, vomiting, diarrhea. *Allergic*: Pruritus, dermatitis, urticaria, tingling, breathing difficulties. *Other*: Hypotension.

Drug Interactions

Interactant	Interaction
Antibiotics Barbiturates Narcotics	Allergic reactions of unknown cause
Succinylcholine	↑ Effect of succinylcholine with respiratory difficulties

Dosage   IM: *prophylaxis or postoperative abdominal distention*: 250–500 mg. Repeat once after 2 hr; **then** q 6 hr until danger of distention has passed. *Paralytic ileus*: 500 mg **IM**; repeat after 2 hr, **then** q 4–6 hr. Continue above regimens until all danger of distention has passed (usually for a period of 48 to 72 hr or longer).

Dexpanthenol can be administered by IV drip when mixed with 5% dextrose or lactated Ringer's solution.

Administration

1. Delay administration of dexpanthenol for 12 hours after administration of neostigmine or similar drug, or for 1 hour after administration of succinylcholine.
2. Do not administer full strength solution into vein.

Nursing Implications

Assess

a. for presence of bowel sounds to evaluate the effectiveness of dexpanthenol.
b. whether patient is passing flatus, an indication of peristaltic activity.
c. for hypokalemia manifested by apathy, muscle weakness, atonia, cardiac arrhythmias, and impaired respirations, and report to medical supervision as dexpanthenol is not effective if the patient is in a hypokalemic state.

METOCLOPRAMIDE   Maxeran,* Reglan (Rx)

Classification   Gastrointestinal stimulant.

Action/Kinetics   Metoclopramide, by increasing sensitivity to acetylcholine, increases motility of the upper GI tract and relaxes the pyloric sphincter and duodenal bulb. This results in shortened gastric emptying and gastrointestinal transit time. It is considered a dopamine antagonist. The drug facilitates intubation of the small bowel and speeds transit of a barium meal. **Onset, IV**: 1–3 min; **IM**, 10–15 min; **PO**, 30–60 min. **Duration**: 1–2 hr. t½: 4 hr. Significant first pass effect following PO use; unchanged drug and metabolites excreted in urine.

Uses PO: Acute and recurrent diabetic gastroparesis, gastroesophageal reflux. **Parenteral**: Facilitate small bowel intubation, stimulate gastric emptying and increase intestinal transit of barium to aid in radiologic examination of stomach and small intestine, prophylaxis of nausea and vomiting in cancer chemotherapy. *Investigational*: Nausea and vomiting due to pregnancy, labor, gastric ulcer, anorexia nervosa. To improve lactation.

Contraindications Gastrointestinal hemorrhage, obstruction, or perforation; epilepsy, patients taking drugs likely to cause extrapyramidal symptoms, such as phenothiazines. Pheochromocytoma. Safe use during pregnancy and lactation not established.

Untoward Reactions *CNS*: Restlessness, drowsiness, fatigue, lassitude, insomnia. Headaches, dizziness, extrapyramidal symptoms, parkinson-like symptoms, dystonia, myoclonus, depression, dyskinesia. *GI*: Nausea, bowel disturbances. *CV*: Hypertension (transient).

Drug Interactions

Interactant	Interaction
Acetaminophen	↑ GI absorption of acetaminophen
Anticholinergics	↓ Effect of metoclopramide
Cimetidine	↓ Effect of cimetidine due to ↓ absorption from GI tract
CNS depressants	Additive sedative effects
Digoxin	↓ Effect of digoxin due to ↓ absorption from GI tract
Ethanol	↑ GI absorption of ethanol
Levodopa	↑ GI absorption of levodopa
Narcotic analgesics	↓ Effect of metoclopramide
Tetracyclines	↑ GI absorption of tetracyclines

Dosage PO. *Diabetic gastroparesis*: 10 mg 30 min before meals and at bedtime for 2–8 weeks (therapy should be reinstituted if symptoms recur). *Gastroesophageal reflux*: 10–15 mg q.i.d. 30 min before meals and at bedtime. **IV.** *Prophylaxis of vomiting due to chemotherapy*: **initial**, 1–2 mg/kg for 2 doses with the first dose 30 min before chemotherapy; **then**, 10 mg or more q 3 hr for 3 doses. Inject slowly over 15 minutes. *Facilitate small bowel intubation*: **Adults**, 10 mg given over 1–2 min; **pediatric, 6–14 years**: 2.5–5 mg; **pediatric, less than 6 years**: 0.1 mg/kg. *Radiologic exams to increase intestinal transit time*: Single dose given over 1–2 min (same dosage as for small bowel intubation).

Administration

1. Inject slowly over 1–2 min to prevent transient feelings of anxiety and restlessness.
2. After oral use, absorption of certain drugs from the GI tract may be affected (see *Drug Interactions*).
3. Metoclopramide is physically and/or chemically incompatible with a number of drugs; check package insert if drug is to be admixed.

Nursing Implications

Teach patient and/or family

a. that metoclopramide will add to sedative effect of any other CNS depressant he is taking (e.g., tranquilizers or a sleeping pill).

b. that operating a car or hazardous machinery should not be attempted, as medication has a sedative effect.

RANITIDINE HYDROCHLORIDE   Zantac (Rx)

Classification H_2-receptor antagonist.

Action/Kinetics   Ranitidine competitively inhibits gastric acid secretion by blocking the effect of histamine on histamine H_2-receptors. Both daytime and noctural basal gastric acid secretion, as well as food- and pentagastrin-stimulated gastric acid are inhibited. **Peak effect: PO**, 1–3 hr; **IM, IV,** 15 min. **t½:** 2.5–3 hr. **Duration:** 9–12 hr. **Serum level to inhibit 50% stimulated gastric acid secretion:** 36–94 ng/ml. Excreted through urine.

Uses   Short-term treatment of duodenal ulcer (4–8 weeks). Pathologic hypersecretory conditions as Zollinger-Ellison syndrome and systemic mastocytosis. *Investigational:* Gastric ulcers, reflux esophagitis, prophylaxis of pulmonary aspiration of acid during anesthesia.

Contraindications   Use with caution in pregnancy and lactation and in decreased hepatic or renal function. Safety and efficacy not established in children.

Untoward Reactions   *GI*: Constipation, nausea, vomiting, diarrhea, abdominal pain. *CNS*: Headache, dizziness, malaise, insomnia, vertigo. *CV*: Bradycardia or tachycardia, premature ventricular beats. *Hematologic*: Thrombocytopenia, granulocytopenia, leukopenia, pancytopenia. *Hepatic*: Hepatotoxicity, jaundice, hepatitis, increase in SGPT. *Allergic*: Bronchospasm, rashes, fever, eosinophilia. *Other*: Arthralgia, alopecia.

Drug Interactions   Antacids may ↓ the absorption of ranitidine.

Dosage   PO. Adults: *Duodenal ulcer*: 150 mg b.i.d. to heal ulcer although 100 mg b.i.d. will inhibit acid secretion. *Hypersecretory conditions*: 50 mg b.i.d. (up to 6 gm/day have been used in severe cases). In impaired renal function (creatinine clearance less than 50 ml/min): 150 mg/day. **IM, IV injection or infusion:** 50 mg q 6–8 hr.

Administration

1. Antacids should be given concomitantly for pain although they may interfere with absorption of ranitidine.

2. About one-half of patients may heal completely within 2 weeks; thus, endoscopy may show no need for further treatment.

Nursing Implications

1. Because complete healing may occur within 2 weeks, be sure to encourage patient to report to physician/radiologist as scheduled.

2. Drug therapy should be terminated as soon as healing is documented.

SIMETHICONE Gas-X, Mylicon, Mylicon-80, Ovol,* Silain (OTC)

Classification Antiflatulent.

Action/Kinetics Simethicone acts as a defoamant, which decreases surface tension of gas bubbles thus facilitating their coalescence and expulsion as flatus or belching. It also prevents the accumulation of mucus enclosed pockets of gas. Excreted in feces unchanged.

Use Relief of pain caused by excess gas in digestive tract. Adjunct in the treatment of postoperative gaseous distention, air swallowing, functional dyspepsia, peptic ulcer, spastic irritable colon, or diverticulitis.

Dosage **PO,** *tablets*: 40–80 mg after each meal and at bedtime; *drops*: 40 mg q.i.d. after meals and at bedtime.

Administration
1. Chew tablets or dissolve in mouth.
2. Use calibrated dropper to administer medication.

SUCRALFATE Carafate (Rx)

Action/Kinetics Sucralfate is the aluminum salt of a sulfurated disaccharide. It acts locally by forming a protein complex at the site of the ulcer that provides a barrier to gastric acid, pepsin, and bile salts which may aggravate an ulcer. May be used in conjunction with antacids.

Use Short-term treatment (up to 8 weeks) of duodenal ulcers. *Investigational*: Hasten healing of gastric ulcers, chronic treatment of gastric or duodenal ulcers.

Contraindications Safety for use with children and in pregnancy and lactation has not been fully established.

Untoward Reactions *GI*: Constipation (most common); also, nausea, diarrhea, indigestion, dry mouth. *Miscellaneous*: Back pain, dizziness, drowsiness, vertigo, rash, pruritus.

Drug Interaction Sucralfate may prevent the absorption of cimetidine, phenytoin, or tetracyclines from the GI tract.

Dosage **Usual**: 1 gm q.i.d. 1 hr before meals and at bedtime (it may also be taken 2 hr after meals). The drug should be taken for 4–8 weeks unless x-ray films or endoscopy have indicated significant healing.

Administration
1. If Antacids are used, they should be taken either ½ hour before or after sucralfate.
2. Even though healing of ulcers may result, the frequency or severity of subsequent attacks is not altered.

Nursing Implications
1. Assess for effectiveness of sucralfate by reduction in signs and symptoms of ulcer.
2. Teach patient and/or family the importance of taking the medication exactly as prescribed.

Chapter Fifty-four

LAXATIVES AND CATHARTICS

General Statement   Difficult or infrequent passage of stools (constipation) is a symptom of many conditions ranging from purely organic causes (obstruction, megacolon) to common functional disorders. Patients confined to bed may often develop constipation. Constipation may also be of psychological origin. The underlying cause of constipation should be elucidated by a physician, especially since a marked change in bowel habits may be a symptom of a pathologic condition.

The cathartics discussed in this section are effective because they act locally either by specifically stimulating the smooth muscles of the bowel or by changing the bulk or consistency of the stools. The cathartics can be divided into four categories:

1. *Stimulant cathartics*: Substances that chemically stimulate the smooth muscles of the bowel so as to increase contractions.
2. *Saline cathartics*: Substances that increase the bulk of the stools by retaining water.
3. *Bulk-forming cathartics*: Nondigestible substances that pass through the stomach and then increase the bulk of the stools.

4. *Emollient laxatives*: Agents that soften hardened feces and facilitate their passage through the lower intestine.

Today cathartics are prescribed less frequently for chronic constipation than in the past. In fact, continued use of laxatives has been held responsible for some cases of chronic constipation and other intestinal disorders because the patient may start to depend on the psychological effect and physical stimulus of the drug rather than on the body's own natural reflexes. Prevention of constipation should include adequate fluid intake and diet as well as daily exercise.

Uses   Cathartics are indicated for the following conditions: anorectal lesions like hemorrhoids; for diagnostic procedures and in conjunction with surgery or anthelmintic therapy; and in cases of chemical poisoning. Short-term treatment of constipation.

Contraindications   Severe abdominal pain that *might* be caused by appendicitis, enteritis, ulcerative colitis, diverticulitis, intestinal obstruction. The administration of cathartics in such cases might cause rupture of the abdomen or intestinal hemorrhage. Children under the age of 2.

Untoward Reactions   Excess activity of the colon resulting in nausea, diarrhea, or vomiting. Dehydration, disturbance of the electrolyte balance. Dependency if used chronically.
Bulk laxatives: Obstruction in the esophogus, stomach, small intestine, or rectum. *Stimulant cathartics:* Chronic abuse may lead to malfunctioning colon.

Drug Interactions

Interactant	Interaction
Anticoagulants, oral	↓ Absorption of vitamin K from GI tract induced by cathartics may ↑ effects of anticoagulants and result in bleeding
Digitalis	Cathartics may ↓ absorption of digitalis
Tetracyclines	↓ Effect of tetracyclines due to ↓ absorption from GI tract

Administration/Storage
1. Administer cathartic at a temperature and in or with a substance that makes it more palatable.
2. Administer a cathartic at a time when it will not interfere with the patient's digestion and absorption of nutrients.
3. Note the length of time it takes for the prescribed cathartic to take effect and administer it in such a manner that the time of its action will not interfere with the patient's rest.

Nursing Implications
1. Promote better bowel function without the use of cathartics by either assisting the patient to the bathroom or by providing a commode at the bedside and ensuring privacy.
2. Keep a record of patient's bowel function and response to cathartics so that they will be given only as needed.
3. Check directions carefully and administer accordingly when cathartics are ordered to prepare the patient for diagnostic studies. Explain how the drug will affect him/her and stress the importance of procedure for accurate diagnostic study.

4. *Teach patient and/or family*
   a. that a daily bowel movement is not essential and that one or two bowel movements may be missed without harm to health.
   b. that rather than relying on cathartics, it would be far better to include more fluids and bulk in the diet and more exercise in daily activity, if such are not contraindicated. Explain that regular use of cathartics can lead to chronic constipation.
   c. with abdominal pain or a sudden change in bowel habits, to obtain medical supervision rather than self-medicating with cathartics.

STIMULANT CATHARTICS

BISACODYL   Apo-Bisacodyl,* Bisco-Lax, Dacodyl, Deficol, Dulcolax, Fleet Bisacodyl, Theralax (OTC)

Classification   Cathartic, stimulant.

Action/Kinetics   Bisacodyl is a local chemical stimulant that acts by increasing the contraction of the muscles of the colon. Bisacodyl is not absorbed systemically and can be administered orally or as a rectal suppository. It produces a gentle bowel movement and soft, formed stools. It usually acts within 6 to 8 hours after PO administration and 15 to 60 minutes after rectal administration.

Uses   Cleansing of colon preoperatively and postoperatively and for diagnostic procedures (radiology, barium enemas, proctoscopy), colostomies and chronic constipation.

   May be used during pregnancy or in the presence of cardiovascular, renal, or hepatic disease.

Contraindications   Acute surgical abdomen or acute abdominal pain.

Additional Untoward Reactions   Suppositories may cause burning sensation.

Drug Interaction   Use of bisacodyl with antacids, milk, or cimetidine may result in premature dissolution of the enteric coating, leading to cramping and vomiting.

Dosage   PO. Adults: 10–15 mg at bedtime or before breakfast; **pediatric, over 6 years:** 5–10 mg at bedtime or before breakfast. **Rectal suppository, adults and children over 2 years**: 10 mg; **under 2 years**: 5 mg. **Enema. Adults:** 37 ml.

Administration/Storage

BISACODYL TABLETS
1. Administer at bedtime for effectiveness in morning.
2. Otherwise administer before breakfast so that drug will not interfere with the patient's rest at night but rather will be effective within 6 hours.
3. Advise patient not to take within one hour of ingesting milk or antacids.
4. Advise patient to swallow tablets whole and not chew them or crush them. Children who cannot swallow pills will be unable to take medication PO.

5. Anticipate for surgery, radiography, or sigmoidoscopy preparation that the drug should be given orally the night before and by rectal suppository in AM.
6. Refrigerate bisacodyl tablets at a temperature not exceeding 30°C (86°F).

BISACODYL SUPPOSITORIES

1. Administer at a time least likely to interfere with patient's rest.
2. Anticipate that the suppository will be effective in 15 minutes to 2 hours and provide for adequate toileting facilities.

BISACODYL TANNEX ENEMA Clysodrast (Rx)

Classification Cathartic, stimulant.

Action/Kinetics Bisacodyl tannate is a complex of bisacodyl (see preceding drug) and tannic acid. The tannic acid increases the solubility of bisacodyl, decreases the mucous secretions of the lining of the large intestine (due to its astringent effects), and improves the adherence of contrast media to the wall of the bowel. Solutions of bisacodyl tannate are stable; however, if mixed with barium sulfate for diagnostic studies, the preparation should be used immediately. Bisacodyl tannate is used only rectally.

Uses Cleansing enema prior to radiologic examination of colon; for sigmoidoscopic and proctoscopic procedures.

Contraindications Extensive ulcerations of colon, children younger than 10 years of age, and pregnancy.

Untoward Reaction If absorbed, tannic acid may be hepatotoxic.

Drug Interactions See Bisacodyl, p. 647.

Dosage *Cleansing enema:* 2.5 gm (1 packet) in 1 liter of warm water. *Barium enema:* 2.5–5 gm (1–2 packets) in 1 liter of barium sulfate suspension; total dosage for one exam should not exceed 7.5 gm with no more than 10 gm given in a 72-hour period.

Administration Anticipate that for radiologic examination or sigmoidoscopic or proctoscopic procedures, the patient will be placed on a residue-free diet 1 day before examination and 30–60 ml castor oil will be ordered for administration 16 hours before the examination. A cleansing enema of bisacodyl tannex may be administered on the day of the examination and may be repeated as necessary.

CASCARA SAGRADA Cascara Sagrada Fluid Extract, Cascara Sagrada Aromatic Fluid Extract (OTC)

Classification Cathartic, stimulant.

Action/Kinetics Cascara sagrada stimulates the contractions of the colon without affecting the small intestine. It produces stools within 6–8 hr. The drug is available as a fluid extract and as a less effective but better-tasting aromatic, debittered fluid extract.

Additional Contraindication The drug gets into breast milk and may cause diarrhea in the infant.

Additional Untoward Reactions Dark pigmentation of the mucosa of the colon (called melanosis coli) which is slowly reversed after the drug is discontinued. Acid urine may be colored yellowish-brown while an alkaline urine may be colored pink, red, or violet.

Dosage PO. *Fluid extract*: 1 ml; *aromatic fluid extract*: 5 ml; *tablets*: 1 (325 mg) at bedtime.

Nursing Implication

Teach patient that cascara may cause urine to appear yellow-brown or reddish.

CASTOR OIL Kellogg's Castor Oil, Purge (OTC)

CASTOR OIL, EMULSIFIED Alphamul, Emulsoil, Fleet Castor Oil Stimulant Laxative, Neoloid (OTC)

Classification Cathartic, stimulant.

Action/Kinetics The active ingredient is ricinoleic acid, which is liberated in the small intestine. This substance inhibits water and electrolyte absorption leading to fluid accumulation and increased peristalsis. Prompt (within 2–6 hr) and complete evacuation of the bowel occurs.

Use Prompt evacuation of bowel.

Contraindications Pregnancy, menstruation, abdominal pain, and intestinal obstruction. Common constipation. Concomitantly with fat-soluble anthelmintics.

Untoward Reactions Severe diarrhea, abdominal pain and colic, altered mucosal permeability in the small intestine, dehydration, and changes in electrolyte balance, including hyperkalemia, acidosis, or alkalosis.

Dosage *Castor oil*: 15–60 ml before diagnostic procedures; **infants**: 1–5 ml; **children over 2 years**: 5–15 ml. *Castor oil emulsified*, **PO**: 15–60 ml; **infants less than 2 years**: 1.25–7.5 ml; **children over 2 years**: 5–30 ml. Dose depends on strength of preparation.

Nursing Implications

1. The more palatable oil-in-water emulsion aromatized with flavoring agents is preferred.
2. Disguise taste of plain castor oil with a glass of orange juice.

DANTHRON Akshun Tablets, Dorbane, Modane, Modane Mild, Roydan* (OTC)

Classification Cathartic, stimulant.

Action/Kinetics Danthron stimulates peristalsis in the large intestine. **Onset:** 6–8 hr. Has been combined with a fecal moistening agent such as docusate sodium.

Contraindications Pregnancy, lactation, nausea, vomiting, or abdominal pain.

Additional Untoward Reactions Severe diarrhea, hyperkalemia, and dehydration. Dark pigmentation of the mucosa of the colon (melanosis coli) which is slowly reversed after drug discontinuance. Alkaline urine may be colored pink, red, or violet.

Drug Interaction Docusate preparations may ↑ toxicity of danthron due to ↑ rate of absorption.

Dosage **PO:** 37.5–150 mg with or 1 hr after evening meal; 300 mg may be required occasionally.

> **Nursing Implication**
> Teach patient that danthron may cause urine to appear pink or red in color.

PHENOLPHTHALEIN Alophen Pills, Correctol, Espotabs, Evac-U-Gen, Evac-U-Lax, Ex-Lax, Feen-A-Mint, Phenolax, Prulet (OTC)

Classification Cathartic, stimulant.

Action/Kinetics The drug primarily acts on the large intestine to produce a semifluid stool with little or no accompanying colic. **Onset:** 4–8 hr. **Duration:** May be 3–4 days due to residual effect.

Use Simple constipation.

Additional Untoward Reactions Hypersensitivity reactions: dermatitis, pruritus; rarely, nonthrombocytopenic purpura or anaphylaxis. Phenolphthalein may color alkaline urine pink-red and acidic urine yellow-brown.

Dosage **PO. Adults:** 30–270 mg/day; **pediatric, over 6 years:** 30–60 mg/day; **pediatric, 2–5 years:** 15–20 mg/day. Usually taken at bedtime.

> **Nursing Implications**
> *Teach patient and/or family*
> a. that phenolphthalein colors alkaline stools or urine red.
> b. to store medication out of children's reach so it will not be ingested as "candy."
> c. that Ex-Lax is a medication and not candy.

SENNA Black Draught, Senexon, Senokot, Senolax (OTC)

SENNOSIDES A AND B, CALCIUM SALTS Nytilax (OTC)

Classification Cathartic, stimulant.

Action/Kinetics   Senna is prepared from the dried leaf or fruit of the *Cassia acutifolia* or *Cassia angustifolia* tree. Senna is similar to cascara although it is more potent. It increases peristalsis of the large intestine and colon; it also alters electrolyte secretion. **Onset:** 6–12 hr.

Uses   Constipation, preoperative and prediagnostic procedures involving the GI tract.

Contraindications   Irritable colon, nausea, vomiting, abdominal pain, and appendicitis or possibility thereof. Administer with caution to nursing mothers.

Untoward Reactions   Abdominal pain, colic, and diarrhea. Senna colors alkaline urine pink, red, or violet and acid urine yellow-brown.

Dosage   *Senna*. **Tablets: Adults,** 2 at bedtime; **pediatric, over 60 lb:** 1 tablet at bedtime. **Suppositories: Adults,** 1 at bedtime; **pediatric, over 60 lb:** ½ suppository at bedtime. **Black-Draught Granules: Adults,** ¼–½ level teaspoon with water (not recommended for children). **Senokot Granules: Adults,** 1 teaspoon; **pediatric, over 60 lb:** ½ teaspoon. Taken at bedtime. **Syrup: Adults,** 10–15 ml at bedtime; **pediatric, 1–12 months:** 1.25–2.5 ml at bedtime; **pediatric, 1–5 years:** 2.5–5 ml; **5–15 years:** 5–10 ml.
   Sennosides A and B. **Adults:** 12–36 mg (1–3 tablets) at bedtime; **children, 6–10 years:** 12 mg (1 tablet) at bedtime.

Nursing Implications
Teach patient and/or family
   a. that gripping pain is a symptom of overdosage. Drug must be omitted when this occurs and patient should check with physician.
   b. that drug imparts a yellowish-brown color to acid urine and a reddish color to alkaline urine.

SALINE CATHARTICS

Action/Kinetics   Saline laxatives increase the bulk of the stools by attracting and holding large amounts of fluids. The increased bulk results in the mechanical stimulation of peristalsis. The saline cathartics should be administered with sufficient fluid so as not to cause dehydration of the patient. **Onset:** 2–6 hr.
   The saline cathartics, which include magnesium sulfate, milk of magnesia (see antacids), magnesium citrate, sodium phosphate, sodium sulfate, potassium sodium tartrate, and potassium phosphate, are very similar in activity, differing mostly with respect to palatability, cost, and efficiency.
   There is always some systemic absorption of the saline cathartics. This presents a problem in the case of magnesium ions, which may cause magnesium intoxication when given to patients with poor renal function. Magnesium intoxication is characterized by drowsiness, dizziness, and other signs of CNS depression. Thirst may be an early sign of magnesium intoxication.
   See Table 27, p. 652 for individual agents.

Use   To empty the bowel prior to diagnostic or surgical procedures; to eliminate parasites following anthelmintic therapy; to remove toxic material following poisoning; collection of stool specimen for parasite examination.

TABLE 27 SALINE CATHARTICS

Drug	Dosage	Remarks
Fleet enema, OTC	**Rectal only: Adults,** 4 oz; **children,** 2 oz.	Contains 16 gm sodium biphosphate and 6 gm sodium phosphate/100 ml.
Magnesium carbonate, OTC	**Rectal only: Adults,** 4 oz; **pediatric, over 2 yrs:** 2 oz.	
Magnesium citrate (Citro-Mag,* Citroma, Citroma Low Sodium, Citro-Nesia), OTC	**PO. Adults:** 240 ml (100 ml contain 1.75 gm magnesium citrate); **pediatric:** ½ the adult dose.	Observe for magnesium intoxication. Do not give in case of poor renal function. *Administration* Store preferably in refrigerator to improve taste. *Nursing Implications* 1. Remain with patient and encourage drinking the entire solution at once. 2. Provide a cold solution of medication for this makes it taste best. 3. Assess for signs of magnesium toxicity. (For characteristics, see Table 37 p. 815.)
Magnesium hydroxide (Milk of Magnesia, M.O.M.), OTC	**PO. Adults and children over 12 yr:** 15–60 ml; **pediatric, 6–12 yr:** 15–30 ml; **pediatric, 2–6 yr:** 5–15 ml.	Suspension should be mixed with water.
Magnesium oxide (Maox, Mag-Ox-400, Par-Mag, Uro-Mag), OTC	**PO. Adults:** 4 gm.	Administer with milk or water.
Magnesium sulfate (Epsom Salt), OTC	**PO. Adults:** 10–15 gm; **pediatric:** 5–10 gm.	Effective in 1–2 hr. *Administration* Dissolve in glassful of ice water or other fluid to lessen the disagreeable taste.
Phospho-soda (Fleet), OTC	**PO. Adults:** 20–30 ml; **pediatric:** 5–15 ml.	Contains 18 gm sodium phosphate and 48 gm sodium biphosphate/100 ml. *Administration* Mix with ½ glass of cold water.
Sodium phosphate, OTC	**PO:** 4 gm. Exsiccated sodium phosphate: 2 gm.	Relatively pleasant tasting. Somewhat less effective than magnesium or sodium sulfate. Available as flavored solution. *Administration* Administer before breakfast dissolved in a glassful of warm water.
Sodium phosphate effervescent, OTC	**PO:** 10 gm. Sodium phosphate solution: 5–10 ml.	Pleasant tasting. Also contains sodium bicarbonate, tartaric, and citric acids. Dry powder liberates carbon dioxide upon addition of water.
Sodium sulfate (Glauber's Sulfate), OTC	**PO:** 15 gm.	Very vile tasting. As effective as magnesium sulfate.

BULK-FORMING LAXATIVES

Action   Bulk-forming cathartics increase the bulk of the feces and stimulate peristalsis by mechanical means. These are the safest of the available laxatives and cathartics.

Untoward Reactions   Obstruction of the esophogus, stomach, small intestine, and rectum.

METHYLCELLULOSE   Cologel, Gonio-Gel* (OTC)

Classification   Cathartic, bulk forming.

Action/Kinetics   Methylcellulose is composed of indigestible fibers that form a colloidal, bulky gelatinous mass on contact with water. The fibers pass through the stomach and increase the bulk of the feces, stimulating peristalsis. The drug is usually effective within 12–24 hours. Several nonprescription laxatives contain methylcellulose.

Uses   Chronic constipation, colostomy. Methylcellulose has also been used in weight control products to induce a sense of fullness.

Contraindications   Intestinal obstruction, ulceration, and severe abdominal pain.

Dosage   PO. 5–20 ml t.i.d. with a glass of water.

Administration   Follow each dose with a glass of water or milk to prevent impaction.

PSYLLIUM HYDROPHILIC MUCILOID   Cillium, Effersyllium Instant Mix, Fiberall, Hydrocil Instant, Karacil,* Konsyl, Konsyl-D, Metamucil, Modane Bulk, Mucilose, Naturacil, Neo-Mucil,* Perdiem, Prodiem,* Prodiem Plain* Pro-Lax, Regacilium, Reguloid, Serutan, Siblin, Syllact, V-Lax (OTC)

Classification   Cathartic, bulk-forming.

Action/Kinetics   This drug is obtained from the fruit of various species of plantago. The powder forms a gelatinous mass with water which adds bulk to the stools and stimulates peristalsis. It also has a demulcent effect on an inflamed intestinal mucosa. These preparations may also contain dextrose, sodium bicarbonate, monobasic potassium phosphate, citric acid, and benzyl benzoate. Dependence may occur.

Contraindications   Severe abdominal pain, or intestinal obstruction.

Drug Interactions   Psyllium should not be used concomitantly with salicylates, nitrofurantoin or cardiac glycosides (e.g., digitalis).

Dosage   Dose depends on the product. General information on adult dosage follows. **Granules/Flakes:** 1–2 teaspoons 1–3 times/day spread on food or with a glass of water. **Powder:** 1 rounded teaspoon in 8 oz of liquid 1–3 times/day. **Effervescent powder:** 1 packet in water 1–3 times/day. **Chewable pieces:** 2 pieces followed by a glass of water 1–3 times/day.

EMOLLIENT CATHARTICS

Action/Kinetics As their name implies, these laxatives promote defecation by softening the feces. These agents are useful when it is desirable to keep the feces soft or when straining at stool is undesirable.

In addition to mineral oil (liquid petrolatum), this group of laxatives includes several surface-active agents that lower the surface tension of the feces and promote their penetration by water and fat. This increases the softness of the fecal mass.

Except for mineral oil, the compounds are not absorbed systemically and do not seem to interfere with the absorption of nutrients.

Uses Constipation associated with dry, hard stools, megacolon, bedridden patients, and cardiovascular and other diseases in which straining at stool should be avoided. After rectal surgery, especially hemorrhoidectomy.

DOCUSATE CALCIUM (DIOCTYL CALCIUM SULFOSUCCINATE)
D-C-S, Pro-Cal-Sof, Surfak (OTC)

DOCUSATE POTASSIUM (DIOCTYL POTASSIUM SULFOSUCCINATE) Dialose, Diocto-K, Kasof (OTC)

DOCUSATE SODIUM (DIOCTYL SODIUM SULFOSUCCINATE)
Lube, Afko-Lube Dioctyl, Bu-Lax 100 and 250, Colace, Dilax 250, Diocto, Dioeze, Diosuccin, Dio-Sul, Disonate, Di-Sosul, Doss 300, Doxinate, D-S-S, Duosol, Laxinate 100, Modane Soft, Molatoc, Pro-Sof, Pro-Sof-100, Regular SS, Regulex,* Regutol, Stulex (OTC)

Classification Cathartic, emollient.

Use To lessen strain of defecation in persons with hernia or cardiovascular diseases, megacolon, or bedridden patients.

Contraindications Nausea, vomiting, abdominal pain, and intestinal obstruction.

Drug Interactions Docusate may ↑ absorption of mineral oil from the GI tract.

Dosage *Docusate calcium*. PO, **Adults**: 240 mg daily; **pediatric, over 6 years**: 50–150 mg daily. *Docusate potassium*. **PO: Adults**, 100–300 mg daily; **pediatric, over 6 years**: 100 mg at bedtime. *Docusate sodium*. **PO, Adults and children over 12 years**: 50–240 mg; **pediatric, under 3 years**: 10–40 mg; **3–6 years**: 20–60 mg; **6–12 years**: 40–120 mg. May also be used as a flushing or retention enema: 50–100 mg.

Administration *Docusate Sodium.* Administer oral solutions with milk or fruit juices to help mask bitter taste.

MINERAL OIL Agoral Plain, Fleet Mineral Oil, Kondremul Plain, Milkinol, Neo-Cultrol, Nujol, Petrogalar Plain, Zymenol (OTC)

Classification Cathartic, emollient.

Action/Kinetics This mixture of liquid hydrocarbons obtained from petroleum softens the stools and lubricates the GI tract. It coats the feces and thus prevents dehydration. **Onset:** 6–8 hr. Mineral oil is available for oral use as a liquid, emulsion, jelly, or suspension and for rectal use as an enema.

Uses Constipation, to avoid straining under certain conditions, such as rectal surgery, hemorrhoidectomy, and certain cardiovascular conditions.

Contraindications Nausea, vomiting, abdominal pain, or intestinal obstruction.

Untoward Reactions Acute or chronic lipid pneumonia due to aspiration of mineral oil; young, elderly, and dysphagic patients are at greatest risk. Pruritus ani which may interfere with healing following anorectal surgery. Use during pregnancy may decrease vitamin K absorption sufficiently to cause hypoprothrombinemia in the newborn.

Drug Interactions

Interactant	Interaction
Anticoagulants, oral	↑ Hypoprothrombinemia by ↓ absorption of vitamin K from GI tract; also, mineral oil could ↓ absorption of anticoagulant from GI tract
Sulfonamides	↓ Effect of nonabsorbable sulfonamide in GI tract
Surface-active laxatives	↑ Absorption of mineral oil
Vitamins A, D, E, K	↓ Absorption following prolonged use of mineral oil

Dosage   **PO. Adults:** 15–30 ml at bedtime, **children:** 5–20 ml at bedtime. **Rectal, adults:** 90–120 ml; **children 2 years and older:** 30–60 ml.

Administration

1. Do not administer with food because oil may delay digestion and prevent absorption of vitamins.
2. Do not administer with vitamin preparation since again the medication will interfere with the absorption, especially of vitamins A, D, E and K.
3. Administer at bedtime and, unless contraindicated, follow with orange juice or give patient a piece of orange to suck on. The emulsion is pleasant tasting and does not require orange to make it palatable. However, when given at bedtime, the risk of lipid pneumonia increases.
4. Store in refrigerator to make medication more palatable.
5. Administer mineral oil to the elderly, debilitated, and to children slowly and carefully to prevent aspiration which may result in lipid pneumonia. Check with physician whether other relief for condition might be utilized if there seems to be a danger of aspiration.
6. For an oil retention enema, administer slowly via catheter. Follow 20 minutes later with cleansing enema as ordered.

Nursing Implications

1. Because mineral oil may cause hypoprothrombinemia in the newborn, warn pregnant women not to take medication to relieve constipation but rather to check with medical supervision for suitable medication.
2. Check perianal area of patients taking more than 30 ml of mineral oil because they are susceptible to leakage of feces through anal sphincter and thus need more frequent cleansing and a perianal pad to prevent soiling of clothes and bedding.

POLOXAMER 188   Alaxin (OTC)

Classification   Cathartic, emollient.

Action/Kinetics   Surface active agent with emulsifying and wetting properties similar to dioctyl sodium sulfosuccinate. This physiologically inert substance permits water and fats to penetrate stools so that they are softer.

Uses   To decrease straining of defecation in presence of hernia or cardiovascular disease. Also megacolon and for bedridden patients with constipation.

Dosage   PO. **Adults**: 480 mg at bedtime; **pediatric**: 240–480 mg at bedtime.

Administration   Administer as a single or divided dose which may be reduced after several days of therapy.

MISCELLANEOUS LAXATIVES

GLYCERIN SUPPOSITORIES   Fleet Babylax, Sani-Supp (OTC)

Classification   Cathartic, miscellaneous.

Action/Kinetics   Glycerin suppositories promote defecation by irritating rectal mucosa as well as by a hyperosmotic action. Glycerin may also soften and lubricate fecal material. The suppository does not have to melt to be effective.

Use   To establish normal bowel function in patients dependent on laxatives.

Contraindications   Should not be used in the presence of anal fissures, fistulas, ulcerative hemorrhoids, or proctitis.

Untoward Reactions   Mucous membrane irritation.

Dosage   **Suppository:** Insert one adult or pediatric suppository high in the rectum and hold for 15 min. **Liquid:** 4 ml inserted gently with the tip of the applicator pointed toward the navel.

Administration/Storage   Store in tight container in refrigerator below 25°C (77°F).

LACTULOSE   Chronulac (Rx)

See *Miscellaneous Drugs*, p. 877.

Chapter Fifty-five

ANTIDIARRHEAL AGENTS

General Statement   Diarrhea accompanies many different disorders and the treating physician should attempt to elucidate the underlying cause of its manifestations. When diarrhea is caused by an infectious organism, the physician may prescribe a specific antibiotic or chemotherapeutic agent to eradicate the causative agent.

Often diarrhea is a self-limiting natural defense reaction by means of which the body rids itself of a toxic or irritating substance. Dehydration and disturbance of the electrolyte balance can be a major complication of diarrhea. Symptomatic antidiarrheal therapy can prevent extreme dehydration.

Most antidiarrheal agents are used for symptomatic relief. Anticholinergic drugs (p. 592), which reduce the excessive motility of the intestine, are also effective constipating agents.

Antidiarrheal agents fall into two categories: those that act locally on the intestine and its contents and those that act systemically.

SYSTEMIC AGENTS

DIPHENOXYLATE HYDROCHLORIDE WITH ATROPINE   Diphenatol, Enoxa, Latropine, Lofene, Lomanate, Lomotil, Lonox, Lo-Trol, Low-Quel, Nor-Mil, SK-Diphenoxylate (C-V) (Rx)

Classification   Antidiarrheal agent, systemic.

Action/Kinetics   Diphenoxylate is a systemic constipating agent chemically related to the narcotic analgesic drug meperidine but without the analgesic properties. Diphenoxylate inhibits GI motility and has a constipating effect. High doses over prolonged periods can, however, cause euphoria and physical dependence. The preparation also contains small amounts of atropine sulfate, which decreases GI motility.

Uses   Symptomatic treatment of chronic and functional diarrhea. Also, diarrhea associated with gastroenteritis, irritable bowel, regional enteritis, malabsorption syndrome, ulcerative colitis, acute infections, food poisoning, postgastrectomy, and for drug-induced diarrhea. Therapeutic results for control of acute diarrhea are inconsistent. Also used in the control of intestinal passage time in patients with ileostomies and colostomies.

Contraindications   Obstructive jaundice, liver disease, diarrhea associated with pseudomembranous enterocolitis after antibiotic therapy, children under the age of 2. Use with caution in pregnancy and lactation and in patients in whom anticholinergics may be contraindicated.

Untoward Reactions   *GI:* Nausea, vomiting, anorexia, abdominal discomfort, paralytic ileus, megacolon. *Allergic:* Pruritus, angioneurotic edema, swelling of gums. *CNS:* Dizziness, drowsiness, malaise, restlessness, headache, depression, numbness of extremities, respiratory depression, coma. *Topical:* Dry skin and mucous membranes, flushing. *Other:* Tachycardia, urinary retention, hyperthermia.

Drug Interactions

Interactant	Interaction
Alcohol	Additive CNS depression
Barbiturates	Additive CNS depression
MAO inhibitors	↑ Chance of hypertensive crisis
Narcotics	↑ Effect of narcotics

Overdosage   Overdosage is characterized by flushing, lethargy, coma, hypotonic reflexes, nystagmus, pinpoint pupils, tachycardia, and respiratory depression.
   Treatment: Gastric lavage and assisted respiration.
   IV administration of a narcotic antagonist, see p. 485. Administration may be repeated after 10 to 15 minutes. Observe patient and readminister antagonist if respiratory depression returns.

Dosage   PO: Adults, initial, 5 mg t.i.d.–q.i.d., **children**: 0.3–0.4 mg/kg/day in divided doses. Contraindicated in children under 2 years of age. See also below.

Pediatric	Total daily dose[a]
2–5 years	6 mg
5–8 years	8 mg
8–12 years	10 mg

[a]Based on 4 ml per teaspoonful, or 2.00 mg of diphenoxylate.

Each tablet or 5 ml of liquid preparation contains 2.5 mg diphenoxylate hydrochloride and 25 μg of atropine sulfate. Dosage should be maintained at initial levels until symptoms are under control; then reduce to maintenance levels.

Nursing Implications

1. *Assess*
   a. patient on combination of Lomotil and other narcotics or barbiturates closely for potentiation of CNS depression.
   b. patient with liver disease who is receiving Lomotil for signs of impending coma such as minor mental aberrations and motor disturbances, untidiness, drowsiness, night wandering, faraway look in eye, and a coarse or "flapping" tremor of the hands.

2. Have naloxone (Narcan) readily available in case of overdosage.
3. *Teach patient and/or family*
   a. to follow the recommended dosage schedule exactly.
   b. to store out of reach of children because accidental overdosage may cause death.

LOPERAMIDE HYDROCHLORIDE Imodium (Rx)

Classification Antidiarrheal agent, systemic.

Action/Kinetics Loperamide is a piperidine derivative that slows intestinal motility by acting on the nerve end receptors embedded in the intestinal wall. The prolonged retention of the feces in the intestine results in reducing volume of the stools, increasing viscosity, and decreasing fluid and electrolyte loss. The drug is reported to be more effective than diphenoxylate.

Uses Symptomatic relief of acute, nonspecific diarrhea, chronic diarrhea associated with inflammatory bowel disease, reduction of volume discharged from ileostomies.

Contraindications Discontinue drug promptly if abdominal distention develops in patients with acute ulcerative colitis. Safe use in pregnancy and children under 12 years of age not established. In patients where constipation should be avoided.

Untoward Reactions *GI:* Abdominal pain, distention, or discomfort. Constipation, dry mouth, nausea, vomiting, epigastric distress. Toxic megacolon in patients with acute colitis. *CNS:* Drowsiness, dizziness, fatigue. *Other:* Allergic skin rashes.

Dosage **PO**, *acute diarrhea*: **initial**, 4 mg, followed by 2 mg after each unformed stool up to maximum of 16 mg/day. *Chronic diarrhea*: 4–8 mg/day as a single or divided dose.

In acute diarrhea discontinue drug after 48 hr if ineffective. In chronic diarrhea discontinue if 16 mg daily for 10 days is ineffective.

PAREGORIC Camphorated Opium Tincture (C-III) (Rx)

Classification Antidiarrheal agent, systemic.

Action/Kinetics The active principle of the mixture is opium (0.04% morphine). The preparation also contains benzoic acid, camphor, and anise oil. Morphine increases the muscular tone of the intestinal tract, decreases digestive secretions, and inhibits normal peristalsis. The slowed passage of the feces through the intestines promotes desiccation, which is a function of the time the feces spend in the intestine.

Uses Acute diarrhea.

Contraindications See Morphine, p. 474. Do not use in patients with diarrhea caused by poisoning until toxic substance has been eliminated.

Untoward Reactions See Morphine, p. 474.

Drug Interactions See Narcotic Analgesics, p. 474.

Dosage PO, adult: 5–10 ml 1 to 4 times daily (4 ml contains 1.6 mg of morphine). **Pediatric**: 0.25–0.5 ml/kg after each loose stool.

Administration/Storage

1. Give paregoric with water to ensure that it will reach stomach.
2. Mixture of paregoric and water will have milky appearance.
3. Store in light-resistant container.

Nursing Implications

1. Assess patient on prolonged use for signs of physical dependence. Even though paregoric contains relatively little morphine, its long-term use may lead to dependence.
2. Read the order, the medicine card and the label of the bottle carefully to ensure that correct medication is being administered. This is extremely important because opium tincture contains 25 times more morphine than paregoric.
3. Preparations containing paregoric are subject to the Controlled Substances Act, and must be charted accordingly.
4. Have naloxone (Narcan) on hand in case of overdosage.
5. *Teach patients and/or family*
   a. to adhere to regimen prescribed by physician.
   b. when diarrhea has abated, check with physician for further instructions. Continued use of drug may result in constipation.

LOCAL AGENTS

General Statement These are only moderately successful in the treatment of diarrhea, and their mode of action is not completely understood. The local agents consist of inert, nonabsorbable material, such as kaolin, charcoal, or bismuth. The individual particles of these preparations have large surface areas that are believed to adsorb fluid and toxic substances.

Some locally acting antidiarrheal agents, such as kaolin and pectin, have demulcent properties that can protect the irritated, inflamed walls of the intestine. Many nonprescription antidiarrheal preparations consist of a mixture of several locally acting agents. See Table 28, p. 661.

Contraindications Pseudomembranous enterocolitis, toxigenic bacteria-induced diarrhea, in the presence of high fever, in children less than 3 years of age unless approved by physician.

Untoward Reactions Prolonged use may result in constipation or interfere with the proper absorption of nutrients.

Administration Local agents should not be given for more than 2 days.

Nursing Implications

1. Maintain a daily record indicating the frequency, character, and number of stools.
2. Analyze the stool record to evaluate the patient's response to medication.
3. Be alert to increased diarrhea or development of constipation, because either may require dosage adjustment.

(*continued on page 663*)

TABLE 28   LOCALLY ACTING ANTIDIARRHEAL AGENTS

Drug	Main Use	Dosage	Remarks
Bismuth subgallate (Devrom), OTC	Antidiarrheal.	**PO:** 200–400 mg t.i.d. with meals.	Also has antacid and demulcent properties. Chew or swallow tablets whole.
Bismuth subsalicylate (Pepto-Bismol), OTC	Antidiarrheal, nausea, indigestion, relief of flatulence and cramps. *Investigational:* Prophylaxis and treatment of traveler's diarrhea.	**PO. Adults:** 2 tablets or 30 ml. **Pediatric, 3–6 years:** ½ tablet or 5 ml; **6–12 years:** 1 tablet or 10 ml.	*Drug Interactions* 1. The salicylate may increase the effect of anticoagulants and sulfonylureas. 2. The salicylate may interfere with the activity of drugs used to treat gout. *Administration* 1. Dose may be repeated q 30–60 min for a total of 8 doses in 24 hr. 2. May cause short-term darkening of the tongue and stools.
Charcoal, activated (CharcolantiDote, Liquid-Antidose), OTC	Emergency treatment of drug poisoning.	**PO. Adults: initial,** 1 gm/kg or 30–100 gm. Mix with 6–8 oz water to form a slurry.	Most valuable single agent for emergency treatment of certain cases of drug poisoning. Part of universal antidote. *Contraindications* Poisoning by cyanide, mineral acids, or alkalis. *Drug Interactions* Charcoal will adsorb and inactivate laxatives and Syrup of Ipecac. *Administration* 1. If induction of emesis is appropriate, do so prior to administration of charcoal. 2. Charcoal should only be given to conscious patients.
Cholestyramine resin (Cuemid, Questran), Rx	See *Hypocholesterolemics*, p. 360.		

TABLE 28 (Continued)

Drug	Main Use	Dosage	Remarks
Donnagel, OTC	Symptomatic treatment of diarrhea.	**Initial**, 30 ml, **then** 15–30 ml q 3 hr. **Infants weighing 10 lb:** 2.5 ml; **20 lb:** 5 ml; **30 lb and over:** 5–10 ml q 3 hr.	Mixture of kaolin, pectin and 3 anticholinergics (atropine, scopolamine, hyoscyamine). For contraindications, etc., see individual agents.
Donnagel-PG, Rx or OTC	Same as Donnagel	Same as Donnagel	Same content as Donnagel plus powdered opium, 24 mg.
Kaolin with pectin (Kaopectate, **Kapectolin, K-Pek**), OTC	Symptomatic relief of diarrhea	**PO. Adults:** 60–120 ml after each bowel movement. **Pediatric, over 12 years:** 60 ml; **6–12 years:** 30–60 ml/dose; **3–6 years:** 15–30 ml/dose.	Kaolin is a clay consisting of aluminum silicate, mainly effective in small intestine. The product contains 5.85 gm kaolin and 130 mg pectin/30 ml.
Lactobacillus cultures (Bacid, DoFus, Lactinex), OTC	Treatment of diarrhea including antibiotic-induced diarrhea.	*Bacid:* 2 capsules 2–4 times/day taken with meals. *Lactinex:* 4 tablets or 1 packet (1 gm) 3–4 times/day with food, milk, juice, or water. *DoFus:* 1 capsule with water before meals.	These bacterial cultures apparently help restore the normal intestinal flora after use of antimicrobial drugs and suppress emergence of some pathogenic staphylococci and *Candida*.
Parepectolin, OTC or Rx	Antidiarrheal.	**PO, adults:** 15–30 ml; **pediatric:** 2.5–10 ml. Dose given after evacuation up to a maximum of 4 doses in 12 hr.	Mixture contains pectin, kaolin, and opium (15 mg). See Kaolin with Pectin.

4. *Teach patient and/or family*
   a. that compliance with the regimen prescribed by the physician is essential for control of diarrhea. Highly spiced foods and foods high in fat should be eliminated from the diet of patient suffering from diarrhea.
   b. (parents of infants and young children under 5 years of age) to consult a doctor rather than to administer antidiarrheal medications on their own because children are more susceptible to the consequences of severe fluid and electrolyte depletion.
   c. to stop taking medication once diarrhea is controlled or constipation will result.
   d. to consult physician should several doses of medication prove ineffective in controlling diarrhea.

Chapter Fifty-six

EMETICS/ANTIEMETICS

EMETICS

General Statement Emetics are used in cases of acute poisoning to induce vomiting when it is desirable to empty the stomach promptly and completely after ingestion of toxic materials.

Vomiting can be elicited either by direct action on the chemoreceptor trigger zone (CTZ) in the medulla, or by indirect stimulation of the GI tract. Some agents act in both ways.

Nursing Implications

1. Do not administer an emetic if patient is comatose or semiconscious, has taken a convulsant poison, such as strychnine, or has ingested a corrosive substance like a strong acid or caustic, or petroleum distillates like kerosene.
2. Have on hand the following for the treatment of poison ingestion: gastric lavage equipment, oxygen, positive pressure apparatus, emergency drugs, and intravenous equipment and fluids.
3. Position the patient on side after administration of emetic to prevent aspiration when patient vomits.
4. Have available 200–300 ml of water at time of administration as emetics are usually administered with water.

APOMORPHINE HYDROCHLORIDE   (Rx)

Classification   Emetic.

Action/Kinetics   Apomorphine is a synthetic derivative of morphine. It produces emesis by stimulating the CTZ. **Onset after SC administration:** 5–15 min. Not effective if given orally.

Use   Emergency use in drug overdose and in certain poisonings.

Contraindications   Shock, drug-induced CNS depression, ingestion of corrosive substances, petroleum distillates, and lye and for patients sensitive to morphine. Use with caution in patients with cardiac decompensation and in children and debilitated persons.

Untoward Reactions   *CNS:* Depression, euphoria, restlessness, tremors. *Other:* Tachypnea, cardiovascular collapse.

Overdosage may result in excessive emesis, cardiac depression, and death.

Dosage   **SC: Adults,** 2–10 mg; **pediatric:** 0.1 mg/kg. **Do not repeat.**

Administration/Storage

1. Before administration, give the patient 300 ml of water.
2. Do not use solutions with emerald-green hue, indicating that drug has disintegrated.
3. Store solution in the dark in a closed container.

Additional Nursing Implications

See also *Nursing Implications*, above.

1. Patient should drink 200–300 ml water immediately before injection.
2. Assess for respiratory distress for at least 1 hour after administration of apomorphine as it may depress the respiratory center.
3. Chart apomorphine given in Narcotic Book in compliance with the Controlled Substances Act.

IPECAC SYRUP   (Rx: 2% Syrup; OTC: 1.5% Syrup)

Classification   Emetic.

Action/Kinetics   The active principle of ipecac, an alkaloid extracted from Brazil root, acts both locally on the gastric mucosa and centrally on the chemoreceptor trigger zone. Vomiting occurs within 15 to 60 minutes in 90% of all patients. In contrast with apomorphine, a second dose may be given if necessary. **Ipecac syrup must not be confused with ipecac fluid extract, which is 14 times as strong.**

Syrup of ipecac can be purchased without a prescription. It has been abused by patients suffering from bulemia.

Uses   Oral poisoning or drug overdose. Expectorant.

Contraindications   With corrosives or in individuals who are unconscious, semi-comatose, severely inebriated or in shock. Infants under six months of age.

Drug Interactions   Activated charcoal adsorbs ipecac syrup thus decreasing its effect.

Dosage   **PO. Syrup. Adults and children over 5 years:** 15–30 ml followed by 360 ml water; **pediatric, 1–5 years:** 15 ml preceded or followed by 240 ml water; **pediatric, 9–11 months:**   10 ml preceded or followed by 120–240 ml water; **pediatric, 6–8 months:** 5 ml.

Administration

1. Check label of medication closely so that the syrup and the fluid extract are not confused.
2. Dosage may be repeated once if vomiting does not occur within 30 min. Gastric lavage should be considered if vomiting does not occur within 15 minutes after the second dose.

Nursing Implications

Teach patient and/or family

a. to purchase ipecac syrup to have available in case of accidental poisoning.

b. the important difference in dosage when drug is used as an expectorant or as an emetic and teach appropriate method of administration.

ANTIEMETICS

General Statement   Nausea and vomiting can be caused by a great variety of conditions, such as infections, drugs, radiation, motion, organic disease, or psychological factors. The underlying cause for the symptoms must be elicited before emesis is corrected.

The act of vomiting is complex. The vomiting center in the medulla responds to stimulation from many peripheral areas as well as to stimuli from the CNS itself, CTZ, vestibular apparatus of the ear, and the cerebral cortex.

The selection of an antiemetic depends on the cause of the symptoms as well as on the manner in which the vomiting is triggered.

Many drugs used for other conditions, such as the antihistamines, phenothiazines, barbiturates and scopolamine, have antiemetic properties and can be so used. (For details see appropriate sections.) These agents often have serious side effects (mostly CNS depression) that make their routine use undesirable. Several miscellaneous antiemetics are treated here.

Drug Interaction Because of their antiemetic and antinauseant activity, the antiemetics may mask overdosage caused by other drugs.

Nursing Implications
1. Assess for other untoward symptoms beside nausea since antiemetic may mask signs of overdosage of other drugs or pathology, such as increased intracranial pressure or intestinal obstruction.
2. Caution the patient against driving or performing hazardous tasks until individual response to the drug has been evaluated. Antiemetics tend to cause drowsiness and dizziness.

BENZQUINAMIDE HYDROCHLORIDE   Emete-Con (Rx)

Classification Antiemetic.

Action/Kinetics This drug has antiemetic, antihistaminic, anticholinergic, and sedative properties. It is a benzoquinoline derivative. **Onset:** rapid (15 min after parenteral administration). t½: 40 min. **Duration of effect:** 3–4 hr. Metabolized in liver, excreted in kidneys.

Uses Prevention and treatment of nausea during anesthesia and surgery.

Contraindications Hypersensitivity to drug. Pregnancy; children under 12 years of age. IV for cardiac patients.

Untoward Reactions *CNS:* Drowsiness, insomnia, restlessness, headache, excitement, nervousness. *GI:* Dry mouth, hiccoughs, salivation, anorexia, nausea. *CV:* Hypertension, hypotension, dizziness, arrhythmias especially after IV use. *Other:* Shivering, sweating, flushing, blurred vision, hyperthermia, muscle twitching/ tremors, urticaria, skin rashes.

Drug Interaction Use lower dose of benzquinamide in patients receiving epinephrine-like drugs or pressor agents.

Dosage   IM: 50 mg or 0.5–1 mg/kg. May be repeated after 1 hr, **then** q 3 to 4 hr. **IV:** 25 mg or 0.2–0.4 mg/kg. Inject slowly (½ to 1 minute); switch to **IM** after one **IV** dose.

Administration/Storage
1. Reconstituted solution stable for 14 days at room temperature.
2. Store solution and unreconstituted powder in light-resistant containers.
3. For prophylaxis give 15 minutes prior to when patient is expected to regain consciousness from anesthesia.

BUCLIZINE HYDROCHLORIDE   Bucladin-S (Rx)

Classification Antiemetic, antihistamine.

Action/Kinetics Buclizine is a piperazine-type antihistamine that primarily suppresses nausea and vomiting through an action on the CNS. **Duration:** 4–6 hr.

Uses Nausea, vomiting, dizziness of motion sickness, Ménière's syndrome, labyrinthitis.

Contraindications Hypersensitivity to drug, pregnancy. Safe use in children not established.

Untoward Reactions Drowsiness, dryness of mouth, headache, nervousness.

Drug Interactions See *Antihistamines*, p. 625.

Dosage **PO: usual**, 50 mg alleviates nausea and prevents motion sickness. May be repeated after 4–6 hr. *Severe nausea*: up to 150 mg. **Maintenance**: 50 mg b.i.d.

Administration
1. Take 30 minutes before departure.
2. Tablet can be chewed, swallowed whole, or dissolved in mouth.

CYCLIZINE HYDROCHLORIDE   Marezine (Rx: Injection; OTC: Tablets)

See *Antihistamines*, p. 628.

Classification Antiemetic, antihistamine.

Action/Kinetics Antiemetic effect due to action on the chemoreceptor trigger zone and reduction of sensitivity of the labyrinthine apparatus.

Dosage **PO.** *Antiemetic*, adults: 50 mg q 4–6 hr, not to exceed 200 mg/day; **pediatric, 6–10 years**: ½ the adult dose up to t.i.d. **IM. Adults**: 50 mg q 4 to 6 hrs.

DIMENHYDRINATE   Calm X, Dimentabs, Dinate, Dommanate, Dramaban, Dramamine, Dramilin, Dramocen, Dramoject, Dymenate, Hydrate, Marmine, Motion-Aid, Reidamine, Wehamine (Rx and OTC)

Remarks Dimenhydrinate consists of both diphenhydramine and chlorotheophylline. Also, see *Antihistamines*, p. 628.

Dosage **PO. Adults**: 50–100 mg q 4 hr not to exceed 400 mg/day; **pediatric, 6–12 years**: 25–50 mg q 6–8 hr not to exceed 150 mg/day; **pediatric, 2–6 years**: 25 mg q 6–8 hr not to exceed 75 mg/day. **IM. Adults**: 50 mg as necessary; **pediatric, 8–12 years**: 1.25 mg/kg up to 300 mg/day. **IV. Adults**: 50 mg in 10-ml sodium chloride injection given over a 2-min period.

DIPHENHYDRAMINE HYDROCHLORIDE   Benadryl, Fenylhist, Valdrene, Others (Rx)

See *Antihistamines*, Table 26, p. 628.

DIPHENIDOL HYDROCHLORIDE   Vontrol (Rx)

Classification Antiemetic.

Action/Kinetics Diphenidol appears to depress labyrinth excitability and may also depress the chemoreceptor trigger zone. The drug is well absorbed from GI tract.

Peak plasma concentrations: 1.5–3 hr. **Onset: PO**, 30–45 min; **IM**, 15 min. **Duration**: 4– 6 hr; **t½**: 4 hr. Metabolized, slowly excreted in urine.

Uses   Nausea, vomiting, and vertigo associated with infectious diseases, malignancies, radiation sickness, general anesthesia, motion sickness, labyrinthitis, and Ménière's disease.

Contraindications   Hypersensitivity to drug, anuria, pregnancy, infants under 6 months or weighing less than 25 pounds. Administer with caution to patients with glaucoma, pyloric stenosis, pylorospasm, obstructive lesions of GI and urinary tract, and sinus tachycardia.

Untoward Reactions   *CNS:* Confusion, disorientation, hallucinations; discontinue drug immediately if any of these symptoms occur. Also, drowsiness, malaise, headache, nervousness, excitation, sleep disturbances, weakness. *GI:* Dry mouth, GI irritation, nausea, indigestion, heartburn. *Other:* Skin rash, urticaria, mild jaundice, slight hypotension.

Symptoms of overdosage should be treated symptomatically with assurance that blood pressure and respiration are maintained. Gastric lavage may be indicated in oral overdosage.

Dosage   PO. Adults: 25–50 mg q 4 hr. **Pediatric.** *Nausea and vomiting only:* 0.4 mg/lb no more often than q 4 hr not to exceed 2.5 mg/lb/day. If symptoms persist after the first dose, a second dose can be given after 1 hr.

Nursing Implications

1. *Assess*
   a. for hallucinations, disorientation, and confusion (especially within first 3 days of starting medication.) Withhold drug and report to physician.
   b. for masking of symptoms related to undiagnosed pathology or toxicity.
   c. intake and output. Report oliguria, which interferes with excretion of drug.
2. Be prepared in case of overdosage to assist with gastric lavage, monitor BP and respiration, and provide supportive measures such as oxygen or mechanical respiration.
3. *Teach patient and/or family*
   a. the necessity for hospitalization or close medical supervision when drug is used.
   b. to withhold drug and report to doctor if untoward CNS symptoms are noted.
   c. not to drive a car or operate other hazardous machinery as drug may cause blurred vision and/or dizziness.

HYDROXYZINE   Atarax, Vistaril (Rx)

See *Antianxiety Agents*, Chapter 31.

MECLIZINE   Antivert, Antivert/25, Bonine, Dizmiss, Motion Cure, Wehvert (Rx and OTC)

See *Antishitamines*, p. 629.

Dosage   PO. *Motion sickness*: 25–50 mg 1 hr prior to travel; repeat dosage daily, if necessary. *Vertigo*: 25–100 mg daily in divided doses.

PHOSPHORATED CARBOHYDRATE SOLUTION   Calm-X, Eazol, Emetrol, Especol, Nausetrol (OTC)

Classification   Antiemetic.

Remark   This preparation is a low-cost, mint-flavored. concentrated carbohydrate syrup with phosphoric acid.

Action   This is a hyperosmolar carbohydrate solution with phosphoric acid. Claimed to relieve nausea and vomiting by direct action on the GI wall leading to a delay in gastric emptying time and a decrease in contraction of smooth muscles.

Uses   Symptomatic relief of nausea and vomiting due to a variety of causes, including vomiting due to psychogenic factors, morning sickness, nausea or vomiting due to drug therapy, and regurgitation in infants.

Contraindications   Diabetes, fructose intolerance.

Dosage   *Morning sickness:* 15–30 ml on arising and q 3 hr thereafter if necessary. *Vomiting due to psychogenic factors:* **Adults,** 15–30 ml at 15 min intervals until vomiting subsides or until 5 doses have been taken; **pediatric,** 5–10 ml at 15 min intervals in same manner as adults. *Motion sickness, vomiting due to drug therapy, inhalation anesthesia:* **Adults and older children:** 15 ml; **young children:** 5 ml. *Regurgitation in infants:* 5–10 ml, 10–15 min before feeding (for refractory cases: 10–15 ml 30 min before feeding).

Administration

1. *Do not* dilute.
2. Do not allow liquids PO for 15 min after administration.
3. In case of nausea, repeat at 15 min intervals until condition is under control.
4. Regurgitating infants: 10 to 15 minutes before each feeding; refractory cases: 10–15 ml ½ hr before feeding.
5. Morning sickness: On arising and q 3 hr thereafter or when nausea threatens.

Nursing Implications

1. Do not administer this concentrated carbohydrate solution to a diabetic.
2. Anticipate that this emetic will not cause toxicity, side effects, or mask symptoms of organic disease.

PROCHLORPERAZINE   Compazine (Rx)

PROCHLORPERAZINE EDISYLATE   Compazine Edisylate (Rx)

PROCHLORPERAZINE MALEATE   Compazine Maleate (Rx)

See *Phenothiazines*, p. 408.

Uses   Postoperative nausea and vomiting, radiation sickness, vomiting due to toxins. Generally not used for patients weighing less than 20 pounds or under 2 yrs of age.

Dosage   *Severe nausea/vomiting in adults.* **PO:** 5–10 mg t.i.d.–q.i.d. or sustained release: 15 mg on arising or 10 mg q 12 hr. **IM:** 5–10 mg q 3–4 hr not to exceed 40 mg/day. **Rectal:** 25 mg b.i.d.

Severe nausea/vomiting in children. **PO, rectal: 20–29 lb:** 2.5 mg 1–2 times daily not to exceed 7.5 mg daily; **30–39 lb:** 2.5 mg b.i.d.–t.i.d. not to exceed 10 mg daily; **40–85 lb:** 2.5 mg t.i.d. or 5 mg b.i.d. not to exceed 15 mg daily. **IM:** 0.13 mg/kg (usually only one dose is needed).

Severe nausea/vomiting in adults undergoing surgery. **IM:** 5–10 mg 1–2 hr before anesthesia or following surgery (may be repeated once). **IV:** 5–10 mg 15–30 min before anesthesia or following surgery (may be repeated once). *IV infusion:* 20 mg/liter of isotonic solution added 15–30 min before anesthesia. Total daily dose should not exceed 40 mg.

SCOPOLAMINE HYDROBROMIDE (Rx and OTC)

See *Anticholinergics*, Chapter 47.

THIETHYLPERAZINE MALEATE   Torecan Maleate (Rx)

Classification   Antiemetic.

Action/Kinetics   Phenothiazine derivative that acts on both the chemoreceptor trigger zone and the vomiting center. **Onset, PO:** 30 min. **Duration:** 4 hr. For details, see *Phenothiazines*, p. 401.

Uses   Control of nausea and vomiting of various origins. Possibly effective to treat vertigo.

Contraindications   Severe CNS depression, comatose states, pregnancy, children under 12 years of age. Administer with caution to patients with liver or kidney disease. IV use (causes hypotension).

Untoward Reactions   Drowsiness, dryness of mouth and nose, restlessness, hypotension, extrapyramidal complications.

Dosage   PO, rectal, IM: 10–30 mg 1 to 3 times daily. Do not use **IV**. Dosage for children not established.

Administration   Administer by deep IM injection.

Additional Nursing Implications

See also *Nursing Implications*, p. 666. Review *General Statement* and *Nursing Implications* for phenothiazines, p. 404.

1. Do not administer to a patient performing hazardous tasks, or to a patient with depressed respiratory rate, or in a comatose state.
2. Assess for postural hypotension manifested by weakness, dizziness, and faintness. Monitor BP.
3. Have available levarterenol and phenylephrine should hypotension occur because epinephrine is contraindicated.
4. Assess for extrapyramidal symptoms, such as torticollis, dysphagia, random movements of the eyes, or convulsions.
5. Have available caffeine sodium benzoate and diphenhydramine hydrochloride (Benadryl) IV for relief of extrapyramidal symptoms.

TRIMETHOBENZAMIDE HYDROCHLORIDE   Tegamide, Tigan (Rx)

Classification   Antiemetic.

General Statement   Trimethobenzamide is an antiemetic related to the antihistamines but with weak antihistaminic properties. The drug is less effective than the phenothiazines but has fewer side effects. Not suitable as sole agent for severe emesis. Can be used rectally.

Action/Kinetics   Trimethobenzamide appears to control vomiting by depressing the chemoreceptor trigger zone of the medulla. **Onset: PO and IM**, 10–40 min. **Duration**: 3–4 hr. 30–50% of drug excreted unchanged in urine in 48–72 hr.

Uses   Emesis during surgery, radiation-induced nausea, and vomiting; pregnancy.

Contraindications   Hypersensitivity to drug, and when suppositories are used, to benzocaine. Do not use suppositories for neonates; do not use IM in children. Use with caution in pregnancy and lacatation.

Untoward Reactions   *CNS:* Depression of mood, disorientation, headache, drowsiness, dizziness, seizures, coma. *Other:* Hypersensitivity reactions, hypotension, Parkinson-like symptoms, blood dyscrasias, jaundice, muscle cramps, opisthotonos, blurred vision. *After IM injection:* Pain, burning, stinging, redness at injection site.

Drug Interactions   Concomitant use with atropine-like drugs and CNS depressants including alcohol should be avoided.

Dosage   **PO. Adults**: 250 mg t.i.d.–q.i.d.; **pediatric, 30–90 lb**: 100–200 mg t.i.d.– q.i.d. **Rectal. Adults**: 200 mg t.i.d.–q.i.d.; **pediatric, under 30 lb**: 100 mg t.i.d.– q.i.d.; **30 to 90 lb**: 100–200 mg t.i.d.–q.i.d. **IM only. Adults**: 200 mg t.i.d.–q.i.d. (IM route not to be used in children).

Administration   Inject drug IM deeply into the upper outer quadrant of the gluteus muscle and be careful to avoid escape of fluid from needle so as to minimize local reaction.

Additional Nursing Implications
See also *Nursing Implications*, p. 666.

1. Assess for skin reaction, the first sign of hypersensitivity to drug.
2. Do not administer suppositories to patients allergic to benzocaine or similar local anesthetics.
3. Ask the patient whether there is any local reaction to suppositories.

Chapter Fifty-seven

DIGESTANTS

General Statement Digestants are agents that replace or supplement one of the many enzymes or other chemical substances that participate in the digestion of food. They are rarely indicated for therapeutic reasons but may be required for elderly patients or those suffering from certain deficiency diseases of the GI tract. They may also be required after GI surgery.

Commonly used digestants include hydrochloric acid, bile salts, and the enzymes produced by the stomach and glands associated with digestion.

Nonprescription preparations also contain many of the same ingredients as prescription drugs; however, these are usually present at levels too low to be effective.

DEHYDROCHOLIC ACID Atrocholin, Cholan DH, Decholin, Dycholium,* Hepahydrin, Neocholan (Rx and OTC)

Classification Digestant, laxative.

Action/Kinetics Dehydrocholic acid is a derivative of bile acids. The drug has some laxative effect and appears to increase the flow of bile and facilitate evacuation of the gall bladder. Also, there is increased emulsification and absorption of fats.

Uses Various conditions involving the biliary tract including recent or repeated surgery for biliary calculi or strictures, cholecystitis, cholangitis, biliary dyskinesia, to promote drainage of an infected bile duct, bile duct obstruction. Laxative.

Contraindications Complete obstruction of the biliary, GI, or genitourinary tracts. Also, hepatic insufficiency, jaundice, cholelithiasis. In presence of abdominal pain, nausea, or vomiting (i.e., symptoms of appendicitis). Use with caution in patients with a history of asthma and allergies as well as in children under 6 years, the elderly, and in prostatic hypertrophy.

Dosage **PO**: 250–500 mg b.i.d.–t.i.d. after meals for 4 to 6 weeks. Bile salts may be given concomitantly. Discontinue drug if no improvement is noted after 4 to 6 weeks.

Nursing Implications

1. Check that skin test was done on patients with a history of allergy or asthma before injection of dehydrocholic acid.
2. Have epinephrine available in case of allergic response to IV administration of drug.

3. Assess after IV injection for extravasation into the perivascular tissue because pain, redness, and swelling may occur. Report and apply warm compresses should extravasation occur.
4. Instruct patient who will be taking medication at home to consult the physician if pain persists or if severe nausea and pain develop.
5. Be prepared to assist the physician in determining circulation time, defined as the time it takes from injection of the drug into the antecubital vein until the patient perceives a bitter taste that passes from the base of the tongue to its tip. The range of normal values is 8 to 16 seconds.

GLUTAMIC ACID HYDROCHLORIDE   Acidulin (OTC)

Classification Digestant.

Action/Kinetics On contact with water this compound releases hydrochloric acid, which acidifies the stomach. Thus, the drug has the same effect as hydrochloric acid but is easier to administer because it comes in capsule form. Also available combined with pepsin.

Uses Hypochlorhydria, achlorhydria, as an adjunct in pernicious anemia or gastric cancer, certain allergies, chronic gastritis.

Contraindications Hyperacidity and peptic ulcer.

Untoward Reaction An overdose may result in systemic acidosis.

Dosage **PO**: 1–3 tablets (325 mg) or capsules (340 mg) t.i.d. before meals.
   Note: 340 mg contains about 1.8 mEq hydrochloric acid.

Nursing Implications
Teach patient and/or family
   a. to keep capsules dry before ingesting.
   b. the symptoms of systemic acidosis, such as stupor, weakness, and deep rapid breathing.
   c. to have available sodium bicarbonate or sodium lactate or other alkaline solution to treat overdosage.

HYDROCHLORIC ACID, DILUTED

Classification Digestant.

Action/Kinetics Replacement of naturally occurring substance by diluted hydrochloric acid (10% w/v).

Uses Hypochlorhydria, hydrochloric acid deficiency often occurring in the elderly (is frequently associated with pernicious anemia or gastric cancer).

Contraindications Hyperacidity and peptic ulcer.

Untoward Reactions Prolonged administration may disturb electrolyte balance (depletion of sodium bicarbonate) and increase the levels of sodium chloride.

Dosage PO: Administer 2–8 ml of a 10% solution copiously diluted. Dilute each milliliter with at least 25 ml of water.

Nursing Implications
Teach patient and/or family
   a. to sip medication with meal through a straw to protect tooth enamel (do not use a metal straw).
   b. to use an alkaline mouth wash if ingestion of hydrochloric acid solution will not be completed until after the meal.

OX BILE EXTRACT (BILE SALTS) Bilron (OTC)

Classification Digestant.

Action/Kinetics Natural dried extract of ox bile, which allegedly increases the flow of bile as well as exerting a laxative effect. Effectiveness has not been shown, however.

Uses Bile deficiency states. Laxative.

Contraindications Complete mechanical biliary obstruction. If symptoms of appendicitis are present (i.e., nausea, vomiting, abdominal pain). Use with caution in patients with obstructive jaundice.

Untoward Reactions Nausea, vomiting, diarrhea, and cramping.

Dosage PO. Administer 150–600 mg.

Administration
   1. Teach patient not to chew tablets because they are bitter.
   2. Take with water with or after meals.

PANCREATIN Viokase (OTC)

Classification Digestant.

Action/Kinetics This mixture of enzymes (mainly lipase, amylase, and trypsin) is obtained from hog pancreas. The preparation increases digestion, or predigestion of food.

Uses Pancreatic deficiency diseases such as pancreatitis, cystic fibrosis of the pancreas, pancreatectomy.

Contraindications Give with caution to patients sensitive to hog protein. Use with caution in pregnancy and lactation.

Untoward Reactions *Allergic:* Rash, sneezing, lacrimation. Inhalation of the powder may cause irritation of the nasal mucosa and bronchospasms in sensitive individuals. Holding the tablets in the mouth may cause ulceration and stomatitis. High doses may cause hyperuricemia and hyperuricosuria.

Dosage PO. *Tablets:* 1–3 with meals. *Powder:* 0.75 gm mixed with food.

Administration

1. Advise patient to swallow and not chew tablets.
2. Do not administer granules alone as the enzymes would be destroyed.
3. Sprinkle granules on food or add to milk or water for those unable to swallow capsules.
4. Do not give with hot foods.

Nursing Implications
1. Check that the patient maintains diet ordered.
2. Assess for constipation and anorexia indicating overdosage.

PANCRELIPASE   Cotazym, Cotazym-S, Ilozyme, Ku-Zyme-HP, Pancrease, Viokase (Rx and OTC)

Classification   Digestant.

Action/Kinetics   Enzyme concentrate from hog pancreas containing lipase (mainly), amylase, and protease, which replace or supplement naturally occurring enzymes.

Uses   Replacement therapy in symptomatic relief of malabsorption syndromes caused by pancreatic deficiency of organic origin as in cystic fibrosis of pancreas, cancer of the pancreas, and chronic inflammation of the pancreas.

Contraindications   Give with caution to patients hypersensitive to hog protein. Use with caution in pregnancy.

Untoward Reactions   *CNS:* Nausea, diarrhea, cramping. Inhalation of the powder is irritating to the skin and mucous membranes. High doses may cause hyperuricemia and hyperuricosuria.

Dosage   **PO:** dosage should be calculated according to fat content of diet. Approximately 300 mg/17 gm dietary fat. Usually the dose is 1–3 tablets or capsules at each meal or 1 with each snack (may be increased to 8 if no GI side effects occur). The dose of powder is 1–2 packets before meals or snacks.

Administration

1. Pediatric: for young children the contents of the capsule can be sprinkled on food. After several weeks of use, dosage should be adjusted according to therapeutic results.
2. Unopened preparations should be stored in tight containers at a temperature not to exceed 25° C.

Nursing Implication
Check that patient maintains prescribed diet.

HORMONES AND HORMONE ANTAGONISTS

Chapter Fifty-eight

INSULIN, ORAL ANTIDIABETICS, AND INSULIN ANTAGONISTS

INSULINS

General Statement   In 1922, the isolation of the hormone insulin, which is naturally produced by the islets of Langerhans in the pancreas, marked the beginning of hormone therapy in individuals who manifest deficient insulin secretion and thus may be diagnosed as having diabetes mellitus. Diabetes mellitus is classified as insulin dependent (Type I; formerly referred to as juvenile-onset) and noninsulin dependent (Type II; formerly referred to as maturity-onset).

There are three sources of commercial insulin to treat Type I diabetes: insulin isolated from cattle or hog pancreas, and human insulin either made semisynthetically or derived from recombinant DNA. The structure of insulin from pork sources more closely resembles human insulin than that from beef sources.

Proinsulin still remains the major impurity in insulin products. Such impurities lead to local or systemic allergic reactions as well as antibody-mediated insulin resistance. In recent years, however, technology has improved so that insulin preparations currently marketed in the United States do not contain more than 25 parts per million (ppm) of proinsulin. Insulin products that contain between 20 and 25 ppm of proinsulin are referred to as "single peak" insulins while those products which contain 10 ppm or less of proinsulin are referred to as "purified insulins."

Insulin preparations having different times of onset, peak activity, and duration of action have been developed. Such products are prepared by precipitating insulin in the presence of zinc chloride to form zinc insulin crystals and/or combining insulin with a protein such as protamine. Based on these modifications, insulin products are classified as fast-acting, intermediate-acting, and long-acting. These preparations permit the physician to select the preparation best suited to the lifestyle of the patient.

RAPID-ACTING INSULIN

1. Insulin injection (Regular Insulin, Crystalline Zinc Insulin, Unmodified Insulin)
2. Prompt insulin zinc suspension (Semilente)

INTERMEDIATE-ACTING INSULIN

1. Isophane insulin suspension (NPH)
2. Insulin zinc suspension (Lente)

LONG-ACTING INSULIN

1. Protamine zinc insulin suspension (PZI)
2. Extended insulin zinc suspension (Ultralente)

Note: Insulin preparations with various times of onset and duration of action are often mixed to obtain optimum control of diabetic patients.

Action/Kinetics   Insulin facilitates the transport of glucose into cardiac and skeletal muscle and adipose tissue. It also increases synthesis of glycogen in the liver. Insulin stimulates protein synthesis and lipogenesis and inhibits lipolysis and release of free fatty acids from fat cells. This latter effect prevents or reverses ketoacidosis sometimes observed in the diabetic. Insulin also causes intracellular shifts in magnesium and potassium.

Since insulin is a protein, it is destroyed in the GI tract. Thus, it must be administered subcutaneously where it is readily absorbed into the bloodstream and distributed throughout the extracellular fluid. Insulin is metabolized mainly by the liver.

Uses   Replacement therapy in Type I diabetes; diabetic ketoacidosis. Insulin is also indicated in Type II diabetes when other measures have failed or in times of surgery, trauma, infection, fever, endocrine dysfunction, pregnancy, gangrene, Raynaud's disease, or kidney or liver dysfunction.

Regular insulin is used in IV hyperalimentation solutions, in IV dextrose to treat severe hyperkalemia, and IV as a provocative test for growth hormone secretion.

Diet   The dietary control of diabetes is as important as medication with appropriate drugs. The role of the nurse in teaching the patient how to eat properly cannot be underestimated.

As a first step the physician must determine the individual patient's dietary requirements. Since there is a very close relationship between carbohydrate (CHO), fat (F), and protein (P) intake of each of these nutrients must be regulated. The prescribed amount of CHO, P, and F eaten at each meal must remain constant.

The nurse must teach the patient how to calculate exchange values of various foods. Food lists and food-exchange values published by the American Diabetes Association and the American Dietetic Association are valuable teaching aids.

Diabetic patients should adhere to a regular meal schedule. Patients taking large amounts of insulin will frequently be better controlled when they have four to six small meals daily rather than three large ones. The frequency of meals and the overall caloric intake vary with the type of drug taken. Diabetic children may be on a less restricted diet, adjusting insulin dosage according to blood and urine glucose readings. Children with negative urine glucose tend to become hypoglycemic rapidly with exercise or decrease in appetite, and many physicians allow for glucose spilling.

Contraindication   Hypersensitivity to insulin.

Untoward Reactions   *Hypoglycemia*: Due to insulin overdose, delayed or decreased food intake, too much exercise in relationship to insulin dose, or when transferring from one preparation to another. Even carefully controlled patients occasionally develop signs of insulin overdosage characterized by hunger, weakness, fatigue, nervousness, pallor or flushing, profuse sweating, headache, palpitations, numbness of mouth, tingling in the fingers, tremors, blurred and double vision, hypothermia, excess yawning, mental confusion, incoordination, tachycardia, and loss of consciousness.

Symptoms of hypoglycemia may mimic psychic disturbances. Severe prolonged hypoglycemia may cause brain damage and in the elderly may mimic stroke.

Allergic: Urticaria, angioedema, lymphadenopathy, bullae, anaphylaxis. Occurs mostly following intermittent insulin therapy or IV administration of large doses to insulin-resistant patients. Antihistamines or corticosteroids may be used to treat these symptoms. Patients who are highly allergic to insulin and cannot be treated with oral hypoglycemics may respond to human insulin products.

At site of injection: Swelling, stinging, redness, itching, warmth. These symptoms often disappear with continued use. Atrophy or hypertrophy of subcutaneous fat tissue (minimize by rotating site of injection).

Insulin resistance: Usual cause is obesity. Acute resistance may occur following infections, trauma, surgery, emotional disturbances, or other endocrine disorders.

Ophthalmologic: Blurred vision, transient presbyopia. Occurs mainly during initiation of therapy or in patients who have been uncontrolled for a long period of time.

Hyperglycemic rebound (Somogyi effect): Usually in patients who receive chronic overdosage.

DIFFERENTIATION BETWEEN DIABETIC COMA AND HYPOGLYCEMIC REACTION (INSULIN SHOCK)

Coma in diabetes may be caused by uncontrolled diabetes (high sugar content in blood or urine, ketoacidosis) or by too much insulin (insulin shock, hypoglycemia).

Diabetic coma and insulin shock can be differentiated in the following manner:

Diagnostic Feature	Hyperglycemia (Diabetic Coma)	Hypoglycemia (Insulin Shock)
Onset	Gradual (days)	Sudden (24–48 hours)
Medication	Insufficient insulin	Excess insulin
Food intake	Normal or excess	Probably too little
Overall appearance	Extremely ill	Very weak
Skin	Dry and flushed	Moist and pale
Infection	Frequent	Absent
Fever	Frequent	Absent
Mouth	Dry	Drooling
Thirst	Intense	Absent
Hunger	Absent	Occasional
Vomiting	Common	Absent
Abdominal pain	Frequent	Rare
Respiration	Increased, air hunger	Normal
Breath	Acetone odor	Normal
Blood pressure	Low	Normal
Pulse	Weak and rapid	Full and bounding
Vision	Dim	Diplopia
Tremor	Absent	Frequent
Convulsions	None	In late stages
Urine sugar	High	Absent in second specimen
Ketone bodies	High	Absent in second specimen
Blood sugar	High	Less than 60 mg/100 ml

Source: Adapted with permission from, *The Merck Manual*, Eleventh Edition.

Diabetic coma is usually precipitated by the patient's failure to take insulin. Hypoglycemia is often precipitated by the patient's unpredictable response, excess exertion, stress due to illness or surgery, errors in calculating dosage, or failure to eat.

TREATMENT OF DIABETIC COMA OR SEVERE ACIDOSIS   Administer 30 to 60 units of insulin. This is followed by doses of 20 units or more every 30 minutes. To avoid a hypoglycemic state, 1 gm of dextrose is administered for each unit of insulin given. Treatment is often supplemented by electrolytes and fluids. Urine samples are collected for analysis, and vital signs monitored as ordered.

TREATMENT OF HYPOGLYCEMIA (INSULIN SHOCK)   Mild hypoglycemia can be relieved by oral administration of carbohydrates such as orange juice, candy, or a lump of sugar. If the patient is comatose, adults may be given 10–30 ml of 50% dextrose solution IV; children should receive 0.5–1 ml/kg of 50% dextrose solution. Epinephrine, hydrocortisone, or glucagon may be used in severe cases to cause an increase in blood glucose.

Drug Interactions

Interactant	Interaction
Alcohol, ethyl	↑ Hypoglycemia → low blood sugar and shock
Anabolic steroids	↑ Hypoglycemic effect of insulin
Beta-adrenergic blocking agents	↑ Hypoglycemia due to insulin
Chlorthalidone	↓ Hypoglycemic effect of antidiabetics
Contraceptives, oral	↑ Dosage of antidiabetic due to impairment of glucose tolerance
Corticosteroids	↓ Effect of insulin due to corticosteroid-induced hyperglycemia
Dextrothyroxine	↓ Effect of insulin due to dextrothyroxine-induced hyperglycemia
Diazoxide	Diazoxide-induced hyperglycemia ↓ diabetic control
Digitalis glycosides	Use with caution, as insulin affects serum potassium levels
Epinephrine	↓ Effect of insulin due to epinephrine-induced hyperglycemia
Estrogens	↓ Effect of insulin due to impairment of glucose tolerance
Ethacrynic acid	↓ Hypoglycemic effect of antidiabetics
Fenfluramine	Additive hypoglycemic effects
Furosemide	↓ Hypoglycemic effect of antidiabetics
Glucagon	Glucagon-induced hyperglycemia ↓ effect of antidiabetics
Guanethidine	↑ Hypoglycemic effect of insulin
MAO inhibitors	MAO inhibitors ↑ and prolong hypoglycemic effect of antidiabetics
Oxytetracycline	↑ Effect of insulin
Phenothiazines	↑ Dosage of antidiabetic due to phenothiazine-induced hyperglycemia
Phenytoin	Phenytoin-induced hyperglycemia ↓ diabetic control

Interactant	Interaction
Propranolol	Propranolol inhibits rebound of blood glucose after insulin-induced hypoglycemia
Salicylates	↑ Effect of hypoglycemic effect of insulin
Tetracyclines	May ↑ hypoglycemic effect of insulin
Thiazide diuretics	↓ Hypoglycemic effect of antidiabetics
Thyroid preparations	↑ Dosage of antidiabetic due to thyroid-induced hyperglycemia
Triamterene	↓ Hypoglycemic effect of antidiabetic

Laboratory Test Interferences Alters liver function tests and thyroid function tests. False + Coombs' test, ↑ serum protein, ↓ serum amino acids, calcium, cholesterol, potassium, and urine amino acids.

Dosage Insulin is usually administered SC. Insulin injection (regular insulin) is the only preparation that may be administered IV. This route should only be used for patients with severe ketoacidosis or diabetic coma.

Dosage for insulin is always expressed in USP units.

Dosage is established and monitored by blood glucose, urine glucose, and acetone tests. Dosage is highly individualized. Furthermore, since the requirements of patients may change with time, dosage must be checked at regular intervals. It is usually advisable to hospitalize patients while their daily insulin and caloric requirements are being established.

In pregnancy, insulin requirements may increase suddenly during the last trimester. After delivery, there may be a sudden drop in requirement to prepregnancy levels. To prevent the development of hypoglycemia, insulin is often discontinued on the day of delivery and glucose is administered IV.

The various insulin preparations can be mixed to obtain the combination best suited for the individual patient. However, mixing must be done according to the directions received from the physician and/or pharmacist.

Administration/Storage

1. Read the product information brochure and any important notes inserted into package of prescribed insulin.
2. Discard open vials that have not been used for several weeks or any whose expiration date has passed.
3. Refrigerate stock supply of insulin but avoid freezing. Freezing destroys the manner in which insulin is suspended in the formulation.
4. Store insulin vial in a cool place avoiding extremes of temperature or exposure to sunlight.
5. The following guidelines should be followed with respect to mixing the various insulins:
   a. Regular insulin may be mixed with NPH, PZI, or lente insulins. However to avoid transfer of the longer-acting insulin into the regular insulin vial, regular insulin should be drawn into the syringe first.
   b. A mixture of regular insulin with NPH, lente, or PZI insulin should be administered within 15 minutes of mixing due to binding of regular insulin by excess protamine and/or zinc in the longer-acting preparations.
   c. Lente, semilente, or ultralente insulins may be mixed with each other in any proportion; however, these insulins should not be mixed with NPH or PZI insulins.
   d. When used in an insulin infusion pump, insulin may be mixed in any proportion with either 0.9% sodium chloride injection or water for injection.

Due to stability changes, such mixtures should be used within 24 hr of their preparation.

6. Store compatible mixtures of insulin for no longer than 1 month at room temperature or 3 months at 2°–8°C (36°–46°F). However, bacterial contamination may occur.

7. To ensure a constant amount of precipitate in each dose, invert the vial several times to mix before the material is withdrawn. Avoid vigorous shaking and frothing of the material. (Regular and globin insulin are the only two insulins that do not have a precipitate.)

8. Discard any vial in which the precipitate is clumped or granular in appearance or which has formed a solid deposit of particles on the side of the vial.

9. In order to prevent dosage error, do not alter the order of mixing insulins or change the model or brand of syringe or needle.

10. Administer at a 90-degree angle when using a ½-inch needle and a 45-degree angle when using a 5/8-inch needle for injection.

11. Provide an automatic injector for patients who are fearful of injecting themselves.

12. Assist the visually impaired diabetic to obtain information and devices for self-administration of insulin by writing to: New York Diabetes Association, 104 East 40th Street, New York, NY 10016, for *Devices for Visually Impaired Diabetics*, and to The Lighthouse, The New York Association for the Blind, 111 East 59th Street, New York, NY 10022, for *An Evaluation of Devices for Insulin Dependent Visually Handicapped Diabetics*.

13. Rotate the sites of SC injections of insulin to prevent local atrophy (appears as mild dimpling of skin to deep pits seen mostly on girls and young women) and hypertrophy (appears as well-developed muscle on anterior and lateral thigh mostly in boys and young men).

   a. If insulin has been refrigerated, allow to warm to room temperature at least 1 hour before injection.

   b. Encourage patient to keep a chart indicating injection sites (see Fig. 6).

   c. Allow 3–4 cm between injection sites.

   d. Do not inject same site for at least 1 month.

   e. Avoid 1 cm around the umbilicus, because area has high vascularity.

   f. Avoid waistline, as area has a sensitive nerve supply.

   g. For self-injection, teach patient to brace arm to be injected against a hard surface, such as a wall or a chair.

   h. See Figure 6 for recommended sites for insulin injection.

   i. Prevent further lipodystrophy by using insulin at room temperature.

14. Always have an extra vial of insulin and equipment for administration on hand when the patient is in the hospital, at home, or traveling.

15. Have regular insulin available for emergency use.

16. Apply pressure for a minute after injection, but do not massage after injection since this may interfere with rate of absorption.

17. Delay administration of insulin if breakfast is delayed for tests.

18. Care of reusable syringes and needles.

   a. Do not use heavily chlorinated water or water with a high chemical content for sterilizing syringes. To sterilize, boil the syringe and needle for 5 minutes.

   b. Needle and syringe can be sterilized by soaking in isopropyl alcohol at least 5 minutes. The alcohol must evaporate from equipment before use to prevent reduction in strength of insulin.

Setting Up An Easy Rotation Cycle

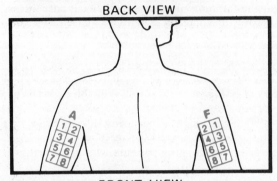

BACK VIEW

FRONT VIEW

Injection Log

SITE		1	2	3	4	5	6	7	8
right arm	A								
right abdomen	B								
right thigh	C								
left thigh	D								
left abdomen	E								
left arm	F								

c. Clean syringes covered by a precipitate with a cotton-tipped swab soaked in vinegar; then, thoroughly rinse syringe in water and sterilize it. Clean needles with a wire, and sharpen with a pumice stone.

Nursing Implications

Applicable to all diabetic patients controlled by medication whether insulin or an oral hypoglycemic.

1. Assess for symptoms of hyperglycemia: thirst, polyuria, drowsiness, flushed skin, fruity odor to breath, and unconsciousness.

2. Obtain medical supervision as rapidly as possible for patient showing signs of hyperglycemic reaction. Have insulin injection available for administration. After administration of insulin, monitor patient closely. As a guide for continued therapy, use clinical observations and laboratory data.

3. Assess for early symptoms of hypoglycemia: fatigue, headache, drowsiness, lassitude, tremulousness, or nausea. More marked late symptoms, such as weakness, sweating, tremor, or nervousness may occur. Observe the patient at night for excessive restlessness and profuse sweating.

4. Administer carbohydrate promptly to a hypoglycemic patient and notify the physician. Orange juice, candy, or a lump of sugar is helpful, if the patient is conscious. If the patient is unconscious, honey or Karo syrup may be applied to the buccal membrane or glucagon administered if available. If the patient is on long-acting insulin, also administer slow digestible carbohydrate, such as bread with corn syrup or honey. Provide additional carbohydrate for the next 2 hours. Milk and crackers would be suitable. In the hospital, have available for IV therapy 10–20 gm of dextrose in a vial.

5. Anticipate reduction in insulin dose if the Symogyi effect occurs in a patient originally being treated for hypoglycemia. The Symogyi effect occurs when hypoglycemia triggers the release of epinephrine, glucocorticoids, and growth hormone (GH), which stimulate glycogenesis and a higher blood sugar level. Reduction in insulin dosage is needed to stabilize patient.

6. Assess juvenile diabetics more closely for hypoglycemia. They are more susceptible to insulin shock and have a more limited response to glucagon.

7. Assess juvenile diabetics closely for infection or emotional disturbances, which may increase insulin requirements. Juvenile diabetics are more susceptible to diabetic coma if requirements are not met.

(continued)

FIGURE 6 Pattern for varying insulin injection sites. If you follow the sketch, you will see that the right arm is marked A, the right side of the abdomen is B, and the right thigh is C. Crossing to the left side of the body, the left thigh is marked D, the abdomen E, and the left arm F. Each of these areas can be thought of as a rectangle which may be divided, as shown, into eight different squares more than one inch on each side. These squares are numbered, starting from the upper and outside corner, which is number one, to the lowest corner, which is number eight, with all even numbers toward the middle of the body. If you select square number one and inject into it at each of the six areas A through F, it will take you six days to return again to A. Then selecting square number two and injecting into it at each of the six areas again rotates you around your body, returning in six days to area A. Follow with square number three, and so forth. It is easy to see that this procedure provides 48 different places in which to make your injections. If you make one injection daily, it will be that many days before you return to the A-1 square . . . almost seven weeks. (Figure and legend courtesy of Becton Dickinson and Company.)

8. Review patient's entire medication regimen for drugs that may enhance or antagonize antidiabetic agents and require dosage adjustment of antidiabetic agents.

9. Refer the patient and family to a public health agency to ensure continued health supervision in the home.

10. *Teach patient and/or family*
    (*Applicable to all diabetic patients controlled by insulin or oral antidiabetics*)

    a. the nature of diabetes mellitus—signs and symptoms.

    b. the necessity for regular medical supervision.

    c. how to test urine for sugar and acetone.

    d. how to administer insulin. Explain equipment, care of equipment, provision and storage of medication, and the technique and time of administration.

    e. the importance of adhering to prescribed diets, with emphasis on weight control and ingestion of food relative to peak period of the medication being taken and the use of the food-exchange list.

    f. how to use home glucose monitoring machine, if prescribed.

    g. the effects of exercise in raising carbohydrate needs.

    h. the necessity for good hygienic practices to prevent infection.

    i. to observe for hypoglycemic symptoms: fatigue, headache, drowsiness, tremulousness, or nausea.

    j. to observe for symptoms of hyperglycemia (leading to ketoacidosis): thirst, polyuria, drowsiness, flushed dry skin, fruity odor to breath, and unconsciousness.

    k. the procedures to follow in hypo- and hyperglycemia and other emergency situations, as noted in the *Nursing Implications* above.

    l. the necessity for the patient to carry candy or a lump of sugar to counteract hypoglycemia.

    m. the importance of reporting hypo- and hyperglycemic reactions to medical supervision for adjustment of dosage of medication.

    n. the advisability of patients carrying a card or wearing a Medic Alert bracelet (see Appendix), indicating that they are diabetic.

    o. that allergic reactions, such as itching, redness, swelling, stinging, or warmth at the injection site, usually disappear after a few weeks of therapy, but to report to doctor, as type of insulin may need to be changed.

    p. that if blurred vision is experienced during initiation of insulin therapy, the condition will subside in 6 to 8 weeks, and to delay eye examination until that time. The effect is caused by the fluctuation of blood glucose levels, which produces osmotic changes in the lens and within the ocular fluids.

    q. that if a meal is omitted because of illness (fever, nausea, or vomiting), to omit the next dose of insulin, unless the urine test indicates that there is sugar present. Test urine every 4 hours and report to physician for insulin regulation.

    r. to replace foods omitted by a similar amount of carbohydrate in the form of orange juice, or some other form of easily absorbed carbohydrate.

    s. that if the supply of insulin is exhausted or equipment unavailable, and the patient must omit medication, to decrease food intake by one-third and drink plenty of fluids. It is most important that supplies be obtained immediately and that the patient continue with dosage and diet.

t. that if the patient becomes ill, to notify the physician. Maintain adequate hydration to prevent coma by providing 1 cup or more/hour of noncaloric fluids (coffee, tea, water, and broth). Test urine more frequently.

u. to test urine for glycosuria with Clinitest Tablets, Tes-Tape, Diastix, or Clinistix, as recommended by the physician. Test a fresh second voided specimen. Instruct patient to empty bladder by urinating about 1 hour before mealtime. As soon as the patient can void again, obtain the specimen and test. Be alert to test interferences if patient is receiving additional drugs. Use appropriate testing procedure if laboratory test interference occurs.

v. to observe for possible drug interactions.

w. not to drink alcohol, as hypoglycemia could result. Excessive alcohol intake may require reduction in insulin dosage because alcohol potentiates the hypoglycemic effect of insulin.

EXTENDED INSULIN ZINC SUSPENSION   Single Peak: Ultralente Iletin I, Ultralente Insulin (OTC)

Classification   Long-acting insulin.

Action/Kinetics   Large crystals of insulin and a high content of zinc are responsible for the slow-acting properties of this preparation. **Onset:** 4–8 hr. **Peak:** 16–18 hr. **Duration:** 36 hr.

Uses   Mild to moderate hyperglycemia in stabilized diabetics. Not suitable for the treatment of diabetic coma or emergency situations.

Dosage   **SC**, *individualized*. **Usual, initial:** 7–26 units as a single dose 30–60 min before breakfast. **Do not administer IV**.

HUMAN INSULIN   Regular: Humulin R, Novolin-R. Insulin Zinc: Novolin-L. Isophane: Humulin N, Novolin N (OTC)

Classification   Human insulin from semisynthetic or recombinant DNA sources.

Action/Kinetics   Human insulin derived from recombinant DNA technology utilizes genetically modified *E. coli*. These organisms synthesize each chain of insulin into the same amino acid sequence as human insulin. The chains are then combined and purified to produce human insulin. Human insulin prepared semisynthetically undergoes a process whereby the terminal amino acid of porcine insulin is enzymatically substituted with an amino acid making the product identical with human insulin. This product is then purified.

Note: Human insulins are available as regular, insulin zinc, and isophane; for the kinetics of these products, please refer to the appropriate products described elsewhere in this chapter.

Human insulins are said to cause fewer allergic reactions and cause less insulin-induced antibody formation than insulins from animal sources.

Uses   Management of Type I diabetes mellitus. At this time, as long as the patient is well controlled on insulin from porcine or beef sources, transfer to human insulin is not recommended. Human insulin may be preferred in the following situations: local or systemic allergic reactions to products from animal sources, lipoatrophy at injection site, Type II diabetics who require short-term insulin treatment, in patients resistant to insulin from animal sources, and in pregnancy.

Dosage Dosage and routes of administration are similar to products from animal sources.

Additional Nursing Implications

Teach patient and/or family that dose may have to be reduced, so it is particularly important to watch for signs and symptoms of hypoglycemia.

INSULIN INJECTION (CRYSTALLINE ZINC INSULIN, UNMODIFIED INSULIN, REGULAR INSULIN) Single peak: Insulin Injection, Regular Iletin I. Purified: Beef Regular Iletin II, Pork Regular Iletin II, Velosulin (OTC)

Classification Rapid-acting insulin.

Action/Kinetics This product is rarely administered as the sole agent due to its short duration of action. Injections of 100 units/ml or less are clear; cloudly, colored solutions should not be used. Regular insulin is the only preparation suitable for IV administration. **Onset:** $1/2$–1 hr. **Peak:** 2–3 hr. **Duration:** 5–7 hr.

Uses Suitable for treatment of diabetic coma, acidosis, or other emergency situations. Especially suitable for the patient suffering from labile diabetes.

During acute phase of diabetic acidosis or for the patient in diabetic crisis, patient is monitored by serum glucose and serum ketone levels.

Dosage **Individualized. SC. Adults: usual, initial:** 5–10 units; **pediatric:** 2–4 units. Injection is given 15–30 min before meals and at bedtime.

INSULIN INJECTION, CONCENTRATED Regular (Concentrated) Iletin II (Rx)

Action/Kinetics This very concentrated preparation (500 units/ml) of Insulin Injection (see above) is indicated for patients with a marked resistance to insulin requiring more than 200 units/day. Patients must be kept under close observation until dosage is established. Depending on response, dosage may be given SC or IM as a single or as 2 or 3 divided doses. Not suitable for IV administration because of possible allergic or anaphylactoid reactions.

Additional Untoward Reactions Deep secondary hypoglycemia 18 to 24 hours after administration.

Administration/Storage

1. Administer only water-clear solutions (concentrated insulin may appear straw colored).

2. Use a tuberculin-type syringe for accuracy of measurement.

3. Keep cool or refrigerated.

Additional Nursing Implications

See *Nursing Implications* for Insulin, p. 685.

1. Assess patients closely for signs and symptoms of hyper- or hypoglycemia during period when correct dosage is being established. Monitor urine q hr.
2. For deep secondary hypoglycemia 18 to 24 hours after injection and/or glucose; have available 10–20% dextrose solution.
3. *Teach patient and/or family*
   a. to monitor urine carefully as ordered by medical supervision.
   b. to be alert to signs of hypoglycemia, which may indicate that responsiveness to insulin has been regained, and that a reduction in dosage is warranted.

INSULIN ZINC SUSPENSION   Single peak: Lente Iletin I, Lente Insulin. Purified: Beef Lente Iletin II, Lentard, Pork Lente Iletin II, Purified Pork Insulin Zinc Suspension (OTC)

Classification   Intermediate-acting insulin.

Action/Kinetics   Contains 30% prompt and 70% extended insulin zinc suspension, which is cloudy or milky in appearance. Principal advantage is the absence of a sensitizing agent such as protamine or globin. **Onset:** 1–2 hr. **Peak:** 8–12 hr. **Duration:** 18–24 hr.

Uses   Useful in patients allergic to other types of insulin, and for patients disposed to thrombotic phenomena in which protamine may be a factor. Zinc insulin is not a replacement for regular insulin and is not suitable for emergency use.

Dosage   SC. Adults, initial: 7–26 units 30–60 min before breakfast. Dosage is then increased by daily or weekly increments of 2 to 10 units until satisfactory readjustment is established. A second smaller dose may be given prior to the evening meal or at bedtime.

Patients on NPH can be transferred to insulin zinc suspension on a unit for unit basis. Patients being transferred from regular insulin should begin zinc insulin at $\frac{2}{3}$–$\frac{3}{4}$ the regular insulin dosage. If being transferred from protamine zinc insulin, the dose of zinc insulin should be about 50% of that required for protamine zinc insulin.

ISOPHANE INSULIN SUSPENSION (NPH)   Single peak: Isophane Insulin, NPH Iletin I. Purified: Beef NPH Iletin II, Insulatard NPH, Pork NPH Iletin II (OTC)

Classification   Intermediate-acting insulin.

Action/Kinetic   Contains zinc insulin crystals modified by protamine appearing as a cloudy or milky suspension. Not recommended for emergency use. Not suitable for IV administration. Not useful in the presence of ketosis. **Onset:** 1–2 hr. **Peak:** 8–12 hr. **Duration:** 18–24 hr.

Dosage   SC, individualized. Adult, usual, initial: 7–26 units as a single dose 30–60 min before breakfast. A second smaller dose may be given, if needed, prior to the evening meal or at bedtime. If necessary, the daily dose may be increased in increments of 2–10 units at daily or weekly intervals until desired control is achieved.

Patients on insulin zinc may be transferred directly to isophane insulin on a unit for unit basis. If being transferred from regular insulin, the initial dose of isophane should be from ⅔–¾ the dose of regular insulin.

ISOPHANE INSULIN SUSPENSION AND INSULIN INJECTION
Mixtard (OTC)

Classification Mixture of insulins to achieve variable duration of action.

Action/Kinetics Contains 30% insulin injection and 70% isophane insulin. This combination allows for a rapid onset (30–60 min) due to insulin injection and a long duration (24 hr) due to isophane insulin.

PROMPT INSULIN ZINC SUSPENSION Single peak: Semilente Iletin I, Semilente Insulin (OTC)

Classification Fast-acting insulin.

Action/Kinetics Contains small particles of zinc insulin in a nearly colorless suspension. Not suitable for emergency use. Cannot be injected IV. **Onset:** ½–1 hr. **Peak:** 4–7 hr. **Duration:** 12–16 hr.

Uses In combination with insulin zinc or extended insulin zinc suspensions to control diabetes. May also be used alone for rapid control when initiating therapy.

Dosage SC. **Individualized. Adults, initial:** 10–20 units ½ hr before breakfast. A second daily dose is usually required.

PROTAMINE ZINC INSULIN SUSPENSION Single peak: Protamine, Zinc, & Iletin I. Purified: Beef Protamine, Zinc & Iletin II (OTC)

Classification Long-acting insulin.

Action/Kinetics Contains protamine, zinc, and insulin in a cloudy or milky suspension. Not suitable for use in emergency situations and not to be given IV. Due to its long onset and duration, this product is not as adaptable to dosage alterations as are other preparations. **Onset:** 4–8 hr. **Peak:** 14–20 hr. **Duration:** 36 hr.

Uses Mild to moderate diabetes.

Dosage SC. **Individualized. Adults, initial:** 7–26 units as a single dose 30–60 min before breakfast. If transferring from regular insulin, the initial dose should be approximately 2/3 that of regular insulin.

ORAL ANTIDIABETIC AGENTS

General Statement Several oral antidiabetics agents are available for patients with the milder forms of diabetes. These agents are sulfonylureas, which are related chemically to sulfonamides; however, they are devoid of antibacterial activity. Oral hypoglycemic drugs are classified as either first or second generation. Generation refers to structural changes in the basic molecule. Second generation oral hypoglycemic drugs are more lipophilic and, as such, have a greater hypoglycemic potency. Also, second generation drugs are bound to plasma protein by covalent bonds whereas first generation drugs are bound to plasma protein by ionic bonds. The implication is that the second generation drugs are potentially less susceptible to displacement from plasma protein by drugs such as salicylates, oral anticoagulants, and others.

These agents are used chiefly for patients with maturity-onset, mild, nonketotic diabetes, usually associated with obesity, when the condition cannot be controlled by diet alone, but the patient does not require insulin. The oral antidiabetics should not be used in unstable or brittle diabetes, whatever the patient's age.

Action/Kinetics   These drugs are believed to act by one or more of the following mechanisms: (1) the sensitivity of pancreatic islet cells is increased; (2) the pancreatic beta-cell membrane is directly depolarized leading to insulin secretion; or (3) the peripheral tissues become more sensitive to insulin due to an increase in the number of insulin receptors or an increased ability of circulating insulin to combine with receptors. The drugs are ineffective in the complete absence of functioning beta-islet cells.

Patients whose condition is to be controlled by oral antidiabetics should be subjected to a 7-day therapeutic trial. A drop in blood sugar level, a decrease in glucosuria, and disappearance of pruritus, polyuria, polydipsia, and polyphagia indicate that the patient can probably be managed on oral antidiabetic agents. These drugs should not be used in patients with ketosis.

If the patient is transferred from insulin to an oral antidiabetic drug, the hormone should be discontinued gradually over a period of several days.

The sulfonylureas have similar pharmacologic actions but differ in their pharmacokinetic properties (see individual agents).

Uses   Maturity-onset diabetes (Type II) that does not respond to diet management alone. As an adjunct to stabilize insulin-dependent maturity-onset diabetes.

Contraindications   Stress before and during surgery, severe trauma, fever, infections, pregnancy, diabetes complicated by recurrent episodes of ketoacidosis or coma, juvenile, growth onset, insulin-dependent, or brittle diabetes; impaired endocrine, renal or liver function. Use with caution in debilitated, malnourished patients. Not indicated for patients whose diabetes can be controlled by diet alone. Relapse may occur with the sulfonylureas in undernourished patients.

Untoward Reactions   Hypoglycemia is the most common side effect. *CV:* Chronic use of oral hypoglycemic drugs has been associated with an increased risk of cardiovascular mortality. *GI:* Nausea, heartburn, diarrhea, full feeling. *CNS:* Fatigue, dizziness, fever, headache, weakness, malaise. *Hepatic:* Cholestatic jaundice, aggravation of hepatic porphyria. *Dermatologic:* Skin rashes, urticaria, erythema, pruritus, eczema, photophobia. *Hematologic:* Thrombocytopenia, leukopenia, anemia, and eosinophilia are the most common. Also, agranulocytosis, hemolytic anemia, pancytopenia, aplastic anemia.

Resistance to drug action develops in a small percentage of patients.

Drug Interactions

Interactant	Interaction
Acetazolamide	↑ Blood sugar in prediabetics and diabetics on oral hypoglycemics
Anabolic steroids	↑ Hypoglycemic effect of oral antidiabetics
Anticoagulants, oral	↑ Effect of oral hypoglycemics by ↓ breakdown by liver and ↓ plasma protein binding

Interactant	Interaction
Barbiturates	Oral hypoglycemics ↑ effects of barbiturates
Beta-adrenergic blocking	↓ Hypoglycemic effect of oral hypoglycemics
Calcium channel blockers	↑ Requirements for sulfonylureas agents
Chloramphenicol	↑ Effect of oral hypoglycemics by ↓ break-down by liver
Clofibrate	↑ Hypoglycemic effect of oral antidiabetics
Corticosteroids	↑ Requirements for sulfonylureas
Diazoxide	Effects of both drugs decreased
Digitoxin	↓ Effect of digitoxin by ↑ breakdown by liver
Ethanol	Disulfiram-type reaction; ↑ hypoglycemia
Fenfluramine	Additive hypoglycemia
Isoniazid	↑ Requirements for sulfonylureas
Methyldopa	↑ Effect of sulfonylureas due to ↓ breakdown by liver
Monoaminne oxidase inhibitors	↑ Hypoglycemic effect of oral antidiabetics
Nonsteroidal anti-inflammatory agents	↑ Hypoglycemic effect of oral antidiabetics
Oral contraceptives	↓ Hypoglycemic effect of oral antidiabetics
Phenothiazines	↑ Requirements for sulfonylureas
Phenylbutazone	↑ Effect of oral hypoglycemics due to ↓ breakdown by liver and ↓ plasma protein binding
Phenytoin	↓ Effect of sulfonylureas
Rifampin	↓ Effect of sulfonylureas due to ↑ breakdown by liver
Salicylates	↑ Effect of oral hypoglycemics by ↓ plasma protein binding
Sulfonamides	↑ Effect of oral hypoglycemics by ↓ plasma protein binding and ↓ breakdown by liver
Sympathomimetics	↑ Requirements for sulfonylureas
Thiazides	↑ Requirements for sulfonylureas
Thyroid hormone	↑ Requirements for sulfonylureas

Laboratory Test Interference ↑ BUN and serum creatinine.

Dosage **PO**: See individual preparations. Adjust dosage according to needs of patient. Exercise and diet are of primary importance in the control of diabetes.

Administration

1. These drugs may be taken with food to decrease GI upset.
2. Withdraw the medication if ketonuria, acidosis, increased glycosuria, or serious side effects occur.

TRANSFER FROM INSULIN

1. Patients receiving 20 or less units of insulin daily: Institute maintenance dosage of oral hypoglycemic agents. Insulin may be discontinued abruptly.
2. Patients receiving 20–40 units of insulin daily: Institute maintenance dosage of oral hypoglycemic agent and reduce insulin dose by 35–50%. Discontinue insulin gradually, using absence of glucose in urine as a guide.
3. Patients receiving more than 40 units of insulin daily: Institute maintenance

dosage and reduce insulin by 20%. Discontinue insulin gradually, using glucose in urine as a guide. It might be advisable to transfer patients on such high doses of insulin while they are hospitalized.

Patients should test their urine for glucose and ketone bodies regularly (1 to 3 times daily) during the transfer period. Positive results must be reported to the physician.

Mild symptoms of hyperglycemia may appear during the transfer period. No transition period is needed when patient is transferred from one sulfonylurea to another. However, if a patient is to be transferred from chlorpropamide, caution should be exercised due to the prolonged duration of action of this drug.

THERAPEUTIC FAILURE OF HYPOGLYCEMIC AGENTS   Diabetic patients who do not respond to the sulfonylureas are said to be primary failures. Patients may respond to the sulfonylureas during the initial months of therapy, yet fail to respond thereafter. These patients are referred to as secondary failures.

Nursing Implications

See *Nursing Implications* for all diabetic patients receiving medication to control the disease, p. 685.

1. Assess very closely during the first 7 days of treatment with a sulfonylurea, because this is a trial period during which the therapeutic response must be evaluated.
2. Be prepared to begin treatment with IV dextrose solution if severe hypoglycemia develops. Close medical supervision will be required during the following 3 to 5 days.
3. *Teach patient and/or family*
   a. to test urine for sugar and ketone bodies at least 3 times a day during transition period.
   b. the need to adhere to prescribed diet for sulfonylurea to be effective. Most secondary failures are due to poor dietary practices.
   c. to know how to self-administer insulin, because this may be necessary should complications occur.
   d. to report to medical supervision when not feeling as well as usual or when pruritus, skin rash, jaundice, dark urine, fever, sore throat, or diarrhea are noted.
   e. to report sulfonylurea medication if scheduled for a thyroid test, because the drug interferes with the uptake of radioactive iodine.
   f. the need for close medical supervision during first 6 weeks of therapy.
   g. to report for periodic laboratory tests as ordered by physician, as these drugs can cause blood dyscrasias.

ACETOHEXAMIDE   Dymelor (Rx)

Classification   First generation sulfonylurea.

Action/Kinetics   **Onset:** 1 hr. **t½:** 6–8 hr **Duration:** 12–24 hr. Changed to active metabolite in liver.

Additional Untoward Reaction   Hair loss.

Dosage   PO Range: 0.25–1.5 gm daily. *Newly diagnosed or elderly*, 250 mg daily before breakfast, adjusting by 250–500 mg increments every 5 to 7 days. *Moderately severe diabetes*, 1.5 gm on day 1; 1.0 gm on day 2, **then** 0.5 gm daily, adjusting dosage thereafter until optimum control is achieved. Doses in excess of 1.5 gm/day not recommended.

Administration   Doses of 1 gm or less can be given once daily.

CHLORPROPAMIDE   Apo-Chlorpropamide,* Chloronase,* Diabinese, Novopropamide* (Rx)

Classification   First generation sulfonylurea.

General Statement   Chlorpropamide may be effective in patients who do not respond well to other antidiabetic agents.

Action/Kinetics   **Onset**: 1 hr. **t½**: 35 hr. **Duration**: 60 hr. 80% metabolized in liver. Long duration due to slow excretion.

Additional Use   *Investigational:* Neurogenic diabetes insipidus.

Additional Untoward Reactions   Untoward reactions occur frequently with chlorpropamide. Severe diarrhea is occasionally accompanied by bleeding in the lower bowel. Severe GI distress may be relieved by dividing total daily dose in half. In older patients hypoglycemia may be severe. May cause inappropriate antidiuretic hormone secretion leading to hyponatremia, water retention, low serum osmolality, and high urine osmolality.

Additional Drug Interactions

Interactant	Interaction
Ammonium chloride	↑ Effect of chlorpropamide due to ↓ excretion by kidney
Probenecid	↑ Effect of chlorpropamide
Sodium bicarbonate	↓ Effect of chlorpropamide due to ↑ excretion by kidney

Dosage   PO: initial, middle-aged patients, 250 mg daily as a single or divided dose; **geriatric: initial,** 100–125 mg daily. **Maintenance, all patients**: 100–250 mg daily as single or divided doses. Severe diabetics may require 500 mg daily; doses greater than 750 mg daily are not recommended. *Neurogenic diabetes insipidus:* 125–250 mg daily.

GLIPIZIDE   Glucotrol (Rx)

Classification   Second generation sulfonylurea.

Action/Kinetics   Glipizide also has mild diuretic effects. **Onset:** 1–1.5 hr. **t½:** 2–4 hr. **Duration:** up to 24 hr. Metabolized in liver to inactive metabolites.

Additional Drug Interaction   Cimetidine may ↑ effect of glipizide due to ↓ breakdown by liver.

Dosage   PO: initial, 5 mg before breakfast; **then,** adjust dosage by 2.5–5 mg q few days until adequate control is achieved. **Maintenance:** 15–40 mg daily. Older patients should begin with 2.5 mg.

Administration
1. Maintenance doses greater than 15 mg daily should be divided.
2. For greatest effect, give 30 min before meals.

GLYBURIDE   Diabeta, Euglucon,* Micronase (Rx)

Classification   Second generation sulfonylurea.

Action/Kinetics   Glyburide has a mild diuretic effect. **Onset:** 2–4 hr. **t½:** 10 hr. **Duration:** 24 hr. Metabolized in liver to inactive metabolites. Excreted in bile and through the kidneys.

Dosage   PO: initial, 2.5–5 mg daily; **then,** increase by 2.5 mg at weekly intervals to desired response. **Maintenance:** 1.25–20 mg daily. Patients sensitive to sulfonylureas should start with 1.25 mg/day.

Administration
1. For best results administer prior to meals.
2. May be given in single or divided daily doses.

TOLAZAMIDE   Tolinase (Rx)

Classification   First generation sulfonylurea.

Action/Kinetics   Drug is effective in some patients who have a history of coma or ketoacidosis. Also, it may be effective in patients who do not respond well to other oral antidiabetic agents. Use with insulin is not recommended for maintenance. **Onset:** 4–6 hr. **t½:** 7 hr. **Duration:** 10–16 hr. Changed in liver to metabolites with minor hypoglycemic activity.

Additional Contraindication   Renal glycosuria.

Additional Drug Interaction   Concomitant use of alcohol and tolazamide may →photosensitivity.

Dosage   PO: initial, 100 mg/day if fasting blood sugar is less than 200 mg/100 ml, or 250 mg/day if fasting blood sugar is greater than 200 mg/100 ml. Adjust dose to response. If more than 500 mg/day required, the dose should be given in 2 divided doses. **Elderly or debilitated patients:** 100 mg/day with breakfast, adjusting dose by increments of 50 mg daily each week. Doses greater than 1 gm daily will probably not improve control.

TOLBUTAMIDE   Apo-Tolbutamide,* Mobenol,* Novobutamide,* Oramide, Orinase (Rx)

TOLBUTAMIDE SODIUM   Orinase Diagnostic (Rx)

Classification   First generation sulfonylurea.

Action/Kinetics   Onset: 1 hr. **t½:** 4–5 hr **Duration:** 6–12 hr. Changed in liver to inactive metabolites. May be used as a supplement to insulin therapy in some cases of labile diabetes. Most useful for patients with poor general physical status who should receive a short-acting compound.

Special Use Tolbutamide sodium is used to diagnose pancreatic islet cell tumors. It causes blood glucose, in presence of a tumor, to drop quickly after IV administration and remain low for 3 hours.

Additional Untoward Reactions Melena (dark, bloody stools) in some patients with a history of peptic ulcer. Relapse or secondary failure may occur a few months after therapy has been started. May cause hyponatremia and a mild goiter.

Additional Drug Interactions

Interactant	Interaction
Alcohol	Photosensitivity reactions
Sulfinpyrazone	↑ Effect of tolbutamide due to ↓ breakdown by liver

Dosage **PO**, administered as a single dose before breakfast or divided doses with meals. **Initial**: 1–2 gm/day; adjust dosage depending on response (range: 0.25–3 gm/day).

INSULIN ANTAGONISTS

DIAZOXIDE ORAL Proglycem (Rx)

Classification Insulin antagonist, hypotensive agent.

Action/Kinetics Diazoxide inhibits the release of insulin from beta-islet cells of the pancreas, leading to an increase in blood glucose levels. Effect is dose related. Diazoxide causes sodium, potassium, uric acid, and water retention. **Onset**: 1 hr. **Duration**: 8 hr. Optimum dosage is usually established within 2 to 3 days. Excreted by kidney.

Uses Hypoglycemia caused by insulin overdosage, or overproduction of insulin by malignant beta cells. The drug is used parenterally as an antihypertensive agent (see p. 344).

Contraindications Functional hypoglycemia, hypersensitivity to drug or thiazides. Use with extreme caution in patients with history of gout or those in whom edema presents a risk (cardiac disease). Safe use in pregnancy not established.

Untoward Reactions *CV:* Sodium and fluid retention (common), palpitations, increased heart rate, hypotension, transient hypertension. *Metabolic:* Hyperglycemia, glycosuria, diabetic ketoacidosis, hyperosmolar nonketotic coma. *GI:* Nausea, vomiting, diarrhea, transient taste loss, anorexia, ileus, abdominal pain. *CNS:* Weakness, headache, insomnia, extrapyramidal symptoms, dizziness, paresthesia, fever. *Hematologic:* Thrombocytopenia, purpura, eosinophilia, neutropenia, decreased hemoglobin. *Dermatologic:* Skin rashes, hirsutism, herpes, loss of hair from scalp, monilial dermatitis. *GU:* Hematuria, proteinuria, decrease in urine production, nephrotic syndrome (reversible). *Ophthalmologic:* Blurred or double vision, lacrimation, transient cataracts, ring scotoma, subconjunctival hemorrhage. *Other:* Pancreatitis, pancreatic necrosis, galactorrhea, gout, premature aging of bone, polyneuritis, enlargement of lump in breast.

Drug Interactions

Interactant	Interaction
Alpha-adrenergic blocking agents	↓ Effect of diazoxidiazoxide
Anticoagulants, oral	↑ Effect of anticoagulant due to ↓ plasma protein binding.
Antihypertensives	Excessive ↓ blood pressure due to additive effects
Phenytoin	↓ Effect phenytoin due to ↑ breakdown by liver
Sulfonylureas	↓ Effect of both drugs
Thiazide diuretics	↑ Hypoglycemic and hyperuricemic effects

Laboratory Test Interference ↑ Serum uric acid, SGOT, alkaline phosphatase; ↓ creatinine clearance.

Dosage *Individualized*, on the basis of blood glucose level and response of patient. **PO**. **Adults and children: initial**, 3 mg/kg/day in 3 equal doses q 8 hr; **maintenance**: 3–8 mg/kg/day divided into 2 or 3 equal doses q 8–12 hr. **Infants and newborns: initial**, 10 mg/kg/day in 3 equal doses q 8 hr; **maintenance**: 15 mg/kg/day divided into 2 or 3 equal doses q 8–12 hr.

Administration Blood glucose levels and urinary glucose and ketones must be monitored carefully until the patient has stabilized, which usually takes 1 week. The drug is discontinued if a satisfactory effect has not been established within 2 to 3 weeks.

Nursing Implications

1. *Assess*
   a. clinical response and laboratory test results, which are the basis for dosage adjustment by the physician.
   b. patient with a history of CHF for fluid retention, which may precipitate failure.
   c. BP for potentiation of antihypertensive effect when patient is already maintained on another antihypertensive agent.
   d. for ecchymosis, petechiae, or frank bleeding—symptoms that will require discontinuance of drug.
   e. closely up to 7 days after overdosage until blood sugar level is within normal range (80–120 mg/100 ml).
2. Reassure patient with hirsutism that the condition will subside with discontinuance of the drug.
3. Have insulin and IV fluids available to counteract possible ketoacidosis.

GLUCAGON (Rx)

Classification Insulin antagonist.

Action/Kinetics Glucagon is a hormone produced by the alpha-islet cells of the pancreas. The hormone increases blood glucose by increasing breakdown of glycogen to glucose, stimulating gluconeogenesis from amino acids and fatty acids, and inhibiting conversion of glucose to glycogen. The drug is effective in overcoming hypoglycemia only if the liver has a glycogen reserve. **Onset**: 5–20 min.

Maximum effect: 30 min. **Duration**: 1–2 hr. **t½**: 3–6 min. Metabolized by the liver.

Uses Used to terminate insulin-induced shock in diabetic or psychiatric patients. Patient usually regains consciousness 5 to 20 minutes after the parenteral administration of glucagon. The drug should only be used under medical supervision or in accordance with strict instructions received from the physician. Failure to respond may be an indication for IV administration of glucose—especially true in the juvenile diabetics. As a diagnostic aid in radiologic examination of the GI tract when a hypotonic state is desirable.

Contraindications Use with caution in patients with renal or hepatic disease, in those who are undernourished and emaciated, and in patients with a history of pheochromocytoma or insulinoma.

Untoward Reactions Nausea, vomiting, circulatory collapse, and hypersensitivity. Stevens-Johnson syndrome when used as diagnostic aid.

Drug Interactions

Interactant	Interaction
Anticoagulants, oral	↑ Effect of anticoagulants by ↑ hypoprothrombinemia
Antidiabetic agents	Hyperglycemic effect of glucagon antagonizes hypoglycemic effect of antidiabetics
Corticosteroids Epinephrine Estrogens Phenytoin	Additive hyperglycemic effect of drugs listed

Dosage *Hypoglycemia*: **IM, IV, SC**, 0.5–1 mg; 1–2 additional doses may be given if necessary. *Insulin shock therapy*: **IM, IV, SC**, 0.5–1 mg after 1 hour of coma; if no response, dose may be repeated. *Diagnostic aid for GI tract*: dose dependent on desired onset of action and duration of effect necessary for the examination: **IV**, 0.25–0.5 mg (onset: 1 min; duration: 9–17 min); 2 mg (onset: 1 min; duration: 22–25 min). **IM**, 1 mg (onset: 8–10 min; duration: 12–27 min); 2 mg (onset: 4–7 min; duration: 21–32 min).

Administration Once the hypoglycemic patient responds, supplemental carbohydates should be given to prevent secondary hypoglycemia.

Nursing Implications

1. Refer to the chart on p. 680 to differentiate between diabetic coma and insulin shock (reaction).
2. Administer carbohydrate after the patient awakens following administration of glucagon. Rapidly available sugar such as that in orange juice and Karo syrup in water should be given. If shock was caused by a long-acting medication, give a more slowly digestible carbohydrate such as bread with honey.
3. *Teach patient and/or family*
   a. how to administer glucagon SC or IM in the event of a hypoglycemic reaction with loss of consciousness by the patient.
   b. the need to inform the physician of hypoglycemic reactions so that the dosage of insulin may be adjusted.

Chapter Fifty-nine

THYROID AND ANTITHYROID DRUGS

General Statement The thyroid manufactures two active hormones: thyroxine and triiodothyronine, both of which contain iodine. These thyroid hormones are released into the bloodstream, where they are bound to protein.

Diseases involving the thyroid fall into two groups:

1. Hypothyroidism or diseases in which little or no hormone is produced. These can be subdivided into cretinism, resulting from a deficiency of thyroid hormone during fetal and early life, and myxedema, a deficiency of thyroid hormone in the adult. Cretinism is characterized by arrested physical and mental development with dystrophy of the bones and soft parts and lowered basal metabolism. Myxedema is characterized by a dry waxy type swelling, with abnormal deposits of mucin in the skin. The edema is nonpitting, and the facial changes are distinctive, with swollen lips and a thickened nose. Primary myxedema results from atrophy of the thyroid gland. Secondary myxedema may result from hypofunction of the pituitary gland or prolonged administration of antithyroid drugs.

2. Hyperthyroidism or conditions associated with an overproduction of hormones as in Graves' or Basedow's disease (diffuse enlargement of the thyroid gland; often characterized by protruding eyes), and Plummer's disease in which extra thyroid hormone is produced by a single "hot" thyroid nodule. These conditions are usually characterized by hypertrophy and hyperplasia of the thyroid and a state of extreme nervousness.

EUTHYROID OR SIMPLE, NONTOXIC GOITER (ENDEMIC GOITER) In these states, a normal or near-normal amount of hormone is produced by an enlarged thyroid gland. This condition can occur when the dietary intake of iodine is below normal.

Today, the disease is much rarer because iodine is added as a matter of routine to cooking salt. The thyroid, in such patients, tends to become enlarged, especially during adolescent growth and pregnancy. Surgery may be necessary to alleviate the pressure on the trachea caused by the enlarged thyroid and to prevent the oxygen supply from being cut off.

Drugs used in the treatment of thyroid disease fall into two groups: (1) thyroid preparations used to correct thyroid deficiency diseases, and (2) antithyroid drugs that cut down production of hormones by an overactive gland.

The external supply of thyroid hormones usually results in a reduction in the amount of natural hormone produced by the thyroid gland.

The accurate determination of thyroid function is crucial for the treatment of thyroid disease. Thyroid function can be evaluated by (1) total levothyroxine (T4), (2) free levothyroxine, (3) serum liothyronine (T3), (4) liothyronine resin uptake (RT3U), (5) free thyroxine index, and (6) thyroid stimulating hormone. The results of some of the tests are at times skewed by medications the patient is taking so that the effect of these drugs must be considered when evaluating the test.

Thyroid conditions are often treated by fixed combinations of levothyroxine sodium and liothyronine sodium in a ratio of 4:1. Such a preparation is liotrix (Euthroid, Thyrolar). For all information regarding these drugs, see drug entries for levothyroxine sodium and liothyronine sodium.

Action/Kinetics The thyroid hormones regulate growth by controlling protein synthesis and regulating energy metabolism by increasing the resting metabolic rate (BMR). Other metabolic effects include increased conversion of cholesterol to bile acids, increase in protein bound iodine (PBI), increased carbohydrate utilization, and participation in the calcification of long bones.

The hormones also have a cardiostimulatory effect and can increase renal blood flow as well as glomerular filtration rate (GFR) (diuresis). The thyroid gland is under the control of the hypothalamus and pituitary gland, which produce thyroid-stimulating hormone releasing factor and thyrotropin (thyroid-stimulating hormone, TSH) respectively. Like other hormone systems, the thyroid, pituitary, and hypothalamus work together in a feedback mechanism. Excess thyroid hormone causes a decrease in TSH and a lack of thyroid hormone causes an increase in the production and secretion of TSH.

THYROID PREPARATIONS

Uses Replacement therapy in primary and secondary myxedema, myxedemic coma, nontoxic goiter, hypothyroidism, some thyroid tumors, chronic thyroiditis, sporadic cretinism, and thyrotropin-dependent tumors. With antithyroid drugs for thyrotoxicosis (to prevent goiter or hypothyroidism).

Contraindications Uncorrected adrenal insufficiency, myocardial infarction, hyperthyroidism, and thyrotoxicosis. Use with extreme caution in the presence of angina pectoris, hypertension, and other cardiovascular disease, renal insufficiency, and ischemic states. Adrenal insufficiency unless treatment with adrenocortical steroids is initiated first. Not to be used to treat obesity or infertility in either males or females.

Untoward Reactions Thyroid preparations have cumulative effects, and overdosage (i.e. symptoms of hyperthyroidism) may occur. *CV:* Arrhythmias, palpitations, angina, increased heart rate and pulse pressure, cardiac arrest, aggravation of congestive heart failure. *GI:* Cramps, diarrhea, nausea, appetite changes. *CNS:* Headache, nervousness, mental agitation, irritability, insomnia, tremors. *Miscel-*

laneous: Weight loss, hyperhidrosis, excessive warmth, irregular menses, heat intolerance, fever, dyspnea.

Drug Interactions

Interactant	Interaction
Anticoagulants	↑ Effect of anticoagulants by ↑ hypoprothrombinemia
Antidepressants, tricyclic	↑ Effect of antidepressant and ↑ effect of thyroid
Antidiabetic agents	Hyperglycemic effect of thyroid preparations may necessitate ↑ in dose of antidiabetic agent
Cholestyramine	↓ Effect of thyroid hormone due to ↓ absorption from GI tract
Corticosteroids	Thyroid preparations increase tissue demands for corticosteroids. Adrenal insufficiency must be corrected with corticosteroids before administering thyroid hormones. In patients already treated for adrenal insufficiency, dosage of corticosteroids must be increased when initiating therapy with thyroid drug
Digitalis compounds	↓ Effect of digitalis with worsening of arrhythmias or congestive heart failuare
Epinephrine	Cardiovascular effects ↑ by thyroid preparations
Estrogens	Estrogens may ↑ requirements for thyroid hormone
Ketamine	Concomitant use may result in severe hypertension and tachycardia
Levarterenol	Cardiovascular effects ↑ by thyroid preparations
Phenytoin	↑ Effect of thyroid hormone by ↓ plasma protein binding
Salicylates	Salicylates compete for thyroid-binding sites on protein

Laboratory Test Interferences Alter thyroid function tests. ↑ Prothrombin time. ↓ Serum cholesterol.

Dosage Thyroid drugs are started with a low dose that is gradually increased until a satisfactory response is achieved within safe dose limits. When necessary, a decrease in dosage and a more gradual upward adjustment relieves severe side effects.

Nursing Implications

1. Anticipate that treatment will be initiated with a small dose that is gradually increased.
2. Be aware the dose for a child may be the same as the full adult dose.
3. Follow specific instructions to prevent overdose or relapse when changing from one thyroid drug to another.
4. *Assess*
   a. for drug interactions when patient is receiving other medications that affect the cardiovascular system.

(continued)

b. patient on anticoagulant therapy for bleeding from any orifice or purpura, since the action of anticoagulants is potentiated by thyroid preparations.

c. for positive results of medication characterized by reduction in weight, improvement in appearance of skin and hair, and increased mental alertness.

5. *Teach patient and/or family*

a. that drug must be taken only with medical supervision and that the drug must be taken regularly, often for life.

b. to report promptly to physician excessive weight loss, palpitations, leg cramps, nervousness, diarrhea, or abdominal cramps, headache, insomnia, intolerance to heat, and fever. Symptoms are most likely to occur from 1 to 3 weeks after therapy for hypothyroidism is started.

c. when patient is diabetic, to test urine at least three times a day for sugar and acetone, because thyroid preparations may require adjustment of insulin dosage.

d. when patient is on anticoagulant therapy to report purpura or bleeding from any orifice since anticoagulants are potentiated by thyroid preparations.

e. to keep most thyroid preparations in a cool dark place away from heat, moisture, and light (not in kitchen or bathroom).

f. to take thyroid drug in a single morning dose to reduce likelihood of nighttime insomnia.

LEVOTHYROXINE SODIUM (T4)   Eltroxin,* Levothroid, Synthroid, Synthrox, Syroxine, L-Thyroxine Sodium (Rx)

Classification   Thyroid preparation.

Action/Kinetics   Levothyroxine is the synthetic sodium salt of the levoisomer of thyroxine (tetraiodothyronine). Levothyroxine is well absorbed from the GI tract and has a slower onset but a longer duration than sodium liothyronine. It is more active on a weight basis than is thyroid. t½: 6–7 days. Is 99% protein bound.

Note: All levothyroxine products are not bioequivalent; thus, changing brands is not recommended.

Dosage   *Individualized.* **PO: initial,** 25–100 µg daily increased by 50–100 µg q 1–4 weeks until desired clinical response is attained; **maintenance:** 100–400 µg daily.
   Myxedematous coma without heart disease. **IV: initial,** 200–500 µg. If there is no response in 24 hr, 100–300 µg may be given on the second day.
   Pediatric. *Congenital hypothyroidism:* **Over 12 years:**   150 µg or more daily; **6–12 years:** 100–150 µg daily; **1–5 years:** 75–100 µg daily; **6–12 months:** 50–75 µg daily; **up to 6 months:** 25–50 µg daily. *Cretinism:* **initial,** 25–50 µg daily; **then,** increase by 50–100 µg q 2 weeks until patient is euthyroid (usual maintenance dose is 300–400 µg daily).
   Transfer from liothyronine to levothyroxine—administer replacement drug for several days before discontinuing liothyronine. Transfer from levothyroxine to liothyronine—discontinue levothyroxine before starting patient on low daily dose of liothyronine.

Administration   Prepare solutions for injection immediately before administration. Solution is made by adding prescribed amount of normal saline to powder and shaking solution until it is clear. Discard unused portion of IV medication.

LIOTHYRONINE SODIUM (T3) Cyronine, Cytomel, Sodium-L-Triiodothyronine, Tertroxin* (Rx)

Classification Thyroid preparation.

Action/Kinetics Synthetic sodium salt of levoisomer of triiodothyronine. Drug has a rapid onset and short duration of action. t½: 12 hr. Is 99% protein bound.

Dosage *Mild hypothyroidism, individualized.* **PO:** 25 μg daily. Increase by 12.5–25 μg q 1–2 weeks until satisfactory response has been obtained. **Usual maintenance:** 25–75 μg daily. Use lower initial dosage (5 μg/day) for the elderly, children, and patients with cardiovascular disease. Increase gradually as adult dosage.

Myxedema, **PO: initial,** 5 μg/day increased by 5–10 μg daily q 1 to 2 weeks until 25 μg/day is reached; **then,** increase q 1–2 weeks by 12.5–50 μg. **Usual maintenance:** 50–100 μg/day.

Nontoxic goiter: **Initial,** 5 μg/day; **then,** increase q 1–2 weeks by 12.5 μg or 25 μg. **Usual maintenance:** 75 μg/day.

Cretinism: **initial,** 5 μg daily; increase by 5 μg q 3–4 days to a total daily dose of 20 μg; 50 μg/day may be required for children 1 year of age; full adult dosage may be necessary for children 3 years of age or older.

Transfer from other thyroid preparations to liothyronine—discontinue old preparation before starting on low daily dose of liothyronine. Transfer from liothyronine to other thyroid preparation—start therapy with replacement drug several days prior to complete withdrawal of sodium liothyronine.

LIOTRIX Euthroid, Thyrolar (Rx)

Classification Thyroid preparation.

General Statement Mixture of synthetic levothyroxine sodium (T4) and liothyronine sodium (T3). The mixture contains the products in a 4:1 ratio by weight and in a 1:1 ratio by biologic activity. The two commercial preparations contain slightly different amounts of each component. Because of this discrepancy, a switch from one preparation to the other must be made cautiously. The dosage content of the two preparations are as follows:

Tablets #	T4		T3		Thyroid Equivalency
		Euthroid			
½	30	μg	7.5	μg	30 mg
1	60	μg	15	μg	60 mg
2	120	μg	30	μg	120 mg
3	180	μg	45	μg	180 mg
		Thyrolar			
¼	12.5	μg	3.1	μg	15 mg
½	25	μg	6.25	μg	30 mg
1	50	μg	12.5	μg	60 mg
2	100	μg	25	μg	120 mg
3	150	μg	37.5	μg	180 mg

Dosage **PO, adults and children: initial,** tablet # ½ (*Euthroid:* 30 μg levothyroxine and 7.5 μg of liothyronine; *Thyrolar:* 25 μg levothyroxine and 6.25 μg of liothyronine). In adults, dosage is increased by tablet # ½ at 1- or 2-week intervals and in children by tablet # ½ at 2-week intervals, until satisfactory response has been attained.

Administration/Storage
1. Give as single dose before breakfast.
2. Protect tablets from light, heat, and moisture.

THYROGLOBULIN   Proloid (Rx)

Classification   Thyroid preparation.

General Statement   Thyroid preparation, containing levothyroxine (T_4) and liothyronine (T_3) in a ratio of 2.5 to 1. Drug is a natural product purified from hog thyroid glands. It has no clinical advantage over thyroid, and has a slow onset of action that makes it unsuitable for the treatment of myxedematous coma.

Dosage   **PO: initial**, 32 mg, increased gradually at 1–2 week intervals until control is established. **Usual maintenance**: 32–200 mg daily.
  Therapy is aimed at maintaining 5–9 $\mu g/100$ ml protein-bound iodine.
  Transfer from and to sodium liothyronine should be made gradually.

THYROID DESICCATED   Armour Thyroid, S-P-T, Thyrar, Thyroid Strong, Thyroid U.S.P., Thyro-Teric (Rx)

Classification   Thyroid preparation.

Action/Kinetics   Thyroid is cleaned, dried, powdered animal (usually hog) thyroid gland. The active ingredients of the powder are mainly levothyroxine and liothyronine. The drug has a slow onset of action that makes it unsuitable for the treatment of myxedematous coma.

Dosage   *Myxedema*: **PO, initial**, 16 mg/day for 14 days; **then**, 32 mg/day for 14 more days; **then**, 65 mg/day and reevaluate patient, increasing daily dosage if necessary. **Maintenance**: 65–195 mg/day. *Adult hypothyroidism*: **PO, initial**, 65 mg/day increasing dosage by 65 mg q 30 days until desired response obtained. *Cretinism*: Dosage is the same as for myxedema in the adult; final maintenance dosage may be higher in a growing child than in adults.
  Transfer from liothyronine: start thyroid several days before withdrawal. When transferring from thyroid, discontinue thyroid before starting with low daily dose of replacement drug.

Administration/Storage   Store protected from moisture and light.

THYROTROPIN   Thytropar, Thyroid Stimulating Hormone, Thyrotron* (Rx)

Classification   Thyroid preparation.

Action/Kinetics   Highly purified thyroid-stimulating hormone from bovine pituitary glands. **Peak effect:** 1–2 days.

Uses   Diagnostic agent to evaluate thyroid function.

Contraindications   Untreated Addison's disease, coronary thrombosis. Safe use in pregnancy, lactation, or children has not been established.

Untoward Effects Tachycardia, nausea, vomiting, swelling of thyroid gland, urticaria, headache, anaphylaxis.

Dosage **IM, SC**: Administer 10 International Units daily for 1–3 days followed by radioiodine uptake study within 24 hours.

Administration Store reconstituted solution in refrigerator for two weeks or less.

IODINE SOURCES

POTASSIUM IODIDE   Thyro-Block* (Rx)

SODIUM IODIDE   (Rx)

STRONG IODINE SOLUTION   Lugol's Solution (Rx)

Classification Source of iodine.

Action/Kinetics Small doses of iodine are concentrated by the thyroid gland resulting in an increased synthesis of thyroid hormones. However, large doses are capable of inhibiting thyroid hormone synthesis and release. This is the basis for the use of these drugs in treating hyperthyroidism. Iodine specifically produces involution of a hyperplastic thyroid gland, making it less friable and less vascular prior to surgery. Iodine also shortens the time required by other antithyroid drugs to reduce the output of natural hormone.
  Onset: 1–2 days. **Peak effects:** 10–15 days. **Duration:** Up to 6 weeks.
  Strong Iodine Solution contains 5% iodine and 10% sodium iodide.

Uses Prophylaxis of simple and colloid goiters, exophthalmic goiter. As adjunct with antithyroid drugs to prepare thyrotoxic patients for thyroidectomy, to treat thyrotoxic crisis, or neonatal thyrotoxicosis. Also, for thyroid blocking in radiation emergency.

Contraindications Iodine is contraindicated in tuberculosis because it may cause breakdown of healing of lesions. Also contraindicated in patients hypersensitive to iodine.

Untoward Reactions *Acute poisoning:* Vomiting, abdominal pain, diarrhea, gastritis, swelling of glottis or larynx, shock syndrome. May be treated by soluble starch gastric lavage followed by milk to relieve irritation. *Chronic toxicity (iodism):* Skin reactions including acneiform, vesicular, bullous, or maculopapular eruptions; swelling and inflammation of mucous membranes. Also, conjunctivitis, edema, erythema, fever, irritability.

Dosage *Sodium Iodide: Thyroid crisis*: **IV**, 1–3 gm/day. *Potassium iodide:* **Adults and children over 1 year,** 130 mg (1 tablet) daily or 6 drops of solution (21 mg/drop) daily in ½ glass of liquid; **infants under 1 year:** 3 drops or ½ tablet daily. *Strong iodine solution*: 2–6 drops t.i.d. for 10 days prior to surgery.

Administration
1. Measure iodine solution very carefully with a dropper because medication is very potent and volume tends to be small.
2. Dilute, preferably in 60 ml of milk or orange juice, because medication is very bitter.
3. Do not store other than in original brown, light-resistant container.

Additional Nursing Implications

See also *Nursing Implications*, below.
Teach patient and/or family

a. the symptoms of acute iodine poisoning (see *General Statement*).
b. to withhold drug and report to doctor if toxicity is noted.
c. to check with doctor whether or not to use iodized salt.

ANTITHYROID DRUGS

Action/Kinetics Antithyroid drugs include thiouracil derivatives and large doses of iodide. These drugs suppress (partially or totally) production of thyroid hormones by the thyroid gland. Since these agents do not affect release of preformed hormone, it may take several weeks for the therapeutic effect to become established.

Uses Hyperthyroidism and preparation for thyroid surgery.

Contraindications Lactation. Use with caution during pregnancy and in the presence of cardiovascular disease.

Untoward Reactions *Hematologic:* Agranulocytosis, thrombocytopenia, granulocytopenia, hypoprothrombinemia. *GI:* Nausea, vomiting, taste loss, epigastric pain. *CNS:* Headache, paresthesia, drowsiness, vertigo. *Dermatologic:* Skin rash, urticaria, alopecia, skin pigmentation, pruritus, exfoliative dermatitis. *Miscellaneous:* Jaundice, arthralgia, myalgia, neuritis, edema, sialadenopathy, lymphadenopathy, vasculitis, lupus-like syndrome, drug fever, periarteritis, hepatitis, nephrotic syndrome.

Nursing Implications

Teach patient and/or family

a. that these drugs may take up to 12 weeks to achieve full effect, and must be taken regularly, exactly as directed. If this is not done, hyperthyroidism may recur, whereas if the drug is taken as ordered for 1 or more years, more than half of the patients achieve permanent remission.
b. to report any symptoms of illness to physician promptly: sore throat, enlargement of cervical lymph nodes, GI disturbances, fever, rash, or jaundice. These symptoms may necessitate either a reduction of dosage or withdrawal of the drug.
c. to increase the use of herbs and nonsodium seasonings if loss of taste occurs.

METHIMAZOLE Tapazole (Rx)

Classification Antithyroid preparation.

Action/Kinetics Onset is more rapid, but effect less consistent than that of propylthiouracil. **Duration:** 2–3 hr. t½: 1–2 hr.

Dosage **PO.** *Mild hyperthyroidism*: **initial**, 15 mg/day; *moderately severe hyperthyroidism*: 30–40 mg/day; *severe hyperthyroidism*: 60 mg/day. **Maintenance:** 5–

15 mg/day. **Pediatric: initial**, 0.4 mg/kg; **maintenance**: approximately one-half the initial dose.

Storage/Administration

1. Store in light-resistant containers.
2. Doses should be administered in 3 equal doses at 8 hour intervals.

PROPYLTHIOURACIL Propyl-Thyracil* (Rx)

Classification Antithyroid preparation.

Action/Kinetics Rapidly absorbed from the GI tract. **Duration:** 2–3 hr. **t½:** 3–5 hr. 80% is protein bound.

Drug Interactions Propylthiouracil may produce hypoprothrombinemia, adding to the effect of anticoagulants.

Dosage **PO. Initial**, 300 mg/day (up to 900 mg/day may be required in some patients with severe hyperthyroidism); **maintenance**: 100– 150 mg/day. **Pediatric, 6–10 years: initial**, 50–150 mg/day; **over 10 years: initial**, 150–300 mg/day. Maintenance for all pediatric use is based on response.

Administration Doses should be administered in 3 equal doses at 8 hr intervals.

RADIOACTIVE AGENT

SODIUM IODIDE ^{131}I Iodotope Therapeutic, Sodium Iodide ^{131}I Therapeutic (Rx)

Classification Radioactive agent.

Action/Kinetics This compound is a radioactive iodide salt that concentrates in the thyroid gland, where it is incorporated into thyroid hormones. **Onset:** Detection of radioactivity in thyroid: minutes. **Duration:** 8–10 weeks for thyroid function to return to normal.

Uses *Diagnosis:* Evaluation of thyroid function and detection of malignancies involving the thyroid gland. *Therapeutic:* Hyperthyroidism, selected cases of thyroid cancer.

Contraindications *Therapeutic:* Extreme tachycardia. Recent episodes of coronary thrombosis, myocardial infarction, or large nodular goiters. Pregnancy, lactation, persons younger than 18 years of age.

Untoward Reactions The most severe effects are seen following use for thyroid carcinoma. *Hematologic:* Anemia, leukemia, bone marrow depression, leukopenia, thrombocytopenia. *Radiation sickness:* Nausea, vomiting. *Miscellaneous:* Acute thyroid crisis, chromosome abnormalities, cough, swelling or tenderness in neck, pain on swallowing, sore throat, alopecia (temporary).

Dosage *Diagnostic,* **PO, IV:** 1–25 microcuries. *Therapeutic,* **PO, IV,** *hyperthyroidism:* 4–10 millicuries. *Thyroid cancer or metastases:* 50–150 millicuries.

Administration/Storage

1. Therapeutic dose only given to hospitalized patients.

2. Upon standing, solution and glass storage containers may darken as a result of radiation. This does not affect efficacy of the product.

Nursing Implication
For radiation protection, observe hospital procedure.

Chapter Sixty

CALCITONIN, CALCIUM SALTS, AND CALCIUM REGULATORS

General Statement Appropriate calcium levels in the body are required for many processes including blood coagulation, regulation of heart rhythm, and skeletal muscle contraction. Maintenance of extracellular calcium levels is controlled by parathyroid hormone utilizing a feedback mechanism.

Dysfunction of the parathyroid may result in hypocalcemic tetany, seizures, and death. Administration of either parathyroid hormone obtained from animal sources or a synthetic compound restores calcium levels toward normal values. Because the response is slow, calcium salts are usually administered concomitantly.

CALCITONIN-SALMON Calcimar (Rx)

Classification Calcium regulator.

General Statement Calcitonin is a polypeptide hormone produced in mammals by the parafollicular cells of the thyroid gland. However, calcitonin isolated from salmon is used therapeutically. This salmon-derived compound has the same therapeutic effect as the human hormone except for a higher potency per milligram and a somewhat longer duration of action. The drug is ineffective when administered orally.

Action/Kinetics Calcitonin decreases serum calcium (i.e., opposes the effects of parathyroid hormone) by inhibiting calcium and phosphorus reabsorption by the renal tubules. It also inhibits bone resorption. **Onset:** 2 hr. **Peak:** 6 hr. **Duration:** 12 hr. Clinical effectiveness: after 1 month. Excreted unchanged in the urine.

Uses Moderate to severe Paget's disease characterized by polyostotic involvement with elevation of serum alkaline phosphatase and urinary excretion of hydroxyproline. For the early treatment of hypercalcemia. Comcomitantly with calcium and vitamin D to treat postmenopausal osteoporosis.

Contraindications Allergy to salmon calcitonin or its gelatin diluent. Pregnancy, lactation. Safe use in children not established.

Untoward Reactions *Allergic:* Due to foreign protein reaction to salmon calcitonin or the gelatin diluent. Skin rashes, systemic allergic symptoms. *GI:* Nausea, vomiting. *Other:* Flushing of hands and face, local inflammation at injection site, antibody formation rendering the drug ineffective.

Laboratory Test Alteration Reduction of alkaline phosphatase and 24-hour urinary excretion of hydroxyproline are indicative of successful therapy. Monitor urine for casts (indicative of kidney damage).

Dosage *Paget's disease:* **SC, IM, initial,** 100 MRC units/day (0.5. ml). In some patients improvement can be maintained by giving 50 MRC units every day or every other day, but effectiveness of such a regimen has not been determined.
  Hypercalcemia: **SC, IM, initial,** 4 MRC units/kg/12 hr; if response not evident after 1–2 days, increase to 8 MRC units/kg/12 hr. If response still unsatisfactory after 2 more days, dose can be increased to maximum of 8 MRC units/kg/6 hr. Use IM route or multiple sites if volume exceeds 2 ml.
  Postmenopausal osteoporosis: **SC, IM,** 100 IU units/day with calcium and vitamin D.

Nursing Implications

1. Ascertain that sensitivity test is negative before administering medication.
2. *Assess*
   a. for systemic allergic reaction, and be prepared to provide emergency care with oxygen, epinephrine, and steroids.
   b. for local inflammatory reaction at the site of injection and report.
   c. for facial flushing, which may occur with treatment.
   d. for hypocalcemic tetany during administration, and have calcium available for emergency use. (Progressive signs of hypocalcemic tetany are muscular fibrillation, twitching, tetanic spasms, and finally convulsions.)
   e. compliance with drug regimen if a relapse occurs.
3. Ascertain that patients who have a good initial clinical response, but who then relapse, are evaluated for antibody formation in response to serum calcitonin.
4. *Teach patient and/or family*
   a. appropriate assessments detailed above.
   b. aseptic method of reconstituting solution, injection technique, and importance of alternating injection sites.

(continued)

    c. that nausea and vomiting, which may occur at the onset of therapy, tend to disappear as treatment is continued.

    d. the importance of returning for periodic urine sediment tests to check for possible kidney damage.

CALCIUM SALTS

Classification   Electrolyte, mineral.

General Statement   Calcium is essential for maintenance of normal function of nerves, muscles, skeletal system and cell membrane and capillary permeability. For example, calcium is necessary for activation of many enzyme reactions and is required for nerve impulses; contraction of cardiac, smooth, and skeletal muscles; renal function; respiration; and blood coagulation. It has a role in the release of neurotransmitters and hormones; in the uptake and binding of amino acids, in vitamin B_{12} absorption, and gastrin secretion.

The normal calcium serum concentration is 9–10.4 mg/dl (4.5–5.2 mEq/L). When the calcium level of the extracellular fluid falls below this level, calcium is first mobilized from bone. However, eventually blood calcium depletion may be so great as to become openly manifest.

Hypocalcemia is characterized by muscular fibrillations, twitching, skeletal muscle spasms, leg cramps, tetanic spasms, cardiac arrhythmias, smooth muscle hyperexcitability, mental depression, and anxiety states. Excessive, chronic hypocalcemia is characterized by brittle, defective nails, poor dentition, and brittle hair.

The Recommended Daily Dietary Allowance for elemental calcium is 0.8 gm/day for adults and children from 1–10 years, 1.2 gm for pregnant or lactating women and children 10–18 years of age, 0.54 gm for children 6–12 months of age, and 0.36 gm for infants less than 6 months of age. Calcium deficiency can be corrected by the administration of various calcium salts.

Calcium is well absorbed from the upper GI tract. However, severe low calcium tetany is best treated by IV administration of calcium gluconate.

The presence of vitamin D is necessary for maximum calcium utilization. The hormone of the parathyroid gland is necessary for the regulation of the calcium level.

Uses   **IV:** Acute hypocalcemic tetany secondary to renal failure, hypoparathyroidism, premature delivery, maternal diabetes mellitus in infants, poisoning due to magnesium, oxalic acid, radiophosphorus, carbon tetrachloride, fluoride, phosphate, strontium, and radium. Also during cardiac resuscitation when epinephrine or isoproterenol has not improved myocardial contraction (may also be given into the ventricular cavity for this purpose). To reverse cardiotoxicity of hyperkalemia.

IM or IV: Reduce spasm in renal, biliary, intestinal, or lead colic. To relieve muscle cramps due to insect bites and to decrease capillary permeability in various sensitivity reactions.

PO: Osteoporosis, osteomalacia, chronic hypoparathyroidism, rickets, latent tetany, hypocalcemia secondary to use of anticonvulsant drugs. Myasthenia gravis, Eaton-Lambert syndrome, supplement for pregnant, postmenopausal, or nursing women. Also, prophylactially for primary osteoporosis.

Investigational: As an infusion to diagnose Zollinger-Ellison syndrome and medullary thyroid carcinoma. To antagonize neuromuscular blockade due to aminoglycosides.

Contraindications Digitalized patients, sarcoidosis, renal or cardiac disease. Use with caution in cor pulmonale, respiratory acidosis, renal disease or failure, ventricular fibrillation, hypercalcemia. Cancer patients with bone metastases.

Untoward Reactions Excess calcium may cause hypercalcemia characterized by lassitude, fatigue, depression of nervous and neuromuscular function (emotional disturbances, confusion, skeletal muscle weakness, and constipation), impairment of renal function (polyuria, polydipsia, and azotemia), renal calculi, arrhythmias, and bradycardia.

Following PO use: GI irritation, constipation.

Following IV use: Venous irritation, tingling sensation, feeling of oppression or heat, chalky taste. Rapid IV administration may result in vasodilation, decreased blood pressure and heart rate, cardiac arrhythmias, syncope, or cardiac arrest.

Following IM use: Burning feeling, necrosis, tissue sloughing, cellulitis, soft tissue calcification.

Note: If calcium is injected into the myocardium rather than into the ventricle, laceration of coronary arteries, cardiac tamponade, pneumothorax, and ventricular fibrillation may occur.

Drug Interactions

Interactant	Interaction
Cephalocin	Incompatible with calcium salts
Corticosteroids	Interfere with absorption of calcium from GI tract
Digitalis	Increased digitalis arrhythmias and toxicity. Death has resulted from combination of digitalis and IV calcium salts
Milk	Excess of either agent may cause hypercalcemia, renal insufficiency with azotemia, alkalosis, and ocular lesions
Tetracyclines	↓ Effect of tetracyclines due to ↓ absorption from GI tract
Vitamin D	Enhances intestinal absorption of dietary calcium

Dosage See Table 29, p. 712.

Note: One mEq of elemental calcium is equivalent to 20 mg.

Administration

ORAL

1. Administer 1–1½ hours p.c. because alkalies and large amounts of fats decrease absorption of calcium.
2. Advise patients who have difficulty swallowing large pills that calcium in water suspension may be obtained from the pharmacist or be made by diluting medication with *hot* water because calcium goes into suspension six times more readily in hot water than cold water. Solution may then be cooled before drinking.

IV

1. Administer very slowly, observing vital signs closely for bradycardia and hypotension.
2. Prevent leakage of medication into tissues because these salts are highly irritating.

IM

1. Rotate sites of injection because medication may cause sloughing.
2. Do not administer IM calcium gluconate to children.

TABLE 29 CALCIUM SALTS[a]

Drug	Uses	Dosage	Percent of Calcium in Preparation, which Indicates Efficacy
Calcium carbonate (BioCal, Cal-Sup, Caltrate,* Caltrate-600, Os-Cal 500), OTC	Mild hypocalcemia, latent hypocalcemic tetany	**PO:** 1-1.5 gm t.i.d. with meals.	40%
Calcium chloride, Rx	Mild hypocalcemia, latent tetany, severe hypocalcemic tetany, magnesium intoxication, cardiac resuscitation to reverse the harmful effects of hyperkalemia	**IV only.** *Hypocalcemia:* 0.5–1 gm q 1–3 days. *Magnesium intoxication:* 0.5 gm; observe for recovery before other doses given. *Cardiac resuscitation:* 0.5–1 gm. *Hyperkalemia:* Sufficient amount to return EEG to normal. **Never administer IM.**	27.2%
Calcium glubionate (Neo-Cal-glucon), OTC	Hypocalcemia, calcium deficiency, tetany of newborn, hypoparathyroidism, pseudohypoparathyroidism, osteoporosis, rickets, osteomalacia	*Dietary supplement:* **Adults and children over 4 yr, PO:** 15 ml t.i.d.–q.i.d. **Pediatric (under 4 yr):** 10 ml t.i.d. **Infants:** 5 ml 5 times/day. *Tetany of newborn:* On the basis of laboratory tests, usually 50–150 mg/kg/day in 3 or more divided doses. *Other calcium deficiencies:*	6.5%

Calcium gluceptate, Rx	Hypocalcemia, tetany, exchange transfusion in newborns	**Adult:** 15–45 ml one to three times daily. **IM:** 2–5ml (0.44–1.1 gm containing 36–90 mg calcium) in gluteal region (for infants: give in lateral thigh). **IV:** 5–20 ml (1.1–4.4 gm containing 90–360 mg calcium). *Newborns for exchange transfusions:* 0.5 ml (0.11 gm) after every 100 ml of blood exchanged.	22%
Calcium gluconate (Kalcinate), Rx (injection) and OTC (tablets)	Latent hypocalcemic tetany severe hypocalcemic tetany	**PO:** 1–2 gm t.i.d.; **children:** 500 mg/kg in divided doses. **IV:** 0.5–2.0 gm. **Children:** 500 mg/kg/day in divided doses. Rate of injection should not exceed 0.5 ml/min.	9%
Calcium lactate, OTC	Latent hypocalcemic tetany, hyperphosphatemia	**PO, adult:** 0.325–1.3 gm t.i.d. with meals. **Pediatric:** 500 mg/kg daily in divided doses.	13%
Dibasic calcium phosphate dihydrate, OTC	Calcium deficiency states, dietary supplement	**PO:** 0.5–1.5 gm b.i.d.–t.i.d.	23%

[a] Other calcium salts may be prescribed as well.

Nursing Implications
1. Prevent patient in hypocalcemic tetany from injury by providing safety precautions.
2. *Teach patient and/or family*
   a. that calcium requirements are best met by milk in diet.
   b. that multivitamin and mineral preparations do not contain sufficient calcium to meet their needs.

MISCELLANEOUS AGENTS

ETIDRONATE DISODIUM (EHDP)   Didronel (Rx)

Classification   Bone growth regulator.

Action/Kinetics   Paget's disease is characterized by bone resorption, compensatory new bone formation, and increased vascularization of the bone. Etidronate disodium slows bone metabolism, thereby decreasing bone resorption, bone turnover, and new bone formation; it also reduces bone vascularization. **Absorption:** Dose dependent; after 24 hr, one-half of absorbed drug is excreted. The drug remaining in the body is adsorbed to bone, where therapeutic effects persist 3–12 months after discontinuation of the drug.

Uses   Paget's disease (osteitis deformans), especially of the polyostotic type accompanied by pain and increased urine levels of hydroxyproline and serum alkaline phosphatase. Heterotopic ossification due to spinal cord injury or total hip replacement.

Contraindications   Use with caution in the presence of renal dysfunction, during pregnancy, and lactation. Safe use in children not established.

Untoward Reactions   *GI:* Nausea, diarrhea, loose bowel movements. *Bones:* Increased incidence of bone fractures and increased or recurrent bone pain. Drug should be discontinued if fracture occurs and not restarted until healing takes place.

Dosage   **PO.** *Paget's disease,* **initial,** 5 mg/kg/day for 6 months or less; 10 mg/kg up to a maximum of 20 mg/kg/day for patients when bone metabolism suppression is highly advisable; treatment at this dose level should not exceed 3 months. Another course of therapy may be instituted after rest period of 3 months.
   Heterotopic ossification due to spinal cord injury: 20 mg/kg/day for 2 weeks; **then** 10 mg/kg/day for 10 weeks.
   Heterotopic ossification complicating total hip replacement: 20 mg/kg/day for 30 days preoperatively; **then,** 20 mg/kg/day for 90 days postoperatively.

Administration
1. Give as single dose 2 hours before meals with juice or water.
2. Advise patient not to eat for 2 hours after taking medication because foods particularly high in calcium may reduce absorption.
3. Patients should maintain adequate intake of calcium and vitamin D.

4. Urinary hydroxyproline excretion and/or serum alkaline phosphatase levels should be determined periodically when the drug is given for Paget's disease.
5. There are no indications that etidronate will affect mature heterotopic bone.

Nursing Implications
1. Monitor urinary hydroxyproline excretion and serum alkaline phosphatase because reduction in these levels are first indication of a beneficial therapeutic response. Reduced levels usually occur 1 to 3 months after initiation of therapy.
2. Teach patient and/or family to maintain a well-balanced diet with adequate intake of calcium and vitamin D.

SODIUM CELLULOSE PHOSPHATE   Calcibind, Calcisorb* (Rx)

Classification   Calcium binding agent.

Action/Kinetics   Sodium cellulose phosphate is a synthetic ion exchange substance that exchanges sodium for calcium and magnesium ions in the GI tract. The bound calcium, from both dietary and endogenous sources, is excreted in the feces. Thus, urinary calcium is decreased. There are small increases in urinary phosphorous and oxalate.

Uses   Absorptive hypercalciuria Type I with excretion of calcium oxalate or calcium phosphate stones.

Contraindications   Primary or secondary hyperparathyroidism, hypocalcemia, hypomagnesemia, enteric hyperoxaluria, osteoporosis, osteomalacia, osteitis, low intestinal absorption or renal excretion of calcium, when hypercalciuria is due to mobilization from bones. Children under age 16. Use with caution in congestive heart failure, ascites, or in pregnancy.

Untoward Reactions   *GI:* Diarrhea, dyspepsia, loose bowel movements. *Other:* Hyperparathyroid bone disease, hyperoxaluria, hypomagnesiuria, loss of copper, zinc, iron.

Dosage   **PO.** *Urinary calcium greater than 300 mg/day:* 5 gm with each meal; *urinary calcium less than 150 mg/day:* 2.5 gm with breakfast and lunch and 5 gm with dinner.

Administration
1. Parathyroid hormone levels should be monitored at least once between two weeks and three months after therapy initiated.
2. A moderate calcium intake is recommended.
3. Mix each dose of sodium cellulose phosphate with water, juice, or soft drink and take within 30 min of the meal.
4. Foods such as dark greens (e.g., spinach), rhubarb, chocolate, and brewed tea should be avoided as they contain oxalate.
5. Sufficient fluid should be taken daily to ensure a minimum urine output of 2 liters.
6. Magnesium gluconate supplements may be given in the following regimens: 1.5 gm magnesium gluconate before breakfast and at bedtime in patients re-

ceiving 15 gm of sodium cellulose phosphate daily; 1 gm magnesium gluconate, as above, in patients taking 10 gm sodium cellulose phosphate daily. To avoid binding, magnesium should be given 1 hr before or after sodium cellulose phosphate.

Nursing Implications
1. Be aware that magnesium, iron, and other trace metal supplements may be ordered.
2. *Teach patient and/or family*
   a. that dose should be taken with a meal to maximize uptake of dietary calcium.
   b. to avoid ingesting calcium-containing foods such as milk, cheese, or ice cream.
   c. to avoid spinach and dark green vegetables, rhubarb, chocolate, and brewed tea.
   d. to avoid Vitamin C supplements, salt, and lightly salted foods.

Chapter Sixty-one

ADRENOCORTICOSTEROIDS AND ANALOGS

ADRENOCORTICOSTEROIDS

General Statement   The adrenocorticosteroids are a group of natural hormones produced by the adrenal cortex (outer shell of the adrenal gland). They are used for a variety of therapeutic purposes. Many slightly modified synthetic variants are available today, and some patients respond better to one substance than to another.

The hormones of the adrenal gland influence many metabolic pathways and all organ systems and are essential for survival.

The release of adrenocorticosteroids is controlled by hormones such as corticotropin releasing factor produced by the hypothalamus and ACTH (corticotropin) produced by the anterior pituitary.

The adrenocorticosteroids play an important role in most major metabolic processes. They have the following effects:

1. **Carbohydrate metabolism.** Deposition of glucose as glycogen in the liver and the conversion of glycogen to glucose when needed. Gluconeogenesis (i.e., the transformation of protein into glucose).
2. **Protein metabolism.** The stimulation of protein loss from many organs (catabolism). This is characterized by a negative nitrogen balance.
3. **Fat metabolism.** The deposition of fatty tissue in facial, abdominal, and shoulder regions.
4. **Water and electrolyte balance.** Alteration of glomerular filtration rate; increased sodium and consequently fluid retention. Also affects the excretion rate of potassium, calcium, and phosphorous. Urinary excretion rate of creatine and uric acid increases.

The hormones also have a marked anti-inflammatory effect and aid the organism to cope with various stressful situations (trauma, severe illness). The adrenocorticosteroids also suppress the lymphatic system, decreasing the number of

*Topical agent, see Table 30, p. 718.

TABLE 30 CORTICOSTEROIDS USED TOPICALLY

Drug	Dosage/Administration
Amcinonide (Cyclocort), Rx	Apply cream (0.1%) or ointment (0.1%) sparingly and rub in.
Betamethasone benzoate (Benisone, Uticort), Rx	Apply cream, gel, lotion, or ointment (each 0.025%) sparingly and rub in.
Betamethasone dipropionate (Alphalex, Diprosone), Rx	Apply aerosol (0.1%), cream (0.05%), lotion (0.05%), or ointment (0.05%) sparingly and rub in.
Betamethasone valerate (Betatrex, Beta-Val, Valisone, Valisone Reduced Strength, Valnac), Rx	Apply cream (0.01%, 0.1%), lotion (0.1%), or ointment (0.1%) sparingly and rub in.
Clocortolone pivalate (Cloderm), Rx	Apply cream (0.1%) sparingly and rub in.
Desonide (DesOwen, Tridesilon), Rx	Apply a thin film of cream or ointment (each 0.05%) b.i.d.–t.i.d.
Desoximetasone (Topicort, Topicort LP), Rx	Apply a thin film of cream (0.25%), gel (0.05%), or ointment (0.25%) b.i.d.
Dexamethasone (Aeroseb-Dex, Decaderm, Decaspray), Rx	Apply cream (0.04%), aerosol (0.01%, 0.04%), or gel (0.1%) b.i.d.–t.i.d.
Dexamethasone sodium phosphate (Decadron Phosphate), Rx	Apply cream (0.1%) and rub in lightly.
Dexamethasone sodium phosphate ophthalmic (AK-Dex Ophthalmic, Decadron Phosphate Ophthalmic, Maxidex Ophthalmic), Rx	**Solution** (0.1%): **initial**, 1–2 drops in conjunctival sac q hr during day and q 2 hr during night; **then**, decrease to 1 drop q 4 hr to 1 drop t.i.d.–q.i.d. **Ointment** (0.05%): **initial**, instill a small amount in conjunctival sac t.i.d.–q.i.d.; **then**, decrease to b.i.d. and then once daily.
Diflorasone diacetate (Flutone,* Maxiflor), Rx	Apply cream (0.05%) or ointment (0.05%) sparingly and rub in.
Fluocinolone Acetonide (Dermophyl,* Fluoderm,* Duolar,* Fluoderm,* Fluolar,* Fluolean,* Fluonid, Flurosyn, Psoranide, Synalar, Synalar-HP, Synamol,* Synemol), Rx	Apply cream (0.01%, 0.025%, 0.2%), ointment (0.025%), or solution (0.01%) b.i.d.–t.i.d.
Fluocinonide (Lidemol,* Lidex, Lidex-E, Lyderm*), Rx	Apply a thin film of cream, gel, ointment, or solution (each 0.05%). Use small amounts by rubbing gently into cleansed affected areas.
Fluorometholone (FML Liquifilm Ophthalmic), Rx	**Suspension (ophthalmic):** 1–2 drops into conjunctival sac q hr during day and q 2 hr at night; **then**, reduce to 1 drop q 4 hr.
Flurandrenolide (Cordran, Cordran SP, Drenison*), Rx	Apply cream (0.025%, 0.05%), lotion (0.05%), or ointment (0.025%, 0.05%) b.i.d.–t.i.d. Tape (4 µg/sq cm) is applied as occlusive dressing; change q 12 hr. Protect from light, heat, and freezing.
Halcinonide (Halog, Halog-E), Rx	Apply cream (0.025%, 0.1%), ointment (0.1%), or solution (0.1%) b.i.d.–t.i.d. Can be used with an occlusive dressing during night (12 hr); use without occlusion during day.
Hydrocortisone (**Creams:** Bactine Hydro-	Apply cream (0.125%, 0.25%, 0.5%, 1%,

TABLE 30   (*Continued*)

Drug	Dosage/Administration
cortisone, Cort-Dome, Cortril, Cortizone-5, Dermacort, DermiCort, Dermolate Anti-Itch, Dermtex HC, Eldecort, H_2Cort, Hi-Cor 1.0 and 2.5, Hydro-tex, Hytone, Nutracort, Penecort, Pro-Cort, Pro-Cort M, Racet SE-½% and 1%, Synacort, Ulcort) OTC (0.5% or less) and Rx	2.5%), gel (1%), lotion (0.25%, 0.5%, 1%, 2.5%), ointment (0.5%, 1%, 2.5%), or spray (0.5%). Medication should be applied sparingly and rubbed in.
(**Gels**: HC-Jel, Nutracort), Rx	
(**Lotions**: Acticort 100, Cetacort, Cort-Dome, Delacort, Dermacort, Dermolate Scalp Itch, Hytone, MyCort, Nutracort, Texacort Scalp Lotion), OTC and Rx	
(**Sprays**: Aeroseb-HC, CaldeCort, Clincort, Cortaid, Dermolate Anti-Itch), OTC and Rx	
Hydrocortisone Acetate	Apply cream (0.5%), foam (1%), lotion (0.5%), or ointment (0.5%, 1%, 2.5%). Apply sparingly and rub in.
(**Creams**: CaldeCort, Clinicort, Cortaid, Gynecort, Lanacort, Pharma-Cort, Resicort, Rhulicort), OTC	
(**Foam**: Epifoam), Rx	
(**Lotions**: Cortaid, Rhulicort), OTC	
(**Ointments**: Cortaid, Cortef Acetate), OTC (0.5%) and Rx (1%, 2.5%)	
Hydrocortisone butyrate (Locoid), Rx	Apply cream (0.1%) or ointment (0.1%) sparingly and rub in.
Hydrocortisone valerate (Westcort), Rx	Apply cream (0.2%) or ointment (0.2%) sparingly and rub in.
Methylprednisolone acetate (Medrol Acetate), Rx	Apply ointment (0.25%, 1%) sparingly and rub in.
Prednisolone acetate ophthalmic (AK-Tate Ophthalmic, Econopred Ophthalmic, Econopred Plus Ophthalmic, Pred Forte Ophthalmic, Pred Mild Ophthalmic, Predulose Ophthalmic), Rx	Instill 1–2 drops of the suspension (0.12%, 0.125%, 0.25%, 1%) into the conjunctival sac q hr during the day and q 2 hr during the night initially; then, after response obtained, decrease dose to 1 drop q 6–8 hr.
Prednisolone sodium phosphate ophthalmic (AK-Pred Ophthalmic, Inflamase Ophthalmic, Inflamase Forte Ophthalmic, Metreton Ophthalmic), Rx	Apply solution (0.125%, 0.5%, 1%) in a manner similar to prednisolone acetate ophthalmic.
Triamcinolone acetonide (Aristocort, Aristocort A, Flutex, Kenac, Kenalog, Kenalog-H, Triacet, Triderm, Trymex), Rx	Apply aerosol (0.2 mg/2 sec spray), cream (0.025%, 0.1%, 0.5%), lotion (0.025%, 0.1%), or ointment (0.025%, 0.1%, 0.5%) sparingly and rub in.

circulating lymphocytes and eosinophils, shrinking the lymph nodes, and atrophying the thymus. The production of immunoglobulins (antibodies) is depressed.

According to their chemical structure and chief physiologic effect, the adrenocorticosteroids fall into two subgroups, which have considerable functional overlap.

1. Those, like cortisone and hydrocortisone, that mainly regulate the metabolic

pathways involving protein, carbohydrate, and fat. This group is often referred to as *glucocorticoids*.

2. Those, like aldosterone and desoxycorticosterone, that are more specifically involved in electrolyte and water balance. These are often referred to as *mineralocorticoids*.

Action/Kinetics   Glucocorticoids are qualitatively similar. Differences between these agents are due to duration of action and half-life (see individual agents).

Uses   When used for anti-inflammatory or immunosuppressant therapy, the corticosteroid should possess minimal mineralocorticoid activity. Therapy with glucocorticoids is not curative and in many situations should be considered as adjunctive rather than primary therapy.

1. **Replacement therapy**. Acute and chronic adrenal insufficiency, including Addison's disease, congenital adrenal hyperplasia, adrenal insufficiency secondary to anterior pituitary insufficiency. However, not all drugs can be used for replacement therapy; some lack glucocorticoid effects, others lack mineralocorticoid effects. For replacement therapy, drugs must possess both effects.

2. **Rheumatic diseases**. Rheumatoid arthritis, bursitis, ankylosing spondylitis, osteoarthritis, tenosynovitis.

3. **Collagen diseases**. Systemic lupus erythematosus, rheumatic carditis, polymyositis, polyarteritis nodosa, dermatomyositis, polychondritis, arteritis.

4. **Dermatologic diseases**. Urticaria, pemphigus, dermatitis herpetiformis, exfoliative dermatitis, psoriasis, seborrheic dermatitis, mycosis fungoides, contact dermatitis, eczema, cutaneous sarcoidosis, lichen planus, erythema multiform.

5. **Allergic manifestations**. Serum sickness, acute allergic rhinitis, angioneurotic edema, intractable hay fever, drug reactions, anaphylaxis, bronchial asthma (including status asthmaticus).

6. **Renal disease**. Acute or chronic glomerulonephritis, nephrotic syndrome due to systemic lupus erythematosus, primary renal disease.

7. **Ocular diseases**. Allergic blepharitis, purulent conjunctivitis, corneal inflammation, uveitis, acute choroiditis, sympathetic ophthalmia, retrolental fibroplasia, iritis, diffuse posterior uveitis, optic neuritis.

8. **Respiratory diseases**. Symptomatic sarcoidosis, berylliosis, tuberculosis (as adjunct only), lipid pneumonitis. *Investigational:* Betamethasone or dexamethasone has been used in threatened premature delivery to prevent hyaline membrane disease.

9. **Hematologic disorders**. Thrombocytopenia, acquired hemolytic anema, erythroblastopenia, congenital hypoplastic anemia.

10. **Gastrointestinal disorders**. Ulcerative colitis, sprue, regional enteritis, celiac disease.

11. **Neoplastic diseases**. Acute lymphocytic leukemia and lymphoma, chronic lymphatic leukemia, Hodgkin's disease, lymphosarcoma, breast carcinoma.

12. **Other uses**. Cerebral edema, myasthenia gravis, as adjunct to prevent organ transplant rejection, inflammation from dental procedures, and exacerbation of multiple sclerosis.

Note: Glucocorticoids have also been used in active and alcoholic hepatitis, certain types of cirrhosis, and to treat shock. However, their effectiveness for these situations remains unclear.

Contraindications   Corticosteroids are contraindicated in any situation where infection may be suspected as these drugs may mask infections. Also peptic ulcer, psychoses, acute glomerulonephritis, herpes simplex infections of the eye, vaccinia or varicella, the exanthematous diseases, Cushing's syndrome, active tuberculosis, myasthenia gravis.

Adrenoglucocorticoids should be used with caution in the presence of diabetes mellitus, hypertension, congestive heart failure, chronic nephritis, thrombophlebitis, osteoporosis, convulsive disorders, infectious diseases, diverticulitis, renal insufficiency, pregnancy.

Topical application in the treatment of eye disorders is contraindicated in dendritic keratitis, vaccinia, chickenpox, or other viral disease that may involve the conjunctiva or cornea. Also tuberculosis and fungal or acute purulent infections of the eye. Topical treatment of the ear is contraindicated in aural fungal infections and perforated eardrum. Topical use in dermatology contraindicated in tuberculosis of the skin, herpes simplex, vaccinia, varicella, and infectious conditions in the absence of anti-infective agents.

Untoward Reactions Small physiologic doses given as replacement therapy or short-term high dosage therapy during emergencies rarely cause side effects. Prolonged therapy may cause a Cushing-like syndrome with atrophy of the adrenal cortex and subsequent adrenocortical insufficiency. A steroid withdrawal syndrome may occur following prolonged use; symptoms include anorexia, nausea, vomiting, lethargy, headache, fever, joint pain, desquamation, myalgia, weight loss, hypotension.

Fluid and electrolyte: Edema, hypokalemic alkalosis, hypokalemia, hypertension, congestive heart failure. *Musculoskeletal:* Muscle wasting, muscle pain or weakness, osteoporosis, vertebral compression fractures, delayed wound healing. *GI:* Nausea, vomiting, anorexia or increased appetite, diarrhea or constipation, abdominal distention, pancreatitis, gastric irritation, ulcerative esophagitis. Development or exacerbation of peptic ulcers. *Endocrine:* Cushing's syndrome, amenorrhea, decreased glucose tolerance, hyperglycemia, diabetes mellitus. *CNS:* Headache, vertigo, insomnia, restlessness, increased motor activity, ischemic neuropathy, EEG abnormalities, seizures. Also, euphoria, mood swings, depression, anxiety, personality changes, psychoses. *Dermatologic:* Skin atrophy and thinning, acne, increased sweating, hirsutism, facial erythema, striae, petechiae, ecchymoses, easy bruising. *Allergic:* Allergic dermatitis, urticaria, angioedema, burning or tingling of perineal area following IV use. *Miscellaneous:* Hypercholesterolemia, atherosclerosis, thrombosis, thromboembolism, fat embolism, thrombophlebitis. **In children:** Suppression of linear growth; reversible pseudo-brain tumor syndrome characterized by papilledema, oculomotor or abducens nerve paralysis, visual loss, or headache.

INTRA-ARTICULAR Postinjection flare, Charcot-like arthropathy. Due to reduction in inflammation and pain, patients may overuse the joint.

EYE THERAPY Application of corticosteroid preparations to the eye may reduce the aqueous outflow and increase ocular pressure, thereby inducing or aggravating simple glaucoma. Ocular pressure therefore should be checked frequently in the elderly or in patients with glaucoma. Stinging, burning, dendritic keratitis (herpes simplex), corneal perforation (especially when the drugs are used for diseases that cause corneal thinning). Posterior subcapsular cataracts, especially in children. Exophthalmos, secondary fungal or viral eye infections.

TOPICAL USE Except when used over large areas, when the skin is broken, or with occlusive dressings, topically applied corticosteroids are not absorbed systemically in sufficiently large quantities to cause the untoward reactions noted in the previous paragraphs. Topically applied corticosteroids, however, may cause atrophy of the epidermis, drying of the skin, or atrophy of the dermal collagen. When used on the face, the agents may cause diffuse thinning and homogenization of the collagen, epidermal thinning, and striae formation. Topical corticosteroids should be used cautiously, or not at all, for infected lesions, and in that case, the use of occlusive dressings is contraindicated. Occasionally, topical corticosteroids may cause a sensitization reaction, which necessitates discontinuation of the drug.

Drug Interactions

Interactant	Interaction
Amphotericin B	Corticosteroids ↑ K depletion caused by amphotericin B
Antacids	↓ Effect of corticosteroids due to ↓ absorption from GI tract
Antibiotics, broad spectrum	Concomitant use may result in emergence of resistant strains leading to severe infection
Anticholinergics	Combination ↑ intraocular pressure; will aggravate glaucoma
Anticoagulants, oral	↓ Effect of anticoagulants by ↓ hypoprothrombinemia; also ↑ risk of hemorrhage due to vascular effects of corticosteroids
Antidiabetic agents	Hyperglycemic effect of corticosteroids may necessitate an ↑ dose of antidiabetic agent
Barbiturates	↓ Effect of corticosteroids due to ↑ breakdown by liver
Bumetanide	Enhanced K loss due to K-losing properties of both drugs
Cholestyramine	↓ Effect of corticosteroids due to ↓ absorption from GI tract
Colestipol	↓ Effect of corticosteroids due to ↓ absorption from GI tract
Contraceptives, oral	Estrogen ↑ anti-inflammatory effect of hydrocortisone by ↓ breakdown by liver
Cyclosporine	↑ Effect of both drugs due to ↓ breakdown by liver
Digitalis glycosides	↑ Chance of digitalis toxicity due to hypokalemia
Estrogens	Estrogens ↑ anti-inflammatory effect of hydrocortisone by ↓ breakdown by liver
Ethacrynic acid	Enhanced K loss due to K-losing properties of both drugs
Furosemide	Enhanced K loss due to K-losing properties of both drugs
Heparin	Ulcerogenic effects of corticosteroids may → ↑ risk of hemorrhage
Indomethacin	↑ Chance of GI ulceration
Isoniazid	↓ Effect of isoniazid due to ↑ breakdown by liver and ↑ excretion
Muscle relaxants, nondepolarizing	↓ Effect of muscle relaxants
Phenobarbital	↓ Effect of corticosteroids due to ↑ breakdown by liver
Phenytoin	↓ Effect of corticosteroids due to ↑ breakdown by liver

Interactant	Interaction
Rifampin	↓ Effect of corticosteroids due to ↑ breakdown by liver
Salicylates	Both are ulcerogenic; also, corticosteroids may ↓ blood salicylate levels
Theophyllines	Corticosteroids ↑ effect of theophyllines
Thiazide diuretics	Enhanced K loss due to K-losing properties of both drugs
Vitamin A	Topical vitamin A can reverse impaired wound healing in patients receiving corticosteroids

Laboratory Test Interferences   ↑ Urine glucose, serum cholesterol, serum amylase. ↓ Serum potassium, triiodothyronine, serum uric acid. Alteration of electrolyte balance.

Dosage   Dosage is highly individualized, according to both the condition being treated and the response of the patient. Although the various adrenocorticosteroids are very similar in their actions, patients may respond better to one type of drug than to another. It is most important that therapy not be discontinued abruptly. Except for replacement therapy, treatment should always be aimed at the minimum effective dosage and shortest period of time. Long-term use often causes severe side effects. If corticosteroids are used for replacement therapy or high doses are used for prolonged periods of time, the dose must be *increased* if surgery is required.

For topical use, ointment, cream, lotion, solution, plastic tape, aerosol suspension and aerosol cream are selected, depending on dermatologic condition to be treated.

Lotions are considered best for weeping eruptions, especially in areas subject to chafing (axilla, feet, and groin). Creams are suitable for most inflammations; ointments are preferred for dry scaly lesions.

Administration

1. Administer PO forms with food, to minimize ulcerogenic effect.
2. When corticosteroids are given chronically, use the smallest dose that will achieve the desired effect. At frequent intervals, the dose should be gradually decreased to determine if symptoms of the disease can be controlled effectively.
3. In certain diseases (e.g., asthma, ulcerative colitis, rheumatoid arthritis), corticosteroids, given every other day, may maintain therapeutic effects but reduce or eliminate undesirable side effects.
4. Whenever feasible, local administration is preferred over systemic therapy in order to minimize systemic side effects.
5. Corticosteroids should be discontinued gradually if used chronically.

Administration of Topical Corticosteroids

1. Cleanse area before application of medication.
2. Apply agent sparingly and rub gently into area.
3. Apply occlusive type dressing, as ordered, to promote hydration of stratum corneum and increase the absorption of the medication. Two methods are used to apply occlusive type dressing:
   a. Apply a heavy application of medication to cleansed area. Cover with a thin, pliable, nonflammable, plastic film, which is then sealed to surrounding tissue with skin tape or held in place with gauze. Change the dressing every 3 to 4 days.

b. Apply a light application of medication and cover with a damp cloth. Then cover with a thin pliable, nonflammable plastic film and seal to surrounding tissue with tape or hold in place with gauze. Change this dressing b.i.d.

Nursing Implications

1. *Assess*
   a. the urine of patients with a history of diabetes before each meal and at bedtime, because drug has a tendency to cause hyperglycemia and consequently glycosuria.
   b. that patients on long-term therapy have blood tests periodically to determine glucose levels.
   c. patient's muscles for weakness and wasting (signs of negative nitrogen balance).
   d. for effects resembling Cushing's syndrome, such as rounding of face, hirsutism, acne, muscular weakness, cervicothoracic hump, hypertension, osteoporosis, edema, amenorrhea, striae and thinning of skin and nails, ecchymosis, impaired glucose tolerance, negative nitrogen balance, alkalosis, and mental disturbances. Report same.
   e. the patient for signs and symptoms of other diseases because adrenocorticosteroids mask the severity of most illnesses.
   f. weight before therapy is instituted and then daily under standard conditions. Anticipate that the patient will have a small weight gain due to increased appetite, but sudden increases are probably due to edema and must be reported. Edema occurs most frequently with cortisone or desoxycorticosterone acetate and less frequently with the new synthetic agents.
   g. BP at least 2 times daily until the patient is stabilized on a maintenance dose. Report increases in BP.
   h. the height and weight of children regularly because growth suppression is a hazard of adrenocorticosteroid administration.
   i. for GI bleeding when patient is on long-term therapy by testing stool for guaiac periodically.

2. *Teach patient and/or family*
   a. to report to physician any symptoms of gastric distress so that antacids, special diet, and possibly diagnostic x-rays may be ordered.
   b. to be particularly careful to avoid falls and other accidents, because steroids may cause osteoporosis, which makes the bones more susceptible to fractures.
   c. to provide supportive measures and reassurance to patients who are having flareups, explaining that symptoms are caused by forced reduction of drug dosage.
   d. *that patients with arthritis should not overuse the now painless joint*. Permanent joint damage may result from overuse because underlying pathology is still present though pain is relieved.
   e. to carry a card identifying the drug and dosage he is taking.
   f. the need for slowly withdrawing the drug when therapy is completed so that his own adrenal cortex will gradually be reactivated to take over the production of hormones.
   g. how to supplement diet with potassium-rich foods if indicated (e.g., citrus juices, bananas).

h. how to maintain a low-salt diet if ordered.

i. that wounds may heal slowly because of delay in development of granulation tissue caused by steroid therapy.

j. that patients on long-term ophthalmic therapy should have frequent eye examinations because steroids may cause cataracts.

k. the need for regular medical supervision because dosage may have to be adjusted frequently.

l. the need to maintain general hygiene with scrupulous cleanliness to avoid infection because antibody production is decreased by adrenocorticosteroids.

m. to delay vaccination during adrenocorticosteroid therapy because there is limited immune response during therapy with steroids.

n. that children who develop vertigo, headache and convulsions due to pseudo-brain tumors will find that these symptoms will disappear when therapy is discontinued.

TOPICAL CORTICOSTEROIDS

1. *Assess*

a. for local sensitivity reaction at site of application. Withhold medication and report should sensitivity reaction be noted.

b. closely for signs of infection because corticosteroids tend to mask infection. Do not apply occlusive dressings when infection is present.

c. temperature of patient with large occlusive dressings q 4 hr, and remove dressing if temperature is elevated.

d. for signs of systemic absorption of medication, such as edema and transient inhibition of pituitary-adrenal function manifested by muscular pain, lassitude, depression, hypotension, and weight loss.

BECLOMETHASONE DIPROPIONATE   INHALANT: Beclovent, Vanceril (Rx). INTRANASAL: Beconase Nasal Inhaler, Vancenase Nasal Inhaler (Rx). TOPICAL: Propaderm*

Classification Adrenocorticosteroid, synthetic, glucocorticoid type.

Action/Kinetics Rapidly inactivated, thereby resulting in few systemic effects.

Note: If a patient is on systemic steroids, transfer to beclomethasone may be difficult, since recovery from impaired renal function may be slow.

Uses Inhalation therapy for chronic use in bronchial asthma. In glucocorticoid-dependent patients, beclomethasone often permits a decrease in the dosage of the systemic agent. Withdrawal of systemic corticosteroids must be carried out very gradually.

Contraindications Status asthmaticus, acute episodes of asthma, hypersensitivity to drug or aerosol ingredients. Safe use in pregnancy, lactation, and children under 6 years of age not established.

Dosage   Inhalation. *Asthma.* **Adults:** 2 inhalations (total of 84 μg beclomethasone) t.i.d.–q.i.d. *Severe asthma:* **initial,** 12–16 inhalations (504–672 μg beclomethasone) daily; **then,** decrease dose according to response. **Maximum daily dose:** 20 inhalations (840 μg beclomethasone). **Pediatric, 6–12 years:** 1–2 inhalations (42–84 μg) t.i.d.–q.i.d., not to exceed 10 inhalations (420 μg) daily.

Intranasal. *Rhinitis.* **Adults and children over 12:** 1 inhalation (42 μg) in each nostril b.i.d.–q.i.d. (i.e., total daily dose: 168–336 μg daily). If no response after three weeks, discontinue therapy.

In patients also receiving systemic glucocorticosteroids, beclomethasone should be started when condition of patient is relatively stable.

Administration

1. Follow these steps for administration of beclomethasone:
   a. Shake metal canister thoroughly immediately prior to use.
   b. Instruct patient to exhale as completely as possible.
   c. Place mouthpiece of inhaler into mouth and instruct patient to tighten lips around it.
   d. Instruct patient to inhale deeply through mouth while pressing metal canister down with forefinger.
   e. Instruct patient to hold breath for as long as possible.
   f. Remove mouthpiece.
   g. Instruct patient to exhale slowly.
2. A minimum of 60 seconds must elapse between inhalations.

Storage   To prevent explosion of contents under pressure, do not store or use near heat or open flame or throw in fire in incinerator. Keep secure from children.

Nursing Implications

1. For initiation of beclomethasone therapy in patients on systemic steroid therapy, withdrawal of systemic steroids must be carried out *very* slowly as ordered by the doctor.
2. *Assess*
   a. for subjective signs of adrenal insufficiency, such as muscular pain, lassitude, and depression. Report to medical supervision even though respiratory function may have improved.
   b. for objective signs of adrenal insufficiency, such as hypotension and weight loss. Signs of adrenal insufficiency necessitate that systemic steroid dose be temporarily boosted and then be withdrawn more gradually.
3. After withdrawal of systemic steroids, anticipate that patient will be provided with a supply of oral glucocorticoids to be taken immediately if he is subjected to unusual stress or is experiencing an asthmatic attack. Physician must be called after steroids are taken.
4. *Teach patient and/or family*
   a. how to use an inhaler correctly. Review printed instructions with them.
   b. drug compliance in patients not receiving systemic steroids, especially since improvement of respiratory function may not be apparent for 1 to 4 weeks.
   c. that inhaler should not be used for treatment of an asthmatic attack.
   d. not to overuse inhaler because more than 1 mg in adults or more than 500 μg in children may precipitate hypothalamic-pituitary axis depression, resulting in adrenal insufficiency.
   e. to be alert to localized fungal infection of mouth, which requires antifungal medication or possible discontinuation of drug.
   f. that patients also receiving bronchodilators by inhalation should use bron-

chodilator at least several minutes before using beclomethasone, to increase penetration of steroid and to reduce the potential toxicity from inhaled flurocarbon propellants of both inhalers.

g. to carry a card indicating his condition, diagnosis, treatment, and the possible need for systemic glucocorticoids, should he be exposed to unusual stress.

BETAMETHASONE   Betnelan,* Celestone (Rx)

BETAMETHASONE ACETATE AND BETAMETHASONE SODIUM PHOSPHATE   Celestone Soluspan (Rx)

BETAMETHASONE BENZOATE   TOPICAL: Beben,* Benisone, Uticort (Rx)

BETAMETHASONE DIPROPIONATE   TOPICAL: Alphatrex, Diprosone (Rx)

BETAMETHASONE SODIUM PHOSPHATE   Betameth, Betnesol,* Celestone Phosphate, Cel-U-Jec, Prelestone, Selestoject (Rx)

BETAMETHASONE VALERATE   TOPICAL: Betacort,* Betaderm,* Beta-Val, Betnovate,* Celestoderm-V,* Celestoderm-V/2,* Ectosone,* Novobetamet,* Valisone, Valisone Reduced Strength (Rx)

Classification   Adrenocorticosteroid, synthetic, glucocorticoid type.

General Statement   Causes low degree of sodium and water retention as well as potassium depletion. The injectible form contains both rapid-acting and repository forms of betamethasone (mixture of betamethasone sodium phosphate and betamethasone acetate). Not recommended for replacement therapy in any acute or chronic adrenal cortical insufficiency, because it does not have strong sodium-retaining effects.

Action/Kinetics   Long-acting. t½: over 300 min.

Additional Use   Prevention of hyaline membrane disease in premature infants.

Dosage   *Betamethasone.* **PO**: 0.6–7.2 mg/day. *Betamethasone sodium phosphate*: **Parenteral (IV, local)**: **initial**, up to 9 mg/day; then, adjust dosage at minimal level to reduce symptoms. *Betamethasone sodium phosphate and betamethasone acetate*: **IM**: initial, 0.5–9 mg/day. **Intrabursal, intra-articular, periarticular, intradermal, intralesional**: 0.75–6 mg, depending on size of joint or area to be injected. For disorders of the foot (bursitis, tenosynovitis, acute gouty arthritis), dosage is given at 3–7-day intervals. *Betamethasone benzoate, betamethasone dipropionate, betamethasone valerate*: **Topical**: Apply sparingly to affected areas and rub in lightly.

Administration Avoid injection into deltoid muscle because SC atrophy of tissue may occur.

CORTICOTROPIN   ACTH, Acthar, Adrenocorticotropic Hormone, Duracton* (Rx)

CORTICOTROPIN REPOSITORY   ACTH Gel, Corticotropin Gel, Cortigel-40 and -80, Cortrophin Gel, Cotropic-Gel-40 and -80, H.P. Acthar Gel (Rx)

CORTICOTROPIN ZINC HYDROXIDE   Cortrophin Zinc (Rx)

Classification Anterior pituitary hormone.

General Statement The overall physiologic effects of corticotropin are similar to those of cortisone. Since the latter is more easily obtainable, is more predictable, and has more prolonged activity, it is usually used for therapeutic purposes. ACTH is, however, very useful for the diagnosis of Addison's disease and other conditions in which the functionality of the adrenal cortex is to be determined.

   Corticotropin cannot elicit a hormonal response from a nonfunctioning adrenal gland.

Action/Kinetics Corticotropin, or ACTH, is extracted from the anterior pituitary gland. The hormone stimulates the functional adrenal cortex to secrete its entire spectrum of hormones, including the corticosteroids.

Uses Diagnosis of adrenal insufficiency syndromes, severe myasthenia gravis, multiple sclerosis. For same diseases as glucocorticosteroids, see p. 720.

Additional Contraindications Cushing's syndrome, psychotic or psychopathic patients, active TB, active peptic ulcers. Use with caution in patients who have diabetes and hypotension.

Additional Untoward Reactions In the treatment of myasthenia gravis, corticotropin may cause severe muscle weakness 2 to 3 days after initiation of therapy. Equipment for respiratory assistance must be on hand for such emergencies. Muscle strength recovers and improves 2 to 7 days after cessation of treatment, and improvement lasts for about 3 months.

Dosage *Highly individualized.* **SC, IM, or slow IV drip.** Usual (*aqueous solution*), **IM or SC**: 20 units q.i.d. **IV**: 10–25 units of aqueous solution in 500 ml 5% dextrose injection over period of 8 hr. Infants and young children require larger dose per body weight than do older children or adults.

   Repository gel (IM, SC) or aqueous suspension with zinc hydroxide (IM only): 40–80 units q 24–72 hours. 12.5 units q.i.d. causes little metabolic disturbance; 25 units q.i.d. causes definite metabolic alterations.

   As a general rule, patients are started on 10–12.5 units q.i.d. If no clinical effect is noted in 72 to 96 hours, dosage is increased by 5 units q few days to a final maximum of 25 units q.i.d.

   Multiple sclerosis, acute exacerbation: **IM,** 80–120 units daily for 2–3 weeks.

Administration Check label carefully for IV administration. **The label must say that**

the product is for intravenous use. IV administration should be slow, taking 8 hours.

Additional Nursing Implications
See also *Nursing Implications*, p. 724.

1. Before beginning IV administration of ACTH, check that patients with a known sensitivity to animal extracts have had sensitivity tests with the brand of corticotropin to be used.
2. Provide potassium intake during IV administration of ACTH either by foods as tolerated, or check with physician regarding administration of potassium by IV.
3. Assess and report exaggerated euphoria or nervousness and pronounced insomnia and depression as these are indications for reducing or discontinuing drug. Sedatives may be ordered as needed.

CORTISONE ACETATE   Compound E, Cortone Acetate (Rx)

Classification   Adrenocorticosteroid, naturally occurring; glucocorticoid type.

Action/Kinetics   Absorption: Slowly absorbed from IM injection site (24–48) hr. Short-acting. **Onset**: More rapid after PO administration. **Duration**: PO shorter than IM (effective 24–48 hr). t½: 90 min.

Uses   Primarily used for replacement therapy in chronic cortical insufficiency. Also inflammatory or allergic disorders, but only for short-term use because the drug has a strong mineralocorticoid effect.

Dosage   **PO or IM, initial** *or during crisis*: 20–300 mg daily . Decrease gradually to lowest effective dose. *Anti-inflammatory*: 25–150 mg daily, depending on severity of the disease. *Acute rheumatic fever*: 200 mg b.i.d. day 1, thereafter 200 mg, daily. *Addison's disease*: **Maintenance, IM:** 0.25–0.35 mg/kg daily; **maintenance, PO:** 0.5–0.75 mg/kg daily.

Administration   Single course of therapy should not exceed 6 weeks. Rest periods of 2 to 3 weeks indicated between treatments.

COSYNTROPIN   Cortrosyn (Rx)

Classification   Synthetic ACTH derivative.

Action/Kinetics   Cosyntropin is a synthetic ACTH derivative that causes effects similar to those of ACTH although fewer hypersensitivity reactions have been noted. The activity of 0.25 mg cosyntropin is equal to 25 units of ACTH.

Uses   Diagnosis of adrenocortical insufficiency.

Dosage   **IM, rapid IV, IV infusion. Adults, Usual, IM:** 0.25 mg dissolved in sterile saline. Range: 0.25–0.75 mg. **Pediatric, under 2 years:** 0.125 mg.

Administration   When given by IV infusion, 0.25 mg cosyntropin is added to dextrose or saline solution, and 40 μg/hr is administered over 6 hr.

DESOXYCORTICOSTERONE ACETATE   DOCA Acetate, Percorten Acetate (Rx)

DESOXYCORTICOSTERONE PIVALATE   Percorten Pivalate (Rx)

Classification   Adrenocorticosteroid, naturally occurring; mineralocorticoid type.

Action/Kinetics   Desoxycorticosterone, a mineralocorticoid, increases sodium and water retention and promotes potassium excretion by altering reabsorption by the renal tubules. It also decreases sodium content of saliva, sweat, and gastric juices. By normalizing electrolyte balance and plasma volume, the hormone increases cardiac output, increases BP, increases fat and glucose absorption from the GI tract, and decreases nitrogen retention. Desoxycorticosterone does not affect protein or carbohydrate metabolism or skin pigmentation.

Uses   Primary and secondary adrenocortical insufficiency in Addison's disease and salt-losing adrenogenital syndrome.

Contraindication   Use with caution in patients with hypertension.

Untoward Reactions   Serious adverse effects may result from excessive dosage or prolonged treatment. These include increased blood volume, edema, increased blood pressure, enlargement of heart, headaches, arthralgia, ascending paralysis, and low potassium syndrome (sudden attacks of weakness, changes in ECG).

Dosage   IM, Maintenance: 2–5 mg daily with either hydrocortisone (10–30 mg daily) or cortisone (10–37.5 mg daily). Also available as a long-acting suspension (25–100 mg IM, q 4 weeks); or as implantable pellets lasting 8–12 months. The latter are implanted surgically under asepsis.
   Acute crisis: 10–15 mg b.i.d. for 1 or 2 days; supportive measures (whole adrenal cortical extract, cortisone or hydrocortisone, infusions of dextrose in isotonic sodium chloride solution, whole blood or plasma) may also be indicated.
   Drug requirements and salt intake are inversely related. The higher the sodium intake, the lower are the requirements for the drug. Most patients need 3 mg of the drug when ingesting 3–6 gm of sodium chloride in addition to a normal diet. Potassium intake has no effect.

Administration   IM: Use a 20-gauge needle and inject into upper outer quadrant of buttock.

DEXAMETHASONE   ORAL: Baycadron, Decadron, Deronil,* Dexasone,* Dexone, Hexadrol, Maxidex,* SK-Dexamethasone (Rx). TOPICAL: Aeroseb-Dex, Decaderm, Decaspray, Hexadrol (Rx). OPHTHALMIC: Maxidex Ophthalmic (Rx)

Classification   Adrenocorticosteroid, synthetic; glucocorticoid type.

Action/Kinetics   Long-acting. Low degree of sodium and water retention. Diuresis may ensue when patients are transferred from other corticosteroids to dexamethasone. Not recommended for replacement therapy in adrenal cortical insufficiency. t½: over 300 min.

Additional Use   In acute allergic disorders, oral dexamethasone may be combined with dexamethasone sodium phosphate injection. This combination is used for 6 days. Used to test for adrenal cortical hyperfunction. Cerebral edema due to brain tumor, craniotomy, or head injury. Diagnosis of depression. Antiemetic in cisplatin-induced vomiting.

Additional Drug Interaction   Ephedrine ↓ the effect of dexamethasone due to ↑ breakdown by the liver.

Dosage   **PO: initial,** 0.75–9 mg/day; **maintenance:** gradually reduce to minimum effective dose (0.5–3 mg/day). *Suppression test, for Cushing's syndrome:* 0.5 mg q 6 hr for 2 days for 24 hr urine collection (or 1 mg at 11:00 PM with blood withdrawn at 8:00 AM for blood cortisol determination). *Suppression test, to determine cause of pituitary ACTH excess:* 2 mg q 6 hr for 2 days (for 24 hr urine collection). **Topical:** Apply to affected areas b.i.d.–t.i.d.

DEXAMETHASONE ACETATE   Dalalone D.P., Dalalone L.A., Decadron-LA, Decaject-L.A., Decameth L.A., Dexacen LA-8, Dexasone-LA, Dexo-LA, Dexon LA, Dexone LA, L.A. Dezone, Solurex-LA (Rx)

Classification   Adrenocorticosteroid, synthetic, glucocorticoid type.

Action/Kinetics   This ester of dexamethasone is practically insoluble and provides the prolonged activity suitable for repository injections. Not for IV use.

Dosage   **Repository injection. IM:** 8–16 mg q 1–3 weeks, if necessary. **Intralesional:** 0.8–1.6 mg. **Soft tissue and intra-articular:** 4–16 mg repeated at 1–3-week intervals.

DEXAMETHASONE SODIUM PHOSPHATE   SYSTEMIC: AK-Dex, Baydex, Dalalone, Decadrol, Decadron Phosphate, Decaject, Decameth, Dexacen-4, Dexasone, Dexon, Dezone, Hexadrol Phosphate, Savacort-D, Solurex (Rx). INHALER: Decadron Phosphate Respihaler (Rx). INTRANASAL: Turbinaire Decadron Phosphate (Rx). OPHTHALMIC: AK-Dex Ophthalmic, Decadron Phosphate Ophthalmic (Rx). TOPICAL: Decadron Phosphate (Rx)

Classification   Adrenocorticosteroid, synthetic; glucocorticoid type.

Additional Uses   For IV or IM use in emergency situations when dexamethasone can not be given PO. Routes of administration include inhalation (especially for bronchial asthma), ophthalmic, topical, intrasynovial, and intra-articular.

Contraindications   Acute infections, persistent positive sputum cultures of *Candida albicans*.

Dosage   *Systemic:* **initial,** 0.5–9 mg daily (usually one-third to one-half the oral dose); **then,** adjust dose if required (some may require high doses in life-threatening situations). *Cerebral edema:* **initial, IV:** 10 mg; **then, IM,** 4 mg q 6 hr until maximum effect obtained. Switch to oral therapy (1–3 mg t.i.d.) as soon as feasible and then slowly withdraw over 5–7 days. **Pediatric: PO** 0.2 mg/kg daily in divided doses. *Shock, unresponsive:* **IV,** either 40 mg q 2–6 hr as long as needed or 1–6 mg/kg as a single dose. *Intralesional, intra-articular, soft tissue injections:* 0.4–6 mg, depending on the site.

Inhalation, *bronchial asthma:* **Adults, initial,** 3 inhalations (84 μg dexamethasone/inhalation) t.i.d.–q.i.d.; **maximum:** 3 inhalations/dose; 12 inhalations/day. **Pediatric: initial,** 2 inhalations t.i.d.–q.i.d.; **maximum:** 2 inhalations/dose; 8 inhalations/day.

Intranasal: *Allergies, nasal polyps:* **Adults,** 2 sprays (total of l68 μg dexamethasone) in each nostril b.i.d.–t.i.d. (maximum: 12 sprays/day); **pediatric, 6–12 years:** 1–2 sprays (total of 84–168 μg dexamethasone) in each nostril b.i.d. (maximum: 8 sprays/day).

Ophthalmic ointment: Instill a small amount into the conjunctival sac t.i.d.– q.i.d. As response is obtained, reduce the number of applications. **Ophthalmic solution:** Instill 1–2 drops into the conjunctical sac q hr during the day and q 2 hr at night until response obtained; **then,** reduce to 1 drop q 6–8 hr. **Topical cream:** Apply sparingly to affected areas and rub in.

Administration   Do not use preparation containing lidocaine IV.

Additional Nursing Implications
See also *Nursing Implications*, p. 724.
Spray only the number of times ordered for nasal spray.

FLUDROCORTISONE ACETATE   Florinef Acetate (Rx)

Classification   Adrenocorticosteroid, synthetic; mineralocorticoid type.

Action/Kinetics   Produces marked sodium retention and inhibits excess adrenocortical secretion. Should not be used systemically for its anti-inflammatory effects. Supplementary potassium may be indicated.

Principal Uses   Addison's disease and adrenal hyperplasia.

Dosage   *Addison's disease,* **PO:** 0.1–0.2 mg daily to 0.1 mg 3 times/week usually in conjunction with hydrocortisone or cortisone. *Salt-losing adrenogenital syndrome:* 0.1–0.2 mg/day.

FLUNISOLIDE   INHALATION: Aerobid (Rx). INTRANASAL: Nasalide, Rhinalar* (Rx)

Classification   Intranasal and inhalation corticosteroid.

Action/Kinetics   Produces anti-inflammatory effects intranasally with minimal systemic effects. Several days may be required for full beneficial effects.

Uses   Seasonal or perennial rhinitis, especially if other treatment has proven unsatisfactory.

Contraindications   Active or quiescent tuberculosis, especially of the respiratory tract. Untreated fungal, bacterial, systemic viral infections. Ocular herpes simplex. Do not use until healing occurs following recent ulceration of nasal septum, nasal surgery, or trauma.

Additional Untoward Reactions   Nasal irritation and dryness. Rarely, *Candida* infections of nose and pharynx. Systemic corticosteroid effects, especially if recommended dose is exceeded.

Dosage   Inhalation. Adults: 2 inhalations (total of 500 μg flunisolide) in AM and PM, not to exceed 4 inhalations b.i.d. (i.e. total daily dose of 2 mg). **Pediatric, 6–15 years:** 2 inhalations b.i.d.

Intranasal. Adults: initial, 50 μg (2 sprays) in each nostril b.i.d.; may be increased to 2 sprays t.i.d. up to maximum of 400 μg (i.e., 8 sprays in each nostril). **Children, 6–14 years: initial,** 25 μg (1 spray) in each nostril t.i.d. or 50 μg (2 sprays) in each nostril b.i.d. Up to maximum of 200 μg (i.e., 4 sprays in each nostril). **Maintenance, adults, children:** smallest dose necessary to control symptoms. Not recommended for children under 6 years of age.

Administration

1. If nasal congestion is present, use a decongestant before administration to ensure the drug reaches the site of action.
2. If beneficial effects do not occur within three weeks, discontinue therapy.

Additional Nursing Implications

Teach patient and/or family how to administer nasal spray. See *Administration of Nasal Spray,* p. 28.

HYDROCORTISONE (CORTISOL) SYSTEMIC: Cortef, Cortef Sterile, Hydrocortone (Rx). **TOPICAL:** Aeroseb-HC, Acticort 100, Bactine Hydrocortisone, Caldecort Anti-Itch, Cetacort, Clinicort, Cortaid, Cortate,* Cort-Dome, Cortril, Cortizone-5, Delacort, Dermacort, Dermicort, Dermolate Anal Itch, Dermolate Anti-Itch, Dermolate Scalp Itch, Dermtex HC, Eldecort, Emo-Cort,* HC-Jel, H-Cort, H2 Cort, Hi-Cor, Hi-Cor-25, Hycort 1/2%, Hydro-Tex, Hytone, Microcort,* Mycort, Nutracort, Pro-Cort, Pro-Cort M, Racet SE-1/2% and 1%, Sensacort, Synacort, Texacort Scalp Lotion, Ulcort, Ulcort 1/2%, Unicort* (Both Rx and OTC). **ANORECTAL:** Dermolate Anal-Itch, Proctocort, Rectocort* (Rx)

HYDROCORTISONE ACETATE SYSTEMIC: Biosone, Cortef Acetate, Fernisone, Hydrocortone Acetate (Rx). **TOPICAL:** Caladryl Hydrocortisone, Caldecort, Caldecort Rectal-Itch, Clinicort, Cortaid, Cortamed,* Cort-Dome High, Cort-Dome Regular, Cortef Acetate, Cortef Feminine Itch, Cortef Rectal Itch, Corticreme,* Cortifoam, Cortiment,* Epifoam, Gynecort, Hyderm,* Lanacort, Novohydrocort,* Pharma-Cort, Resicort, Rhulicort (Both Rx and OTC)

HYDROCORTISONE BUTYRATE Locoid (Rx)

HYDROCORTISONE CYPIONATE Cortef (Rx)

HYDROCORTISONE RETENTION ENEMA Cortenema (Rx)

HYDROCORTISONE SODIUM PHOSPHATE Hydrocortone Phosphate (Rx)

HYDROCORTISONE SODIUM SUCCINATE A-Hydrocort, Lifocort-100, S-Cortilean,* Solu-Cortef (Rx)

HYDROCORTISONE VALERATE Westcort (Rx)

Classification Adrenocorticosteroid, naturally occurring; glucocorticoid type.

Action/Kinetics Short-acting. t½: 90 min.

Dosage *Hydrocortisone.* **PO:** 20–240 mg/day, depending on disease. **IM only:** one-third to one-half the oral dose q 12 hr. **Rectal:** 100 mg in retention enema nightly for 21 days. **Topical (ointment, cream, gel, spray, lotion):** Apply sparingly to affected area and rub in lightly t.i.d.–q.i.d. **Ophthalmic: Solution,** 1–2 gtt in the conjunctival sac q hr during day and q 2 hr during night initially; **then,** reduce to 1 gtt q 4 hr when response obtained (may be further reduced to 1 gtt t.i.d.–q.i.d.); **Ointment:** insert thin coating in lower conjunctival sac t.i.d.–q.i.d.; when favorable response noted, reduce to b.i.d. and then once/day.

Hydrocortisone acetate. **Intralesional, intra-articular, soft tissue**: 5–50 mg, depending on condition. **Topical and ophthalmic**: See Hydrocortisone, above.

Hydrocortisone butyrate. **Topical:** See Hydrocortisone, above.

Hydrocortisone cypionate (as suspension): 20–240 mg/day, depending on the severity of the disease.

Hydrocortisone sodium phosphate. **IV, IM, SC: initial,** 15–240 mg/day depending on use and severity of the disease. Usually, one-half to one-third the oral dose is given q 12 hr. *Adrenal insufficiency, acute*. **IV, adults, initial,** 100 mg ; **then,** 100 mg q 8 hr in an IV fluid; **older children: initial, IV bolus,** 1–2 mg/kg; **then,** 150–250 mg/kg daily **IV,** in divided doses; **infants: initial, IV bolus,** 1–2 mg/kg; **then,** 25–150 mg/kg daily in divided doses.

Hydrocortisone sodium succinate. **IM, IV, initial:** 100–500 mg; **then,** adjust dosage depending on response and severity of condition.

Hydrocortisone valerate: **Topical (cream):** See Hydrocortisone, above.

Administration Check labels of parenteral hydrocortisone to verify route that can be used for a particular preparation, because IM and IV routes are not necessarily interchangeable.

METHYLPREDNISOLONE   Medrol (Rx)

METHYLPREDNISOLONE ACETATE   Baymep-40, Depmedalone 40 and 80, Depoject, Depo-Medrol, Depopred-40 and -80, D-Med 80, Duralone-40 and -80, Dura-Meth, Med-Depo, Medralone-40 and -80, Medrone-40 and -80, Mepred-40 and -80, Methylone, M-Prednisol-40 and -80, Pre-Dep-40 and -80, Rep-Pred 40 and 80 (Rx). ENEMA: Medrol Enpak (Rx). TOPICAL: Medrol Acetate (Rx)

METHYLPREDNISOLONE SODIUM SUCCINATE   A-Methapred, Solu-Medrol (Rx)

Classification Adrenocorticosteroid, synthetic, glucocorticoid type.

Action/Kinetics Low incidence of increased appetite, peptic ulcer, and psychic stimulation. Also low degree of sodium and water retention. May mask negative nitrogen balance. **Onset:** Slow, 12–24 hr. **Duration:** Long, up to 1 week.

Additional Drug Interactions

Interactant	Interaction
Erythromycin	↑ Effect of methylprednisolone due to ↓ breakdown by liver
Troleandomycin	↑ Effect of methylprednisolone due to ↓ breakdown by liver

Laboratory Test Interference ↓ Immunoglobulins A, G, M.

Dosage *Highly individualized. Methylprednisolone,* **PO:** *Rheumatoid arthritis,* 6–16 mg daily. Decrease gradually when condition is under control. **Pediatric:** 6–10 mg daily. *Systemic lupus erythematosus:* **acute:** 20–96 mg daily; **maintenance:** 8–20 mg daily. *Acute rheumatic fever,* 1 mg/kg body weight daily. Drug is always given in 4 equally divided doses after meals and at bedtime.

Methylprednisolone acetate, **not for IV use. IM:** *Adrenogenital syndrome:* 40 mg q 2 weeks. *Rheumatoid arthritis:* 40–120 mg/week. *Dermatologic lesions, dermatitis:* 40–120 mg/week for 1–2 weeks; for severe cases, a single dose of 80–

120 mg should provide relief. *Seborrheic dermatitis:* 80 mg/week. *Asthma, rhinitis:* 80–120 mg. **Intra-articular, soft tissue and intralesional injection:** 4–80 mg depending on site. **Retention enema:** 40 mg 3 to 7 times/ week for 2 or more weeks. **Topical, ointment:** 0.25–1% applied sparingly b.i.d.–q.i.d.

Methylprednisolone sodium succinate. **IV: initial,:** 10–40 mg depending on the disease; **then,** adjust dose depending on response with subsequent doses given either **IM** or **IV**. *Severe conditions:* 30 mg/kg infused IV over 10–20 min; may be repeated q 4–6 hr for 2–3 days only. **Pediatric:** not less than 0.5 mg/kg/day.

Administration Solutions of methylprednisolone sodium succinate should be used within 48 hours after preparation.

PARAMETHASONE ACETATE Haldrone (Rx)

Classification Adrenocorticosteroid, synthetic.

Action/Kinetics Approximately two and one-half times as potent as prednisone. **Onset:** (rapid), 30 min. **Duration:** 8–10 hr.

Dosage **PO. Initial:** 2–24 mg daily; **maintenance:** 1–8 mg daily.

PREDNISOLONE SYSTEMIC: Cortalone, Delta-Cortef, Fernisolone-P, Sterane (Rx). TOPICAL: Meti-Derm (Rx)

PREDNISOLONE ACETATE SYSTEMIC: Articulose 50, Key-Pred-25, -50 and -100, Niscort, Predaject-50, Predcor-25 and -50, Savacort-50 (Rx). OPHTHALMIC: AK-Tate Ophthalmic, Econopred Ophthalmic, Econopred Plus Ophthalmic, Pred Forte Ophthalmic, Pred Mild Ophthalmic, Predulose Ophthalmic (Rx)

PREDNISOLONE ACETATE AND PREDNISOLONE SODIUM PHOSPHATE Duapred (Rx)

PREDNISOLONE SODIUM PHOSPHATE SYSTEMIC: Hydeltrasol, Key-Pred-SP, PSP-IV, Solupredalone (Rx). OPHTHALMIC: AK-Pred Ophthalmic, Inflamase Ophthalmic, Inflamase Forte Ophthalmic, Metreton Ophthalmic (Rx)

PREDNISOLONE TEBUTATE Hydeltra-T.B.A., Metalone T.B.A., Nor-Fred T.B.A., Predcor-TBA, Prednisol TPA, TPA-Pred (Rx)

Classification Adrenocorticosteroid, synthetic.

Action/Kinetics Intermediate-acting. Prednisolone is five times more potent than hydrocortisone and cortisone. Side effects are minimal except for GI distress. **t½:** over 200 min.

Contraindications Use with particular caution in diabetes.

Dosage   *Prednisolone*. **PO**: 5–60 mg/day, depending on disease being treated. *Multiple sclerosis (exacerbation):* 200 mg/day for 1 week; **then,** 80 mg on alternate days for 1 month. **Topical** (0.5% cream): Apply sparingly to affected areas b.i.d.–q.i.d. and rub in lightly.

Prednisolone acetate. **IM**: 4–60 mg. **Not for IV use. Intralesional, intra-articular, soft tissue injection**: 5–100 mg (larger doses for large joints). *Multiple sclerosis (exacerbation): See Prednisolone.* **Ophthalmic** (0.12–1% suspension): 1–2 drops in the conjunctival sac q hr during the day and q 2 hr during the night; **then,** after response obtained, decrease dose to 1 drop q 6–8 hr.

Prednisolone acetate and prednisolone sodium phosphate. *Systemic*. **IM only**: 10–80 mg acetate and 5–10 mg sodium phosphate q several days for 3 to 4 weeks. **Intra-articular, intrasynovial**, same as IM.

Prednisolone sodium phosphate. **IM, IV**: 4–60 mg/day. *Multiple sclerosis (exacerbation): See Prednisolone.* **Intralesional, intra-articular, soft tissue injection**: 4–30 mg, depending on site and severity of disease. **Ophthalmic** (0.125–1% solution): See Prednisolone acetate.

Prednisolone tebutate. **Intra-articular, intralesional, soft tissue injection**: 4–30 mg, depending on site and severity of disease.

Additional Nursing Implications
See also *Nursing Implications*, p. 724.
Ask the physician if drug should be administered with an antacid.

PREDNISONE   Apo-Prednisone,* Cortan, Deltasone, Liquid Pred, Meticorten, Orasone, Panasol, Prednicen-M, SK-Prednisone (Rx)

Classification   Adrenocorticosteroid, synthetic.

Action/Kinetics   Drug is three to five times as potent as cortisone or hydrocortisone. May cause moderate fluid retention. Prednisone is metabolized in the liver to prednisolone, the active form.

Dosage   *Highly individualized*. **PO (acute, severe conditions): initial,** 5–60 mg daily, in 4 equally divided doses after meals and at bedtime. Decrease gradually by 5–10 mg q 4 to 5 days to establish minimum maintenance dosage (5–10 mg) or discontinue altogether until symptoms recur. **Pediatric:** *Replacement,* 0.1–0.15 mg/kg daily.

TRIAMCINOLONE   Aristocort, Kenacort (Rx)

TRIAMCINOLONE ACETONIDE   SYSTEMIC: Acetospan, Baytac-40, Cenocort A-40, Kenaject, Kenalog-10 and-40, Kenalone, Tramacort-40, Triam-A, Triamonide 40, Tri-Kort, Trilog (Rx). INHALATION: Azmacort (Rx). TOPICAL: Aristocort, Aristocort A, Cremocort,* Flutex, Kenac, Kenalog, Kenalog-H, Triaderm,* Trianide,* Trymex (Rx)

TRIAMCINOLONE DIACETATE   Amcort, Aristocort Forte, Aristocort Intralesional, Articulose L.A., Baytac-D, Cenocort Forte, Cino-40, Tracilon, Triacin 40, Triacort, Triam-Forte, Triamolone 40, Trilone, Tristoject (Rx)

TRIAMCINOLONE HEXACETONIDE   Aristospan Intra-Articular, Aristospan Intralesional (Rx)

Classification   Adrenocorticosteroid, synthetic.

Action/Kinetics   More potent than prednisone. Intermediate-acting. **Onset**: several hours; **Duration**: 1 or more weeks. **t½**: over 200 min.

Additional Uses   Pulmonary emphysema accompanied by bronchospasm or bronchial edema. Diffuse interstitial pulmonary fibrosis. With diuretics to treat refractory CHF or cirrhosis of the liver with ascites. Multiple sclerosis. Inflammation following dental procedures. Triamcinolone hexacetonide is restricted to intra-articular or intralesional treatment of rheumatoid arthritis and osteoarthritis.

Additional Contraindications   Use with special caution in patients who have decreased renal function or renal disease.

Additional Untoward Reactions   Intra-articular, intrasynovial, or intrabursal administration may cause transient flushing, dizziness, local depigmentation, and rarely, local irritation. Exacerbation of symptoms has also been reported. A marked increase in swelling and pain and further restricted joint movement may indicate septic arthritis. Intradermal injection may cause local vesicular ulceration and persistent scarring.

Syncope and anaphylactoid reactions have been reported with triamcinolone regardless of route of administration.

Dosage   *Highly individualized. Triamcinolone.* **PO**. *Adrenocortical insufficiency (with mineralocorticoid therapy)*: 4–12 mg/day. *For treating other disease states*: 8–60 mg/day. *Acute leukemias (children)*: 1–2 mg/kg. *Acute leukemia or lymphoma in (adults)*: 16–40 mg daily (up to 100 mg daily may be necessary). *Edema*: 16–20 mg (up to 48 mg may be required). *Tuberculosis meningitis*: 32–48 mg.

Triamcinolone acetonide. **IM only (not for IV use)**: *Systemic*, 2.5–60 mg daily depending on the disease and its severity. **Intra-articular, intrabursal, tendon sheaths**: 2.5–5 mg for smaller joints and 5–15 mg for larger joints, although up to 40 mg has been employed. **Intradermal**: 1 mg/injection site (use 10 mg/ml suspension only). **Topical** (0.025%, 0.1%, 0.5% ointment or cream; 0.025%, 0.1% lotion; 0.1% gel, spray): Apply sparingly to affected area b.i.d.–q.i.d. and rub in lightly.

Triamcinolone diacetate. *Systemic*: **IM**, 40 mg weekly. **Intra-articular/intra-**

synovial: 5–40 mg. **Intralesional/sublesional**: 5–48 mg (no more than 12.5 mg/injection site and 25 mg/lesion).

  Triamcinolone hexacetonide. **Intra-articular**: 2–6 mg for small joints and 10–20 mg for large joints. **Intralesional/sublesional**: up to 0.5 mg/square inch of affected area. **Not for IV use.**

Additional Nursing Implications
See also *Nursing Implications*, p. 724.
  Teach patient and/or family
  a. to ingest a liberal amount of protein because there is a tendency with this drug toward gradual weight loss, associated with anorexia, muscle wasting, and weakness.
  b. to lie down if feeling faint.
  c. to try to counteract drug-induced depression by encouragement and reassurance.

MISCELLANEOUS AGENTS

AMINOGLUTETHIMIDE Cytadren (Rx)

Action/Kinetics This drug decreases the synthesis of glucocorticoids and mineralocorticoids in the adrenal cortex by inhibiting the enzymatic conversion of cholesterol to delta-5-pregnenolone (a precursor to the steroids). $t\frac{1}{2}$: 5–9 hr (after 1–2 wk use).

Uses Cushing's syndrome. To decrease steroid levels in adrenal carcinoma or ectopic ACTH-producing tumors. *Investigational:* Advanced breast carcinoma in postmenopausal patients; metastatic prostate carcinoma.

Contraindications Hypersensitivity to aminoglutethimide or glutethimide (Doriden). Can cause harm to the fetus if administered to pregnant women. Safety and effectiveness in children not known.

Untoward Reactions *Most common:* Drowsiness, morbilliform skin rash, nausea, anorexia. *GI:* Vomiting. *CNS:* Headache, dizziness. *Hematologic:* Rarely, anemia, pancytopenia, thrombocytopenia. *Endocrine:* Adrenal insufficiency, hypothyroidism, masculinization and hirsutism in females, precocious sex development in males. *CV:* Hypotension including orthostatic, tachycardia. *Dermatologic:* Rash, pruritus, urticaria. *Miscellaneous:* Fever, myalgia, cholestatic jaundice (due to hypersensitivity).

Drug Interaction Aminoglutethimide ↑ biotransformation of dexamethasone.

Laboratory Test Interferences Abnormal liver function tests. ↑ SGOT, alkaline phosphatase.

Dosage **PO. Initial**: 250 mg q 6 hr; if response inadequate (as judged by plasma steroid assays), increase by 250 mg daily at 1–2 week intervals to a maximum of 2 gm/day.

Administration
  1. Dosage should be initiated in a hospital setting until a stable regimen is reached.

2. Therapy may have to be discontinued or modified in the event of adverse reactions. For example, terminate therapy if skin rash persists for more than 5 to 8 days.
3. It may be necessary to initiate mineralocorticoid or glucocorticoid (e.g., hydrocortisone, 20–30 mg PO in the morning) replacement therapy.

Nursing Implications
1. *Assess*
   a. for suppression of adrenal cortical function especially when used in presence of surgery, trauma, or acute illness.
   b. for hypotension resulting from suppression of aldosterone production.
   c. for hypothyroidism manifested by thyroid enlargement and reduced plasma level of hormone.
2. Be prepared to administer hydrocortisone rather than dexamethasone if glucocortoid therapy is required.
3. *Teach patient and/or family*
   a. to be alert to symptoms of hypotension, such as weakness, dizziness, and headaches. Sit down or lie down if symptoms occur.
   b. to report to doctor drowsiness, nausea, anorexia, headache, dizziness, weakness, or rash.
   c. to use caution when driving a car or operating other machinery as drowsiness or dizziness may occur.

METYRAPONE   Metopirone (Rx)

Classification   Adrenocorticosteroid inhibitor, synthetic.

Action   Metyrapone inhibits cortisol synthesis by the adrenal cortex at the 11-β-hydroxylation step. This results a compensatory increase in ACTH release in persons who have normal hypothalamic-pituitary function followed by a two- to fourfold increase in 17-hydroxycorticoids and a twofold increase in 17-ketosteroid excretion. In hypopituitarism, a subnormal response to metyrapone is seen.

Use   To test for hypothalamicopituitary function.

Contraindications   Adrenocortical insufficiency; hypersensitivity to drug. Safe use in pregnancy not established.

Untoward Reactions   *GI:* Nausea, abdominal discomfort. *CNS:* Sedation, headache, dizziness. *Dermatologic:* Rashes.

Drug Interactions

Interactant	Interaction
Cyproheptadine	Erroneous results for pituitary function up to 2 weeks following cessation of cyproheptadine therapy
Estrogens	↓ Response to metyrapone
Phenytoin	Erroneous results for pituitary function up to 2 weeks following cessation of phenytoin therapy

Dosage   PO. Adults: 750 mg q 4 hr for 6 doses. **Pediatric**: 15 mg/kg q 4 hr for 6 doses (minimal single dose: 250 mg). After a 24-hr control measurement of 17-hydroxycorticoids and 17-ketosteroids (day 1) followed by administration of ACTH to assess cortical function (day 2), metyrapone is given on day 5. On day 6, another 24-hr steroid determination is made.

Administration
1. Corticosteroid therapy must be discontinued before and during testing.
2. Administer with milk or food, to decrease gastric irritation.

TRILOSTANE   Modrastane (Rx)

Classification   Adrenal corticosteroid inhibitor.

Action/Kinetics   Trilostane inhibits the synthesis of steroids by the adrenal cortex resulting in a decrease in circulating levels of corticosteroids. The drug is effective following the first few days of therapy. Response to the drug is not uniform among patients and is not curative.

Uses   Cushing's syndrome, especially for initial therapy until other approaches can be undertaken.

Contraindications   Adrenal insufficiency. Kidney or liver disease, pregnancy. Use with caution during lactation and in patients receiving other drugs that suppress adrenocortical activity. Safety and efficacy in children have not been established.

Untoward Reactions   *GI:* Diarrhea (common), nausea, GI upset, abdominal pain or discomfort, bloated feeling, flatulence, belching. *CNS:* Headache, fever, fatigue, fainting. *Dermatologic:* Skin rash, erythema, numbness, tingling. *Other:* Flushing, burning sensation of nasal or oral membranes, pain in muscles and joints, lacrimation, rhinorrhea, nasal stuffiness.

Drug Interaction   Use with aminoglutethimide or mitotane may result in severe hypofunction of the adrenal cortex.

Dosage   PO. Initial: 30 mg q.i.d.; **then,** slowly increase the dose q 3–4 days up to usual of 360 mg/day. Doses above 480 mg/day are not recommended. If no response within 2 weeks, therapy should be discontinued.

Administration
1. To establish a dosage regimen, therapy should be started in the hospital.
2. In times of severe stress (i.e., illness, surgery), administration of corticosteroids may be necessary.
3. The patient must be carefully monitored for corticosteroid levels and plasma electrolytes.

Nursing Implications
Teach patient and/or family

   a. that barrier-type or other nonhormonal contraception should be practiced during treatment.
   b. to consult with physician immediately if pregnancy is suspected.

Chapter Sixty-two

ESTROGENS, PROGESTINS, AND ORAL CONTRACEPTIVES

ESTROGENS

General Statement The estrogens are a group of natural female hormones first produced in large quantities during puberty. They are responsible for the development of primary and secondary female sex characteristics. From puberty on, estrogens are secreted primarily by the ovarian follicles during the early phase of the menstrual cycle. Their production decreases sharply at menopause, but small quantities continue to be produced. Men also produce some estrogens.

During each cycle, estrogens trigger the proliferative phase of the endometrium, affect the vaginal tract mucosa and breast tissue, and increase uterine tone. During adolescence, estrogens cause closure of the epiphyseal junction. Large doses inhibit the development of the long bones by causing premature closure and inhibiting endochondral bone formation. In adult women, estrogens participate in bone maintenance by aiding the deposition of calcium in the protein matrix of bones. They increase elastic elements in the skin, tend to cause sodium and fluid retention, and have an anabolic effect by enhancing the turnover of dietary nitrogen and other elements into protein. Furthermore, they tend to keep plasma cholesterol at relatively low levels.

All natural estrogens, including estradiol, estrone, and estriol, are steroids. These compounds are either obtained from the urine of pregnant mares or are prepared synthetically. Nonsteroidal estrogens, including diethylstilbestrol, and chlorotrianisene, are always prepared synthetically.

Action/Kinetics   Estrogens combine with a receptor in the cytoplasm of the cell, resulting in an increase in protein synthesis. For example, estrogens are required for secondary sex characteristics, development and maintenance of the female genital system and breasts, as well as effects in the pituitary and hypothalamus. Natural estrogens are generally administered parenterally because they are either destroyed in the GI tract or have a significant first-pass effect, hence adequate plasma levels are never reached. Synthetic derivatives can be given PO and are rapidly absorbed, distributed, and excreted. Estrogens are metabolized in the liver and excreted in urine (major portion) and feces.

Uses   Primary ovarian failure, female hypogonadism or castration, menopausal symptoms (especially flushing, sweating, chills), atrophic vaginitis, kraurosis vulvae, abnormal uterine bleeding (progestins are preferred), postpartum breast engorgement. Adjunct to diet and calcium for prophylaxis of osteoporosis. Palliative treatment in advanced, inoperable, metastatic breast carcinoma in postmenopausal women and in men. Advanced inoperable carcinoma of the prostate. Certain estrogens are used as postcoital contraceptives. Mestranol or ethinyl estradiol in combination with a progestin are components of oral contraceptives.

Contraindications   Cancerous or precancerous lesions of the breast (until 5 years past menopause) and of the genital tract. Administer with caution to patients with a history of thrombophlebitis, thromboembolism, asthma, epilepsy, migraine, cardiac failure, renal insufficiency, and diseases involving calcium or phosphorus metabolism, or a family history of mammary or genital tract cancer. Estrogen therapy may be contraindicated in patients with blood dyscrasias, hepatic disease, or thyroid dysfunction. Prolonged therapy is inadvisable in women who plan to become pregnant. Undiagnosed abnormal genital bleeding.

Estrogens also are contraindicated in patients who have not yet completed bone growth.

Estrogens should be used with caution during pregnancy because they may masculinize the female fetus.

Untoward Reactions   Untoward reactions to estrogens are dose-dependent. *CV:* The potentially most serious side effects involve the cardiovascular system. Thromboembolism, thrombophlebitis, myocardial infarction, pulmonary embolism, retinal thrombosis, mesenteric thrombosis, subarachnoid hemorrhage, postsurgical thromboembolism. Hypertension, edema, stroke. *GI:* Nausea, vomiting, abdominal cramps, bloating, diarrhea, changes in appetite. *Dermatologic:* Most common are chloasma or melasma. Also, erythema multiforme, erythema nodosom, hirsutism, alopecia, hemorrhagic eruptions. *Hepatic:* Cholestatic jaundice, aggravation of porphyria, benign (most common) or malignant liver tumors. *Genitourinary:* Breakthrough bleeding, spotting, changes in amount and/or duration of menstrual flow, amenorrhea (following use), dysmenorrhea, premenstrual-like syndrome. Increased incidence of *Candida* vaginitis. *CNS:* Mental depression, dizziness, changes in libido, chorea, headache, aggravation of migraine headaches, fatigue, nervousness. *Ocular:* Steepening of corneal curvature resulting in intolerance to contact lenses. Optic neuritis or retinal thrombosis resulting in sudden or gradual, partial or complete loss of vision, double vision, papilledema. *Hematologic:* Increase in prothrombin and blood coagulation factors VII, VIII, IX, and X. Decrease in antithrombin III. *Miscellaneous:* Breast tenderness, enlargement, or secretions. Increased risk of gall bladder disease. Premature closure of epiphyses in children. Increased frequency of benign or malignant tumors of the cervix, uterus, vagina, and other organs. Weight gain. Increased risk of congenital abnormalities. Hypercalcemia in patients with metastatic breast carcinoma.

In males, estrogens may cause gynecomastia, loss of libido, decreased spermatogenesis, testicular atrophy, and feminization. Prolonged use of high doses may inhibit the function of the anterior pituitary. Estrogen therapy affects many laboratory tests.

Drug Interactions

Interactant	Interaction
Anticoagulants, oral	↓ Anticoagulant response by ↑ activity of certain clotting factors
Anticonvulsants	Estrogen-induced fluid retention may precipitate seizures. Also, contraceptive steroids ↑ effect of anticonvulsants by ↓ breakdown in liver and ↓ plasma protein binding
Antidiabetic agents	Estrogens may impair glucose tolerance and thus change requirements for antidiabetic agent
Barbiturates	↓ Effect of estrogen by ↑ breakdown by liver
Phenytoin	See Anticonvulsants
Rifampin	↓ Effect of estrogen due to ↑ breakdown by liver
Succinylcholine	Estrogens may ↑ effects of succinylcholine
Tricyclic antidepressants	Possible increased effects of tricyclic antidepressants

Laboratory Test Interferences Alter liver function tests and thyroid function tests. False + urine glucose test. BSP retention and serum glucose. ↓ Serum cholesterol and total serum lipids. ↑ Serum triglyceride levels and thyroxine-binding globulin.

Dosage   PO, IM, SC, intravaginal, topical, or by implantation.

Most orally administered estrogens are metabolized rapidly and, with the exception of chlorotrianisene, must be administered daily.

Parenterally administered estrogens are released more slowly from their aqueous suspensions or oily solutions. Both types of preparations are suitable for treatment of estrogen deficiency states, requiring cyclic therapy.

Estrogens in pellet form can be implanted under the skin or in muscle tissue, providing a fairly uniform release of estrogens for periods up to several months. This form of administration is suitable for long-term treatment of prostatic and mammary carcinoma.

Dosage of estrogens is highly individualized and is aimed at the minimal effective amount.

Cyclic therapy (3 weeks on, 1 week off) is usually recommended for women to avoid continuous stimulation of reproductive tissue.

To reduce postpartum breast engorgement, doses are administered during the first few days after delivery.

Nursing Implications

Teach patient and/or family

a. that medical supervision is essential during prolonged estrogen therapy.
b. when on cyclic therapy, to take the medication for 3 weeks and then to omit it for 1 week. Menstruation may then occur, but not pregnancy, because ovulation was suppressed.

c. to report unusual vaginal bleeding, which may be caused by excessive amounts of estrogen.

d. that nausea, when present, usually disappears with continuation of therapy. Nausea can be relieved by taking medication with meals, or, if only one daily dose is required, by taking medication at bedtime.

e. how to assess for presence of edema and to report positive findings.

f. to weigh herself at least twice a week and to report sudden weight gain.

g. how to assess for phlebitis and to report positive findings.

h. in the case of a diabetic patient, that estrogen can alter glucose tolerance. Symptoms of hyperglycemia and glycosuria should be reported promptly, because dosage of antidiabetic medication might have to be altered.

i. that in the case of a male patient on estrogen therapy who might be developing feminine characteristics or suffering from impotence, he will find that these symptoms will disappear when the course of estrogen therapy has been completed.

j. how to apply estrogen ointments locally. Explain what symptoms may occur in a systemic reaction to estrogen ointment.

k. how to insert intravaginal estrogen suppository. Also, advise women to use a perineal pad if vaginal discharge increases during treatment and to store suppositories in the refrigerator.

l. in the case of a mother planning to breast-feed, not to take estrogens. She should consult with medical supervision for an alternative form of contraception if she so desires.

CHLOROTRIANISENE   Tace (Rx)

Classification   Estrogen, synthetic, nonsteroidal.

Action/Kinetics   The long-lasting effect of this synthetic estrogen is attributed to its storage in adipose tissue, which then acts as a reservoir.

Dosage   PO. *Prostatic cancer*: 12–25 mg daily. *Breast engorgement*: 72 mg b.i.d. for 2 days with first dose within 8 hr after delivery. *Atrophic vaginitis, kraurosis vulvae*: 12–25 mg daily given cyclically for 30 to 60 days. *Female hypogonadism*: 12–25 mg/day cyclically for 21 days; give PO progestin for last 5 days of therapy or IM progesterone (100 mg). Begin next course on day 5 of menstrual flow.

DIENESTROL   DV, Estraguard, Ortho Dienestrol (Rx)

Classification   Estrogen, synthetic.

Use   Dienestrol is available only in suppositories or creams and is used for atrophic vaginitis and kraurosis vulvae.

Dosage   Suppositories: 1–2 daily; some require cyclic therapy for several years. **Vaginal cream: initial,** 1–2 applicatorfuls daily; **maintenance,** 1 applicatorful 1–3 times/week once vaginal mucosa is restored.

DIETHYLSTILBESTROL DES, Stilbestrol (Rx)

DIETHYLSTILBESTROL DIPHOSPHATE Honvol,* Stilphostrol (Rx)

Classification Estrogen, synthetic, nonsteroidal.

Note: Potent nonsteroidal estrogen. **Not to be used during pregnancy because of the possibility of vaginal cancer in female offspring.**

Additional Use Postcoital contraceptive (emergency use only).

Contraindication Pregnancy.

Dosage *Diethylstilbestrol.* **PO.** *Menopausal symptoms, atrophic vaginitis, kraurosis vulvae:* 0.2–0.5 mg up to 2 mg daily, given cyclically. *Estrogen deficiency states:* 0.2–0.5 mg daily, given cyclically. *Palliative treatment of prostatic cancer,* **PO:** 1–3 mg daily with increases in advanced cases. *Mammary cancer in males and females:* 15 mg daily. *Postcoital contraceptive (emergency treatment only):* 25 mg b.i.d. for 5 consecutive days, beginning within 24 hr (and not later than 72 hr) after exposure. **Vaginal suppository.** *Atrophic vaginitis or kraurosis vulvae:* 1–2 suppositories daily, usually at bedtime. Some may require up to 2 mg daily (four 0.5 mg suppositories). *Diethylstilbestrol Diphosphate. Palliative treatment of prostatic carcinoma,* **PO:** 50 mg t.i.d. up to 200 mg t.i.d.; **IV:** 500 mg on day 1 followed by 1 gm daily for 5 days. **Maintenance, IV:** 250–500 mg 1 to 2 times weekly.

ESTRADIOL Estrace (Rx)

Classification Estrogen, naturally derived, steroidal.

Dosage **PO.** *Vasomotor symptoms, kraurosis vulvae, atrophic vaginitis, hypogonadism, primary ovarian failure:* **initial,** 1–2 mg daily; **then,** adjust dosage to control symptoms. Give cyclically (3 weeks on, 1 week off). *Prostatic carcinoma:* 1–2 mg t.i.d. chronically. *Breast carcinoma in males and females:* 10 mg t.i.d. for a minimum of 3 months.

ESTRADIOL CYPIONATE IN OIL Depanate, Depestro, Depgynogen, Depo-Estradiol Cypionate, Depogen, Dura-Estrin, E-Ionate P.A., Estra-D, Estro-Cyp, Estroject-L.A. (Rx)

Dosage **IM only.** *Menopause:* 1–5 mg q 3–4 weeks. *Hypogonadism:* 1.5–2.0 mg at monthly intervals. Supplied in cottonseed oil.

Storage Injectable solutions of the esters should be protected from light and stored at room temperature to prevent separation of crystals from oil solutions.

ESTRADIOL VALERATE IN OIL Delestrogen, Dioval, Dioval XX, Dioval 40, Duragen-10, -20, and -40, Estradiol L.A. 20 and 40, Estra-L-20 and -40, Estraval P.A., Estraval 2X and 4X, Feminate-10, -20, and -40, Gynogen L.A. 10 and 20, L.A.E. 20, Valergen-10, 20-, and -40 (Rx)

Dosage **IM.** *Menopause, atrophic vaginitis, kraurosis vulvae, hypogonadism, primary ovarian failure:* 10–20 mg q 4 weeks. *Postpartum breast engorgement:* 10–

25 mg at end of first stage of labor. *Prostatic carcinoma*: 30 mg (or more) q 1–2 weeks. Supplied in sesame oil.

ESTROGENIC SUBSTANCES, AQUEOUS   Estaqua, Estrofol, Estroject-2, Foygen Aqueous, Gravigen Aqueous, Gynogen, Hormogen-A, Kestrin Aqueous, Theogen, Unigen Aqueous, Wehgen (Rx)

Classification   Estrogen, steroidal.

Note: These preparations contain a mixture of steroidal estrogens, mostly estrone, in an aqueous suspension.

Dosage   IM only. *Menopause, kraurosis vulvae, atrophic vaginitis*: 0.1–0.5 mg 2–3 times/week. *Hypogonadism, primary ovarian failure, castration*: **initial**, 0.1–1 mg/week in single or divided doses. Up to 2 mg/week may be necessary. *Prostatic carcinoma (inoperable)*: 2–4 mg 2–3 times/week. Response to therapy should become apparent within 3 months after initiation of therapy.

ESTROGENS COMBINED, AQUEOUS   (Rx)

Classification   Estrogen, steroidal.

Note: Combination of water-soluble and water-insoluble forms of estrone provides both rapid and prolonged estrogenic effects.

Dosage   IM only. *Replacement therapy*: 0.1–1.0 mg weekly in single or divided doses, up to 2 mg weekly. Dose must be individualized. *Atrophic vaginitis, kraurosis vulvae:* 0.1–0.5 mg 2–3 times/week. *Abnormal uterine bleeding (hormonal imbalance)*: 2–5 mg for several days. *Prostatic carcinoma (inoperable)*: 2–4 mg 2–3 times/week; response should be apparent within 3 months of initiating therapy. *Breast carcinoma (inoperable, in men and postmenopausal women)*: 5 mg 3 or more times/week.

ESTROGENS CONJUGATED (CONJUGATED ESTROGENIC SUBSTANCES)   C.E.S.,* Oestrilin,* Premarin, Premarin Intravenous (Rx)

ESTERIFIED ESTROGENS   Climestrone,* Estratab, Estromed,* Menest, Neo-Estrone* (Rx)

Classification   Estrogen, natural.

Note: Mixture of sodium salts of sulfate esters of natural estrogenic substances: 50% to 65% estrone sodium sulfate and 20% to 35% equilin sodium sulfate. Isolated from urine of pregnant mares. Less potent than estrone.

Uses   Parenteral preparation: Abnormal uterine bleeding. **Oral preparation**: Replacement therapy, primary ovarian failure, hypogonadism, prostatic or breast carcinoma, menopausal symptoms. **Vaginal cream:** Atrophic vaginitis, kraurosis vulvae.

Dosage   PO. *Menopausal symptoms:* 0.3–1.25 mg daily, up to 3.75 mg daily if necessary. Given cyclically. *Atrophic vaginitis, kraurosis vulvae:* 0.3–1.25 mg/day; use cyclically for short-term. *Hypogonadism:* 2.5–7.5 mg/day in divided doses for 20–21 days followed by a 7–10 day rest period. *Primary ovarian failure, castration:*

2.5–7.5 mg/day in divided doses for 20 days with the addition of a progestin the last 5 days. *Prostatic carcinoma:* 1.25–2.5 mg t.i.d. for several weeks. *Breast carcioma in men and postmenopausal women:* 10 mg t.i.d. for 3 months. *Osteoporosis:* 1.25 mg daily; give cyclically. *Postpartum breast engorgement:* 3.75 mg q 4 hr for 5 doses or 1.25 mg q 4 hr for 5 days.

IM, IV: 25 mg; repeat in 6–12 hr, if necessary. **Vaginal cream:** 1–2 applicatorfuls daily; then, reduce dose gradually.

Administration

1. Parenteral solution is compatible with normal saline, invert sugar solutions, and dextrose. It is not compatible with acid solutions or protein hydroylsates.
2. Reconstituted parenteral solutions should be used within a few hours although the solution is stable for 60 days if refrigerated.

ESTRONE, AQUEOUS SUSPENSION   Bestrone, Estrone "5," Estronol, Kestrone-5, Theelin Aqueous (Rx)

ESTROPIPATE (PIPERAZINE ESTRONE SULFATE)   Ogen (Rx)

Classification   Estrogen, steroidal, natural or synthetic.

Dosage   *Estrone*. **IM only**. *Menopausal symptoms, atrophic vaginitis, kraurosis vulvae:* 0.1–0.5 mg 2 to 3 times/week. *Hypogonadism, primary ovarian failure, castration:* 0.1–1 mg/week in single or divided doses (up to 2 mg/week may be necessary). *Prostatic carcinoma (inoperable):* 2–4 mg 2 to 3 times/week; response should be apparent within 3 months of initiating therapy.

Estropipate. **PO**. *Menopause, atrophic vaginitis, kraurosis vulvae:* 0.625–5 mg/day for short-term therapy (give cyclically). *Hypogonadism, primary ovarian failure, castration:* 1.25–7.5 mg/day for first 3 weeks; **then**, rest period of 8–10 days. Duration depends on responsiveness of patient. **Vaginal cream:** 1–2 applicatorsful/day; then, reduce dose gradually.

ETHINYL ESTRADIOL   Estinyl, Feminone (Rx)

Classification   Estrogen, steroidal, synthetic.

Action/Kinetics   This synthetic steroid is a derivative of estradiol. It is effective orally and is a component of many oral contraceptives.

Dosage   **PO**. *Menopausal symptoms:* 0.02 or 0.05 mg daily. Give cyclically (3 weeks on followed by a 7 day rest period); a progestin may be added during last 5 days of cycle. *Replacement therapy:* 0.05 mg 1–3 times/day for first 2 weeks of theoretical menstrual cycle; then, administer progesterone for the second half of the cycle. Continue for 3–6 months. *Carcinoma of the female breast (inoperable):* 1 mg t.i.d. chronically. *Carcinoma of prostate:* 0.15–2 mg daily, given chronically.

POLYESTRADIOL PHOSPHATE   Estradurin (Rx)

Classification   Estrogen, steroidal, natural or synthetic.

Use   Principal use is palliation of cancer of the prostate.

Dosage   Deep IM (only): 40–80 mg q 2–4 weeks. Response should be manifested within 3 months.

Administration   Injection is painful and may require concomitant administration of local anesthetic.

QUINESTROL   Estrovis (Rx)

Classification   Estrogen, steroidal.

Action/Kinetics   Orally active estrogen is stored in body fat, is slowly released, and is subsequently metabolized in the blood to the active ethinyl estradiol. Ethinyl estradiol is excreted unchanged in the feces and by the kidneys.

Dosage   PO. Initial, 100 μg daily for 7 days; **then,** 100 μg weekly beginning 2 weeks after starting therapy. Some patients may require 200 μg/week. At 3–6 month intervals, attempts should be made to discontinue or reduce the dosage of the drug.

PROGESTERONE AND PROGESTINS

General Statement   Progesterone is a natural female ovarian steroid hormone produced in large amounts during pregnancy. It is chiefly secreted by the corpus luteum during the second half of the menstrual cycle. During pregnancy, it is also produced by the placenta.

   The hormone acts on the thick muscles of the uterus (myometrium) and on its lining (endometrium). It prepares the latter for the implantation of the fertilized ovum. Under the influence of progesterone, the estrogen-primed endometrium enters its "secretory phase," during which it thickens and secretes large quantities of mucus and glycogen. The myometrium relaxes under the effect of progesterone. During puberty, progesterone participates in the maturation of the female body, acting on the breasts and the vaginal mucosa.

   Progesterone interacts, by feedback mechanism, with the hormones FSH and LH produced by the anterior pituitary. When progesterone and estrogen are high there is a decrease in the production of FSH and LH. This inhibits ovulation and accounts for the fact that progesterone is an effective contraceptive. Natural progesterone has to be injected, but a whole series of compounds with progesterone-type activity (collectively called progestins) can be taken orally. These substances are now routinely substituted for natural progesterone. Progesterone is essential for the maintenance of pregnancy.

   Although progesterone stimulates the development of alveolar mammary tissue during pregnancy, it does not initiate lactation. On the contrary, it suppresses the lactogenic hormone; lactation starts postpartum only when progesterone and estrogen levels have decreased.

   Progesterone, like estrogen, can be used to relieve postpartum breast engorgement.

Action/Kinetics   Physiologic doses are used for replacement therapy and to suppress gonadotropin production, which inhibits ovulation. Pharmacologic doses have several uses (see below). Progesterone must be administered parenterally because of major inactivation in liver (first-pass effect). The hormones are metabolized in the liver and a major portion excreted in the urine (urinary analysis is used to monitor progesterone levels).

Uses   Functional uterine bleeding, primary or secondary amenorrhea (used with an estrogen), endometriosis, premenstrual tension. Alone or with an estrogen for contraception. May also be used in combination with an estrogen for endometriosis and hypermenorrhea.

Note: Not to be used to prevent habitual abortion or to treat threatened abortion.

Contraindications   Genital malignancies, thromboembolic disease, vaginal bleeding of unknown origin, impaired liver function. Use with caution in case of asthma, epilepsy, depression, and migraine.

Untoward Reactions   Occasionally noted with short-term dosage, frequently observed with prolonged high dosage. *Genitourinary:* Spotting, irregular periods, amenorrhea, changes in amount and/or duration of menstrual flow, changes in cervical secretion and cervial erosion, breast tenderness or secretions. *Dermatologic:* Allergic rashes, pruritus, acne, melasma, chloasma, alopecia, hirsutism. *CNS:* Depression, pyrexia, insomnia. *Miscellaneous:* Weight gain or loss, cholestatic jaundice, masculinization of the female fetus, nausea, edema, precipitation of acute intermittent porphyria, photosensitivity.

Drug Interactions   Rifampin and possibly phenobarbital ↓ the effect of progesterone by ↑ breakdown by the liver.

Dosage   Progesterone must be administered parenterally. Other progestins can be administered PO and parenterally.

The usual schedule of administration for *functional uterine bleeding, amenorrhea, infertility, dysmenorrhea, premenstrual tension and contraception*: is days 5 through 25 of menstrual cycle with day 1 being the first day of menstrual flow.

Nursing Implications

1. *Assess*
    a. for thrombic conditions, such as thrombophlebitis, pulmonary embolism, and cerebrovascular alterations.
    b. for edema.
    c. for yellowing of sclera.
2. *Teach patient and/or family*
    a. to observe for symptoms of thrombic disease and to report if noted.
    b. to check weight at least twice weekly and to report sudden weight gain, because it may indicate edema. Also, to observe for swelling of extremities and report if noted.
    c. to report yellowing of sclera.
    d. that GI distress may subside with use (after the first few cycles).
    e. to report episodes of bleeding.
    f. that progestins may reactivate or worsen a psychic depression.
    g. that when administered to diagnose pregnancy, menstruation will occur 3–7 days after withdrawal of medication, if she is not pregnant.
    h. in the case of a diabetic patient that progesterone may alter glucose tolerance, and to report positive urine tests promptly because dosage of antidiabetic medication may have to be adjusted.
    i. to recognize and report early symptoms of ophthalmic pathology, such as headaches, dizziness, blurred vision, or partial loss of vision.

ETHYNODIOL DIACETATE   (Rx)

Classification   Progestational hormone, synthetic.

Use   Used only for oral contraception. See Table 31.

TABLE 31   COMBINATION ORAL CONTRACEPTIVE PREPARATIONS AVAILABLE IN THE UNITED STATES

Trade Name	Estrogen	Progestin
	MONOPHASIC	
Brevicon 21-day	Ethinyl estradiol (35 μg)	Norethindrone (0.5 mg)
Brevicon 28-day	Ethinyl estradiol (35 μg)	Norethindrone (0.5 mg)
Demulin 1/35-21	Ethinyl estradiol (35 μg)	Ethynodiol diacetate (1 mg)
Demulin 1/35-28	Ethinyl estradiol (35 μg)	Ethynodiol diacetate (1 mg)
Demulin 1/50-21	Ethinyl estradiol (50 μg)	Ethynodiol diacetate (1 mg)
Demulin 1/50-28	Ethinyl estradiol (50 μg)	Ethynodiol diacetate (1 mg)
Enovid-E 21	Mestranol (100 μg)	Norethynodrel (2.5 mg)
Loestrin 21 1.5/30	Ethinyl estradiol (30 μg)	Norethindrone acetate (1.5 mg)
Loestrin 21 1/20	Ethinyl estradiol (20 μg)	Norethindrone acetate (1 mg)
Loestrin Fe 1.5/30 (28 day)	Ethinyl estradiol (30 μg)	Norethindrone acetate (1.5 mg)
Loestrin Fe 1/20 (28 day)	Ethinyl estradiol (20 μg)	Norethindrone acetate (1.0 mg)
Lo Ovral-21	Ethinyl estradiol (30 μg)	Norgestrel (0.3 mg)
Lo-Ovral-28	Ethinyl estradiol (30 μg)	Norgestrel (0.3 mg)
Modicon 21	Ethinyl estradiol (35 μg)	Norethindrone (0.5 mg)
Modicon 28	Ethinyl estradiol (35 μg)	Norethindrone (0.5 mg)
Nordette-21	Ethinyl estradiol (35 μg)	Levonorgestrel (0.15 mg)
Nordette-28	Ethinyl estradiol (35 μg)	Levonorgestrel (0.15 mg)
Norinyl 1 + 35 21-day	Ethinyl estradiol (35 μg)	Norethindrone (1 mg)
Norinyl 1 + 35 28-day	Ethinyl estradiol (35 μg)	Norethindrone (1 mg)
Norinyl 1 + 50 21-day	Mestranol (50 μg)	Norethindrone (1 mg)
Norinyl 1 + 50 28-day	Mestranol (50 μg)	Norethindrone (1 mg)
Norinyl 1 + 80 21-day	Mestranol (80 μg)	Norethindrone (1 mg)
Norinyl 1 + 80 28-day	Mestranol (80 μg)	Norethindrone (1 mg)
Norinyl 2 mg (20 day)	Mestranol (100 μg)	Norethindrone (2 mg)
Norlestrin 21 1/50	Ethinyl estradiol (50 μg)	Norethindrone acetate (1 mg)
Norlestrin 28, 1/50	Ethinyl estradiol (50 μg)	Norethindrone acetate (1 mg)
Norlestrin Fe 1/50	Ethinyl estradiol (50 μg)	Norethindrone acetate (1 mg)
Norlestrin 21, 2.5/50	Ethinyl estradiol (50 μg)	Norethindrone acetate (2.5 mg)
Norlestrin Fe 2.5/50	Ethinyl estradiol (50 μg)	Norethindrone acetate (2.5 mg)
Ortho Novum 1/35-21	Ethinyl estradiol (35 μg)	Norethindrone (1 mg)
Ortho Novum 1/35-28	Ethinyl estradiol (35 μg)	Norethindrone (1 mg)
Ortho Novum 1/50-21	Mestranol (50 μg)	Norethindrone (1 mg)
Ortho Novum 1/50-28	Mestranol (50 μg)	Norethindrone (1 mg)
Ortho Novum 1/80-21	Mestranol (80 μg)	Norethindrone (1 mg)
Ortho Novum 1/80-28	Mestranol (80 μg)	Norethindrone (1 mg)
Ovcon-50	Ethinyl estradiol (50 μg)	Norethindrone (1 mg)
Ovcon-35	Ethinyl estradiol (35 μg)	Norethindrone (0.4 mg)
Ovral (21 day)	Ethinyl estradiol (50 μg)	Norgestrel (0.5 mg)
Ovral-28	Ethinyl estradiol (50 μg)	Norgestrel (0.5 mg)
Ovulen-21	Mestranol (100 μg)	Ethynodiol diacetate (1 mg)
Ovulen-28	Mestranol (100 μg)	Ethynodiol diacetate (1 mg)
	BIPHASIC	
Ortho-Novum 10/11-21	Ethinyl estradiol (35 μg in each tablet)	Norethindrone (10 tablets of 0.5 mg followed by 11 tablets of 1 mg)
Ortho-Novum 10/11-28	See Ortho-Novum 10/11-21	

TABLE 31   *(Continued)*

Trade Name	Estrogen	Progestin
	TRIPHASIC	
Ortho-Novum 7/7/7 (21 or 28 day)	Ethinyl estradiol (35 μg in each tablet)	Norethindrone (0.5 mg the first 7 days, 0.75 the next 7 days, and 1 mg the last 7 days).
Tri-Norinyl (21 or 28 day)	Ethinyl estradiol (35 μg in each tablet)	Norethindrone (0.5 mg the first 7 days, 1 mg the next 9 days, and 0.5 mg the last 5 days).
Triphasil-21 (21 or 28 day)	1st 6 days: Ethinyl estradiol (30 μg)	Levonorgestrel (0.05 mg)
	Next 5 days: Ethinyl estradiol (40 μg)	Levonorgestrel (0.075 mg)
	Last 10 days: Ethinyl estradiol (30 μg)	Levonorgestrel (0.125 mg)

All combination oral contraceptives are Rx.

HYDROXYPROGESTERONE CAPROATE IN OIL   Delalutin, Duralutin, Gesterol L.A.250, Hy-Gesterone, Hylutin, Hydrogest 250, Hyproval P.A., Hydroxon, Pro-Depo (Rx)

Classification   Progestational hormone, synthetic.

Action/Kinetics   Hydroxyprogesterone is a synthetic progestin devoid of androgenic effects. It is suitable for prolonged therapy; priming with estrogens may be necessary to obtain desired response. **Duration:** 9–17 days.

Additional Untoward Reactions   Rarely, dyspnea, chest constriction, coughing, allergic reactions.

Dosage   IM. *Amenorrhea and other menstrual disorders*: 375 mg, anytime. If no menses after 21 days, cyclic therapy should be initiated repeating every 4 weeks and stopping after 4 cycles. Wait for 2–3 cycles after cessation of therapy to determine whether normal cyclic function has occurred. *Adenocarcinoma of uterine corpus (advanced)*: 1–7 gm/week. If no response after 12 weeks, therapy should be terminated. *Test for endogenous estrogen production*: 250 mg, anytime; repeat after 4 weeks.

Storage
1. Store at room temperature.
2. Wet syringe and needle may cause solution to become cloudy but this does not affect potency.

INTRAUTERINE PROGESTERONE CONTRACEPTIVE SYSTEM
Progestasert (Rx)

Classification   Contraceptive system (intrauterine device).

General Statement   Progestasert is an intrauterine contraceptive device (IUD) impregnated with a reservoir of 38 mg progesterone. Its contraceptive effectiveness is 12 months and it is considered superior to conventional IUDs, because of its smaller size. It can, however, be expelled from the uterine cavity inadvertently.

Action/Kinetics   Uncertain. Believed to change uterine milieu to prevent nidation and/or alter capacitation (ability of sperm to fertilize egg). Releases 65 μg progesterone/day into the uterine cavity.

Uses   Contraception in parous and nulliparous women.

Contraindications   Pregnancy or suspicion thereof, previous ectopic pregnancy, presence or history of pelvic inflammatory disease (PID), venereal disease, postpartum endometriosis, previous pelvic surgery, suspicion of malignant uterine disease, genital bleeding of unknown origin, acute cervicitis. Use with caution in presence of coagulopathy.

Untoward Reactions   Increased incidence of septic abortion; increased likelihood of ectopic pregnancy occurs with device in place. Transitory bleeding and cramps during initial weeks after insertion. Also, endometriosis, spontaneous abortion, septicemia, perforation of uterus and cervix, pelvic infection, cervical erosion, vaginitis, leukorrhea, uterine embedment, difficult removal, intermenstrual spotting, increased duration of menstruation, anemia, amenorrhea, delayed menses, dysmenorrhea, backaches, dyspareunia (painful coitus), neurovascular episodes including bradycardia and syncope following insertion, perforation of abdomen resulting in abdominal adhesions, intestinal penetration, intestinal obstruction, cystic masses in the pelvis.

Drug Interaction   Use with caution in patients receiving anticoagulants.

Dosage   One Progestasert system inserted into the uterine cavity; must be replaced once a year after insertion.

Administration   Should be inserted during or shortly after menses, since the system may cause fetus to abort if woman is pregnant.

Nursing Implications
1. Be prepared to support women with a history of syncope, bradycardia, or other neurovascular episodes, as such episodes might occur during insertion or removal of IUD.
2. Ascertain that Papanicolaou (Pap) smear, gonococcus culture, and other VD tests thought appropriate are done before insertion of IUD.
3. *Teach patient*
   a. to review package insert and instructions.
   b. to plan for insertion during or shortly after menstruation to reduce possibility of insertion when pregnancy exists.
   c. that bleeding and cramping may occur for a few weeks after insertion.
   d. the examination and replacement time schedule, that is,
      (1) preferably after first menses following insertion, definitely by third month after insertion.
      (2) annual examination.
      (3) annual replacement, if continuation of this form of contraception is desired (progesterone supply of device will then have been depleted).
   e. recognition and need for reporting ectopic pregnancy and/or septicemia:
      (1) that ectopic pregnancy is characterized by delayed menses, excessive menstrual bleeding, pelvic pain, weakness, and fatigue.
      (2) that septicemia is characterized by flulike symptoms, fever, abdominal cramping, pain, bleeding, or abnormal vaginal discharge.
   f. to return for removal or replacement of IUD if partial expulsion is suspected (as when threads of IUD do not protrude from cervix after menses).

MEDROXYPROGESTERONE ACETATE   Amen, Colprone,* Curretab, Depo-Provera, Provera (Rx)

Classification   Progestational hormone, synthetic.

Action/Kinetics   Medroxyprogesterone acetate, a synthetic progestin, is devoid of estrogenic and androgenic activity. Also available in depot form. Priming with estrogen is necessary before response is noted.

Additional Uses   Endometrial or renal carcinoma. *Investigational*: Perimenopausal and menopausal symptoms (injection). To stimulate respiration in obesity–hypoventilation syndrome (oral).

Dosage   **PO.** *Secondary amenorrhea:* 5–10 mg/day for 5–10 days with therapy beginning at any time. If endometrium has been estrogen primed: 10 mg medroxyprogesterone/day for 10 days. *Abnormal uterine bleeding with no pathology:* 5–10 mg/day for 5–10 days with therapy beginning on day 16 or 21 of the menstrual cycle. If endometrium has been estrogen primed: 10 mg/day for 10 days beginning on day 16 of the menstrual cycle. Bleeding usually begins within 3–7 days. **IM.** *Endometrial or renal carcinoma:* **initial,** 400–1000 mg weekly; **then, if improvement noted,** 400 mg monthly.

MEGESTROL ACETATE   Megace, Pallace (Rx)

Classification   Progestational hormone, synthetic.

General Statement   The mechanism through which this synthetic progestin exerts its antineoplastic effect is unknown.

Use   Palliative treatment of endometrial or breast cancer.

Dosage   **PO.** *Breast cancer:* 40 mg q.i.d. *Endometrial carcinoma:* 40–320 mg/day in divided doses. Administer for at least 2 months before assessing beneficial effects.

NORETHINDRONE   Norlutin (Rx)

NORETHINDRONE ACETATE   Aygestin, Norlutate (Rx)

Classification   Progestational hormone, synthetic.

Action/Kinetics   Norethindrone is twice as potent and norethindrone acetate is four times as potent as parenteral progesterone. Both synthetic progestins have estrogenic and androgenic properties and should not be used during pregnancy (masculinization of female fetus).

Norethindrone or norethindrone acetate, in combination with mestranol or ethinyl estradiol, is widely used for oral contraception.

Dosage   **PO.** *Norethindrone: Menstrual disorders,* 5–20 mg daily beginning on day 5 and ending on day 25 of menstrual cycle. *Endometriosis:* 10 mg/day for 2 weeks; **then,** increase in 5-mg increments every 2 weeks until a dose of 30 mg/day is reached (therapy maintained for 6–9 months).

Norethindrone acetate: Menstrual disorders, 2.5–10 mg daily beginning on day

5 and ending on day 25 of menstrual cycle. *Endometriosis*: 5 mg/day for 2 weeks; then, increase in 2.5-mg increments q 2 weeks until a dose of 15 mg/day is reached (therapy maintained for 6–9 months).

NORETHYNODREL (Rx)

Classification Progestational hormone, synthetic.

Use A synthetic progestin only used for oral contraception and menstrual abnormalities (see Table 31).

NORGESTREL (Rx)

Classification Progestational hormone, synthetic.

Uses Used only for oral contraceptives. See Table 31.

PROGESTERONE AQUEOUS (Rx)

PROGESTERONE IN OIL BY Progest, Femotrone in Oil, Gesterol 50 (Rx)

PROGESTERONE POWDER Bay Progest (Rx)

Classification Progestational hormone, natural.

General Statement This natural progestational hormone has minimal androgenic effects. IM injection of an oil solution acts more rapidly than SC injection of aqueous suspension. Pain and swelling at injection site are common.

Dosage **IM**. *Amenorrhea*, 5–10 mg for 6 to 8 consecutive days. *Functional uterine bleeding*: 5–10 mg daily for 6 days. After 6 days, bleeding should stop.

Administration
1. If progesterone is used with estrogen, begin progesterone after 2 weeks.
2. When menses begins, therapy should be terminated.

ORAL CONTRACEPTIVES: ESTROGEN–PROGESTERONE COMBINATIONS

General Statement The majority of oral contraceptives contain both an estrogen and a progestin in each tablet; such products are referred to as combination oral contraceptives. There are three types of combination products: (a) Monophasic—contain the same amount of estrogen and progestin in each tablet; (b) Biphasic—contain the same amount of estrogen in each tablet but the progestin content is

lower for the first 10 days of the cycle and higher the last 11 days; (c) Triphasic—
the estrogen content may be the same or may vary throughout the medication
cycle; the progestin content varies (see Table 31). The purpose of the biphasic and
triphasic products is to provide hormones in a similar manner as that seen physiologically. This is said to decrease breakthrough bleeding during the medication
cycle.

The other type of oral contraceptive is the progestin-only ("mini-pill") product,
which contains small amounts of a progestin in each tablet (see Table 33).

Action/Kinetics The combination oral contraceptives are thought to act by inhibiting ovulation due to an inhibition (through negative feedback mechanism) of
LH and FSH, which are required for development of ova. These products also act
to alter the cervical mucus so it is not conducive to sperm penetration as well as
to render the endometrium less suitable for implantation of the blastocyst should
fertilization occur.

The progestin-only products do not consistently inhibit ovulation. However,
these products also alter the cervical mucus, render the endometrium unsuitable
for implantation, and may alter tubal transport of the ovum. This method of
contraception is less reliable than combination therapy.

Uses Contraception, menstrual irregularities, menopausal symptoms. High doses
are used for endometriosis and hypermenorrhea (see Table 32).

Contraindications History of cerebrovascular disease, thrombophlebitis, and/or
pulmonary embolism, hypertension, ocular proptosis, partial or complete loss of
vision, defects in visual field, diplopia, carcinomatous condition of the breast or
genital tract, adolescents with incomplete epiphyseal closure, impaired hepatic
function, undiagnosed genital bleeding. Use with caution in patients with asthma,
epilepsy, migraine, diabetes, metabolic bone disease, renal or cardiac disease, and

TABLE 32   ORAL CONTRACEPTIVES USED FOR HYPERMENORRHEA OR ENDOMETRIOSIS

Trade Name	Content	Dosage
Enovid 5 mg, Rx	Mestranol: 75 μg Norethynodrel: 5 mg	*Endometriosis*: **initial**, 5–10 mg norethynodrel/day for 2 weeks; **then**, increase by 5–10 mg norethynodrel q 2 weeks up to 20 mg/day. Continue without interruption for 6–9 months. In severe cases, norethynodrel, 40 mg/day, can be used. *Hypermenorrhea*: **initial**, beginning on day 5 of cycle, 20–30 mg norethynodrel/day until bleeding is controlled; **then**, decrease to 10 mg/day until day 24 of cycle and withdraw medication.
Enovid 10 mg, Rx	Mestranol: 150 μg Norethynodrel: 9.85 mg	
Norinyl 2 mg, Rx	Mestranol: 100 μg Norethindrone: 2 mg	*Hypermenorrhea:* 1 tablet/day from day 5–24 of the cycle for a total of 3 cycles. Discontinue treatment to assess need for further therapy.
Ortho-Novum 2 mg, Rx	Mestranol: 100 μg Norethindrone: 2 mg	Same dosage as Norinyl 2 mg.

TABLE 33   PROGESTIN-ONLY CONTRACEPTIVE PREPARATIONS AVAILABLE IN THE UNITED STATES

Trade Name	Manufacturer	Progestin
Micronor	Ortho	Norethindrone (0.35 mg)
Nor QD	Syntex	Norethindrone (0.35 mg)
Ovrette	Wyeth	Norgestrel (0.075 mg)

Dosage: 1 tablet daily every day of the year. These products are Rx.

history of mental depression. Smoking. Use with caution in patients taking ampicillin, antiepileptic drugs, phenylbutazone, and rifampin, since intermittent bleeding (spotting) and unwanted pregnancy may result.

Untoward Reactions   The oral contraceptives have wide-ranging effects. These are particularly important, since the drugs are given for long periods of time to healthy women. Many authorities have voiced concern about the long-term safety of these agents. Some advise discontinuing therapy after 18–24 months' continuous use. The majority of untoward reactions of oral contraceptives are due to the estrogen component. These are listed under Estrogens, p. 743.

Other untoward reactions include: Auditory disturbances, Raynaud's syndrome, pancreatitis, rhinitis, hemolytic uremic syndrome, possible association with systemic lupus erythematosus. Also, there is an increased risk of congenital abnormalities if oral contraceptives are given to pregnant women. Oral contraceptives decrease the quantity and quality of breast milk.

Drug Interactions

Interactant	Interaction
Acetaminophen	↓ Effect of acetaminophen due to ↑ breakdown by liver
Anticoagulants, oral	↓ Effect of anticoagulants by increasing levels of certain clotting factors
Ascorbic acid	↑ Effect of oral contraceptives due to ↓ breakdown by liver
Barbiturates	↓ Effect of oral contraceptives due to ↑ breakdown by liver
Benzodiazepines	↑ or ↓ Effect of benzodiazepines due to changes in breakdown by liver
Caffeine	↑ Effect of caffeine due to ↓ breakdown by liver
Carbamazepine	↓ Effect of oral contraceptives due to ↑ breakdown by liver
Corticosteroids	↑ Effect of corticosteroids due to ↓ breakdown by liver
Griseofulvin	Griseofulvin may ↓ effect of oral contraceptives
Guanethidine	↓ Effect of guanethidine
Hypoglycemics	Oral contraceptives ↓ effect of hypoglycemics
Insulin	Oral contraceptives may ↑ insulin requirements
Isoniazid	↓ Effect of oral contraceptives due to ↑ breakdown by liver
Metoprolol	↑ Effect of metoprolol due to ↓ breakdown by liver
Neomycin	↓ Effect or oral contraceptive due to ↑ breakdown by liver
Penicillins	Penicillins may ↓ effect of oral contraceptives
Phenylbutazone	↓ Effect of contraceptives due to ↑ breakdown by liver

Interactant	Interaction
Phenytoin	↓ Effect of oral contraceptives due to ↑ breakdown by liver
Rifampin	↓ Effect of contraceptives due to ↑ breakdown by liver
Tetracyclines	↓ Effect of contraceptives due to tetracycline-induced inhibition of gut bacteria that hydrolyze steroid conjugates
Tricyclic antidepressants	Oral contraceptives ↓ effect of antidepressants
Troleandomycin	↑ Chance of jaundice

Laboratory Test Interferences Alter liver and thyroid function tests. ↓ Prothrombin time, 17-hydroxycorticosteroids, 17-ketosteroids, and 17-ketogenic steroids. (Therapy with ovarian hormones should be discontinued 60 days before performance of laboratory tests.) ↑ Gamma globulins.

Dosage See Tables 31 (p. 751), 32 (p. 756), and 33 (p. 757).

Administration

1. Tablets should be taken at approximately the same time each day (e.g. with a meal or at bedtime).
2. Spotting or breakthrough bleeding may occur for the first 1–2 cycles; if it continues past this time, consult the physician.
3. For the initial cycle, an **additional** form of contraception should be used for the first week.
4. The type of oral contraceptive preparation will determine the precise manner in which the drug is taken:
   a. For 20 or 21 day regimen, one tablet is taken daily beginning on day 5 of menses (day 1 is the first day of menstrual flow). No tablets are taken for 7 or 8 days.
   b. For a 28-day regimen, hormone-containing tablets are taken for the first 21 days followed by 7 days of inert or iron-containing tablets.
   c. Certain products, including the biphasic and selected triphasic oral contraceptives, are termed Sunday start. The first tablet should be taken the Sunday following the beginning of menses (if menses begins on Sunday, the first tablet should be taken that day).

Note: The biphasic and triphasic products have varying amounts of estrogen and/or progestin depending on the stage of the cycle; the patient should understand fully how these preparations are to be taken.

   d. For progestin-only products, the first tablet is taken on the first day of menses; thereafter, one tablet is taken every day of the year.
5. Currently, it is recommended that for a women beginning combination oral contraceptive therapy, a product be chosen that contains 50 μg estrogen or less.
6. If a woman fails to take one or more tablets, the following recommendations should be followed:
   a. If one tablet is missed, it should be taken as soon as it is remembered. Or, two tablets can be taken the following day.
   b. If two tablets are missed, two tablets can be taken each day for two days; or, two tablets can be taken on the day the missed tablets are remembered with the second missed tablet being discarded.
   c. If three tablets are missed, a new medication cycle should be initiated 7 days after the last tablet was taken and an additional form of contraception should be used until the start of the next menstrual period.

Note: With each succeeding tablet missed, the possibility increases that ovulation will occur.

Nursing Implications

1. Patients on combination therapy are susceptible to any of the untoward effects of estrogen and progesterone noted in the *General Statement*. See *Nursing Implications* for estrogen and progesterone, p. 744 and p. 750 respectively.

2. *Teach patient*

   a. to take tablets exactly as prescribed to prevent pregnancy.

   b. to take one missed tablet as soon as remembered. If two consecutive tablets are missed, the dosage must be doubled for the next 2 days. The regular schedule can then be resumed, but it is advisable to use additional contraceptive measures for the remainder of the cycle. If three tablets are missed, therapy should be discontinued and a new course started as indicated by the type of medication. Alternative contraceptive measures should be used when tablets are not taken and for 7 days after new course has been started.

   c. to discontinue therapy and consult her physician if she experiences symptoms of a thrombotic disorder, such as pain in legs, pain in chest, respiratory distress, unexplained cough, severe headache, dizziness, or blurred vision.

   d. that oral contraceptives decrease viscosity of the cervical mucus and increase susceptibility to vaginal infections, which are more difficult to treat successfully. Good hygienic practices are essential.

   e. to consult with her physician for possible adjustment of dosage or a different combination if minor side effects, such as nausea, edema, and skin eruptions, persist after four cycles.

   f. to report symptoms of eye pathology, such as headache, dizziness, blurred vision, or partial loss of sight.

   g. to report missed menstruation. If two consecutive menstrual periods are missed, therapy should be discontinued until pregnancy is ruled out.

   h. to have a yearly physicial examination and a Pap smear.

   i. not to take tablets for longer than 18 months without consulting physician.

   j. to request from her physician another form of contraception, if she is receiving ampicillin, antiepileptics, phenylbutazone, rifampin, or tetracycline, as intermittent bleeding and unwanted pregnancy might result due to effect of drug interactions.

   k. to limit caffeine consumption. Insomnia, irritability, tremors, and cardiac irregularities may occur because contraceptive interferes with caffeine elimination.

   l. if she is a lactating mother, to use another form of contraception until lactation is well established.

Chapter Sixty-three

OVARIAN STIMULANTS

Chorionic Gonadotropin 760   Menotropins 762
Clomiphene Citrate 761

General Statement   Ovarian stimulants are potent drugs to be used only in carefully selected patients. The fertility of the husband must be established prior to the treatment of the wife. A thorough clinical evaluation must also precede each new course of treatment.

CHORIONIC GONADOTROPIN (HCG)   Android-HCG, A.P.L. Secules, Chorex, Corgonject-5, Follutein, Glukor, Gonic, Libigen, Pregnyl, Profasi HP (Rx)

Classification   Gonadotropic hormone.

Action/Kinetics   The actions of human chorionic gonadotropin (HCG), produced by the trophoblasts of the fertilized ovum and then by the placenta, resemble those of luteinizing hormone (LH).

    In males, HCG stimulates androgen production by the testes, the development of secondary sex characteristics, and testicular descent when no anatomic impediment is present. In women, HCG stimulates progesterone production by the corpus luteum and completes expulsion of the ovum from a mature follicle.

Uses   *Males*: Prepubertal cryptorchidism, hypogonadism due to pituitary insufficiency. *Females*: Corpus luteum insufficiency, infertility (together with menotropins).

Contraindications   Precocious puberty, prostatic cancer or other androgen-dependent neoplasm, hypersensitivity to drug. Development of precocious puberty is cause for discontinuance of therapy. Since HCG increases androgen production, drug should be used with caution in patients in whom androgen-induced edema may be harmful (epilepsy, migraines, asthma, cardiac or renal diseases).

Untoward Reactions   *CNS:* Headache, irritability, restlessness, depression, fatigue. *Miscellaneous:* Edema, precocious puberty, gynecomastia, pain at injection site.

Dosage   **IM only.** *Prepubertal cryptorchidism*: various regimens including (1) 4,000 USP units 3 times/week for 3 weeks; (2) 5,000 USP units q other day for 4 injections; (3) 15 injections over a period of 6 weeks of 500–1,000 units/injection; (4) 500 USP units 3 times/week for 4–6 weeks. *Hypogonadism in males*: 500–1,000 USP units 3 times/week for 3 weeks; then, 500–1,000 USP units twice a week for 3 weeks. Or, 4,000 USP units 3 times/week for 6–9 months; then, 2,000 USP units 3 times/week for 3 more months. *Induction of ovulation (used with menotropins)*: 5,000–10,000 USP units one day after the last dose of menotropins.

Administration/Storage Reconstituted solutions are stable for 1–3 months, depending on manufacturer, when stored at 2°–8°C (35.6°–46.4°F).

Nursing Implications

1. Assess prepubescent male patient for appearance of secondary sex characteristics indicating sexual precocity, which necessitates withdrawal of medication.
2. Arrange to have patient with cryptorchidism examined for testicular descent 1 time/week to evaluate response to therapy.
3. Withhold chorionic gonadotropin and report if bleeding occurs in female patients after 15th day of administration, if therapy is for corpus luteum deficiency.
4. Teach patient and/or family how to assess for edema and to report if noted.

CLOMIPHENE CITRATE Clomid, Serophene (Rx)

Classification Ovarian stimulant.

Action/Kinetics The drug acts by combining with estrogen receptors thus decreasing the number of available receptor sites. Through negative feedback, the hypothalamus and pituitary are thus stimulated to increase secretion of LH and FSH. Under the influence of increased levels of these hormones, an ovarian follicle develops followed by ovulation and corpus luteum development. Most patients ovulate after the first course of therapy. Further treatment may be inadvisable if pregnancy fails to occur after ovulatory responses. It is readily absorbed from the GI tract and is excreted in the feces.

Uses Selected cases of female infertility in which normal endogenous estrogen levels have been observed. *Investigational*: Oligospermia.

Contraindications Pregnancy, liver disease or history thereof, abnormal bleeding of undetermined origin. Ovarian cysts. The absence of neoplastic disease should be established before treatment is initiated. Therapy is ineffective in patients with ovarian or pituitary failure.

Untoward Reactions *Ovarian:* Ovarian overstimulation and/or enlargement and subsequent symptoms resembling premenstrual syndrome. *Ophthalmologic:* Blurred vision, spots or flashes probably due to intensification of after images. *GI:* Abdominal distention, pain, or soreness; nausea, vomiting. *GU:* Abnormal uterine bleeding, breast tenderness. *CNS:* Insomnia, nervousness, headache, depression, fatigue, lightheadedness, dizziness. *Miscellaneous:* Hot flashes, increased urination, allergic symptoms, weight gain, alopecia (reversible).

Laboratory Test Interference ↑ Serum thyroxine and thyroxine-binding globulin.

Dosage **PO**, *First course*: 50 mg daily for 5 days. *Second course*: same dosage. In absence of ovulation, dose may be increased to 100 mg/day for 5 days.

Therapy may be started any time in patients who had no recent uterine bleeding. Otherwise, on fifth day of cycle; after 30 days in patients who did not respond to previous course.

Note: Most patients will respond following the first course of therapy. Further therapy is not recommended if pregnancy does not result following 3 ovulatory responses.

Nursing Implications

Teach patient to

a. take basal body temperature and chart on graph.

b. continue taking basal body temperature in AM and charting it to ascertain whether ovulation has occurred.

c. discontinue drug and check with medical supervision if abdominal symptoms or pelvic pain occur because these indicate ovarian enlargement and/or ovarian cyst.

d. discontinue drug and report to medical supervision should visual problems occur because retina may be affected and ophthalmologic examination may be required.

e. avoid performing hazardous tasks involving body coordination or mental alertness because drug may cause lightheadedness, dizziness, or visual disturbances.

f. discontinue medication and check with medical supervision if she suspects that she is pregnant, because drug may have teratogenic effect.

MENOTROPINS   Pergonal (Rx)

Classification   Ovarian stimulant.

Action/Kinetics   Menotropins is a mixture of follicle-stimulating hormone (FSH) and luteinizing hormone (LH), which cause growth and maturation of ovarian follicles. For ovulation to occur, HCG is administered the day following menotropins. In men, menotropins with HCG given for a minimum of 3 months induces spermatogenesis.

Uses   In combination with HCG for infertility caused by primary or secondary amenorrhea (including galactorrhea), polycystic ovary syndrome, and anovulatory cycles. In combination with HCG to induce spermatogenesis in males with secondary hypogonadotropic hypogonadism.

Contraindications   *Women:* Pregnancy. Primary ovarian failure as indicated by high levels of urinary gonadotropins, ovarian cysts, intracranial lesions, including pituitary tumors. *Men:* Normal gonadotropin levels, primary testicular failure, disorders of fertility other than hypogonadotropic hypogonadism. Thyroid or adrenal dysfunction. Absence of neoplastic disease should be established before treatment is initiated.

Untoward Reactions   *Women:* Ovarian overstimulation, hyperstimulation syndrome (maximal 7 to 10 days after discontinuance of drug), ovarian enlargement (20% of patients), ruptured ovarian cysts, hemoperitoneum, thromboembolism, multiple births (20%). Fever. *Men:* Erythrocytosis-HCT, gynecomastia.

Dosage   **Women, IM**, *individualized*: **initial**, 75 IU of FSH and 75 IU of LH for 9 to 12 days, followed by 10,000 USP units of HCG on day after last dose of menotropins. *Subsequent courses*: same dosage schedule. In absence of ovulation, dose may be increased to 150 IU of FSH and 150 IU of LH for 9 to 12 days, followed by HCG as above for 2 or more courses.

Men, IM: To increase serum testosterone levels, it may be necessary to give HCG alone, 5,000 IU 3 times weekly, for 4–6 months prior to menotropins; **then,**

75 IU FSH and 75 IU LH 3 times weekly and HCG 2,000 IU 2 times weekly for at least 4 months. If no response after 4 months, double each dose of menotropins with the HCG dose unchanged.

Administration   Use reconstituted solution immediately. Discard unused portion.

Nursing Implications

1. *Withhold HCG* and inform doctor if daily urinary estrogen excretion level is greater than 100 μg or daily estriol excretion is greater than 50 μg. These are signs of impending hyperstimulation syndrome.

2. *Teach patient*
   a. that she must be examined at least every other day for signs of excessive ovarian stimulation during therapy and for 2 weeks thereafter.
   b. to collect 24-hr urine daily, to be analyzed for estrogen. Provide her with a suitable container for collection.
   c. to deliver this sample to appropriate laboratory facility.
   d. to take basal body temperature and chart on graph.
   e. signs and tests that indicate time of ovulation, such as increase in basal body temperature, and increase in the appearance and volume of cervical mucus, spinnbarkeit, and ferning of cervical mucus. Also explain significance of the urinary excretion of estriol.
   f. that daily intercourse is advisable from the day before chorionic gonadotropin is administered and ovulation occurs.
   g. to abstain from intercourse in case of significant ovarian enlargement because this increases chance of rupturing ovarian cysts.

3. Should hyperstimulation syndrome occur,
   a. explain to patient that hospitalization is necessary for close monitoring.
   b. maintain intake and output and weigh daily to assist in monitoring hemoconcentration. Assess specific gravity of urine, hematocrit, and serum and urinary electrolytes.
   c. anticipate that sodium heparin will be ordered if hematocrit rises to critical levels.
   d. explain to patient the need for bed rest, fluid, and electrolyte replacement and the availability of analgesics if needed.

Chapter Sixty-four

ABORTIFACIENTS

Prostaglandins

Other Agents

General Statement   Several agents are used to induce abortions during the second trimester of pregnancy. These include the prostaglandins F_2 alpha and E_2 or highly concentrated solutions of sodium chloride (20%) or urea (40–50%).

After administration, most of these agents induce evacuation of the uterus within a predictable number of hours. If uterine contractions fail to start or are not strong enough to expel the fetus, the same aborifacient is readministered. If this measure is again unsuccessful, the pregnancy must be terminated by another means, such as the administration of a different abortifacient, oxytocin, or surgery.

Second-trimester abortions are usually carried out by a physician trained in amniocentesis and in a hospital in which intensive care and surgical facilities are available.

Dinoprost tromethamine, sodium chloride, and urea are administered intra-amniotically while carboprost is given only IM and dinoprostone by vaginal suppository. Oxytocin is sometimes administered concurrently, with both prostaglandins and hypertonic abortifacients.

Administration (Intra-amniotic)

1. Have patient void before procedure to prevent injection of abortifacient into bladder.
2. Prepare abdomen with antiseptic solution.
3. Be prepared to assist while physician administers local anesthetic and inserts needle through abdominal wall (14-gauge spinal needle with stylet) suitable for amniocentesis. One milliliter of amniotic fluid is withdrawn to check on position of needle.
4. If fluid withdrawn contains blood, needle must be repositioned. Otherwise, a Teflon catheter is threaded beyond needle top; the needle is withdrawn and administration of abortifacient started.
5. An amount of amniotic fluid approximately equivalent to the volume of the abortifacient to be injected is removed through the catheter.
6. The abortifacient is injected slowly, especially at first, to determine the sensitivity of the patient.
7. The catheter may be left in place for 24–48 hours to facilitate repeat administration of drug.
8. Be prepared to administer antibiotics prophylactically through catheter.
9. A small surgical dressing is applied to abdomen when the catheter is withdrawn.

Nursing Implications

1. Provide emotional support to patient receiving an abortifacient because she is in great need of reassurance and acceptance and often lacks a good support system.
2. Explain abortion procedure, including administration of drug, labor, and delivery. Provide an opportunity for questions, and answer these appropriately.
3. Have antiemetics available to administer before procedure to minimize vomiting.
4. Remain close to patient and provide support as needed during administration of abortifacient.
5. Assess for onset of labor.
6. Monitor progress of labor, assessing frequency, length, and strength of contractions.
7. Monitor BP, temperature, pulse rate, and respirations per minute, to assess for hypertension, hemorrage, dyspnea, bradycardia, and alterations in function of central nervous system.
8. Assess for nausea, vomiting, and diarrhea both to minimize discomfort and to prevent electrolyte imbalance.
9. If oxytocin is also to be administered, assess that contractions have ceased before initiating therapy. Use Y-tubing system in which one bottle contains IV solution and oxytocin and another contains only IV solution. In this manner, the drug can be discontinued but patency of the vein can be maintained when the switch to the drug-free infusion bottle is made. To prevent uterine rupture and cervical lacerations, discontinue oxytocin and notify doctor if contractions exceed 50 mm of Hg as measured on an electric monitor or last longer than 70 seconds without a period of complete relaxation of uterus in between contractions. Remain with patient receiving oxytocin for induction of labor.
10. Monitor patient during fourth stage of labor.
11. Assess patient for hemorrhage, fever, and signs of infection, which may indicate that placenta was retained after delivery of fetus.
12. Observe perineal area for trickle of blood from vagina, which may be indicative of undetected cervical laceration.
13. Have RhoGam available for administration after delivery to unsensitized RH-negative women.
14. *Teach patient to*
    a. observe for signs and symptoms of infection and hemorrhage.
    b. avoid vaginal intercourse, use of tampons, and douches for 2 weeks post-delivery.
    c. return for reexamination in 2 to 4 weeks.
    d. recognize symptoms of depression, common after delivery.
    e. wear a supporting bra, if lactation occurs after abortion.
    f. use one of several suggested methods of contraception after postpartum examination if family planning is desired or medically indicated.

PROSTAGLANDINS

Action/Kinetics Prostaglandins are becoming the drugs of choice for the induction of late second-trimester abortions. These hormone-like substances induce uterine contractions similar to normal labor, usually resulting in expulsion of the fetus in 12–48 hr. The drugs also facilitate dilation and softening of the cervix. Due to their effect on smooth muscle, prostaglandins may also increase GI tract motility, cause bronchospasms, vasocontriction, and changes in blood pressure. The drugs differ with respect to route of administration, number of weeks after gestation when they can be used, and the intensity of side effects.

Uses See individual drugs.

Contraindications Hypersensitivity to drug. Acute pelvic inflammatory disease. Use with caution for patients with history of asthma, epilepsy, hypo- or hypertension, cardiovascular, renal, or hepatic disease, anemia, jaundice, diabetes, cervicitis, infected endocervical lesions, acute vaginitis, history of uterine surgery (e.g., cesarean section).

Untoward Reactions *GI:* Nausea, vomiting, diarrhea, hiccoughs, fever, chills. *CNS:* Headache, weakness, anxiety, drowsiness, dizziness, weakness, lethargy. *GU:* Laceration or perforation of uterus or cervix, rupture of uterus, endometritis, urinary tract infections, profuse bleeding, pain. *CV:* Chest tightness or pain, hypo- or hypertension, cardiac arrhythmias. *Respiratory:* Wheezing, dyspnea, coughing, hyperventilation, epistaxis. *Other:* Sweating, backache, skin rash, breast tenderness, eye pain.

Note: Since prostaglandins do not directly affect the fetal placental unit, it is possible that a live fetus may be born.

Dosage See individual drugs.

Additional Nursing Implications

See also *Nursing Implications*, p. 765.

1. Monitor patient for pyrexia for at least three days after abortion.
2. Assess patient with postabortion pyrexia to determine whether endometritis or prostaglandin-induced pyrexia is occurring. Drug-induced pyrexia is usually manifested 1–16 hours after the first injection, after which temperature returns to pretreatment level after discontinuation of therapy. With endometritis, the pyrexia usually occurs the third day after the abortion and continues with infection, unless treated.
3. If patient has drug-induced pyrexia, sponge with water or alcohol and maintain adequate hydration.

CARBOPROST TROMETHAMINE   Prostin/15 M (Rx)

Action/Kinetics Synthetic analog of prostaglandin F2 alpha. Carboprost may be preferred over other prostaglandin abortifacients since IM injection is less difficult to administer and it may be used without fear of expulsion of vaginal suppositories in presence of excess vaginal bleeding. **Mean time to abortion:** 16 hr.

Uses To induce abortion from weeks 13–20 of pregnancy.

Dosage **IM only: initial,** 0.25 mg deep in the muscle; **then,** repeat at intervals of 1.5 and 3.5 hr depending on response. Dose may be increased to 0.5 mg if response inadequate after several 0.25 mg doses. Total dose should not exceed 12 mg.

Administration Pretreatment or concurrent use of an antiemetic and/or antidiarrheal decreases GI side effects.

DINOPROST TROMETHAMINE   Prostin F$_2$ Alpha (Rx)

Action/Kinetics Oxytocin may be used as an adjunct with caution. **Mean time to abortion:** 20 hr. Rapidly metabolized.

Uses Intra-amniotically to induce abortion between weeks 16–20 of gestation. *Investigational:* Induction of labor, stimulation of contractions in early rupture of membranes, missed abortion, intrauterine fetal death, hydatidiform mole.

Additional Untoward Reactions Bronchospasm, breast engorgement, lactation, tonic-clonic seizures in patients prone to epilepsy, A-V conduction disturbances, paresthesia, hyperesthesia, dysuria.

Dosage Intra-amniotically. After removal of 1 ml of amniotic fluid, 40 mg (8 ml) is instilled with a spinal needle slowly if fluid is not bloody. The first 1 ml should be injected slowly over 1–2 min to assess sensitivity. If there is minimal or no response after 24 hr, a second 10–20 mg dose may be given.

Administration The patient should be placed in lithotomy position for vaginal examination before each dose to ensure that intra-amniotic catheter has not prolapsed into the vagina.

DINOPROSTONE   Prostin E$_2$ (Rx)

Action/Kinetics Dinoprostone is a naturally occurring prostaglandin derivative. **Mean time to abortion:** 17 hr.

Uses To induce labor in intrauterine fetal death, hydatidiform mole, anencephalic fetus, missed abortion, elective abortion (from weeks 12–20), and in uterine perforation before completion of suction curettage. *Investigational:* Low doses to initiate labor and to induce cervical ripening before induction of labor.

Dosage Vaginal suppository: one 20 mg suppository inserted high in the vagina. Repeat, if necessary, q 3–5 hr until abortion occurs. Should not be given for more than 2 days.

Administration
1. Patient should remain supine for 10 min after insertion.
2. The number of suppositories used should be determined by patient tolerance and uterine contractility.
3. Suppositories should be stored at −20° C or below.
4. Allow suppositories to warm to room temperature before unwrapping and inserting.

OTHER AGENTS

SODIUM CHLORIDE 20% SOLUTION   (Rx)

Classification Abortifacient.

Action/Kinetics Hypertonic sodium chloride may release prostaglandins, which cause uterine contractions. Abortion may be incomplete in 25–40% of all cases and must be completed by other means. Usually induces termination of pregnancy within 48 hr (97% abort within 72 hr). IV oxytocin may be used concomitantly to decrease time to abortion.

Uses Termination of pregnancy during second trimester (weeks 16 to 24).

Contraindications Increased intra-amniotic pressure, as in actively contracting or hypertonic uterus. Suspected pelvis adhesions. Patients sensitive to sodium chloride overload (cardiovascular and renal disorders, hypertension and epilepsy), or suffering from blood disorders. Previous uterine surgery.

Untoward Reactions *CV:* Flushing, circulatory failure, hypervolemia, intravascular coagulation (decrease in platelets, hematocrit, fibrinogen, factors V and VIII; increase in plasma volume, fibrin, thrombin, prothrombin). *GU:* Cervical laceration and perforation, uterine rupture, cervicovaginal fistula. If placenta is retained, infection, endometritis, sepsis, hemorrhage, and fever are possible. *Other:* Pulmonary embolism, pneumonia, renal cortical necrosis, ascites, severe electrolyte imbalance.

If hypertonic sodium chloride is inadvertently injected intravascularly, severe, life-threatening reactions may occur.

Drug Interactions Terbutaline may prolong the time to abortion when used with hypertonic sodium chloride.

Dosage **Transabdominal intra-amniotic:** 45–250 ml of 20% sodium chloride solution. If labor has not begun within 48 hr after instillation, the patient should be reassessed by the physician.

Additional Administration

1. During instillation of saline pay close attention to complaints of patient (sensation of heat, thirst, severe headache, mental confusion, vague distress, lower back, pelvic or abdominal pain, tingling sensations, numbness of fingertips, a feeling of warmth about the lips and tongue, extreme nervousness, or tinnitus) that may indicate that drug is not being instilled into amniotic sac. Be prepared to assist with 5% dextrose infusion and other supportive therapy to prevent hypernatremic shock.

2. Observe patient for 1 to 2 hr after instillation of hypertonic saline for untoward reactions and onset of labor.

Nursing Implications

See also *Nursing Implications* on *Abortifacients*, p. 765.

1. Encourage patient to drink at least 2 liters of water on the day of the procedure to facilitate the excretion of salt.

2. Assess for and report symptoms of hypernatremia following injection, such as thirst, rough dry tongue, flushed skin, elevated temperature, excitement, hypo- or hypertension, tachycardia, and numbness of fingertips.

3. Have available 5% dextrose injection and IV administration set to use, should hypernatremia occur.

UREA 40–50% INJECTION   (Rx)

Classification Abortifacient.

Action/Kinetics Hypertonic urea is believed to exert its abortifacient effect by damaging cells that release prostaglandins; the prostaglandins, in turn, induce uterine smooth muscle contractions. The average induction period is 18–30 hr. Eighty percent of patients abort within 76 hours. In 30–40% of patients, the uterine evacuation must be completed by surgical or other means.

Uses   Second-trimester (beyond week 16) termination of pregnancy. Usually used concomitantly with oxytocin.

Contraindications   History of pelvic adhesions or pelvic surgery. Severely impaired renal function, frank liver failure, active intracranial bleeding, marked dehydration, and major systemic disease.

Untoward Reactions   *GI:* Nausea, vomiting, diarrhea. *GU:* Cervical laceration and perforation, myometrial necrosis. If placenta is retained, infection, endometritis, fever, or hemorrhage may occur. *Electrolytes:* Dehydration, hyponatremia, hypokalemia. *Other:* Intravascular coagulation, headaches, decrease in platelets and fibrinogen.

Intravascular, intramyometrial, or intraperitoneal injection can lead to myometrial necrosis, dehydration, hyponatremia, hypokalemia, or hyperkalemia.

Dosage   Intra-amniotically: 200–250 ml (equal to amount of amniotic fluid removed) of 40–50% urea solution (approximately 80 gm urea) given over 20–30 min. If response is inadequate after 48 hr, an additional 80 gm urea may be given.

Additional Administration/Storage
1. All amniotic fluid should be removed first to prevent sudden increases in intra-amniotic pressure.
2. Warm diluent in waterbath to 60°C (140°F) before mixing with urea. Administer at body temperature.
3. Urea solution should be used within a few hours after reconstitution, if stored at room temperature, and within 48 hours, if stored at 2°–8°C (35.6°–46.4°F).
4. Administer urea over period of 20 to 30 minutes.
5. Drug should be discontinued, if patient manifests symptoms of lower abdominal pain.

Additional Nursing Implications
See also *Nursing Implications* on *Abortifacients*, p. 765.

1. Encourage fluids to prevent dehydration and to promote urea excretion.
2. Assess for muscle weakness and lethargy, signs of electrolyte imbalance.
3. Ascertain that blood chemistries are performed and results evaluated. Have IV fluids available to correct electrolyte imbalance.

Chapter Sixty-five

ANDROGENS AND ANABOLIC STEROIDS

Androgens/Anabolic Steroids

Miscellaneous Agent

ANDROGENS/ANABOLIC STEROIDS

General Statement The principal male hormone manufactured by the interstitial cells of the testes is testosterone. Testosterone, its degradation products, and synthetic substitutes are collectively referred to as the androgens (from the Greek *andros*, man). Like the primary female hormones estrogen and progesterone, the production of testosterone is controlled by the gonadotropins, follicle-stimulating hormone (FSH), and the interstitial cell-stimulating hormone (ICSH), both of which are produced by the anterior pituitary.

At puberty, these gonadotropins initiate the production of testosterone, which in turn stimulates the development of primary sex organs and secondary sexual characteristics. Testosterone also stimulates bone and skeletal muscle growth, increases the retention of dietary protein nitrogen (anabolism), and slows down the breakdown of body tissues (catabolism). Androgens promote retention of sodium, potassium, nitrogen, and phosphorus and the excretion of calcium. Toward the end of puberty, testosterone hastens the conversion of cartilage into bone, thereby terminating linear growth.

Treatment with testosterone and its congeners is complicated by the fact that the exogenous supply of the hormone may depress secretion of the natural hormone through inhibitory effects on the pituitary. Too large a dose may cause permanent damage. Treatment is usually associated with a feeling of well being. In addition to testosterone and its various esters, several synthetic variants are available commercially.

Uses Replacement therapy in males for congenital or acquired primary hypogonadism, congenital or acquired hypogonadotropic hypogonadism, delayed puberty. In postmenopausal females to treat inoperable metastatic breast carcinoma or in premenopausal females following oophorectomy. Postpartum breast engorgement.

Anabolic steroids are indicated for weight gain following illness or catabolic states, as an adjunct in senile or postmenopausal osteoporosis, certain types of anemia (aplastic anemia, red cell aplasia, hemolytic anemias), and to promote a positive nitrogen balance in chronic corticosteroid therapy.

Contraindications Prostatic or breast (males) carcinoma. Pregnancy (masculinization of female fetus). Use with caution in young boys who have not completed their growth (because of premature epiphyseal closure) or in patients with cardiac, renal, or hepatic disorders (because of edema caused by androgen administration). Discontinue if hypercalcemia occurs.

Untoward Reactions *Hepatic:* Liver toxicity is the most serious side effect. Jaundice, cholestasis, alterations in BSP retention, SGOT, and SPGT. Rarely, hepatic necrosis, hepatocellular neoplasms, peliosis hepatis. *GI:* Nausea, vomiting, diarrhea, anorexia, symptoms of peptic ulcer. *CNS:* Headache, anxiety, increased or decreased libido, insomnia, excitation, paresthesia, sleep apnea syndrome, CNS hemorrhage, chills, choreiform movements, habituation, confusion (toxic doses). *GU:* Testicular atrophy with inhibition of testicular function, impotence, chronic priapism, epididymitis, irritable bladder, oligospermia, prepubertal phallic enlargement, decreased volume of ejaculate. *Electrolyte:* Retention of sodium, chloride, calcium, potassium, phosphates. Edema. *Miscellaneous:* Acne, flushing, suppression of clotting factors (II, V, VII, X), polycythemia, leukopenia, rashes, dermatitis, anaphylaxis (rare), muscle cramps. Hypercalcemia, especially in immobilized patients or those with metastatic breast carcinoma.

   In females, menstrual irregularities, virilization, clitoral enlargement, hirsutism, increased libido, baldness (male pattern), virilization of external genitalia of female fetus. **In children,** disturbances of growth, premature closure of epiphyses, precocious sexual development.

   Buccal preparations may cause stomatitis. Inflammation and pain at site of IM or SC injection.

Drug Interactions

Interactant	Interaction
Anticoagulants, oral	Anabolic steroids ↑ effect of anticoagulants
Antidiabetic agents	Additive hypoglycemia
Barbiturates	↓ Effect of androgens due to ↑ breakdown by liver
Corticosteroids	Chance of edema
Phenylbutazone	Certain androgens ↑ effect of phenylbutazone

Laboratory Test Interferences Alter thyroid function tests. False + or ↑ BSP, alkaline phosphatase, bilirubin, cholesterol, and acid phosphatase (in women). Alteration of glucose tolerance tests.

Dosage Androgens are given **PO, deep IM,** and by the **buccal** and **sublingual** route. See Table 34, p. 773, for individual compounds. Diuretics may be given to control edema.

Nursing Implications
1. *Assess*
    a. children closely for signs of precocious puberty and growth retardation.
    b. for edema; weigh the patient at least 2 times/week. Check I & O.
    c. sclera, mucous membranes, and skin for signs of jaundice.
    d. for pruritis, which may occur before jaundice is noted.

(continued)

2. Report whether GI upset is due to medication. Report onset of permanent signs of virilization, such as deepening of the voice and clitoral enlargement.
3. Alert the physician to reports by female patients of increased libido. Such manifestations may require explanation and emotional support. Increased libido may be an early sign of serious toxicity.
4. Reassure female patients that growth of facial hair and development of acne are reversible once the drug is withdrawn.
5. Explain to female patients that medication may cause menstrual cycle irregularities in premenopausal women and withdrawal bleeding in postmenopausal women.
6. Report priapism in male patients because this necessitates at least temporary withdrawal of drug.
7. Provide a diet high in calories, proteins, vitamins, minerals, and other nutrients unless contraindicated.
8. In patients who have high serum calcium levels, the drug will have to be withdrawn and fluids administered to prevent renal calculi (normal: 4.5–5.5 mEq/L). If hypercalcemia is due to metastases, other appropriate therapy may be instituted. Hypercalcemia is characterized by relaxed skeletal muscles, deep bony pain caused by honeycombing of bones, flank pain caused by kidney stones resulting from excessively high serum calcium levels.

MISCELLANEOUS AGENT

DANAZOL Cyclomen,* Danocrine

Classification Androgen, synthetic.

Action/Kinetics This synthetic androgen inhibits the release of gonadotropins (FSH and LH) by the anterior pituitary. In women this action results in arrest of ovarian function, induces amenorrhea, and causes atrophy of normal and ectopic endometrial tissue. **Onset** (amenorrhea, anovulation): 6 to 8 weeks. $t^{1/2}$: 29 hr. **Duration**: Ovulation and menstruation usually resume 60 to 90 days after cessation of therapy.

Uses Endometriosis amenable to hormonal management in patients who cannot tolerate other drug therapy or who have not responded to other drug therapy. Fibrocystic breast disease. Hereditary angioedema in males and females. *Investigational*: Gynecomastia, menorrhagia, precocious puberty.

Contraindications Undiagnosed genital bleeding, markedly impaired hepatic, renal, and cardiac function, pregnancy and lactation.

Untoward Reactions *Androgenic:* Acne, decrease in breast size, oily hair and skin, weight gain, deepening of voice and hair growth, clitoral hypertrophy, testicular atrophy. *Estrogen deficiency:* Flushing, sweating, vaginitis, nervousness, changes in emotions. *GI:* Nausea, vomiting, constipation, gastroenteritis. *Hepatic:* Jaundice, dysfunction. *CNS:* Fatigue, tremor, headache, dizziness, sleep problems, paresthesia, anxiety, depression, appetite changes. *Miscellaneous:* Allergic reactions, muscle cramps or spasms, joint swelling or lock-up, hematuria, increased blood pressure, chills, pelvic pain, carpal tunnel syndrome, hair loss, change in libido.

TABLE 34 ANDROGENS AND ANABOLIC STEROIDS

Drug	Uses	Dosage	Remarks
Dromostanolone propionate (Drolban), Rx	Antineoplastic; inoperable metastatic cancer of breast in women	**IM:** 100 mg 3 times weekly. May take 8 to 12 weeks for beneficial effects to be noted.	Synthetic. The regression produced by drug usually only lasts 1 year.
Ethylestrenol (Maxibolin), Rx	Anabolic agent: to offset catabolic effects of corticosteroids and in certain forms of cancer, prolonged immobilization, retarded growth, osteoporosis, anemias	**PO, initial, adults:** 4–8 mg daily; **usual,** 4 mg daily. **Children under 12 years:** 1–3 mg daily.	Synthetic. Do not exceed 6 weeks therapy. Reinstitute if necessary after 4-week rest period. Fewer androgenic effects than methyltestosterone. However, these may be particularly marked in children. Drug may affect liver function; hence periodic liver function tests are indicated. Growth may occur for up to 6 months after drug has been terminated.
Fluoxymesterone (Android-F, Halotestin, Ora-Testryl), Rx	Androgen deficiency states in males (when hypogonadism starts in adult life); metastatic breast carcinoma in women; postpartum breast engorgement	*Delayed puberty:* **initial,** 2 mg/day; **then,** increase dose gradually depending on response. *Hypogonadism, testicular hypofunction,* **PO:** 2–10 mg daily. *Inoperable mammary cancer:* 15-30 mg daily in divided doses. Continue for 2–3 months. *Postpartum breast engorgement:* **initial,** 2.5 mg at time of labor; **then,** 5–10 mg daily for 4–5 days.	Synthetic. Drug does not result in full sexual maturation in patients with prepubertal testicular function. Five times more potent than long-acting esters of testosterone or testosterone pellets when used as replacement therapy in males and androgen deficiency. GI disturbances more frequent than with other androgens.
Methyltestosterone (Android-5, -10, -25, Metandren, Oreton Methyl, Testred, Virilon), Rx	Androgen deficiency states, anabolic agent, breast cancer in women, postpartum breast engorgement, cryptorchidism	*Androgen deficiency, eunuchoidism, eunuchism.* **PO:** 10–40 mg daily in divided doses. **Buccal:** 5–20 mg daily. *Breast cancer in women.* **PO:** 200 mg daily. **Buccal:** 100 mg daily. *Postpartum breast engorgement.* **PO:** 80 mg daily. **Buccal:** 40	Semisynthetic. Ineffective in producing full sexual maturation in patients with prepubertal testicular failure. Buccal use provides twice the androgenic effect as oral tablets. *Administration* 1. Place linguet under tongue or in lower buccal pouch.

773

TABLE 34 (*Continued*)

Drug	Uses	Dosage	Remarks
		mg for 3–4 days. *Postpubertal cryptorchidism.* **PO**: 30 mg daily. **Buccal**: 15 mg daily.	2. Avoid eating, drinking, chewing, or smoking during dissolution process, as swallowing is detrimental to absorption. 3. Oral hygiene measures indicated after absorption of linguet.
Nandrolone decanoate (Anabolin LA 100, Analone-50 and -100, Androlone-D 50 and 100, Deca-Durabolin, Hybolin Decanoate), Rx	Osteoporosis, anemias, debilitated states, metastatic breast cancer	**IM. Adults**: 50–100 mg q 3–4 weeks for 4 months. **Children 2 to 13 years**: 25–50 mg q 3–4 weeks. *Metastatic breast cancer*: 100–200 mg/week.	Synthetic. A rest period of 6 to 8 weeks is suggested after a 4-month course of therapy.
Nandrolone phenpropionate (Androlone, Androlone 50, Anabolin I.M., Durabolin, Hybolin Improved, Nandrobolic), Rx	Anabolic agent: growth retardation, osteoporosis, in corticosteroid therapy, inoperable mammary cancer in females	**IM. Adults: initial**, 25–50 mg once weekly. **Children 2–13 years**: 12.5–25 mg q 2–4 weeks. *Metastatic breast cancer*: 50 - 100 mg/week depending on response.	Synthetic. Children under 7 yr are particularly sensitive to the drug. Observe 3-month rest period after 3-month course of therapy.
Oxandrolone (Anavar), Rx	Anabolic agent: reverses negative nitrogen balance, excess calcium and nitrogen excretion. Muscle wasting due to chronic corticosteroid therapy. Patients recovering from surgery, infections, burns, severe traumatic injuries	**PO, adults**: 2.5 mg b.i.d. to q.i.d., **range**: 2.5–20 mg daily. **Children under 12 years**: 0.25 mg/kg daily.	Synthetic. Drug has low androgenic properties. Children may be particularly sensitive to the androgenic effects of oxandrolone. Therapy usually continued 2 to 4 weeks. Do not exceed 3 months.
Oxymetholone (Anadrol-50, Anapolon 50*), Rx	Anemias	*Anemias.* **Adults and children, individualized**, 1–5 mg/kg/day. Minimum of 3–6	Continuous therapy is usually indicated in congenital aplastic anemia.

Stanozolol (Winstrol), Rx	Aplastic anemia, osteoporosis, muscle wasting in chronic corticosteroid therapy	months therapy usually indicated. **PO, adults:** 2 mg t.i.d. before or with meals or 2 mg daily in young women; **children up to 6 years:** 1 mg b.i.d.; **6–12 years:** up to 2 mg t.i.d.	Synthetic. May cause premature epiphyseal closure in children. Patients should be placed on high protein, high calorie diet. Periodic liver function studies required.
Testosterone Aqueous Suspension (Andro 100, Android T, Bay Testone-50, Histerone 50 and 100, Testaqua, Testoject-50), Rx	Male sex hormone deficiency states, eunuchoidism, castration. Females: selected menstrual disorders, lactation suppression, advanced mammary cancer. Aplastic anemia, hypoplastic anemias	*Testosterone and testosterone propionate,* **IM only** . *Replacement therapy:* 10–25 mg 2 to 3 times/week. *Postpartum breast engorgement:* 25–50 mg daily for 3 to 4 days beginning at the time of delivery. *Breast cancer:* 100 mg 3 times/week. *Testosterone enanthate and cypionate,* **IM only.** *Hypogonadism:* 50–400 mg q 2–4 weeks. *Delayed puberty:* 50–200 mg q 2–4 weeks. *Breast cancer in women:* 200–400 mg q 2–4 weeks.	Natural hormone and salts of natural hormone. Continue therapy for at least 2 months for satisfactory response and 5 months for objective response. Observe for priapism, virilization, hypercalcemia. Testosterone propionate is more effective than testosterone for parenteral injection because it is released more slowly. Priapism (persistent erection) may be a sign of overdosage.
Testosterone Cypionate in Oil (Andro-Cyp 100 and 200, Andronate 100 and 200, depo-Andro 100 and 200, Depo-Testosterone, Duratest-100 and -200, Testa-C, Testionate, Testoject L.A., T-Ionate P.A.), Rx			
Testosterone Enanthate (Android-T, Andro L.A. 200, Andryl 200, Anthatest, Delatestryl, Everone, Testone LA 100 and 200, Testrin PA, Testoject-E.P.), Rx			
Testosterone Propionate in Oil (Testex), Rx			

Drug Interactions

Interactant	Interaction
Insulin	Danazol ↑ insulin requirements
Warfarin	Danazol ↑ prothrombin time in warfarin-stabilized patients

Dosage   PO. *Endometriosis*: 400 mg b.i.d. for 3–6 months (up to 9 months may be required in some patients). Begin therapy during menses, if possible, to be sure patient is not pregnant. *Fibrocystic breast disease*: 100–400 mg/day in 2 divided doses. *Hereditary angioedema*: **Initial**, 200 mg b.i.d.–t.i.d.; after desired response, decrease dosage by 50% (or less) at 1–3-month intervals. Subsequent attacks can be treated by giving up to 200 mg/day.

Nursing Implications
1. *Assess*
   a. closely for signs of virilization, such as hirsutism, reduced breast size, deepening of voice, acne, increased oiliness of skin, weight gain, edema, and clitoral enlargement because some androgenic side effects may not be reversible and may necessitate change in dosage or discontinuance of drug.
   b. observe patients with epilepsy, migraine, or cardiac or renal dysfunction for edema because drug may cause fluid retention.
2. *Teach patient and/or family*
   a. to report signs of virilization noted above because physician may adjust dosage.
   b. that hypoestrogenic side effects usually disappear after drugs are discontinued.
   c. that ovulation will resume 60 to 90 days after drug is discontinued.

Chapter Sixty-six

POSTERIOR PITUITARY HORMONES AND RELATED DRUGS/GROWTH HORMONE

Posterior Pituitary Hormone

Antidiuretic Hormone and Analogs

Growth Hormone

   The two important hormones secreted by the posterior pituitary are oxytocin and vasopressin (ADH, antidiuretic hormone), each of which contain eight amino acids. Oxytocin is formed in the paraventricular nuclei of the hypothalamus while vasopressin is formed in the supraoptic nuclei. Once synthesized the hormones are carried by a protein, named neurophysin, down nerve endings to the posterior pituitary where they are stored.
   Oxytocin acts on the smooth muscle of the uterus and alveoli of the breast. Vasopressin controls reabsorption of water from the glomerular filtrate and increases blood pressure by causing contraction of the vascular bed and increased peripheral resistance (pressor effect).
   Except for posterior pituitary injection, which has oxytocic, vasopressor, and ADH activity, the drugs belonging to this group are used either for obstetric or antidiuretic purposes.

POSTERIOR PITUITARY HORMONE

POSTERIOR PITUITARY INJECTION   Pituitrin, Pituitrin-(S) (Rx)

Classification   Posterior pituitary hormone.

General Statement   The natural extract of the posterior pituitary has oxytocic, vasopressor, and antidiuretic hormone properties. The rapid pressor effect of this drug may make its use hazardous. Most physicians now use more refined agents with specific oxytocic or antidiuretic properties.

Uses   Postoperative ileus, to stimulate expulsion of gas prior to pyelography, to achieve hemostasis in presence of esophageal varices, adjunct in the treatment of shock, diabetes insipidus, uterine stimulation after complete expulsion of placenta. Enuresis of diabetes insipidus.

Contraindications   Toxemia of pregnancy, cardiac disease, hypertension, epilepsy, advanced arteriosclerosis, first stage of labor. Use with great caution at any stage of delivery.

Untoward Reactions   *Common*: Facial pallor, increased GI motility, uterine cramps. *Allergic:* Urticaria, angioneurotic edema, anaphylaxis. *Miscellaneous:* Tinnitus, anxiety, albuminuria, unconsciousness, eclamptic attacks, mydriasis, anaphylaxis, angioneurotic edema, urticaria.

Drug Interactions

Interactant	Interaction
Barbiturates	↑ Risk of coronary insufficiency and cardiac arrhythmias
Carbamazepine	↑ Antidiuretic effect of posterior pituitary hormones
Chlorpropamide	↑ Antidiuretic effect of posterior pituitary hormones
Clofibrate	↑ Antidiuretic effect of posterior pituitary hormones

Dosage   IM (preferred) and SC: 5–20 units (usual: 10 units). *Postpartum hemorrhage*: 10 units.

Nursing Implications

1. Assess closely for allergic reaction following administration of medication and have emergency supportive medications and oxygen readily available.
2. Monitor BP closely for $1/2$ hour following administration of medication, because it reduces cardiac output and may diminish coronary blood flow.
3. Consult with doctor about supplementation with another drug after primary use of posterior pituitary injection for control of postpartum hemorrhage since the posterior pituitary injection is short acting.

OXYTOCICS

General Statement The uterus consists mainly of two types of tissues: (1) the *endometrium* or mucous membrane lining the inner surface whose function is governed chiefly by the ovarian hormones, and (2) the *myometrium*, a thick wall of smooth muscle heavily interlaced with blood vessels. The latter are necessary to supply the placenta and fetus with oxygen and nutrients.

An understanding of the different stages of labor is essential for the judicious use of drugs in obstetrics. Premature use of any agent might be harmful to mother and child.

Labor is divided into 3 stages. Stage I is characterized by the onset of strong regular contractions of the myometrium and complete dilatation of the cervix. Stage II begins with the complete dilatation of the cervix and ends with the delivery of the baby. Stage III begins after delivery, involves placental separation, and terminates with birth of the placenta.

Immediately after delivery, the smooth muscles of the uterus are completely relaxed (uterine atony), and during this time the patient may bleed heavily. This period of smooth muscle relaxation is followed by renewed contractions, which produce placental separation and also clamp shut the countless blood vessels exposed when the placenta separates from the uterus. The average amount of blood lost during this stage is 200–300 ml.

The drugs discussed in this section assist the uterus during the various stages of labor. The oxytocic drugs, like oxytocin and ergotamine, promote contraction.

Oxytocic agents are used occasionally to induce labor and to promote incomplete abortions.

As a rule, oxytocic agents are not used during the first or second stage of labor. The premature use of oxytocic agents may cause severe laceration and trauma to the mother (rupture of the uterus), and trauma—even death—to the infant.

Action/Kinetics Oxytocics cause contraction of uterine musculature by combining with specific receptors in the myometrium. Although the exact mechanism is not known, it may involve calcium, prostaglandins, and cyclic AMP. Uterine sensitivity to oxytocics increases gradually during gestation with a sharp increase in sensitivity just before parturition. Oxytocics also cause contraction of the myoepithelium of the lacteal glands resulting in lactation.

Drug Interactions

Interactant	Interaction
Anesthetics, local	See vasoconstrictors
Cyclophosphamide	↑ Effect of oxytocics

Interactant	Interaction
Vasoconstrictors (e.g., in anesthetics)	May have synergistic and additive effectswith oxytocics. Concomitant use may result in severe, persistent hypertension and rupture of cerebral blood vessels

ERGONOVINE MALEATE   Ergotrate Maleate (Rx)

METHYLERGONOVINE MALEATE   Methergine (Rx)

Classification   Oxytocic agent.

Action/Kinetics   Ergonovine is a natural alkaloid obtained from ergot (a fungus that grows on rye) while methylergonovine is a closely related synthetic drug. These drugs stimulate the rate, tone, and amplitude of uterine contractions. Ergonovine maleate also stimulates smooth muscle surrounding certain blood vessels by interacting with adrenergic, dopaminergic, and tryptaminergic receptors. *Ergonovine.* **Onset** (uterine contractions): **PO**, 5–15 min; **IM**, 7–8 min; **IV**, immediate. **Duration: PO, IM**, 3 or more hr; **IV**, 45 min. *Methylergonovine.* **Onset** (uterine contractions): **PO**, 5–10 min; **IM**, 2–5 min; **IV:** immediate.

Uses   Management and prevention of postpartum and postabortal hemorrhage by producing firm uterine contractions and decreasing uterine bleeding. Migraine headaches. *Investigational:* Ergonovine has been used to diagnose Prinzmetal's angina (variant angina).

Contraindications   Pregnancy. Should be given with caution in sepsis, obliterative vascular disease, impaired renal or hepatic function. To induce labor or threatened spontaneous abortions. Toxemia, hypertension. Ergot hypersensitivity.

Untoward Reactions   *Ergonovine. GI:* Nausea, vomiting, diarrhea. *Miscellaneous:* Allergic reactions, headache, increased blood pressure. *Ergotism:* In overdosage. Nausea, vomiting, diarrhea, changes in blood pressure, chest pain, hypercoagulability, numb and cold extremities, gangrene of fingers and toes, dyspnea, weak pulse, excitability to convulsions, delirium, hallucinations, death. Treatment is symptomatic and to decrease drug absorption. *Methylergonovine. GI:* Nausea, vomiting. *CNS:* Dizziness, headache, tinnitus. *Miscellaneous:* Sweating, tinnitus, chest pain, dyspnea, palpitations.

Note: Use of these agents during labor may result in uterine tetany with rupture, cervical and perineal lacerations, embolism of amniotic fluid as well as hypoxia and intracranial hemorrhage in the infant.

Dosage   *Ergonovine.* **IM, IV (emergencies only):** 0.2 mg q 2–4 hr. **PO:** 0.2–0.4 mg q 6–12 hr for 48 hr or until danger of uterine atony has passed.

Note: Severe cramping is indicator of effectiveness. IV calcium salts may be required to enhance effectiveness in calcium-deficient patients. *Methylergonovine.* **IM, IV (emergencies only):** 0.2 mg q 2–4 hr following delivery of placenta, of the anterior shoulder, or during the puerperium. **PO:** 0.2 mg t.i.d.–q.i.d. for maximum of 1 week.

Administration/ Storage

1. Ergonovine ampules must be stored in a cold place. If kept in the delivery room, they must be discarded after 60 days due to loss of potency.

2. Discolored methylergonovine ampules should be discarded. Drug should be protected from heat and light during storage.
3. IV methylergonovine should be administered slowly over 1 min.

Nursing Implications
1. *Assess*
   a. height, consistency, and location of fundus of obstetric patient.
   b. lochia of postpartum patient.
   c. for severe cramping as this may suggest reduction in dose.
   d. for early signs of accidental ergotism: nausea, vomiting, cramps, diarrhea, drowsiness, dizziness, headache and confusion, as drug is a derivative of lysergic acid. GI and CNS effects may occur before circulatory disturbances to hand and feet.
2. Monitor vital signs for shock or hypertension after administration. Have appropriate drugs available.

OXYTOCIN, PARENTERAL   Pitocin, Syntocinon (Rx)

OXYTOCIN SYNTHETIC, NASAL   Syntocinon (Rx)

Classification   Oxytocic agent.

Action/Kinetics   These products are synthetic compounds identical to the natural hormone isolated from the posterior pituitary. Oxytocin has uterine stimulant, vasopressive, and antidiuretic properties. It acts by increasing the number of contracting myofibrils in the endometrium. **Onset:** Buccal, 30 min; **IM**, 3–7 min; **IV**, 1 min. **t½:** 1–6 min. Buccal absorption is erratic.

Uses   Induction or stimulation of labor at term. Used to overcome true primary or secondary uterine inertia. Induction of labor with oxytocin is only indicated under certain *specific* conditions and is not usual because serious toxic effects can occur. Oxytocin is indicated

1. for uterine inertia.
2. for induction of labor in cases of erythroblastosis fetalis, maternal diabetes mellitus, preeclampsia, and eclampsia.
3. for induction of labor after premature rupture of membranes in last month of pregnancy when labor fails to develop spontaneously within 12 hours.
4. for routine control of postpartum hemorrhage and uterine atony.
5. to hasten uterine involution.
6. to complete inevitable abortions after the 20th week of pregnancy.
7. intranasally for initial letdown of milk.
   Investigational: Breast engorgement, oxytocin challenge test for determining antepartum fetal heart fate.

Contraindications   Hypersensitivity to drug, cephalopelvic disproportion, malpresentation of the fetus, undilated cervix, overdistention of the uterus, hypotonic uterine contractions, and history of caesarean section, or other uterine surgery. Also, predisposition to thromboplastin and amniotic fluid embolism (dead fetus, abruptio placentae), history of previous traumatic deliveries, or patients with four or more deliveries. Oxytocin should never be given IV undiluted or in high concentrations. Oxytocin citrate is contraindicated in severe toxemia, cardiovascular or renal disease. Intranasal oxytocin is contraindicated in pregnancy.

Untoward Reactions   *Mother*: Tetanic uterine contractions, rupture of the uterus, hypertension, tachycardia, and electrocardiographic changes after IV administration of concentrated solutions. Also, rarely, anxiety, dyspnea, precordial pain, edema, cyanosis, or reddening of the skin, and cardiovascular spasm. Water intoxication from prolonged IV infusion, maternal deaths due to hypertensive episodes, subarachnoid hemorrhage, or uterine rupture.

Fetus: Death, premature ventricular contractions, bradycardia, tachycardia, hypoxia, intracranial hemorrhage due to overstimulation of the uterus during labor leads to uterine tetany with marked impairment of uteroplacental blood flow.

Remarks: Hypersensitivity reactions occur rarely. When they do, they occur most often with natural oxytocin administered IM or in concentrated IV doses and least frequently after IV infusion or diluted doses. Accidental swallowing of buccal tablets is not harmful.

Oxytocin citrate (see also *Oxytocin*): Nausea, vomiting, premature ventricular contractions, fetal cardiac arrhythmias, tetanic contractions of the uterus during induction of labor, and local vasoconstriction of the oral mucosa.

Drug Interactions   Severe hypertension and possible stroke when used with sympathomimetic pressor amines.

Dosage   *Induction or stimulation of labor*: **IV infusion**, dilute 10 units (1 ml) to 1,000 ml isotonic saline or 5% dextrose. **Initial**: 0.001–0.002 units/min (0.1–0.2 ml/min); dose can be gradually increased by 0.001 units/min (0.1 ml/min) to maximum of 0.02 units/min (2 ml/min). *Reduction of postpartum bleeding*: **IV infusion**, dilute 10–40 units (1–4 ml) to 1,000 ml with isotonic saline or 5% dextrose. Administer at a rate to control uterine atony. **IM**: 10 units after placental delivery. *As adjunct to prostaglandin or hypertonic abortifacient*: **IV infusion**, dilute 10 units (1 ml) to 500 ml with isotonic saline or 5% dextrose. Infuse at rate 20–40 drops/min. **Synthetic, nasal** (*for milk letdown*): one spray into one or both nostrils 2–3 min before nursing or pumping breasts.

Administration
1. *IV*: Use Y-tubing system, with one bottle containing IV solution and oxytocin and another containing only IV solution. In this manner, the drug can be discontinued, but patency of the vein can be maintained when the switch to the drug-free infusion bottle is made. Use electric infusion pump when possible to regulate flow for induction or stimulation of labor.
2. *Nasal spray*: Sit patient upright and hold bottle upright. Apply gentle pressure while spraying medication into nostril.
3. The nasal spray may be administered in drop form by applying gentle pressure to bottle.

Nursing Implications
(For Induction, Stimulation of Labor and/or Oxytocin Challenge Test)

1. Ascertain that physician is always readily available during administration.
2. Remain with the patient. During induction or stimulation of labor, patient must be attended by trained personnel.

(continued)

3. *Assess*
   a. resting uterine tone and uterine contractions for frequency, length, and strength.
   b. fetal heart rate and rhythm.
4. Prevent uterine rupture and fetal damage by clamping off IV oxytocin, starting medication-free IV fluids, providing oxygen, and notifying the doctor when the following occur:
   a. contractions occurring more frequently than every 2 minutes and lasting longer than 60 seconds with absence of a period of uterine relaxation between contractions.
   b. contractions that are excessively strong and/or exceed 50 mm Hg, as measured on either an external monitor or an internal uterine catheter with electronic monitor.
   c. fetal heart rate indicating bradycardia, tachycardia, or irregularities of rhythm, as measured by fetuscope, Dopptone, or other type of electric monitor.
5. Assess for water intoxication following prolonged administration of oxytocin characterized by lethargy, confusion, stupor, and coma. Neuromuscular hyperexcitability with increased relexes, muscular twitching, and convulsions may occur if water intoxication is acute. Monitor intake and output.
6. Assess vital signs at least hourly.

Nursing Implications
(During the Fourth Stage of Labor When Oxytocin Is Administered for Prevention or Control of Hemorrhage)

1. *Assess*
   a. location, size, and firmness of uterus. Report displaced or boggy uterus and follow protocol of hospital.
   b. lochia for amount and color. Report bright red lochia, excessive bleeding, and/or passage of clots of blood.
   c. vital signs until stabilized.
   d. for water intoxication characterized by lethargy, stupor, and coma. Neuromuscular hyperexcitability, with increased reflexes, muscular twitching, and convulsions may occur following prolonged administration. Monitor I & O.

ANTIDIURETIC HORMONE AND ANALOGS

Vasopressin, the antidiuretic hormone, controls the reabsorption of water from the glomerular filtrate. Its deficiency causes diabetes insipidus or polyuria.

Patients suffering from a mild form of the disease can be treated by intranasal application of suitable substances (desmopressin, lypressin), whereas patients with severe disease may require systemic treatment with posterior pituitary injection, vasopressin, or vasopressin tannate.

Treatment requires individual dosage adjustment. Overdosage may cause fluid retention and hypernatremia. Another common adverse reaction is contraction of the smooth muscles of the intestine, uterus, and blood vessels. Animal proteins that may be present in the extracts of the pituitary glands may result in allergic reactions. Thus, synthetic preparations are preferred.

DESMOPRESSIN ACETATE   DDAVP, Stimate (Rx)

Classification   Antidiuretic hormone, synthetic.

Action/Kinetics   Desmopressin is a synthetic antidiuretic devoid of vasopressor and oxytocic effects. **Onset:** 1 hr. **Peak:** 1–5 hr. **Duration:** 8–20 hr. **t½:** initial, 8 min; final: 75 min. Effect ceases abruptly. It also increases factor VIII levels (**onset:** 30 min min; **peak:** 1½–2 hr).

Uses   *Parenteral:* Neurogenic diabetes insipidus, hemophilia A with factor VIII levels more than 5%, Type I von Willebrand's disease with factor VIII levels greater than 5%. *Intranasal:* Diabetes insipidus.

Contraindications   Hypersensitivity to drug. Children under 3 months for hemophilia A or von Willebrand's disease. Parenteral desmopressin for diabetes insipidus in children under 12 years and intranasal in children less than 3 months. Safety in pregnancy and lactation not established.

Untoward Reactions   Rare. High doses may cause dose-dependent transient headaches, nausea, nasal congestion, rhinitis, flushing, mild abdominal cramps and vulval pain. Side effects can be reduced by a reduction in dosage.

Drug Interaction   Chlorpropamide, clofibrate, and carbamazepine may potentiate the effects of desmopressin.

Dosage   *Diabetes insipidus.* **SC, direct IV: Adults, usual,** 0.5–1 ml/day in 2 doses. Then, adjust dosage depending on response. **Intranasal: Adults,** 0.1–0.4 ml/day in one or more doses depending on diurnal rhythm of water turnover. **Pediatric, 3 months–12 years:** 0.05–0.3 ml/day in one or more doses. *Hemophilia A, von Willebrand's disease.* **IV, Adults and children weighing more than 10 kg:** 0.3 µg/kg diluted in 50 ml physiologic saline; **children weighing less than 10 kg:** 0.3 µg/kg diluted in 10 ml saline. Administer slowly over 15–30 min.

Administration/ Storage

1. Refrigerate solution and injection at 4°C (39.2°F).
2. Note carefully the three graduation marks on the soft flexible plastic nasal tube: 0.2, 0.1, and 0.05 ml. The 0.05 is not designated by number.
3. Cleanse and dry tube appropriately.
4. Measure dosage exactly because drug is very potent.
5. When used for hemophilia A or von Willebrand's disease, tachyphylaxis may occur if used more frequently than every 2 days.

Nursing Implications

1. Assess for early signs of water intoxication, such as drowsiness, headache, and vomiting.
2. Anticipate that fluid intake should be adjusted to avoid water intoxication and hyponatremia, especially in the very young and very old.
3. Anticipate that excessive fluid retention may be treated with a saluretic such as furosemide to induce diuresis.

(continued)

4. Monitor duration of sleep and daily I & O because these parameters are used to estimate response.
5. *Teach patient and/or family*
    a. administration technique.
    b. to report to doctor if drowsiness, listlessness, headache, shortness of breath, heartburn, nausea, abdominal cramps, vulval pain, or severe nasal congestion and/or irritation occurs.
    c. recommendations for fluid intake.
    d. how to monitor I & O.

LYPRESSIN   Diapid (Rx)

Classification   Antidiuretic hormone, synthetic.

Action/Kinetics   Lypressin is a synthetic antidiuretic, similar to vasopressin, for intranasal use only. It has minimal vasopressor or oxytocic effects. **Onset:** immediate. **Peak:** 30–60 min. **Duration:** 3–8 hr. t½: 15 min. The drug is metabolized in the kidney and liver; excreted in urine.

Uses   Diabetes insipidus of neurohypophyseal origin. Particularly suitable for patients allergic or refractory to vasopressin of animal origin.

Untoward Reactions   *Nasal:* Congestion, pruritus, irritation, or ulceration of nasal passages. Rhinorrhea. *GI:* Increased bowel movements, abdominal cramps. *Miscellaneous:* Periorbital edema with itching. Fluid retention (overdose). Heartburn (due to dripping into pharynx). Headache, conjunctivitis, hypersensitivity. Inhalation has resulted in coughing, transient dyspnea, substernal tightness.

Drug Interaction   Chlorpropamide, clofibrate, or carbamazepine may potentiate the effects of lypressin.

Dosage   **Topical (intranasal), adults and children**: 1 (2 USP units) or more sprays 3 to 4 times daily. Two or three sprays in each nostril is maximum that can be absorbed at any one time. (Each spray contains approximately 7 μg lypressin.)

Administration
1. Encourage the patient to clear nasal passage before use.
2. Hold the bottle upright and insert the nozzle into the patient's nostril with the head in a vertical position.
3. Apply gentle pressure to bottle while spraying medication into nostril.

Nursing Implications
1. *Assess*
    a. for dehydration by checking turgor of skin, condition of mucous membranes, and presence of thirst.
    b. for early signs of water intoxication, such as drowsiness, headache, and vomiting.
2. *Teach patient and/or family*
    a. administration technique.

 b. not to increase the number of sprays at one time, but rather to check with the physician if more frequent administration is needed. Usually the frequency of administration is increased, rather than the number of sprays at one time.

 c. to report to doctor if drowsiness, listlessness, headache, shortness of breath, heartburn, nausea, abdominal cramps, vulval pain, or severe nasal congestion or irritation occur.

 d. recommendations for fluid intake.

 e. how to monitor I & O.

VASOPRESSIN Pitressin Synthetic (Rx)

VASOPRESSIN TANNATE INJECTION Pitressin Tannate in Oil (Rx)

Classification Pituitary (antidiuretic) hormone.

Action/Kinetics The antidiuretic hormone ADH, more often referred to as vaso-pressin, is released from the anterior pituitary gland. The hormone regulates water conservation by promoting reabsorption of water by the distal portion of the renal tubules.

 Insufficient output of ADH results in neurohypophyseal diabetes insipidus, characterized by the excretion of large quantities of normal but very dilute urine and excessive thirst. These symptoms result from primary (no organic lesion) or secondary (injury) malfunction of posterior pituitary. Vasopressin is effective in the treatment of the condition. It is ineffective when the diabetes insipidus is of renal origin (nephrogenic diabetes insipidus).

 In addition to its diuretic properties, vasopressin also causes vasoconstriction (pressor effect) and increases the smooth muscular activity of the bladder, GI tract, and uterus. *Vasopressin*. **IM, SC: Onset**, variable; **duration**, 2–8 hr. t½: 10–20 min. **Effective plasma levels**: 4.5–6 microunits. *Vasopressin tannate*. **Duration**: 24–96 hr. Hormone metabolized by the liver and kidney.

Use Vasopressin: Neurogenic diabetes insipidus, relief of postoperative intestinal gaseous distention, to dispel gas shadows in abdominal roentgenography. *Investigational:* Bleeding esophageal varices. **Vasopressin tannate:** Neurogenic diabetes insipidus.

Contraindications Vascular disease, especially when involving coronary arteries; angina pectoris. Chronic nephritis until reasonable blood nitrogen levels are attained. Caution in presence of asthma, epilepsy, migraine, and congestive heart failure. Never give the tannate IV.

Untoward Reactions *GI:* Nausea, vomiting, increased intestinal activity (e.g., belching, cramps, urge to defecate), flatus. *Miscellaneous:* Facial pallor, tremor, sweating, allergic reactions, vertigo, bronchoconstriction, anaphylaxis, "pounding" in head, water intoxication (drowsiness, headache, coma, convulsions).

 IV use of vasopressin may result in severe vasoconstriction; local tissue necrosis if extravasation occurs. IM use of tannate may cause pain and sterile abscesses at site of injection.

Drug Interactions Carbamazepine, chlorpropamide, or clofibrate may ↑ antidiuretic effects of vasopressin.

Dosage   **Vasopressin.** *Diabetes insipidus.* **IM, SC:** 5–10 units b.i.d.–t.i.d. **Intranasal:** Individualize. *Abdominal distention.* **IM: Adults, initial,** 5 units; **then,** 10 units q 3–4 hr; **pediatric:** 2.5–5 units. *Abdominal roentgenography.* **IM, SC:** 2 injections of 10 units each 2 hr and ½ hr before films exposed.

   Vasopressin tannate: IM only, 0.3–1 ml administered as needed.

Administration

1. Administer intranasally using cotton pledgets, spray, or dropper.
2. Administration of 1–2 glasses of water prior to use for diabetes insipidus will reduce side effects as nausea, cramps, blanching of skin.
3. Shake vial of vasopressin tannate in oil before withdrawing dose.

Nursing Implications

1. *Assess*
   a. I & O to aid in evaluation of response to drug.
   b. for dehydration by checking turgor of skin, condition of mucous membranes, and presence of thirst.
   c. for increased continence and decreased urinary frequency after drug is administered to improve bladder activity.
   d. for bowel sounds, passage of flatus, and resumption of bowel movements after drug is administered to improve peristalsis in the GI tract.
   e. BP at least 2 times daily while the patient is on a regimen of vasopressin, and report untoward reactions, such as an excessive elevation of BP or lack of response to drug as characterized by lowering of BP.

GROWTH HORMONE

SOMATROPIN (SOMATOTROPIN)   Asellacrin, Crescormon (Rx)

Classification   Pituitary growth hormone.

Action/Kinetics   Somatotropin is extracted from human pituitary glands. It is an anabolic agent that stimulates intracellular transport of amino acids and retention of nitrogen, phosphorus, and potassium. It also stimulates linear growth. The hormone stimulates both intestinal absorption and urinary excretion of calcium. The hormone also inhibits intracellular glucose metabolism, and decreases the response to insulin. Other effects of this hormone include increased serum levels of phosphorus and alkaline phosphatase, increased synthesis of chondroitin sulfate and collagen, stimulation of intracellular lipolysis and fatty acid oxidation, and stimulation of urinary excretion of hydroxyproline.

   Patients who fail to respond to somatotropin should be tested for somatotropin antibodies. During therapy the bone age should be monitored annually, especially in pubertal patients or those who receive concurrent thyroid hormone or androgen therapy.

Uses   Linear growth failure due to deficiency of pituitary growth hormone ascertained by failure of the latter to increase to above 5 to 7 ng/ml after administration of two of the following stimuli: hypoglycemia, arginine (IV), levodopa (PO), glucagon (IM).

Contraindications Closed epiphyses. Use with caution in patients with diabetes or family history thereof, or intracranial lesions.

Untoward Reactions Few. Antibodies to somatotropin, which interfere with treatment in 5% of the cases, pain at injection site. SC use may result in local lipoatrophy or lipodystrophy. These increase the likelihood of the production of antibodies to somatotropin. Hypothyroidism, hyperglycemia, ketosis. SC use may result in lipoatrophy or lipodystrophy.

Drug Interactions Glucocorticoid therapy inhibits the effect of somatropin.

Dosage **IM, SC**: Miniumum of 2–5 IU 3 times/week at minimum intervals of 48 hr. If growth rate is less than 2.5 cm during any 6-month period, dose may be doubled for the next 6 months. If there is still no response, therapy should be discontinued and re-evaluated.

Administration/Storage

1. Administer IM or SC (Asellacrin only) and rotate injection sites.
2. Unreconstituted vials may be stored at room temperature. Store reconstituted vials in refrigerator and use within 1 month.
3. Reconstitute with bacteriostatic water for injection.
4. Therapy should be ceased if satisfactory height has been reached, when the patients fails to respond to therapy, and when epiphyseal closure has occured.

Nursing Implications

1. Measure height monthly.
2. Withhold drug and check with medical supervision if concomitant glucocorticoid therapy is ordered because steroids tend to inhibit response to somatotropin.
3. Check with medical supervision for frequency of glycosuria determinations.
4. Assess diabetic patients and those with family history thereof for symptoms of hyperglycemia and acidosis.

Part Eleven

AGENTS AFFECTING WATER AND ELECTROLYTES

Chapter Sixty-seven

DIURETICS

Thiazides and Related Diuretics

General Statement   The kidney is a complex organ with three main functions:

1. Elimination of waste materials and return of useful metabolites to the blood.
2. Maintenance of the acid-base balance.
3. Maintenance of an adequate electrolyte balance, which in turn governs the amount of fluid retained in the body.

Malfunction of one or more of these regulatory processes may result in the retention of excessive fluid by various tissues (edema). The latter can be an important manifestation of many conditions, for example, congestive heart failure, pregnancy, and premenstrual tension.

Action   Diuretic drugs increase the urinary output of water and sodium (prevention or correction of edema) mostly through one of the following mechanisms:

1. Increasing the glomerular filtration rate.
2. Decreasing the rate at which sodium is reabsorbed from the glomerular filtrate by the renal tubules.
3. Promoting the excretion of sodium by the kidney.

Some of the commonly used diuretics, especially the thiazides, also have an antihypertensive effect. Diuretic drugs can enhance the normal function of the kidney but cannot stimulate a failing kidney into action. According to their mode of action and chemical structure, the diuretics fall into the following classes: the thiazides (benzothiadiazines); the carbonic anhydrase inhibitors (used mainly for glaucoma); the organic mercurial diuretics; osmotic diuretics; loop diuretics, and potassium-sparing drugs.

Uses   Edema, congestive heart failure, hypertension, pregnancy, and premenstrual tension.

Nursing Implications

1. Administer in the morning if drug is to be given daily so that the patient will have major diuretic effect before bedtime.
2. Dilute liquid potassium preparations with fruit juice or milk to make them more palatable, because they are bitter.
3. Have bedpan or commode readily available for the patient. Patients who are usually ambulatory may feel weak because of diuresis and may require bedpans. Use safety measures for patients affected by ataxia, confusion, or disorientation. Support ambulatory ataxic patients.
4. *Assess*
   a. weight each morning under standard conditions, that is, after patient has voided and before patient has eaten or taken fluids.
   b. intake and output of fluids. Report absence of or decrease in diuresis.
   c. for edema: ambulatory patients may have edema of the lower extremities, whereas patients on bedrest are more likely to have edema of the sacral area. Measure for edema of the lower extremities 5 cm above the medial malleolus and at the level of the umbilicus for ascites.
   d. *for signs of electrolyte imbalance*:
      (1) *Hyponatremia* (low-salt syndrome)—characterized by muscle weakness, leg cramps, dryness of mouth, dizziness, and GI disturbances.
      (2) *Hypernatremia* (excessive sodium retention in relation to body water)—characterized by CNS disturbances, such as confusion, loss of sensorium, stupor, and coma. Poor skin turgor or postural hypotension are not as prominent as when there are combined deficits of sodium and water.
      (3) *Water intoxication* (caused by defective water diuresis)—characterized by lethargy, confusion, stupor, and coma. Neuromuscular hyperexcitability with increased reflexes, muscular twitching, and convulsions may occur if water intoxication is acute.
      (4) *Metabolic acidosis* —characterized by weakness, headache, malaise, abdominal pain, nausea, and vomiting. Hyperpnea occurs in severe metabolic acidosis. Signs of volume depletion, such as poor skin turgor, soft eyeballs, and a dry tongue, may be observed.
      (5) *Metabolic alkalosis* —characterized by irritability, neuromuscular hyperexcitability, and in severe cases, tetany.
      (6) *Hypokalemia* (deficiency of potassium in blood)—characterized by muscular weakness, failure of peristalsis, postural hypotension, respiratory embarrassment, and cardiac arrhythmias.
      (7) *Hyperkalemia* (excess of potassium in blood)—characterized by early signs of irritability, nausea, intestinal colic and diarrhea; by later signs of weakness, flaccid paralysis, dyspnea, difficulty in speaking, and arrhythmias. Signs of electrolyte imbalance should be reported to the physician and physical safety for the patient should be provided.
   e. patients on enteric-coated potassium tablets for abdominal pain, distention, or GI bleeding because such tablets can cause small bowel ulceration. Discontinue tablets if such symptoms appear.
   f. patients also receiving antihypertensive drugs for excessively low blood pressure, as diuretics potentiate antihypertensive agents. Caution patients to rise slowly from bed and to sit down or lie down should they feel dizzy or faint.

(continued)

g. urine of diabetic patient and observe patients for signs of hyperglycemia since diuretics may precipitate symptoms of diabetes in latent or mild diabetic patients.

h. apical pulse of patient also receiving digitalis, as hyper- or hypokalemia associated with diuretic therapy may potentiate toxic effects of digitalis and precipitate cardiac arrhythmias.

i. for symptoms of sore throat, skin rash, or jaundice, which are signs of blood dyscrasias due to drug hypersensitivity.

j. patients with a history of liver disease for electrolyte imbalance, which may cause stupor, coma, and death.

k. for increased frequency of acute attacks of gout (pain in single joint) precipitated by diuretics in patients with history of the disease.

5. *Teach patient and/or family*

a. that drug may cause frequent urination in large amounts so that the patient may plan activities and not be alarmed by diuresis.

b. that patients for whom additional potassium intake is desirable should ingest foods high in potassium since this is preferable to potassium chloride tablets. Foods high in potassium are citrus, grape, cranberry, apple, pear, and apricot juices, bananas, meat, fish, fowl, cereals, and tea and cola beverages. Patients receiving diuretics and requiring potassium supplementation are encouraged to drink a large glass of orange juice daily unless it is contraindicated because of another preexisting condition such as diabetes or gastric ulcer.

c. to use caution in driving car or operating other hazardous machinery, because weakness and/or dizziness may occur with diuresis.

THIAZIDES AND RELATED DIURETICS

General Statement　The thiazide diuretics are related chemically to the sulfonamides. They are devoid of anti-infective activity but can cause the same hypersensitivity reactions as the sulfonamides. In addition to their diuretic effect, they exert some antihypertensive activity. The drugs can be used for patients with some degree of kidney impairment. They must, however, be used with caution because they can aggravate renal insufficiency. The thiazides potentiate several antihypertensive agents, especially the rauwolfia alkaloids (See Chapter 26).

The thiazides are apt to induce electrolyte imbalance, especially hypokalemia, which can cause cardiac arrhythmias and render the heart more sensitive to the toxic effects of digitalis. Salt intake is usually not restricted, and potassium supplementation (nutritional or otherwise) may be indicated. Patients resistant to one type of thiazide may respond to another.

Action/Kinetics　The thiazides and related diuretics promote diuresis by decreasing the rate at which sodium and chloride are reabsorbed by the distal renal tubules of the kidney. By increasing the excretion of sodium and chloride, they force excretion of additional water. They also increase the excretion of potassium and, to a lesser extent, bicarbonate. Sodium and chloride are excreted in approximately equal amounts. The thiazides do not affect the glomerular filtration rate.

The antihypertensive mechanism of action of the thiazides is attributed to a direct dilation of the arterioles, as well as to a reduction in the total fluid volume of the body. *Diuretic effect*: Usual, **Onset**: 1–2 hr. **Peak**: 4–6 hr. **Duration**: 6–24 hr. *Antihypertensive effect*: **Onset**: several days. *Optimal therapeutic effect*: 3–4 weeks.

Most thiazides are absorbed from GI tract; a large fraction is excreted unchanged in urine.

Additional Uses   Edema due to congestive heart failure, nephrosis, nephritis, renal failure, premenstrual syndrome, hepatic cirrhosis, corticosteroid therapy. Hypertension. *Investigational:* Alone or in combination with allopurinol (or amiloride) for prophylaxis of calcium nephrolithiasis. Nephrogenic diabetes insipidus.

Contraindications   Hypersensitivity to drug. Impaired renal function and advanced hepatic cirrhosis. Administer with caution to debilitated or elderly patients, or to those with a history of hepatic coma, or precoma, gout, diabetes mellitus, during pregnancy and lactation.

Drugs should not be used indiscriminately in patients with edema and toxemia of pregnancy even though they may be therapeutically useful because the thiazides may have adverse effects on newborn (thrombocytopenia and jaundice).

Thiazides and related diuretics may precipitate myocardial infarctions in elderly patients with advanced arteriosclerosis, especially if patient is also receiving therapy with other antihypertensive agents.

Patients with advanced heart failure, renal disease, or hepatic cirrhosis are most likely to develop hypokalemia.

Particular care must be exercised when thiazides are administered concomitantly with drugs that also cause potassium loss, such as digitalis, corticosteroids, and some estrogens.

Thiazides may activate or worsen systemic lupus erythematosus.

Untoward Reactions   *Electrolyte imbalance:* Hypokalemia (most frequent) characterized by cardiac arrhythmias. Hyponatremia characterized by weakness, lethargy, epigastric distress, nausea, vomiting. Hypokalemic alkalosis. *GI:* Dry mouth, thirst, stomach pain or upset, sore throat, diarrhea, anorexia. *CNS:* Mood changes, tiredness, fever, dizziness. *CV:* Irregular heart rate, orthostatic hypotension. *Allergic:* Skin rashes, urticaria, photosensitivity. *Hematologic:* Agranulocytosis, thrombocytopenia. *Endocrine:* Hyperglycemia, aggravation of preexisting diabetes mellitus, hyperuricemia. *GU:* Renal colic, hematuria, crystalluria. *Miscellaneous:* Muscle cramps, impaired liver function, necrotizing vasculitis of skin and kidney, pancreatitis, jaundice, hepatic coma.

Drug Interactions

Interactant	Interaction
Anticholinergic agents	↑ Effect of thiazides due to ↑ amount absorbed from GI tract
Anticoagulants, oral	↓ Effect of anticoagulants by concentrating circulating clotting factors and ↑ clotting factor synthesis in liver
Antidiabetic agents	Thiazides antagonize hypoglycemic effect of antidiabetic agents
Antihypertensive agents	Thiazides potentiate the effect of antihypertensive agents
Cholestyramine	↓ Effect of thiazide due to ↓ absorption from GI tract
Colestipol	↓ Effect of thiazide due to ↓ absorption from GI tract
Corticosteroids	Enhanced K loss due to K-losing properties of both drugs

Interactant	Interaction
Diazoxide	Enhanced hypotensive effect. Also, ↑ hyperglycemic response
Digitalis glycosides	Thiazides produce ↑ K and Mg loss with ↑ chance of digitalis toxicity
Ethanol	Additive orthostatic hypotension
Fenfluramine	↑ Antihypertensive effect of thiazides
Guanethidine	Additive hypotensive effect
Indomethacin	↓ Effect of thiazides possibly by inhibition of prostaglandin
Lithium	Increased risk of lithium toxicity due to ↓ renal excretion
Norepinephrine	Thiazides ↓ arterial response to norepinephrine
Quinidine	↑ Effect of quinidine due to ↑ renal tubular reabsorption
Reserpine	Additive hypotensive effect
Sulfonamides	↑ Effect of thiazides due to ↓ plasma protein binding
Tetracyclines	↑ Risk of azotemia
Tubocurarine	↑ Muscle relaxation and ↑ hypokalemia
Vasopressors (sympathomimetics)	Thiazides ↓ responsiveness of arterioles to vasopressors

Laboratory Test Interferences Alteration of potassium, other electrolytes, BUN, uric acid. False + or ↑ serum glucose (fasting) and amylase. ↓ Serum PBI levels (no signs of thyroid disturbance).

Dosage See Table 35, p. 795. Drugs are preferentially given **PO**, but some preparations can be given parenterally. They are usually given in the morning so the peak effect occurs during the day.

Additional Nursing Implications

See also *Nursing Implications* for *Diuretics*, p. 791.

1. Anticipate that thiazide will be stopped at least 48 hours before surgery, because drug inhibits pressor effect of epinephrine.
2. Evaluate dietary potassium intake since potassium chloride supplement should only be given when dietary measures are inadequate. Liquid potassium preparations should be used since these do not produce ulcerations as tablets may.
3. *Teach patient and/or family*
   a. not to ingest alcohol, since this causes severe hypotension with thiazides.
   b. that the patient should not eat licorice when on thiazide therapy, because severe hypokalemia and paralysis may be precipitated.
   c. to include foods high in potassium, such as orange juice and bananas.

TABLE 35   THIAZIDES AND RELATED DIURETICS

Drug	Dosage	Onset	Peak	Duration
Bendroflumethiazide (Naturetin), Rx	*Edema, hypertension,* **PO: initial,** 5 mg daily in AM, may be increased to 20 mg daily; **maintenance:** 2.5–15 mg daily, **Pediatric, initial,** 0.1 mg/kg daily in 1 or 2 doses; **maintenance:** 0.05–0.3 mg/kg daily in 1 or 2 doses.	1–2 hr	4–6 hr	6–12 hr; **t½:** Approximately 3.5 hr. Risk of electrolyte imbalance reduced by alternate day or 3–5 day/week dosage. Divide daily doses in excess of 20 mg.
Benzthiazide (Aquatag, Exna, Hydrex, Marazide, Proaqua), Rx	*Edema,* **PO: initial:** 50–200 mg daily; **maintenance:** 50–150 mg daily. Divide dose when daily dose exceeds 100 mg. **Pediatric, all cases:** 1–4 mg/kg daily in 3 doses. *Hypertension:* **initial:** 25–50 mg b.i.d. after breakfast and lunch; **maintenance:** according to patient response, up to 50 mg q.i.d.	2 hr	4–6 hr	6–12 hr
Chlorothiazide (Diachlor, Diuril, SK-Chlorothiazide), Rx Chlorothiazide sodium (Sodium Diuril), Rx	*Edema,* **PO:** 0.5–1 gm 1–2 times daily. **IV:** direct dissolve 500 mg in 18 ml isotonic solution b.i.d. Avoid extravasation of liquid into **SC** tissue. May be given **IV** in dextrose or NaCl solutions. *Hypertension:* **PO only:** 250 mg b.i.d.–500 mg q.i.d. **Pediatric:** 22 mg/kg daily in divided doses; infants under 6 months of age may require 33 mg/kg in 2 divided doses.	1–2 hr	4 hr	6–12 hr; **t½:** 1–2 hr. Incompletely absorbed from the GI tract. Produces a greater diuretic effect if given in divided doses. Also found in Diupres (Appendix 3).
Chlorthalidone (Apo-Chlorthalidone,* Hygroton, Hylidone, Novothalidone,* Thalitone, Uridon*), Rx	*Edema,* **PO: initial,** 50–100 mg daily or 100 mg 3 times/week. **Maximum daily dose:** 200 mg. **Pediatric:** all uses, 2 mg/kg 3 times weekly. *Hypertension:* **initial,** 25–50 mg once daily up to 100 mg daily (doses greater than 25 mg/day do not increase effectiveness but do increase K excretion); **maintenance:** usually lower than initial but determined by patient response.	2 hr	Within 2–6 hr	24–72 hr; **t½:** 46 hr. Give in AM with food. Particularly good for potentiation and reducing dosage of other anti-hypertensive agents. Also found in Regroton (Appendix 3).
Cyclothiazide (Anhydron, Fluidil), Rx	*Edema,* **Adults, PO: initial,** 1–2 mg once daily; **maintenance:** 1–2 mg q 2–3 days. *Hypertension:* **PO: usual,** 2 mg once daily (some may require 4–6 mg daily). **Pediatric, all uses:** 0.02–0.04 mg/kg/day. **Maximum effective dose:** 8 mg. Divide dose if daily dosage exceeds 8 mg.	slow: < 6 hr Give in AM.	7–12 hr	18–24 hr
Hydrochlorothiazide (Apo-Hydro,* Aquazide H, Chlorzide, Diaqua, Diuchlor H,* Diu-Scrip, Esidrex, Hydro-Chlor, Hydro-Diuril, Hydromal, Hydro-T, Hydro-Z-50, Mictrin,	**PO. Adults,** *Edema:* 25–100 mg daily (or as needed); some require up to 200 mg daily. *Hypertension:* **Adults, initial,** 50–100 mg/day; **maintenance;** 25–100 mg, up to 200 mg/day. **Pediatric, 2–12 years:** 18.75–50 mg b.i.d.; **6 mo–2 years:** 6.25–18.75 mg b.i.d.; **up to 6 mo:** 3.3 mg/kg/day in 2 doses.	2 hr	4–6 hr	6–12 hr; **t½:** Approximately 10 hr. Divide daily doses in excess of 100 mg. Give b.i.d. at 6–12 hr intervals. Also found in Aldactazide, Aldoril, Apresazide, Dyazide, Hydropres, and Ser-Ap-Es (Appendix 3).

TABLE 35 (*Continued*)

Drug	Dosage	Remarks		
		Onset	Peak	Duration
Natrimax,* Neo-Codema,* Novohydrazide,* Oretic, SK-Hydrochlorothiazide, Thiuretic, Urozide,* Zide), Rx	**PO:** *Edema:* **initial,** 50 mg 1–2 times/day; **maintenance:** 25–200 mg, depending on response (divide dosage if over 100 mg daily). *Hypertension:* **initial,** 50 mg b.i.d.; **maintenance:** 50–100 mg daily not to exceed 200 mg/day.	1–2 hr	3–4 hr	6–12 hr
Hydroflumethiazide (Diucardin, Saluron), Rx				
Indapamide (Lozol), Rx	**PO.** *Edema, hypertension.* **Adults:** 2.5 mg in the AM. If necessary, may be increased to 5 mg daily.	1–2 hr t½: 14 hr.	2 hr	Up to 36 hr
Methyclothiazide (Aquatensen, Duretic,* Enduron, Ethon), Rx	*Edema, hypertension,* **PO:** 2.5–10 mg daily initially; **maintenance:** 2.5–5 mg once daily. **Pediatric, all uses:** 0.05–0.2 mg/kg daily.	2 hr	6 hr	24 hr

Drug	Dosage	Onset	Peak	Duration
Metolazone (Diulo, Zaroxylyn), Rx	Edema, PO: 5–20 mg once daily. Hypertension: 2.5–5 mg once daily. Reduce all doses if possible when patient has stabilized.	1 hr	2 hr	12–24 hr

t½: 8 hr.

Additional Contraindications

Prehepatic and hepatic coma. Use for children.

Additional Untoward Reactions

Bloating, palpitations, chest pain, chills.

Drug	Dosage	Onset	Peak	Duration
Polythiazide (Renese), Rx	Edema, hypertension, PO: 1–4 mg daily. Initial doses up to 12 mg daily in divided doses may be required. Pediatric, all uses: 0.02–0.08 mg/kg daily.	2 hr	6 hr	36 hr

t½: Approximately 24 hr.

Drug	Dosage	Onset	Peak	Duration
Quinethazone (Aquamox,* Hydromox), Rx	PO: 50–100 mg/day (some may require 150–200 mg/day); maintenance: adjust to patient response.	2 hr	6 hr	18–24 hr

Drug	Dosage	Onset	Peak	Duration
Trichloromethiazide (Aquazide, Metahydrin, Mono-Press, Naqua, Niazide, Trichlorex), Rx	Edema; PO: 1–4 mg daily, up to 16 mg may be required. Hypertension: 2–4 mg daily initial dose; maintenance: 2–4 mg daily. Pediatric, all cases: 0.07 mg/kg daily.	2 hr	6 hr	24 hr

Additional Uses

Edema associated with premenstrual tension and menopausal syndrome.

CARBONIC ANHYDRASE INHIBITOR DIURETICS

General Statement   The carbonic anhydrase inhibitor diuretics are related chemically to sulfonamides, but they are devoid of anti-infective activity. They may, however, cause the same hypersensitivity reactions as other sulfonamides. The carbonic anhydrase inhibitors promote the excretion of bicarbonate and sodium, which mandates excretion of additional fluid. The drugs also increase potassium excretion.

The usefulness of the drugs is limited, because they promote metabolic acidosis, which inhibits their diuretic action. This difficulty is partially circumvented by giving the drugs on alternate days or alternating them with other diuretics, especially the mercurial diuretics. The latter tend to become less active because of their self-induced alkalosis.

The carbonic anhydrase inhibitors are mild, safe diuretics. They are particularly useful in the treatment of glaucoma, as they reduce intraocular pressure, and in maintenance therapy, for mild drug-induced edema (corticosteroids) or water retention associated with menstruation, pregnancy, and certain chronic conditions.

Patients may respond to one carbonic anhydrase inhibitor and not to another. Failures in therapy may result from overdosage or from too frequent use.

Action/Kinetics   Inhibition of the enzyme carbonic anhydrase. In the eye, this results in decrease of secretion of aqueous humor by the ciliary body. In the kidney, this enzyme inhibition increases electrolyte excretion and, therefore, induces diuresis. The agents also have a mild antiepileptic activity.

Uses   Glaucoma (open-angle, secondary). Acetazolamide is used for edema due to congestive heart failure, edema due to drugs, and absence seizures. *Investigational:* Acetazolamide is used for prophylaxis of high altitude mountain sickness.

Contraindications   Idiopathic renal hyperchloremic acidosis, renal failure, hepatic insufficiency, and conditions associated with depressed sodium and potassium levels, such as Addison's disease and all other types of adrenal failure. Use with caution in the presence of mild acidosis, hepatic cirrhosis, advanced pulmonary disease, and pregnancy.

Untoward Reactions   *Electrolyte imbalance*: Metabolic acidosis characterized by nausea; dizziness; numbness of fingers, toes, and lips; fatigue; drowsiness; headache; dry mouth; irritability; diarrhea; tinnitus; disorientation; dysuria; ataxia; and weight loss. *Hypersensitivity*: Like other sulfonamides, drug can cause blood dyscrasias, skin rashes, and fever. Also crystalluria and renal calculi.

Untoward reactions may be dose related and are often relieved by decrease in dosage. Alternate day therapy or rest periods allow kidney to recover.

Drug Interactions

Interactant	Interaction
Amphetamine	↑ Effect of amphetamine by ↑ renal tubular reabsorption
Ephedrine	↑ Effect of ephedrine by ↑ renal tubular reabsorption
Lithium carbonate	↓ Effect of lithium by ↑ renal excretion
Methotrexate	↓ Effect of methotrexate due to ↑ renal excretion
Primidone	↓ Effect of primidone due to ↓ GI absorption
Pseudoephedrine	↑ Effect of pseudoephedrine by ↑ renal tubular reabsorption
Quinidine	↑ Effect of quinidine by ↑ renal tubular reabsorption
Salicylates	↓ Effect of salicylates by ↑ renal excretion

Dosage   See Table 36.

Administration

1. Because of the self-inhibitory metabolic acidosis produced by the carbonic anhydrase drugs, they are usually administered for 3 consecutive days each week or every other day. Since kidney recovery does not play a role, intermittent administration is not necessary when drugs are used for glaucoma or epilepsy.
2. Due to possible differences in bioavailability, brands should not be interchanged.
2. Take with food if GI upset occurs.

Additional Nursing Implication

See also *Nursing Implications* for *Diuretics*, p. 791.
   Caution the patient to maintain dosage and schedule prescribed by physician to maintain effectiveness of the drug and prevent metabolic acidosis.

Nursing Implications for Treatment of Glaucoma

1. Report if the patient complains of eye pain because drug may not be effective and intraocular pressure may be unrelieved or increasing.
2. Anticipate that carbonic anhydrase inhibitors should be administered at least once daily for treatment of glaucoma or epilepsy whereas in treatment of edema the drug is administered intermittently.

LOOP DIURETICS

BUMETANIDE   Bumex (Rx)

Classification   Loop diuretic.

Action/Kinetics   Bumetanide inhibits reabsorption of both sodium and chloride in the ascending loop of Henle. It may also have some activity in the proximal tubule especially to promote phosphate excretion. **Onset (PO):** 30–60 min. **Peak effect (PO):** 1–2 hr. **Duration (PO):** 4–6 hr (dose dependent). **Onset (IV):** Several minutes. **Peak effect (IV):** 15–30 min. **t½ (PO, IV):** 1–1.5 hr.

Uses   Edema associated with congestive heart failure, nephrotic syndrome, hepatic disease.

Contraindications   Anuria, heaptic coma, severe electrolyte depletion, hypersensitivity to the drug. Safety in pregnancy, lactation, and children under age 18 has not been established.

Untoward Reactions   *Electrolyte and fluid changes:* Excess water loss, dehydration, electrolyte depletion including hypokalemia, hypochloremia, hyponatremia; hypovolemia, thromboembolism, circulatory collapse. *Otic:* Hearing loss, ear discomfort, ototoxicity. *GI:* Nausea, abdominal pain, vomiting, dry mouth, diarrhea, gastric upset. *CNS:* Dizziness, headache, vertigo, fatigue. *Allergic:* Pruritus, urticaria, rashes. *Miscellaneous:* Hypotension, encephalopathy, hyperglycemia, ECG

TABLE 36 CARBONIC ANHYDRASE INHIBITORS

Drug	Uses	Dosage	Remarks			
			Onset	Peak	Duration	
Acetazolamide (Acetazolam,* Ak-Zol, Apo-Acetazolamide,* Dazamide, Diamox), Rx	Edema, epilepsy, glaucoma, congestive heart failure	**PO, IV, IM.** *Edema:* 250–375 mg daily for 1–2 days followed by a 1 day rest period. *Epilepsy:* Usual, 0.372–1 gm daily (if used with other anticonvulsants, initial dose is 0.25 gm once daily). *Glaucoma, simple open angle:* 0.25–1 gm daily in divided doses. *Glaucoma, closed angle prior to surgery or secondary:* 0.25 gm q 4 hr, 0.25 gm b.i.d., or 0.5 gm followed by 0.125–0.25 gm q 4 hr. May be given IV for rapid relief.	**Tablets** 60–90 min **Sustained release capsules** 2 hr **Injection (IV)** 2 min	2–4 hr 8–12 15 min	8–12 hr 18–24 hr 4–5 hr	1. Tolerance after prolonged use may necessitate dosage increase. 2. Solutions diluted for IV use should be used within 24 hrs. 3. **IV** route preferred to **IM** because of alkalinity of solution. 4. Sustained release should not be used for seizures.
Acetazolamide Sodium (Diamox), Rx						
Dichlorphenamide (Daranid), Rx	Glaucoma	**PO, priming dose, adults:** 100–200 mg followed by 100 mg q 12 hr until desired response manifested. **Maintenance, adults:** 25–50 mg 1 to 3 times/day.	3 hr	2–4 hr	6–12 hr	
Methazolamide (Neptazane), Rx	Glaucoma	**PO:** 50–100 mg b.i.d. or t.i.d. Used with miotic or osmotic agents.	2–4 hr	6–8 hr	10–18 hr	

changes, weakness, joint and muscle pain, chest pain, sweating, hyperventilation, renal failure, premature ejaculation, difficulty in maintaining an erection.
Cross-sensitivity may be seen in patients allergic to sulfonamides.

Drug Interactions

Interactant	Interaction
Aminoglycosides	Additive ototoxicity
Antihypertensive drugs	Potentiation of antihypertensive effect
Digitalis glycosides	Bumetanide produces excess K loss with ↑ chance of cardiac arrhythmias
Indomethacin	↓ Effect of bumetanide
Lithium	↑ Risk lithium toxicity due to ↓ renal excretion
Probenecid	↓ Effect of bumetanide

Laboratory Test Interferences Alterations in LDH, SGOT, SGPT, alkaline phosphatase, creatinine clearance, total serum bilirubin, serum proteins.

Dosage **PO:** 0.5–2 mg once daily; if response inadequate, a second or third dose may be given at 4–5 hr intervals up to a maximum of 10 mg daily. **IV, IM:** 0.5–1 mg; if response inadequate, a second or third dose may be given at 4–5 hr intervals up to a maximum of 10 mg daily. Oral dosing should be started as soon as possible.

Administration

1. IV doses should be given slowly over 1–2 minutes.
2. The recommended oral dosing schedule is on alternate days or for 3–4 days with a 1–2 day rest period in between.
3. In patients allergic to furosemide, bumetanide may be substituted at a 1:40 ratio of bumetanide to furosemide.
4. Solutions for IM or IV use should be prepared fresh and used within 24 hours.
5. Ampuls may be reconstituted with 5% dextrose in water, 0.9% sodium chloride, or lactated Ringer's solution.

Nursing Implications

Assess

a. blood pressure and pulse regularly because a rapid diuresis may cause dehydration and circulatory collapse. Hypotension may also occur when drug is administered with antihypertensive drugs.
b. for ototoxicity, especially if patient is receiving other ototoxic drugs.

ETHACRYNIC ACID   Edecrin (Rx)

ETHACRYNATE SODIUM   Sodium Edecrin (Rx)

Classification Loop diuretic.

Action/Kinetics Ethacrynic acid inhibits the reabsorption of sodium and chloride by the renal tubule (mainly by acting on ascending loop of Henle). Large quantities of sodium and chloride and smaller amounts of potassium and bicarbonate ion are excreted during the diuresis. **Onset: PO**, 30 min; **IV**, 5–15 min. **Peak: PO**, 2 hr; **IV**; 30 min. **Duration: PO**, 6–8 hr. **IV**, 2 hr.

Diuresis and electrolyte loss are more pronounced with ethacrynic acid than with thiazide diuretics. Ethyacrynic acid is ofen effective in patients refractory to other diuretics. Careful monitoring of the diuretic effects is necessary.

Uses Of value in patients resistant to less potent diuretics. Congestive heart failure, pulmonary edema, edema associated with nephrotic syndrome, ascites due to idiopathic edema, lymphedema, malignancy. Short-term use in pediatric patients with nephrotic syndrome or congenital heart disease. *Investigational.* **Ethacrynic acid:** Nephrogenic diabetes insipidus unresponsive to vasopressin; **Ethacrynate sodium:** Hypercalcemia, bromide intoxication, and with mannitol in ethylene glycol poisoning.

Contraindications Anuria and severe renal damage. Patients with history of gout should be watched closely. To be used with caution in diabetic subjects and also in patients with hepatic cirrhosis. The latter are particularly susceptible to electrolyte imbalance.

Untoward Reactions Electrolyte imbalance (hypokalemia). The drug may also cause dehydration, reduction in blood volume, vascular complications, tetany, and metabolic alkalosis. *GI* (frequent): Anorexia, nausea, diarrhea, vomiting, acute pancreatitis, jaundice. Severe, watery diarrhea is an indication for permanent discontinuance of drug. GI bleeding, especially in patients on IV therapy or receiving heparin concomitantly. *CNS*: Tinnitus, hearing loss (permanent), vertigo, headache, blurred vision, apprehension, confusion, fatigue. *Hematologic*: Agranulocytosis, thrombocytopenia, neutropenia. *Miscellaneous*: Skin rashes, abnormal liver function tests in seriously ill patients, fever, chills, hematuria. Ethacrynic acid increases uric acid levels and may precipitate attacks of gout. The drug may also produce changes in glucose metabolism (hyperglycemia and glycosuria).

Drug Interactions

Interactant	Interaction
Alcohol	↑ Orthostatic hypotension
Aminoglycoside antibiotics	Additive ototoxicity and nephrotoxicity
Anticoagulants, oral	↑ Effect of anticoagulants by ↓ plasma protein binding
Antidiabetic agents	Ethacrynic acid antagonizes hypoglycemic effect of antidiabetics
Antihypertensive agents	↑ Antihypertensive effect
Barbiturates	↑ Orthostatic hypotension
Cephaloridine	↑ Risk of ototoxicity and nephrotoxicity
Cisplatin	↑ Risk of ototoxicity
Corticosteroids	Enhanced K loss due to K-losing properties of both drugs
Digitalis glycosides	Ethacrynic acid produces excess K and Mg loss with ↑ chance of cardiac arrhythmias
Furosemide	Combination may result in hypokalemia, tachycardia, deafness, hypotension—**do not use together**
Lithium	↑ Risk of lithium toxicity due to ↓ renal clearance
Narcotics	↑ Orthostatic hypotension

Interactant	Interaction
Skeletal muscle relaxants, nondepolarizing	↑ Muscle relaxation
Warfarin	↑ Effect of warfarin due to ↓ plasma protein binding

Dosage *Ethacrynic acid* is administered **PO**; *sodium ethacrynate* is given **IV**. Because of local pain or irritation, **the drug should not be given SC or IM.** *Individualized* according to response. **Typical PO regimen:** *day 1*: 50 mg; *day 2*: 50 mg b.i.d.; *day 3*: 100 mg AM, 50–100 mg PM. **Maximum daily dose:** 400 mg. Drug is always given after meals. If used with other diuretics, the initial dose should be 25 mg with subsequent increments of 25 mg.

 Pediatric: initial, 25 mg given AM. May be increased by 25 mg daily. After desired response, dose may be reduced to minimum maintenance dose.

 IV, adult: initial, 50 mg or 0.5–1.0 mg/kg, injected slowly directly or through IV tubing. Usually one dose is sufficient to initiate diuresis, but dose may be repeated at other injection site.

Administration/Storage Reconstitute sodium ethacrynate according to directions on vial. Do not use hazy or opalescent solutions, and do not administer simultaneously with whole blood or its derivatives. Use dilutions within 24 hours.

Additional Nursing Implications

See also *Nursing Implications*, p. 791.

1. *Assess*
    a. for excessive diuresis (2 pounds daily) because electrolyte imbalance is more likely to occur at higher rates of diuresis.
    b. patient having rapid excessive diuresis for pain in calves, pelvic area, or in chest because rapid hemoconcentration may cause thromboembolic effects.
    c. for GI effects that may necessitate discontinuation of drug. Severe diarrhea mandates permanent discontinuation of ethacrynic acid.
    d. stools for blood.
    e. urine for hematuria.
    f. for vestibular disturbances and do not administer IV concomitantly with another ototoxic agent.
2. Consult with physician regarding need for supplementary potassium.

FUROSEMIDE Apo-Furosemide,* Furoside,* Lasix, Neo-Renal,* Novosemide,* SK-Furosemide, Uritol* (Rx)

Classification Loop diuretic.

Action/Kinetics Furosemide inhibits the reabsorption of sodium and chloride in the ascending loop of Henle, resulting in the excretion of sodium, chloride and, to a lesser degree, potassium and bicarbonate ions. The resulting urine is more acid. Diuretic action is independent of changes in patients' acid-base balance. Furosemide has a slight antihypertensive effect. **Onset: PO, IM:** 1 hr; **IV:** 5 min. **Peak: PO, IM:** 1–2 hr; **IV** 30 min. **Duration: PO, IM:** 4–8 hr; **IV** 2 hr.

The drug may be effective for patients resistant to thiazides and for those with reduced glomerular filtration rates. Furosemide can be used in conjunction with spironolactone, triamterene, and other diuretics *except* ethacrynic acid. **Never use with ethacrynic acid.**

Uses   Edema associated with coronary heart failure, nephrotic syndrome, hepatic cirrhosis, and ascites. Hypertension alone or as an adjunct. Adjunct in treatment of acute or chronic renal failure. IV for acute pulmonary edema, severe hypercalcemia and as adjunt for hypertensive crisis.

Contraindications   Anuria, hypersensitivity to drug, severe renal disease associated with azotemia and oliguria, hepatic coma associated with electrolyte depletion, pregnancy, and pediatric patients. Only use in pregnancy when benefits clearly outweigh risks.

Untoward Reactions   *Electrolyte and fluid effects:* Fluid and electrolyte depletion leading to dehydration, hypovolemia, thromboembolism. Hypokalemia and hypochloremia may cause metabolic alkalosis. *GI:* Nausea, GI irritation, vomiting, anorexia, diarrhea (especially in children) or constipation, cramps. *Otic:* Tinnitus, hearing impairment (may be reversible or permanent), reversible deafness. Usually following rapid IV or IM administration of high doses. *CNS:* Vertigo, headache, dizziness, lightheadedness, blurred vision, weakness, restlessness, paresthesias. *Hematologic:* Anemia, thrombocytopenia, neutropenia, leukopenia. Rarely, agranulocytosis. *Allergic:* Rashes, pruritus, urticaria, photosensitivity, exfoliative dermatitis, purpura, vasculitis, erythema multiforme. *Miscellaneous:* Hyperglycemia, glycosuria, exacerbation of systemic lupus erythematosus, increased perspiration, muscle spasms, urinary bladder spasm, urinary frequency.

Following IV use: Thrombophlebitis, cardiac arrest. Following IM use: Pain at injection site, cardiac arrest.

Because this drug is resistant to the effects of pressor amines and potentiates the effects of muscle relaxants, it is recommended that oral drug be discontinued one week before surgery and IV drug two days before surgery.

Drug Interactions

Interactant	Interaction
Adrenergic blocking agents	Potentiation of effects
Alcohol	↑ Orthostatic hypotension
Aminoglycoside antibiotics	Additive ototoxicity and nephrotoxicity
Anticoagulants	↑ Effect of anticoagulant due to ↓ plasma protein binding
Antidiabetic agents	Furosemide antagonizes hypoglycemic effect of antidiabetics
Antihypertensive agents	Potentiation of antihypertensive effect
Barbiturates	↑ Orthostatic hypotension
Cephalosporins	↑ Renal toxicity of cephalosporins
Corticosteroids	Enhanced K loss due to K-depleting properties of both drugs
Digitalis glycosides	Furosemide produces excess K and Mg loss with ↑ chance of cardiac arrhythmias
Ethacrynic acid	Combination may result in hypokalemia, tachycardia, deafness, hypotension—**do not use together**
Ganglionic blocking agents	Potentiation of effects

Interactant	Interaction
Indomethacin	Indomethacin ↓ diuretic and antihypertensive effect of furosemide
Lithium	↓ Renal clearance of lithium leading to ↑ risk of toxicity
Narcotics	↑ Orthostatic hypotension
Phenytoin	↓ Diuretic effect of furosemide due to ↓ absorption
Salicylates	↑ Risk of salicylate toxicity due to ↓ renal excretion
Succinylcholine	Furosemide potentiates the action of succinylcholine
Theophylline	Furosemide may ↑ or ↓ the effect of theophyllines
d-Tubocurarine	Furosemide antagonizes the action of tubocurarine

Dosage **PO.** *Edema*: **initial**, 20–80 mg daily as a single dose. For resistant cases, dosage can be increased by 20–40 mg q 6–8 hr until desired diuretic response is attained. *Hypertension*: 40 mg b.i.d. Adjust dosage depending on response. **Pediatric: initial**, 2 mg/kg; if response unsatisfactory, increase by 1–2 mg/kg no sooner than after 6–8 hr. Dose should not exceed 6 mg/kg. **IV, IM.** *Edema:* **initial**, 20–40 mg; if response inadequate after 2 hr, increase dose in 20 mg increments. **Pediatric: initial**, 1 mg/kg; if response inadequate after 2 hr, increase dose by 1 mg/kg. Doses greater than 6 mg/kg should not be given. **IV.** *Acute pulmonary edema*: 40 mg slowly over 1–2 min; if response inadequate after 1 hr, give 80 mg slowly over 1–2 min. Concomitant oxygen and digitalis may be used.

Administration/Storage

1. Discoloration by light does not affect potency.
2. Store in light-resistant container.
3. The drug should be given 2–4 days per week.
4. If used IV, furosemide should not be mixed with solutions with a pH below 5.5.

Additional Nursing Implications
See also *Nursing Implications*, p. 791.

1. *Assess*
   a. BP closely when drug is administered for hypertension, especially initially.
   b. patient having rapid diuresis for dehydration and circulatory collapse. Monitor BP and pulse.
   c. for ototoxicity, when patient has renal impairment or is receiving other ototoxic drugs.
   d. for signs of vascular thrombosis and embolism, particularly in the elderly.
2. Assure the patient that pain after IM injection is transient and will pass.
3. Caution patient to consult with his physician about taking aspirin, because salicylate intoxication occurs at lower level because of competitive renal excretory sites.

MERCURIAL DIURETIC

MERSALYL AND THEOPHYLLINE   Mercutheolin, Theo-Syl-R (Rx)

Classification   Diuretic, mercurial.

Action/Kinetics   Diuresis is induced by decreasing reabsorption of sodium and chloride in the renal tubules (ascending limb of the loop of Henle). The release of mercury ions is pH dependent and occurs more efficiently in an acid medium. Since chloride is excreted more rapidly than sodium, hypochloremic alkalosis may occur; slight increase in potassium excretion. Not widely used due to toxicity. Low glomerular filtration rates can cause refraction to the drug. Acidifying salts (e.g., ammonium chloride) potentiate the mercurial diuretics in the presence of alkalosis. **Onset:** 1–2 hr. **Peak:** 6–9 hr. **Duration:** 12–24 hr. Rapidly excreted by the kidney, minimizing the risk of mercury intoxication.

Each milliliter contains 100 mg mersalyl and 50 mg theophylline.

Uses   Edema due to congestive heart failure, nephrotic stages of glomerulonephritis, ascites due to hepatic cirrhosis or portal obstruction, chronic nephrosis.

Contraindications   Hypersensitivity to drug (mercury ion), acute nephritis, ulcerative colitis, and malignant hypertension. Extreme caution must be exercised for other states of renal insufficiency and for patients with cardiac arrhythmias, those on digitalis, and after a recent myocardial infarction. Use extreme caution during pregnancy and lactation. IV administration should be reserved for extreme emergencies.

Untoward Reactions   *Immediate fatal reactions following IV use* (very rare): Precipitous fall in blood pressure, cardiac irregularities, cyanosis, dyspnea, and irregular, gasping respiration.

Allergic: Fever, flushing, pruritus, urticaria, dermatitis. *Hematologic:* Agranulocytosis, neutropenia. *GI:* Nausea, vomiting. *GU:* Exacerbation of azotemia, acute urinary retention. *Miscellaneous:* Thromboembolism, induration, ecchymoses, dehydration, hyperuricemia, muscle pain, weakness, somnolence.

Systemic mercury poisoning: Characterized by hypochloremic alkalosis, hyponatremia, hypokalemia, stomatitis, dermatitis, colitis, renal tubular necrosis, gastric pain, cardiac arrhythmias.

Drug Interactions   Mercurial diuretics potentiate the toxic effects of digitalis due to potassium loss. May lead to severe cardiac arrhythmias.

Dosage   **IM, SC, or slow IV: initial (test dose),** 0.5 ml. In severe edema, 1–2 ml daily or q other day; **maintenance,** individualized depending on response.

Administration

1. IM administration is preferred. Administer deep into the muscle and massage well to minimize local irritation and pain.
2. SC administration may be painful.
3. The drug should be administered in the morning.
4. Prior administration of 4–8 gm of an acid-producing diuretic such as ammonium chloride given in divided doses for 2 to 3 days before mercurial diuretic will potentiate diuresis.

Additional Nursing Implications

See also *Nursing Implications* for *Diuretics*, p. 791.

1. *Assess*
   a. results of a sensitivity test dose of mercurial diuretics administered 24 hr before administration of full dose.
   b. urine for albumin, blood cells, and casts, which may indicate renal irritation.
   c. mouth for stomatitis and encourage good oral care.
   d. rectum of patients receiving mercury suppositories for local irritation.
   e. pulse after IV injection because ventricular arrhythmias may occur.
   f. for symptoms of systemic mercury poisoning (see Untoward Reactions) and have dimercaprol available for treatment of toxicity.

OSMOTIC DIURETICS

General Statement As opposed to other diuretics, the osmotic diuretics maintain their effectiveness even when renal circulation is acutely compromised, such as in hypovolemic shock, trauma, and dehydration.

Action/Kinetics Osmotic diuretics (mannitol and urea) increase the osmotic pressure of the glomerular filtrate inside the renal tubules. This decreases the amount of fluid and electrolytes that are reabsorbed by the tubules, thereby increasing the loss of fluid, chloride, sodium, and, to a lesser extent, potassium.

Additional Nursing Implications

See also *Nursing Implications*, p. 791.

1. Maintain strict intake and output. Measure output hourly and record.
2. Anticipate insertion of Foley catheter if patient is comatose, incontinent, or unable to void into a receptacle because therapy is based on very strict evaluation of intake and output.
3. *Assess*
   a. particularly for symptoms of water intoxication and for other types of electrolyte imbalance. See p. 815.
   b. at site of IV administration for edema due to extravasation into SC tissue and for thrombophlebitis due to local irritation of drug.
   c. vital signs at least hourly while patient is being treated for acute episode.
   d. for pulmonary edema characterized by coughing, wheezing, dyspnea, cyanosis, and frothy sputum.

ISOSORBIDE Ismotic (Rx)

Classification Diuretic, osmotic.

Action/Kinetics This solution is rapidly absorbed after PO administration. **Onset:** 30 min. **Peak effect:** 1–1½ hr. **Duration:** 5–6 hr. Is excreted unchanged by the kidney.

Uses   To decrease intraocular pressure before and after glaucoma or cataract surgery. Chronic simple glaucoma, primary angle glaucoma, secondary glaucoma (certain types).

Isosorbide dinitrate oral and sublingual tablets are used as a coronary vasodilator (see p. 301).

Contraindications   Acute pulmonary edema, anuria, hemorrhagic glaucoma, severe hydration, severe cardiac decompensation. Use with caution in patients with salt-retaining diseases.

Untoward Reactions   *GI:* Gastric discomfort, thirst, nausea, vomiting. *CNS:* Syncope, lethargy, vertigo, dizziness, irritability, headache, confusion, lightheadedness. *Electrolyte:* Hypernatremia, hyperosmolality. *Miscellaneous:* Rash, hiccoughs.

Dosage   **PO only. Initial,** 1.5 gm/kg; usual range: 1–3 gm/kg b.i.d.–q.i.d.

Administration   To improve palatability, administer poured over cracked ice and advise patient to sip.

Additional Nursing Implications
See also *Nursing Implications* for *Diuretics*, p. 791.
Teach patient and/or family
a. to report untoward reactions.
b. to maintain adequate intake of fluid to promote kidney function.
c. to report decreasing urinary output.
d. how to assess for edema and to report edema if noted.

MANNITOL   Mannitol, Osmitrol (Rx)

Classification   Diuretic, osmotic.

Action/Kinetics   **IV:** *Diuresis,* **onset:** 1–3 hr; *Intraocular pressure,* **onset:** 30–60 min, **duration:** 4–6 hr; *cerebrospinal fluid,* **onset:** 15 min, **duration:** 3–8 hr. Mostly excreted unchanged in urine. A test dose is usually administered.

Uses   Acute renal failure, cerebral edema, reduction of intracranial pressure, glaucoma when other measure have failed. Determination of glomerular filtration rate. It is discontinued when urine flow is greater than 100 ml/hr. *Mannitol is not used for chronic edema.*

Contraindications   Anuria, pulmonary edema, dehydration, intracranial bleeding (except during craniotomy). Pregnancy and children under 12 years of age. Withdraw drug if renal damage, renal dysfunction, heart failure, or pulmonary congestion are observed.

Untoward Reactions   *Electrolyte:* Hypernatremia, acidosis, loss of electrolytes, dehydration. *GI:* Nausea, vomiting, thirst, dry mouth. *CV:* Edema, hypotension or hypertension, increase in heart rate, angina-like chest pain, thrombophlebitis. *Miscellaneous:* Urinary retention, pulmonary congestion, rhinitis, chills, fever, urticaria, pain in arm.

Drug Interaction   May cause deafness when used in combination with kanamycin.

Laboratory Test Interferences ↑ or ↓ Inorganic phosphorus. ↑ Ethylene glycol values, because mannitol also is oxidized to an aldehyde during test.

Dosage **Always by IV infusion.** *Test dose (oliguria or possible reduced renal function):* Either 50 ml of 25% solution, 75 ml of 20% solution, or 100 ml of 15% solution in 3–5 min. If urine flow is 30 to 50 ml/hr, therapeutic dose can be given. If no response, give a second test dose; if still no response, patient must be reevaluated. *Prevention of oliguria:* 50–100 gm (5–25% solution). *Treatment of oliguria:* Up to 100 gm of a 15–20% solution. *To reduce intracranial pressure and brain mass:* 1.5–2.0 gm/kg (use 15–25% solution) infused over 30–60 min. *To reduce intraocular pressure:* 1.5–2.0 gm/kg (15–25% solution) infused over 30 min (if used preoperatively, give 1–1½ hr before surgery). *Diuresis during intoxication:* maximum of 200 gm infused as 5–10% solution. *Measurement of glomerular filtration rate:* 100 ml of 20% solution diluted with 180 ml of sodium chloride injection—infuse at rate of 20 ml/min.

Additional Nursing Implications
See also *Nursing Implications* for *Diuretics*, p. 791.

1. Provide mouth care to relieve thirst and provide fluids if allowed.
2. Report chest pain and pulmonary edema manifested by dyspnea, cyanosis, and frothy sputum.

UREA Ureaphil (Rx)

Classification Diuretic, osmotic.

Action/Kinetics **IV,** *Diuresis, intraocular, intracranial, cerebrospinal fluid pressure:* **Peak:** 1–2 hr. *Diuresis, intracranial pressure:* **Duration:** 3–10 hr. *Intraocular pressure:* **Duration:** 5–6 hr.

Uses To decrease intraocular and intracranial pressure. Abortifacient (given by intra-amniotic injection).

Contraindications Impaired renal function, dehydration, liver failure, intracranial bleeding. Not for use in lower extremities of geriatric patients due to possible phlebitis and thrombosis. Safety in pregnancy and lactation not established.

Untoward Reactions *CNS:* Disorientation, headaches, syncope, confusion, nervousness. *GI:* Nausea, vomiting, dehydration. *Miscellaneous:* Hypotension, hyperthermia, pain, skin irritation.
Note: Phlebitis, thrombosis, infection, or estravasation at the injection site may be observed.

Drug Interactions

Interactant	Interaction
Anticoagulants	↑ Effect of anticoagulants
Lithium carbonate	↓ Lithium effect by ↑ renal excretion

Dosage **Slow IV infusion** (not to exceed 4 ml/min of 30% solution) to prevent hemolysis and increased capillary bleeding. **Adults:** 1–1.5 gm/kg. **Pediatric: up**

to 2 years of age, 0.1 gm/kg; **over 2 years of age**: 0.5–1.5 gm/kg. The total daily dose should not exceed 120 gm.

Additional Nursing Implications

See also *Nursing Implications*, p. 791.

1. Do not administer urea into lower extremities of elderly patients because drug has a fibrinolytic effect.
2. Assess patients with congestive heart failure closely, monitoring vital signs since increase in plasma volume by injection of the drug itself may precipitate pulmonary edema.
3. Assess for signs of personality change and report.
4. Provide close supervision and safety measures, such as side rails, because patient may be mentally confused and hypotensive.

POTASSIUM-SPARING DIURETICS

AMILORIDE HYDROCHLORIDE   Midamor (Rx)

Classification   Diuretic, potassium-sparing.

Action/Kinetics   Acts in the proximal and distal tubules by inhibiting sodium-potassium ATPase. Amiloride is a potassium-sparing drug with weak diuretic and antihypertensive activity. **Onset**: 2 hr. **Peak effect**: 6–10 hr. **Duration**: 24 hr. **t½**: 6–9 hr. Approximately 50% is excreted unchanged by kidney and feces.

Uses   Adjunct with thiazides or other kaliuretic diuretics in the treatment of hypertension or congestive heart failure to help restore normal serum potassium or prevent hypokalemia. Rarely used alone.

Contraindications   Hyperkalemia (greater than 5.5 mEq potassium/liter). In patients receiving other potassium-sparing diuretics or potassium supplements. Impaired renal function. Diabetes mellitus. Use with caution in metabolic or respiratory acidosis or in pregnancy.

Untoward Reactions   *Electrolyte:* Hyperkalemia, hyponatremia and hypochloremia if used with other diuretics. *CNS:* Headache, dizziness, encephalopathy. *GI:* Nausea, anorexia, vomiting, diarrhea, changes in appetite, gas, abdominal pain, bleeding, thirst, dyspepsia, heartburn, activation of preexisting peptic ulcer. *Respiratory:* Dyspnea, cough. *Musculoskeletal:* Weakness, muscle cramps, fatigue. *GU:* Impotence, polyuria, dysuria, bladder spasms, urinary frequency. *CV:* Angina, palpitations, arrhythmias, orthostatic hypotension. *Miscellaneous:* Aplastic anemia, neutropenia, visual disturbances, nasal congestion, tinnitus, increased intraocular pressure, visual disturbances.

Drug Interactions

Interactant	Interaction
Captopril	↑ Risk significant hyperkalemia
Lithium	↓ Renal excretion of lithium → ↑ chance of toxicity
Spironolactone ⎫ Triamterene ⎭	Hyperkalemia, hyponatremia, hypochloremia

Dosage *As single agent or with other diuretics*: **PO, initial**, 5 mg/day; 10 mg/day may be necessary in some patients. Doses as high as 20 mg/day may be used, if needed, with careful monitoring of electrolytes.

Administration Take with food to reduce chance of GI upset.

Additional Nursing Implications

See also *Nursing Implications* for *Diuretics*, p. 791.

1. Assess for hyperkalemia (see p. 815) and for indications for withdrawal of drug, because cardiac irregularities may be precipitated.
2. Do not encourage potassium supplementation or foods rich in potassium because drug does not promote potassium excretion.
3. Do not administer with other potassium-sparing diuretics.

SPIRONOLACTONE Alatone, Aldactone, Novospiroton* (Rx)

Classification Diuretic, potassium-sparing.

Action/Kinetics Spironolactone is a mild diuretic that antagonizes (blocks) the sodium-retaining effects of the hormone aldosterone. This results in increased elimination of sodium and fluid, but not of potassium. The drug also manifests a slight antihypertensive effect. **Onset**: Urine output increases over 3 days. **Peak**: On day 3. **Duration**: 2–3 days, and declines thereafter.

Spironolactone is also found in Aldactazide (Appendix 3).

Uses ·Edema due to congestive heart failure, cirrhosis of the liver, nephrotic syndrome, idiopathic edema, primary hyperaldosteronism, and essential hypertension. Frequently used as adjunct with potassium-losing diuretics when it is important to avoid hypokalemia. *Investigational:* Hirsutism.

Contraindications Acute renal insufficiency, progressive renal failure, hyperkalemia, and anuria. Patients receiving potassium supplements.

Untoward Reactions *Electrolyte:* Hyperkalemia, hyponatremia (characterized by lethargy, dry mouth, thirst, tiredness). *GI:* Diarrhea, cramps. *CNS:* Drowsiness, ataxia, lethargy, confusion, headache. *Endocrine:* Gynecomastia, menstrual irregularities, impotency, bleeding in postmenopausal women, deepening of voice. *Miscellaneous:* Skin rashes, drug fever, urticaria, breast carcinoma, hyperchloremic metabolic acidosis in hepatic cirrhosis (decompensated).

Note: Spironolactone has been shown to be tumorigenic in chronic rodent studies.

Drug Interactions

Interactant	Interaction
Anesthetics, general	Additive hypotension
Anticoagulants, oral	Inhibited by spironolactone
Antihypertensives	Potentiation of hypotensive effect of both agents. Reduce dosage, especially of ganglionic blockers, by one-half
Captopril	↑ Risk of significant hyperkalemia
Digitalis	The potassium-conserving effect of spironolactone may decrease effectiveness of digitalis. Though severe con-

Interactant	Interaction
	sequences have occurred in patients with impaired kidney function, drugs are often given concomitantly. Monitor closely
Diuretics, others	Often administered concurrently because of potassium-sparing effect of spironolactone. Severe hyponatremia may occur. Monitor closely
Lithium	↑ Chance of lithium toxicity due to ↓ renal clearance
Norepinephrine	↓ Responsiveness to norepinephrine
Potassium salts	Since spironolactone conserves potassium excessively, hyperkalemia may result. Rarely used together
Salicylates	Large doses may ↓ effects of spironolactone
Triamterene	Hazardous hyperkalemia may result from combination

Dosage **PO**. *Edema*: **Adults, initial**, 100 mg/day (range: 25–200 mg/day); **maintenance**: dosage dependent on patient response. **Pediatric**: 3.3 mg/kg/day. *Hypertension*: **Adults, initial**, 50–100 mg/day; maintenance dosage depends on patient response. *Hypokalemia*: 25–100 mg/day. *Diagnosis of primary hyperaldosteronism*: 400 mg/day for either 4 days or 3–4 weeks (depending on test used). *Hyperaldosteronism, prior to surgery:* 100–400 mg/day.

Administration Protect drug from light.

Additional Nursing Implications

See also *Nursing Implications* for *Diuretics*, p. 791.

1. Do not encourage supplemental potassium, because drug is potassium–sparing.
2. Warn patients on large doses against driving a car or operating dangerous machinery, because drowsiness or ataxia may occur.
3. Assess patient for tolerance to drug, which may be characterized by edema and reduced urine output.
4. Assess patient with a history of liver disease for stupor.

TRIAMTERENE   Dyrenium (Rx)

Classification Diuretic, potassium-sparing.

General Statement Triamterene is most valuable when combined with other diuretics. Long onset makes drug unsuitable for initiation in patients with severe congestive heart failure.

Withdraw drug slowly as an excessive excretion of potassium may occur with abrupt withdrawal. Patients with hepatic cirrhosis and ascites are more susceptible to hypokalemia.

Lab work to check BUN, creatinine, and serum electrolytes should be done periodically.

Triamterene is also found in Dyazide (p. 900).

Action/Kinetics Triamterene is a mild diuretic that acts directly on the renal tubule. It promotes the excretion of sodium—which is exchanged for potassium or hydrogen ions— bicarbonate, chloride, and fluid. The drug increases urinary pH. It is also a weak folic acid antagonist. **Onset:** 2 hr. **Peak:** 6–8 hr. **Duration:** 12–16 hr.

Uses Congestive heart failure, idiopathic edema, edema associated with hepatic cirrhosis, nephrotic syndrome, steroid therapy, late pregnancy, and secondary hyperaldosteronism. Hypertension (in combination with a thiazide).

Contraindications Hypersensitivity to drug, severe renal insufficiency, and severe hepatic disease, anuria, hyperkalemia. Pregnancy.

Untoward Reactions *Electrolyte:* Hyperkalemia, electrolyte imbalance. *GI:* Nausea, vomiting (may also be indicative of electrolyte imbalance), diarrhea, dry mouth. *CNS:* Dizziness, drowsiness, weakness, headache. *Miscellaneous:* Anaphylaxis, photosensitivity, blood dyscrasias, hypotension, muscle cramps, rash.

Drug Interactions

Interactant	Interaction
Antihypertensives	Potentiated by triamterene
Captopril	↑ Risk of significant hyperkalemia
Digitalis	Inhibited by triamterene
Lithium	↑ Chance of lithium toxicity due to ↓ renal clearance
Potassium salts	Additive hyperkalemia
Spironolactone	Additive hyperkalemia

Laboratory Test Interference Triamterene may impart blue fluorescence to urine, interfering with fluorometric assays (e.g., lactic dehydrogenase, quinidine).

Dosage *Edema*, **initial**; 100 mg 1 to 2 times daily after meals; **maximum daily dose**: 300 mg. **Maintenance**: 100 mg q other day.
    Hypertension (usually given in combination with a thiazide): 100 mg b.i.d. after meals.
    Triamterene dosage usually reduced by one-half when another diuretic is added to regimen.

Administration Minimize nausea by giving drug after meals.

Additional Nursing Implications

See also *Nursing Implications* for *Diuretics*, p. 791.

1. *Assess*
   a. for hyperkalemia (see p. 815), an indication for withdrawal of drug, since irregularities may result.
   b. for signs of blood dyscrasias demonstrated by fever, sore throat, and rash.
   c. for signs of uremia characterized by lethargy, headache, drowsiness, vomiting, restlessness, mental wandering, and foul breath.
2. Do not encourage potassium supplementation, as drug is potassium–sparing.

Chapter Sixty-eight

ELECTROLYTES AND CALORIC AGENTS

General Statement   Water, electrolytes, and nutrients are used as adjuncts in the management of a great variety of disorders and conditions. Since there is a close link between fluid volume and electrolyte balance, these two subjects will be discussed together.

The electrolyte concentration of the body varies within extremely narrow limits (see Appendix 1). Any major deviation from normal quickly results in physiologic changes manifested by dehydration, fluid retention, and disturbance of the acid-base balance. Severe illness (chronic or acute), shock, trauma, poisoning, burns, and certain medications often affect the fluid and electrolyte balance of the body. The administration of suitable replacements to prevent or correct disequilibration of the fluid and electrolyte balance is an important aspect of patient care.

Fluid and electrolytes can be supplied orally, subcutaneously (rare), or intravenously. The oral route should be chosen whenever possible. Parenteral therapy should be discontinued at the earliest point feasible.

Numerous single and multiple electrolyte replacement solutions with or without carbohydrates are commercially available.

Drugs are often added to parenterally administered solutions, and the nurse must be aware of possible interactions and incompatibilities. Unless specifically instructed to do otherwise, it is advisable to add only one drug at a time to the intravenous assembly.

Fluid balance can also be manipulated with diuretics. These are discussed in Chapter 67. Calcium, an electrolyte, is discussed in Chapter 60. Blood volume expanders are discussed in Chapter 21.

TABLE 37   CLINICAL SYMPTOMS OF ELECTROLYTE IMBALANCE

Calcium

Hypocalcemia
CNS: Mental depression, anxiety states
CV: Arrhythmias
GI: Abdominal cramps
Neuromuscular: Peripheral numbness, tingling of fingers, muscular fibrillations, facial muscle cramping, skeletal muscle cramps, leg cramps, tetany, smooth muscle irritability
Other: Abnormal blood coagulation, fractures

Hypercalcemia (Acute Crisis)
CNS: Stupor, coma
CV: Cardiac arrest
GI: Nausea, vomiting, dehydration
Neuromuscular: Weakness
           (Long-term)
GU: Flank pain (renal calculi)
Other: Deep pain over bony areas

Magnesium

Hypomagnesemia
CV: Arrhythmias, vasodilation, ↓ BP
Neuromuscular: Hyperirritability, leg and food cramps, ↑ deep tendon reflexes, involuntary muscle twitching and movements, weakness spacticity, tetany, tremors, convulsions

Hypermagnesemia
CNS: Depression, lethargy, slow, shallow breathing
CV: Deep tendon reflexes
CV: ↓ BP, Slow weak pulse
Neuromuscular: ↓ Deep tendon reflexes
Other: Flushing of skin

Potassium

Hypokalemia
CNS: Dizziness, mental confusion
CV: Arrhythmias; weak, irregular pulse, hypotension, cardiac arrest
GI: Abdominal distention, anorexia
Neuromuscular: Weakness, paresthesia
Other: Malaise

Hyperkalemia
CV: Bradycardia, then tachycardia, cardiac arrest
GI, GU: Abdominal cramps, oliguria or anuria, nausea, diarrhea
Neuromuscular: Weakness, tingling, paralysis

Sodium

Hyponatremia
CNS: Anxiety, lassitude
GI, GU: Rough, dry tongue; abdominal cramps, ↓ specific gravity of urine
Neuromuscular: Tremors, progressing to convulsions

Hypernatremia
CNS: Headaches, convulsions, ↑ body temperature
GI, GU: Nausea, vomiting, ↓ specific gravity of urine
Neuromuscular: ↓ Reflexes, weakness
Other: Thirst, restlessness, dry mucous membranes

Chloride

Hypochloremia
CNS: ↓ Respiration
Neuromuscular: Hypertonicity, tetany

Hyperchloremia
CNS: Stupor; rapid, deep breathing; weakness leading to coma

Characteristic clinical symptoms of electrolyte imbalance are summarized in Table 37, above.

Please note that the dosage of IV solutions is highly individualized especially for infants, children, elderly, or debilitated patients and those suffering from cardiovascular diseases.

Action/Kinetics Supplementary electrolytes and nutrients are indistinguishable by the body from the same elements supplied in the diet and are metabolized in the same manner.

ELECTROLYTES

MAGNESIUM SULFATE (Rx)

Classification   Electrolyte.

General Statement   Magnesium is an important cation present in the extracellular fluid at a concentration of 1.5–2.5 mEq/liter. Magnesium is an essential element for muscle contraction, certain enzyme systems, and nerve transmission. For symptoms of hypomagnesemia and hypermagnesemia see Table 37, p. 815. Large doses of magnesium manifest pharmacologic effects such as CNS depression and hypotension. Magnesium is excreted by the kidneys.

Uses   Replacement therapy in magnesium deficiency. Adjunct in total parenteral nutrition (TPN). Anticonvulsant in toxemia of pregnancy (see p. 466). Cathartic (see p. 652).

Contraindications   Use with caution in patients with renal disease because magnesium is removed from the body solely by the kidneys; in the presence of heart block or myocardial damage.

Untoward Reactions   Magnesium intoxication. *CNS:* Depression. *CV:* Flushing, hypotension, circulatory collapse, depression of the myocardium. *Other:* Sweating, hypothermia, muscle paralysis, respiratory paralysis.

Treatment of Magnesium Intoxication

1. Use artificial ventilation immediately.
2. Have 5–10 mEq of calcium (e.g., 10–20 ml of 10% calcium gluconate) readily available for IV injection.

Drug Interactions

Interactant	Interaction
CNS depressants (anesthetics, hypnotics, narcotics)	Additive CNS depression
Digitalis preparations	Alteration in cardiac conduction and heart block if treating magnesium toxicity with calcium
Neuromuscular blocking agents	Additive neuromuscular blockade

Dosage   *Hypomagnesemia, mild,* **IM**: 1 gm q 6 hr 4 times total (or total of 32.5 mEq/24 hr). *Severe,* **IM**: up to 2 mEq/kg over 4 hr or, **IV**: 5 gm (40 mEq) in 1,000 ml dextrose 5% or sodium chloride solution by **slow** infusion over period of 3 hr. *Hyperalimentation,* **adults**: 8–24 mEq/day; **infants**: 2–10 mEq/day. *Anticonvulsant:* **Adults, IV**: 1–4 gm of a 10–20% solution; **IM**: 1–5 gm of a 25–50% solution 6 times daily as required; **IV infusion**: 4 gm in 250 ml of 5% dextrose at a rate not exceeding 3 ml/min.

Administration

1. IM: deep injection of 50% concentrate is appropriate for adults. A 20% solution should be used for children. IV: dilute as specified by manufacturer.
2. Administer slowly and cautiously at a rate not exceeding 1.5 ml of a 10% concentrate/minute.

Nursing Implications
1. Withhold drug and check with doctor before administration if
    a. patellar reflexes are absent.
    b. respirations are below 16/minute.
    c. urinary output was less than 100 ml during past 4 hours.
    d. there is flushing, sweating, hypotension, or hypothermia, early signs of hypermagnesemia.
    e. there is a previous history of heart block or myocardial damage.
2. Do not administer magnesium sulfate for 2 hours preceding delivery of baby.
3. Assess newborn for neurologic and respiratory depression if mother received continuous IV therapy with magnesium sulfate during 24 hours preceding delivery.
4. Be prepared to assist with emergency treatment of magnesium intoxication. Have available equipment for artificial ventilation and calcium gluconate IV.

POTASSIUM SALTS CAPSULES/TABLETS: Kalium Durules,* Kaon, Kaon-Cl, Kaon Cl-10, Kao-Nor, K-Forte Regular And Maximum Strength, K-Long,* Klotrix, K-Tab, Micro-K, Micro-K 10, Osto-K, Novolente-K,* Slow-K, Slow-Pot 600.* (Rx and OTC) EFFERVESCENT TABLETS: Effer-K, Kaochlor-Eff, Klorvess, K-Lyte, K-Lyte/Cl, K-Lyte/Cl 50, K-Lyte DS (Rx). LIQUIDS: Bayon, Bl-K, Cena-K, Duo-K, EM-K-10%, K-10 Solution,* Kaochlor 10%, Kaochlor 20,* Kaochlor S-F, Kaon, Kaon-Cl 20%, Kay Ciel, Kaylixir, K-G Elixir, Klor-10%, Klor-Con, Klorvess 10%, Kolyum, Potachlor 10% And 20%, Potasalan, Potassine, Potassium Chloride, Potassium Gluconate, Roychlor,* Rum-K, SK-Potassium Chloride, Tri-K, Trikates, Twin-K, Twin-K-Cl (Rx). POWDERS: Kato, Kayciel, K-Lor, Klor-Con, Klor-Con/25, Klorvess Effervescent Granules, Koyum, K-Lyte/Cl, Potage (Rx). PARENTERAL: Potassium Acetate, Potassium Chloride (Rx).

Classification Electrolyte.

General Statement Potassium is the major cation of the body's intracellular fluid. It is essential for the maintenance of important physiologic processes, including cardiac, smooth, and skeletal muscle function, acid-base balance, gastric secretions, renal function, protein and carbohydrate metabolism. Symptoms of hypokalemia include weakness, cardiac arrhythmias, fatigue and in severe cases flaccid paralysis and inability to concentrate urine.

The usual adult daily requirement of potassium is 40–80 mg. In adults, the normal plasma concentration of potassium ranges from 3.5 to 5 mEq/liter. Concentrations up to 5.6 mEq/liter are normal in children.

Both hypokalemia and hyperkalemia, if uncorrected, can be fatal; thus, potassium must always be administered very cautiously.

Potassium is readily and rapidly absorbed from the gastrointestinal tract. Though a number of salts can be used to supply the potassium cation, potassium chloride is the agent of choice since hypochloremia frequently accompanies potassium deficiency. Dietary measures (bananas, orange juice) can often prevent and even correct potassium deficiencies.

Potassium is excreted by the kidney and is partially reabsorbed from the glomerular filtrate.

Uses   Correction of potassium deficiency caused by vomiting, diarrhea, excess loss of gastrointestinal fluids, hyperadrenalism, malnutrition, debilitation, prolonged negative nitrogen balance, dialysis, metabolic alkalosis, diabetic acidosis, certain renal conditions, cardiac arrhythmias, cardiotonic glycoside toxicity, and myasthenia gravis (experimentally).

Long-term electrolyte replacement regimen or total parenteral nutrition with potassium-free solutions. Correction of potassium deficiency possibly caused by certain drugs, including many diuretics, adrenal corticosteroids, testosterone or corticotropin.

Prophylaxis after major surgery when urine flow has been reestablished.

Contraindications   Severe renal function impairment, postoperatively before urine flow has been reestablished. Crush syndrome, Addison's disease, hyperkalemia, heat cramps, acute dehydration. Administer with caution in the presence of cardiac and renal disease and in patients receiving potassium-sparing drugs. Safety in pregnancy, lactation, and children has not been established.

Untoward Reactions   For symptoms of hypokalemia and hyperkalemia see Table 37, p. 815.

GI: Nausea, vomiting, diarrhea, abdominal discomfort, GI bleeding or obstruction. Ulceration or perforation of the small bowel from enteric-coated potassium chloride tablets. *Other:* Skin rashes, hyperkalemia.

Treatment of Overdosage   (Plasma potassium levels greater than 6.5 mEq/liter.) All measures must be monitored by electrocardiogram. Measures consist of actions taken to shift potassium ions from plasma into cells by

1. **Sodium bicarbonate**: IV infusion of 40–160 mEq over period of 5 minutes. May be repeated after 10 to 15 minutes if ECG abnormalities persist.
2. **Dextrose**: IV infusion of 300–500 ml of 10–25% injection over period of 1 hour. Insulin is sometimes added to dextrose (5–10 units per 20 gm of dextrose) or given separately.
3. **Calcium gluconate—or other calcium salt**: (only for patients not on digitalis or other cardiotonic glycosides): IV infusion of 0.5–1 gm (5–10 ml of a 10% solution) over period of 2 minutes. Dosage may be repeated after 1 to 2 minutes if ECG remains abnormal. When ECG is approximately normal, the excess potassium should be removed from body by administration of polystyrene sulfonate, hemo- or peritoneal dialysis (patients with renal insufficiency) or other means.

Drug Interactions

Interactant	Interaction
Digitalis glycosides	Cardiac arrhythmias
Potassium-sparing diuretics	Severe hyperkalemia

Dosage   Highly individualized. Oral administration is preferred because the slow absorption from the GI tract prevents sudden, large increases in plasma potassium levels. Dosage is usually expressed as mEq/liter of potassium. The bicarbonate, chloride, citrate, and gluconate salts are usually administered orally. The chloride, acetate, and phosphate may be administered by **slow IV** infusion.

IV infusion. *Serum K less than 2.0 mEq/L:* 400 mEq/day at a rate not to exceed 40 mEq/hr. *Serum K more than 2.5 mEq/L:* 200 mEq/day at a rate not to exceed 20 mEq/hr.

PO. *Prophylaxis of hypokalemia:* 16–24 mEq/day. *Potassium depletion:* 40–100 mEq/day.

Note: Usual dietary intake of potassium is between 40 and 250 mEq/day.

For patients with accompanying metabolic acidosis, an alkalinizing potassium salt (potassium bicarbonate, potassium citrate, or potassium acetate) should be selected.

Administration

PO

1. Dilute or dissolve liquid potassium in fruit or vegetable juice if not already in flavored base.
2. Chill to increase palatability.
3. Instruct patient to swallow enteric-coated tablets and not dissolve them in mouth.
4. Give oral doses 2–4 times daily. Hypokalemia should be corrected slowly over a period of 3–7 days to minimize hyperkalemia.
5. Salt substitutes should not be used concomitantly with potassium preparations.
6. Administer dilute liquid solutions of potassium rather than tablets to patients with esophageal compression.

PARENTERAL

1. Administer very slowly as ordered for individual patient by the doctor.
2. Potassium should not be administered IV undiluted. Usual is to administer by slow IV infusion in dextrose solution at a concentration of 40–80 mEq/L.
3. Ensure uniform distribution of potassium by inverting container during addition of potassium solution and then by agitating container. Squeezing the plastic container will not prevent potassium chloride from settling to the bottom.
4. Check site of administration frequently for pain and redness because drug is extremely irritating.

Nursing Implications

1. Discontinue ingestion of potassium-rich foods and oral potassium medication when parenteral potassium administration is initiated.
2. Withhold oral potassium medication if abdominal pain, distention, or GI bleeding occurs.
3. Be alert to symptoms of hypokalemia, such as weakness, cardiac arrhythmias, and fatigue, which indicate a low intracellular potassium level even though the serum potassium level is within normal limits.
4. Assess that urinary flow is adequate before starting administration of potassium because impaired renal function can lead to hyperkalemia.
5. Withhold potassium medication from patients with oliguria, anuria, or azotinuria, chronic adrenal insufficiency, or extensive tissue breakdown as in burns.
6. Do not administer potassium medication to patients receiving potassium-sparing diuretics, such as spironolactone or triamterene.
7. Monitor ECG when patient is on parenteral potassium for signs of hyperkalemia as noted in *Untoward Reactions*.
8. Monitor serum potassium while patient is receiving parenteral potassium. (Norm: 3.6–5.5 mEq/L.)
9. Assess for signs of hyperkalemia, such as listlessness, mental confusion, weakness or heaviness of legs, flaccid paralysis, cold skin, gray pallor, hypotension, cardiac arrhythmias, and heart block.

(continued)

10. Be prepared to assist with emergency treatment of hyperkalemia. Have available sodium bicarbonate, calcium gluconate, and regular insulin for parenteral use.
11. *Teach patient and/or family*
    a. the importance of potassium to other medications in regimen to promote compliance.
    b. symptoms of hypokalemia and hyperkalemia and the need to report these.
    c. to ingest potassium-rich food, such as citrus juices, bananas, apricots, raisins, and nuts, after parenteral potassium is discontinued.

SODIUM CHLORIDE Slo-Salt (OTC)

Classification Electrolyte.

General Statement Sodium is the major cation of the body's extracellular fluid. It plays a crucial role in maintaining the fluid and electrolyte balance. Excess retention of sodium results in overhydration (edema, hypervolemia), which is often treated with diuretics. Abnormally low levels of sodium result in dehydration. Normally, the plasma contains 136–145 mEq sodium and 98–106 mEq chloride/liter. The average daily requirement of salt is approximately 5 gm.

For symptoms of hyponatremia and hypernatremia see Table 37.

Uses PO: Prophylaxis of heat prostration or muscle cramps, chloride deficiency due to diuresis or salt restriction. **Parenteral:** Fluid and electrolyte replacement.

Contraindications Congestive heart failure, severely impaired renal function. Administer with caution to patients with cardiovascular, cirrhotic, renal disease, in presence of hyperproteinemia, and in patients receiving corticosteroids or corticotropin.

Untoward Reactions Hypernatremia, postoperative intolerance of sodium chloride characterized by cellular dehydration, asthenia, disorientation, anorexia, nausea, oliguria, and increased BUN levels.

Dosage PO: *Heat cramps/dehydration:* 0.5–1 gm with 8 oz water up to 10 times/day; total daily dose should not exceed 4.8 gm. **IV:** *individualized* as required. *Hypotonic* (0.11–0.45% NaCl) solutions are used when fluid losses exceed electrolyte depletion. *Isotonic* (0.9% NaCl) provides approximately physiologic concentrations of sodium and chloride ions. *Hypertonic* (3% or 5%) when sodium loss exceeds fluid loss.

Administration Hypertonic injections of NaCl must be given slowly and cautiously in a volume not to exceed 100 ml/hr. Plasma electrolyte levels should be determined before additional sodium chloride is given.

Nursing Implications
1. Assess patient for signs of hypernatremia, such as flushed skin, elevated temperature, rough dry tongue, edema, hypertension or hypotension, tachycardia, urine specific gravity above 1.02, and serum sodium above 146 mEq/liter.
2. Interrupt IV and report condition of patient to doctor should these signs occur.

CALORIC AGENTS

Carbohydrates

Classification Caloric agents.

General Statement The simplest and most easily absorbed caloric agents are dextrose (D–glucose) and fructose, or an equimolar mixture of the two—invert sugar. Fructose and dextrose are monosaccharides. They can replace and supplement orally absorbed food and water. They decrease excess ketone formation, spare body proteins and electrolytes.

One liter of a 10% solution of any of the above provides 340–380 calories. Five percent solutions are approximately isotonic. Both 5% and 10% solutions are used to correct dehydration and supply calories. More concentrated solutions also have a diuretic effect.

Remark: Solutions without NaCl should not be used as diluents for blood.

Contraindications Do not use concentrated (hypertonic) solutions in the presence of intracranial or intraspinal hemorrhages or delirium tremens in dehydrated patients.

Administration
1. The amount of fluid to be received in a specific time is to be ordered by the doctor. The amount is highly individualized, especially in children.
2. Administer concentrated solution into large, central vein to prevent irritation.

Nursing Implications
1. Iso-osmolar (isotonic) parenteral therapy: Assess for signs of cerebral edema manifested by slow pulse rate, high blood pressure, and headaches. *Reduce* rate of flow markedly should these symptoms occur and report to doctor.
2. Hyperosmolar (hypertonic) parenteral therapy:
   a. Assess for signs of dehydration manifested by rapid pulse rate, low BP, and restlessness. *Reduce* rate of flow markedly should these symptoms occur, and report to doctor.
   b. Determine that hyperosmolar solution does not run faster than 3–4 ml/min to prevent further electrolyte imbalance and local irritation.
   c. Assess site of infusion for redness and pain because hyperosmolar solutions can cause sclerosis and thrombophlebitis.
   d. Anticipate that a 5% dextrose solution will be administered following abrupt withdrawal of hypertonic dextrose solution to prevent hypoglycemia.

DEXTROSE (D–Glucose) (Rx)

Classification Caloric agent, carbohydrate.

Action/Kinetics Dextrose may result in decreased nitrogen and protein loss, cause increased glycogen storage, and prevent or reduce ketosis. It may also cause diuresis. Dextrose, 5% solution, is isotonic.

Uses To supply calories and water when nonelectrolytic fluid and caloric replacement are necessary. Also, to spare proteins and minimize loss of electrolytes. Toxemia of pregnancy, renal failure (use 20% solution), diabetic acidosis (use 2.5% dextrose and 0.45% NaCl), reduction of cerebrospinal fluid pressure and to maintain blood volume (use 50% solution). To correct insulin reaction (hypoglycemia), use 50% solution.

Additional Contraindications Hyperglycemia.

Untoward Reactions Hyperglycemia and glycosuria (especially with rapid injection of hypertonic solutions). *CNS:* Fever, mental confusion, unconsciousness. *CV:* Thrombosis or phlebitis from site of injection, extravasation, hypo- or hypervolemia.

Dosage *Individualized,* depending on the age, weight, and condition of the patient. *Hypoglycemia:* **adults and children, IV, usual,** 20–50 ml of dextrose, 50%, at a rate of 3 ml/min; **neonates/infants, IV, usual,** 2 ml/kg of dextrose, 10–25%. *Diabetic, hypoglycemia in conscious patients:* **PO,** 10–20 gm; may be repeated in 10–20 min if required. *Fluid replacement:* 1–3 liters of 5% solution daily.

Administration

1. Maximum rate of administration to avoid hyperglycemia: 0.5 gm/kg/hr.
2. Concentrated solutions should not be given IM or SC.
3. Dextrose solutions are available in percentages ranging from 2.5–70%. These solutions should only be used if clear; they should not be frozen or exposed to extreme heat.
4. Concentrations of glucose over 20% should only be administered by a central vein after appropriate dilution.

FRUCTOSE   Levulose (Rx)

Classification Caloric agent, carbohydrate.

Action/Kinetics More rapidly metabolized and converted to glycogen than dextrose. When necessary can be administered more quickly than dextrose (100 gm in 1 hour). Suitable for diabetic patients because it does not require insulin to be metabolized.

Uses To supply calories, water; to spare body proteins and electrolytes.

Contraindications Acute hypoglycemia (use dextrose instead), hereditary fructose intolerance. Gout.

Untoward Reactions *CNS:* Fever. *CV:* Hypervolemia, venous thrombosis or phlebitis.
   In infants, rapid administration has caused an increase in pulse and respiratory rate and liver size, accompanied by a decrease in blood pH value and CO_2.

Dosage **IV:** *individualized,* **usual daily dose,** 1–3 liters of 10% solution. **Infants:** 100–1,000 ml of 10% solution; **children:** 200–2,000 ml of 10% solution. Each 10 ml of solution contain approximately 1 gm of fructose.

Administration IV only. Unless otherwise instructed, administer slowly, especially in children (rate should not exceed 1 gm/kg/hr).

INVERT SUGAR   Travert (Rx)

Classification Caloric agent, carbohydrate.

Remarks Equimolar mixture of dextrose and fructose; the combination is more rapidly utilized than dextrose alone. A 5% solution is sometimes administered together with amino acids.

Dosage *Individualized*. **IV: usual**, 1–3 liters of 10% solution daily.

Administration The rate is determined by the reaction of patient.

INTRAVENOUS NUTRITIONAL THERAPY

General Statement Intravenous nutrition is an important treatment regimen for patients in whom oral feeding is not possible or is inadequate. There are a large number of products available that provide one or more of the following nutrients: dextrose, electrolytes, amino acids, fat emulsion, vitamins, minerals, and fluids. These preparations are administered intravenously either peripherally or via a central venous catheter. Such regimens are often referred to as total parenteral nutrition (TPN). The success of TPN is gauged by weight gain and positive nitrogen balance.

The proper administration of TPN products requires a thorough knowledge of the nutritional needs of the patients, as well as of their fluid and electrolyte balance. Patients receiving TPN must be frequently evaluated by means of complete laboratory tests.

Uses In situations where gastrointestinal absorption of nutrients is impaired due to disease, obstruction, or other drug therapy (e.g., cancer chemotherapy). Following GI surgery or in situations where nutrient requirements are increased as in trauma, burns, or severe infections.

Special preparations are available for use in renal failure, hepatic failure or encephalopathy, or in acute metabolic stress.

Peripheral administration is indicated for short-term therapy (up to 12 days), in situations where the caloric requirements are not excessive, or as a supplement to oral feeding. These solutions are isotonic in nature. Central parenteral administration is indicated in patients requiring hypertonic dextrose.

Contraindications Hypersensitivity to specific proteins or inborn errors of amino acid metabolism. Products for general nutritional purposes (e.g., crystalline amino acid infusions) should not be used in severe kidney or liver disease, hyperammonemia, or encephalopathy. Also, severe uncorrected acid-base imbalance. Use with caution in pregnancy.

Sodium-containing products should be used with caution in patients with congestive heart failure, renal insufficiency, or edema. Potassium-containing products should be used cautiously in patients with severe renal failure or hyperkalemia. Products containing acetate should be used with care in alkalosis and hepatic insufficiency.

Untoward Reactions *Metabolic:* Hyperchloremic metabolic acidosis, hyperammonemia, ketosis, glucose intolerance, acid-base imbalance, dehydration, hypo- or hypervitaminosis, elevated hepatic enzymes, hypophosphatemia, hypocalcemia, osteoporosis. Rapid withdrawal of concentrated dextrose solutions may result in hypoglycemia. Essential fatty acid deficiency following long-term use of products that are fat free (symptoms include dry, scaly skin, rash resembling eczema, alopecia, slow wound healing, and fatty infiltration of the liver). *Dermatologic:* Skin rashes, flushing, sweating. *Other:* Nausea, vertigo, fever, headache, dizziness. *At site of catheter:* Venous thrombosis, phlebitis.

Drug Interactions

Interactant	Interaction
Folic acid	Precipitation of calcium as calcium folate
Sodium bicarbonate	Precipitation of calcium and magnesium carbonate; ↓ effect of insulin and vitamin B complex with C
Tetracyclines	↓ Effect of amino acids to conserve protein

Dosage The dose, route of administration, and content of the infusion is determined individually for each patient depending on the nutritional need, physical state, and length of therapy anticipated.

Administration

1. Appropriate laboratory monitoring with baseline values and evaluation are required before and during administration.
2. Dextrose, 12.5% or greater should not be utilized in peripheral venous infusions.
3. Blood should not be administered through the same infusion site.
4. Solutions must be prepared aseptically under a laminar flow hood in the pharmacy.
5. Solutions should be used as soon as possible after preparation. No more than 24 hours should elapse for administration of a single bottle.
6. The IV administration set should be replaced daily.
7. Appropriate guidelines must be followed for patients in whom indwelling catheters will be in place for a long period of time.

Nursing Implications

See *Nursing Implications* for Central Parenteral Administration in Chapter 6, p. 36.

1. Assess for allergic reaction to protein hydrolysate characterized by pruritus, urticaria, and wheals. Report positive observations to doctor.
2. Report blood sugar determinations over 200 mg/100 ml indicating need for insulin to be added to TPN.
3. Report fractional urine determinations of 3+–4+, indicating need for insulin to be added to TPN.
4. Discontinue TPN if blood sugar exceeds 1,000 mg/100 ml and substitute a hypoosmolar solution to prevent neurologic dysfunction and coma.

CRYSTALLINE AMINO ACID INFUSION Aminosyn 3.5%, 5%, 7%, 8.5%, and 10%; Aminosyn 3.5% M, Aminosyn 7% and 8.5% With Electrolytes, Freamine III 8.5% and 10%, Freamine III 3% With Electrolytes, Novamine 8.5% and 11.4%, Procalamine, Travasol 5.5%, 8.5%, and 10%, Travasol 5.5% and 8.5% With Electrolytes, 3.5% Travasol M With Electrolyte 45, Veinamine 8% (Rx)

Classification Nutritional agent.

General Statement These products contain both essential and nonessential amino acids as well as various electrolytes. Dextrose, IV fat emulsion, vitamins, and minerals may be added as required. Percentage refers to the amino acid concentration. The amino acids present in the products either conserve protein or induce protein synthesis by providing the necessary amino acids.

Administration The initial rate of infusion should not exceed 2 ml/min. The rate may then be increased slowly depending on laboratory values of urinary and blood glucose.

AMINO ACID FORMULATION FOR HEPATIC FAILURE OR HEPATIC ENCEPHALOPATHY   Hepatamine (Rx)

Classification Nutritional agent.

General Statement This product contains both essential and nonessential amino acids with high levels of branched chain amino acids as leucine, isoleucine, and valine. Fat emulsion, dextrose, electrolytes, and vitamins may be added if required.

Use To normalize amino acid levels and improve nitrogen balance in patients with cirrhosis and hepatitis who manifest hepatic encephalopathy.

Additional Contraindication Anuria.

Administration
1. The total daily fluid intake is usually 2–3 liters given over a period of 8–12 hrs.
2. Infusion rates should be slow to start and gradually increased to 60–125 ml/ hr.
3. The product may be given either peripherally or by central venous indwelling catheter.

AMINO ACID FORMULATION FOR HIGH METABOLIC STRESS Freamine HBC (Rx)

Classification Nutritional agent.

General Statement This preparation has similar content as that for hepatic failure.

Use Acute metabolic stress characterized by increased urinary excretion of nitrogen, hyperglycemia, and decreased concentration or plasma branched chain amino acids.

Additional Contraindications Anuria, electrolyte imbalance, acid-base imbalance, hepatic coma.

Administration This product may be administered either peripherally or by central venous indwelling catheter.

AMINO ACID FORMULATIONS FOR RENAL FAILURE Aminosyn-RF, Nephramine, Renamin (Rx)

Classification Nutritional agent.

General Statement The nutritional requirements for patients with renal disease are different than patients with normal renal function. Administration of minimal amounts of essential amino acids enhances utilization of urea. Administration of nonessential amino acids should be restricted.

Use Uremia patients requiring parenteral nutrition.

Additional Contraindications Acid-base imbalance, electrolyte imbalance, hyperammonemia. Use with caution in children with acute renal failure and in infants with low birth weight.

Administration These products should be given through a central venous catheter at an initial rate not to exceed 20–30 ml/hr for the first 6–8 hr. Then the rate can be increased by 10 ml/hr each 24 hours to a maximum of 60–100 ml/hr.

INTRAVENOUS FAT EMULSION   Intralipid 10% And 20%, Liposyn 10% And 20%, Soyacal 10% And 20%, Travamulsion 10% And 20% (Rx)

Classification Nutritional agent.

General Statement These products contain either soybean oil or safflower oil in a concentration of 10% or 20%, egg yolk phospholipids (1.2%), glycerin (2.21%–2.5%), and water for injection. The fatty acids present in these preparations (linoleic, linolenic, oleic, palmitic, and stearic) provide essential fatty acids to maintain normal cellular membrane function. The products provide from 1.1 cal/ml (10% oil) to 2.0 cal/ml (20% oil). Since it is isotonic, it can be administered into a peripheral vein. The preparation increases heat production, oxygen consumption, and decreases the respiratory quotient (ratio of CO_2/O_2; normal: 0.77–0.90).

Use Source of calories and essential fatty acids for prolonged parenteral nutrition (longer than 5 days). Fatty acid deficiency.

Contraindications Disturbances of fat metabolism (e.g., lipoid nephrosis, pathologic hyperlipidemia, acute pancreatitis with hyperlipemia). Sensitivity to egg yolk. Use with caution in patients with hepatic damage, anemia, respiratory disease, coagulation problems, or possibility of fat embolism. Caution should be exercised when used in premature or jaundiced premature infants. Safe use in pregnancy not established.

Untoward Reactions *Premature infants:* Deaths due to intravascular fat accumulation in the lungs. **Acute untoward reactions.** *GI:* Nausea, vomiting. *CNS:* Headache, fever, drowsiness, dizziness. *Other:* Hyperlipemia, dyspnea, increased coagulation, flushing, sweating, cyanosis, back and chest pain, pressure over eyes, hypersensitivity reactions with urticaria, increases in liver enzymes (transient). Neonates may manifest thrombocytopenia. **Long-term untoward reactions.** *Hepatic:* Jaundice, hepatomegaly, alterations in liver function tests. *Overloading syndrome:* Splenomegaly, seizures, fever, leukocytosis, shock. *Other:* Deposition of pigment (brown) in reticuloendothelial system. **Sepsis and thrombophlebitis due to contamination or procedure.**

Dosage **IV**, as part of total parenteral nutrition regimen. **Maximum:** 3 gm/kg/day. **Pediatric maximum:** 4 gm/kg/day. The product should not exceed 60% of daily caloric intake. *Fatty acid deficiency:* Approximately 8–10% of caloric intake.

Administration/Storage

1. Discard if oiling out occurs before administration.
2. May be given parenterally or centrally using a separate line, though it can be administered into same peripheral vein as carbohydrate-amino acid solutions using a Y connection located near infusion site. Flow rate of each solution should be controlled separately by infusion pump. Do not use filters.
3. May be mixed with certain nutrient solutions (check package insert).
4. The rate of infusion should be: **Adults: 10% products, initial,** 1 ml/min for first 15–30 min; **then,** if no untoward reactions, increase to 83–125 ml/hr up to 500 ml the first day. Amount may be increased the second day. **Adults: 20% products, initial,** 0.5 ml/min for first 15–30 min; **then,** if no untoward reactions, increase to 62 ml/hr up to 250–500 ml (depending on product) the first day. Amount may be increased the second day. Total daily dose should not exceed 3 gm/kg. **Pediatric: 10% products, initial,** 0.1 ml/min for first 10–15 min; **then,** if no untoward reactions, increase to maximum of 100 ml/hr. **Pediatric: 20% products, initial,** 0.05 ml/min; **then,** if no untoward reactions, increase to maximum of 50 ml/hr. Total daily dose should not exceed 4 gm/kg.
5. Store in refrigerator at 4°–8°C (39.2°– 46.4°F).

Nursing Implications

Assess closely for first 10 to 15 minutes of administration for allergic reaction to medication.

Chapter Sixty-nine

ACIDIFYING AND ALKALINIZING AGENTS

General Statement   Acidifying and alkalinizing agents are used to alter the pH of the system, stomach, or the urine for the purpose of correcting acid-base balance, increasing or decreasing the absorption or excretion of certain drugs, or as an adjunct in drug therapy. Caution must be exercised to prevent excesses in changes in pH.

ACIDIFYING AGENT

AMMONIUM CHLORIDE   Ammonium Muriate* (Rx)

Classification   Urinary acidifying agent, diuretic.

Action/Kinetics   The ammonium ion is metabolized to urea liberating hydrogen ions that acidify the urine. Ammonium chloride also induces diuresis. Ammonium chloride is rapidly absorbed from the GI tract even though the full effect of the drug becomes apparent only after several days.

Uses   Systemic acidifier used for the prevention or correction of metabolic alkalosis due to chloride ion loss caused by vomiting (especially in infants with pyloric obstruction), gastric fistula drainage, gastric suction; to acidify the urine to decrease or promote the excretion of certain drugs. Urinary calculi to promote solubility of calcium and phosphate. Diuretic in premenstrual edema or Ménière's syndrome. Expectorant.

Contraindications   Marked renal and hepatic impairment. Respiratory acidosis. Administration by the SC, rectal, or IP route.

Untoward Reactions   Symptoms are due to overdosage. Severe metabolic acidosis especially in patients with impaired renal function. *Electrolyte:* Hypokalemia, hyperchloremic acidosis. *CV:* Arrhythmias, bradycardia. *GI:* Nausea, vomiting, thirst. *CNS:* Headache, drowsiness, confusion, tonic seizures, twitching, coma.

Other: Sweating, pallor.

Rapid IV: Pain, irritation at site or along the vein.

Treatment of Overdosage Sodium bicarbonate or sodium lactate, IV, is used to reverse acidosis or loss of electrolytes. Potassium supplements, PO, will reverse hypokalemia.

Drug Interactions

Interactant	Interaction
Aminosalicylic acid	↑ Chance of aminosalicylic acid crystalluria
Amphetamine	↓ Effect of amphetamine by ↓ renal tubular reabsorption
Antidepressants, tricyclic	↓ Effect of tricyclics by ↓ renal tubular reabsorption
Salicylates	↑ Effect of salicylates by ↑ renal tubular reabsorption

Dosage **PO**: 4–12 gm daily in divided doses q 4–6 hr; **pediatric**: 75 mg/kg daily in 4 divided doses. Drug is more effective as diuretic when rest periods of a few days are part of regimen (i.e., 3 days on, 2 days off). *Premenstrual edema*: 1.5 gm b.i.d. for 4 to 5 days, premenstrually.

IV *(metabolic alkalosis): Highly individualized* and based on blood chemistry determinations (CO_2 combining power or chloride ion deficit). Always start with minimal dosage. **Usual, adults and children**: 10 ml/kg of 2.14% solution at a rate of 0.9–1.3 ml/minute up to 2 ml/minute.

Administration

1. PO: To minimize GI effects, give after meals or as enteric-coated tablets.
2. Administer liquid with acid juices, raspberry, or cherry syrup to mask saline taste.
3. Do not administer with milk or any other alkaline solution, because these are incompatible with ammonium chloride.
4. Parenteral: Carbon dioxide combining power and serum electrolytes should be monitored prior to and periodically during IV infusion so as to avoid serious acidosis.

Nursing Implications

1. Have on hand sodium bicarbonate or sodium lactate for treatment of electrolyte loss or acidosis.
2. Anticipate administration of potassium supplements if hypokalemia occurs.
3. Assess for untoward reactions.
4. Do not administer to patients with a history of liver impairment.
5. Anticipate intermittent administration of drug to maintain diuresis.
6. Discontinue administration at site of hypodermoclysis if pain occurs.

ALKALINIZING AGENTS

SODIUM BICARBONATE   Bell/ans, Soda Mint (Rx and OTC)

Classification   Alkalinizing agent, antacid, electrolyte.

Action/Kinetics   Sodium bicarbonate neutralizes hydrochloric acid by forming sodium chloride and carbon dioxide (1 gm of sodium bicarbonate provides 11.9 mEq each of sodium and bicarbonate). See also Chapter 52.

Uses   As adjunct in sulfonamide therapy, treatment of metabolic acidosis, antacid, increases excretion of drugs by alkalinizing the urine, severe diarrhea. Gastric and systemic alkalinizer.

Contraindications   Renal impairment, congestive heart failure, patients on restricted sodium diet, edema, cirrhosis of the liver, metabolic or respiratory alkalosis, toxemia of pregnancy. Use with extreme caution for patients losing chloride through vomiting or continuous GI suction and in those in whom diuretics produce hypochloremic alkalosis.

Untoward Reactions   Systemic alkalosis characterized by dizziness, abdominal cramps, thirst, anorexia, nausea, vomiting, hyperirritatbility, tetany, diminished breathing, convulsions.

    Extravasation following IV use may manifest ulceration, sloughing, cellulitis, or tissue necrosis at the site of injection.

Drug Interactions

Interactant	Interaction
Amphetamine	↑ Effect of amphetamine by ↑ renal tubular reabsorption
Antidepressants, tricyclic	↑ Effect of tricyclics by ↑ renal tubular reabsorption
Ephedrine	↑ Effect ephedrine by ↑ renal tubular reabsorption
Erythromycin	↑ Effect of erythromycin in urine due to ↑ alkalinity of urine
Lithium carbonate	Excretion of Li is proportional to amount of sodium ingested. If patient on sodium-free diet, may develop Li toxicity since less Li is excreted
Methenamine compounds	↓ Effect of methenamine due to ↑ alkalinity of urine
Nitrofurantoin	↓ Effect of nitrofurantoin due to ↑ alkalinity of urine
Procainamide	↑ Effect of procainamide due to ↓ excretion by kidney
Pseudoephedrine	↑ Effect of pseudoephedrine due to ↑ tubular reabsorption
Quinidine	↑ Effect of quinidine by ↑ renal tubular reabsorption
Tetracyclines	↓ Effect of tetracyclines due to ↑ excretion by kidney

Dosage   *Metabolic acidosis*, **IV infusion: Adults and older children**, 2–5 mEq/kg over a 4–8 hr period; **then**, assess clinical response of patient before additional bicarbonate administered. *Cardiac arrest*, **rapid IV: Adults**, 200–300 mEq (use 7.5 or 8.4% solution); **infants, up to 2 years**: up to 8 mEq/kg/day as a 4.2% solution.

Systemic and urinary alkalinizer, antacid: **PO**, 0.325–2 gm up to q.i.d. (not to exceed 16 gm/day in patients under 60 and 8 gm/day in patients over 60).

Administration
1. Hypertonic solutions must be administered by the physician.
2. IV dose should be determined based on arterial blood pH, pCO₂, and determination of base deficit.
3. Isotonic solutions should be administered slowly as ordered as too rapid administration may result in death due to cellular acidity.
4. Check rate of flow frequently.

Nursing Implications
Assess

a. acidotic patients being treated with sodium bicarbonate for relief of dyspnea and hyperpnea and report because the drug must be discontinued when these conditions are relieved.
b. acidotic patients being treated with sodium bicarbonate for edema, since this may necessitate a change to potassium bicarbonate.

SODIUM LACTATE   (Rx)

Classification   Systemic alkalinizing agent.

Action/Kinetics   Metabolism of sodium lactate to bicarbonate in the liver with removal of both lactate and hydrogen. The lactate ion is eventually metabolized to carbon dioxide and water. Sodium bicarbonate is usually preferred as an alkalinizing agent.

Uses   Metabolic acidosis.

Contraindications   Congestive heart failure, edema, oliguria, anuria, in patients receiving cortcosteroids, pulmonary edema, metabolic or respiratory alkaloisis, severe hepatic insufficiency, shock, hypoxia, hypernatremia. Lactic acidosis.

Untoward Reactions   Metabolic acidosis (from overtreatment). Reactions at the injection site including infection, thrombosis, phlebitis, extravasation.

Dosage   **IV**. *Highly individualized* and based on blood level of sodium ion. The following formula can be used to estimate correct dose:

$$\begin{array}{l} \text{Dose in ml of 1/6 M sodium} \\ \text{lactate (167 mEq/liter each} \\ \text{of sodium and lactate ions)} \end{array} = \begin{array}{l} (60 - \text{plasma CO 2}) \times \\ (0.8 \text{ body weight in pounds}) \end{array}$$

Alkalinization of urine: **PO**, 30 ml/kg/day in divided doses.

Administration   Administration rate should not exceed 300 ml/hour of 1/6 M solution.

Nursing Implications
Assess patient by observing clinical signs and laboratory results for electrolyte balance.

TROMETHAMINE Tham, Tham-E (Rx)

Classification Systemic alkalinizing agent.

Action/Kinetics Tromethamine, an organic buffering substance and systemic alkalinizing agent, actively binds hydrogen ions, decreasing and correcting acidosis. It promotes the excretion of acids, carbon dioxide, and electrolytes and is thought to be able to neutralize some intracellular acid. It acts as an osmotic diuretic, increasing urine flow. Seventy-five percent of the drug is eliminated within 8 hr, the remainder within 3 days.

Uses Prevention and correction of systemic acidosis, especially that accompanying cardiac bypass surgery and cardiac arrest.

Contraindications Uremia and anuria, pregnancy. Administer with caution to patients with renal disorders.

Untoward Reactions Transient decrease of blood glucose, respiratory depression, alkalosis, fever, hypervolemia. At injection site: extravasation, phlebitis, venous thrombosis, infection. *In newborn:* Hemorrhagic liver necrosis when given by umbilical vein.

Dosage **IV**: Minimum amount to correct acid–base imbalance. The amount of tromethamine can be estimated using the following formula:

$$\frac{\text{ml of 0.3 M tromethamine}}{\text{solution required}} = \frac{\text{body weight (kg)} \times \text{base}}{\text{deficit (mEq/liter)} \times 1.1}$$

Acidosis in cardiac bypass surgery: 500 ml (150 mEq). Severe cases may require 1,000 ml. *Acidosis in cardiac arrest* (given at the same time as other standard procedures are being applied): **if chest is open,** 65–185 ml (2–6 gm) into the ventricular cavity; **if chest closed,** 111–333 (3.6–10.8 gm) into a large peripheral vein.

Administration

1. Tests on blood pH, pCO_2, bicarbonate, glucose, electrolytes should be determined before, during, and after administration of tromethamine.
2. Concentration of solution administered *must not* exceed 0.3 M.
3. Prepare a 0.3 M solution of tromethamine by adding 1,000 ml of sterile water for injection to 36 gm of lyophilized tromethamine.
4. Infuse slowly.
5. Administer into the largest antecubital vein through a large needle or indwelling catheter and elevate limb.
6. For treatment of cardiac arrest, the drug may be injected into the ventricular cavity if the chest is open. If the chest is not open, the drug may be injected into a large peripheral vein.
7. Do not administer longer than 1 day unless acute life-threatening situation exists.
8. Discontinue administration *immediately*, if extravasation occurs. The treatment for extravasation is administration of 1% procaine hydrochloride with hyaluronidase to reduce venospasm and dilute drug in local tissues. Phentolamine mesylate (Regitine) has been used for local infiltration for its adrenergic blocking properties. If necessary, a nerve block of the autonomic fibers may be done.

Nursing Implications

1. *Assess*

   a. for respiratory depression and have equipment for mechanical ventilation readily available.

   b. for weakness, moist pale skin, tremors, and a full bounding pulse, symptoms of hypoglycemia after rapid or high dosage of drug.

   c. for nausea, diarrhea, tachycardia (later bradycardia), oliguria, weakness, numbness or tingling, symptoms of hyperkalemia, more likely to occur in patients with impaired renal function.

2. Ascertain that blood chemistries are done before, during, and after administration of drug and monitor results.

POTASSIUM-REMOVING RESIN

SODIUM POLYSTYRENE SULFONATE   Kayexalate, SPS (Rx)

Classification   Ion exchange resin (potassium).

Action/Kinetics   Sodium polystyrene sulfonate is a resin that exchanges sodium ions for potassium ions. The exchange takes place primarily in the large intestine. Treatment with the resin is not very quantitative; excess amounts of potassium, calcium, and magnesium may be removed. Therapy is governed by daily monitoring of serum potassium levels. Therapy is to be discontinued when serum potassium levels have reached 4–5 mEq/liter. Serum calcium determinations are indicated when therapy exceeds 3 days. Sorbitol is often administered concurrently to prevent constipation. **Onset, PO:** 2–12 hrs.

Uses   Hyperkalemia.

Contraindications   Use with caution for patients sensitive to sodium overload (cardiovascular diseases) or for those receiving digitalis preparations since the action of these agents is potentiated by hypokalemia.

Untoward Reactions   *GI:* Nausea, vomiting, constipation, anorexia, diarrhea. Fecal impaction in geriatric patients. *Electrolyte:* Sodium retention, hypokalemia, hypocalcemia, hypomagnesemia. *Other:* Overhydration, pulmonary edema.

Drug Interactions

Interactant	Interaction
Aluminum hydroxide	↑ Chance of intestinal obstruction
Aluminum or magnesium-containing antacids or laxatives	Systemic alkalosis and ↓ effect of exchange resin laxatives

Dosage   **PO (preferred). Adults:** 15 gm suspended in 150–200 ml water 1 to 4 times daily (1 gm resin contains 4.1 mEq sodium). Sorbitol: 10–20 ml of 70% solution q 2 hr initially; then, adjust so two diarrheal stools are produced daily. **Children:** For calculation of dosage, use exchange ratio of 1 mEq of potassium per gram of resin. *High retention enema*: 30–50 gm q 6 hr suspended in 100 ml of 1% methylcellulose solution, 20% dextrose, or 25% sorbitol solution.

Administration/ Storage

1. Give resin suspended in a small amount of water or syrup (3–4 ml/gm resin). If necessary, resin can be administered through a nasogastric tube, either as aqueous suspension, mixed with dextrose, or as a peanut or olive oil emulsion.
2. Rectal administration:
   a. First administer cleansing enema.
   b. To administer medication insert soft large-size rubber tube (French 28) into rectum for distance of 20 cm until well into sigmoid colon and tape in place.
   c. Suspend resin into 100 ml or less of vehicle (see *Dosage*) at body temperature. Administer by gravity while stirring suspension.
   d. Flush suspension that remains in container with 50–100 ml fluid, clamp tube, and leave in place.
   e. Elevate hips—or ask patient to assume knee-chest position (for a short time)—if there is back leakage.
   f. Enema should be kept in colon as long as possible (3 to 4 hours).
   g. Resin is removed by colonic irrigation with 2 quarts of a *nonsodium*-containing solution warmed to body temperature. Returns are drained constantly through a Y tube.
3. Use freshly prepared solutions within 24 hours. Do not heat resin.

Nursing Implications

1. Assess for clinical signs of electrolyte imbalance related to magnesium, calcium, sodium, and potassium, and monitor blood chemistries.
2. Monitor intake and output.
3. Report increased urinary output because this may be an indication of increased potassium excretion, and the use of sodium polystyrene sulfonate may be contraindicated.
4. Encourage patient to retain medication rectally for several hours.

Chapter Seventy

VITAMINS

General Statement Vitamins are divided into fat-soluble (A, D, E, K) and water-soluble (B complex, C) vitamins. Vitamins are necessary for the normal metabolic functioning of the body. Although a normal diet usually provides sufficient vitamins, supplemental vitamins are of value in certain disease states (e.g., malabsorption syndrome, blood dyscrasias), during pregnancy, and for children during maximum periods of growth. However, there is no advantage of giving patients excessive amounts of vitamins and, in fact, may be dangerous if fat-soluble vitamins are given in excess.

The minimum daily requirement (MDR) for most vitamins has been determined and is often used as a standard. The abbreviations RDDA (recommended daily dietary allowance) or RDA are also used.

The body also requires small amounts of certain minerals as iodine, magnesium, iron, calcium, phosphorous, copper, zinc, and manganese.

Nursing Implications

1. Assess particularly the young and elderly, for symptoms of vitamin deficiencies, such as an inflamed tongue or cracks at the corner of the mouth and refer them to medical supervision. (See Table 38 for deficiency symptoms.)

2. *Teach patient and/or family*

   a. to eat a nutritionally sound diet.

   b. the composition of a nutritious diet and foods that may be substituted on low cost diets, as well as how a diet may be adapted to meet a patient's particular physiologic and cultural needs. (See Table 38 for foods high in specific vitamins and minerals.)

   c. how to read labels of vitamin preparations to ascertain that the RDA is met and explain that such vitamins are usually satisfactory for supplementation, unless the physician orders larger doses of a vitamin.

   d. not to overdose with vitamins.

   e. to store vitamins in a cool place in a light-resistant container to minimize loss of potency.

   f. not to take mineral oil at the same time that they ingest fat-soluble vitamins, such as A, D, E, and K because the vitamins will be dissolved in the oil and not be absorbed by the body.

VITAMIN A   Acon, Alphalin, Aquasol A, Dispatabs, Sust-A (Rx and OTC)

Classification Fat-soluble vitamin.

TABLE 38 VITAMINS AND RELATED SUBSTANCES: FUNCTION, U.S. RDA FOR ADULTS, AND FOOD SOURCE

Substance[a]	Use	Good Food Source	Usual Therapeutic Dose
Vitamin A 4,000–5,000 IU Retinol equivalents (RE) 800–1,000 µg	Helps form and maintain healthy function of eyes, skin, hair, teeth, gums, various glands, and mucous membranes. It is also involved in fat metabolism. *Deficiency symptoms:* night blindness, hyperkeratosis of skin, xerophthalmia.	Whole milk, eggs, green leafy vegetables (e.g., spinach, kale, broccoli; turnip greens, brussels sprouts).	Up to 100,000 units/day
Vitamin B$_1$ (thiamine) 1.0–1.5 mg	Helps get energy from food by promoting proper metabolism of sugars. *Deficiency symptoms:* beriberi, peripheral neuritis, cardiac disease	Milk, chicken, fish, red meat, liver, whole grain bread, green leafy vegetables.	5–30 mg/day
Vitamin B$_2$ (riboflavin) 1.2–1.7 mg	Functions in the body's use of carbohydrates, proteins and fats, particularly to release energy to cells. *Deficiency symptoms:* cheilosis, angular stomatitis, dermatitis, photophobia.	Milk, eggs, red meat, liver, whole grain, enriched bread, green leafy vegetables.	10–30 mg/day
Vitamin B$_6$ (pyridoxine) 1.8–2.0 mg	Has many important roles in protein metabolism. It also aids in the formation of red blood cells and proper function of the nervous system, including brain cells. *Deficiency symptoms:* seborrhea-like skin lesions; nerve inflammations, anemias, epileptiform convulsions in infants.	Green leafy vegetables, red meat, whole grains, green beans.	25–100 mg/day
Vitamin B$_{12}$ (cyanocobalamin) 3.0 µg	Helps to build vital genetic material (nucleic acids) for cell nuclei, and to form red	Milk, fish (salt water), red meat, liver, oysters, kidneys.	1–2 µg/day

TABLE 38 (*Continued*)

Substance[a]	Use	Good Food Source	Usual Therapeutic Dose
	blood cells. Essential for normal function of all body cells, including brain and other nerve cells as well as tissues that make red cells. *Deficiency symptoms*: pernicious anemia.		
Folacin 0.4 mg	Assist in the formation of certain body proteins and genetic materials for the cell nucleus, and in the formation of red blood cells. *Deficiency symptoms*: macrocytic anemia (nutritional).	Green leafy vegetables, liver.	1–15 mg/day
Pantothenic acid 10.0 mg	A key substance in body metabolism involved in changing carbohydrates, fats, and proteins into molecular forms needed by the body. Also required for formation of certain hormones and nerve regulating substances. *Deficiency symptoms* (rare): Fatigue, malaise, headache, sleep disturbance, cramps.	Eggs, green leafy vegetables, nuts, liver, kidneys	Unknown
Niacin (niacinamide B₃) 13–19 mg	Present in all body tissues and is involved in energy-producing reactions in cells. *Deficiency symptom*: pellagra	Eggs, red meat, liver, whole grain, whole grain enriched bread.	100–1,000 USP units/day
Biotin 0.30 mg	It is involved in the formation of certain fatty acids and the production of energy from the metabolism of glucose. It is essential for the working of many chemical systems in the body.	Eggs, green leafy vegetables, string beans, kidneys, liver.	

| Vitamin C
60 mg	To help form and keep bones, teeth and blood vessels healthy. It is also important in the formation of collagen, a protein that helps support body structures such as skin, bone and tendon. *Deficiency symptoms:* scurvy (hemorrhage, loose teeth, gingivitis).	Potatoes, green leafy vegetables, lemons, tomatoes, oranges, green peppers, strawberries, cantaloupes.	100–1,000 mg/day
Vitamin D
(including D_2 and D_3)
200–400 I.U.
5–10 μg cholecalciferol | For strong teeth and bones. To help the body use calcium and phosphorus properly. *Deficiency symptoms:* infantile rickets, infantile tetany, osteomalacia. | Milk, egg yolks, tuna, salmon, cod liver oil. | 400–1,600 USP units/day |
| Vitamin E
(tocopherol) 12–15 I.U. | To help normal red blood cells, muscle and other tissues. Protects fat in the body's tissue from abnormal breakdown. *Deficiency symptoms:* abnormal fat deposits, creatinuria, macrocytic anemia (when associated with protein deficiency). | Vegetable oil, whole grains. | Not established |
| Vitamin K (need in human nutrition established but levels have not yet been determined) | For normal blood clotting. *Deficiency symptoms:* hemorrhages, prolonged clotting time. | Green leafy vegetables. | See drug entry |
| Iron
10–18 mg | An essential part of hemoglobin, the protein substance which enables red cells to carry oxygen throughout the body. It is also part of certain important enzymes. | Red meat, egg yolk, liver, green vegetables (e.g., spinach, kale, broccoli, chard, turnip greens, brussels sprouts). | |
| Calcium
800–1,200 mg | To help build strong bones and teeth. Also required for activity of nerve and muscle | Milk, egg yolk, tuna, salmon, cheese. | |

TABLE 38 (Continued)

Substance[a]	Use	Good Food Source	Usual Therapeutic Dose
	cells, including the heart, and for normal blood clotting.		
Phosphorus 800–1,200 mg	Essential in building and maintaining strong teeth and bones, in quick release of energy, in muscle contraction, and in nerve function.	Milk, fish, meat, whole grain.	
Iodine 150 μg	Forms an integral part of hormones produced by the thyroid gland, which is involved in the regulation of cell metabolism.	Seafood (shrimp, oysters, fish) and iodized salt.	
Copper 2.0 mg	Is present in many organs, including the brain, liver, heart and kidneys. It occurs as part of important proteins, including certain enzymes involved in brain and red cell function. Also needed for making red blood cells.	Kidneys, nuts, raisins, chocolate, mushrooms.	
Magnesium 300–400 mg	Is an important constituent of all soft tissues and bones. It helps trigger many vital enzyme reactions in humans.	Broccoli, whole grain enriched bread, meat.	
Zinc 15 μg; Fluorine, Cobalt, Chromium, Selenium, Manganese, Molybdenum	Zinc considered essential every day for normal skeletal growth and tissue repair. Fluorine makes the teeth harder. Cobalt is an integral part of the vitamin B_{12} molecule. The others are needed in a wide variety of body functions.	Whole grains, broccoli, liver, meat, strawberries, oranges.	

[a] Values given are *Recommended Daily Allowances* for individuals over 11 years of age. National Academy of Sciences, 1979.

General Statement The active principle of vitamin A is retinol. One international unit or U.S.P. unit of vitamin A is equivalent to 0.3 μg of retinol or 0.6 μg of beta-carotene; retinol equivalents (RE) are now often used as the standard. Beta-carotene, known as provitamin A, is converted to retinol after absorption from the GI tract. Vitamin A has an important role in night vision, the physiology of the epithelial tissue (prevention of follicular keratosis), and bone growth and regeneration. Vitamin A deficiency can result in night-blindness (xerophthalmia), blindness, growth retardation, thickening of bone, lowered resistance to infection, hyperkeratinization, and tooth malformation. Excess vitamin A can result in hypervitaminosis A, which can be reversed by withdrawal of the vitamin. Regular intake of normal doses of vitamin A or its precursors seems to increase protection from cancer.

Action/Kinetics Retinol combines with opsin (red protein moiety of visual pigment), forming rhodopsin, necessary for darkness adaptation. Absorption of Vitamin A requires bile acids, dietary fat, and pancreatic lipase. It is stored in the liver (Kupffer cells).

Uses Vitamin A deficiency and prophylaxis during periods of high requirement, such as infancy, pregnancy, and lactation. Supplements may also be required in patients with steatorrhea, severe biliary obstruction, cirrhosis of the liver, total gastrectomy and xerophthalmia, nyctalopia, certain hyperkeratoses of the skin, and lowered resistance to infection.

Untoward Reactions Hypervitaminosis A, characterized by the following symptoms: *CNS:* Increased intracranial pressure/pseudotumor cerebri manifested by bulging fontanels, exophthalmos, papilledema, headache, vertigo, irritability, fatigue, malaise, lethargy. *GI:* Anorexia, vomiting, abdominal discomfort. *Dermatologic:* Inflammation of the tongue, lips, and gums; pruritus, erythema, alopecia, drying and cracking of skin, lip fissures, desquamation, increased pigmentation. *Skeletal:* Slow growth, bone pain, premature epiphyseal closure, arthralgia. *Miscellaneous:* Night sweats, hypomenorrhea, jaundice, hepatosplenomegaly, edema of lower extremities. High plasma levels also manifest hypercalcemia, polydipsia, and polyuria.

Drug Interactions

Interactant	Interaction
Corticosteroids	Impairment of wound healing in patients receiving topical vitamin A—systemic vitamin A may inhibit anti-inflammatory effect of systemic corticosteroids
Mineral oil	↓ Absorption of vitamin A from intestine
Oral contraceptives	Oral contraceptives ↑ plasma vitamin A levels

Dosage PO. Adults and children over 8 years: *Severe deficiency with xerophthalmia*, 500,000 IU/day for 3 days; **then**, 50,000 IU/day for 2 weeks; *severe deficiency*: 100,000 IU/day for 3 days; **then**, 50,000 IU/day for 2 weeks. *Follow-up therapy*: 10,000–20,000 IU/day for 2 months. **IM. Adults**: 100,000 IU/day for 3 days; **then**, 50,000 IU/day for 2 weeks. **Pediatric, 1–8 years**: 17,500–35,000 IU/day for 10 days; **infants**, 7,500–15,000 IU/day for 10 days.

VITAMIN B COMPLEX

General Statement This large, assorted group of vitamins is usually considered together because all members are water soluble and all can be obtained from the same sources, such as yeast and liver. Since the individual vitamins have different functions, they shall be considered separately.

Action/Kinetics The B vitamins are *coenzymes*; they have a crucial role in the tricarboxylic (TCA, Krebs or citric acid) cycle—the main metabolic pathways that convert "food" (glucose) to energy (high-energy phosphate bonds).

Drug Interaction Anticoagulants (oral) may interact with B complex vitamins and cause hemorrhage.

CALCIUM PANTOTHENATE (VITAMIN B₅)   Durasil, Pantholin (OTC)

Classification Vitamin B complex.

Action/Kinetics Pantothenic acid acts as a part of coenzyme A, which is a cofactor required for oxidative metabolism of carbohydrates, synthesis and breakdown of fatty acids, sterol synthesis, gluconeogenesis, and steroid synthesis. Pantothenic acid is found in many foods; thus, deficiency in humans has not been observed.

Uses Although specific indications are absent, the drug has been used for the treatment of peripheral neuritis, muscular cramps, during pregnancy, for delirium tremens, systemic lupus erythematosus, and acute cataract disorders.

Contraindication Hemophilia.

Untoward Reaction Allergic symptoms have occurred occasionally.

Dosage PO: 10 mg/day for approximate daily allowance; 20–100 mg/day for experimental purposes.

CYANOCOBALAMIN (VITAMIN B₁₂)   Anacobin,* Bedoz,* Cyanabin,* Redisol, Rubion* (OTC)

CYANOCOBALAMIN CRYSTALLINE (VITAMIN B₁₂)   Bay Bee-12, Berubigen, Betalin 12, Cabadon-M, Cobex, Crystimin-1000, Cyanoject, Cyomin, Dodex, Kaybovite-1000, Pernavit, Redisol, Rubesol-1000, Rubramin PC, Sytobex, Vibal (Rx and OTC)

Classification Vitamin B₁₂.

Action/Kinetics Cyanocobalamin (vitamin B₁₂) is a cobalt-containing substance produced by certain microorganisms, such as *Streptomyces griseus*. The vitamin can also be isolated from liver and is identical to that of the antianemic factor of liver. This vitamin is essential for hematopoiesis, cell reproduction, nucleoprotein and myelin synthesis.

Intrinsic factor is required for adequate absorption of oral vitamin B₁₂ and in pernicious anemia and malabsorption diseases intrinsic factor is administered simultaneously. This vitamin is rapidly absorbed following IM or SC administration. Following absorption, vitamin B₁₂ carried by plasma proteins to the liver where it is stored until required for various metabolic functions.

Products containing less than 500 μg vitamin B₁₂ are nutritional supplements and are not to be used for the treatment of pernicious anemia.

Uses   Pernicious anemia, tropical and nontropical sprue, nutritional macrocytic anemia due to vitamin B_{12} deficiency, certain types of megaloblastic anemia of infancy. Also, in conditions with an increased need for vitamin B_{12} such as thyrotoxicosis, hemorrhage, malignancy, pregnancy, and in liver and kidney disease. Vitamin B_{12} is particularly suitable for the treatment of patients allergic to liver extract.

Note: Folic acid is not a substitute for vitamin B_{12} although concurrent folic acid therapy may be required.

Contraindications   Hypersensitivity to cobalt. Safety and efficacy in pregnancy, lactation, and in children have not been established.

Untoward Reactions   Untoward reactions are manifested following parenteral use. *Allergic:* Urticaria, itching, exanthema, anaphylaxis, shock, death. *Other:* Polycythemia vera, optic nerve atrophy in patients with hereditary optic nerve atrophy, diarrhea, peripheral vascular thrombosis, congestive heart failure, pulmonary edema.

Note: Benzyl alcohol, which is present in certain products, may cause a fatal "gasping syndrome" in premature infants.

Drug Interactions

Interactant	Interaction
Alcohol	↓ Vitamin B_{12} absorption
Aminosalicyclic acid	↓ Vitamin B_{12} absorption
Chloramphenicol	Chloramphenicol ↓ response to vitamin B_{12} therapy
Colchicine	↓ Vitamin B_{12} absorption
Neomycin	↓ Vitamin B_{12} absorption

Dosage   *Cyanocobalamin*, **PO, adults,** *nutritional vitamin B_{12} deficiency*: 25–250 μg daily. *Cyanocobalamin crystalline, vitamin B_{12} deficiency*, **PO**: 1,000 μg/day. *Patients with normal intestinal absorption*: 15 μg/day. **IM**: 30 μg/day for 5 to 10 days; **then** 100–200 μg/month **IM** or **SC** until remission is complete. Higher doses may be necessary in the presence of neurologic or infectious disease, or hyperthyroidism. *Schilling test*: 1,000 μg **IM** (flushing dose).

Administration   Cyanocobolamin crystalline injection should be protected from light and should not be frozen.

Additional Nursing Implications

See also *Nursing Implications*, p. 836.
Teach patient and/or family

a. that repository vitamin B_{12} will provide medication for at least 4 weeks and that additional injections are not required during that period.
b. that the stinging, burning sensation that may occur after injection is transient.

FOLIC ACID   Apo-Folic,* Folvite (Rx and OTC)

LEUCOVORIN CALCIUM (CITROVORUM FACTOR, FOLINIC ACID) Novofolacid,* Wellcovorin (Rx)

Classification   Vitamin B complex.

General Statement Folic acid is required for nucleoprotein synthesis (DNA) and the maintenance of normal levels of mature red cells (erythropoiesis). The vitamin is readily available in a great variety of foods, including liver, kidney, and leafy green vegetables.

Uses Megaloblastic and macrocytic anemia resulting from folic acid deficiency; nutritional macrocytic anemia, megaloblastic anemias of pregnancy, infancy and childhood, and megaloblastic anemia associated with primary liver disease, intestinal obstruction, anastomoses, or sprue. Supplemental folic acid may also be required by patients on renal dialysis or receiving drugs that interfere with folic acid metabolism, such as methotrexate, phenytoin, and barbiturates.

Folic acid is sometimes administered in conjunction with vitamin B_{12} for the treatment of refractory or aplastic anemia.

Contraindication Vitamin B_{12}-deficiency anemias (e.g., pernicious, aplastic, or normocytic anemias).

Untoward Reactions *Allergic:* Erythema, skin rash, itching, malaise, respiratory difficulties, bronchospasms. High doses may cause: *GI:* Anorexia, nausea, distention, flatulence, bad taste in mouth. *CNS:* Excitement, altered sleep patterns, difficulty in concentration, irritability, overactivity, mental depression, confusion, and impaired judgement.

Note: Pernicious anemia may be obscured with doses of folic acid of 1 mg or more daily.

Drug Interactions

Interactant	Interaction
Aminosalicylic acid	↓ Effect of folic acid due to ↓ absorption from GI tract
Phenytoin	↓ Effect of phenytoin due to ↑ rate of breakdown by liver; also, phenytoin may ↓ plasma folate levels
Sulfasalazine	↓ Effect of folic acid due to ↓ absorption from GI tract

Dosage *Folic acid.* **PO, usual:** 0.25–1 mg daily. **Maintenance (per day), infants:** 0.1 mg; **children 4 years and less:** 0.3 mg; **adults and children over 4 years:** 0.4 mg; **pregnancy or lactation:** 0.8 mg. The dose may need to be increased in alcoholics, and patients with hemolytic anemia, chronic infections, or anticonvulsant therapy. Folic acid should be administered by **deep IM, SC, or IV** in the presence of severe malabsorption.

Leucovorin calcium. **IM:** *Megaloblastic anemia:* 1 mg/day. *Overdose of folic acid antagonists:* **usual for methotrexate effects, IM or PO,** 10 mg/m²; **then, PO,** 10 mg/m² q 6 hr for 3 days. **For trimethoprim or pyrimethamine effects: PO,** 5–15 mg/day.

Administration/Storage

1. Store folic acid solutions in a cold place.
2. Leucovorin calcium injection diluted with bacteriostatic water for injection should be used within one week. If water for injection is employed, the solution should be used immediately.

HYDROXOCOBALAMIN Acti-B12,* Alphamin, Alpha Redisol, Codroxomin, Droxomin, Hybalamin, Hydrobexan, Hydro-Cobex, Hydroxo-12, LA-12, Vibal L.A. (Rx)

Classification Vitamin B complex.

General Statement This synthetic compound can be converted to cyanocobalamin by the body and has the same therapeutic function as cyanocobalamin. Hydroxocobalamin is absorbed more slowly from the injection site and its action is thought to be more prolonged.

Uses Same as cyanocobalamin. *Investigational:* Prophylaxis and treatment of cyanide toxicity due to sodium nitroprusside.

Untoward Reactions Pain at injection site, transient diarrhea; rarely allergic reaction.

Dosage *Hydroxocobalamin crystalline,* **IM only. Adults:** 30 μg/day for 5 to 10 days; **then,** 100–200 μg/month. **Pediatric:** 100 μg doses up to a total of 1–5 mg over 2 or more weeks; **then,** 30–50 μg q 4 weeks. Concurrent folic acid therapy may be required.

NICOTINAMIDE (NIACINAMIDE)   (Rx: Injection; OTC: Tablets)

NICOTINIC ACID (NIACIN)   Niac, Nico-400, Nicobid, Nicolar, Nico-Span, Nicotinex, Span-Niacin-150, Tega-Span (Rx and OTC)

Classification Vitamin B complex.

Action/Kinetics Nicotinic acid and nicotinamide are water-soluble, heat-resistant vitamins prepared synthetically. Niacin is a component of the coenzymes NAD and NADP, which are essential for oxdiation-reduction reactions involved in lipid metabolism, glycogenolysis, and tissue respiration. Deficiency of niacin results in pellagra, the most common symptoms of which are dermatitis, diarrhea, and dementia. In high doses niacin also produces vasodilation and a reduction in serum lipids. **Peak serum levels:** 45 min; **t½:** 45 min.

Uses *Nicotinic acid:* Pellagra or prophylaxis thereof. Hyperlipidemia. It has been used as a vasodilating agent but its value has not been well documented. Megadoses have been used to treat schizophrenia although there is no evidence for effectiveness.
   Nicotinamide: Pellagra and prophylaxis thereof.

Contraindications Hypotension, hemorrhage, liver dysfunction, peptic ulcer. Use with caution in diabetics, gall bladder disease, and patients with gout.

Untoward Reactions *GI:* Nausea, vomiting, diarrhea, peptic ulcer activation, abdominal pain. *Dermatologic:* Flushing, warm feeling, skin rash, pruritus, dry skin, itching and tingling feeling, keratosis nigricans. *Other:* Hypotension, headache, macular cystoidedema, amblyopia.

Note: Megadoses are accompanied by serious toxicity including the symptoms listed above as well as liver damage, hyperglycemia, hyperuricemia, arrhythmias, tachycardia, and dermatoses.

Drug Interaction

Interactant	Interaction
Sympathetic blocking agents	↑ Vasodilatory effect → postural hypotension

Dosage *Nicotinic acid.* **PO.** *Niacin deficiency:* 10–20 mg daily. *Pellagra:* up to 500 mg daily. *Hyperlipidemia:* 1.0–2.0 gm t.i.d. up to maximum of 6 gm/day. **IV (pre-**

ferred), **IM, SC.** *Vitamin deficiency* **only:** 0.1–3 gm daily depending on severity of deficiency. The length of parenteral therapy depends on patient response and on how soon oral therapy and a well-balanced diet can be instituted.

Nicotinamide. **PO, IM:** 50 mg 3–10 times/day.

Administration

1. Nicotinic acid should be taken orally only with cold water (no hot beverages).
2. Can be taken with meals if GI upset occurs.

Nursing Implications

1. Explain to patients that flushing is a frequent side effect.
2. Advise patients who feel weak and dizzy after taking niacin to lie down until they are feeling recovered and then to inform physician.

PYRIDOXINE HYDROCHLORIDE (VITAMIN B₆)   Beesix, Hexa-Betalin, Nestrex, Pyroxine, Vitabee-6 (Rx: Injection; OTC: Tablets)

Classification   Vitamin B complex.

Action/Kinetics   Pyridoxine hydrochloride is a water-soluble, heat-resistant vitamin. It is destroyed by light. It is prepared synthetically. It acts as a coenzyme in the metabolism of protein, carbohydrates, and fat. As the amount of protein increases in the diet, the pyridoxine requirement increases. **t½:** 2–3 weeks.

Uses   Irradiation sickness. Prophylaxis of isoniazid-induced peripheral neuritis. Infants with epileptiform convulsions. Hypochromic anemias due to familial pyridoxine deficiency, some cases of hypochromic or megaloblastic amemias.

Drug Interactions

Interactant	Interaction
Cycloserine	↑ Pyridoxine requirements
Hydralazine	↑ Pyridoxine requirements
INH (isoniazid)	↑ Pyridoxine requirements
Levodopa	Daily doses exceeding 5 mg pyridoxine antagonize the therapeutic effect of levodopa
Oral contraceptives	↑ Pyridoxine requirements
Penicillamine	↑ Pyridoxine requirements

Dosage   *Dietary deficiency,* **PO, IM, IV:** 10–20 mg daily for 3 weeks; **then,** 2–5 mg/day for several weeks. *Adjunct in the administration of isoniazid to prevent neuropathy:* 6–25 mg/day (up to 50 mg daily may be used); *established neuropathy:* 50–200 mg/day. *Vitamin B₆ dependency syndrome:* **initial,** up to 600 mg/day; **then** 30 mg/day for life.

Additional Nursing Implications

See also *Nursing Implications* for *Vitamins,* p. 836.

1. Consult with doctor for orders for pyridoxine supplementation when patient is receiving cycloserine, isoniazid, or oral contraceptives.
2. *Teach patient and/or family*

a. those foods high in B_6. See Table 38, p. 837.
b. that a patient only on levodopa therapy should not take vitamin supplements containing vitamin B_6, because more than 5 mg antagonizes effect of levodopa.
c. that pyridoxine may inhibit lactation.

RIBOFLAVIN (VITAMIN B₂)   Riobin-50 (Rx: Injection; OTC: Tablets)

Classification   Vitamin B complex.

General Statement   Riboflavin is a water-soluble, heat-resistant substance. It is sensitive to light. Riboflavin acts as a coenzyme for various tissue respiration reactions. Riboflavin deficiency is characterized by characteristic lesions of the tongue, lips and face, photophobia, itching, burning and keratosis of the eyes. Riboflavin deficiency often accompanies pellagra.

Uses   Riboflavin deficiency. Adjunct, with niacin, in the treatment of pellagra.

Drug Interactions

Interactant	Interaction
Chloramphenicol	Riboflavin may counteract bone marrow depression and optic neuritis due to chloramphenicol
Tetracyclines	Antibiotic activity ↓ by riboflavin

Dosage   **PO.** *Dietary supplement:* **Adults and children over 12 years of age**: 5–10 mg/day. **IM.** *Deficiency:* **usual,** 50 mg.
Note: The urine may show a yellow discoloration.

THIAMINE HYDROCHLORIDE (VITAMIN B₁)   Baybee-1, Biamine (Rx: Injection; OTC: Tablets/Elixir)

Action/Kinetics   Water-soluble vitamin, stable in acid solution. The vitamin is decomposed in neutral or acid solutions. Thiamine is required for the synthesis of thiamine pyrophosphate a coenzyme required in carbohydrate metabolism.

Uses   Thiamine deficiency states and associated neurologic and cardiovascular symptoms. Prophylaxis and treatment of beriberi. Alcoholic neuritis, neuritis of pellagra, and neuritis of pregnancy. To correct anorexia due to thiamine insufficiency.

Untoward Reaction   Serious hypersensitivity reactions can occur; thus, intradermal testing is recommended if sensitivity is suspected. *Dermatologic:* Pruritus, urticaria, sweating, feeling of warmth. *CNS:* Weakness, restlessness. *Other:* Nausea, tightness in throat, angioneurotic edema, cyanosis, hemorrhage into the GI tract, pulmonary edema, cardiovascular collapse. Death has been reported.

Drug Interaction   Since vitamin B_1 is unstable in neutral or alkaline solutions, the vitamin should not be used with substances as citrates, barbiturates, or carbonates that yield alkaline solutions.

Dosage   **PO.** *Dietary supplement:* 5–30 mg/day. **IM.** *Beriberi:* 10–20 mg t.i.d. for 2 weeks; **then, PO:** 5–10 mg/day for 1 month. **IV.** *Wet beriberi with myocardial failure:* 30 mg t.i.d.

Additional Nursing Implication

See also *Nursing Implications*, p. 836.
   Be prepared with epinephrine to treat anaphylactic shock should it occur after a large parenteral dose of thiamine.

VITAMIN C

ASCORBATE CALCIUM   (OTC)

ASCORBATE SODIUM   Cenolate, Cevita (Rx: Injection; OTC: Oral products)

ASCORBIC ACID   Arco-Cee, Ascorbicap, Best-C, C-Caps 500, Cecon, Ceebate, Cemill, Cetane, Cevalin, Cevi-Bid, Ce-Vi-Sol, Cevita, C-Long Granucaps, C-Span, Dull-C, Flavorcee, Redoxon,* Schiff Effervescent Vitamin C, Vita-C (Rx: Injection; OTC: Oral products)

General Statement   Vitamin C (ascorbic acid) is a specific antiscorbutic, substance. The vitamin is unstable and easily destroyed by air, light, and heat. Vitamin C is essential to the maintenance of the connective and supporting tissue of the body.
   Vitamin C deficiency leads to scurvy, which is characterized by changes in the fibrous tissues, the matrix of dentine, bone, cartilage, and the vascular endothelium.
   The stores of vitamin C in the body are depleted very rapidly and patients on IV feeding may develop ascorbic acid deficiency. This may cause a delay in healing in patients who have undergone surgery. Due to an increased rate of oxidation during infectious diseases, the daily requirements of vitamin C rise.

Uses   Treatment of scurvy and prophylaxis thereof. Vitamin C supplementation is indicated for burn victims, debilitated patients, and as an adjunct in iron therapy and in patients on prolonged IV feedings.
   Large doses of vitamin C have been indicated for treating cancer and to prevent the common cold; however, current data do not support these uses.

Untowards Reactions   *Large or megadoses*: Diarrhea, renal stones (oxalate, urate). Rapid IV administration may cause transitory faintness and dizziness.

Drug Interactions

Interactant	Interaction
Acidic drugs	Large doses of ascorbic acid ↑ reabsorption of acid drugs in kidney → ↑ effect

Interactant	Interaction
Amphetamine	↓ Effect of amphetamine by ↓ renal tubular reabsorption
Antidepressants, tricyclic	↓ Effect of tricyclics by ↓ renal tubular reabsorption
Basic drugs	Large doses of ascorbic acid ↓ reabsorption of basic drugs in kidney → ↑ effect
Dicoumarol	Ascorbic acid may influence the intensity and duration of action
Digitalis	Calcium ascorbate may cause cardiac arrhythmias in patients receiving digitalis
Disulfiram	Ascorbic acid may interfere with the action of disulfiram
Ethinyl estradiol	↑ Effect of ethinyl estradiol
Salicylates	↑ Effect of salicylates by ↑ renal tubular reabsorption
Smoking	↑ Need for vitamin C
Sulfonamides	↑ Chance of crystallization of sulfonamides in urine
Warfarin	Ascorbic acid ↓ effect of warfarin

Laboratory Test Interference Megadoses may cause false − urine glucose determinations (glucose oxidase method) or false + (copper reductase or Benedict's solution).

Dosage **PO, IM, IV.** *Prophylaxis:* **Adults,** 70–150 mg/day; **infants,** 30 mg. *Scurvy:* **Adults,** 0.3–1 gm/day; **infants,** 0.1–0.3 gm/day. *Enhance wound healing:* **Adults,** 0.3–0.5 gm/day for 7–10 days both pre- and postoperatively. *Burns:* **Adults,** individualized; *severe burns:* 1–2 gm/day.

Administration
1. Sodium ascorbate can be administered IM or IV.
2. Calcium ascorbate should never be injected SC. IM injection may cause tissue necrosis in infants.

Additional Nursing Implications
See also *Nursing Implications*, p. 836.
  Be alert to the many drug interactions with vitamin C.

VITAMIN D

Classification Fat-soluble vitamin.

General Statement Vitamin D, the antirachitic factor, has a key role in controlling calcium and phosphorus metabolism. The regulating (homeostatic) effect on calcium serum levels is such that it is now considered to have hormonal activity.
  In the presence of sunlight (UV irradiation) humans can synthesize vitamin D

in the skin from a variety of plant and animal sterols. Under ideal circumstances intake of exogenous vitamin D may not be necessary. Irradiated milk and fish liver oils, however, are excellent sources of the vitamin.

Vitamin D deficiency is characterized by inadequate absorption of calcium and phosphate. During periods of active growth, vitamin D deficiency may lead to rickets. In adults, vitamin D deficiency may result in osteomalacia (adult rickets).

Several compounds have vitamin D activity. The most important of these are calcitriol, calcifediol, cholecalciferol (D_3), dihydrotachysterol, and ergocalciferol (D_2).

Action/Kinetics   Vitamin D analogs, along with parathyroid hormone and calcitonin, regulate serum calcium levels by increasing absorption of calcium (and phosphorous), increasing resorption of calcium by bone, and increasing reabsorption of calcium and phosphate by the kidney. In addition, dihydrotachysterol increases absorption of calcium from the intestine and mobilizes calcium in the absence of parathyroid hormone.

Uses   See individual agents.

Contraindications   Impaired renal or cardiac function, arteriosclerosis, concomitantly with digitalis glycosides, hypercalcemia. Vitamin D toxicity.

Untoward Reactions   Physiologic doses are virtually without adverse effects. However, excessive doses produce severe toxicity due to hypercalcemia. *GI:* Anorexia, dry mouth, nausea, vomiting, cramps, diarrhea or constipation, metallic taste, weight loss. *CNS:* Fatigue, weakness, drowsiness, headache, vertigo, ataxia, irritability, decreased libido, seizures. *CV:* Arrhythmias, hypertension. *Other:* Tinnitus, exanthema, muscle and bone pain, rhinorrhea, pruritus, nephrocalcinosis, impaired renal function, osteoporosis (adults), anemia, photophobia, decreased growth in children, pancreatitis, calcification of blood vessels.

Treatment of Overdose   Immediate discontinuation of therapy, institution of a low calcium diet, and withdrawal of any calcium supplements. To increase excretion of calcium, give IV fluids, acidify urine, or administer a loop diuretic (e.g., ethacrynic acid, furosemide, others).

In acute accidental overdosage, induction of emesis or gastric lavage is beneficial if the overdose is discovered within a short time; also, administration of mineral oil may increase fecal excretion of the drug.

Drug Interactions

Interactant	Interaction
Antacids (magnesium-containing)	↑ Risk hypermagnesemia
Cholestyramine	↓ Effect vitamin D due to ↓ absorption from GI tract
Corticosteroids	↓ Effects of vitamin D
Digitalis	Hypercalcemia may ↑ risk of arrhythmias
Phenobarbital	↓ Effect of vitamin D due to ↑ breakdown by liver
Phenytoin	↓ Effect of vitamin D due to ↑ breakdown by liver
Thiazides	↑ Risk of hypercalcemia
Verapamil	Hypercalcemia may ↑ risk of atrial fibrillation

Laboratory Test Interference   Toxic doses of vitamin D analogs may ↑ urinary calcium, phosphate, albumin: also, ↑ BUN, serum cholesterol, SGOT, SGPT. ↓ Serum alkaline phosphatase.

Dosage   See individual agents.

Nursing Implications

See also *Nursing Implications* for *Vitamins,* p. 836.
Teach patient and/or family

a. to have blood and urine tests performed periodically as ordered to evaluate calcium, magnesium, phosphorus, and alkaline phosphatase levels.

b. to avoid magnesium-containing antacids.

c. to withhold drug and report to medical supervision if weakness, nausea, vomiting, dry mouth, constipation, muscle pain, bone pain, or a metallic taste (early symptoms of vitamin D intoxication) occur.

d. to take medication in dosage prescribed since the dosage for each patient is highly individualized.

e. to adhere to diet and calcium supplementation recommended.

f. to avoid nonprescription medications unless prescribed by medical supervision.

g. the necessity for light diet, plenty of fluids, and laxatives to facilitate elimination of excessive calcium from the body.

CALCIFEDIOL   Calderol (Rx)

Action/Kinetics   Absorbed from the intestine. t½: 16 days. **Duration:** 15–20 days. Excreted mainly by the bile.

Uses   Metabolic bone disease, hypocalcemia in patients on chronic renal dialysis.

Dosage   PO: 300–350 μg/week in divided daily or alternate daily dosage; if no response, increase at 4-week intervals. Patients with normal serum calcium may respond to 20 μg q other day.

CALCITRIOL   Rocaltrol (Rx)

Action/Kinetics   Onset: 2 hr. **Peak effect:** 10 hr. **Duration:** 3–5 days. t½: **7–12 hr.**

Uses   Hypocalcemia in patients on chronic renal dialysis. Hypoparathyroidism or pseudohypoparathyroidism. *Investigational:* Vitamin D dependent rickets (especially in children), Vitamin D resistant rickets, hypocalcemia in premature infants.

Dosage   PO. *Hypocalcemia in renal dialysis:* **Adults, initial,** 0.25 μg/day; **then,** if necessary, increase by 0.25 μg/day at 4–8 week intervals. Some may respond to 0.25 μg on alternate days. *Hypoparathyroidism/pseudohypoparathyroidism:* **Adults and children over 1 year, initial,** 0.25 μg/day; **maintenance, adults and children over 6 years of age:** 0.5–2 μg/day; **children, 1–5 years:** 0.25–0.75 μg/day.

CHOLECALCIFEROL (VITAMIN D₃)   Delta-D (OTC)

Action/Kinetics   Bile is necessary for maximum absorption. Excreted primarily by the bile.

Uses Prophylaxis or treatment of Vitamin D deficiency (i.e., osteomalacia, rickets), dietary supplement.

Dosage Recommended daily dietary allowances: **Adults,** 5–10 μg; **pregnancy/lactation:** 10–15 μg; **pediatric:** 10 μg.

DIHYDROTACHYSTEROL DHT, Hytakerol (Rx)

Action/Kinetics **Onset:** slow, 7–10 days. Maximum effect occurs up to 2 weeks after daily administration. **Duration:** 2 weeks. One milligram dihydrotachysterol equals 3 mg ergocalciferol.

Uses Hypophosphatemia, hypocalemia due to chronic renal disease, hypoparathyroidism, pseudohypoparathyroidism, osteoporosis (with sodium fluoride).

Dosage **PO.** *Hypophosphatemia:* **Adults and children, initial:** 0.5–2 mg/day until bones heal; **then,** 0.2–1.5 mg/day. Phosphate salts may also be given. *Hypoparathyroidism or pseudohypoparathyroidism:* **Adults, initial:** 0.75–2.5 mg/day for several days; **maintenance:** 0.2–1 mg/day. Some patients may require 1.5 mg/day. **Pediatric: initial,** 1–5 mg/day for 4 days; **maintenance:** 0.5–1.5 mg/day. *Chronic renal failure:* 0.1–0.6 mg/day. *Osteoporosis:* 0.6 mg/day with calcium and fluoride.

ERGOCALCIFEROL (VITAMIN D₂) Calciferol, Deltalin, Drisdol, Ostoforte* (Rx and OTC)

Action/Kinetics Serum calcium levels should be maintained between 9–10 mg/dl. **Onset (PO, IM):** 10–24 hr. **Peak effect:** 4 weeks after daily dosage. **Duration:** 2 months or longer. **t½:** 24 hr. Bile is required for absorption. Excreted mainly by the bile. One milligram ergocalciferol is equivalent to 40,000 USP units.

Uses Rickets, osteomalacia, hypophosphatemia, hypocalcemia due to chronic renal disease, hypoparathyroidism, pseudohypoparathyroidism, osteoporosis, dietary supplement.

Dosage *Rickets/osteomalacia,* **PO:** 25 μg/day, although up to 125 μg/day have been given. *Severe malabsorption or deficiency,* **PO,** 0.25–7.5 mg/day or **IM,** 0.25 mg/day. **Pediatric: PO,** 0.25–0.625 mg/day. *Hypophosphatemia:* **PO, initial,** 1–2 mg/day with phosphate salts; **then,** increase daily dose at 3–4 month intervals by 0.25–0.5 mg. **Maintenance, adults:** 0.25–1.5 mg/day. *Osteoporosis:* **PO,** 0.025–0.25 mg/day or 1.25 mg 2 times/week; use with calcium and fluoride supplements. *Hypoparathyroidism or pseudohypoparathyroidsim:* **PO, adults,** 0.625–5 mg/day with calcium supplements and/or parathyroid hormone; **pediatric:** 1.25–5 mg with calcium. To prevent toxicity, reduce dosage as soon as serum calcium approaches normal levels. *Renal failure:* **PO, initial,** 0.5 mg; **then,** adjust depending on serum calcium levels (range: 0.25–7.5 mg daily). **Pediatric: maintenance,** 0.1–1 mg daily. *Dietary supplement:* **PO, adults, healthy children, infants,** 10 μg/day. **Premature infants:** For normal bone development, 12–20 μg/day, although doses up to 750 μg/day may be necessary.

VITAMIN E

VITAMIN E (TOCOPHEROL, TOCOPHEROL ACETATE)   Aquasol E, Cen-E, E-Ferol, E-Ferol Succinate, Epsilan-M, E-Vital, Pheryl-E, Viterra E (Rx: Injection; OTC: Oral products)

General Statement   Vitamin E refers to a group of fat-soluble substances, including the powerful antioxidants alpha-, beta-, gamma-, and delta-tocopherol. The exact physiologic function of vitamin E is difficult to ascertain. Deficiency symptoms have been studied mainly in animals.

The usefulness of the vitamin for therapeutic purposes is questionable. However, it is consumed in large amounts by food faddists.

Uses   Prophylaxis and treatment of vitamin E deficiency. *Topical:* Minor skin disorders such as burns, diaper rash, sunburn, abrasions, itching; deodorant. *Investigational:* Premature infants to reduce toxicity of oxygen therapy on the lung parenchyma and retina. Decrease severity of hemolytic anemia in infants.

Contraindications   None known.

Untoward Reactions   Large doses over prolonged periods may cause skeletal muscle weakness, disturbances of reproductive functions, and GI upset.

Drug Interactions

Interactant	Interaction
Anticoagulants, oral	Vitamin E ↑ effect of anticoagulants
Iron Therapy	Vitamin E ↓ response to iron therapy

Dosage   **PO, Parenteral: Usual**, RDA, **children 4–6 years**: 9 IU; **adult males**: 15 IU, **adult females**: 12 IU; **pregnancy or lactation**: 15 IU.

Note: Potencies of products differ widely; thus, dosage should be based on equivalent international units. **Topical**: Apply as needed and rub in lightly.

Administration   Topical products are available as creams, liquids, oils, and ointments.

VITAMIN K

Classification   Fat-soluble vitamin, blood clotting factor.

Action/Kinetics   Vitamin K is essential for the hepatic synthesis of prothrombin and factors VII, IX, and X, all of which are essential for blood clotting. The chief manifestation of vitamin K deficiency is an increase in bleeding tendency. This is demonstrated by ecchymoses, epistaxis, hematuria, GI bleeding, postoperative and intracranial hemorrhage.

Vitamin K is available as phytonadione (vitamin K_1) and menadione (vitamin K_3), both of which are synthetic lipid-soluble analogs. In addition, menadiol sodium diphosphate (vitamin K_4), a water-soluble synthetic analog, is available.

Uses   Primary and drug-induced hypoprothrombinemia, especially that caused by anticoagulants of the coumarin and phenindione type. Vitamin K cannot reverse the anticoagulant activity of heparin.

Parenteral use for Vitamin K malabsorption syndromes. Adjunct during whole blood transfusions. Preoperatively to prevent the danger of hemorrhages in surgical patients who may require anticoagulant therapy.

Certain forms of liver disease. Hemorrhagic states associated with obstructive jaundice, celiac disease, ulcerative colitis, sprue, and GI fistulas.

Contraindications Severe liver disease. Use with caution in neonates.

Untoward Reactions *Allergic:* Rash, urticaria, anaphylaxis. *After PO use:* Nausea, vomiting, stomach upset, headache. *After parenteral use:* Flushing, alteration of taste, sweating, hypotension, dizziness, weak pulse, dyspnea, cyanosis, delayed skin reactions. Hyperbilirubinemia and fatal kernicturus may occur in the newborn.

Drug Interactions

Interactant	Interaction
Antibiotics	Antibiotics may inhibit the body's production of vitamin K and may lead to bleeding. Vitamin K supplements should be given
Anticoagulants, oral	Vitamin K antagonizes anticoagulant effect
Cholestyramine	↓ Effect of phytonadione and menadione due to ↓ absorption from GI tract
Mineral oil	↓ Effect of phytonadione and menadione due to ↓ absorption from GI tract

MENADIOL SODIUM DIPHOSPHATE (K₄)   Synkayvite (Rx)

MENADIONE (K₃)   (Rx)

Classification Vitamin K.

Action/Kinetics Precursors of blood-clotting factors. Menadiol sodium diphosphate is water soluble and is converted to menadione in the body; it is one-half as potent as menadione. Menadione is lipid soluble. Both may be absorbed directly into the bloodstream even in the absence of bile. Menadiol sodium diphosphate: **Onset, IM, SC**: 1–2 hr. **Duration** (normal prothrombin time): 8–24 hr. **IV**, onset faster than IM, SC, **duration**: shorter.

Contraindications Last weeks of pregnancy or during labor as a prophylaxis against hypoprothrombinemia or hemorrhagic disease of the newborn. Use in infants.

Additional Untoward Reaction Hemolysis of red blood cells in patients with glucose 6-phosphate dehydrogenase deficiency.

Laboratory Test Interference Falsely elevated urinary 17-hydroxycorticosteroid levels (Reddy, Thorn, and Jenkins procedure).

Dosage *Menadione*. **PO**: 5–10 mg/day. Not for use in infants.
   Menadiol sodium diphosphate. **PO**: *Hypoprothrombinemia due to obstructive jaundice and biliary fistulas*: 5 mg/day; *hypoprothrombinemia due to antibacterial/salicylate use:* 5–10 mg/day. **IM, IV, SC**: *Hypoprothrombinemia*, **adults**: 5–15 mg, 1–2 times/day; **children**: 5–10 mg, 1–2 times/day.

PHYTONADIONE (VITAMIN K₁)   Aqua-Mephyton, Konakion, Mephyton (Rx)

Classification Fat soluble vitamin.

Action/Kinetics Phytonadione is similar to natural vitamin K. It has a more rapid and more prolonged effect than menadione and menadiol sodium diphosphate and is generally more effective. GI absorption requires the presence of bile salts. Heparin may be used to reverse overdosage of phytonadione. Frequent determinations of prothrombin time are indicated during therapy. **Onset: PO,** 6–12 hr; **IM, IV:** 1–2 hr. *Control of bleeding:* Parenteral, 3–8 hr. Normal prothrombin time: 12–14 hr.

Additional Uses Prothrombin deficiency due to oral anticoagulants, hemorrhagic disease of the newborn.

Additional Untoward Reactions IV administration may cause severe reactions leading to death. May be transient flushing of the face, sweating, a sense of constriction of the chest, and weakness. Cramplike pain, weak and rapid pulse, convulsive movements, chills and fever, hypotension, cyanosis, or hemoglobinuria have been reported occasionally. Shock, cardiac, and respiratory failure may be observed.

Dosage PO, IM, IV, SC. IV administration is reserved for emergency situations; rate of **IV** administration should not exceed 1 mg/min. **IM and SC** administration are indicated for patients unsuitable for **PO** therapy.

Anticoagulant-induced hypoprothrombinemia: (1) In the absence of bleeding, **PO, IM, or SC:** 2.5–10 mg or more (up to 25 mg). Repeat after 12 to 48 hr if prothrombin time has not reached normal levels. (2) In the presence of hemorrhage or threatened hemorrhage, **IV:** 10–50 mg; **children:** 5–10 mg. *Preoperatively to offset effects of anticoagulant therapy,* **PO, IM, SC** (given 24 hr before surgery): 5–25 mg; **IV** (12 hr before surgery): 10–25 mg or more.

Prophylaxis of hemorrhagic disease of the newborn, **IM, to mother:** 1–5 mg 12 to 24 hr prior to delivery; or, **IM, to newborn:** 0.5–2 mg. *Treatment of acute hemorrhagic disease of newborn:* **SC, IM,** 1–2 mg for several days. *Hypoprothrombinemia from other causes:* 2–25 mg (up to 50 mg may be necessary in some); route of administration and duration of treatment depends on severity of the condition.

Administration/Storage

1. Store injectable emulsion or colloidal solutions in cool, 5°–15°C (41°–59°F), dark place.
2. Do not freeze.
3. Protect vitamin K from light. IV should be completed within 2 to 3 hours.
4. Do not administer faster than 1 mg/minute by IV.
5. Mix emulsion only with water or D₅W.
6. Mix colloidal solution with D₅W, isotonic sodium chloride injection, or dextrose and sodium chloride injection.

Additional Nursing Implications

See also *Nursing Implications* for *Vitamins*, p. 836.

1. Check that prothrombin times are being done while the patient is on therapy and have therapy evaluated.
2. Assess patient, during parenteral administration, for sweating, transient flushing of face, a sense of constriction of chest, weakness, tachycardia, hypotension which may progress to shock, cardiac arrest, and respiratory failure.

Chapter Seventy-one

HEAVY METAL ANTAGONISTS

General Statement   Heavy metals are toxic because they bind to reactive sites, thus inactivating important substances, such as enzymes. Heavy metal antagonists have the ability to bind (chelate) the metal ions to form a nontoxic complex that is eliminated by the kidneys.

Heavy metal poisoning occurs as a consequence of overdosage from drugs such as gold compounds (used to treat rheumatoid arthritis) and iron (used to treat anemias) as well as accidental ingestion of substances such as lead-containing paint, arsenic-containing weed-killers, and pesticides.

DEFEROXAMINE MESYLATE   Desferal Mesylate (Rx)

Classification   Heavy metal antagonist (iron chelator).

Action/Kinetics   Deferoxamine, a complex organic molecule, binds to iron thus preventing iron from entering various chemical reactions. The resulting chelate is water soluble and is excreted by the kidneys as well as in the feces via the bile. Adequate renal function is necessary for effectiveness.

Uses   Adjunct in treatment of acute iron intoxication. Chronic iron overload including thalessemia. *Investigational:* Accumulation of aluminum in renal failure and in encephalopathy due to aluminum.

Contraindications   Severe renal disease, anuria. Use with caution for patients with pyelonephritis. Should not be used in children under the age of 3 years unless mobilization of 1 mg iron/day or more can be shown. Should *not* be used to treat primary hemochromatosis.

Untoward Reactions   *Allergic:* Rash, itching, wheal formation, anaphylaxis. *GI:* Abdominal discomfort, diarrhea. *Other:* Dysuria, blurred vision, leg cramps, fever, tachycardia.

Following rapid IV use: Hypotension, urticaria, erythema. *Following SC use:* Local pain, erythema, swelling, pruritus, skin irritation.

Dosage   *Acute iron intoxication*: **IM (preferred), initial,** 1 gm; **then,** 0.5 gm q 4 hr for 2 doses; if necessary, then give 0.5 gm q 4–12 hr, not to exceed 6 gm/day. **IV infusion** (*only in emergencies as cardiovascular collapse*): Same as IM at a rate not to exceed 15 mg/kg/hr. Begin IM therapy as soon as possible. *Chronic iron overload*: **IM,** 0.5–1.0 gm/day; **SC,** 1–2 gm (20–40 mg/kg/day) given by mini-infusion pump over 8–24-hr period; **IV,** 2 gm (given separately but at same time as each unit of blood); IV rate not to exceed 15 mg/kg/hr. **Pediatric: IM, IV,** 50 mg/kg q 6 hr or **continuous IV,** 15 mg/kg/hr to a maximum of 6 gm/day or 2 gm/dose.

Administration

1. Dissolve deferoxamine mesylate by adding 2 ml of sterile water to each ampule.
2. For IV administration use physiologic saline, or Ringer's lactated solution and administer *slowly* at a rate not exceeding 15 mg/kg/hour.
3. Discard dissolved drug if not used within 1 week.
4. Pain and induration may occur at IM injection site.

Nursing Implications

1. *Assess*
   a. for adequate urine flow before initiating therapy.
   b. patient with a history of pyelonephritis for pain and hematuria caused by deferoxamine, which may induce an exacerbation of the disease.
   c. patient in shock and report. Physician may transfer to IM administration after recovery from shock.
2. Have epinephrine readily available for allergic-type reactions.
3. In the presence of iron intoxication and/or acidosis, be prepared to assist with induction of emesis, gastric lavage, suction, maintenance of airway, and administration of IV fluid and blood.
4. Teach patient and/or family that drug may give urine a reddish color.
5. Anticipate that pain and induration at the site of administration may occur.

DIMERCAPROL   Bal In Oil (Rx)

Classification Heavy metal antagonist.

Action/Kinetics Dimercaprol forms a chelate with arsenic, mercury, and gold. Since arsenic has a greater affinity for dimercaprol than sulfhydryl-containing enzymes, toxicity is prevented. To be fully effective, the drug should be administered as soon after poisoning is noted. **Peak plasma concentration: IM**, 30–60 min. Mostly distributed to extracellular fluid. Rapidly metabolized to inactive product and completely excreted in urine and feces in 4 hr.

Uses Acute arsenic, mercury and gold poisoning, resulting from overdosage with mercurial diuretics, arsenicals, gold salts, accidental ingestion of mercury, arsenic, or gold-containing salts. Wilson's disease. With EDTA in acute lead poisoning.

Contraindications Iron, cadmium, or selenium poisoning. Hepatic insufficiency. Use with caution in the presence of renal insufficiency and in patients with glucose 6-phosphate dehydrogenase deficiency.

Untoward Reactions *CV:* Most common including hypertension and tachycardia. *GI:* Nausea, vomiting, salivation, abdominal pain, burning feeling of the lips, mouth and throat. *CNS:* Anxiety, weakness, restlessness. *Other:* Constriction and pain in the throat, chest, or hands; sweating, conjunctivitis, blepharal spasm, lacrimation, rhinorrhea, tingling of hands, burning feeling in the penis, sterile abscesses.

Children may also develop fever. At very high doses dimercaprol may cause coma or convulsions and metabolic acidosis.

Drug Interactions

Interactant	Interaction
Cadmium salts	
Iron salts	Dimercaprol may increase toxicity
Selenium salts	of these heavy metal salts
Uranium salts	

Laboratory Test Interference Iodine-131 thyroidal uptake ↓ during and immediately after dimercaprol therapy.

Dosage **Deep IM only.** *Mild arsenic and gold poisoning*: 2.5 mg/kg q.i.d. for days 1 and 2; b.i.d. on day 3; once daily for 10 days thereafter or until recovery is complete. *Severe arsenic or gold poisoning*: 3 mg/kg q 4 hr for days 1 and 2; q.i.d. on day 3; b.i.d. for 10 days. *Mercury poisoning*: **initial**, 5 mg/kg, **then** 2.5 mg/kg 1 or 2 times daily for 10 days. *Acute lead encephalopathy*: 4 mg/kg alone initially; **then** q 4 hr in combination with EDTA administered in a separate site.

Administration

1. Check with physician whether a local anesthetic may be given with IM injection to minimize pain at injection site.
2. Inject IM deeply into muscle and massage after injection.
3. Anticipate that the medication has an unpleasant garliclike odor.
4. Do not allow fluid to come in contact with skin as it may cause a skin reaction.
5. Urine should be kept alkaline to reduce possibility of kidney damage.

Nursing Implications

1. *Assess*
   a. for adequate urine flow before initiating therapy.
   b. BP, pulse, and temperature to assist in evaluating response to medication.
2. Reassure patient experiencing untoward GI or CNS symptoms that these effects will pass within 30–90 minutes. Provide supportive care.
3. Have ephedrine and/or an antihistamine available for premedication or for later use if patient should experience an untoward reaction.

EDETATE CALCIUM DISODIUM (CALCIUM EDTA) Calcium Disodium Versenate, Calcium EDTA (Rx)

Classification Heavy metal antagonist.

Action/Kinetics Calcium disodium edetate displaces lead and cadmium from biologic molecules and body tissues. It is used primarily for lead poisoning, but also for zinc, copper, chromium, manganese, and nickel. It is ineffective in mercury or arsenic poisoning. It also combines with free heavy metal ions in the extracellular fluid. Lead excretion: **Onset:** 1 hr after IV therapy. **Peak lead excretion:** 24–48 hr. EDTA is mainly distributed in extracellular fluid and excreted unchanged or as metal chelate in urine. t½, **IV**, 20–60 min; **IM**, 1.5 hr.

Uses Acute lead poisoning and lead encephalopathy (sometimes in conjunction with dimercaprol); diagnosis of lead poisoning. Effective in reducing the incidence of residual neurologic damage. Chronic lead poisoning.

Contraindication   Anuria. Women of child-bearing age, pregnancy.

Untoward Reactions   Few side effects are noted when drug is administered at prescribed dosage levels. The greatest danger is renal tubular necrosis that may occur when drug is given at too high dosage and increased intracranial pressure following rapid IV administration in patients with cerebral edema.

Other side effects include: malaise, fatigue, excessive thirst, numbness and tingling, followed by sudden fever and shaking chills, myalgia, arthralgia, headache, GI disturbances, and transitory allergic manifestations. Thrombophlebitis.

Prolonged administration may cause kidney damage, transient bone marrow depression, GI disturbances, and mucocutaneous lesions.

Dosage   **IV. Adults**: for mild symptoms or asymptomatic, give 1,000 mg (5 ml amp) diluted with 250–500 ml normal saline or 5% dextrose over a period of 1 hr. Can be given twice/day for 5 days; **then** rest period of 2 days followed by 5 more days of treatment. **IM (route of choice for children)**: 0.5 gm/30 lb b.i.d. (equivalent to 75 mg/kg/day); for milder cases, do not exceed 50 mg/kg/day; pediatric dosage should be given in divided doses q 8–12 hr for 3–5 days; a second course can be given after a rest period of 4 or more days.

Administration

1. **IV.** Administer to asymptomatic adults over a period of 1 hour b.i.d. and to symptomatic adults over a period of 2 hours b.i.d. For symptomatic adults, excess fluids should be avoided.

2. **IM.** Procaine, to achieve a concentration of 0.5%, can be added to IM injections to reduce pain at the injection site.

3. If the patient is dehydrated from vomiting, urine flow should be established by IV infusion prior to the initiation of EDTA therapy. Once the drug has been administered, fluids should be kept to basal levels.

4. If administered together for lead encephalopathy, EDTA calcium and dimercaprol should be given at separate deep IM sites.

Nursing Implications

1. **Never exceed the recommended daily dose, because edetate calcium disodium may produce toxic and potentially fatal reactions**.

2. *Assess*
   a. for adequate urine flow before initiating therapy.
   b. intake and output. Withhold drug and report to physician if anuria occurs.
   c. results of daily urine analysis for proteinuria, hematuria, and renal casts. Should these occur, withhold drug and report to physician.
   d. pulse regularly for cardiac arrhythmias that may be caused by medication.

3. Provide large amounts of milk orally to facilitate removal of lead salts from the gut if lead has been ingested. Enemas are also administered to hasten removal of lead.

4. Check that x-ray film is taken before initiation of EDTA therapy to ascertain that all lead has been removed from gut.

5. Unless contraindicated, encourage fluid intake to facilitate excretion of lead.

6. Avoid contact of calcium EDTA with contaminated skin of patient, because contact increases systemic absorption.

7. Check that tests for BUN are done periodically to detect renal damage.

8. Check that serum lead levels are performed periodically to evaluate drug response. Children with lead levels above 40 μg/100 ml of blood require treatment.

EDETATE DISODIUM (EDTA)   Chealamide, Disotate, Endrate (Rx)

Classification   Heavy metal antagonist.

Action/Kinetics   Edetate disodium has a great affinity for calcium, forming a soluble chelate that is rapidly excreted by the kidneys. It also forms chelates with magnesium, zinc, and other trace elements. In addition, it increases the excretion of potassium although a chelate is not formed.

Uses   Emergency treatment of hypercalcemia. Ventricular arrhythmias in digitalis toxicity.

Contraindications   Use with caution in patients with heart disease or hypokalemia. Anuric patients; patients with ventricular arrhythmias. Safety in pregnancy has not been established.

Untoward Reactions   Electrolyte imbalance including hypocalcemia, hypokalemia, hypomagnesemia may occur during treatment. *CV:* Decrease in both systolic and diastolic pressure, thrombophlebitis, anemia. *GI:* Nausea, vomiting, diarrhea. *CNS:* Headache, numbness, circumoral paresthesia, fever. *Other:* Hyperuricemia, exfoliative dermatitis, nephrotoxicity, hemorrhagic tendencies.

Rapid injection may produce hypocalcemic tetany and convulsions, respiratory arrest, and severe arrhythmias.

Laboratory Test Interference   ↓ Alkaline phosphatase levels.

Dosage   **IV**: Individualized and depending on degree of hypercalcemia. **Recommended maximum dose, adult**: 50 mg/kg up to a total of 3 gm daily for a period of 5 days, followed by a rest period of 2 days. Course may be repeated, if necessary, to a total of 15 doses. **Children**: 40 mg/kg up to a maximum of 70 mg/kg/day.

Administration

1. Administer to patient in Fowler's position.
2. Check label on vial carefully that drug is disodium edetate and not calcium disodium edetate.
3. Dilute medication in 500 ml of 5% dextrose solution or isotonic saline solution as ordered.
4. Infuse slowly over 3 to 4 hours.
5. Do not extend the recommended dose, concentration, or rate of administration.

Nursing Implications

1. Record which vein is used for site of administration as repeated use of the same vein is likely to result in thrombophlebitis. Greater dilution of the solution and slower administration reduces the incidence of thrombophlebitis if the same vein must be used.
2. Monitor BP during infusion as a transitory hypotension may occur, which would necessitate lowering the patient until hypotension has passed and blood pressure stabilized.
3. Be alert to a generalized systemic reaction that may occur from 4 to 8 hours after infusion of the drug and usually subsides within 12 hours. Report such a reaction and provide supportive care for fever, chills, back pain, vomiting, muscle cramps, or urinary urgency should they occur.
4. Teach diabetic patients that drug may cause hypoglycemia and that physician should be consulted whether to reduce insulin or increase food intake should patient feel hypoglycemic or urine test be negative for sugar.

PENICILLAMINE   Cuprimine, Depen (Rx)

Classification   Heavy metal antagonist, antiarthritic, to treat cystinuria. See Chapter 39, p. 510.

Chapter Seventy-two

MISCELLANEOUS DRUGS

ADENOSINE PHOSPHATE (ADENOSINE 5-MONOPHOSPHATE, AMP)
Adeno Cobalasine, Soraden (Rx)

Action/Kinetics   The adenosine phosphates are essential to the energy economy of muscle tissue. The therapeutic effects of adenosine phosphate in reducing tissue edema and inflammation are believed to result from increasing levels of adenosine triphosphate (ATP) or from its vasodilator effect and ability to decrease edema and inflammation.

Uses   Adjunct in treatment of varicose vein ulcers, stasis dermatitis, and chronic thrombophlebitis (pre- and postoperatively). Tenosynovitis, intractable pruritus, and multiple sclerosis, when other measures fail.

Contraindications   Myocardial infarction, cerebral hemorrhage. Use with caution in patients with a history of asthma and in pregnancy. Safe use in children has not been determined.

Untoward Reactions   *CNS:* Dizziness, headaches. *GI:* Nausea, epigastric distress, diarrhea. *Other:* Flushing, diuresis, palpitations, rash, hypotension, dyspnea, increased symptoms of bursitis or tendinitis. Local reaction at injection site.

Dosage   IM only. Initial: 25–50 mg/day or 50 mg three times/week; **maintenance:** 25 mg 2–3 times/week.

Nursing Implications

1. Be alert to complaints of dyspnea and tightness in chest after injection, indications of an allergic reaction. Discontinue medication and promptly treat with epinephrine, oxygen, and corticosteroids.
2. Assess patient for reduction of edema.
3. Assess patient for reduction of inflammation.

ALPROSTADIL   Prostin VR Pediatric (Rx)

Classification   Prostaglandin.

Action/Kinetics   Alprostadil is one of the prostaglandins that are naturally occuring acidic lipids. Alprostadil relaxes smooth muscle of the ductus arteriosus leading to increased pulmonary blood flow with increased blood oxygenation and lower body perfusion. Patients with low pO_2 values respond best. The drug may also cause vasodilation, inhibit platelet aggregation, and stimulate both intestinal and uterine smooth muscle. Alprostadil is rapidly metabolized by oxidation in the lung, and metabolites are excreted by the kidney.

Uses   For temporary maintenance of patency of the ductus arteriosus (until surgery can be performed) in neonates with congenital heart defects.

Contraindications   Respiratory distress syndrome (hyaline membrane disease). Use with caution in neonates with bleeding tendencies.

Untoward Effects   *CNS:* Apnea, especially in neonates less than 2 kg at birth, fever, seizures, hypothermia, jitteriness, lethargy, cerebral bleeding, stiffness, hyperextension of the neck. *CV:* Flushing, especially after intra-arterial dosage, bradycardia, hypotension, tachycardia, cardiac arrest and edema, congestive heart failure, shock, arrhythmias. *Respiratory:* Respiratory depression or distress, wheezing, hypercapnea, bradypnea. *GI:* Diarrhea, hyperbilirubinemia, gastric regurgitation. *Renal:* Hematuria, anuria. *Skeletal:* Cortical proliferation of long bones. *Hematologic:* Disseminated intravascular coagulation, thrombocytopenia, anemia, bleeding. *Miscellaneous:* Sepsis, peritonitis, hypoglycemia, hypokalemia, or hyperkalemia.

Dosage   Continuous IV infusion or umbilical artery: Initial, 0.1 μg/kg/min; **then,** after response achieved, decrease infusion rate to lowest dose that will maintain response (e.g., 0.1 to 0.05 to 0.025 to 0.01 μg/kg/min).

Note: If 0.1 μg/kg/min is insufficient, dosage can be increased up to 0.4 μg/kg/min.

Administration/Storage

1. Administer only in pediatric intensive care facilities.
2. Dilute with either sodium chloride injection or dextrose injection in volumes appropriate for infant's fluid intake and suitable for type of infusion pump available. Use a "Y" set up.

3. Discard unused solution and prepare a fresh infusion solution every 24 hours.
4. Store ampules at 2–8°C (36–46°F).

Nursing Implications
1. Assess cardiac function, blood pressure, and respiratory function by electric monitor.
2. Remain with infant during first hour of infusion when apnea is most likely to occur.
3. Have respirator available at bedside.
4. Monitor arterial pressure intermittently by umbilical artery catheter, auscultation, or with a Doppler transducer. Reduce rate of infusion immediately if arterial pressure falls significantly. Obtain guidelines for arterial pressures from physician.
5. Assess for overdosage manifested by apnea, bradycardia, pyrexia, hypotension, and flushing.
   a. if apnea or bradycardia occur, stop drug administration and switch to unmedicated solution. Start resuscitation if indicated and report to physician.
   b. if pyrexia or hypotension occur, reduce IV flow rate and report to physician. Anticipate that IV flow rate will be reduced until temperature and blood pressure return to at least baseline values.
   c. if flushing occurs, report to physician as this is an indication of incorrect intra-arterial placement of the catheter. The catheter may require repositioning.
6. Evaluate response of infant with restricted pulmonary blood flow by monitoring blood gases. A positive response to alprostadil would be indicated by at least a 10 mm Hg increase in blood pO_2.
7. Evaluate response of infant with restricted systemic blood flow by monitoring systemic blood pressure and blood pH. A positive response to alprostadil would be indicated by an increased pH in acidotic infants, increase in blood pressure, and decreased ratio of pulmonary artery pressure to aortic pressure.

AZATHIOPRINE Imuran (Rx)

Classification Immunosuppressant.

Action/Kinetics Antimetabolite that is quickly split to mercaptopurine. To be effective, the drug must be given during the induction period of the antibody response. Precise mechanism in depressing the immune response is unknown but it suppresses cell-mediated hypersensitivities causing changes in antibody production. Is readily absorbed from the GI tract. The anuric patient manifests increased effectiveness and toxicity (up to twofold).

Uses Prophylaxis to prevent rejection of kidney transplants. Rheumatoid arthritis (adults only). *Investigational:* Chronic ulcerative colitis.

Contraindications Treatment of rheumatoid arthritis in pregnancy or in patients previously treated with alkylating agents. Pregnancy.

Untoward Reactions *Hematologic:* Leukopenia, thrombocytopenia. *GI:* Nausea, vomiting, diarrhea, steatorrhea. *Other:* Increased risk of carcinoma, severe infections, and hepatotoxicity are major side effects. Less frequent: Skin rashes, fever, alopecia, arthralgias, negative nitrogen balance.

Drug Interactions

Interactant	Interaction
Allopurinol	Allopurinol ↑ pharmacologic effect of azathioprine due to ↓ breakdown in liver
Corticosteroids	With azathioprine, it may cause muscle wasting after prolonged therapy
Tubocurarine	Azathioprine ↓ effect of tubocurarine

Dosage *Kidney transplantation*. **PO, IV**: *individualized*, **Initial** (usual): 3–5 mg/kg daily; **maintenance**: 1–3 mg/kg daily. *Rheumatoid arthritis*. **PO: initial**, 50–100 mg (about 1 mg/kg) 1–2 times/day. After 6–8 weeks and thereafter every 4 weeks, increase 0.5 mg/kg/day up to maximum of 2.5 mg/kg/day; maintenance therapy: lowest effective dose. Dosage should be reduced in patients with renal dysfunction.

Administration

1. When used for rheumatoid arthritis, the patient should be considered refractory if no beneficial effect is seen after 12 weeks.
2. The injection is for IV use only. It should be reconstituted with sterile water for injection and used within 24 hr.

Nursing Implications

1. *Assess*
   a. for liver dysfunction. Drug may have to be discontinued if jaundice appears.
   b. intake and output.
   c. daily weight.
   d. for signs of rejection of kidney transplant, manifested by decrease in urine volume and creatinine clearance.
2. Report oliguria.
3. Encourage increased fluid intake.

BETA-CAROTENE   Solatene (Rx)

Classification Vitamin A precursor.

Action/Kinetics Beta-carotene eliminates the photosensitivity reaction (burning sensation, edema, erythema, pruritus, and/or cutaneous lesions) in patients suffering from erythropoietic protoporphyria (edema produced by exposure to sunlight). Patients receiving beta-carotene develop yellowing of the skin, but not of the sclera. The protective effect of the drug becomes apparent 2 to 6 weeks after initial administration and persists 1 to 2 weeks after discontinuance.

Uses Erythropoietic protoporphyria (EPP).

Contraindications Hypersensitivity to drug, pregnancy. Use with caution in patients with impaired renal and hepatic function and in pregnancy.

Untoward Reactions Yellowing of skin starting with palms of hands, soles of feet and face. Loose stools.

Dosage **PO**: *individualized*, **Adults**, 30–300 mg daily as single or divided dose; **children under 14 years**: 30–150 mg daily.

Administration
1. Administer with meals.
2. Mix contents of capsule with orange juice or tomato juice for those unable to swallow capsules.

Nursing Implications
1. *Teach patient and/or family*
   a. not to ingest additional vitamin preparations of vitamin A, since beta-carotene fills normal vitamin A requirements.
   b. not to increase exposure to sun for 2 to 6 weeks after initiation of therapy (until palms and soles turn yellow, as patient becomes carotemic), and to expose himself to the sun gradually, because protective effect is not complete, and each individual must establish limits of exposure.

BROMOCRIPTINE MESYLATE   Parlodel (Rx)

Classification   Prolactin secretion inhibitor; dopamine receptor agonist.

Action/Kinetics   Bromocriptine is a nonhormonal agent that inhibits the release of the hormone prolactin by the pituitary. The drug should be used only when prolactin production by pituitary tumors has been ruled out. Its effect in parkinsonism is due to a direct stimulating effect on dopamine receptors in the corpus striatum.

Less than 30% of the drug is absorbed from the GI tract. **Peak plasma concentration**: 1–1.5 hr. **t½ (biphasic)**: first t½, 4–4½ hr; **second t½**: 45–50 hr. Metabolized in liver, excreted mainly through bile and thus the feces.

Uses   Short-term treatment of amenorrhea/galactorrhea associated with hyperprolactinemia. Prevention of physiologic lactation. Parkinsonism. Female infertility. *Investigational*: Acromegaly.

Contraindications   Sensitivity to ergot alkaloids. Pregnancy, lactation, children under 15 years of age. Peripheral vascular disease, ischemic heart disease. Use with caution in liver disease.

Untoward Reactions   *GI:* Nausea, vomiting, abdominal cramps, diarrhea, constipation. *CNS:* Headache, dizziness, fatigue, lightheadedness, syncope. When used for parkinsonism: Abnormal voluntary movements, hallucinations, confusion, asthenia, ataxia, insomnia, depression, vertigo, nightmares, seizures. *CV:* Hypotension. *Other:* Nasal congestion, shortness of breath.

Drug Interactions

Interactant	Interaction
Alcohol	↑ Chance of GI toxicity; alcohol intolerance
Antihypertensives	Additive effects decrease BP
Diuretics	Should be avoided during bromocriptine therapy
Phenothiazines	Should be avoided during bromocriptine therapy

Laboratory Test Interference   ↑ BUN, SGOT, SGPT, GGPT, CPT, alkaline phosphatase, uric acid.

Dosage   **PO**. *Amenorrhea/galactorrhea/female infertility*: 2.5 mg b.i.d.–t.i.d. with meals. For amenorrhea/galactorrhea, do not use for more than 6 months. To reduce side effects, start with 2.5 mg/day and increase to full dose within 1 week. *Prevention of lactation* (begin no sooner than 4 hr after delivery): 2.5 mg b.i.d. with meals; therapy should be continued for 14–21 days. *Parkinsonism*: **Initial**, 1.25 mg (one-half tablet) b.i.d. with meals while maintaining dose of levodopa, if possible. Dosage may be increased q 14–28 days by 2.5 mg/day with meals. Dose should not exceed 100 mg/day.

Administration

1. During treatment contraception (other than oral contraceptives) should be practiced.
2. The first dose should be taken lying down due to the possibility of fainting or dizziness.

Nursing Implications

1. Advise use of contraceptive measures other than "the pill" while patient is receiving bromocriptine.
2. Schedule for pregnancy tests every 4 weeks during period of amenorrhea and after resumption of menses when a menstrual period is missed.
3. Alert patient to signs and symptoms of pregnancy and advise withholding drug and reporting to medical supervision, should these occur, since pregnancy tests may fail to diagnose early pregnancy, and the medication may harm the fetus.

CHENODIOL (CHENODEOXYCHOLIC ACID)   Chenix (Rx)

Classification   Naturally occurring human bile acid.

Action/Kinetics   Chenodiol, by reducing hepatic synthesis of cholesterol and cholic acid, replaces both cholic and deoxycholic acids in the bile acid pool. This effect helps desaturation of biliary cholesterol and leads to dissolution of radiolucent cholesterol gallstones. The drug is ineffective on calcified gallstones or on radiolucent bile pigment stones. Fifty percent of patients have stone recurrence within 5 years.

Chenodiol is well absorbed following oral administration. It is metabolized by bacteria in the colon to lithocholic acid, most of which is excreted in the feces.

Uses   Patients with radiolucent cholesterol gallstones in whom surgery is a risk due to age or systemic disease. The drug is ineffective in some patients and has potential liver toxicity. The best results have been seen in thin females with a serum cholesterol not higher than 227 mg/dl and who have a small number of radiolucent cholesterol gallstones.

Contraindications   Known hepatic dysfunction or bile ductal abnormalities. Pregnancy or in those who may become pregnant. Safety and efficacy in lactation and children have not been established.

Untoward Reactions   Hepatotoxicity including increased SGPT in one-third of patients, intrahepatic cholestasis. *GI:* Diarrhea (common), anorexia, constipation, dyspepsia, flatulence, heartburn, cramps, epigastric distress, nausea/vomiting, abdominal pain. *Hematologic:* Decreased white cell count. Chenodiol may contribute to colon cancer in susceptible patients.

Drug Interactions

Interactant	Interaction
Antacids, aluminum	↓ Effect of chenodiol due to ↓ absorption from GI tract
Cholestyramine	See Antacids
Clofibrate	↓ Effect of chenodiol due to ↑ biliary cholesterol secretion
Colestipol	See Antacids
Estrogens, oral contraceptives	↓ Effect of chenodiol due to ↑ biliary cholesterol secretion

Dosage **PO. Initial:** 250 mg b.i.d. for 2 weeks; **then,** increase by 250 mg weekly until maximum tolerated or recommended dose is reached (13–16 mg/kg/day in 2 divided doses morning and night).

Note: Doses less than 10 mg/kg are usually ineffective and may result in increased risk of cholecystectomy.

Administration

1. Periodic liver function tests and monitoring for stone dissolution should be performed.
2. Diarrhea may be relieved by reducing the dose temporarily or by using anti-diarrheal agents.
3. The physician should be informed immediately of symptoms of gallstone complications: severe, sudden upper quadrant pain radiating to shoulder; nonspecific abdominal pain; or, nausea/vomiting.

Nursing Implications

Teach patient and/or family

1. that drug may be taken for 24 months before gallstones dissolve.
2. that gallstones may recur, even when the drug treatment has been successful.
3. to notify physician if there is any question that conception has occurred while on drug.
4. that while pregnancy should be avoided during drug therapy, oral contraceptives may decrease the effectiveness of the drug.
5. the importance of periodic visits to the physician for liver function tests and possibly cholocystograms.
6. not to use antacids without consultation with physician; most antacids have an aluminum base, which adsorbs the drug.

CHYMOPAPAIN FOR INJECTION   Chymodiactin, Discase (Rx)

Classification Proteolytic enzyme.

General Statement Chymopapain is a proteolytic enzyme derived from the crude latex of *Carica papaya*. The nanoKatal (nKat) is used as the unit of chymopapain activity (1 mg of chymopapain is equivalent to at least 0.52 nKat units). The preparation also contains sodium L-cysteinate hydrochloride as a reducing agent to keep the sulphur in the sulphydryl form.

Chymopapain should be used only in a hospital setting by physicians and supportive personnel trained in the diagnosis and treatment of lumbar disc disease as well as in the management of potential side effects from chymopapain.

Action/Kinetics Chymopapain is injected into the herniated lumbar intervertebral disc (nucleus pulposus) where it hydrolyzes the noncollagenous proteins or polypeptides that maintain the structure of the chondromucoprotein of the nucleus pulposus. As a result of hydrolysis, the osmotic activity is decreased leading to a reduction of intradiscal pressure and a decrease in fluid absorption.

Although chymopapain acts locally in the disc, it does appear in the plasma where it is inactivated. Small amounts are excreted in the urine.

Uses Treatment of herniated lumbar intervertebral discs that have not responded to more conservative therapy.

Contraindications Sensitivity to chymopapain, papaya, or its derivatives. Severe spondylolisthesis, spinal cord tumor or a cauda equina lesion, or in progressing paralysis manifested by rapidly progressing neurologic dysfunction. Patients previously treated with chymopapain. Injection into any location other than lumbar area.

Untoward Reactions *Neuromuscular:* Back pain, stiffness, soreness, back spasm, paraplegia, acute transverse myelitis or myelopathy characterized by onset of paraplegia or paraparesis (without prior symptoms) within 2–3 weeks. Also, sacral burning, leg pain, hyperalgesia, leg weakness, tingling/numbness in legs/toes, cramping in both calves, paresthesia, pain in opposite leg. *Allergic:* Anaphylaxis (more common in females). Complications secondary to anaphylaxis including staphylococcal meningitis with disc abscess. Rash, itching, urticaria. *Other:* Cerebral hemorrhage, nausea, paralytic ileus, urinary retention, headache, dizziness.

Drug Interactions Possible arrhythmias if used with halothane or epinephrine.

Dosage A single injection of 2–5 nKat units/disc (maximum dose with multiple disc herniation is 10 nKat units).

Administration

1. An open IV line must always be available in the event of anaphylaxis. Epinephrine is the drug of choice to treat anaphylaxis.
2. Sterile water for injection should be used for reconstitution as bacteriostatic water for injection inactivates the enzyme.
3. Automatic filling syringes should not be used since a residual vacuum is present in the vial.
4. Alcohol should be used to cleanse the vial stopper before inserting the needle; since alcohol inactivates the enzyme, it should be allowed to dry before continuing with reconstitution.
5. The package literature should be consulted for specific procedures for administration.

Nursing Implications

1. Assess blood pressure and respiratory status since drug can cause hypotension and bronchospasms.
2. *Teach patient and/or family*
   a. that back pain and muscle spasms may occur several days to several weeks after treatment.
   b. that paraplegia and paresis may occur suddenly several weeks after treatment. Report immediately to physician.

CYCLOSPORINE   Sandimmune (Rx)

Classification   Immunosuppressant.

Action/Kinetics   Cyclosporine is an immunosuppressant thought to act by inhibiting the immunocompetent lymphocytes in the G_0 or G_1-phase of the cell cycle. T-lymphocytes are specifically inhibited. Cyclosporine also inhibits interleukin 2 or T-cell growth factor production and release. **Peak plasma levels:** 3.5 hr. **t½:** Approximately 19 hr. Metabolized by the liver.

Uses   In combination with corticosteroids for prophylaxis of rejection in kidney, liver, and heart transplants.

Contraindications   Hypersensitivity to cyclosporine or polyoxyethylated castor oil. Lactation. Use with caution in pregnancy.

Untoward Reactions   *GI:* Nausea, vomiting, diarrhea, gum hyperplasia, anorexia, gastritis, hiccoughs, peptic ulcer, abdominal discomfort. *Hematologic:* Leukopenia, lymphoma, thrombocytopenia. *Allergic:* Anaphylaxis (rare). *CV:* Hypertension, edema. *CNS:* Headache, tremor, confusion, fever, seizures. *Other:* Nephrotoxicity, hepatotoxicity, acne, hirsutism, flushing, paresthesia, sinusitis, gynecomastia, conjunctivitis, brittle fingernails, hearing loss, tinnitus, hyperglycemia, muscle pain, infections.

Drug Interactions

Interactant	Interaction
Amphotericin B	↑ Plasma level of cyclosporine due to ↓ breakdown by liver
Cimetidine	↑ Plasma level of cyclosporine due to ↓ breakdown by liver
Ketoconazole	↑ Plasma level of cyclosorine due to ↓ breakdown by liver
Nephrotoxic drugs	Additive nephrotoxicity
Phenobarbital	↓ Plasma level of cyclosporine due to ↑ breakdown by liver
Phenytoin	↓ Plasma level of cyclosporine due to ↑ breakdown by liver
Rifampin	↓ Plasma level of cyclosporine due to ↑ breakdown by liver
Sulfatrimethoprim	↓ Plasma level of cyclosporine due to ↑ breakdown by liver

Laboratory Test Interference   ↑ Serum creatinine, BUN, total bilirubin, alkaline phosphatase, serum potassium.

Dosage   **PO. Adults and children, initial:** 15 mg/kg/day given 4–12 hr prior to transplantation; **then,** 15 mg/kg/day postoperatively for 1–2 weeks followed by 5% decrease in dose per week to maintenance of 5–10 mg/kg/day. **IV (only in patients unable to take PO medication):** 5–6 mg/kg/day 4–12 hr prior to transplantation and postoperatively until patient can be switched to PO dosage.
Note: Steroid therapy must be used concomitantly.

Administration

1. The oral solution may be diluted with milk, chocolate milk, or juice immediately before being administered.
2. The IV concentration should be diluted 1 ml in 20–100 ml 0.9% sodium chloride injection or 5% dextrose injection. The IV solution is given by slow IV infusion over 2–6 hr.

3. Due to variable absorption of the oral solution, blood levels of cyclosporine should be monitored.

4. Due to the possibility of anaphylaxis, patients receiving IV cyclosporine should be closely monitored for 30 min following the initiation of the infusion. Epinephrine (1:1,000) should be available at the bedside for treating anaphylaxis.

5. Patients with malabsorption from the GI tract may not achieve appropriate blood levels.

Nursing Implications

1. Because this drug is so important to a patient with a transplant, patient and family should have a written list of all possible side effects of drugs and know which need to be reported to the physician.

2. Oral solutions need to be mixed with milk or juice to make more palatable and should be drunk immediately after mixing.

DIMETHYLSULFOXIDE (DMSO)   Kemsol,* Rimso-50 (Rx)

Classification   Organic solvent.

Action/Kinetics   DMSO is a clear liquid miscible with both water and most organic solvents. It is widely used as an industrial solvent and has many pharmacologic effects, including nerve blockade, bacteriostasis, diuresis, inhibition of cholinesterase, muscle relaxation, and vasodilation. It also penetrates membranes readily. The drug is currently indicated only for symptomatic relief of interstitial cystitis. Its use for musculoskeletal disorders is widely debated, and conclusive evidence for its efficacy is lacking. DMSO is used for these disorders on an investigational basis; the compound is distributed by certain clinics outside the United States, and is available through mail order houses in the United States.

Widely distributed after topical administration. **Onset:** rapid. DMSO and its metabolite are excreted through the urine and feces; DMSO is also excreted through the skin and lungs and gives off a garlic-type odor.

Uses   Symptomatic relief of interstitial cystitis. *Investigational*: Musculoskeletal disorders, collagen diseases as scleroderma, and as a carrier to increase the percutaneous absorption of other drugs.

Contraindications   Pregnancy, lactation. Safety in children not established.

Untoward Reactions   *After topical use:* Nausea, vomiting, sedation, headache, rashes, burning or aching eyes. Garliclike taste and breath. Transient chemical cystitis. Discomfort following administration (usually subsides with repeated use).

Drug Interaction   ↓ Effect of sulindac due to ↓ rate of conversion to active metabolite.

Dosage   *Cystitis*. Instillation of 50 ml of DMSO every 2 weeks until symptomatic relief is achieved. *Musculoskeletal disorders*: Application of 50–90% solution or gel to skin.

Administration

1. Use analgesic lubricant, such as lidocaine jelly, in urethra before inserting catheter to prevent spasms.

2. Dilute DMSO immediately before instillation in glass vessel. Use 1 part DMSO to 1 part of sterile water.

3. Solution is to be retained by patient for 15 min and then expelled by voiding.

4. For patient who is not relieved by the usual treatment, the doctor may order the following: Distend the bladder gently by gravity instillation of 500 ml of 1 part DMSO and 1 part sterile water mixed in a glass delivery container before instilling the standard 50 ml undiluted dose of DMSO. Instruct patient to retain fluid for 15 min and then void.

5. A patient with a sensitive bladder may require administration of an oral analgesic, a belladonna and opium suppository, or anesthesia.

Nursing Implications

1. Explain to patient that instillation may cause moderately severe discomfort that will lessen with repeated administration.

2. Report if patient experiences an unusual amount of discomfort or increased discomfort; doctor may plan to provide analgesia or anesthesia.

3. Ensure that ophthalmic examination is done prior to and periodically during course of therapy.

4. Ensure that liver and kidney function tests are done every 6 months.

5. Inform patient that he may note a garliclike taste after instillation and that a garliclike odor may persist on the breath and skin for 72 hr after treatment.

DISULFIRAM   Antabuse (Rx)

Classification   Treatment of alcoholism.

Action/Kinetics   Disulfiram (Antabuse) produces severe hypersensitivity to alcohol. It is used as an adjunct in the treatment of alcoholism. The toxic reaction to disulfiram appears to be due to the inhibition of liver enzymes that participate in the normal degradation of alcohol. When alcohol and disulfiram are both present, acetaldehyde accumulates in the blood. High levels of acetaldehyde produce a series of symptoms referred to as the disulfiram-alcohol reaction or syndrome. The specific symptoms are listed under *Untoward Reactions.* The symptoms vary individually and are dose–dependent, both with respect to alcohol and disulfiram and persist for 30 minutes to several hours, and a single dose of disulfiram may be effective for 1 to 2 weeks.

Uses   To prevent further ingestion of alcohol in chronic alcoholics. Disulfiram should only be given to cooperating patients fully aware of the consequences of alcohol ingestion.

Contraindications   Alcohol intoxication; severe myocardial or occlusive coronary disease. Use with caution in narcotic addicts or patients with diabetes, goiter, epilepsy, psychosis, hypothyroidism, hepatic cirrhosis or nephritis. Use of paraldehyde or alcohol-containing products such as cough syrups.

Untoward Reactions   **In the absence of alcohol,** the following symptoms have been reported: Drowsiness (most common), headache, restlessness, fatigue, psychoses, peripheral neuropathy, dermatoses, hepatotoxicity, metallic or garlic taste, arthropathy, impotence.

In the presence of alcohol, the following symptoms may be manifested. *CV:* Flushing, chest pain, palpitations, tachycardia, hypotension, syncope, arrhythmias, cardiovascular collapse, myocardial infarction, acute congestive heart failure. *CNS:* Throbbing headaches, vertigo, weakness, uneasiness, confusion, unconsciousness, seizures, death. *GI:* Nausea, severe vomiting, thirst. *Respiratory:* Respiratory difficulties, dyspnea, hyperventilation, respiratory depression. *Other:* Throbbing in head and neck, sweating.

In the event of an Antabuse-alcohol interaction, measures should be undertaken to maintain blood pressure and treat shock. Oxygen, antihistamines, ephedrine, and/or vitamin C may also be used.

Drug Interactions

Interactant	Interaction
Anticoagulants, oral	↑ Effect of anticoagulants by ↑ hypoprothrombinemia
Barbiturates	↑ Effect of barbiturates due to ↓ breakdown by liver
Chlordiazepoxide ⎱ Diazepam ⎰	↑ Effect of chlordiazepoxide or diazepam due to ↓ plasma clearance
Izoniazid	↑ Side effects of isoniazid (especially CNS)
Metronidazole	Acute toxic psychosis
Paraldehyde	Concomitant use produces Antabuse-like effect
Phenytoin (Dilantin)	↑ Effect of phenytoin due to ↓ breakdown by liver

Dosage   **Initial** (after alcohol-free interval of 12–48 hr): 500 mg daily for 1–2 weeks; **maintenance:** *usual,* 250 mg daily (range: 120–500 mg daily). Dose should not exceed 500 mg/day.

Nursing Implications

1. Be prepared to treat disulfiram–alcohol reactions symptomatically with oxygen, pressor agents, and antihistamines.
2. Emphasize to family that disulfiram must never be given to the patient without his knowledge.
3. *Teach patient and/or family*
   a. the effects of disulfiram and emphasize the necessity for close medical and psychiatric treatment when on disulfiram.
   b. that as little as 30 ml of 100-proof alcohol ingested while on therapy with disulfiram may cause severe symptoms and possibly death.
   c. not to take or use alcohol in disguised forms such as in foods, sauces, or vinegar; medications: paregoric, cough syrups, tonics; liniments or lotions.
   d. that side effects of disulfiram, such as drowsiness, fatigue, impotence, headache, peripheral neuritis, and a metallic or garliclike taste tend to subside after about 2 weeks of therapy.
   e. to report skin eruptions should they occur, since physician may order antihistamines.
   f. to carry an identification card stating that he is on disulfiram therapy and describing the symptoms and treatment should an Antabuse–alcohol reaction occur. The name of his physician should also be on the card. Cards may be obtained from the Ayerst Laboratories, 685 Third Avenue, New York, NY 10017.

GUANIDINE HYDROCHLORIDE   (Rx)

Classification   Cholinergic muscle stimulant.

Action/Kinetics   Guanidine hydrochloride increases the release of acetylcholine at the synapses following nerve impulse transmission; it slows the rate of depolarization and repolarization of the muscle cell membrane therefore acting as a cholinergic muscle stimulant. It is ineffective in the treatment of myasthenia gravis.

Uses Reduction of muscle weakness and relief of fatigue associated with Eaton-Lambert syndrome.

Contraindications Hypersensitivity to and intolerance of drug. Safe use in pregnancy or in children not established.

Untoward Reactions *CNS:* Nervousness, tremors, irritability, lightheadedness, ataxia, psychoses, confusion, changes in mood and emotions, hallucinations. *GI:* Nausea, cramps, diarrhea, anorexia, dry mouth. *Dermatologic:* Rashes, petechiae, ecchymoses, sweating, dry skin, scaling of skin, folliculitis. *CV:* Hypotension, atrial fibrillation, tachycardia, palpitations. *Other:* Paresthesia, cold sensation in extremities, nephritis, tubular necrosis, sore throat, fever.

Laboratory Test Interferences Increase in blood creatinine, uremia, abnormal liver function tests.

Dosage PO: *individualized*, **initial**, 10–15 mg/kg/day in 3 or 4 divided doses. Increase dose gradually to 35 mg/kg/day or up to the development of side effects.

Nursing Implications

1. Verify that baseline blood, renal, and liver function tests are performed prior to initiation of therapy and then periodically while patient is receiving the drug because damage may be dose-related.
2. *Assess*
   a. for anorexia, increased peristalsis, or diarrhea, which are early warnings that suggest the drug should be discontinued.
   b. for signs of intoxication manifested by hyperirritability, tremors, and convulsive contractions of muscles, salivation, vomiting, diarrhea, and hypoglycemia.
   c. patient who has had primary neoplastic lesion removed for improvement of symptoms that would permit discontinuance of drug, since the latter is highly toxic and treatment should continue only as long as necessary.
3. Have calcium gluconate available to control neuromuscular and convulsive symptoms.
4. Have atropine available to reduce GI symptoms, circulatory disturbances, and changes in blood sugar level.

HEMIN Panhematin (Rx)

Classification Iron-containing metalloporphyrin.

Action/Kinetics This drug possibly inhibits biosynthesis of porphyrin by inhibition of the rate-limiting enzyme delta-aminolevulinic acid synthetase.

Uses Acute intermittent porphyria, porphyria variegata, hereditary coproporphyria.

Contraindications Porphyria cutanea tarda, hypersensitivity to hemin. Safe use in pregnancy, lactation, and in children not established.

Untoward Reactions *Renal:* Oliguria, increased retention of nitrogen, renal shut down. *Other:* Phlebitis with or without leucocytosis, pyrexia.

Drug Interactions

Interactant	Interaction
Anticoagulants	↑ Effect of anticoagulants
Barbiturates	↓ Effect of hemin
Estrogens	↓ Effect of hemin

IV infusion only: 1–4 mg/kg daily for 3–14 days (determined by clinical response). In severe cases up to 6 mg/kg/day may be given.

Administration

1. Before initiating hemin therapy, glucose, 400 gm/day, should be first tried for 1–2 days.
2. Administer hemin over a period of 10–15 min.
3. To reconstitute, add 43 ml of sterile water for injection and shake for 2–3 min. Use immediately.
4. A filtered IV system should be used, since reconstituted solution is not transparent and undissolved particles may not be visible.

Nursing Implications

Teach patient and/or family that drug is not a cure for porphyria, but that symptomatic improvement is highly likely.

HYALURONIDASE   Hyalase,* Wydase (Rx)

Classification   Enzyme, miscellaneous.

Action/Kinetics   Hyaluronidase, an enzyme that hydrolyzes hyaluronic acid, a constituent of connective tissue, acts to promote the diffusion of injected liquids. The purified enzyme has no effect on blood pressure, respiration, temperature, and kidney function. It will not result in spread of localized infection as long as it is not injected into the infected area.

Uses   Adjunct to promote absorption and dispersion of liquids and drugs, for hypodermoclysis, adjunct in urography to improve resorption of radiopaque agents, administration of local anesthetics. (Hyaluronidase can be added to primary drug solution or injected prior to administration of primary drug solution.)

Contraindications   Do not inject into acutely infected or cancerous areas.

Untoward Reactions   Rarely, sensitivity reactions. Hypovolemia.

Dosage   *Drug and fluid dispersion* **(usual), adults and older children**: 150 units (this facilitates absorption of 1,000 ml fluid). *Subcutaneous urography* (when IV injection cannot be used) *with patient in prone position*: 75 units **SC** over each scapula, followed by contrast medium in same site.

Administration

1. Conduct a preliminary skin test for sensitivity by injecting 0.02 ml of the solution intradermally. A positive reaction occurs within 5 minutes when a wheal with pseudopods appears and persists for 20 to 30 minutes and is accompanied by localized itching. The appearance of erythema alone is not a positive reaction.

2. Methods for administering hyaluronidase:
   a. inject hyaluronidase under skin before clysis is started.
   b. after the clysis has been started, inject solution of hyaluronidase into rubber tubing close to needle.
3. Limit clysis for child under 3 years of age to 200 ml; in neonates or premature infants, volume should not exceed 25 ml/kg/day. Rate of infusion for infants: no more than 2 ml/minute.
4. Control rate and volume of fluid for the older patient so that it will not exceed those used for IV administration.

Nursing Implications
1. Do not inject hyaluronidase into an area that is infected or cancerous.
2. Check doctor's orders for dosage of hyaluronidase, type and amount of parenteral solution, rate of flow, and site of injection.
3. Monitor area receiving clysis for pale color, coldness, hardness, and pain. Should untoward signs occur, reduce rate of flow and check with doctor.

HYDROXYPROPYL CELLULOSE OPHTHALMIC INSERT   Lacrisert (Rx)

Classification   Wetting agent, hydrophilic.

Action/Kinetics   Lacrisert contains 5 mg of hydroxypropyl cellulose in a rod-shaped (1.27 mm diameter; 3.5 mm long), water-soluble preparation. It contains no preservatives or other ingredients. This preparation stabilizes and thickens precorneal tear film and prolongs the breakup time for tear film. It also lubricates and protects the eye.

Use   Moderate to severe dry eye syndrome including keratoconjunctivitis sicca. Also exposure keratitis, decreased corneal sensitivity, and recurrent corneal lesions.

Contraindications   Hypersensitivity to hydroxypropyl cellulose.

Untoward Reactions   Transient blurring of vision, ocular discomfort or irritation, photophobia, edema of eyelids, eyelids mat or become sticky, hyperemia.

Dosage   One 5 mg insert daily placed into the conjunctinal sac of the eye. Some patients may require two inserts daily.

Nursing Implications
1. Review instructions in package insert on how to insert and remove Lacrisert; follow them carefully.
2. Assess whether signs and symptoms resulting from dry eye syndrome, such as conjunctival hyperemia, exudation, itching, burning, foreign body sensation, smarting, photophobia, dryness, and blurred or cloudy vision, are relieved by the medication.
3. *Teach patient and/or family*

(continued)

a. how to insert and remove Lacrisert. Review instructions in package insert. Observe practice of insertion and removal of insert.

b. to avoid rubbing eye; this prevents dislodging Lacrisert.

c. that if Lacrisert is accidentally expelled, another Lacrisert may be inserted, if needed.

d. that there is need for regular ophthalmic examinations.

e. that untoward reactions noted above should be reported to ophthalmologist.

f. to use caution while operating a car or other hazardous machinery as drug may cause transient blurring of vision.

g. that medication may retard, stop, or reverse progressive visual deterioration.

ISOTRETINOIN Accutane (Rx)

Classification Vitamin A metabolite.

Action/Kinetics Isotretinoin reduces sebaceous gland size, decreases sebum secretion, and inhibits keratinization. **Peak plasma levels:** 3 hr. **Effective plasma levels;** 160 ng/ml. **t½:** 10 hr.

Uses Severe recalcitrant cystic acne unresponsive to other therapy. *Investigational:* Cutaneous disorders of keratinization.

Contraindications Due to possibility of fetal abnormalities or spontaneous abortion, women who are pregnant or intend to become pregnant should not use the drug. Lactation.

Untoward Reactions *Skin:* Dry skin, facial skin desquamation, skin fragility, pruritus, rash, nail brittleness, skin infections, peeling of palms and soles, photosensitivity. *Ocular:* Cheilitis, conjunctivitis, eye irritation, corneal opacities. *GI:* Nausea, vomiting, abdominal pain, anorexia, mild GI bleeding, inflammatory bowel disease. *CNS:* Lethargy, insomnia, fatigue, headache. *GU:* White cells in urine, proteinuria, hematuria, abnormal menses. *Neuromuscular:* Arthralgia, pain and stiffness of muscles, joints, bones. *Other:* Epistaxis, dry nose and mouth, drying of mucous membranes, temporary thinning of hair, benign intracranial hypertension, respiratory infections.

Drug Interactions

Interactant	Interaction
Alcohol	Potentiation of ↑ in serum triglycerides
Tetracycline	↑ Risk of benign intracranial hypertension
Vitamin A supplements	Additive toxicity

Laboratory Test Interferences ↑ Plasma triglycerides and cholesterol. ↓ High density lipoproteins.

Dosage **PO. individualized. Usual:** 1–2 mg/kg daily, divided in 2 doses for 15–20 weeks. Dose should be adjusted based on toxicity and clinical response; if cyst count decreases by 70% or more, drug may be discontinued. If necessary, a second course of therapy may be instituted after a rest period of 2 months. Doses of 0.05–0.5 mg/kg daily are effective but result in higher frequency of relapses.

Administration The drug should be taken with meals.

Nursing Implications

Teach patient and/or family

1. Not to take vitamin A tablets or multivitamins containing vitamin A.
2. To discontinue the drug if visual disturbances of any kind occur and to consult an ophthalmologist immediately.
3. That pregnancy is to be avoided and that contraception should be used for at least 1 month prior to initial therapy, and continue for at least 1 month after therapy ceases.
4. To discontinue the drug and report to physician any abdominal pain, diarrhea, or rectal bleeding.
5. To keep all appointments with physician for further evaluation and possible dose reduction.
6. To avoid prolonged exposure to the sun.
7. That the acne may worsen during initial therapy.

LACTULOSE   Cephulac, Chronulac (Rx)

Classification   Ammonia detoxicant, laxative.

Action/Kinetics   Lactulose a disaccharide containing both lactose and galactose causes a decrease in the blood concentration of ammonia in patients suffering from portal-systemic encephalopathy. The mechanism involved is attributed to the bacteria-induced degradation of lactulose in the colon, resulting in an acid medium. Ammonia will then migrate from the blood to the colon to form ammonium ion, which is trapped and cannot be absorbed. A laxative action due to increased osmotic pressure from lactic, formic, and acetic acids then expels the trapped ammonium. The decrease in blood ammonia concentration improves the mental state, EEG tracing, and diet protein tolerance of patients. The increased osmotic pressure also results in a laxative effect, which may take up to 24 hr. The drug is partly absorbed from the GI tract.

Uses   Prevention and treatment of portal-systemic encephalopathy (PSE), including hepatic and prehepatic coma. Chronic constipation.

Contraindications   Patients on galactose-restricted diets. Use with caution in presence of diabetes mellitus. Safe use in pregnancy, lactation, and children has not been established.

Untoward Reactions   *GI:* Nausea, vomiting, diarrhea, cramps, flatulence, gaseous distention, belching.

Drug Interaction   Neomycin may cause ↓ degradation of lactulose due to neomycin-induced ↑ in elimination of certain bacteria in the colon.

Dosage   **PO.** *Encephalopathy:* **Adults, initial,** 30–45 ml (20–30 gm) t.i.d.–q.i.d.; adjust q 2–3 days to obtain 2 or 3 soft stools daily. Long-term therapy may be required in portal-systemic encephalopathy; **pediatric, infants:** 2.5–10 ml/day (1.6–6.6 gm/day) in divided doses; **older children and adolescents:** 40–90 ml/day (26.6–60 gm/day) in divided doses. *During acute episodes:* 30–45 ml (20–30 gm) q 1–2 hr to induce rapid initial laxation. *Retention enema:* 300 ml (200 gm), diluted to 1,000 ml with water or saline and retained for 30–60 min; may be repeated q 4–

6 hr. *Chronic constipation*: **Adults and children**, 15–30 ml/day (10–20 gm/day) as a single dose after breakfast (up to 60 ml/day may be required).

Administration/Storage

1. To minimize sweet taste, dilute with water or fruit juice, or add to desserts.
2. When given by gastric tube, dilute well to prevent vomiting and the possibility of aspiration pneumonia.
3. Store below 30°C (86°F). Avoid freezing.

Nursing Implications

1. Report GI distress, which may subside as therapy is continued, but could necessitate a dose reduction.
2. *Assess*
   a. serum potassium levels of patients with portal-systemic encephalopathy to evaluate whether drug is causing further potassium loss that will intensify symptoms of PSE.
   b. for dry flushed skin, dry mouth, intense thirst, abdominal pain, fruity breath, and low blood pressure, symptoms of hyperglycemia more likely to occur in diabetic patients because the medication contains carbohydrate.

MORRHUATE SODIUM   (Rx)

Classification   Sclerosing agent.

Action/Kinetics   Morrhuate sodium is derived from cod liver oil. When injected into a vein, it initiates the formation of a thrombus, followed by fibrous tissue which then obliterates the particular blood vessel. After injection, 2 to 4 inches of the vein harden immediately. The entire vein becomes hard and firm within 24 hr. Injection is followed by a mild feeling of stiffness, which persists for 48 hr. The skin above the vein assumes a bronze discoloration that disappears gradually and which usually does not cause cramping pain.

Uses   Obliteration of small, uncomplicated varicose veins of the legs.

Contraindications   Hypersensitivity to drug. Obliteration of superficial varicose veins in patients suffering from deep varicose veins. Acute superficial thrombophlebitis, underlying arterial disease, varicosities resulting from tumors, uncontrolled diabetes, asthma, bedridden patients, hyperthyroidism, tuberculosis, respiratory diseases, skin diseases, sepsis, blood dyscrasias, incompetence of valves or deep veins. Safe use in pregnancy not established.

Use with particular caution in patient previously treated with morrhuate sodium.

Untoward Reactions   *GI:* Nausea, vomiting. *CNS:* Weakness, dizziness, headache, drowsiness. *Allergic:* Anaphylaxis, urticaria. *Other:* Asthma, respiratory depression, postoperative sloughing, cardiovascular collapse, pulmonary embolism.

Dosage   **IV** *small or medium veins*: 50–100 mg (1–2 ml of 5% solution); *large veins*: 150–250 mg (3–5 ml of 5% solution). Treatment may be repeated after 5 to 7 days. No more than 5 ml should be administered during any one day.

Administration

1. To test sensitivity of patient, injection of test dose (0.25–1 ml of 5% solution) may be requested by medical supervision 24 hours before treatment.

2. Morrhuate sodium is usually administered by a physician familiar with the injection technique.
3. Assist in emptying vein for injection by elevating limb and applying digital pressure or a tourniquet for *only 2 to 3 minutes* after injection to prevent dilution of drug by backflow of blood.
4. The normal coloration of injection is yellow to light brown. Only use clear solution for injection.
5. Submerge ampule in hot water to warm medication, if ampule is cold, contains solid matter, or if medication is to be injected into a small vein.
6. Solution froths easily. Use large-gauge needle to fill syringe but change to small-gauge needle for actual injection by doctor.
7. Place a dry sterile dressing over site of injection.
8. Examine site of injection before patient leaves office for allergic reaction, sloughing, bleeding, or other untoward reaction.

Nursing Implications

Assess

a. for several hours after sensitivity test is done for a hypersensitivity reaction.
b. for hypersensitivity if the patient had received therapy previously, because sensitivity to morrhuate sodium may have developed in the interim.
c. for symptoms of anaphylactoid reactions (see *Untoward Reactions*) when drug is administered and have pressor drugs (epinephrine 1:1,000), antihistamines, corticosteroids, and O_2 available.

NICOTINE RESIN COMPLEX   Nicorette (Rx)

Classification   Gum used as substitute for smoking.

Action/Kinetics   Following chewing, nicotine is released from an ion exchange resin in the gum product providing blood nicotine levels approximating those produced by smoking cigarettes. The amount of nicotine released is dependent on the rate and duration of chewing. Following repeated administration every 30 minutes, nicotine blood levels reach 25–50 ng/ml. If the gum is swallowed, only a minimum amount of nicotine is released. Nicotine is metabolized mainly by the liver with about 10–20% excreted unchanged in the urine.

Uses   Adjunct with behaviorial modification in smokers wishing to give up the smoking habit. Is considered only as an initial aid with the ultimate goal of abstention from all forms of nicotine.

Contraindications   Pregnancy, lactation, nonsmokers, serious arrhythmias, angina, vasospastic disease, active temporomandibular joint disease. Use with caution in hypertension, peptic ulcer, gastritis, stomatitis, hyperthyroidism, insulin-dependent diabetes, and pheochromocytoma.

Untoward Reactions   *CNS:* Dizziness, irritability, headache. *GI:* Nausea, vomiting, indigestion, GI upset, salivation, eructation. *Other:* Sore mouth or throat, hiccoughs, sore jaw muscles.
 Overdosage may cause symptoms of nicotine poisoning including *GI:* Nausea, vomiting, diarrhea, salivation, abdominal pain. *CNS:* Headache, dizziness, confusion, weakness, fainting, seizures. *Respiratory:* Labored breathing, respiratory

paralysis (cause of death). *Other:* Cold sweat, disturbed hearing and vision, hypotension, and rapid, weak pulse.

Treatment of overdosage includes ipecac syrup if vomiting has not occurred, saline cathartic, gastric lavage followed by activated charcoal (if patient is unconscious), maintainence of respiration, maintenance of cardiovascular function.

Drug Interactions Nicotine may increase levels of catecholamines and cortisol.

Dosage **PO. Initial:** one piece of gum chewed whenever the urge to smoke occurs; **maintenance:** about 10 pieces of gum daily during the first month not to exceed 30 pieces daily.

Administration
1. The individual must want to stop smoking and should do so immediately.
2. Each piece of gum should be chewed slowly for about 30 min.
3. Patients should be evaluated monthly and if the individual has not smoked for 3 months, the gum should be slowly withdrawn. Nicotine should not be used for longer than 6 months.

PENTOXIFYLLINE Trental (Rx)

Classification Agent affecting blood viscosity.

Action/Kinetics By an unknown mechanism, pentoxifylline and its active metabolites decrease the viscosity of blood. This results in increased blood flow to the microcirculation and an increase in tissue oxygen levels.

Peak plasma levels: 1 hr. t½: pentoxifylline, 0.4–0.8 hr; metabolites, 1–1.6 hr.

Uses Peripheral vascular disease including intermittent claudication. The drug is not intended to replace surgery.

Contraindications Intolerance to caffeine, theophylline, or theobromine. Pregnancy. Use with caution in lactation. Safety and efficacy in children less than 18 years of age not established.

Untoward Reactions *CV:* Angina, chest pain, arrhythmias, palpitation, flushing. *GI:* Abdominal pain, flatus, diarrhea, dyspepsia, nausea/vomiting. *CNS:* Dizziness, drowsiness, headache, insomnia, nervousness, tremor, blurred vision.

Dosage **PO:** 400 mg t.i.d. with meals. Treatment should be continued for at least 8 weeks. If side effects occur, dosage can be reduced to 200 mg b.i.d.

Nursing Implications
Teach patient and/or family

a. to clarify with physician those untoward reactions which should be reported, such as angina and palpitations.

b. to continue treatment for at least 8 weeks, even though effectiveness is not yet apparent.

Pigmenting Agents—Psoralens

Action/Kinetics The appearance of areas of skin discoloration, characteristic of vitiligo, is associated with a defect in the formation of the dark pigment melanin from a precursor. Special drugs (pigmenting agents) can initiate the formation of melanin. The transformation is enhanced by ultraviolet radiation from natural or artificial sources.

Two substances, methoxsalen and trioxsalen, collectively referred to as psoralens, are used to promote color development and sun protection in affected skin areas. The agents are also useful for selected patients with unusually low tolerance to sun exposure. Methoxsalen is for both topical and systemic use; trioxsalen is for systemic use only. The psoralens have been used on an investigational basis for the treatment of psoriasis and mycosis fungoides.

The agents are more rapidly effective on fleshy areas, such as the face, abdomen and buttocks, then on bony areas, such as the dorsum of the hands and feet. The drugs are only effective in conjunction with functioning pigment-producing cells (melanocytes). Use of pigmenting agents is difficult. Excess exposure to ultraviolet radiation results in erythema and severe burns; overdosage results in blistering and serious burning.

Peak plasma levels: 2–3 hr. Ingestion with food increases blood levels.

Uses Vitiligo. Also see individual drugs.

Contraindications Hepatic insufficiency, familial sun sensitivity, melanoma, aphakia, invasive squamous cell carcinoma, diseases associated with photosensitivity (porphyria, systemic lupus erythematosus, hydroa [a seasonally recurring rash triggered by exposure to sunlight], polymorphic light eruptions), leukoderma of infectious origin, albinism, children under 12 years of age. Safety in pregnancy and lactation has not been established. Use with caution in patients with tartrazine sensitivity.

Untoward Reactions *Skin:* Burning, blistering, erythema. *GI:* Gastric discomfort, nausea. *Other:* Cataracts, premature aging of skin, basal cell epitheliomas.

Treatment of Overdosage In acute oral overdosage, discontinue therapy, empty stomach by inducing emesis. Place patient in dark room for 8 hours or until cutaneous reaction subsides. Supportive measures for treatment of burns should be instituted.

Drug Interactions Use with care in patients receiving drugs that cause photosensitivity (e.g., phenothiazines, griseofulvin, thiazides, sulfonamides, tetracyclines).

Dosage See individual agents.

Nursing Implications

1. Read package insert with information supplied by manufacturer before assisting doctor or instructing patient about psoralens.
2. Administration of psoralens is to be performed by an experienced physician in his office.
3. Ascertain that liver function tests are performed before initiation of therapy, and then for the first few months of treatment.
4. Be prepared to provide burn therapy for patient who has had an overdose or overexposure to sun.
5. *Teach patient and/or family*
   a. to maintain dosage schedule.
   b. the procedure for measured exposure to sun after treatment to prevent severe burns:

(continued)

(1) After oral therapy, protect skin from sun for at least 8 hours, except for metered exposure time instituted 2 hours after ingestion of medication.

(2) After topical therapy, protect skin from sun for 12 to 48 hours, except for metered exposure time instituted 2 hours after application of unguentine. To determine sun-exposure time, use guide provided by the manufacturer of the medication.

c. to wear sunglasses during exposure to the sun.

d. to protect lips with a light-screening lipstick during exposure to the sun.

e. that sunlamp exposure should be carried out under the direction of an experienced physician. Inform doctor what type of sunlamp the patient has at home, so that appropriate recommendations can be made.

f. that results may be delayed, beginning anywhere between a few weeks or 6 to 9 months.

g. that periodic treatments may be required to maintain pigmentation.

h. to check with doctor about any medication taken concomitantly because these may increase susceptibility to burns. If this medication also causes photosensitivity, the susceptibility to burns may be greater.

i. not to ingest the chemical substance furocoumarin contained in certain foods, such as limes, figs, parsley, parsnips, mustard, carrots or celery, because more severe reactions to the sun may occur.

METHOXSALEN TOPICAL Oxsoralen (Rx)

Classification Pigmenting agent.

General Statement Topical administration produces more intensive photosensitivity reactions than systemic administration. Topical usage is only indicated for small well-defined lesions (less than 10 sq cm).

Dosage One percent suspension, applied once a week.

Administration

1. Lotion is applied to well-defined vitiliginous lesions only by physician. Never give to patient for home application.

2. Expose after application to natural sunlight as follows: 1 minute initially, increase exposure time with caution. Decrease exposure time to half when light source is artificial.

3. Decrease frequency of treatment if marked erythema is produced.

4. Keep treated areas protected from light with bandages or a sun screening agent. Patient should not sunbathe for 48 hr after therapy.

METHOXSALEN ORAL Oxsoralen (Rx)

Classification Pigmenting agent.

Additional Use Severe, recalcitrant psoriasis.

Additional Untoward Reactions *CNS:* Headache, dizziness, depression, malaise, nervousness, insomnia, depression. *Dermatologic:* Hypopigmentation, rashes, vesicle formation, herpes simplex, urticaria, folliculitis. *Other:* Edema, leg cramps, hypotension.

When used with ultraviolet light: Pruritus, erythema.

Dosage   *Vitiligo:* **Adults and children over 12 years:** 20 mg in a single dose on alternate days (minimum time between doses) 2–4 hr before ultraviolet light exposure. Exposure to sunlight should be limited to times detailed in package insert. The dose of methoxsalen should not exceed 0.6 mg/kg. *Psoriasis:* 20 in a single dose on alternate days 2 hr before exposure to ultraviolet light. Dose may be increased by 10 mg following 15th treatment.

Administration

1. Administer oral preparation with milk or meals to prevent gastric distress.
2. Follow light exposure times indicated in guide provided by manufacturer.
3. The patient should not sunbathe 24 hr prior to or 48 hr after methoxsalen ingestion and ultraviolet light exposure.
4. Wrap-around sun glasses should be worn for 24 hr after methoxsalen ingestion.

TRIOXSALEN   Trisoralen (Rx)

Classification   Pigmenting agent.

Action/Kinetics   Trioxsalen is more potent but produces fewer side effects than methoxsalen. The dosage of trioxsalen or exposure time following the drug should not be increased.

Additional Uses   Increase tolerance to sunlight, enhance skin pigmentation.

Dosage   *Systemic.* **PO.** *Vitiligo:* **Adults and children over 12 years:** 10 mg/day 2–4 hr before exposure to sun. *To increase tolerance to sunlight and/or enhance pigmentation:* Same as vitiligo but not for longer than 14 days.

Administration   See Methoxsalen, oral.

PIMOZIDE   Orap (Rx)

Classification   Neuroleptic agent.

Action/Kinetics   Pimozide blocks dopamine receptors in the CNS thus decreasing motor and phonic tics in Tourette's syndrome. **Peak serum levels:** 6–8 hr. **t½:** 55 hr. Significant first-pass effect; excreted through the kidneys.

Uses   Tourette's disorder to suppress motor and phonic tics.

Contraindications   Tics other than Tourette's disorder. Cardiac arrhythmias, concomitantly with drugs which prolong the QT interval, severe CNS depresssion. Safety in pregnancy, lactation, and in children under 12 years has not been established. Use with caution in liver or kidney disease.

Untoward Reactions   *CNS:* Headache, drowsiness, seizures, dizziness, insomnia, sedation, akinesia, akathisia, tremors, fainting, parkinsonism, extrapyramidal symptoms, persistent tardive dyskinesia, transient dyskinetic symptoms after abrupt withdrawal, speech disorders, changes in handwriting, depression, excitement, nervousness. *GI:* Nausea, vomiting, diarrhea, constipation, thirst, anorexia, increased appetite, increased salivation, dry mouth. *CV:* Hypotension, hypertension, tachycardia, palpitations. Prolongation of the QT interval with possible ventricular arrhythmias. *Other:* Hyperpyrexia, visual disturbances, changes in taste, muscle tightness, impotence, nocturia, urinary frequency, loss of libido, weight gain or loss, rash or skin irritation, sweating, chest pain, asthenia, periorbital edema.

Note: Sudden death has occurred in some patients especially with doses above 20 mg/day.

Drug Interactions

Interactant	Interaction
Alcohol	↑ CNS depressant effect
Antianxiety agents	↑ CNS depressant effect
Anticonvulsants	↑ Risk of seizures
Antiarrhythmics	Additive effect on QT interval
Narcotics	↑ CNS depressant effect
Phenothiazines	Additive effect on QT interval
Sedative-hypnotics	↑ CNS depressant effect
Tricyclic antidepressants	Additive effect on QT interval

Dosage   PO. Initial: 1–2 mg/day in divided doses; **then,** increase dose every other day to maintenance dose of the lesser of 10 mg/day or 0.2 mg/kg/day. Doses should not exceed 20 mg/day or 0.3 mg/kg/day.

Administration

1. The drug should be introduced slowly and gradually.
2. Gradually withdraw drug periodically to assess need to continue therapy.

Nursing Implications

1. Be sure that baseline ECG has been done and results reported before initiating therapy.
2. Because untoward reactions are so numerous and paradoxical, nurse must assess all body systems regularly and document findings.
3. *Teach patient and/or family* to inspect mouth at least weekly for fine vermiform movements of the tongue, an early sign of tardive dyskinesia. Drug should be discontinued and physician notified.

POLYETHYLENE GLYCOL-ELECTROLYTE SOLUTION   Golytely (Rx)

Classification   Colonic lavage.

Action/Kinetics   Polyethylene glycol acts as an osmotic agent with little net absorption or secretion of ions. The preparation also contains sodium sulfate, sodium and potassium chloride. **Onset:** 30–60 min. **Duration:** 4 hr.

Uses   Prior to GI examination to clean the bowel.

Contraindictions   Gastric retention, bowel perforation, GI obstruction. Use with caution in pregnancy. Safety and efficacy in children not established.

Untoward Reactions   *GI:* Nausea, vomiting, bloating, cramps, abdominal fullness.

Dosage   PO or nastogastric tube. Adults: 4 liters prior to GI exam (8 ounces consumed rapidly every 10 min).

Administration

1. The patient should fast 3–4 hr prior to taking the solution.
2. Only clear liquids should be consumed 2 hours before and after the solution is given and prior to the examination.
3. When preparing the solution, the container should be shaken several times to ensure complete dissolution of powder.
4. Reconstituted solution should be refrigerated and used within 48 hr. Refrigeration enhances palatability.

PRALIDOXIME CHLORIDE   2-Pam Chloride, Protopam Chloride (Rx)

Classification   Cholinesterase inhibitor antidote.

General Statement   The enzyme cholinesterase is inhibited by phosphate esters such as insecticides (e.g., sarin, parathion). Pralidoxime, an antidote for cholinsterase inhibitors, is sometimes given prophylactically to persons exposed to insecticides or to correct overdosage with cholinergic drugs. Pralidoxime is less effective in antagonizing carbamate type cholinesterase inhibitors (e.g., neostigmine); it may even aggravate symptoms of carbamate pesticide poisoning.

The drug should be administered immediately after poisoning. It is ineffective when given more than 36 hours after exposure. Administration as antidote should be combined with gastric lavage (after PO ingestion) and (after skin contamination) thorough washing of skin with alcohol or sodium bicarbonate.

Since GI absorption of the poison is slow, and possible fatal relapses may occur, patient should be watched for 48 to 72 hours after poisoning.

Laboratory determinations of RBC (depressed to 50% of normal), plasma cholinesterase and urinary para-nitrophenol (parathion poisoning only) measurements are desirable to confirm diagnosis and follow progress of the patient.

Action/Kinetics   Pralidoxime competes with cholinesterase for the carbamate or phosphorus group of the inhibitor. When displaced, the enzyme reassumes its physiologic role. Variably absorbed from GI tract. **Peak plasma concentrations: PO**, 2–3hr; **IM**, 10–20 min; **IV**, 5–15 min. t½: 0.8–2.7 hr. Partially metabolized in liver, excreted in urine.

Uses   Parathion and other organophosphate poisoning, prophylaxis of agricultural workers. Relieves paralysis of respiratory muscle. Overdosage in treatment of myasthenia gravis.

Untoward Reactions   *CNS:* Dizziness, headache, drowsiness. *Ophthalmologic:* Diplopia, impaired accommodation. *CV:* Tachycardia, increased blood pressure. *Other:* Nausea, hyperventilation, muscle weakness. Use at reduced dosage in patients with impaired renal function.

Drug Interactions

Interactant	Interaction
Barbiturates	↑ Effect of barbiturates
Aminophylline	
Morphine	
Phenothiazines	**These drugs should be avoided in patients with organo-**
Reserpine	**phosphate poisoning**
Succinylcholine	
Theophylline	

Dosage   *Organophosphate poisoning*. **Adults, IV infusion**: 1–2 gm in 100 ml saline given over 15–30 min, or can give by slow IV injection, 5% solution in water over 5 min; if response is poor, repeat after 1 hr. **Pediatric**: 20–40 mg/kg/dose given as for adults. *Anticholinergic overdosage* (as with drugs used to treat myasthenia gravis): **IV**, 1–2 gm followed by increments of 250 mg q 5 min. *Organophosphate poisoning with no severe GI symptoms*: **PO**, 1–3 gm q 5 hr.

Administration

1. In case of severe poisoning, establish patent airway before initiating therapy.
2. Pretreat patient with atropine sulfate (adults, IV 2–4 mg atropine sulfate; pediatric, **IV** or **IM**: 0.5–1 mg atropine sulfate; these doses are repeated every 10 to 15 minutes until signs of atropine toxicity appear).
3. Pralidoxime is infused in adults in 100 ml NaCl injection over 30 minutes or injected at rate of 200 mg/min. Pediatric: Give as 5% solution.
4. If atropine is used together with pralidoxime, the symptoms of atropine will appear earlier than when atropine is used alone.

Nursing Implications

1. Assess the patient closely for desired and undesired response to therapy. Desired effects—reduction of muscle weakness, cramps, and paralysis. Undesired effects—dizziness, headaches, hypertension, drowsiness. Assess for 48–72 hr after poisoning.
2. Make every effort to determine what insecticide the patient was exposed to since pralidoxime is ineffective or contraindicated in the treatment of poisoning by carbamate insecticides.
3. Report any history of asthma or peptic ulcer to the physician since these conditions contraindicate the use of cholinergic drugs.
4. Have atropine available to use in conjunction with pralidoxime.
5. Be alert to signs of atropine poisoning such as flushing, tachycardia, dry mouth, blurred vision or "atropine jag" demonstrated by excitement, delirium, and hallucinations.
6. Check that respirator, tracheostomy set, and other supportive measures are available when patient is being treated for insecticide poisoning.
7. After administration of pralidoxime as an antidote be prepared to assist with gastric lavage after PO poisoning or to assist with thorough washing of skin with alcohol or sodium bicarbonate after skin contamination with poison.
8. Alert the public to the possible hazards of using insecticides and caution adherence to instructions on container.
9. Caution the patient to avoid contact with insecticides for several weeks after poisoning.
10. Assess patients with myasthenia gravis being treated for overdose of cholinergic drugs, as they may rapidly weaken and pass from a cholinergic crisis to a myasthenic crisis when they will require more cholinergic drugs to treat myasthenia. Call the physician immediately should a patient weaken rapidly. Have edrophonium (Tensilon) on hand to use for diagnostic purposes in such a situation.

RITODRINE HYDROCHLORIDE   Yutopar (Rx)

Classification   Uterine relaxant.

Action/Kinetics   Stimulates beta$_2$ receptors of smooth muscle of the uterus, which results in inhibition of uterine contractility. It may also directly inhibit the actin-myosin interaction. **Peak plasma concentration**: 5–15 ng/ml 30–60 min after PO ingestion of 10 mg q.i.d. Ninety percent of drug excreted within 24 hr.

When indicated, therapy with ritodrine should be initiated as early as possible after diagnosis. However, decision to use ritodrine should include determination of fetal maturity.

Uses   Preterm labor in selected patients.

Contraindications   Before 20th week of pregnancy and when continuation of pregnancy is hazardous to mother. Also, antepartum hemorrhage, eclampsia, and severe preeclampsia, intrauterine fetal death, chorioamnionitis, maternal cardiac disease, pulmonary hypertension, maternal hyperthyroidism, uncontrolled diabetes mellitus, uncontrolled hypertension, and medical conditions requiring treatment with drugs that interact with ritodrine (See *Drug Interactions*).

Untoward Reactions   All effects are related to the stimulation of beta receptors by the drug. **IV.** *CV:* Increase in maternal and fetal heart rate, increase in maternal systolic and marked decrease in diastolic blood pressure (widening of pulse pressure), tachycardia, palpitations, arrhythmias, angina, heart murmur, myocardial ischemia. Sinus bradycardia following drug withdrawal. *GI:* Nausea, vomiting, bloating, ileus, GI upset, diarrhea or constipation. *CNS:* Headache, tremors, malaise, nervousness, restlessness, anxiety, emotional changes, drowsiness, weakness. *Metabolic:* Transient increases in insulin and blood glucose, increases in cAMP and free fatty acids, decrease in potassium, glycosuria, lactic acidosis. *Other:* Erythema, anaphylaxis, rash, dyspnea, hemolytic icterus, sweating, chills, hyperventilation.

PO use. *CV:* Increase in heart rate of mother, palpitations, arrhythmias. *Other:* Tremors, nausea, rashes, restlessness.

In the neonate: Hypoglycemia and ileus are infrequently observed; also hypocalcemia and hypotension in neonates whose mothers also received other beta-receptor agonists.

Drug Interactions

Interactant	Interaction
Anesthetics, general	Additive hypotension
Beta-adrenergic blocking agents	↓ Effect of ritodrine
Corticosteroids	↑ Risk of pulmonary edema
Sympathomimetics	Additive effects of sympathomimetics

Laboratory Test Interferences   ↑ Plasma glucose and insulin; ↓ plasma potassium.

Dosage   **IV: initial**, 0.1 mg/min (20 microdrops/min using microdrip chamber); **then**, depending on response, increase by 0.05 mg/min (10 microdrops/min) q 10 min until desired response occurs. **Effective dose range**: 0.15–0.35 mg/min (30–70 microdrops/min). Continue infusion antepartum for a minimum of 12 hr after contractions cease. **PO therapy following initial IV treatment**: 10 mg 30 min before cessation of IV therapy; **then**, for first 24 hr, 10 mg q 2 hr; **maintenance**: 10–20 mg q 4–6 hr, not to exceed 120 mg/day. Dosage is determined by uterine activity and incidence of side effects.

Administration/Storage

1. Dilute according to directions of manufacturer. Final dilution will contain 0.3 mg/ml ritodrine.
2. To minimize hypotension, administer IV dose while patient is in left lateral position.
3. Use Y set up, infusion pump and microdrip chamber (60 microdrops/ml).
4. Do not use discolored solutions or those containing precipitate. Use diluted solution within 48 hr.
5. PO maintenance is usually initiated 30 min before discontinuing IV therapy.

Nursing Implications

1. Assess patient to rule out preeclampsia, hypertension, or diabetes before initiating therapy.
2. Assist with sonogram and amniocentesis to establish fetal maturity, which determines whether ritodrine can be used.
3. Do not use before the 20th week of pregnancy.
4. Avoid coadministration of beta-adrenergic blocking drugs, such as propranolol, because they inhibit the action of ritodrine.
5. Assess response to IV therapy with ritodrine by evaluating strength and frequency of contraction and fetal heart rate. Be alert to increased fetal heart rate.
6. Maintain blood pressure by positioning patient in left lateral position and monitoring appropriate IV hydration. Be alert to increase in systolic and decrease in diastolic pressure and tachycardia.
7. Prevent circulatory overload by careful monitoring of IV flow rate and volume during administration. Check for infiltration.
8. Assess for respiratory dysfunction that may precede pulmonary edema, especially when patient is also receiving corticosteroids.
9. Assess for signs and symptoms of electrolyte imbalance. Be particularly alert to hypokalemia, hyperglycemia, and acidosis in diabetic patients.
10. Assess postpartum patient who has received both ritodrine and general anesthesia for potentiation of hypotensive effects of both agents.
11. Assess neonate of mother who has received ritodrine for hyper- or hypoglycemia, hypocalcemia, hypotension, and ileus. Have emergency medication available to support neonate.

SODIUM TETRADECYL SULFATE   Sotradecol, Trombovar* (Rx)

Classification   Sclerosing agent.

Action/Kinetics   On injection, this surface-active agent (detergent) causes sufficient irritation to the intima of the vein to result in a thrombus, followed by fibrous tissue which causes obliteration.

Uses   Obliteration of primary varicose veins of legs. *Investigational:* Esophageal varices.

Contraindications   Hypersensitivity to drug. Obliteration of superficial varicose veins in patients suffering from deep varicose veins. Acute superficial thrombophlebitis, underlying arterial disease, varicosities resulting from tumors, uncontrolled diabetes, asthma, bedridden patients, hyperthyroidism, tuberculosis, respiratory diseases, skin diseases, sepsis, blood dyscrasias, incompetence of valves or deep veins. Safe use in pregnancy not established.

Untoward Reactions   *GI:* Nausea, vomiting. *CNS:* Weakness, dizziness. *Allergic:* Anaphylaxis, urticaria. *Other:* Asthma, respiratory depression, postoperative sloughing, cardiovascular collapse; burning or small, permanent discoloration at injection site.

Dosage   **IV**, *small veins*: 5–20 mg (0.5–2 ml of 1% injection). *Medium-large veins*: 15–60 mg (0.5–2 ml of 3% injection). Treatment may be repeated after 5 to 7 days.

Administration

1. To test sensitivity of patient, injection of test dose (0.2–0.5 ml of 1% injection) may be requested by medical supervision several hours before treatment.
2. Sodium tetradecyl sulfate is usually administered by a physician familiar with injection technique.
3. Inject only small amounts (2 ml maximum in a single varicose vein) and no more than 10 ml of 3% injection during 1 treatment.
4. Inject very slowly.
5. Avoid extravasation.
6. Do not use if product is precipitated.

Nursing Implications

1. Assess injection site for allergic reaction for several hours after administration of test dose.
2. Have available epinephrine 1:1,000 solution for treatment of allergic reaction.

APPENDICES

Appendix 1

COMMONLY USED NORMAL PHYSIOLOGIC VALUES

Hematology

Red blood cells (erythrocytes)	$4,500,000-5,000,000/mm^3$
White blood cells (leukocytes)	$5,000-10,000/mm^3$
Polymorphonuclear neutrophils	60–70%
Lymphocytes	25–30%

Monocytes	2–6%
Eosinophils	1–3%
Basophils	0.25–0.5%
Platelets	200,000–300,000/mm³
Hemoglobin (men and women)	14–16 gm/100 ml blood
Hematocrit	
Men	40–54%
Women	37–47%
Bleeding time	1–3 min (Duke); 1–5 min (Ivy)
Coagulation time	6–12 min
Prothrombin time (Quick)	10–15 sec
Sedimentation rate (Wintrobe)	
Men	0–9 mm/hr
Women	0–20 mm/hr
Thrombin time	Within 5 sec of control

Blood Chemistry

Electrolytes (serum)	
Bicarbonate	24–31 mEq/L
Calcium	4.5–5.5 mEq/L
Chloride	95–106 mEq/L
Magnesium	1.5–3.0 mEq/L
Phosphorus	1–1.5 mEq/L
Potassium	3.6–5.5 mEq/L
Sodium	136–145 mEq/L
Enzymes (serum)	
Amylase	80–180 Somogyi units/100 ml less than 1.5 units (ml of n/20 NaOH)
Lipase	
Acid phosphatase	0.5–2.0 Bodansky units
Alkaline phosphatase	2–4.5 Bodansky units
SGOT	5–40 units/ml
SGPT	5–35 units/ml
Proteins (serum)	
Total	6.2–8.5 gm/100 ml
Albumin	3.5–5.5 gm/100 ml
Fibrinogen (plasma)	0.2–0.4 gm/100 ml
Globulin	1.5–3.0 gm/100 ml
Nonprotein nitrogenous substances (serum except where noted)	
Bilirubin	0.3–1.1 mg/100 ml
Blood urea nitrogen (BUN)	10–20 mg/100 ml
Creatinine	0.7–1.5 mg/100 ml
Nonprotein Nitrogen (NPN)	15–35 mg/100 ml
Uric Acid	
Male	2.1–7.8 mg/100 ml
Female	2.0–6.4 mg/100 ml
Other (serum, except where noted)	
Cholesterol, total	158–230 mg/100 ml

Cholesterol, esterified	100–180 mg/100 ml (70% of total)
Icterus index (jaundice)	3–8 units
Iron	75–175 μg/100 ml
Glucose (blood, plasma)	80–120 mg/100 ml
Lipids, total (serum, plasma)	450–1,000 mg/100 ml
Protein bound iodine	3.5–8 μg/100 ml
pH, arterial (plasma)	7.35–7.45

Blood Gases

Whole blood O_2 capacity	17–21 vol %
Arterial	
pCO_2	35–45 mm Hg
pO_2	75–100 mm Hg
pH	7.38–7.44
Venous	
pCO_2	40–54 mm Hg
pO_2	20–50 mm Hg
pH	7.36–7.41
HCO_3, normal range	22–28 mEq/L

Urinalysis

General	
Specific gravity	1.005–1.025
pH	6.0 (av 4.7–8.0)
Volume	600–2,500 ml/24 hours
Total solids	55–70 gm/24 hr (elderly 30 gm/24 hr)
Electrolytes (per 24 hr)	
Calcium	7.4 mEq
Chloride	70–250 mEq
Magnesium	15–300 mg
Phosphorus, inorganic	0.9–1.3 gm
Potassium	25–100 mEq
Sodium	130–260 mEq
Nitrogenous constituents (per 24 hr)	
Ammonia	30–50 mEq
Creatinine	
Men	1.0–1.9 gm
Women	0.8–1.7 gm
Protein	10–50 mg (up to 100 mg)
Urea	6–17 gm
Uric acid	0.25–0.75 gm
Steroids (per 24 hr)	
17-Hydroxycorticosteroids	4.9–14.5 mg
17-Ketosteroids	
Men	8–21 mg
Women	4–14 mg

APPENDIX 2

TOXIC AGENTS AND THEIR ANTAGONISTS

General Measures

1. Remove as much of the poison as possible by appropriate means, such as gastric lavage, induced emesis, washing of eyes, or skin.

    Never induce emesis if patient is unconscious, comatose, if poison is corrosive, a petroleum distillate (e.g., kerosone), or a convulsant.

    Emesis can often be induced by giving a glass of milk and then placing tongue depressor at back of patient's throat. Emesis can also be induced by ipecac syrup.

    When vomiting begins, place patient face down, with head lower than hips so that vomitus does not become aspirated.

2. If poison has been injected (insect, snake) retard absorption of poison by

    a. applying a constricting bandage between injection site and heart. Bandage should not be so tight that it suppresses pulse in affected area completely; remove for 1 minute every 15 minutes.

    b. applying ice pack to affected area.

    c. sucking out poison by suction cup.

3. Administer specific antidote if available.

4. Administer a suitable nonspecific antidote listed in the following table.

5. Institute supportive measures to maintain patient's vital functions.

Poisoning   For immediate information on the content of toxic ingredients of commercial preparations and their antidotes, record the telephone number of your regional poison control center:

Poison Control Center _____

TOXIC AGENTS AND THEIR ANTAGONISTS

Agent or Toxic Reaction	Symptoms	Antagonist or Treatment
Acetaminophen	Nausea, vomiting, sweating, anorexia, hepatotoxicity	Gastric lavage followed by activated charcoal. To prevent hepatotoxicity: N-acetyl-cysteine, **PO, initial,** 140 mg/kg; **then,** 70 mg/kg q 4 hr for 17 doses.
Acids	GI symptoms: nausea, vomiting, diarrhea	Milk of magnesia or lime water, followed by milk and demulcents. Do not induce vomiting.

TOXIC AGENTS AND THEIR ANTAGONISTS (*Continued*)

Agent or Toxic Reaction	Symptoms	Antagonist or Treatment
Alcohol, wood (methyl alcohol)	Blurred vision	Gastric lavage within 3 hours; ethyl alcohol (grain alcohol) **IV**: 0.75–1.0 ml/kg, then 0.5 ml/kg q 4 hr; sodium bicarbonate PO.
Alkali (lye)	GI symptoms: nausea, vomiting, diarrhea	Acetic acid, dilute vinegar, tartaric acid **PO**. Do not induce vomiting.
Anaphylaxis	Circulatory collapse, asphyxia	Epinephrine **SC**: 1:1,000 aqueous (0.01 ml/kg), repeated for total of 3 doses.
Anesthetics	Respiratory depression, coma	See *CNS depressants*
Antidepressants, tricyclic	Arrhythmias, convulsions, coma	To treat cardiovascular effects including arrhythmias: Sodium bicarbonate, 0.5–2 mEq/kg by **IV** bolus; then, **IV** infusion to reach blood pH of 7.5. Vasopressor, phenytoin (100 mg, **IV**, over 3 min), or physostigmine, 1–3 mg **IV**, if other means are ineffective.
Amphetamines	Tachycardia, delirium, seizures	Gastric lavage and emesis followed by activated charcoal and a saline cathartic. Acidification of urine should increase rate of excretion. Diazepam to treat excess stimulation.
Anticoagulants, coumarin type	Hemorrhage	Viatmin K **IM**: 5–10 mg/kg
Arsenic	See *Heavy metals* below	Dimercaprol (BAL in Oil), **IM**, 12.5–3 mg/kg q.i.d. for 2 days; then, decrease dose depending on severity of poisoning.
Aspirin	Hyperthermia, fluid loss, disturbance of acid-base balance, excitement	Gastric lavage and emesis followed by activated charcoal. Sodium bicarbonate to treat acidosis and to increase rate of excretion of aspirin. Diazepam or short-acting barbiturate to treat excess excitement. Supportive therapy to treat hyperthermia.
Atropine anticholinergics	Hyperthermia, dilated pupils, blurred vision, delirium	Emesis and gastric lavage followed by activated charcoal. Physostigmine, 1–3 mg **IV**, or neostigmine, 0.5–2 mg **IV**. Diazepam or short-acting barbiturate to treat excess excitement.

TOXIC AGENTS AND THEIR ANTAGONISTS (*Continued*)

Agent or Toxic Reaction	Symptoms	Antagonist or Treatment
Barbiturates	Respiratory depression, coma	See *CNS depressants*
Black widow spider bites	Hypocalcemic tetany	Calcium gluconate **IV:** 10–20 ml of 10% solution
Carbon monoxide	Respiratory depression and coma	Oxygen (100% O_2 for 30 minutes), artificial respiration, rest.
Carbon tetrachloride	Coma, oliguria, jaundice, abdominal pain, decrease in blood pressure	Remove by gastric lavage or emesis; artificial respiration; maintain BP. **Do not give stimulants.**
CNS depressants	Respiratory depression and coma	Supportive therapy including artificial respiration and oxygen. Maintain blood pressure and kidney function. Use of CNS stimulants is not recommended.
CNS stimulants	Tachycardia, delirium, seizures	Diazepam or a short-acting barbiturate.
Cocaine	Dilated pupils, blurred vision, delirium, hallucinations	Anti-anxiety agent.
Codeine	Respiratory depression, coma	See *Narcotics.*
Cough medication containing narcotics	Respiratory depression	If containing codeine, see *Narcotics.*
Cyanide	Respiratory depression, cyanosis	Sodium nitrite **IV:** 3% solution at 2.5–5.0 ml/min; followed by sodium thiosulfate **IV:** 50 ml of a 25% solution at 2.5–5.0 ml/min.
Heavy metals (lead, mercury)	GI symptoms: Nausea, vomiting, and diarrhea; discoloration of gums; increased salivation	Dimercaprol, **IM, initial,** 4 mg/kg; **then,** dimercaprol, 4 mg/kg q 4 hr with edetate calcium disodium, **IM or IV,** 50–75 mg/kg/day in divided doses.
Heroin	See *Narcotics,* below	See *Narcotics.*
Insecticide (Organophosphate ester type)	Convulsions, GI symptoms: nausea, vomiting, and diarrhea	Atropine: **IV,** up to 1.2 mg; repeat q 20 min until secretions controlled. Up to 10 mg may be necessary. Also pralidoxime chloride (2-PAM, Protopan Cl), **IV:** 1–2 gm over 15–30 min; then, if no significant improvement after 1 hr, give a second 1–2 dose. **Pediatric:** 20–40 mg/kg/dose.
Iron	Gastritis (may be severe), cyanosis, pallor diarrhea, drowsiness, shock, acidosis	Deferoxamine, **IM:** 1 gm; **then,** 0.5 gm q 4 hr for 2 doses and 0.5 gm q 4–12 hr up to 6 gm daily.

TOXIC AGENTS AND THEIR ANTAGONISTS (*Continued*)

Agent or Toxic Reaction	Symptoms	Antagonist or Treatment
Kerosene	Irritation of mouth, throat, stomach; vomiting, pulmonary irritation; CNS depression	Supportive treatment including artificial respiration.
Lead	Convulsions, also see *Heavy metal poisoning,* above	See *Heavy metal poisoning,* above.
LSD (Lysergic acid diethylamide)	Dilated pupils, hallucinations	Sedatives or antianxiety agents. Do not give chlorpromazine.
Methemoglobinemia	Cyanosis	Methylene blue **IV:** 1–2 mg/kg as a 1% solution repeated after 4 hours.
Narcotics	Respiratory depression, constricted pupils	Naloxone: **Adults, initial,** 0.4–2 mg, **IV,** followed by additional doses q 2–3 min. **Pediatric, initial,** 0.01 mg/kg, **IV,** followed by 0.1 mg/kg if needed.
Nicotine	Respiratory stimulation; GI hyperactivity, convulsions; increased blood pressure	Emesis or lavage; activated charcoal; atropine **IM:** 2 mg every 3–8 minutes until atropinization occurs, or phentolamine **IM** or **IV:** 1–5 mg.
Nitrites	Cyanosis	See *Methemoglobinemia,* above.
Petroleum distillates	See *Kerosene*	See *Kerosene,* above.
Phenothiazines	Arrhythmias, CNS stimulation, hypotension, extrapyramidal symptoms, respiratory depression	Monitor respiration. Gastric lavage or emesis (may be ineffective due to antiemetic effects of certain phenothiazines). Maintain blood pressure with norepinephrine or phenylephrine. Phenytoin, 1 mg/kg, **IV,** to treat arrhythmias. Pentobarbital or diazepam to control seizures or excess stimulation.
Sleeping pills	Respiratory depression, coma	See *CNS depressants,* above.
Strychnine	Convulsions	Short-acting barbiturates or diazepam, muscle relaxants; keep patient very quiet.

Appendix 3

COMMONLY PRESCRIBED COMBINATION DRUGS

Trade Name	Generic Name(s)	Amount (mg)	Pharmacologic Classification	Use	Dose/Other Information	Location in Text (p)
Actified (Capsules, Tablets), OTC Syrup contains ½ amount of tablet/5 ml	Pseudoephedrine HCl Triprolidine HCl	2.5 60	Sympathomimetic Antihistamine	Colds, allergies, upper respiratory tract problems	**Adults and children over 12 years:** 1 tablet or 10 ml. syrup t.i.d.–q.i.d.; **pediatric:** 1.25–5 ml syrup t.i.d.–q.i.d.	569 630
Aldactazide, Rx	Spironolactone Hydrochlorothiazide	25 25	Diuretic Diuretic	Diuretic/Antihypertensive	**Adults:** 2–4 tablets/day.	811 795
Aldoril, Rx	Hydrochlorothiazide Methyl-DOPA	15–50 250–500	Diuretic Antihypertensive	Antihypertensive	**Adults:** 1 tablet b.i.d.–t.i.d. for 48 hr; **then,** adjust dose to desired response.	795 325
Azo-Gantrisin, Rx	Sulfisoxazole Phenazopyridine HCl	500 50	Sulfonamide Urinary antiseptic	Urinary anti-infective	**Adults:** 4–6 tablets initially; **then,** 2 q.i.d. for up to 3 days. After 3 days, use only sulfisoxazole.	144 191
Bactrim (Oral Suspension, Tablets), Rx Bactrim DS (Double Strength), Rx contains 160 mg Trimethoprim and 800 mg Sulfamethoxazole	Trimethoprim Sulfamethoxazole	40–80 200–400	Anti-infective Sulfonamide	Anti-infective	*Urinary tract infections, shigellosis, acute otitis media:* 2 tablets q 12 hr for 14 days. *Pneumocytitis carinii pneumonitis;* **adults:** 20 mg/kg trimethoprim and 100 mg/kg sulfamethoxazole/day in divided doses for 14 days.	a 143

Product	Ingredients	Amount	Class	Indication	Dosage	Page
Chlor-Trimeton Decongestant Tablets, OTC	Chlorpheniramine maleate	6	Antihistamine	Colds, allergies, upper respiratory tract problems	**Adults:** 1 tablet q 12 hr.	627
	Pseudoephedrine sulfate	120	Decongestant			569
Chlor-Trimeton Expectorant, OTC	Chlorpheniramine Maleate	2	Antihistamine	Colds, allergies, upper respiratory tract problems	**Adults:** 5 ml. q.i.d.; **children, 6–12 years:** 2.5 ml q.i.d.	627
	Phenylephrine HCl	10	Decongestant			567
	Ammonium Chloride	100	Expectorant			a
	Sodium citrate	50	Expectorant			a
	Guaifenesin	50	Expectorant			620
Darvocet-N, Rx	Acetaminophen	325–650	Nonnarcotic analgesic	Analgesic	1 tablet q 4 hr.	494
	Propoxyphene napsylate	50–100	Analgesic			497
Darvon Compound-65, Rx	Aspirin	227	Nonnarcotic analgesic	Analgesic	1 capsule q 4 hr. This is a C-IV scheduled drug.	490
	Propoxyphene HCl	65	Analgesic			497
Dimetane-DC Cough Syrup (C-V), Rx	Brompheniramine maleate	2/5 ml	Antihistamine	Colds, allergies, upper respiratory tract problems	**Adults:** 5–10 ml q.i.d.	627
	Codeine phosphate	10/5 ml	Narcotic antitussive			478
	Phenylpropanolamine	12.5/5 ml	Decongestant			568
Dimetane Decongestant Elixir, OTC	Brompheniramine maleate	2/5 ml	Antihistamine	Colds, allergies	**Adults:** 10 ml q 4 hr.	627
	Phenylephrine HCl	5/5ml	Decongestant			567
Dimetane Decongestant Tablets, OTC	Brompheniramine maleate	4	Antihistamine	Colds, allergies	**Adults:** 1 tablet q 4 hr.	627
	Phenylephrine HCl	10	Decongestant			567
Dimetapp Tablets, Rx	Brompheniramine maleate	12	Antihistamine	Colds, allergies, upper respiratory tract problems	**Adult:** 1 tablet b.i.d. *Elixir,* **adults:** 5–10 ml t.i.d.–q.i.d.; **children 4 to 12 years:** 5 ml; **2 to 4 years:** 3.75 ml; **7 months to 2 years:** 2.5 ml; **1 to 6 months:** 1.25 ml. Pediatric dose given t.i.d.–q.i.d.	627
	Phenylephrine HCl	15	Decongestant			567
	Phenylpropanolamine HCl	15	Decongestant			568

Trade Name	Generic Name(s)	Amount (mg)	Pharmacologic Classification	Use	Dose/Other Information	Location in Text (p)
Diupres, Rx	Chlorothiazide Reserpine	250–500 0.125	Diuretic Antihypertensive	Antihypertensive	1–2 tablets 1 to 2 times/day. Not indicated for initial therapy.	795 319
Donnatal (Capsules, Tablets, Elixir), all Rx Elixir contains ⅓ amount of tablet/5 ml, Rx	Atropine sulfate Hyoscine HBr Hyoscyamine HBr Phenobarbital	0.0194 0.0065 0.1037 16	Anticholinergic Anticholinergic Anticholinergic Sedative	GI problems	*Tablets, Capsules:* **adult:** 1–2 t.i.d.–q.i.d. *Elixir:* 5–10 ml t.i.d.–q.i.d., **pediatric:** Give elixir. Dose depends on weight.	596 600 597 373
Drixoral, OTC	Dexbrompheniramine maleate Pseudoephedrine Sulfate	6 120	Antihistamine Decongestant	Colds, allergies, upper respiratory tract problems	1 tablet b.i.d.	a 569
Dyazide, Rx	Hydrochlorothiazide Triamterene	25 50	Diuretic Diuretic	Diuretic/antihypertensive	1 to 2 capsules b.i.d.	795 812
Empirin with Codeine No. 2, 15 mg* No. 3, 30 mg* No. 4, 60 mg* (C-III), Rx *Codeine phosphate	Aspirin Codeine phosphate	325 15–60	Nonnarcotic analgesic Narcotic analgesic	Analgesic	*Usual,* **adult:** 1–2 tablets q 4 hr. Depends on severity of pain. This is a C-III Scheduled drug.	490 478
Entex LA, Rx	Guaifenesin Phenylpropanolamine HCl	400 75	Expectorant Decongestant	Colds, allergies, upper respiratory tract problems	**Adults:** 1 tablet b.i.d.	620 568
Equagesic, Rx	Aspirin Meprobamate	325 200	Nonnarcotic analgesic Antianxiety agent	Analgesic	**Adults and children over 12:** 1–2 tablets t.i.d.–q.i.d. **Not recommended for children 12 years and younger.**	490 399
Fiorinal (Capsules, Tablets), Rx	Aspirin Butalbital Caffeine	200 50 40	Nonnarcotic analgesic Sedative barbiturate Stimulant	Analgesic	1–2 tablets or capsules q 4 hr. Daily dose should not exceed 6 tablets or capsules.	490 371 529

Product	Ingredients	Amount	Class	Use	Dosage	Page
Fiorinal/Codeine No. 1, 7.5 mg* No. 2, 15 mg* No. 3, 30 mg* (C-III), Rx *Codeine phosphate	Aspirin Butalbital Caffeine Codeine phosphate	325 50 40 7.5–30	Nonnarcotic analgesic Sedative barbiturate Stimulant Narcotic analgesic	Analgesic	1–2 capsules up to 6 capsules/day as required. This is a C-III Scheduled drug.	490 371 529 478
Gelusil Liquid, OTC	Aluminum hydroxide Magnesium hydroxide Simethicone	200 mg/5 ml 200 mg/5 ml 25 mg 5 ml	Antacid Antacid Antiflatulent	Hyperacidity, peptic ulcer, gastritis, hiatal hernia, esophagitis	Dosage depends on use.	633 635 644
Gelusil II Liquid, OTC	Aluminum hydroxide Magnesium hydroxide Simethicone	400 mg/5 ml 400 mg/5 ml 30 mg/5 ml	Antacid Antacid Antiflatulent	Same as Gelusil	Same as Gelusil	633 635 644
Inderide-80/25, Rx	Hydrochlorothiazide Propranolol HCl	25 80	Diuretic Beta-adrenergic blocking agent	Antihypertensive		795 337
Inderide-40/25, Rx	Hydrochlorothiazide Propranolol HCl	25 40	Diuretic Beta-adrenergic blocking agent	Antihypertensive		795 337
Librax, Rx	Chlordiazepoxide HCl Clidinium Bromide	5 2.5	Antianxiety agent Anticholinergic	GI problems	*Usual:* 1–2 capsules t.i.d.–q.i.d. before meals and at bedtime.	394 597
Lomotil (Liquid, Tablets) (C-V), Rx	Diphenoxylate HCl Atropine sulfate	2.5 0.025	Narcotic antidiarrheal Anticholinergic	Antidiarrheal	**Adults:** 5 mg diphenoxylate q.i.d.; children 2 to 12 years: 0.3–0.4 mg/kg/day of diphenoxylate in divided doses. Use liquid only. Do not use in children under 2 years.	a 596
Moduretic, Rx	Amiloride HCl Hydrochlorothiazide	5 50	Diuretic Diuretic	Diuretic	**Adults:** 1–2 tablets/day with meals.	810 795
Naldecon Syrup, Rx	Chlorpheniramine maleate Phenylephrine HCl Phenylpropanolamine HCL	2.5/5 ml 5/5 ml 20/5 ml	Antihistamine Decongestant Decongestant	Colds, allergies, upper respiratory tract problems	**Adults:** *Syrup,* 5 ml q 3–4 hr. *Tablet:* 1 t.i.d.	627 567 568

Trade Name	Generic Name(s)	Amount (mg)	Pharmacologic Classification	Use	Dose/Other Information	Location in Text (p)
	Phenyltoloxamine citrate	7.5/5 ml	Antihistamine			a
Tablets contain twice the amount as in 5 ml of syrup						
Naldecon Pediatric Syrup, Rx	Chlorpheniramine maleate	0.5/5 ml	Antihistamine	Colds, allergies, upper respiratory tract problems	**Pediatric:** 2.5–10 ml q 3–4 hr.	627
	Phenylephrine HCl	1.25/5 ml	Decongestant			567
	Phenylpropanolamine HCl	5/5 ml	Decongestant			568
	Phenyltoloxamine citrate	2/5 ml	Antihistamine			a
Ornade, Rx	Chlorpheniramine	12	Antihistamine	Upper respiratory tract problems	Sustained release. **Adults and children over 6 years:** 1 capsule b.i.d. **Not indicated in children less than 6 years.**	627
	Phenylpropanolamine HCl	75	Decongestant			568
Parafon Forte, Rx	Acetaminophen	300	Nonnarcotic analgesic	Skeletal muscle relaxant	2 tablets q.i.d.	494
	Chlorzoxazone	250	Skeletal muscle relaxant			445
Percocet (C-II), Rx	Acetaminophen	325	Nonnarcotic analgesic	Analgesic	1–2 tablets q 4–6 hr for pain.	494
	Oxycodone HCl	5	Narcotic analgesic			483
Percodan (C-II), Rx	Oxycodone HCl	4.5	Narcotic analgesics	Analgesic	1–2 tablets q 4–6 hr for pain.	483
	Oxycodone terephthalate	0.38				483
	Aspirin	325	Nonnarcotic analgesic			490
Phenaphen/Codeine No. 2, 15 mg* No. 3, 30 mg* No. 4, 60 mg* (C-III), Rx *Codeine Phosphate	Acetaminophen	325	Nonnarcotic analgesic	Analgesic	Adjust dose for severity of pain and response of patient. *Usual:* **No. 2 or No 3:** 1–2 capsules q 4 hr. **No. 4:** 1 cap. q 4 hr. This is a C-III scheduled drug.	494
	Codeine phosphate	15–60	Narcotic analgesic			478

Product	Ingredients	Strength	Class	Use	Dosage	Page
Phenergan with Codeine Syrup (C-V), Rx	Codeine phosphate	10/5 ml	Narcotic antitussive	Antitussive/antihistamine	**Adults:** 5 ml q 4–6 hr. This is a C-V scheduled drug.	478
	Promethazine HCl	6.25/5 ml	Antihistamine			629
Phenergan with Dextromethorphan, Rx	Dextromethorphan HCl	15/5 ml	Antitussive	Antitussive/antihistamine	**Adults:** 5 ml q 4–6 hr not to exceed 30 ml in 24 hr. **Pediatric: 6–12 years:** 2.5–5 ml q 4–6 hr; **2–6 years:** 1.25–2.5 ml q 4–6 hr.	620
	Promethazine HCl	6.25/5 ml	Antihistamine			629
Phenergan VC with Codeine Syrup (C-V), Rx	Codeine phosphate	10/5 ml	Narcotic antitussive	Antitussive/antihistamine/decongestant	**Adults:** 5 ml q 4–5 hr. This is a C-V scheduled drug.	478
	Phenylephrine HCl	5/5 ml	Decongestant			567
	Promethazine HCl	6.25/5 ml	Antihistamine			629
Phenergan VC Syrup, Rx	Phenylephrine HCl	5/5 ml	Decongestant	Antihistamine/decongestant	**Adults:** 5 ml q 4–6 hr. **Pediatric: 6–12 years:** 2.5–5 ml q 4–6 hr. **2–6 years:** 1.25–2.5 ml q 4–6 hr.	567
	Promethazine HCl	6.25/5 ml	Antihistamine			629
Rondec-DM Oral Drops, Rx	Carbinoxamine maleate	2/1 ml	Antitussive	Colds, allergies, upper respiratory tract problems	**Pediatric:** 0.25–1 ml q.i.d.	a
	Dextromethorphan HBr	4/1 ml	Decongestant			620
	Pseudoephedrine HCl	25/1 ml				569
Rondec-DM Syrup, Rx	Carbinoxamine maleate	4/5 ml	Antihistamine	Colds, allergies, upper respiratory tract problems	**Adults:** 5 ml q.i.d.	a
	Dextromethorphan HBr	15/5 ml	Antitussive			620
	Pseudoephedrine HCl	60/5 ml	Decongestant			569
Septra (Oral Suspension, Tablets), Rx	Trimethoprim	40–80	Anti-infective	Anti-infective	*Urinary tract infections, shigellosis, acute otitis media:* 2 tablets q 12 hr for 14 days. *Pneumocytitis carinii pneumonitis,* **adults:** 20 mg/kg trimethoprim and 100 mg/kg sulfamethoxazole per day in divided doses for 14 days.	a
	Sulfamethoxazole	200–400	Sulfonamide			143
Septra DS (Double Strength), Rx	Contains 160 mg trimethoprim and 800 mg sulfamethoxazole					
Ser-Ap-Es, Rx	Hydralazine HCl	25	Antihypertensive	Antihypertensive	*Individualized, usual,* **adult:** 1–2 tablets t.i.d.	345
	Hydrochlorothiazide	15	Diuretic			795
	Reserpine	0.1	Antihypertensive			319

Trade Name	Generic Name(s)	Amount (mg)	Pharmacologic Classification	Use	Dose/Other Information	Location in Text (p)
Synalgos-DC (C-III), Rx	Aspirin	356.4	Nonnarcotic analgesic	Analgesic	Dose individualized according to severity of pain and response of patient. *Usual, adult:* 2 caps q 4 hr. This is a C-III scheduled drug.	490
	Caffeine	30	Stimulant			529
	Dihydrocodeine bitartrate	16	Narcotic analgesic			a
Talwin NX (C-IV), Rx	Naloxone HCl	0.5	Narcotic antagonist	Analgesic	**Adults:** 1 tablet q 3–4 hr up to a total daily dose not to exceed 600 mg for pentazocine. The naloxone is included to prevent parenteral abuse.	486
	Pentazocine HCl	50	Narcotic analgesic			484
Tavist-D, Rx	Clemastine fumarate	1.34	Antihistamine	Colds, allergies, upper respiratory tract problems	**Adults:** 1 tablet q 12 hr.	628
	Phenylpropanolamine HCl	75	Decongestant			568
Tedral Tablets, OTC	Ephedrine HCl	24	Sympathomimetic	Antiasthmatic	**Adults:** 1–2 tabs q 4 hr; **children over 60 lb:** ½ adult dose.	558
	Phenobarbital	8	Sedative			373
	Theophylline	130	Sympathomimetic		**Adults:** 15–30 ml q 4 hr; **children:** 5 ml/30 lb body weight q 4–6 hr.	614
Elixir: 5 ml is equivalent to one-quarter Tedral Tablet, OTC						
Suspension: 5 ml is equivalent to one-half Tedral Tablet, OTC					**Adults:** 10–20 ml q 4 hr; **children:** 5 ml/60 lb body weight q 4 to 6 hr.	
Triavil, Rx	Amitriptyline HCl	10–50	Antidepressant	Psychotherapeutic	*Initial:* 2–4 mg perphenazine with 10–50 mg amitriptyline t.i.d.-q.i.d. Then adjust dose to smallest amount to control symptoms.	422
	Perphenazine	2–4	Antipsychotic			408
Trinalin, Rx	Azatadine maleate	1	Antihistamine	Colds, allergies, upper respiratory tract problems	1 tablet q 12 hr.	627
	Pseudoephedrine sulfate	120				569

Product	Ingredients	Amount (mg or ml)	Type	Use	Dosage	Page
Tussi-Organidin (C-V), Rx	Iodinated glycerol / Codeine phosphate	30/5 ml / 10/5 ml	Expectorant / Narcotic antitussive	Colds, upper respiratory tract problems	**Adults:** 5–10 ml q 4 hr.	a / 478
Tussionex (Capsules, Elixir, Tablets) (C-III), Rx	Phenyltoloxamine / Hydrocodone	10 / 5	Antihistamine / Narcotic	Antitussive	**Adults:** 1 capsule or 1 tsp. elixir q 8–12 hr. This is a C-III scheduled drug.	a / a
Tuss-Ornade Capsules, Rx	Caramiphen edisylate / Phenylpropanolamine HCl	40 / 75	Antitussive / Decongestant	Colds, upper respiratory tract problems	*Sustained release capsule:* 1 q 12 hr. (Age 12 years and older only).	a / 568
Tuss-Ornade Liquid, Rx	Caramiphen edisylate / Phenylpropanolamine HCl	6.7/5 ml / 12.5/5 ml	Antitussive / Decongestant	Colds, upper respiratory tract problems	**Adults:** *liquid,* 5–10 ml t.i.d.-q.i.d.; **children over 25 lb:** 5 ml t.i.d.-q.i.d.; **15–25 lb,** 2.5 ml t.i.d.-q.i.d.	a / 568
Tylenol/Codeine Capsules No. 3, 30 mg* No. 4, 60 mg* (C-III), Rx *Codeine phosphate	Acetaminophen / Codeine phosphate	300 / 30–60	Nonnarcotic analgesic / Narcotic analgesic	Analgesic	**Adults: No. 3 Capsule,** 1–2 q 4 hr as needed for pain; **No. 4 Capsule,** 1 q 4 hr as needed for pain.	494 / 478
Tylenol/Codeine Tabs No. 1, 7.5 mg* No. 2, 15 mg* No. 3, 30 mg* No. 4, 60 mg* (C-III), Rx *Codeine phosphate The Elixir contains 12 mg codeine phosphate and 120 mg acetaminophen/5 ml (C-V), Rx	Acetaminophen / Codeine Phosphate	300 / 7.5–60	Nonnarcotic analgesic / Narcotic analgesic	Analgesic	**Adults: Tablets, no. 1, no. 2, no. 3:** 1–2 q 4 hr; **No. 4:** 1 q 4 hr. **Elixir, adults:** 15 ml q 4 hr; **pediatric 7 to 12 years:** 10 ml t.i.d.-q.i.d.; **3 to 6 years;** 5 ml t.i.d.-q.i.d.	494 / 478
Tylox (C-II), Rx	Acetaminophen / Oxycodone HCl	500 / 5	Nonnarcotic analgesic / Narcotic analgesic	Analgesic	1–2 capsules q 4–6 hr for pain.	494 / 483
Vicodin (C-III), Rx	Acetaminophen / Hydrocodone bitartrate	500 / 5	Nonnarcotic analgesic / Narcotic analgesic	Analgesic	1 tablet q 4–6 hr for pain.	494 / a

[a] Available only in combination products.

Appendix 4

FOOD-DRUG INTERACTIONS AND NURSING IMPLICATIONS

I Drug	II Food Interactant	III Interaction (Effect and Mechanism)	IV Nursing Implications Teach patient and/or family to:
Acetaminophen	High carbohydrate foods	↓ Absorption rate of acetaminophen ↑ Onset of therapeutic effect, by altering GI motility and emptying rate	1. Restrict intake of foods high in CHO. 2. Take on an empty stomach with a full glass of water.
Aminoglycosides	Urinary alkalizers, (see Appendix 6) Urinary acidifiers	↓ Antibacterial activity of aminoglycosides ↑ Antibacterial activity of aminoglycosides	1. Restrict foods that are urinary alkalizers (see Appendix 6). 2. Maintain adequate intake of foods that are acidifiers, see Appendix 6.
Acetylsalicylic acid	Acidic foods, such as coffee, cola drinks, citrus fruits, pickles, tomatoes Food	↑ Acid gastricity that corrodes stomach lining and may cause ulcers ↓ Absorption rate	1. Avoid acidic foods (see column II). 2. For rapid onset of action take drug on an empty stomach with a full glass of water.
Barbiturates	Alcohol Protein-deficient diet	↑ Absorption ↑ Duration of action of drug by inhibiting cytochrome (P-450) enzyme, which degrades barbiturates	1. Do not drink alcohol when taking barbiturates. 2. Eat a well-balanced diet to prevent protein deficiency. 3. Be alert to toxicity, which is more likely to occur in patients with a protein deficiency.

Drug	Food	Effect	Recommendation
Bisacodyl	Dairy foods and antacids	Wears away enteric coating of drugs too early causing abdominal cramping	1. Avoid dairy foods and antacids at time of administration. 2. Do not use chewed or broken tablets.
Carbamazepine	Food	↑ Absorption of carbamazepine by increasing dissolution	Take with food.
Cephalosporins (oral)	Food	Delays absorption rate by altering GI motility and emptying rate	Preferably take on an empty stomach.
Chlorpropamide	Alcoholic beverages, over-the-counter tonics, formulas, etc.	↑ Hypoglycemia by reducing activity of chlorpropamide, and by the additive hypoglycemic effect of alcohol. Possible Antabuse-like reaction (abdominal cramps, vomiting, flushing of skin)	Restrict use of alcohol.
Cimetidine	Food	Delayed absorption helps maintain effective blood concentration between doses	Take with food.
Clindamycin	Pectin, found in the peel of citrus fruits and apple pulp	↓ Absorption by the formation of insoluble compounds	Avoid use of peel of citrus fruits, apple pulp, or any other pectin-containing food.
Digoxin	Prune juice, bran cereals, and other foods high in fiber	↓ Cardiovascular activity of digoxin by delaying absorption rate	Avoid taking prune juice, bran cereals, and other foods high in fiber.
Diuretics	Monosodium glutamate (MSG) used in seasoned salts, meat tenderizers, frozen vegetables, and oriental cuisine	↑ Removal of excess water from tissue. In combination with diuretic, can deplete vitamin C and B complex and minerals, sodium, calcium, and potassium. Adverse effects of MSG can occur, (tightening of chest, flushing of face)	Do not use MSG with diuretics.
	Licorice (natural)	↑ Salt and water retention	Do not eat natural licorice when on diuretic therapy.

I Drug	II Food Interactant	III Interaction (Effect and Mechanism)	IV Nursing Implications Teach patient and/or family to:
Erythromycin	Acidic foods such as coffee, cola drinks, citrus fruits, pickles, and tomatoes	↓ Antibacterial activity	Avoid acidic foods.
	Food	↓ Absorption rate by altering GI motility and emptying rate	Take on an empty stomach with a full glass of water.
Ethyl alcohol	Food	↓ Absorption by delaying gastric emptying	Take with food to reduce degree of intoxication; milk is particularly effective.
Furazolidine	Food high in tyramine	Possible hypertensive reaction due to inhibition of metabolism of tyramine (6 mg of tyramine may cause hypertensive crisis)	Do not eat foods high in tyramine. See Nursing Implications under MAO inhibitors.
	Alcohol	Possible Antabuse-like reaction (abdominal cramps, vomiting, flushing of skin)	Restrict use of alcohol.
Griseofulvin	Food with high fat content	↑ Absorption due to greater solubilization by increased bile secretions	Take griseofulvin with diet high in fats.
Hydralazine	Food	↑ Absorption because of bioavailability	Take with food. Maintain consistency of administration, preferably with meals.
Indomethacin	Food	↓ Absorption and ↑ time to reach peak serum levels	Nevertheless, take drug with food to avoid GI irritation.
Iron sulfate or chloride	Dairy foods, eggs, cereals, starches and clays	↓ Absorption by formation of insoluble salts	1. Do not take or give to children with foods or substances in column II this entry. 2. Take with citrus juices.
Isoniazid	Citrus juices	↑ Absorption	
	Food	↓ Absorption	Take on an empty stomach with a full glass of water.
Levodopa	Foods high in protein	↓ Absorption rate by compet-	1. Avoid high-protein diets or diets

Drug	Food/Substance	Effect	Recommendations
		...ing for intestinal absorption, change in pH, or gastric emptying time. This results in ↓ peak plasma concentrations and therapeutic effect	in which the protein intake fluctuates.
	Foods high in pyridoxine (B6)	↓ Therapeutic effect by accelerating conversion of levodopa to dopamine	2. Avoid foods high in pyridoxine, such as yeast, whole grains (especially corn), brown rice, meats (especially organ meats), salmon, tuna, lentils, beans, peanuts, tomatoes, sweetpotatoes and yams, walnuts. Smaller amounts of B6 in milk, eggs, and vegetables.
Lincomycin	Food	↓ Absorption and therapeutic effect by altering GI motility and emptying time	1. Take on an empty stomach with a full glass of water.
	Pectin found in the peel of citrus fruits and apple pulp.	↓ Absorption by formation of insoluble compounds	2. Avoid peel of citrus fruits, pulp of apple, or any other pectin-containing foods.
Lithium	Food	↑ Absorption rate by delaying gastric emptying and transition	1. Take with food.
	Low-salt diets	↓ Renal clearance	2. Be alert to signs of toxicity. Withhold drug and report to physician should diarrhea, vomiting, drowsiness, muscular weakness, and lack of coordination occur.
Methenamine mandelate	Urinary alkalizers (see Appendix 6)	↓ Antibacterial activity	1. Restrict alkalizers (see Appendix 6).
	Urinary acidifiers (see Appendix 6)	↑ Antibacterial activity	2. Include acidifiers in diet (see Appendix 6). 3. Encourage vitamin C intake to promote acid urine.
Metronidazole	Alcoholic beverages, wines, beers, tonics, cough formulas.	Possible Antabuse-like reaction (abdominal cramps, vomiting, flushing of skin)	Do not drink alcoholic beverages when on therapy with metronidazole.
Monoamine oxidase inhibitors	Food high in tyramine	Hypertensive effect by inhibiting metabolism of tyramine (6 mg of tyramine may cause hypertensive crisis)	Do not eat foods high in tyramine, such as beer, broad beans, cheeses (brie, cheddar, Camembert, Stilton), Chianti wine, chicken liver, caffeine, cola

I Drug	II Food Interactant	III Interaction (Effect and Mechanism)	IV Nursing Implications Teach patient and/or family to:
			drinks, figs, licorice, liver, pickled or kippered herring, tea, cream, yogurt, yeast extract, and chocolate.
Nitrofurantoin	Food	↑ Bioavailability due to greater dissolution in gastric juices and decreased gastric emptying rate	1. Take with food to minimize gastric irritation.
Penicillin (Amoxicillin and Pen Vee are less affected by food)	Low-protein diets, dairy product foods, and urinary alkalizers (Appendix 6)	↑ Drug excretion due to alkalinization of urine	2. Restrict alkalizers (see Appendix 6). Ensure adequate amounts of protein.
Phenacetin	Food	↓ Therapeutic effect delayed or reduced by absorption or altering gastric motility and emptying rate	Take on an empty stomach with a full glass of water.
	Charcoal-broiled beef	↓ Therapeutic effect by increasing drug metabolism	Avoid ingestion of charcoal-broiled beef, cabbage, and brussels sprouts.
	Cabbage, brussels sprouts	↓ Therapeutic effect by increasing first pass effect and increasing biotransformation in GI tract	
Phenytoin	Monosodium glutamate	↑ Absorption rate of MSG leading to generalized weakness, numbness at back of neck, and palpitations	Do not eat foods prepared with MSG.
Propranolol	Food	↑ Absorption by reducing first pass hepatic metabolism	Take with food.
Propantheline	Food	↓ Therapeutic effect by reducing rate of absorption	Take on an empty stomach with a full glass of water.
Quinidine	Urinary alkalizers (see Appendix 6)	↓ Excretion of drug and may cause quinidine intoxication	1. Restrict alkalizers (see Appendix 6).

Drug	Effect	Food	Recommendation
	manifested by cardiac, respiratory, and CNS alteration in function		2. Preferably take on an empty stomach with a full glass of water. 3. Take with food or milk if necessary to reduce gastric irritation.
Riboflavin	↑ Absorption by food delays gastric emptying or transit time	Food	Take with food.
Rifampin	↓ Serum levels and decreases peak levels due to reduced rate of absorption	Food	Take on an empty stomach with a full glass of water.
Spironolactone	↑ Bioavailability by increasing absorption	Food	Take with food.
Sulfadiazine, Sulfisoxazole	Delays absorption rate by altering GI motility and emptying time	Food	Take on an empty stomach with a full glass of water.
Tetracycline	↓ Absorption by formation of insoluble salts with nutrients	Milk, dairy products, foods high in iron	1. Do not take with dairy products and foods high in iron. 2. Do not take iron supplements or antacids with tetracyclines.
Theophylline	↓ Plasma half-life by increasing levels of cytochrome P-450 enzyme leading to more rapid oxidation	Low carbohydrate and high-protein diet	1. Eat a well-balanced diet, avoiding significant diet changes involving carbohydrate and protein. 2. Take on an empty stomach for faster absorption. 3. Use a liquid form if faster absorption is needed. 4. Take with food only to reduce gastric irritation if necessary.
Thiamine	↓ Absorption rate by altering GI motility and transit time but extent of absorption is unchanged	Food	Take with food.
Thyroid	↓ Thyroid hormone activity and interferes with drug activity	Kale, cabbage, carrots, cauliflower, spinach, peaches, brussels sprouts, turnips	Avoid excessive consumption of foods noted in column II.

I Drug	II Food Interactant	III Interaction (Effect and Mechanism)	IV Nursing Implications Teach patient and/or family to:
Tolbutamide	Alcohol (chronic intake or acute intoxication)	↑ Hypoglycemia by decreasing drug metabolism and additive effect of alcohol. Possible Antabuse-like reaction (abdominal cramps, vomiting, flushing of skin)	Restrict use of alcohol.
Warfarin	Leafy green vegetables, potatoes, citrus juices, vegetable oil, egg yolk, green tea.	↓ Drug activity by presence of vitamin K that antagonizes warfarin	1. Consult with physician regarding diet while on anticoagulant therapy. 2. Avoid excessive use of foods noted in column II.
	Cooking oil with silicone additives	↓ Drug activity by formation of insoluble salts that are not absorbed	3. Do not use cooking oil with silicone additives.

DRUGS THAT AFFECT UTILIZATION OF NUTRIENTS

Drug	Effect
Alcohol	Malabsorption of folic acid and vitamin B_{12}
Aminopterin	Antagonizes folic acid; interferes with absorption of vitamin B_{12}
Antacids	Cause phosphate depletion, muscle weakness, and vitamin D deficiency
Anti-infectives	Decrease utilization of folic acid and malabsorption of vitamin B_{12}, calcium, and magnesium; decrease bacterial synthesis of vitamin K; inactivation of pyridoxine; impair transfer of amino acids
Anticonvulsants	Cause deficiencies of vitamin D, folic acid and vitamin B_{12} by increasing the turnover rate of vitamins in the body
Aspirin	Causes folate deficiency
Atropine	Alters pancreatic or intestinal digestive function
Cathartics	Diminish nutrient absorption
Clofibrate	Alters taste sensation; may suppress appetite and reduce nutrient intake; malabsorption of folic acid and vitamin B_{12}, electrolytes, and sugar
Colchicine	Impairs absorption of vitamin B_{12}, fat, lactose, and electrolytes
Cortisone	Alters pancreatic or intestinal digestive function
Cycloserine	Causes folate deficiency
Digitoxin	Alters pancreatic or digestive function
Diuretics	Cause potassium depletion
Epinephrine	Alters pancreatic or digestive function
Ethacrynic acid	Alters pancreatic or intestinal function
Ganglionic blockers	Cause potassium depletion
Griseofulvin	See Clofibrate
Hydralazine	Depletes vitamin B_6 by inhibiting production of enzymes needed to convert it into a form the body can use or by combining to form a compound that is excreted
Isoniazid	See Hydralazine
Lincomycin	See Clofibrate
Methotrexate	Antagonizes folic acid
Mineral oil	Hinders absorption of vitamins D, E, and K, and carotene
Neomycin	Impairs absorption of vitamin B_{12}; alters pancreatic or digestive function; interferes with bile activity
Oral antidiabetic agents	Impair absorption of vitamin B_{12}
Oral contraceptives	Deplete folic acid and vitamin B_6
Phenobarbital	Causes folate deficiency

Drug	Effect
Phenothiazine	Stimulates appetite, results in increased food intake and weight gain
Surface-active agents	Alter absorption of nutrients by affecting fat dispersion
Thorazine	Induces hypercholesteremia
Tricyclic antidepressants	Stimulate appetite, which results in increased food intake and weight gain

Appendix 6

ACIDIC, ALKALINE, AND NEUTRAL FOODS

Acidifiers: Acid Ash Foods	Alkalizers: Alkaline Ash Foods	Neutral Foods
Dairy foods cheeses (all types)	Dairy foods milk, cream, buttermilk	Butter or margarine Beverages coffee and tea
Eggs	Fruits except cranberries, plums, and prunes	Cooking oils and fats
Fish (including shell fish)		Starches corn and arrowroot
Fruits cranberries, plums, and prunes	Jams, jellies, honey	Sugars
	Molasses	Syrup
Grains breads, cakes, crackers, cereals, cookies	Nuts almonds, chestnuts, co- conut	Tapioca
Macaroni (spaghetti, noo- dles)	Olives	
Mayonnaise	Vegetables except corn and lentils	
Meats		
Nuts Brazil, peanuts, wal- nuts, filberts		
Poultry		
Vegetables corn and lentils		

Foods yielding an acid ash are urinary acidifiers; foods yielding an alkaline ash are urinary alkalinizers.

Appendix 7

LABORATORY TEST INTERFERENCES

GENERAL CONSIDERATIONS

Laboratory tests play a crucial role in diagnosis and medical care. During drug therapy, they are used to monitor the therapeutic efficacy and the side effects of a particular drug. Such tests may or may not be related to the condition for which the drug is prescribed. Thus, penicillins given for an infection may affect the urine glucose determination performed for other reasons.

Drugs, however, can also interfere with the actual measurement on which the diagnostic test is based (methodologic interference). Such interferences may result in false-positive (false +) or abnormally high (↑) values, as well as false-negative (false −) or abnormally low (↓) values. It is often difficult to distinguish between the real changes attributable to the therapeutic agent and interference with the method itself. Furthermore, since a particular drug may affect one method of performing a given laboratory procedure and not another, it is important to consider the specific testing method used in each particular instance.

The interference with laboratory tests can be subdivided as follows:

PHYSICAL INTERFERENCE   For example, coloration of urine is affected by the excretion of a drug or its metabolite, which, in turn, may mask abnormal colors contributed by bile, blood, or porphyrins, and interfere with their determinations by fluorometric, colorimetric, and photometric tests. For example, tetracyclines interfere with the fluorometric methods for porphyrin determination.

BIOLOGIC INTERFERENCE   For example, the drug or its metabolites may stimulate or suppress the enzyme system on which the test is based.

CHEMICAL INTERFERENCE   For example, there may be interference with the oxidation–reduction reactions that are the basis of Benedict's urinary glucose tests.

Most laboratory interferences give rise to false-positive results. Altered liver function tests are often grouped together, and they may include one or several of the following: *False + or ↑ values* —serum alkaline phosphatase, serum bilirubin (icterus index), serum BSP, serum cephalin flocculation, SGOT, SGPT, thymol turbidity, urinary bilirubin. *False− or ↓ values* —blood glucose and serum cholesterol. Most methodologic errors can be avoided when tests are performed on a sample taken 12–24 hr after withholding all medication or food, or by switching to another test. However, this is not always possible. There is also still some inconsistency in the reports by experts on the effects of various drugs on laboratory tests. Therefore, the listings of *Laboratory Test Interferences* should be used only as a general guide.

As in the case of the drug interactions, laboratory tests may be affected by all the drugs a patient is taking, including nonprescription agents.

The agents that most often interfere with laboratory test values are the *anti-*

EFFECTS OF DRUG ON LABORATORY TEST VALUES[a,b]

	Hepatotoxicity	Nephrotoxicity	Intest. Malabs.	Creatinine	BUN	Uric Acid	Bilirubin	SGOT/ SGPT	Serum Glucose	Cholesterol	Prothrombin time	Urine Color	Urine Glucose	Comments
Acetazolamide						I								
Acetohexamide (sulfonylurea)	X			I										
ACTH						D			I					
Allopurinol	X					D								
Aminosalicyclic acid (PAS)	X												+	
Amphotericin B	X	X												
Ampicillin		X												
Anabolic steroids and androgens	X													
Antihistamines											D			
Antimony compounds	X	X												
Arsenicals	X	X												
Ascorbic acid						I	I	I	I				+	
Caffeine							D		I					
Cephaloridine		X		I									+	
Cephalothin													+	
Chloral hydrate					I						D		+	
Chloramphenicol (Chloromycetin)	X				X								+	
Chlordiazepoxide (Librium)	X													

Chlorpromazine (Thorazine)	X					D			I					May cause + pregnancy test
Chlorpropamide (Diabenese)	X													
Chlorprothixene (Taractan)	X					D								
Chlorthalidone (Hygroton)		X							I		I			
Cholinergics							I	I						I—BSP. Changes due to spasm, sphincter of Oddi
Clofibrate (Atromid-S)	X					D				D	I			D—triglycerides, total lipids, LDH
Codeine							I	I						
Colchicine	X		X								D			On coumarins
Colistin		X												
Corticosteroids						D			I	I			+	
Coumarins	X					D					I			
Cyclophosphamide	X													
Dextran					I	I	I		I					
D-Thyroxine									I	D	I			
Erythromycin	X							I					*	*Colorimetric method
Estrogens	X								I	D			+	
Ethacrynic acid (Edecrin)	X					I			I		I		+	
Furosemide (Lasix)					I	I			I					
Gentamicin	X	X												
Gold	X	X												
Griseofulvin	X	X												

EFFECTS OF DRUG ON LABORATORY TEST VALUES[a, b] *(Continued)*

	Hepato-toxicity	Nephro-tox-icity	In-test. Malabs.	Cre-ati-nine	BUN	Uric Acid	Bili-rubin	SGOT/ SGPT	Serum Glu-cose	Cho-les-terol	Pro-throm-bin time	Urine Color	Urine Glu-cose	Comments
Guanethidine analogs					I				D		I			
Heparin											I			Alters turbidity tests (e.g., thymol) and lipo-protein electrophoresis pattern. May interfere with BSP and calcium.
Hydralazine	X					I		I	I		I			
Imipramine (Tofranil)	X												+	
Indomethacin (Indocin)	X											X		
Isoniazid	X	X						I					+	
Kanamycin	X	X	X											
Levodopa						I						X	+	
Lincomycin	X													
MAO inhibitors	X		X											
Meperidine (Demerol)							I	I						
Methicillin		X												
Methotrexate	X					I*								*In gout
Methyldopa (Aldomet)	X			I		I					I	X	+	
Nalidixic acid (Neg Gram)	X	*							I†				+	*Nitrogen retention †Copper reduction method

Drug									
Neomycin	X								
Nicotinic acid (large doses)	X	X	X		I				+
Nitrofurantoin (Furadantin)	X	X						X	
Novobiocin	X								
Oleandomycin	X						D		
Oral contraceptives	X								
Oxacillin	X	X							
Penicillin									+*
Phenobarbital							D		
Phenylbutazone (Butazolidin)	X						I		
Polymyxin B	X	X							
Phenytoin sodium (Dilantin)	X	X				I		X	
Probenecid (Benemid)	X	X	D						+
Procainamide	X								
Propylthiouracil	X		I				I		
Quinacrine	X							X	
Quinine, quinidine							I	X	
Radiopaque contrast media		X	D	X			D		+
Reserpine						I			
Rifampin	X	X					X	X	

*Large doses, PSP-D with massive doses

I—BSP and protein. Serum protein electrophoresis pattern cannot be interpreted

EFFECTS OF DRUG ON LABORATORY TEST VALUES[a][b] (*Continued*)

	Hepa-totox-icity	Ne-phro-tox-icity	In-test. Malabs.	Cre-ati-nine	BUN	Uric Acid	Bili-rubin	SGOT/SGPT	Serum Glu-cose	Cho-les-terol	Pro-throm-bin time	Urine Color	Urine Glu-cose	Comments
Salicylates	X	X				I*							+	*High doses decrease uric acid
Streptomycin		X			D								+	
Sulfonamides	X	X			I							X	+	
Tetracyclines	X	X											+	
Theophylline						I	I							I—ESR
Thiazides	X					I			I				+	D—PSP and creatinine tolerance
Thiothixene	X													
Tolbutamide (Orinase)	X							I						
Vitamin A							I			I				
Vitamin D		*								I				*With hypervitaminosis D
Vitamin K											D			

Source: Adapted with permission from Wallach J: *Interpretation of Diagnostic Tests*. Boston, Little Brown, 1974.

[a]Includes both toxic reactions and methodologic interference. Tests cited are incomplete. Hepatoxicity refers to liver damage that can be reflected in the alteration of one or more tests, including alkaline phosphatase, bilirubin, transaminases, cephalin flocculation, thymol turbidity, BSP retention. Nephrotoxicity refers to renal damage causing changes in BUN, creatinine, presence of urine protein casts or cells.

[b]X = change in laboratory tests; + = positive, including false positives; I = increase; D = decrease.

coagulants, anticonvulsants, antihypertensives, anti-infectives, oral hypoglycemics, hormones, and *central nervous system drugs*.

The uncovering of laboratory test interferences is a relatively new field, and new "errors" are constantly being discovered. A few of the major interferences are listed in Appendix 7. Some of the better known *Laboratory Test Interferences* are listed in the specific drug entries either as part of the *Nursing Implications* or as separate entries.

Appendix 8

DRUGS AND DRUG CLASSES THAT WARRANT SPECIAL MONITORING IN THE GERIATRIC PATIENT

Drug/Drug Class	Age-Induced Changes	Symptoms
Antacids	Increased chance of decreased GI absorption of various drugs	Lack of or reduced response to drug
	Antacids with a high sodium content may aggravate renal or cardiac insufficiency	Edema; intensification of congestive heart failure
Barbiturates	Intensification of action of the drug	Increased CNS depression, disorientation, delirium, forgetfulness
	Paradoxic stimulant effects	Excitement, apprehension, CNS stimulation
Digitalis preparations	Enhanced drug toxicity due to changes in body mass, obesity, etc.	Early signs of digitalis toxicity: changes in mental status, anorexia, blurred vision, halos (white or yellow) around bright objects, cardiac palpitations, nausea, vomiting
	Also serum half-life is prolonged	
Methylphenidate	Methylphenidate-induced decrease in hepatic metabolism of phenytoin, phenothiazines, tricyclic	Intensification of drug response

Drug/Drug Class	Age-Induced Changes	Symptoms
	antidepressants, coumarin anticoagulants	
Narcotic analgesics	Mental confusion and an increase of coexisting mental impairment	Morphine: respiratory depression Codeine: constipation, urinary retention Meperidine: nausea, hypotension, respiratory depression
Penicillin	Enhanced CNS toxicity due to decreased renal elimination	CNS stimulation; possibility of seizures, coma
Phenothiazines	Increased incidence of orthostatic hypotension	Dizziness, lightheadedness when arising from a sitting or lying position; fainting
	Increased chance of Parkinson-like symptoms and extrapyramidal effects	Twitching, lip smacking, pill-rolling of fingers, restlessness, sudden jerking movements of hands and legs
	Increased anticholinergic side effects	Aggravation of glaucoma, urinary retention
	Cholestatic jaundice	Abdominal pain, hyperpigmentation, pruritis, prolonged fever
	Aggravation of epilepsy or mental depression	
Phenylbutazone	Increased frequency of agranulocytosis, aplastic anemia, and sodium retention	Unusual fatigue, cardiac palpitations, exertional dyspnea, recurrent high fever, skin rash, ulcers of the mouth prolonged sore throat, edema
Phenytoin	Increased incidence of neurologic and hematologic toxicity in patients with hypoalbuminemia or renal disease	Intensification of the effects of phenytoin
	Increased chance of folate deficiency	Skin pallor, tiredness, glossitis, nausea and anorexia—signs of megaloblastic anemia
Propranolol	Increased incidence of adverse reactions	Bradycardia, dizziness, headache, drowsiness, heart block, hypotension
Reserpine	Increased incidence of adverse reactions	Peptic ulcer, bradycardia, increased parasympathomimetic activity, mental depression (abnormal irritability, frequent early morning awakening and/or nightmares)
Sulfonamides	Increased chance of hypoglycemic reaction especially if used with oral hypoglycemics	Signs of hypoglycemia: hunger, weakness, sweating, tremors

Drug/Drug Class	Age-Induced Changes	Symptoms
Thiazide diuretics	Increased chance of hypoglycemic reactions especially if used with oral hypoglycemics	Signs of hypoglycemia: hunger, weakness, sweating, tremors
	Alteration of urinary elimination of uric acid	Goutlike attacks
	More troublesome orthostatic hypotension	Lightheadedness, dizziness, fainting when arising from sitting or prone position
	Increased incidence of cardiac arrhythmias especially if patient is also digitalized; hypokalemia more frequent	Signs of potassium depletion: tiredness, leg cramps, muscle weakness, dehydration, constipation
Tricyclic antidepressants	Increased incidence of anticholinergic side effects	Aggravation of glaucoma, urinary retention, dry mouth
	Increased incidence of confusion	Restlessness, agitation, sleep disturbances, disorientation, delusions, forgetfulness
Warfarin sodium	Enhanced anticoagulant effect due to decrease in plasma protein binding	Bleeding, hemorrhage

Appendix 9

REPORTED EFFECTS OF MATERNAL DRUG INGESTION ON THE EMBRYO, FETUS, AND NEONATE[a]

Drug	Possible Effect
Acetazolamide	Limb defects
Alcohol	Teratogenesis, somatic growth, low birth weight, hypoglycemia, hemorrhage, anemia, mental retardation, fetal alcohol syndrome
Aminopterin, amethopterin	Gross deformity, death of fetus
Aminophylline	Abnormal adaptation to extrauterine life
Amitriptyline	Withdrawal symptoms[b]
Amphetamines	Fetal thrombocytopenia, transposition of great vessels, cleft palate
Ampicillin	Decreased maternal urinary and plasma estriol levels; can produce candidiasis and diarrhea in the neonate
Androgens	Labioscrotal fusion before 12th week; after 12th week phallic enlargement; anomalies; increased bilirubin
Anesthetic agents	
Conduction	Convulsions, acidosis, bradycardia, myocardial depression, fetal hypotension, death
General	Methemoglobinemia, increased anomalies, chromosomal abnormality, apnea, respiratory depression
Local paracervical	Methemoglobinemia, fetal acidosis, bradycardia, neurologic and myocardial depression, convulsions, ↓ BP (large doses)
Antacid	Electrolyte imbalance ↑ Major and minor abnormalities
Anticonvulsants (cyclizine, diphenidol, thiethylperazine not recommended during pregnancy)	Teratogenesis, somatic growth, hemorrhage, withdrawal symptoms, mental retardation
Antidepressants	Poor sucking reflex, hypotonia
Antihistamines	Hallucinations, convulsions, excitement, sedation, death
Antineoplastics	Cytotoxicity, teratogenesis, impaired sexual reproductive capacity, increased susceptibility to infection, hypoplasia, growth retardation
Aspirin	Fetal bleeding, premature closing of ductus arteriosus, hemorrhage, prolonged gestation; may interfere with neonatal platelet function

Drug	Possible Effect
Atropine	Fetal tachycardia, dilated nonreacting pupils; inhibits lactation
Barbiturates	Increased anomalies, neonatal bleeding, withdrawal symptoms[b]
Benzodiazepines	Cardiac defects, neonatal withdrawal syndrome[b]
Benzthiazide	Acidosis, thrombocytopenia, hemorrhage, respiratory distress, electrolyte imbalance hemolysis, convulsions, death
Bishydroxycoumarin	Skeletal and facial anomalies, mental retardation
Bromides	Growth failure, lethargy, dilated pupils, dermatitis, hypotonia, mental retardation
Cannabis	Increase in anomalies
Carbon monoxide	Mental retardation
Cephaloridine	False-positive Coombs' test
Chloral hydrate (large doses)	Fetal death
Chloramphenicol	Neonatal "gray baby syndrome" associated with collapse and death
Chlordiazepoxide	Withdrawal symptoms[b]
Chloroquine	Retinal damage, eighth cranial nerve damage
Chlorpromazine	Hypoglycemia
Chlorpropamide	Hypoglycemia, fetal death
Cholinesterase inhibitors	Abnormal adaptation to extrauterine life
Cigarettes	See *Nicotine*
Clomiphene	Anomalies, neural tube defects, Down's syndrome
Corticosteroids	Placental insufficiency, teratogenesis, birth weight anomaly, electrolyte imbalance
Coumarin	Hemorrhage, calcifications, fetal death
Curare	Fetal curarization
Diazepam	Teratogenesis, abnormal adaptation to extrauterine life, withdrawal symptoms[b]
Diazoxide	Teratogenesis, hyperglycemia, alopecia, perinatal mortality, prolonged beta-adrenergic blockade
Dicoumarol	Teratogenesis, hemorrhage, anemia, mental retardation, fetal death
Diethylstilbestrol (DES)	Adenocarcinoma of vagina and cervix of female offspring, genital tract anomalies, congenital heart defect, tracheoesophageal fistula and atresia, carcinoma; diminished lactation
Diphenhydramine	Withdrawal symptoms[b]
Diphenylhydantoin	See *Phenytoin*
Diuretics	Electrolyte imbalance, uterine inertia, meconium, staining, fetal death
Drugs of abuse	Somatic growth, ↓ birth rate, withdrawal symptoms[b]
Edetate calcium disodium (EDTA)	↑ Anomalies
Ergot	Fetal death
Ergotamine	Vomiting and diarrhea, ↓ prolactin levels, multiple doses may inhibit lactation.
Erythromycin	Possible hepatic injury; ↑ neonatal bilirubinemia
Estrogens	See *Diethylstilbestrol*

Drug	Possible Effect
Ethanol	See *Alcohol*
Ethacrynic acid	Jaundice, thrombocytopenia
Ethchlorvynol	CNS depression, withdrawal symptoms[b]
Ether	Apnea, respiratory depression
Fluoride (excess)	Mottled teeth, disturbances in ossification
Ganglionic blockers	Paralytic ileus
Gentamicin	Damage to eighth cranial nerve
Glucocorticoids	Cleft palate, cardiac defects
Glutethimide	Withdrawal symptoms[b]
Hallucinogenics	Teratogenesis
Haloperidol	↑ Limb anomalies
Halothane	Apnea, respiratory depression
Heroin	See *Narcotics*
Hexamethonium	Hypotension, paralytic ileus, abnormal adaptation to extrauterine life
Hydralazine	↑ Anomalies (data not statistically significant)
Hydroxyzine HCl	Withdrawal symptoms[b]
Hypotonic IV fluids	Electrolyte imbalance
Idoxuridine	↑ Anomalies
Imipramine	CNS, ↑ limb anomalies
Immunologic agents (liver virus vaccines)	Viral infection of fetus
Indomethacin	↑ Anomalies, premature closure of ductus arteriosus
Insecticides	Affect enzyme induction
Insulin	Hypoglycemia, skeletal malformations
Intravenous fluids	Excessive fluids, hyponatremia, seizures
Iodides	Hyper- or hypothyroidism, mental retardation, thrombocytopenia, respiratory distress due to tracheal compression
Iodine	Abnormal thyroid function, fetal malformations (data still scant)
Kanamycin	Damage to eighth cranial nerve
Lead	Teratogenesis, fetal death, mental retardation
Levallorphan	No effect unless large doses of narcotics administered to mother—acts as a respiratory depressant if cause of depression is other than a narcotic; may precipitate fetal withdrawal reaction in fetus/neonate
Lithium	Teratogenesis, ↓ immediate adaptation to extra-uterine life, thyroid function, eye anomalies, cleft palate, electrolyte imbalance
Lysergic acid diethylamide	Chromosomal damage, ↑ anomalies
Magnesium sulfate	↓ Immediate adaptation to extrauterine life, convulsions
Meclizine	↑ Anomalies
Menadione (vitamin K)	Hematologic changes, hemorrhage, anemia, jaundice
Meprobamate	Withdrawal symptoms[b]
Mercury	Teratogenesis, mental retardation
Methadone	Withdrawal symptoms[b]
Methotrexate (MTX)	Multiple anomalies
Methyldopa	Neonatal meconium ileus
Mineral oil	↓ Absorption of fat soluble vitamins (A, D, E, K), hypoprothrombinemia

Drug	Possible Effect
Nalidixic acid	Hemolysis
Narcotics	↓ Immediate adaptation to extrauterine life, ↑ respiratory depression, apnea, withdrawal symptoms,[b] hypothermia
Nicotine	↓ Fetal growth, placenta abruptio, placenta previa
Nitrofurantoin	Hyperbilirubinemia, hemolytic anemia
Novobiocin	Thrombocytopenia, hyperbilirubinemia
Oral hypoglycemics	Hypoglycemia, thrombocytopenia
Ovulatory agents	Teratogenesis, ↓ birth weight
Oxytocin	↓ Immediate adaptation to extrauterine life, jaundice, electrolyte imbalance
Paracetamol	Renal failure
Paraldehyde	↓ Immediate adaptation to extrauterine life
Paramethadione (Paradione)	↑ Multiple anomalies, ↓ intrauterine growth, congenital heart disease, mental retardation, fetal death
D-Penicillamine	Connective tissue defects
Pentazocine	Withdrawal symptoms[b]
Phenmetrazine	Teratogenesis, skeletal and visceral anomalies
Phenothiazines	↓ Immediate adaptation to extrauterine life
Phenytoin	Teratogenesis, phenytoin (fetal hydantoin) syndrome, including cleft lip, palate, or gum, syndactyly, polydactyly, microencephaly, anencephaly (data open to question because often used in epileptics who receive more than one drug); hemorrhage, anemia
Pilocarpine	Convulsions
Podophyllin	↑ Multiple anomalies
Primidone	Hemorrhage
Progestins	Masculinization of female fetus
Promethazine	Hemorrhage, anemia
Propranolol	Bradycardia, ↓ cardiac output, hypoglycemia, ↑ embryotoxic
Propylthiouracil	Goiter, mental retardation
Psychotropic drugs	↑ Anomalies, lethargy, cyanosis
Pyridoxine	↓ Immediate adaptation to extrauterine life, convulsions
Pyrimethamine	↑ Anomalies
Quinine	Teratogenesis, deafness, hemorrhage
Radiation	Teratogenesis, carcinogenesis, mental retardation
Radioactive drugs	Abnormal thyroid function
Radioactive dyes	Abnormal thyroid function
Radioisotopes	See *Radiation*
Reserpine	Teratogenesis, ↓ immediate adaptation to extra-uterine life, ↑ respiratory secretions, nasal congestion, lethargy, cyanosis, anorexia
Rifampin	Spina bifida, cleft palate
Salicylates	↓ Immediate adaptation to extrauterine life; salicylate intoxication; fetal death (excessive doses); CNS, GI, skeletal malformation; bleeding
Scopolamine	Hyperpyrexia (from large repeated therapeutic doses), fetal tachycardia
Seratonin	↑ Anomalies
Sodium bisulfate	Hemorrhage, anemia, jaundice
Stilbestrol	See *Diethylstilbestrol*

Drug	Possible Effect
Streptomycin	Damage to eighth cranial nerve, micromelia, multiple skeletal anomalies
Sulfonamides	Hemorrhage, anemia, facial and skeletal defects, hyperbilirubinemia, jaundice and kernicterus (one combination drug, Bactrim [sulfamethoxazole and trimethroprim], has been associated with increased incidence of cleft palate)
Testosterone	Masculinization of the female fetus; see *Androgens*
Tetracyclines	Depression of bone growth, discoloration of primary teeth, micromelia, multiple skeletal anomalies
Thalidomide	Teratogenesis; limb, eye, and GI malformations
Thiazides	Thrombocytopenia, jaundice, hyponatremia, diabetogenic effect, hyperuricemia, ↓ birth weight
Thiouracil	Goiter, hypothyroidism, mental retardation
Thiourea	Thyroid function, hemorrhage, anemia, ↓ mental ability
Tolbutamide	↑ Anomalies, metabolism
Trichloroethylene	Apnea, respiratory depression
Trifluoperazine	Withdrawal symptoms[b]
Trimethadione	Facial and cardiac defects, cleft palate, intrauterine growth retardation (IUGR)
Trycyclic antidepressants	CNS and limb anomalies
Vitamin A (excess)	Congenital anomalies, renal and CNS anomalies
Vitamin B$_6$	Withdrawal seizures
Vitamin C (excess)	Rebound scurvy (in neonate)
Vitamin D (excess)	Congenital anomalies; excess: predisposition to hypercalcemia
Vitamin K	Icterus, kernicterus, anemia
Warfarin	Fetal hemorrhage, stillbirth

[a]Drugs listed also refer to drugs of abuse (street drugs), social drugs (alcohol, cigarettes), environmental pollutants—insecticides, lead, others).

[b]Withdrawal symptoms demonstrated by the newborn of addicted mothers include hyperactivity, tremors, frequent sneezing, a shrill high-pitched cry, hyperactive Moro reflex, hypertonicity, seizures, vomiting diarrhea, and frantic fist sucking. Though these symptoms usually appear within the first 24 hours of life, they may occur as late as 7 days of age in heroin addiction, 2 weeks of age in methadone addiction, and 2 months of age in phenobarbital addiction.

Appendix 10

FORMULAS FOR CALCULATING DOSAGE FOR ADMINISTRATION OF MEDICATIONS AND IV FLOW RATE

1. Formula for calculating dosage for administration of medications:

$$\frac{D \text{ (dose required)}}{X \text{ (units to be administered)}} = \frac{H \text{ (dose available)}}{\text{(no. units containing dose available)}}$$

Example: The physician orders 20 mg of elixir of phenobarbital. The dose on hand is 5 mg/5 ml. How many milliliters should be administered?

$$\frac{20 \text{ mg}}{X \text{ ml}} = \frac{5 \text{ mg}}{5 \text{ ml}}$$
$$5X = 100$$
$$X = 20 \text{ ml}$$ *Ans.*: 20 ml

Example: The physician orders prednisone 20 mg. The tablets on hand are 5 mg each. How many tablets should be administered?

$$\frac{20 \text{ mg}}{X \text{ tabs}} = \frac{5 \text{ mg}}{1 \text{ tab}}$$
$$5X = 20$$
$$X = 4 \text{ tablets}$$ *Ans:* 4 tablets

2. *Clark's rule*, used for computation of pediatric dosage:

$$\frac{\text{Weight in pounds} \times \text{adult dose}}{150^*} = \text{safe dosage for individual child}$$

3. *Fried's rule*, used for computation of pediatric dosage for infant or child up to 2 years of age:

$$\frac{\text{Child's age in months} \times \text{adult dose}}{150} = \frac{\text{safe dosage for individual}}{\text{infant or child}}$$

4. *Young's rule*, used for computation of pediatric dosage for child over 2 years of age:

$$\frac{\text{Age in years} \times \text{adult dose}}{\text{Age in years} + 12} = \text{safe dosage for child}$$

*Average adult weight in pounds.

APPENDIX 10   BODY SURFACE AREA OF CHILDREN—NOMOGRAM FOR DETERMINATION OF BODY SURFACE AREA FROM HEIGHT AND WEIGHT[a]

Height	Body Surface Area	Weight

```
cm 120 ┌ 47 in          ┌ 1.10 m²        kg 40.0 ┌ 90 lb
       ┤ 46             ┤ 1.05                   ┤ 85
   115 ┤ 45             ┤ 1.00            35.0 ┤ 80
       ┤ 44             ┤ 0.95                   ┤ 75
   110 ┤ 43             ┤ 0.90                   ┤ 70
       ┤ 42             ┤ 0.85            30.0 ┤ 65
   105 ┤ 41             ┤ 0.80                   ┤ 60
       ┤ 40                                      ┤ 55
   100 ┤ 39             ┤ 0.75            25.0 ┤
       ┤ 38             ┤ 0.70                   ┤ 50
    95 ┤ 37                                      ┤ 45
       ┤ 36             ┤ 0.65            20.0 ┤ 40
    90 ┤ 35             ┤ 0.60
       ┤ 34                                      ┤ 35
    85 ┤ 33             ┤ 0.55            15.0 ┤
       ┤ 32                                      ┤ 30
    80 ┤ 31             ┤ 0.50
       ┤ 30                                      ┤ 25
    75 ┤ 29             ┤ 0.45
       ┤ 28
    70 ┤ 27             ┤ 0.40            10.0 ┤
    65 ┤ 26                                9.0 ┤ 20
       ┤ 25             ┤ 0.35             8.0 ┤
    60 ┤ 24                                7.0 ┤ 15
       ┤ 23             ┤ 0.30             6.0 ┤
    55 ┤ 22
       ┤ 21             ┤ 0.25             5.0 ┤
    50 ┤ 20                                4.5 ┤ 10
       ┤ 19                                4.0 ┤ 9
    45 ┤ 18             ┤ 0.20             3.5 ┤ 8
       ┤ 17             ┤ 0.19                   ┤ 7
       ┤ 16             ┤ 0.18             3.0 ┤ 6
    40 ┤ 15             ┤ 0.17             2.5 ┤ 5
       ┤ 14             ┤ 0.16
    35 ┤ 13             ┤ 0.15             2.0 ┤ 4
       ┤ 12             ┤ 0.14
    30 ┤ 11             ┤ 0.13             1.5 ┤ 3
       ┤ 10 in          ┤ 0.12
cm 25 └                 ┤ 0.11         kg 1.0 └ 2.2 lb
                        ┤ 0.10
                        ┤ 0.09
                        ┤ 0.08
                        └ 0.074 m²
```

Source: From the formula of Du Bois and Du Bois: *Arch Intern Med* 17:863, 1916: $S = W^{0.425} \times H^{0.725} \times 71.84$, or $\log S = \log W \times 0.425 + \log H \times 0.725 + 1.8564$ (S = body surface in cm², W = weight in kg, H = height in cm).
Reproduced from Documenta Geigy Scientific Tables, 8th edition.
Courtesy CIBA-GEIGY Limited, Basle, Switzerland
[a] A straight edge is placed from the patient's height in the left column to his weight in the right column; this intersect on the body surface area column indicates body surface area.

APPENDIX 10 BODY SURFACE AREA OF ADULTS—NOMOGRAM FOR DETERMINATION OF BODY SURFACE AREA FROM HEIGHT AND WEIGHT[a]

Height	Body Surface Area	Weight

```
cm 200 ─ 79 in          ─ 2.80 m²       kg 150 ─ 330 lb
        78                                   145    320
   195 ─ 77              ─ 2.70             140    310
        76                                         300
   190 ─ 75              ─ 2.60             135    290
        74                                   130
   185 ─ 73              ─ 2.50             125    280
        72                                          270
   180 ─ 71              ─ 2.40             120
        70                                   115    260
   175 ─ 69              ─ 2.30                     250
        68                                   110    240
   170 ─ 67              ─ 2.20             105    230
        66                                   100    220
   165 ─ 65              ─ 2.10              95    210
        64                                   90    200
   160 ─ 63              ─ 2.00             85     190
        62                ─ 1.95                   180
   155 ─ 61              ─ 1.90             80
        60                ─ 1.85                   170
   150 ─ 59              ─ 1.80             75
        58                ─ 1.75                   160
   145 ─ 57              ─ 1.70             70     150
        56                ─ 1.65             65    140
   140 ─ 55              ─ 1.60             60     130
        54                ─ 1.55
   135 ─ 53              ─ 1.50             55     120
        52                ─ 1.45
   130 ─ 51              ─ 1.40             50     110
        50                ─ 1.35                   105
   125 ─ 49              ─ 1.30             45     100
        48                ─ 1.25                    95
   120 ─ 47              ─ 1.20             40      90
        46                ─ 1.15                    85
   115 ─ 45              ─ 1.10             35      80
        44                ─ 1.05                    75
   110 ─ 43              ─ 1.00                     70
        42                ─ 0.95           30      66 lb
   105 ─ 41              ─ 0.90        kg
        40                ─ 0.86 m²
cm 100 ─ 39 in
```

Source: From the formula of Du Bois and Du Bois: *Arch Intern Med* 17:863, 1916: $S = W^{0.425} \times H^{0.725} \times 71.84$, or $\log S = \log W \times 0.425 + \log H \times 0.725 + 1.8564$ (S = body surface in cm², W = weight in kg, H = height in cm).
Reproduced from Documenta Geigy Scientific Tables, 8th edition.
Courtesy CIBA-GEIGY Limited, Basle, Switzerland
[a]A straight edge is placed from the patient's height in the left column to his weight in the right column; this intersect on the body surface area column indicates body surface area.

5. Formula using *Surface Area of Child* for computation of pediatric dosage for child:

$$\frac{\text{Surface area of child (in square meters)} \times \text{adult dose}}{1.7 \text{ M}^2*} = \text{safe dosage for individual child}$$

See nomogram on p. 930 to determine surface area for child.

6. Formula based on *Recommended Pediatric Dosage per Kilogram of Body Weight*:

Milligrams × kilograms of child's body weight = safe dosage for child

Example: John weighs 88 lb. The recommended pediatric dosage for chlorpheniramine maleate is 2 mg/kg/24 hr. What would be a safe dose for John for the total 24 hr?

$$88 \text{ lb}/2.2 \text{ lb/kg} = 40 \text{ kg}$$
$$40 \text{ kg} \times 2 \text{ mg/kg} = 80 \text{ mg} = \text{safe dosage for 24 hr for John}$$

Total doses for 24 hr are to be divided and administered at appropriate intervals as indicated by the physician.

7. Formula for calculation of IV flow rate:

$$\frac{\text{Total volume infused} \times \text{drops/ml}}{\text{Total time for infusion in minutes}} = \text{drops/min}$$

Check the directions with the IV set for the number of drops per milliliter it delivers because different brands and types vary.

Example: The order reads, "Give 240 ml of 5% D/W in 4 hr." What would be the rate of flow?

The directions on the set indicate that the number of drops per milliliter is 15.

$$X = \frac{240 \text{ ml} \times 15 \text{ drops/ml}}{4 \text{ hr} \times 60 \text{ min/hr}}$$
$$X = \frac{60 \times 1}{x \times 4}$$
$$X = 15 \qquad \textit{Ans. The rate of flow} = 15 \text{ drops/min}$$

Example: The order reads, "Ampicillin 0.5 gm IV." After adding the reconstituted ampicillin, the Volutrol chamber has 30 ml of fluid. Directions on the ampicillin vial indicate that the medication must be given in 1 hr. What would the rate of flow be for this medication to be received in 1 hr? The drop factor is 60 microgtts/ml.

$$X = \frac{30 \text{ ml} \times 60 \text{ microgtts}}{1 \text{ hr} \times 60 \text{ min/hr}}$$
$$X = 30 \qquad \textit{Ans. The rate of flow} = 30 \text{ microgtts/min}$$

*Average adult surface area

Appendix 11

FEDERAL CONTROLLED SUBSTANCES ACT (U.S.)

Federal Controlled Substances Act   The Federal Controlled Substances Act of 1970 placed drugs controlled by the Act into five categories or schedules based on their potential to cause psychological and/or physical dependence and their potential for abuse.

SCHEDULE I   Includes substances for which there is a high abuse potential and no current approved medical use. Substances in this category include heroin, marijuana, LSD, peyote, mescaline, psilocybin, tetrahydrocannabinols, certain opiates, opium derivatives, and hallucinogens.

SCHEDULE II   Includes drugs that have a high abuse potential, high ability to produce physical and/or psychological dependence, and a current approved or acceptable medical use. Drugs in this category include narcotics, such as morphine, codeine, hydromorphone, methadone, meperidine, oxycodone, anileridine, and oxymorphine; stimulants, such as cocaine, amphetamine, methylphenidate, and phenmetrazine; depressants, such as amobarbital, pentobarbital, and secobarbital, and methaqualone; and phencyclidine.

SCHEDULE III   Includes drugs for which there is less potential for abuse than drugs in Schedule II and for which there is a current approved medical use. Certain drugs in this category are preparations containing limited quantities of codeine, such as Empirin Compound with Codeine, Tylenol with Codeine, and Phenaphen with Codeine. Other drugs include depressants, such as the barbiturates not listed in other schedules, glutethimide, methyprylon, and other sedative-hypnotics; stimulants, such as benzphetamine, chlorphentermine, clortermine, mazindol, and phendimetrazine; and, the narcotic paregoric.

SCHEDULE IV   Includes drugs for which there is a relatively low abuse potential and for which there is a current approved medical use. Drugs in this category include depressants, such as chloral hydrate, ethchlorvynol, ethinimate, meprobamate, methohexital, chlordiazepoxide, diazepam, oxazepam, chlorazepate, flurazepam, clonazepam, prazepam, lorazepam, and mebutamate; stimulants, such as fenfluramine, diethylpropion, and phentermine; and dextropropoxyphene.

SCHEDULE V   Drugs in this category consist mainly of preparations containing limited amounts of certain narcotic drugs for use as antitussives and antidiarrheals. Federal law provides that limited quantities of these drugs (e.g., codeine) may be bought without a prescription by an individual at least 18 years of age. The product must be purchased from a pharmacist who must keep appropriate records. However, state laws do vary and in certain states these products do require a prescription.

Appendix 12

CONTROLLED SUBSTANCES (CANADA)

In Canada, drugs that are considered subject to abuse, which have an approved medical use, that are not narcotics, are governed by Schedule G of the Canadian Food and Drug Act. These drugs include the following:

Amphetamine and its salts (e.g., amphetamine sulfate, dexamphetamine sulfate)

Barbituric acid and its salts and derivatives (e.g., amobarbital, pentobarbital, secobarbital)

Benzphetamine and its salts (e.g., Didrex)

Butorphanol and its salts (e.g., Stadol)

Chlorphentermine and its salts (e.g., Pre-Sate)

Diethylpropion and its salts (e.g., Nobesine, Regibon, Tenuate)

Methamphetamine and its salts (e.g., Desoxyn, Methedrine)

Methaqualone and its salts (e.g., Rouqualone-300, Triador, Tualone-300)

Methylphenidate and its salts (e.g., Methidate, Ritalin)

Pentazocine and its salts (e.g., Talwin)

Phendimetrazine and its salts (e.g., Plegine)

Phenmetrazine and its salts (e.g., Preludin)

Phentermine and its salts (e.g., Ionamin, Fastin, Pronidin)

Thiobarbituric acid and its salts and derivatives (e.g., thiopental sodium, methohexital, thiamylal sodium)

Narcotics (e.g., morphine, codeine, meperidine) are governed by the Narcotics Control regulations.

Drugs that have no approved medical use are governed by Schedule H of the Canadian Food and Drug Act and include substances such as LSD, DET, DMT, DOM, PCP, psilocin, psilocybin, and a large number of other hallucinogenic substances.

Appendix 13

MEDIC ALERT SYSTEMS

WHO NEEDS MEDIC ALERT? Persons with any medical problem or condition that cannot be easily seen or recognized need the protection of Medic Alert. Heart conditions, diabetes, severe allergies and epilepsy are common problems. Others are listed on the application form under this page. About one in every five persons has some special medical problem.

WHY MEDIC ALERT? Tragic or even fatal mistakes can be made in emergency medical treatment unless the special problem of the person is known. A diabetic could be neglected and die because he was thought to be intoxicated. A shot of penicillin could end the life of one who is allergic to it. Persons dependent on medications must continue to receive them at all times.

WHEN IS MEDIC ALERT IMPORTANT? Whenever a person cannot speak for himself — because of unconsciousness, shock, delirium, hysteria, loss of speech, etc. — the Medic Alert emblem speaks for him.

HOW DOES MEDIC ALERT WORK? The Medic Alert emblem —worn on the wrist or neck — is recognized the world over. On the back of the emblem is engraved the medical problem and the file number of the wearer, and the telephone number of Medic Alert's Central File. Doctors, police, or anyone giving aid can immediately get vital information — addresses of the personal physician and nearest relative, etc. — via collect telephone call (24 hours a day) to the Central File.

WHAT IS MEDIC ALERT? It is a charitable, nonprofit organization. Its services are maintained by a one-time-only membership fee and by voluntary contributions from friends, corporations and foundations. Additional services such as replacement of lost emblems and up-dating of records are charged to members at cost. Membership is tax deductible as a medical expense, and contributions are always deductible on income tax returns.

WHERE IS MEDIC ALERT? Medic Alert Foundation International was founded in Turlock, California in 1956, after a doctor's daughter almost died from reaction to a sensitivity test for tetanus antitoxin. The Foundation is endorsed by over 100 organizations including the American Academy of General Practice (and many more national and state medical organizations) the International Associations of Fire Chiefs, Police Chiefs, the National Sheriffs' Association, and the National Association of Life Underwriters.

For further information, write to:

Medic Alert Foundation International
Turlock, CA 95380
Phone (209) 632-2371.

John D. McPherson, President

Produced internally by Medic Alert Foundation

MEDIC ALERT EMBLEMS ARE SHOWN IN ACTUAL SIZE

BRACELETS:

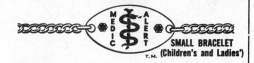

STANDARD BRACELET
T.M.

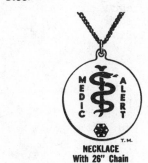

SMALL BRACELET
T.M. (Children's and Ladies')

DISC:

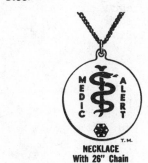

NECKLACE
With 26" Chain

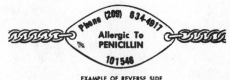

EXAMPLE OF REVERSE SIDE
OF MEDIC ALERT
EMBLEM

ALL MEMBERSHIP FEES AND DONATIONS ARE TAX-DEDUCTIBLE

Reprinted with permission from Medic Alert Foundation International, Turlock CA.

Appendix 14

COMMONLY USED ABBREVIATIONS

A, aa	of each	noct.	night
a.c.	before meals	no.	number
ad	to, up to	O	pint
ad lib	as desired, at pleasure	o.d.	every day
aq	water	O.D.	right eye
aq dest.	distilled water	o.h.	every hour
a.u.	each ear, both ears	ol	oil
a.d.	right ear	O.L.	left eye
a.l.	left ear	o.m.	every morning
b.i.d.	two times daily	o.n.	every night
b.i.n.	two times nightly	O.S.	left eye
c̄	with	os	mouth
Caps	capsule	oz.	ounce
collyr.	an eyewash	p.c.	after meals
D., det.	give, let be given	per	by, through
d.	day	pil	pill
dil.	dilute	PO, p.o.	by mouth
dr.	dram	PR	by rectum
D.t.d.	Let such doses be given.	PRN, p.r.n.	when necessary
emuls.	emulsion	q	every
elix	elixir	q.d.	every day
ext.	extract	q.h.	every hour
F, Ft.	and make	q.i.d.	four times daily
g, gm	gram	q.o.d.	every other day
gr	grain	q.s.	as much as required
gtt	a drop, drops	Rept.	let it be repeated
h, hr	hour	s̄	without
h.s.	at bedtime	ss	one-half
IA	intra-arterial	SC	subcutaneous
IM	intramuscular	Sig, S.	mark on label
IV	intravenous	s.o.s.	if necessary
kg	kilogram	sp	spirits
l, L	liter	stat	immediately, first dose
m.	minim	syr	syrup
M.	mix	tab	tablet
m², M²	square meter (of body surface area)	t.i.d.	three times daily
		t.i.n.	three times nightly
max	maximum	tr	tincture
mC	millicurie	μ	micron
mcg, μg	microgram	μCi	microcurie
mEq	milliequivalent	μg	microgram
mist.	mixture	ung	ointment
ml	milliliter	ut dict	as directed
non rep.	do not repeat		

Appendix 15

COMMONLY USED APPROXIMATE EQUIVALENTS

These equivalents may be used for prepared dosage forms; consult a pharmacist for exact equivalents.

Liquids

Metric	Apothecary	Household
1 ml	15 minims	
5 ml		1 teaspoon
15 ml	[1/2] fl. oz.	1 tablespoon
30 ml	1 fl. oz.	2 tablespoons (6 teaspoons)
250 ml	8 fl. oz.	1 measuring cup (240 ml)
500 ml	1 pint (16 fl. oz)	
1,000 ml	1 quart (32 fl. oz)	
4,000 ml	4 quarts (1 gallon)	

(*Note:* 1 ml is approximately equivalent to 1 cc).

Weight

1 mg (1,000 µg)	1/60 grain
60 mg	1 grain
1 gm	15.4 grains
30 gm	1 oz.
454 gm	1 lb.
1,000 gm (1 kg)	2.2 lb.

Length

1 meter = 39.4 inches
1 inch = 2.5 cm

Rules for Conversion of Degrees Celsius and Fahrenheit

To convert degrees Celsius to Fahrenheit:

$$\frac{9 \times C}{5} + 32 = F$$

To convert degrees Fahrenheit to Celsius:

$$(F - 32) \times 5/9 = C$$

GLOSSARY

Achlorhydria. Absence of hydrochloric acid in the stomach.

Acidosis. Increased acidity of body fluids.

Acrocyanosis. Cyanosis (blueness) of the extremities.

Acromegaly. Overgrowth of bones of extremities and head in adults due to excess secretion of growth hormone.

Acroparesthesia. Tingling, prickling, or numbness of extremities.

Addison's disease. Condition due to deficiency of adrenal cortex.

Adrenergic. Pertaining to the sympathetic portion of the autonomic nervous system.

Agranulocytosis. Low white blood cell count especially neutropenia—characterized by fever, ulceration of mucous membranes, and prostration.

Akathisia. Extreme restlessness, increased motor activity.

Akinesia. Partial or complete loss of muscle movement.

Alopecia. Absence or loss of hair (especially on the head).

Amblyopia. Reduced or dimness of vision.

Amenorrhea. Absence of menses.

Anabolic, anabolism. The building up of body tissues.

Anaphylaxis. Allergic hypersensitivity reaction of the body due to a drug or foreign protein.

Androgenic. Causing masculine characteristics.

Angina, anginal. Usually refers to angina pectoris—severe pain in the heart usually due to insufficient oxygenation.

Angioedema. Allergic reaction resulting in edematous areas of the skin, viscera, or mucous membranes.

Anorexia. Loss of appetite.

Anuria. Absence of urine formation.

Aphakia. Absence of the crystalline lens of the eye.

Aphasia. Loss or impairment of speech.

Aplastic anemia. Anemia due to impairment of the bone marrow.

Apnea. Temporary cessation of breathing.

Arthralgia. Joint pain.

Ascites. Fluid accumulation in the peritoneal cavity.

Asthenia. Muscle weakness; decreased or loss of muscle strength.

Atopic. Out of place, displaced.

Azotemia. Increased urea or nitrogen in the blood.

Bactericidal. Agent that kills bacteria.

Bacteriostatic. Decreasing or inhibiting growth of bacteria.

Blepharospasm. Twitching of the eyelid(s).

Bradycardia. Slow heart rate.

Bruxism. Grinding of the teeth (usually during sleep).

Buerger's disease.   Also called thromboangiitis obliterans. Chronic inflammatory disease especially the peripheral arteries and veins of the extremities—may cause paresthesia or gangrene.

Catabolism.   Breakdown of complex body substances with the usual release of energy.

Cellulitis.   Inflammation of cellular or connective tissue.

Cheilitis.   Inflammation of the lip(s).

Cheilosis.   Condition where lips become reddened with fissures at the angles—usually due to riboflavin deficiency.

Chloasma.   Skin discoloration, usually yellow brown in color.

Cholangitis.   Inflammation of the bile ducts.

Cholecystitis.   Inflammation of the gall bladder.

Cholelithiasis.   Presence of stones or calculi in the gallbladder or bile ducts.

Cholestasia.   Decrease or stoppage of bile excretion.

Cholinergic.   Pertaining to the parasympathetic portion of the autonomic nervous system.

Chorea.   Involuntary muscle twitches of the face or limbs.

Cirrhosis.   A chronic, degenerative disease of the liver.

Claudication.   Limping or lameness.

Colitis.   Inflammation of the colon.

Conjunctivitis.   Inflammation of the conjunctiva of the eye.

Cretinism.   Congenital deficiency of thyroid hormone resulting in arrested physical and mental development.

Crystalluria.   Appearance of crystals in the urine.

Cyanosis.   Abnormal amounts of reduced hemoglobin in the blood resulting in a blue-gray discoloration of the skin.

Cycloplegia.   Paralysis of the ciliary muscles of the eye.

Diaphoresis.   Heavy perspiration.

Diathesis.   Predisposition to a certain condition or disease.

Diplopia.   Double vision.

Dysarthria.   Difficulty or deficiency of speech.

Dyscrasia.   A synonym for disease—usually refers to an abnormal condition of the blood cells.

Dyskinesia.   Impairment of voluntary muscle movement.

Dysmenorrhea.   Painful or difficult menstruation.

Dyspareunia.   Painful sexual intercourse.

Dyspepsia.   Disturbed digestion.

Dysphagia.   Difficulty or inability to swallow.

Dysphonia.   Hoarseness. Difficulty in speaking.

Dyspnea.   Labored or difficult breathing.

Dystonia.   Impairment of muscle tone.

Dysuria.   Painful or difficult urination.

Ecchymosis.   Hemorrhagic areas of the skin producing discoloration ranging from blue-black to green-brown or yellow.

Ectopic.   At a site other than normal. Often refers to pregnancy or heart beat.

Emesis.   Vomiting.

Encephalopathy.   Any dysfunction of the brain.

Endarteritis. Inflammation of the intima of an artery.

Enteritis. Inflammation of the intestines.

Enuresis. Urinary incontinence.

Eosinophilia. Increase in the number of circulating eosinophils.

Epistaxis. Bleeding from the nose.

Eructation. Belching.

Erythema. Redness of the skin.

Erythema multiforme. A skin rash characterized by dark red papules, vesicles, and bullae usually on the extremities.

Erythema nodosum. Red, painful nodules on the legs usually from arthritis.

Exanthema. Any skin eruption with inflammation.

Exfoliative dermatitis. Chronic inflammation of the skin characterized by itchy, scaling, and flaking skin.

Exophthalmus. Protrusion of the eyeball(s).

Flatus. Gas in the GI tract. Expelling of gas from the body.

Florid. Bright red coloration of the skin.

Galactorrhea. Excessive flow of milk.

Gastritis. Inflammation of the stomach.

Gingivitis. Inflammation of the gums.

Glaucoma. Disease of the eye manifested by increased intraocular pressure.

Glossitis. Inflammation of the tongue.

Glycosuria. Presence of glucose in the urine.

Gynecomastia. Enlargement of the mammary glands in the male.

Hematemesis. Vomiting of blood.

Hematuria. Blood in the urine.

Hemoglobinemia. Presence of hemoglobin in the plasma.

Hemoglobinuria. Presence of hemoglobin in the urine.

Hemolytic. Destruction of red blood cells.

Hemoptysis. Coughing up or spitting of blood caused by bleeding in the respiratory tract.

Hepatoxicity. Damage to the liver.

Hirsutism. Excessive growth or presence of hair.

Hypercalcemia. Excessive calcium in the blood.

Hypercapnia. Increased carbon dioxide in the blood.

Hyperglycemia. Increased blood sugar.

Hyperhidrosis. Excessive sweating.

Hyperkalemia. Increased potassium in the blood.

Hypernatremia. Increased sodium in the blood.

Hyperplasia. Excessive growth of normal cells of an organ.

Hyperpyrexia. Increased body temperature.

Hypersensitivity. Increased response to a drug or other substance.

Hypertrichosis. Excess growth of hair.

Hyperuricemia. Increased amount of uric acid in the blood.

Hypocapnia. Decrease in amount of carbon dioxide in the blood.

Hypochlorhydria. Decreased secretion of hydrochloric acid.

Hypoglycemia. Decrease in the amount of glucose in the blood.

Hypokalemia. Deficiency of potassium in the blood.

Hyponatremia. Decrease in the amount of sodium in the blood.

Hypoprothrombinemia. Deficiency of prothrombin in the blood.

Idiopathic. Disease state of unknown origin.

Ileus. Obstruction of the intestine.

Ischemic. Reduction of blood supply to an organ or tissue.

Jaundice. Skin, mucous membranes, whites of eyes, and body fluids become yellow due to excess bilirubin.

Ketosis. Accumulation of ketone bodies.

Kraurosis. Drying and atrophy of any mucous membrane (usually refers to the vulva).

Lacrimation. Secretion of tears.

Lethargic, lethargy. Drowsiness, sluggishness, stupor.

Leukopenia. Abnormal decrease in white blood cells.

Leukorrhea. Mucous discharge from the vagina or cervical canal.

Libido. Sexual drive.

Lipodystrophy. Usually refers to atropy of subcutaneous fat following insulin injections.

Lithiasis. Formation of calculi in the body.

Lochia. Blood, mucus, and tissue discharge from the uterus during the puerperal period.

Lupus erythematosus. Chronic inflammatory disease of connective tissue affecting nervous system, mucous membranes, skin, kidneys, and joints. Manifested by a characteristic rash, fever, joint pain, malaise. Occurs most often in young women.

Lymphadenopathy. Disease involving the lymph nodes.

Melasma. Discoloration or pigmentation of the skin.

Melena. Black, tarry stools due to presence of blood.

Menorrhagia. Excessive bleeding at time of menses.

Methemoglobinemia. Condition in which an excessive amount of hemoglobin is converted to methemoglobin causing cyanosis.

Miosis. Constriction of pupils of the eye.

Myalgia. Muscle pain or tenderness.

Mycosis. Any disease caused by a fungus.

Mydriasis. Dilation of the pupils of the eye.

Myopathy. Disease or abnormal condition of skeletal muscle.

Myxedema. Hypofunction of the thyroid gland in adults.

Narcolepsy. Uncontrollable attacks of desire to sleep.

Necrosis. Areas of tissue or bone which die.

Nephrotoxicity. Damage to the kidneys.

Neuritis. Inflammation of nerve(s).

Neuropathy. Any disease involving the nerves or nervous system.

Neutropenia. Abnormal decrease in the number of neutrophils in the blood.

Nocturia. Excessive urination during the night.

Nystagmus. Involuntary oscillatory movement of the eyeballs.

Obstructive jaundice. Jaundice due to a decrease in the flow of bile from the liver to the duodenum (usually caused by mechanical obstruction).

Oligospermia. Deficiency in the number of spermatozoa in seminal fluid.

Oliguria. Decrease in the amount of urine formed.

Onycholysis. Detachment or loosening of nail from the nailbed.

Ophthalmic. Referring to the eye.

Opisthotonus. Body in the dorsal position becomes arched with head and feet touching the surface.

Orchitis. Inflammation of the testes.

Orthostatic hypotension. Drop in blood pressure when standing up quickly from a reclining or sitting position.

Osteitis. Inflammation of a bone.

Osteomalacia. Softening of the bones.

Osteoporosis. Bones become porous and may break more easily.

Otic. Pertaining to the ear.

Otitis. Inflammation of the ear.

Palpitations. Rapid or throbbing pulsation (often refers to the heart).

Pancreatitis. Inflammation of the pancreas.

Pancytopenia. Abnormal decrease in all formed cells in the blood.

Papilledema. Inflammation and edema of the optic nerve where it enters the eyeball.

Paraparesis. Partial paralysis of the legs.

Paresis. Partial paralysis.

Paresthesia. Sensation of numbness, tingling, or prickling.

Petechiae. Purplish red spot(s) on the skin, mucous membranes, or serous membranes caused by intradermal or submucosal bleeding.

Peyronie's disease. Hardening of the erectile tissue of the penis causing distortion.

Pharyngitis. Inflammation of the pharynx.

Phlebitis. Inflammation of a vein.

Photophobia. Intolerance of light.

Piloerection. Erection of hair—referred to as "hair standing on end."

Polydipsia. Excessive thirst.

Polyphagia. Excessive appetite.

Polyuria. Excessive formation and discharge of urine.

Porphyria. Disorder in which increased amounts of porphyrin are synthesized. Characterized by abdominal pain, psychological, GI, and neurologic disturbances.

Presbyopia. Loss of accomodation of the eye with advancing age.

Priapism. Painful and continuous erection of the penis due to disease.

Proteinuria. Appearance of protein (usually albumin) in the urine.

Pruritus. Severe itching.

Psoriasis. Skin disease of genetic origin manifested by pink or light red lesions and scaling.

Purpura. Hemorrhage occuring in the skin and mucous membranes.

Rales. An abnormal sound of the chest due to passage of air through bronchi containing secretions or which are constricted.

Raynaud's phenomenon. Peripheral vascular disease manifested by cold, cyanotic, painful fingers and hands due to vasoconstriction.

Rhinitis. Inflammation of the mucosa of the nose.

Scleroderma. Disease characterized by induration of the skin in localized or diffuse areas.

Sclerosis. Hardening of a tissue or organ.

Seborrheic. Referring to glands that secrete sebaceous matter.

Sepsis. Febrile reaction due to microorganisms or their poisonous byproducts.

Sialorrhea. Excessive salivation.

Siderosis. Chronic inflammation of the lungs due to prolonged inhalation of dust of iron salts.

Splenomegaly. Enlargement of the spleen.

Steatorrhea. Fatty stools.

Stenosis. Narrowing of any duct or orifice.

Stevens-Johnson syndrome. Extreme inflammatory eruption of skin and mucosa of mouth, pharynx, anogenital region, and conjunctiva with high fever. May be fatal.

Stomatitis. Inflammation of the mouth.

Superinfection. Overgrowth of bacteria different from those causing the original infection.

Syncope. Fainting.

Tachycardia. Abnormal increase in heart rate.

Tamponade. Usually refers to the heart where there is excess accumulation of fluid around the heart.

Tetany. Sudden, intermittent, tonic spasms most often involving the extremities.

Thalassemia. Hereditary anemia occuring in Mediterraneans and Southeast Asians.

Thrombocytopenia. Abnormal decrease in the number of circulating blood platelets.

Thrombophlebitis. Inflammation of a vein with accompanying thrombus formation.

Thrombosis. Formation or existance of a blood clot within the vascular system.

Tinnitus. Ringing of the ears.

Torticollis. Spasms of the neck muscles causing a stiff neck and the head is drawn to one side with chin pointing to the other side.

Urticaria. Hives characterized by severe itching and rash.

Uveitis. Inflammation of the iris, choroid, and/or ciliary body of the eye.

Vasculitis. Inflammation of a lymph or blood vessel.

Vertigo. Term usually used to describe dizziness, lightheadedness, and/or giddiness.

Xerophthalmia. Dryness of the conjunctiva with epithelial keratinization. Usually due to vitamin A deficiency.

Xerostomia. Dryness of mouth resulting from lack of normal salivation.

BIBLIOGRAPHY

Albanese JA. *Nurses' Drug Reference.* New York, McGraw-Hill, 1979.
AMA Drug Evaluations, ed 5. Chicago, American Medical Association, 1983.
American Hospital Formulary Service. American Society of Hospital Pharmacists. Current.
Beaumont E. The New IV Infusion Pumps. *Nursing '77,* pp 31–34, July 1977.
Brunner LS, Suddarth DM. *Textbook of Medical-Surgical Nursing.* Philadelphia, Lippincott, 1984.
Burns N. Cancer chemotherapy. A systemic approach, *Nursing '78,* pp 56–63, February 1978.
Burnside IM. *Nursing and the Aged.* New York, McGraw-Hill, 1974.
Cape R. *Aging: Its Complex Management.* New York, Harper & Row, 1978.
Chemotherapy and You. U.S. Dept. of Health and Human Services, NIH Publication 81-1136. November 1980.
Coblio NA. *Nursing '81,* pp 48–49, 1981.
Compendium of Pharmaceuticals and Specialties, ed 20. Ottawa, Ontario, Canada, Canadian Pharmaceutical Association, 1985.
Craig CR, Stitzel RE. *Modern Pharmacology.* Boston, Little, Brown, 1982.
Daniels L. How can you improve patient compliance? *Nursing '78,* pp 39–47, May 1978.
Drug Information 85. Bethesda, MD, American Society of Hospital Pharmacists, 1985.
Drug Information for the Health Care Provider, ed 5. U.S. Pharmacopeia Drug Information, 1985.
Drug Therapy and Pregnancy: Maternal, Fetal and Neonatal Considerations. (Symposium) *Obstetrics and Gynecology* 58(5) (suppl), November 1981.
Elipoulos C. *Gerontological Nursing.* New York, Harper & Row, 1979.
Facts and Comparisons. St. Louis, Lippincott, Facts and Comparisons Division. Current.
Food and Drug Interactions. *FDA Consumer,* U.S. Dept. of Health, Education and Welfare, U.S. Government Printing Office Publication 311-254/3. March 1978.
Fredette SL, et al. Nursing diagnosis in cancer chemotherapy: In theory. *Am J Nursing,* pp 2013–2020, November 1981.
Fredette SL, et al. Nursing diagnosis in cancer chemotherapy: In practice. *Am J Nursing,* pp 2021–2022, November 1981.
Geuer H. Brompton's mixture. *Nursing '80,* p 57, May 1980.
Gilman AG, Goodman LS, Gilman A. *Goodman and Gilman's The Pharmacological Basis of Therapeutics.* New York, Macmillan, 1980.
Golbus M. Teratology for the Obstetrician: Currrent Status. *Obstetrics and Gynecology* 55(3), pp 269–277, 1979.
Gotch, P. Teaching patients about adrenal corticosteroids. *Am J Nursing.* pp 78–81, January 1981.
Govoni LE, Hayes JE. *Drugs and Nursing Implications,* ed 4. New York, Appleton-Century-Crofts, 1982.
Graef JW. *Manual of Pediatric Therapeutics.* Boston, Little Brown, 1974.
Grant J. The nurses' role in parenteral hyperalimentation. *RN,* July 1973.
Greenwald E. *Cancer Chemotherapy.* Garden City, NY, Medical Examination Publishing Company, 1973.
Hahn AB, Barkin RL, Oestreich SJK. *Pharmacology in Nursing.* St. Louis, Mosby, 1982.
Hansen M, Woods S. Nitroglycerin ointment, where and how to apply it. *Am J Nursing,* pp 112–114, June 1980.
Hansten PD. *Drug Interactions,* ed 5. Philadelphia, Lea & Febiger, 1985.
Hawken M, Ozuna J. Practical aspects of anticonvulsant therapy. *Am J Nursing* pp 1062–1067, June 1979.
Hill R, Stern L. Drugs in pregnancy: Effects on the fetus and newborn. *Drugs* 17, March 1979.
Howard F, Hill J. Drugs in Pregnancy. *Obstetrical and Gynecological Survey* 34(9), pp 643–652, 1979.

Jackson P. Digitoxin therapy at home, keeping the child safe. *Maternal Child Nursing*, pp 105–109, March/April 1979.

Jensen M, Bobak I. *Handbook of Maternity Care*. St. Louis, Mosby, 1980.

Jones D, Dunbar C, Jirovec M. *Medical Surgical Nursing*. New York, McGraw-Hill, 1978.

Kee J. *Fluids and Electrolytes with Clinical Applications*. New York, Wiley, 1978.

King E, Wieck L, Dyer M. *Illustrated Manual of Nursing Techniques*. Philadelphia, Lippincott, 1977.

Kozier B, Erb B. *Fundamentals of Nursing*. Boston, Addison-Wesley, 1979.

Lambert M. Drug and diet interactions. *Am J Nursing*, pp 402–406, March 1975.

Lamy P. How your patient's diet can affect drug response. *Drug Therapy*, pp 82–88, August 1980.

Langslet J, Habel M. The aminoglycoside antibiotics. *Am J Nursing*, pp 1144–1146, June 1981.

Levitt D. Cancer chemotherapy. *RN*, pp 56–59, February 1981.

Luckmann J, Sorensen K. *Medical-Surgical Nursing*. Philadelphia, Saunders, 1980.

Mangini RJ (ed). *Drug Interaction Facts*. St. Louis, Lippincott, Facts and Comparisons Division. Current.

Martin EW. *Hazards of Medication*. Philadelphia, Lippincott, 1978.

Martin L. *Health Care of Women*. Philadelphia, Lippincott, 1978.

Mehl B. Food-drug interactions. *Primary Cardiology*, pp 128–137, September 1981.

Millam A. Final inline filters. *Am J Nursing*, pp 1272–1273, July 1979.

Morris M. Intravenous drug incompatabilities. *Am J Nursing*, pp 1288–1291, July 1979.

Pilliterri A. *Nursing Care of the Growing Family, A Maternal–Newborn Text*. Boston, Little, Brown, 1980.

Physicians Desk Reference, ed 39. 1985.

Postotnik P. Drugs and pregnancy. *FDA Consumer*. U.S. Government Printing Office, October 1978.

Purcell JA, Holder CK. Intravenous nitroglycerin. *Am J Nursing*, pp 254–259, February 1982.

Rayburn WF, Zuspan FP. *Drug Therapy in Obstetrics and Gynecology*. Norwalk, CT, Appleton-Century-Crofts, 1982.

Rissi L, Elliott A. Calcium channel blockers: New treatment for cardiovascular disease. *Am J Nursing*, pp 382–387, March 1983.

Sheridan E, Patterson HR, Gustafson EA. *Falconer's The Drug, The Nurse and The Patient*. Philadelphia, Saunders, 1982.

Skitklorius C. Toward impeccable IV techniques. *RN*, pp 37–40, April 1981.

Spencer RT, Nichols NW, Waterhouse HP, West FW, Bankert EG. *Clinical Pharmacology and Nursing Management*. Philadelphia, Lippincott, 1983.

Symposium on Drugs in Pregnancy. *Obstetrics and Gynecology* 58(supplement), 1981.

Wallach J. *Interpretation of Diagnostic Tests*. Boston, Little, Brown, 1978.

Weeks J. Administering medication to children. *Maternal Child Nursing*, 5, pp 63–64, January/February 1980.

Whitson B, McFarlane J. *The Pediatric Nursing Skills Manual*. New York, Wiley, 1980.

Willis J. Drugs that take the joy out of sex. *FDA Consumer*, pp 31–32, July/August 1981.

Wolff L, Weitzel MH, Zornow Ra, Zsohar H. *Fundamentals of Nursing*. Philadelphia, Lippincott, 1983.

Wong D, Whaley L. *Clinical Handbook of Pediatric Nursing*. St. Louis, Mosby, 1981.

INDEX

Generic names of drugs and general topics appear in **boldface** type.
Trade names of drugs appear in regular type.

A

Abbokinase, 289
Abbreviations, commonly used, 936
Abortifacients, 764–769
  administration (intra-amniotic), 764
  general statement, 764
  nursing implications, 764
Absorbable gelatin sponge, 273
Absorbable sterile gelatin film, 273
Absorption of drugs, factors affecting, 8
Accurbron, 614
Accutane, 876
Acebutolol, 573
  hydrochloride, 335
A'Cenol, 494
  D.S., 494
Acephen, 494
Aceta, 494
Acet-Am*, 615
Acetaminophen, 494
  buffered, 494
Acetazolam*, 800
Acetazolamide:
  as anticonvulsant, 461
  as diuretic, 800
Acetazolamide sodium, 800
Acetohexamide, 693
Acetohydroxamic acid, 183
Acetophenazine maleate, 405
Acetospan, 738
Acetylcarbromal, 380
Acetylcholine chloride, ocular, 588
Acetylcysteine, 621
Acetylsalicylic acid, 490
  buffered, 490
Achromycin:
  IM, 86
  IV, 86
  Ophthalmic, 86
  V, 86
Acidic foods, table of, 914
Acidifying agent, 828
Acidulin, 673
Acon, 836
Acrisorcin, 126
ACT, 233
Actamin, 494
  Extra, 494

ACTH, 728
Acthar, 728
ACTH Gel, 728
Acti-B12*, 844
Acticort 100, 719, 734
Actidil, 630
Actifed, 898
Actinomycin D, 202, 233
Actrapid, 688
Acu-Dyne, 182
Acutrim Maximum Strength, 528, 568
Acycloguanosine, 192
Acyclovir, 192
Adalat*, 307
Adapin, 423
Adeno Cobalasine, 861
Adenosine 5-monophosphate, 861
Adenosine phosphate, 861
Adipex-P, 528
Adipost, 527
Administration of drugs, 6–8
Administration of drugs by various routes, 24–38
  central parenteral, 36
  dermatologic preparations, 30
  ear drops, 29
  extracorporeal perfusion, 38
  eye drops, 29
  eye medication, 29
  eye ointment, 29
  gargles, 27
  hypodermoclysis, 31
  inhalation, 26, 27
  intermittent positive pressure breathing, 27
  intra-arterial infusion, 37
  intra-articular injection, 31
  intramuscular injection, 31
  intrasynovial injection, 31
  intravenous injection, 32
  irrigations, 27
  isolation perfusion, 38
  nasal general, 28
  nasal jelly, 28
  nasal spray, 28
  nasogastric tube, 25
  nebulization, 26
  nose drops, 28
  nursing implications for, 24–38
  oral, 25
  parenteral, 31–38
  rectal, 30
  subcutaneous injection, 32

  urethral, 31
  vaginal, 31
Adphen, 527
ADR, 235
Adrenalin*, 559
Adrenalin Chloride, 559, 571
  Solution, 559
Adrenergic blocking drugs, 573–581
  general statement, 573
Adrenergic drugs, *see* **Sympathomimetic drugs**
Adrenocorticosteroids and analogs, 716–739
  action/kinetics, 720
  administration:
    systemic, 723
    topical, 723
  contraindications, 720
  dosage, 723
  drug interactions, 722
  general statement, 717
  laboratory test interferences, 723
  metabolic effects, 717
  nursing implications, 724
  topical agents, table of, 718
  untoward reactions:
    following eye therapy, 721
    following general use, 721
    following intra-articular use, 721
    following topical use, 721
  uses, 720
Adrenocorticotropic hormone, 728
Adriamycin, 235
Adrin, 313, 517
Adrucil, 227
Adsorbocarpine, 590
Advil, 502
Aerobid, 732
Aerodine, 182
Aerolate, 614
Aerolone, 562
Aeroseb-Dex, 718, 730
Aeroseb-HC, 719, 734
Aerosporin, 106
Afko-Lube, 654
  Dioctyl, 654
Afrin, 571
  Pediatric, 571
Afrinol, 569
Aftate, 137